Pediatric Vitreoretinal Surgery

Your bonus with the purchase of this book

With the purchase of this book, you can use our "SN Flashcards" app to access questions free of charge in order to test your learning and check your understanding of the contents of the book. To use the app, please follow the instructions below

1. Go to https://flashcards.springernature.com/login
2. Create an user account by entering your e-mail adress and assiging a password.
3. Use the link provided in one of the first chapters to access your SN Flashcards set.

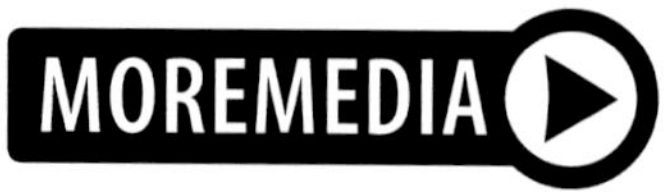

Your personal SN Flashcards link is provided in one of the first chapters.

If the link is missing or does not work, please send an e-mail with the subject **"SN Flashcards"** and the book title to customerservice@springernature.com.

Şengül Özdek • Audina Berrocal •
Ulrich Spandau

Editors

Pediatric Vitreoretinal Surgery

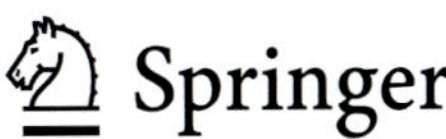
Springer

Editors
Şengül Özdek
Department of Ophthalmology
Gazi University School of Medicine
Ankara, Turkey

Audina Berrocal
Bascom Palmer Eye Institute
Miami University
Florida, FL, USA

Ulrich Spandau
Department of Ophthalmology
University of Uppsala
Uppsala, Sweden

ISBN 978-3-031-14508-7   ISBN 978-3-031-14506-3   (eBook)
https://doi.org/10.1007/978-3-031-14506-3

This Springer imprint is published by the registered company Springer Nature Switzerland AG
The registered company address is: Gewerbestrasse 11, 6330 Cham, Switzerland

Dedicated to;
My beloved family for their patience and support during my whole career,
My dearest husband for tolerating my endless study periods,
My son Egemen and daughter Elif for sharing me with patients, students and residents through all of their life…
To my mentors, teachers, patients, friends, coworkers and colleagues…

Şengül Özdek

Foreword

Pediatric vitreoretinal surgery is among the most interesting, complex, and gratifying subspecialties in the field of ophthalmology. Developmental and hereditary retinal disorders during infancy, childhood, and adolescence are some of the most challenging problems seen in clinical ophthalmic practice. Interest in pediatric retinal diseases has blossomed over the last three decades, and ophthalmology conferences routinely include symposia dedicated to recent advances in pediatric vitreoretinal surgery.

Many pediatric retinal conditions are uncommon, with a broad range of clinical presentations. Consequently, it can take decades to develop a meaningful experience in their diagnosis and management. The goal of *Pediatric Vitreoretinal Surgery* is to provide a comprehensive up-to-date text with succinct authoritative reviews on the evaluation and treatment of a complete list of both commonly encountered and rare pediatric retinal disorders. This text interweaves the expertise of field leaders and is packed with the clinical wisdom needed for tackling our complex field.

Beginning with general guidelines for pediatric vitreoretinal surgery, the text features dedicated chapters on all major disorders and conditions likely to be encountered in the pediatric population. Chapters include current information on incisional and non-incisional procedures, epidemiology, clinical manifestations, diagnosis, and approaches to management for each condition, along with information on anterior segment considerations, pediatric ocular oncology, and visual rehabilitation. In addition, narrated surgical videos enrich the didactic content and multiple-choice questions underscore salient points in each chapter. *Pediatric Vitreoretinal Surgery* will be an invaluable reference resource for house-staff, pediatricians, pediatric ophthalmologists, adult ophthalmologists, and vitreoretinal surgeons at all levels of experience who care for children and adolescents with retinal disease.

Michigan, USA   Antonio Capone, Jr. MD

Preface

If you have knowledge, let others light their candles in it.
Margaret Fuller

It is very well known that ophthalmological examination of children is very difficult and requires more experience, energy, time, and patience than adults. Especially during the preverbal ages, they cannot express themselves with words but only with their behavior. Both the parents and the ophthalmologist need to be very careful to catch those differences in their visual behavior which may reflect their visual acuity and quality. They are usually non-cooperative to most parts of the examination, and we need to find a way to attract their attention to make them more cooperative. It becomes even more difficult when it comes to retinal examination. Ophthalmologist dealing with pediatric retina needs to be very experienced in using indirect ophthalmoscopy to overcome this difficulty. Especially retinopathy of prematurity is a very important public health issue since it may result in "severe irreversible but preventable visual loss." It is our responsibility to learn how to examine and manage the immature retina in these tiny babies to prevent addition of one more blind child to the community.

Not only examination but the treatment of pediatric retinal diseases is also more complex and difficult. These small eyes have very big retinal problems which need to be helped. Most of them are congenital, developmental, or inherited pathologies usually associated with some multisystem disorders and sometimes with mental and motor retardation which makes it even more difficult to manipulate.

Pediatric vitreoretinal surgery is very challenging and unforgiving surgery which has its own rules and its own complications. The philosophy is totally different from adults and needs additional education after becoming an experienced surgeon in adult vitreoretinal surgery. Pediatric vitreoretinal surgery training is not present or takes only a very small part of the training in most of the routine residency and fellowship programs. This book has aimed to fill a gap in the field of practical points in pediatric vitreoretinal surgery. Although there are so many surgical videos available on the Internet, there is no such source providing both the theoretical information about the pediatric retinal diseases together with the practical points for the surgical treatment of them. There are only a few specialists on this subject in all over the world. We expect to help to the training of those ophthalmologist who cannot reach such a training.

The most important features of this book are as follows:

- It covers almost all topics of pediatric vitreoretinal diseases treated surgically in 12 sections with 72 chapters.
- Each chapter includes case scenarios to lead the readers by epitomizing the management of a real case.
- Practical surgical tips are defined step by step by bullets to be understood smoothly.
- Most of the chapters have narrated surgical videos (58 videos) explaining the main steps of the surgery.
- There are multiple-choice questions with the answers at the end of each chapter to review and emphasize the main topics of the chapter.

We expect to change the adult surgical standpoint to pediatric point of view with this book. Our mission would be complete if we can assist the correct management of babies and children with vitreoretinal problems by their surgeons.

Live as if you were to die tomorrow. Learn as if you were to live forever.

Mahatma Gandhi

Ankara, Turkey   Şengül Özdek
Florida, USA   Audina Berrocal
Uppsala, Sweden   Ulrich Spandau

Acknowledgements

I have started this book project when I had COVID-19 at the end of March 2021 which was the second year of the COVID pandemic. It was like a mild flu, but I had a strict home restriction which gave me a lot of time to think about this book project in my head.

I have special thanks to Dr. Michael Trese and Dr. Antony Capone Jr. for teaching me the philosophy of *Pediatric Vitreoretinal Surgery* and to Dr. Capone for his invaluable support in this book project.

Hearty thanks to my co-editors, Dr. Audina M. Berrocal and Dr. Ulrich Spandau for their invaluable work and support in our project.

I would like to thank all the contributors of the book who had written chapters together with awesome narrated videos, very demonstrative cases and figures, all of which added a lot of working hours to their routine daily busy schedule.

Thanks to Springer editing team for their support on every step of the publication procedure.

Many thanks to my mentors, patients, referring colleagues, my coworkers in Gazi University and my private clinic for their trust and support. This project could not be achieved without them.

Şengül Özdek

List of Videos

- **Video 3:** Severe mixed PFV with closed funnel RD
- **Video 4:** PFV-Anterior Retinal Elongation

Chapter 31: Video: PPV for RRD associated with choroidal coloboma by Shunji Kusaka

Chapter 32: Optic Nerve Head Maculopathy surgical videos by Wei Chi Wu

- **Video 1:** Repair of a secondary macular hole with Autologus Fibrin related to optic pit maculopathy
- **Video 2:** Morning glory related RD

Chapter 33: Genetic diseases causing RRD (Caroline Baumal)

- **Video 1:** Marfan related RRD: PPV for giant retinal break RD by Şengül Özdek
- **Video 2:** Stickler related RRD: Encircling Scleral Buckle, external drainage, cryotherapy by Şengül Özdek

Chapter 34: Video on traumatic vitreous hemorrhage, giant retinal break RRD repair with combined scleral buckle, Lensectomy and PPV with silicone oil by Nimesh Patel

Chapter 35: ROP related late RRD

- Video of combined scleral buckle, lens sparing vitrectomy with silicone oil in an 11 year old ROP survivor by Şengül Özdek

Chapter 36: CXLR

- **Video 1:** CXLR related retinal complications: Composite video by Şengül Özdek
- **Video 2:** Bullous retinoschisis repair by Şengül Özdek

Chapter 37: Congenital glaucoma related RD

- Trabeculotomy related PVR-RRD treated with PPV with C3F8 gas tamponade by Şengül Özdek

Chapter 38: Nonsyndromic pathologic myopia associated RRD by H. Mortada

- **Video 1:** Recurrent pediatric RRD, post SB by H. Mortada
- **Video 2:** GRT, Bimanual dissection of post hyaloid by H. Mortada

Chapter 39: Video: Pediatric Giant retinal tear by A. Berrocal

Chapter 41: Video: Combined surgery with buckle and vitrectomy for PVR-RD by Şengül Özdek

Chapter 42: Pneumatic Retinopexy

- **Video 1:** Case 3 Pediatric pneumatic retinopexy cryo by Rajeev Muni
- **Video 2:** Case 4 Pediatric pneumatic retinopexy by Rajeev Muni

Chapter 43: Closed globe injuries by H. Durukan

- **Video:** Closed globe injury chandelier assisted scleral buckle surgery by Hakan Durukan

Chapter 45: Posttraumatic Endophtalmitis by G. Gini

- **Video 1:** PPV for endophthalmitis by G. Gini
- **Video 2:** Endophthalmitis Posterior Hyaloid fenestration by G. Gini
- **Video 3:** Posttraumatic endophthalmitis with IOFB: Vitrectomy and IOFB removal by Şengül Özdek

Chapter 46: IOFB removal by N. Yannuzzi

- **Video 1:** Pencil tip extraction from pars plana in a phakik eye with full vision by Şengül Özdek
- **Video 2:** IOFB-RD: Combined encircling buckle with PPV, metallic IOFB extraction with silicone oil tamponade by Sarah Read

Chapter 47: PVR by G. Gürelik

- **Video:** Mitomycin C use for PVR by G. Gürelik

Chapter 49: Shaken baby syndrome by K. Tran

- **Video:** Shaken baby GRT Macular tear RD by Şengül Özdek

Chapter 50: Vitreous hemorrhage by. P Ferone

- **Video:** Vitreous Hemorrhage in a Buphthalmic eye (FEVR) by Şengül Özdek

Chapter 51: Ocular toxoplasmosis by P. Çakar Özdal

- **Video:** Toxoplasmozis associated TRD with ROP by Şengül Özdek

Chapter 52: Ocular toxocariasis by M. Hasanreisoglu

- **Video:** ocular toxocariasis surgery by Şengül Özdek

Chapter 53: Pars Planitis by Lisa Faia

- **Video:** Vitreous hemorrhage in a pars planitis case by L. Faia

Chapter 54: Other Inflammatory Diseases by Stephanie Llop

- **Video:** Pediatric Lensectomy and Vitrectomy for Cataract and Vitritis by A. Berrocal

Chapter 56: General Guidelines for Lens Surgery at Pediatric Age by Serena Wang

- **Video 1:** Limbal lensectomy-posterior capsulorexis-anteriro vitrectomy: bimanual technique by S. Wang
- **Video 2:** Anterior-posterior capsulotomy-anterior vitrectomy-IOL in the bag by S. Wang
- **Video 3:** Anterior-posterior capsulotomy-anterior vitrectomy-IOL in the bag by S. Wang
- **Video 4:** Limbal lensectomy-anterior vitrectomy in an Anterior PFV case by S. Wang

Chapter 57: Complications of Lens Surgery by Camila Ventura

- **Video:** opacification of Visual Axis surgery by H. Tuba Atalay

Chapter 58: Secondary IOL implantation at pediatric age by Parveen Sen

- **Video 1:** Secondary IOL implantations in sulcus by P. Sen
- **Video 2:** SFIOL with Macular hole surgery by P. Sen

Chapter 59: Management of Aphakia by. Huban Atilla

- **Video:** Fitting aphakic contact lens in babies by H. Atilla.

Chapter 64: Nanophthalmos in children. S. Agarkal

- **Video:** Nanophthalmos retinal detachment-Scleral Window surgery by Şengül Özdek

Contents

Contributors

Abdussalam M. Abdullatif Department of Ophthalmology, Kasr El Aini Hospital, Cairo University, Cairo, Egypt

Luis Acaba-Berrocal Illinois Eye and Ear Infirmary, University of Illinois at Chicago, Chicago, IL, USA

Dhariana Acón Retina and Pediatric Retina Specialist: National Children Hospital Costa Rica, Asociados de Macular Vitreo y Retina de Costa Rica, San Jose, Costa Rica
Universidad de Ciencias Médicas, San Jose, Costa Rica
National Children Hospital, San Jose, Costa Rica

Sumita Agarkar Department of Pediatric Opthalmology and Adult Strabismus, Medical Research Foundation, Chennai, India

Komal Agarwal Srimati Kanuri Santhamma Centre for Vitreoretinal Diseases, and Jasti V. Ramanamma Childrens' Eye Care Centre, L V Prasad Eye Institute, Hyderabad, India

Ishrat Ahmed Retina Service, Massachusetts Eye and Ear, Harvard Medical School, Boston, MA, USA

Janet Alexander School of Medicine, University of Maryland, Baltimore, MD, USA

H. Tuba Atalay School of Medicine, Ophthalmology Department, Gazi University, Ankara, Turkey

Huban Atilla Prof of Ophthalmology, Faculty of Medicine, Department of Ophthalmology, Ankara University, Ankara, Turkey

Grace Baldwin Harvard Medical School, Boston, MA, USA

Alay S. Banker Banker's Retina Clinic and Laser Centre, Ahmedabad, India

Deepa Banker NHL Municipal Medical College, Ahmedabad, India

Caroline R. Baumal Professor, Department of Ophthalmology, New England Eye Center, Tufts University School of Medicine, Boston, MA, USA

Audina M. Berrocal Medical Director of Pediatric Retina and Retinopathy of Prematurity, Vitreoretinal Fellowship Director Retina Department, Bascom Palmer Eye Institute, Miami, FL, USA

Jesse L. Berry The Vision Center at Children's Hospital Los Angeles, Los Angeles, CA, USA
USC Roski Eye Institute, Keck School of Medicine of the University of Southern California, Los Angeles, CA, USA
Norris Comprehensive Cancer Center, Keck School of Medicine, University of Southern California, Los Angeles, CA, USA
The Saban Research Institute, Children's Hospital Los Angeles, Los Angeles, CA, USA

Cagri G. Besirli Department of Ophthalmology and Visual Sciences, Kellogg Eye Center, University of Michigan, Ann Arbor, MI, USA

Muna Bhende Medical Research Foundation, Shri Bhagwan Mahavir Vitreoretinal Services, Chennai, India

Pramod S. Bhende Medical Research Foundation, Shri Bhagwan Mahavir Vitreoretinal Services, Chennai, India

Michael P. Blair Retina Consultants, LTD, Des Plaines, Illinois, United States
Department of Ophthalmology and Visual Science, University of Chicago, Chicago, IL, USA
Retina Consultants, Ltd., Des Plaines, IL, USA

Marie-Christine Bruender Department of Ophthalmology, University Medicine Greifswald, Greifswald, Germany

J. Peter Campbell Department of Ophthalmology, Casey Eye Institute, Oregon Health and Science University, Portland, OR, USA

Antonio Capone Jr. Department of Ophthalmology, Oakland University William Beaumont School of Medicine, Royal Oak, Rochester, MI, USA
Oakland University William Beaumont Hospital School of Medicine, Auburn Hills, MI, USA
Associated Retinal Consultants PC, Royal Oak, MI, USA

Kara M. Cavuoto Bascom Palmer Eye Institute, Pediatric Ophthalmology, University of Miami, Miami, FL, USA

Linda A. Cernichiaro-Espinosa Asociación Para Evitar La Ceguera en México IAP, CDMX, Mexico

Melissa Chandler Department of Ophthalmology and Visual Sciences, Moran Eye Center, University of Utah, Salt Lake City, Utah, USA

Zahed Chehab School of Medicine, Ophthalmology Department, Koç University, Istanbul, Turkey

Michael F. Chiang National Eye Institute, National Institutes of Health, Bethesda, MD, USA

Aaron Coyner Casey Eye Institute, Oregon Health and Science University, Portland, OR, USA

Adrienne Csutak Department of Ophthalmology, Medical School, University of Pécs, Pécs, Hungary

Abhishek Das Department of Pediatric Retina and Ocular Oncology, Aravind Eye Hospital and Post Graduate Institute of Ophthalmology, Coimbatore, Tamilnadu, India

Marcela Raposo Vieira de Oliveira Altino Ventura Foundation, Recife, Brazil

Fernando Del Valle-Nava Hospital Luis Sanchez Bulnes, Asociación Para Evitar La Ceguera en Mexico, Coyoacan, Ciudad de Mexico, Mexico

Maura Di Nicola Department of Ophthalmology, University of Cincinnati College of Medicine, Cincinnati, OH, USA

J. Daniel Diaz Bascom Palmer Eye Institute, Department of Ophthalmology, University of Miami, Miami, FL, USA

Kimberly A. Drenser Department of Ophthalmology, Oakland University William Beaumont School of Medicine, Royal Oak, MI, USA
Pediatric Retinal Research Foundation, Birmingham, MI, USA
Eye Research Institute, Oakland University, Rochester, MI, USA

Ali Hakan Durukan University of Health Sciences, Gulhane School of Medicine, Department of Ophthalmology, Ankara, Turkey

Jared J. Ebert Department of Ophthalmology, University of Cincinnati College of Medicine, Cincinnati, OH, USA

Sonja Katharina Eilts Department of Ophthalmology, University Medicine Greifswald, Greifswald, Germany

Ehab N. El Rayes Chairman of Retina Department – Research Institute of Ophthalmology, Giza, Egypt

Ana Bety Enriquez Clínica Oftalmológica Durango, Hospital de Especialidades AMCCI, Durango, México

Lisa J. Faia Ophthalmology, Oakland University William Beaumont School of Medicine, Royal Oak, MI, USA

Philip J. Ferrone Vitreoretinal Consultants of New York, Great Neck, NY, USA

Alistair R. Fielder FRCP, Department of Optometry and Visual Science, City, University of London, London, UK

Giampaolo Gini University Hospitals Sussex, Worthing, UK

Milena Grundel Department of Ophthalmology, University Medicine Greifswald, Greifswald, Germany

Gökhan Gürelik Faculty of Medicine, Gazi University, Ankara, Turkey

Clio Armitage Harper III University of Texas at Austin, Austin, TX, USA
University of Texas Health San Antonio, San Antonio, TX, USA
Austin Retina Associates, Austin, TX, USA

M. Elizabeth Hartnett Department of Ophthalmology and Visual Sciences, Moran Eye Center, University of Utah, Salt Lake City, Utah, USA

Murat Hasanreisoglu School of Medicine, Ophthalmology Department, Koç University, Istanbul, Turkey

Sandra Hoyek Department of Ophthalmology, Massachusetts Eye and Ear, Harvard Medical School, Boston, MA, USA

S. Tammy Hsu Duke Ophthalmology, Durham, NC, USA

G. Baker Hubbard Emory Eye Center, Emory University School of Medicine, Atlanta, GA, USA
Children's Hospital of Atlanta, Atlanta, GA, USA

Julia Hudson Department of Ophthalmology, Bascom Palmer Eye Institute, Miller School of Medicine, University of Miami, Miami, FL, USA

Aysun İdil Ophthalmologist, Department of Ophthalmology, School of Medicine, Low Vision Rehabilitation and Research Center, Ankara University, Ankara, Turkey

Deborah Im The Vision Center at Children's Hospital Los Angeles, Los Angeles, CA, USA
USC Roski Eye Institute, Keck School of Medicine of the University of Southern California, Los Angeles, CA, USA

Subhadra Jalali Network Director Newborn Eye Health Alliance (NEHA) and Consultant, Srimati Kanuri Santhamma Centre for Vitreoretinal Diseases, and Jasti V. Ramanamma Childrens' Eye Care Centre, L V Prasad Eye Institute, Hyderabad, India

Grant Justin Duke Ophthalmology, Durham, NC, USA

Umut Karaca Suleyman Demirel University, School of Medicine, Department of Ophthalmology, Isparta, Turkey

Erin Kenny Pennsylvania College of Optometry, Salus University, Philadelphia, PA, USA

Saira Khanna Department of Ophthalmology and Visual Science, University of Chicago, Chicago, IL, USA

Hussain Ahmad Khaqan Post-Graduate Medical Institute, Ameer-Ul-Din Medical College, Lahore, Pakistan

Hayyam Kıratlı Ocular and Periocular Oncology Unit, Department of Ophthalmology, Hacettepe University School of Medicine, Ankara, Turkey

İrem Koç Ocular and Periocular Oncology Unit, Department of Ophthalmology, Hacettepe University School of Medicine, Ankara, Turkey

James Kohler University of Minnesota, Minneapolis, MN, USA

Onur Konuk Gazi University Medical School Department of Ophthalmology, Oculoplastic and Orbital Unit, Beşevler Ankara, Turkey

Murat Kucukevcilioglu University of Health Sciences, Gulhane School of Medicine, Department of Ophthalmology, Ankara, Turkey

Ferenc Kuhn Helen Keller Foundation for Research and Education, Birmingham, AL, USA
Department of Ophthalmology, Medical School, University of Pécs, Pécs, Hungary

Anne L. Kunkler Bascom Palmer Eye Institute, Department of Ophthalmology, University of Miami, Miami, FL, USA

Shunji Kusaka Faculty of Medicine, Kindai University, Osakasayama, Osaka, Japan

Eric Wei Chen Lai School of Medicine, University of Maryland, Baltimore, MD, USA

Wei Wei Lee Department of Ophthalmology and Vision Sciences, University of Toronto, Toronto, Canada

Jessica G. Lee Vitreoretinal Consultants of New York, Great Neck, NY, USA

Mahmoud Leila Retina Department – Research Institute of Ophthalmology, Giza, Egypt

Moran Roni Levin University of Maryland School of Medicine, Baltimore, MD, USA

Stephanie M. Llop Clinical Ophthalmology, Bascom Palmer Eye Institute, University of Miami, Miami, FL, USA

Allison R. Loh Department of Ophthalmology, Oregon Health and Science University, Portland, USA

Tamer A. Macky Department of Ophthalmology, Kasr El Aini Hospital, Cairo University, Cairo, Egypt

María Ana Martínez-Castellanos Hospital Luis Sanchez Bulnes, Asociación Para Evitar La Ceguera en Mexico, Coyoacan, Ciudad de Mexico, Mexico

Debahuti Midya Department of Pediatric Opthalmology and Adult Strabismus, Medical Research Foundation, Chennai, India
School of Medicine, Gazi University, Ankara, Turkey

Sandra R. Montezuma University of Minnesota, Minneapolis, MN, USA
Department of Ophthalmology and Visual Neurosciences, Minneapolis, MN, USA

Nallely Morales-Mancillas UT Southwestern Medical Center, Dallas, TX, USA

Hassan A. Mortada Department of Ophthalmology, Kasr El Aini Hospital, Cairo University, Cairo, Egypt

Rusdeep Mundae University of Minnesota, Minneapolis, MN, USA

Rajeev H. Muni Department of Ophthalmology and Vision Sciences, University of Toronto, Toronto, Canada

Sofía M. Muns Department of Ophthalmology, University of Puerto Rico, San Juan, Puerto Rico, USA

Timothy G. Murray Miami Ocular Oncology and Retina, Miami, FL, USA

Muthumeena Muthumalai Department of Pediatric Opthalmology and Adult Strabismus, Medical Research Foundation, Chennai, India

Ameay Naravane University of Minnesota, Minneapolis, MN, USA

Kavitha Kalaivani Natarajan Department of Pediatric Ophthalmology and Strabismus, Sankara Nethralaya, Chennai, India

Eric Nudleman Shiley Eye Institute, Rady Children's Hospital, University of California, San Diego, La Jolla, CA, USA

Ahmed Hamdy Oreaba Eye World Hospital, Giza, Egypt

Alejandro Ortega-Desio Hospital Luis Sanchez Bulnes, Asociación Para Evitar La Ceguera en Mexico, Coyoacan, Ciudad de Mexico, Mexico

Carla J. Osigian Bascom Palmer Eye Institute, Pediatric Ophthalmology, University of Miami, Miami, FL, USA

Ihab Saad Othman Eye World Hospital, Dokki, Giza, Egypt
Cairo University, Cairo, Egypt
Cairo University, Giza, Egypt

Pınar Çakar Özdal Department of Ophthalmology, University of Health Sciences, Ulucanlar Eye Training and Research Hospital, Ankara, Turkey

Şengül Özdek Department of Ophthalmology, School of Medicine, Gazi University, Ankara, Turkey

Hüseyin Baran Özdemir School of Medicine, Ophthalmology Department, Gazi University, Ankara, Turkey

Ece Özdemir Zeydanlı Gazi University, Ankara, Turkey

Seyhan B. Özkan Pediatric Ophthalmology and Strabismus, Private Eye Clinic, Aydın, Turkey

Cemal Özsaygılı Ophthalmology Department, Kayseri City Training and Research Hospital, Kayseri, Turkey

Gayathri J. Panicker Department of Pediatric Ophthalmology and Strabismus, Sankara Nethralaya, Chennai, India

M. Margarita Parra Department of Ophthalmology and Visual Sciences, Moran Eye Center, University of Utah, Medellin, Antioquia, Colombia

Nimesh A. Patel Department of Ophthalmology, Massachusetts Eye and Ear, Harvard Medical School, Boston, MA, USA

R. V. Paul Chan Illinois Eye and Ear Infirmary, University of Illinois at Chicago, Chicago, IL, USA

Luis Gilberto Pérez-Chimal Asociación Para Evitar La Ceguera en México IAP, CDMX, Mexico

Johanna Madeleine Pfeil Department of Ophthalmology, University Medicine Greifswald, Greifswald, Germany

Amy E. Pohodich Department of Ophthalmology, Oregon Health and Science University, Portland, USA

Supalert Prakhunhungsit Faculty of Medicine Siriraj Hospital, Department of Ophthalmology, Mahidol University, Bangkok, Thailand

Graham E. Quinn Children's Hospital of Philadelphia, University of Pennsylvania, Philadelphia, PA, USA

Safa Rahmani Vitreoretinal Surgery, Northwestern University, Chicago, IL, USA Pediatric Vitreoretinal Surgery, Ann and Robert H. Lurie Children's Hospital of Chicago, Chicago, IL, USA

Sarah Read Department of Ophthalmology, Miller School of Medicine, Bascom Palmer Eye Institute, Miller School of Medicine, University of Miami, Miami, FA, USA
Retinal Consultants of Hawaii, Honolulu, HI, USA

Hailey Robles-Holmes University of Miami Miller School of Medicine, Miami, FL, USA

Linnet Rodriguez Virginia Commonwealth University, Richmond, VA, USA

Sarah Hilkert Rodriguez Department of Ophthalmology and Visual Science, University of Chicago, Chicago, IL, USA

Luca Rosignoli University of Texas Health San Antonio, San Antonio, TX, USA

Esra Şahli Ophthalmologist, Department of Ophthalmology, School of Medicine, Low Vision Rehabilitation and Research Center, Ankara University, Ankara, Turkey

Adrienne W. Scott Retina Division, Wilmer Eye Institute, Johns Hopkins University School of Medicine, Baltimore, MD, USA

Brittni A. Scruggs Department of Ophthalmology, Mayo Clinic, Rochester, MN, USA

Parveen Sen Shri Bhagwan Mahaveer Department of Vitreoretinal Services, Sankara Nethralaya, Chennai, India

Parag K. Shah Department of Pediatric Retina and Ocular Oncology, Aravind Eye Hospital and Post Graduate Institute of Ophthalmology, Coimbatore, Tamilnadu, India

Sejal H. Shah Banker's Retina Clinic and Laser Centre, Ahmedabad, India

Sona Shah The Vision Center at Children's Hospital Los Angeles, Los Angeles, CA, USA
USC Roski Eye Institute, Keck School of Medicine of the University of Southern California, Los Angeles, CA, USA

Abdulla Shaheen Department of Ophthalmology, Bascom Palmer Eye Institute, Miller School of Medicine, University of Miami, Miami, FL, USA

Michael J. Shapiro Retina Consultants, LTD, Des Plaines, Illinois, United States
Univerity of Illinois at Chicago, Chicago, Illinois, United States
Ann & Robert H. Lurie Children's Hospital, Chicago, Illinois, United States

Lincoln T. Shaw Department of Ophthalmology and Visual Science, University of Chicago, Chicago, IL, USA

Shreya Sirivolu The Vision Center at Children's Hospital Los Angeles, Los Angeles, CA, USA
USC Roski Eye Institute, Keck School of Medicine of the University of Southern California, Los Angeles, CA, USA

Ethan K. Sobol Emory Eye Center, Emory University School of Medicine, Atlanta, GA, USA
Children's Hospital of Atlanta, Atlanta, GA, USA

Lucia Sobrin Charles Edward Whitten Professor of Ophthalmology, Harvard Medical School, Boston, MA, USA

Christa Soekamto University of Texas Health San Antonio, San Antonio, TX, USA

Ulrich Spandau St Eriks Eye Hospital, University of Stockholm, Stockholm, Sweden

Janani Sreenivasan Medical Research Foundation, Shri Bhagwan Mahavir Vitreoretinal Services, Chennai, India

Andreas Stahl Department of Ophthalmology, University Medicine Greifswald, Greifswald, Germany

S. Tammy Hsu Department of Ophthalmology, Duke University, Durham, NC, USA

Merve İnanç Tekin Ulucanlar Eye Training and Research Hospital, Ankara, Turkey

Cynthia A. Toth Department of Ophthalmology, Duke University, Durham, NC, USA

Kimberly D. Tran Sanford University of South Dakota Medical Center, Sioux Falls, SD, USA

Matthew G. J. Trese Department of Ophthalmology, Oakland University William Beaumont School of Medicine, Royal Oak, MI, Rochester, USA

Michael T Trese Department of Ophthalmology, Oakland University William Beaumont School of Medicine, Royal Oak, MI, Rochester, USA

Ahmet Yücel Üçgül Department of Ophthalmology, Training and Research Hospital, Ahi Evran University, Kırşehir, Turkey

Camila V. Ventura Altino Ventura Foundation, Recife, Brazil
HOPE Eye Hospital, Recife, Brazil

Lejla Vajzovic Department of Ophthalmology, Duke University, Durham, NC, USA
Ophthalmology, Adult and Pediatric Vitreoretinal Surgery and Disease, Duke Ophthalmology, Durham, NC, USA

Nita Valikodath Department of Ophthalmology, Duke University, Durham, NC, USA

Shobhit Varma Shri Bhagwan Mahaveer Department of Vitreoretinal Services, Sankara Nethralaya, Chennai, India

Victor M. Villegas Department of Ophthalmology, University of Puerto Rico, San Juan, Puerto Rico, USA
Bascom Palmer Eye Institute, University of Miami Miller School of Medicine, Miami, FL, USA

Taku Wakabayashi Wills Eye Hospital, Mid Atlantic Retina, Thomas Jefferson University School of Medicine, Philadelphia, PA, USA

Serena Wang UT Southwestern Medical Center, Dallas, TX, USA

Wu Wei-Chi Department of Ophthalmology, Chang Gung Memorial Hospital, Taoyuan, Taiwan
College of Medicine, Chang Gung University, Taoyuan, Taiwan

Basil K. Williams Department of Ophthalmology, University of Cincinnati College of Medicine, Cincinnati, OH, USA

Nicolas Yannuzzi Department of Ophthalmology, Bascom Palmer Eye Institute, Miller School of Medicine, University of Miami, Miami, FL, USA

Chen Yen-Ting Department of Ophthalmology, Chang Gung Memorial Hospital, Taoyuan, Taiwan
College of Medicine, Chang Gung University, Taoyuan, Taiwan

Yoshihiro Yonekawa Wills Eye Hospital, Mid Atlantic Retina, Thomas Jefferson University School of Medicine, Philadelphia, PA, USA

Benjamin K. Young Department of Ophthalmology and Visual Sciences, Kellogg Eye Center, University of Michigan, Ann Arbor, MI, USA

General Guidelines for Pediatric Vitreoretinal Surgery

Embryology of Developmental Surgical Disorders of the Posterior Segment

1

Ihab Saad Othman and Ahmed Hamdy Oreaba

Abstract

The retina and retinal pigment epithelium develop from the inner and outer layers of the optic cup respectively. Blood supply during embryogenesis comes from the choroidal circulation and the hyaloid system. The development of the vitreous passes through stages whereby the primary vitreous develops from the surface ectoderm and neuroectoderm and is vascularized by the hyaloid system, then it regresses by 30 weeks of gestation and is replaced by an acellular secondary vitreous derived from the neuroectoderm. Tertiary vitreous forms the zonular fibers holding the lens in position. Understanding the embryogenic background of the development of the eye helps in better correlation of different pathological entities in retinal disease. For instance, retinopathy of prematurity is related to defect in retinal vasculogenesis, that will end up in an angiogenesis process with all its sequelae. Failure of regression of the fetal vessels results in persistent fetal vasculature with all its variations. Failure of closure of the embryonic optic fissure results in a whole range of optic nerve defects. In this

Supplementary Information The online version contains supplementary material available at https://doi.org/10.1007/978-3-031-14506-3_1.

I. S. Othman (✉) · A. H. Oreaba
Eye World Hospital, Giza, Egypt
e-mail: ihabsaad@hotmail.com

I. S. Othman
Cairo University, Cairo, Egypt

Ş. Özdek et al. (eds.), *Pediatric Vitreoretinal Surgery*,
https://doi.org/10.1007/978-3-031-14506-3_1

chapter, we review the embryological origin of the eye and correlates different congenital pathologic entities to the development of the retina, optic nerve and ocular vasculature.

Keywords

Retinal embryogenesis · Optic nerve development · Hyaloid system · Primary vitreous · Secondary vitreous · Tertiary vitreous · Persistent fetal vasculature · Retinopathy of prematurity · Optic nerve defects · Coloboma · Microphthalmos · Microphthalmos with cyst

Introduction

The human eye develops from tissues with different embryological origins, namely: the neural ectoderm, the surface ectoderm, and the periocular mesenchyme [1]. During the 3rd week of gestation, the neural tube folds forming three dilatations; the forebrain (Prosencephalon), the midbrain (Mesencephalon), and the hindbrain (Rhombencephalon). The wall of the diencephalon undergoes thickening and depression forming the optic sulcus [2–4] (Fig. 1.1).

During the 4th week of gestation, the neural tube closes anteriorly. Meanwhile, two outpouchings of the neural tube at the lateral aspect of the forebrain grow laterally to form the primary optic vesicles as they progress towards the surface ectoderm (Fig. 1.2B) [2–4].

Invagination of the distal part of the optic vesicle will form a double-walled optic cup (Fig. 1.2). This invagination is not limited to the optic cup but extends to the inferior surface forming the embryonic fissure. Whilst invagination occurs, the

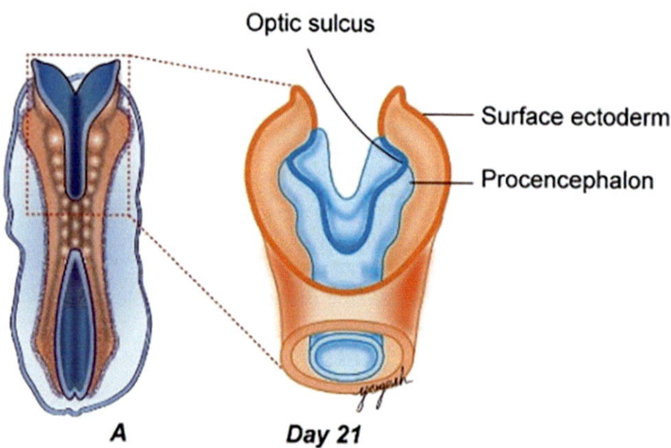

Fig. 1.1 Dilatation of the neural tube with development of the optic vesicle. With permission from: Textbook of Human Embryology, Yogesh Sontakke, CBS Publishers & Distributors Private Limited, 2019, Delhi, India. ISBN 938810837X, 9789388108379

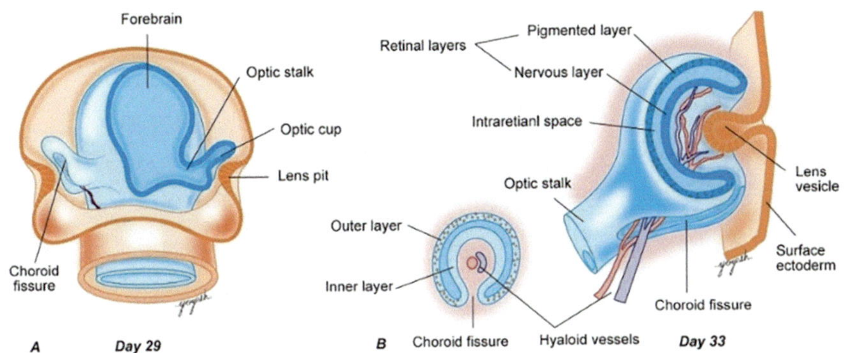

Fig. 1.2 **A** Optic Cup formation **B** Development of the Retina and Hyaloid vessels. Development of the optic nerve from the optic stalk. With permission from: Textbook of Human Embryology, Yogesh Sontakke, CBS Publishers & Distributors Private Limited, 2019, Delhi, India. ISBN 938810837X, 9789388108379

proximal part of the optic vesicle undergoes constriction to form the optic stalk which connects the neural tube to the optic cup [2–5].

Eventually, the outer layer of the optic cup will form the retinal pigment epithelium while the inner layer of the optic cup will form the neural retina. The embryonic fissure within the optic stalk will allow entry of the hyaloid vessels to nourish the developing eye (Fig. 1.2) [2–5].

The developing retina is supported by two types of vascular networks, the first is choroidal blood vessels which supports the development of the Retinal Pigment Epithelial layer and outer retina, while the second is the hyaloid system which is a transient vascular system that supports the growth of the retina, primary vitreous and anterior segment structures [6] (Fig. 1.3A, B).

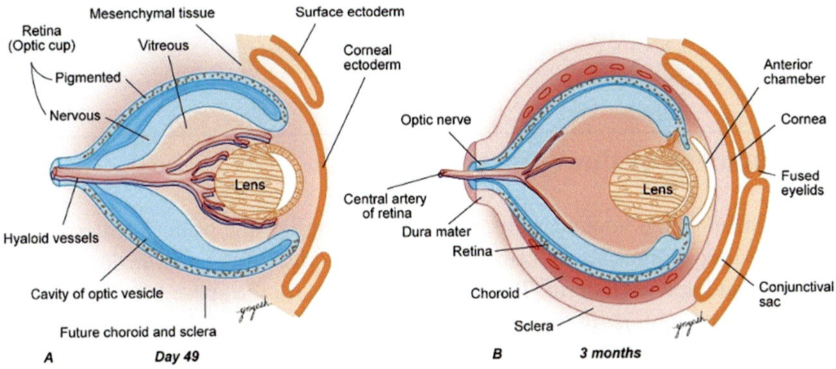

Fig. 1.3 **A** Formation of hyaloid vessels **B** Regression of hyaloid vessels. With permission from: Textbook of Human Embryology, Yogesh Sontakke, CBS Publishers & Distributors Private Limited, 2019, Delhi, India. ISBN 938810837X, 9789388108379

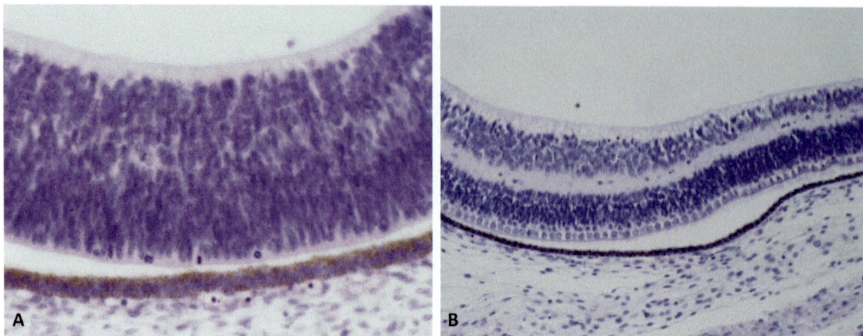

Fig. 1.4 Retinal Development. **A** 8th week of gestation showing the inner neuroblastic layer and the outer neuroblastic layer. **B** Maturation of the retinal cells into its full layers. With permission from: Textbook of Human Embryology, Yogesh Sontakke, CBS Publishers & Distributors Private Limited, 2019, Delhi, India. ISBN 938810837X, 9789388108379

Development of the Retina

As mentioned above, the Retinal Pigment Epithelial layer develops from the outer layer of the optic cup while the neural retina develops from the inner layer of the optic cup. In the 7th week of gestation, differentiation of retinal cells is initiated by the division of the inner layer of the optic cup into the outer marginal zone and inner nuclear zone. After this stage, repopulation of progenitor retinal cells will result in two distinctive zones; the inner neuroblastic layer and the outer neuroblastic layer (Fig. 1.4A). Definitive cells and layers of the mature retina are formed from the two neuroblastic layers; From the inner neuroblastic zone, there will be differentiation of the ganglion cells, the nuclei of the fibers of Müller's, and the amacrine cells (Fig. 1.4B). The outer neuroblastic layer forms the bipolar nuclei, the nuclei of the rods and cones, and the horizontal cells (Fig. 1.4B). Both neuroblastic layers are separated by a narrow interval called the transient layer of Chievitz, which forms the inner plexiform layer [7].

Development of the Vitreous

Development of the vitreous starts with the formation of the primary vitreous. The primary vitreous consists of cells of ectodermal origin arising from lens surface ectoderm and neuroectoderm. These cells migrate to fill the space between the lens plate and optic vesicle. In the meantime, the optic vesicle will be transformed into the optic cup.

Vascularization of the primary vitreous ensues via the hyaloid system, which is derived from the dorsal nasal artery. The hyaloid vessels will pass through the optic fissure till they emerge from the optic papilla, then they reach the central vitreous

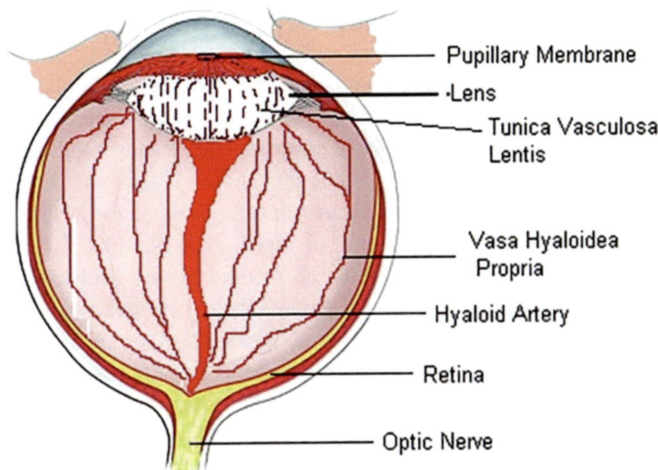

Fig. 1.5 Schematic diagram of the hyaloid vascular systems. With permission from Zhang C, Gehlbach P, Gongora C, Cano M, Fariss R, Hose S, et al. A potential role for β- and γ-crystallins in the vascular remodeling of the eye. Dev Dyn. 2005;234(1):36–47

and enclose the lens then reach the anterior segment. Throughout this journey, the hyaloid system can be subdivided into three separate anatomical entities (Fig. 1.5).

- Vasa Hyaloidea propria (VHP): Tributaries of the hyaloid artery in the vitreous that is located close to the retina.
- Tunica Vasculosa Lentis (TVL): A capillary network that is derived from the hyaloid system and encloses the lens. It has an anterior attachment to the pupillary frill of the iris and anterior lens surface and has a posterior attachment to the ciliary body.
- Pupillary Membrane: It represents the anterior TVL and represents branches supplying the anterior surface of the lens.

Later on, the primary vitreous is replaced by acellular secondary vitreous. The secondary vitreous is derived from the neuroectoderm and will represent the definitive vitreous. The tertiary vitreous will form the zonular system.

Primary vitreous normally starts to regress by 28–30 weeks gestational age, the order of regression starts posteriorly by VHP followed by TVL then the pupillary membrane and finally the hyaloid stalk. Complete obliteration occurs normally before birth leaving only acellular hyaloid canal called the Canal of Cloquet. Failure of spontaneous obliteration of the hyaloid vascular system will give rise to the spectrum of Persistent Fetal Vasculature [10, 11].

Development of the Optic Nerve

The optic nerve develops from the optic stalk, which connects the diencephalon to the developing eye. The optic stalk shows the embryonic fissure on its inferior surface, The Hyaloid blood vessels lie within the embryonic fissure together with the axons of the ganglion cells (Fig. 1.2A, B) [2–4].

By the 5th week, the embryonic fissure edges approximate towards each other and proceed anteriorly and posteriorly to close in a zip like fashion. As the embryonic fissure is closing, it encloses the hyaloid vessels and axons of retinal ganglion and the optic stalk becomes vacuolated to accommodate for the developing fibers of retinal ganglion cells (Fig. 1.2B) [2–4].

By the 7th week, the process of closure of the embryonic fissure is completed. Over time, the inner layer and outer layer of the optic stalk will fuse due to an increase in the number of retinal nerve fibers. Eventually, the optic stalk will be transformed into the optic nerve. The junction of the optic nerve and the developing eye is represented by the optic papilla which allows passage of axons of retinal ganglion cells from the retina to the optic nerve and passage of hyaloid vessels from the optic nerve to the retina and vitreous (Fig. 1.3A) [2–4].

Retinopathy of Prematurity

Retinopathy of prematurity is a proliferative retinal disease that affects preterm babies with a wide spectrum of clinical manifestations ranging from spontaneous regression to total blindness. Two mechanisms have been postulated to explain retinal vascular development. The first phase (vasculogenesis) starts between 14 weeks till 21 weeks of gestation. During this phase, vascular precursor cells of mesenchymal origins leave the optic nerve to form the retinal arcades of the posterior retina. The second phase (angiogenesis) is which there is formation of new vessels by budding from existing vessels forming capillary networks [13, 14].

Retinal blood vessels start to grow from the center towards the periphery between 15 and 18 weeks of gestation. By 36 weeks of gestation, the nasal retina becomes fully vascularized while the temporal retina becomes completely vascularized at term between 36 and 40 weeks of gestation. That is why preterm babies suffer from incomplete retinal vascularization. The avascular retina becomes more hypoxic after a preterm baby is exposed to supplemental oxygen. This hyperoxia will result in delayed retinal vascularization and release of angiogenic factors. Consequently, aberrant retinal and vitreal neovascularization ensue [14–16].

Persistent Fetal Vasculature

Persistent Fetal Vasculature, previously known as Persistent Hyperplastic Primary Vitreous is a congenital anomaly characterized by failure of regression of fetal vessels [17].

The disease was first described as Persistent Hyperplastic Primary Vitreous to refer to the persistent anterior portion of the primary vitreous [17]. Yet, the term Primary Vitreous is limited only to the hyaloid vessels. Consequently, Persistent Fetal Vasculature nomenclature was adopted and widely accepted as it is more relevant to the disease entity including both the hyaloid system and TVL (Fig. 1.5).

The spectrum of Persistent fetal vasculature includes.

Anterior PFV:

- Persistent Pupillary Membranes: due to failure of regression of anterior TVL (Fig. 1.6).
- Persistent Iridohyaloid Blood Vessels: due to failure of regression of anterior TVL (Fig. 1.7).
- Retrolental Membrane: due to failure of regression of posterior TVL (Fig. 1.8).
- Mittendorf dot: a small dot on the posterior surface of the lens representing communication between the hyaloid artery and TVL.

Posterior PFV:

- Bergmeister Papilla: due to failure of regression of posterior part of the hyaloid artery. It may be combined with epiretinal membranes (Fig. 1.9).
- Retinal Folds: Falciform retinal septum (Fig. 1.10).

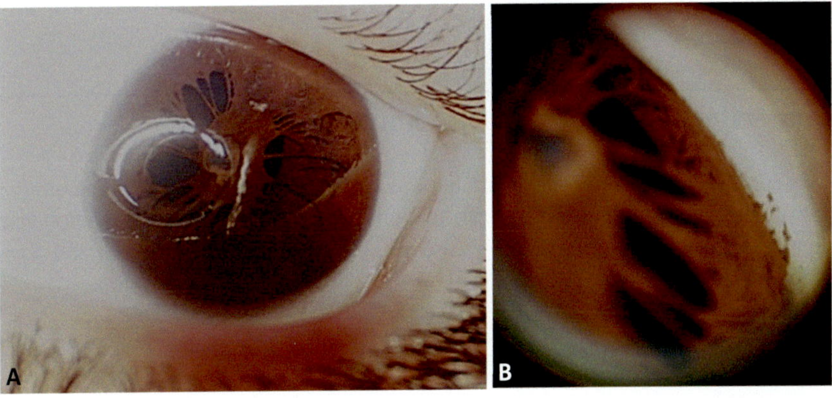

Fig. 1.6 **A** Anterior segment photograph showing persistent pupillary membrane. **B** Retcam angle view showing origin of the membrane at the anterior pupil surface and angle anomalies

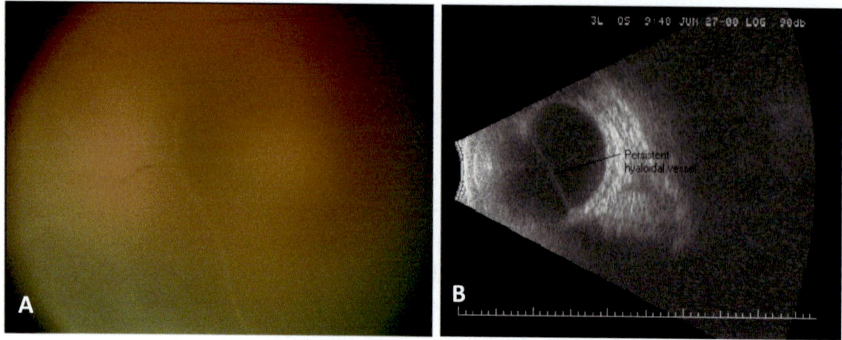

Fig. 1.7 **A** Retcam view showing a Y-shaped persistent fetal vasculature. **B** scan image showing a hyperdense echoe bridging from the optic nerve to the retinal periphery

Fig. 1.8 Persistent retrolenticular membrane

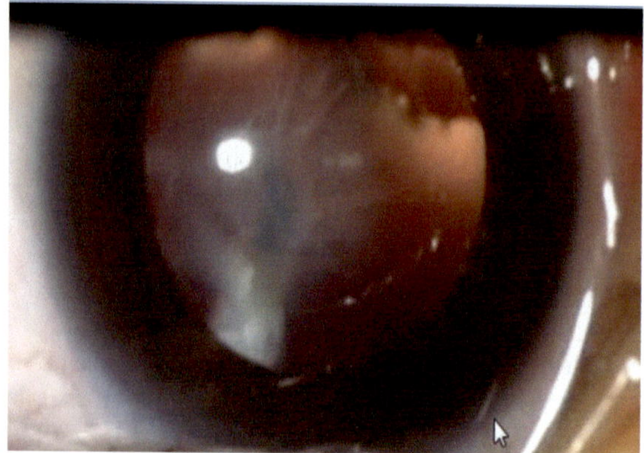

Combined Persistent Fetal Vasculature: the most common and complicated form [11, 18].

Congenital Cavitary Optic Disc Anomalies

Congenital cavitary optic disc anomalies are a group of diseases that share common embryological pathogenesis and association with maculopathy, these anomalies include optic disc coloboma, optic disc pit, morning glory syndrome, and focal peripapillary choroidal cavitation [19].

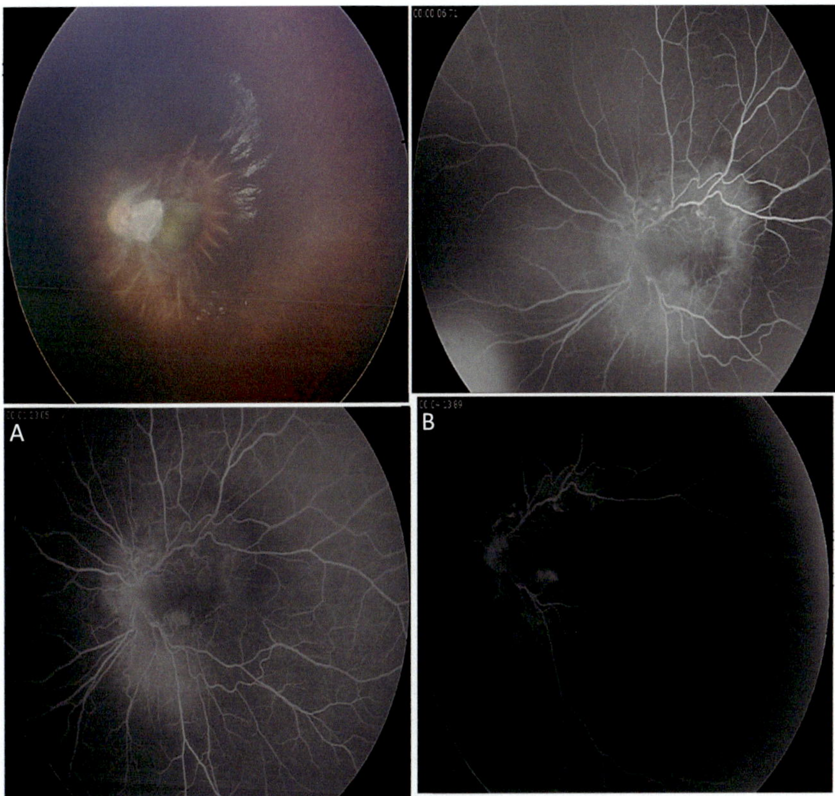

Fig. 1.9 Retcam view of posterior type persistent fetal vasculature showing. **A** Fundus view of a posterior persistent Bergmeister's papilla, with epiretinal fibrous tissue formation. **B–D** fundus fluorescein angiography showing straightening of the retinal vessels and retinal folding due to the effect of persistent posterior portion of primary vitreous

Optic Nerve Coloboma

Colobomas are defects in ocular tissues that result from failure of closure of embryonic fissure between 5 to 7th week. This loss of ocular tissue may affect the optic stalk or optic cup or both resulting in an inferior nasal defect in the optic disc (Fig. 1.11), choroid, retina, ciliary body, or iris. Colobomas of the optic nerve could be isolated finding or commonly associated with CHARGE syndrome [20]. Optic nerve coloboma could also be associated with serous macular detachment [21].

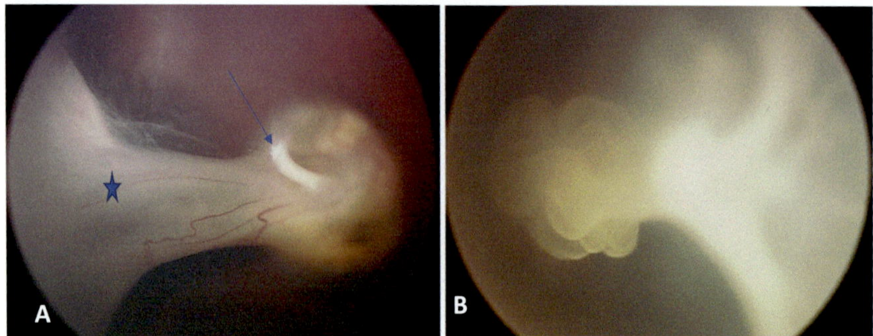

Fig. 1.10 Retcam fundus view showing, **A** Persistent primary vitreous fold bridging from the optic nerve head through canal of Cloquet, and a retinal fold bridging to the retinal periphery (asterisk). **B** Extreme form of posterior persistent retinal fold with crumbling of the retina due to traction by persistent vitreous

Fig. 1.11 Fundus view showing optic nerve coloboma OD, with a persistent optic nerve rim (Arrows). The retina is flat

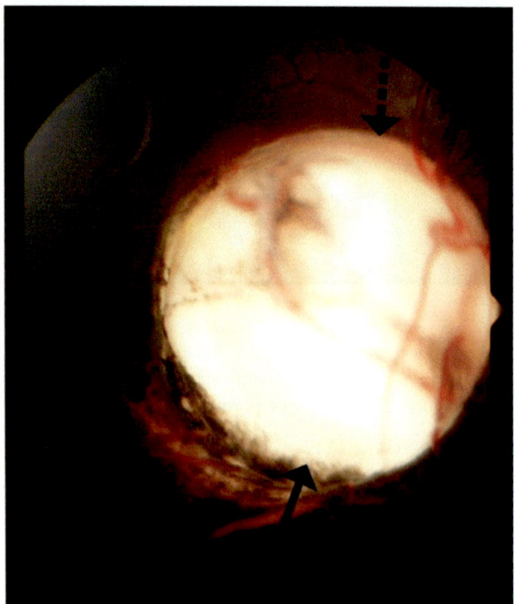

Optic Disc Pit

An optic disc pit is a congenital excavation of the optic disc (Fig. 1.12). While it is argued that optic disc pit is a milder form of coloboma which occurs due to incomplete closure of the embryonic fissure at the optic nerve head, others refute this hypothesis by the fact that the optic disc pit is usually temporal and doesn't show the systemic manifestations that might occur with optic disc coloboma [20].

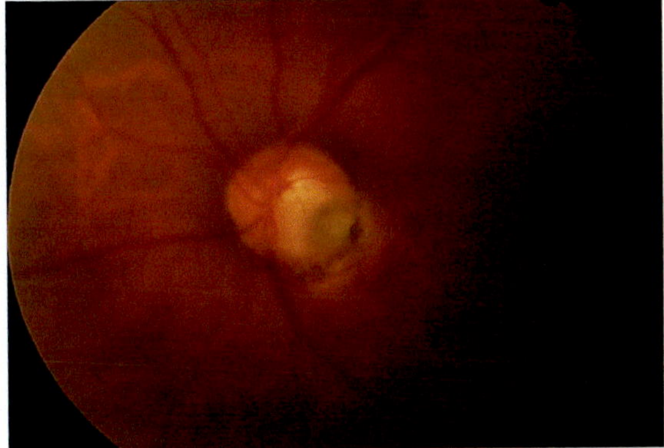

Fig. 1.12 Fundus photograph showing optic disc pit OS

Another theory for optic disc pit embryogenesis is that; it results from abnormal differentiation of primitive epithelial papilla leading to communication between the pit and subarachnoid space [22]. Optic disc pit could be associated with macular edema, retinoschisis, or serous macular detachment [23].

Morning Glory Optic Disc

Morning Glory Optic Disc is a large excavated optic disc with radial peripapillary blood vessels and central white tuft (Fig. 1.13). One theory suggests that it results from failure of closure of embryonic fissure while this theory could be argued by the presence of retinal pigment epithelium denoting effective closure of neuroectoderm of embryonic fissure [20]. another theory postulates that it could be due to mesenchymal failure that results in defective development of posterior sclera and

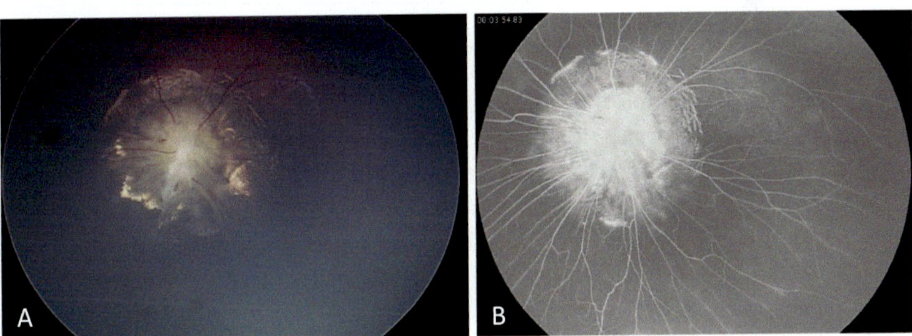

Fig. 1.13 Retcam view OS showing: **A** Morning Glory syndrome with central white tuft on the optic nerve head with straightening of the retinal vessels. **B** Fluorescein angiography showing late staining of the optic nerve head with marked straightening of the retinal vessels

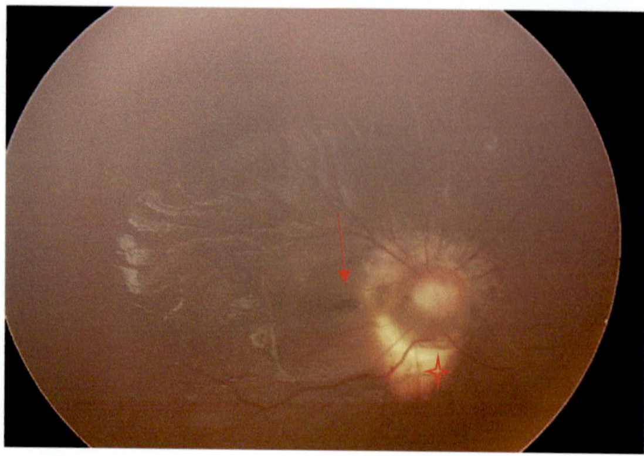

Fig. 1.14 Retcam view OD, showing peripapillary intrachoroidal cavitation (Asterisk), with macular hole (arrow) and associated serous retinal detachment

lamina cribrosa [24]. Morning glory syndrome could be associated with serous macular detachment due to abnormal communication between subarachnoid space around the optic nerve and subretinal space [25].

Peripapillary Intrachoroidal Cavitation

Peripapillary Intrachoroidal Cavitation is a peripapillary lobular yellowish thickening that is frequently underdiagnosed (Fig. 1.14). OCT is of extreme value in diagnosis [26]. One theory for embryogenesis is that it is caused by outer traction by abnormal choroidal vasculature that results from developmental failure of the choroid [27]. Another theory is that unexplained choroidal excavation will lead to ischemia of retinal pigment epithelium [28]. Peripapillary Intrachoroidal Cavitation could be associated with pigment epithelial detachment [26].

Retinochoroidal Coloboma

Retinochoroidal coloboma is a defect in the retina and choroid due to failure of closure of embryonic fissure (Fig. 1.15). In a normal situation, the inner layer of the embryonic fissure should meet the inner layer while the outer layer corresponding to RPE should meet the outer layer. When complete fusion doesn't occur, this will result in the inner layer will override the outer layer, leading to sequestration of non-pigmented tissue in the retinal pigment epithelium. Consequently, the colobomatous region shows the absence of retinal pigment epithelium with choroidal and scleral underdevelopment. Choroidal Coloboma are commonly associated with extensive rhegmatogenous retinal detachment [19, 29].

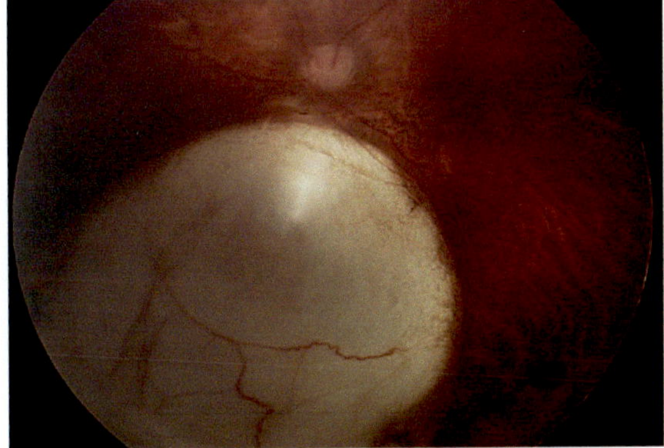

Fig. 1.15 Retcam fundus picture OS showing inferonasal retinochoroidal coloboma

Microphthalmos

Microphthalmos is an abnormally small eye with abnormal ocular structures (Fig. 1.16) in contrast to nanophthalmos in which the eye is small but without anatomical abnormalities [30]. Many theories were suggested to explain the development of microphthalmos including small optic cups, abnormal volume or contents of secondary vitreous, low intraocular pressure, and abnormal growth factors. On some occasions, microphthalmos is associated with a rudimentary cyst which results from failure of closure of embryonic fissure (Fig. 1.16) [31, 32].

Nanophthalmos

Nanophthalmos is a small eye with normal ocular structures [30]. It is caused by the stagnation of eyeball development after the embryonic fissure closes [33].

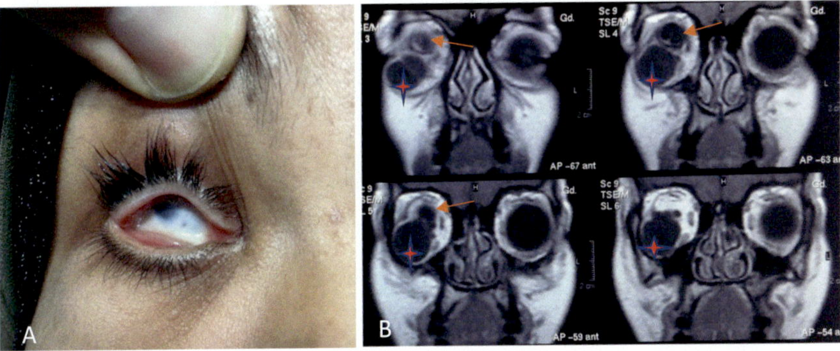

Fig. 1.16 **A** Photomicrograph OD showing an anomalous microphthalmic eye (arrow). **B** MRI, T1-weighted images with contrast showing the anomalous eye in superior orbit, connected to an inferior cyst (asterisk)

Review Questions

1. A neonate presented with this fundus picture (Fig. 1.17). **Which developmental mechanism is associated with this picture?**

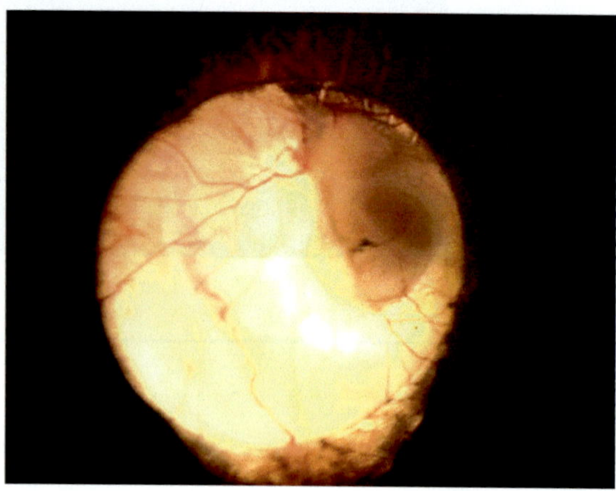

A. Failure of closure of embryonic fissure
B. Abnormal migration of neural crest cells
C. Abnormal proliferations of glial tissues
D. Abnormalities in retinal differentiation

2. All of the following are true regarding the embryologic development of retinal vessels, except:

A. Start by vasculogenesis followed by angiogenesis
B. Start to develop by 16 weeks of gestation
C. Reach to nasal ora by 36 weeks gestation
D. Reach to temporal ora by 34 weeks gestation

3. Which one of these conditions does not fall under the spectrum of Persistent Fetal Vasculature

A. Mittendorf dot
B. Berigmeister Papilla
C. Persistant pupillary membrane
D. Persistent canal of Cloquet

Answers

1. (A) Incomplete closure of embryonic fissure

The patient shown has a chorioretinal and optic disc coloboma, which occurs due to incomplete closure of the embryonic fissure. Colobomas are defects in ocular tissues that may involve the optic nerve, choroid, retina, and iris. Abnormal migration of neural crest cells leads to anterior segment dysgenesis. Abnoral proliferation of glial tissue is a feature of Morning Glory Anomaly. Abnormalities in retinal differentiation occurs in retinal dysplasia.

2. (D) Reach to temporal ora by 34 weeks gestation

Normal retinal vasculature begins to develop at the optic nerve around 16 weeks gestational age and continues throughout pregnancy. This process is considered complete when the retinal vessels reach the boundary between the retina and ciliary body, known as the Ora Serrata. In normal fetal development, the retinal vascularization reaches the nasal Ora Serrata by 36 weeks gestational age and the temporal Ora Serrata by 40 weeks gestational age.

3. (D) Persistent canal of Cloquet

The Cloquet's canal is the remnant of the primary vitreous. During embryonic development, hyaloid vessels pass through this acellular canal to support and nourish the developing eye. It doesn't fall within the spectrum of persistent fetal vasculature which includes.

- Anterior PFV: includes Mittendorf dot, Persistent Pupillary Membranes, Persistent Iridohyaloid Blood Vessels, and Retrolental Membrane.
- Posterior PFV: includes Bergmeister Papilla and Retinal Folds.
- Combined Persistent Fetal Vasculature.

SN Flashcard

Test your learning and check your understanding of this book's contents: use the "Springer Nature Flashcards" app to access questions.

To use the app, please follow the instructions below:

1. Go to https://flashcards.springernature.com/login
2. Create a user account by entering your e-mail address and assigning a password.
3. Use the following link to access your SN Flashcards set: https://sn.pub/NNcpeM

If the link is missing or does not work, please send an e-mail with the subject "**SN Flashcards**" and the book title to customerservice@springernature.com

References

1. Heavner W, Pevny L. Eye development and retinogenesis. Cold Spring Harb Perspect Biol. 2012;1:4(12).
2. Fuhrmann S. Eye morphogenesis and patterning of the optic vesicle. Curr Top Dev Biol. 2010;93:61–84.
3. Graw J. Genetic aspects of embryonic eye development in vertebrates. Dev Genet. 1996;18(3):181–97.
4. Rosen DA, Mahabadi N. Embryology, Optic Cup. In 2019.
5. Graw J. Eye development. Curr Top Dev Biol. 2010;90:343–86.
6. Saint-Geniez M, D'Amore PA. Development and pathology of the hyaloid, choroidal and retinal vasculature. Int J Dev Biol. 2004;48(8–9):1045–58.
7. Mann IC. The process of retinal differentiation in man. Proc R Soc Med. 1927;21(1):110.
8. Gupta MP, Herzlich AA, Sauer T, Chan C-C. Retinal anatomy and pathology. Dev Ophthalmol. 2016;55:7–17.
9. Yang S, Zhou J, Li D. Functions and diseases of the retinal pigment Epithelium. Front Pharmacol. 2021;12:1976.
10. Chen C, Xiao H, Ding X. Persistent fetal vasculature. Asia-Pac J Ophthalmol Phila Pa. 2019;8(1):86–95.
11. Sang DN. Embryology of the vitreous. Congenital and developmental abnormalities. Bull Soc Belge Ophtalmol. 1987;223 Pt 1:11–35.
12. Zhang C, Gehlbach P, Gongora C, Cano M, Fariss R, Hose S, et al. A potential role for β- and γ-crystallins in the vascular remodeling of the eye. Dev Dyn. 2005;234(1):36–47.
13. Flynn JT, Chan-Ling T. Retinopathy of prematurity: two distinct mechanisms that underlie zone 1 and zone 2 disease. Am J Ophthalmol. 2006;142(1):46–59.
14. Dogra MR, Katoch D, Dogra M. An update on Retinopathy of Prematurity (ROP). Indian J Pediatr. 2017;84(12):930–6.
15. Ashton N, Ward B, Serpell G. Role of oxygen in the genesis of retrolental fibroplasia; a preliminary report. Br J Ophthalmol. 1953;37(9):513–20.
16. Qayyum S. Development of retinopathy of prematurity. Commun Eye Health. 2018;31(101):S3.
17. Reese A. Persistent hyperplastic primary vitreous. Trans Am Acad Ophthalmol Otolaryngol Am Acad Ophthalmol Otolaryngol. 1955;59(3):271–95.
18. Goldberg MF. Persistent fetal vasculature (PFV): an integrated interpretation of signs and symptoms associated with persistent hyperplastic primary vitreous (PHPV) LIV Edward Jackson Memorial Lecture. Am J Ophthalmol. 1997;124(5):587–626.
19. Jain N, Johnson MW. Pathogenesis and treatment of maculopathy associated with cavitary optic disc anomalies. Am J Ophthalmol. 2014;158(3):423–35.
20. Nicholson B, Ahmad B, Sears JE. Congenital optic nerve malformations. Int Ophthalmol Clin. 2011 Winter;51(1):49–76.
21. Hotta K, Hirakata A, Hida T. Retinoschisis associated with disc coloboma. Br J Ophthalmol [Internet]. 1999;83. Available from: https://doi.org/10.1136/bjo.83.1.123b.
22. Abe RY, Iguma CI, Wen LC. A hybrid coloboma and optic disc pit associated with macular retinoschisis. BMC Ophthalmol. 2019;19(1):212.
23. Georgalas I, Ladas I, Georgopoulos G, Petrou P. Optic disc pit: a review. Graefes Arch Clin Exp Ophthalmol [Internet]. 2011;249. Available from: https://doi.org/10.1007/s00417-011-1698-5.
24. Dempster AG, Lee WR, Forrester JV, McCreath GT. The "morning glory syndrome" - a mesodermal defect? Ophthalmol J Int Ophtalmol Int J Ophthalmol Z Augenheilkd. 1983;187(4):222–30.

25. Steinkuller PG. The morning glory disk anomaly: case report and literature review. J Pediatr Ophthalmol Strabismus. 1980;17.
26. Nassar S, Tarbett AK, Browning DJ. Choroidal Cavitary disorders. Clin Ophthalmol Auckl NZ. 2020;14:2609–23.
27. Kumano Y, Nagai H, Enaida H, Ueno A, Matsui T. Symptomatic and morphological differences between choroidal excavations. Optom Vis Sci Off Publ Am Acad Optom. 2013;90(4):e110-118.
28. Suzuki M, Gomi F, Hara C, Sawa M, Nishida K. Characteristics of central serous chorioretinopathy complicated by focal choroidal excavation. Retina Phila Pa. 2014;34(6):1216–22.
29. Jesberg DO, Schepens CL. Retinal detachment associated with Coloboma of the choroid. Arch Ophthalmol. 1961;65(2):163–73.
30. Verma AS, FitzPatrick DR. Anophthalmia and microphthalmia. Orphanet J Rare Dis. 2007;2(1):47.
31. Weiss AH, Kousseff BG, Ross EA, Longbottom J. Simple microphthalmos. Arch Ophthalmol. 1989;107(11):1625–30.
32. Weiss AH, Kousseff BG, Ross EA, Longbottom J. Complex microphthalmos. Arch Ophthalmol. 1989;107(11):1619–24.
33. Nguyen ATQ, Johnson MA, Hutcheson KA. Good visual function in posterior microphthalmos. J Am Assoc Pediatr Ophthalmol Strabismus. 2000;4(4):240–2.
34. Lingam G, Sen AC, Lingam V, Bhende M, Padhi TR, Xinyi S. Ocular coloboma—a comprehensive review for the clinician. Eye. 2021;35(8):2086–109.

Surgical Anatomy of Pediatric Eyes: Differences from Adults

2

Brittni A. Scruggs and J. Peter Campbell

Abstract

In this chapter, we review the unique surgical anatomy of the pediatric eye and complex needs of pediatric patients requiring vitreoretinal surgery. There are many differences in the care of these patients, affecting everything from preoperative risk assessment, choice of anesthesia, to surgical approach and the goals of intervention. Using a number of representative cases, we provide an overview of some of the considerations that should be made when approaching some common surgical conditions in this population, including pitfalls to avoid and best practices where there is consensus. Where there may be widespread variation in practice, we try to highlight the diversity of approaches that can be successful as well, based on personal preference and training differences. Most of the topics here are covered elsewhere within this textbook, and elsewhere, in more detail, and we would direct the reader to additional resources to be fully prepared to tackle these challenging cases.

Keywords

Pediatric eye · Pars plana · Pediatric lens · Axial length · Pediatric retinal vasculature · Persistent fetal vasculature · Pediatric vitreous · ROP

B. A. Scruggs
Department of Ophthalmology, Mayo Clinic, Rochester, MN, USA
e-mail: scruggs.brittni@mayo.edu

J. P. Campbell (✉)
Department of Ophthalmology, Casey Eye Institute, Oregon Health and Science University, Portland, OR, USA
e-mail: campbelp@ohsu.edu

Introduction

Pediatric retinal diseases represent a wide range of pathologies, each with unique anatomy, biochemistry, and physiology. Operating on a less developed eye, especially one with retinal dysplasia and/or other anomaly, leaves minimal room for error. Understanding the main differences between pediatric and adult eyes allows modification of surgical techniques for improved safety. Thus, pediatric vitreoretinal surgeons must adapt their surgical approach based on the ocular development and individual anatomy of every child.

This chapter reviews the anterior and posterior segment anatomical differences in children compared to adults that should be considered when performing pediatric vitreoretinal surgery. Surgical modifications related to pars plana width, crystalline lens size and shape, sclera composition, and vitreoretinal adhesions in the developing eye will be discussed.

Anterior Segment Differences

Palpebral dimensions (e.g., palpebral fissure) are influenced by age, and limited exposure in neonates and infants often increases vitreoretinal surgery difficulty. An appropriate pediatric eyelid speculum should be used. It can be advantageous to operate temporally in cases that predominantly involve relieving temporal traction, such as Stage 4 retinopathy of prematurity (ROP) cases (Fig. 2.1). Such positioning increases space for instruments and decreases risk of lens touch, especially when there are tractional forces that need to be relieved inferiorly.

Similar to the eyelid, the anterior segment differs in size between neonates, infants, children, and adults. Often pediatric vitreoretinal surgeons must perform limbal-based surgery, and these anterior segment differences must be understood fully. The major anterior differences include:

- The horizontal and vertical corneal diameters are 9.8–10.1 mm and 10.4–10.7 mm at birth, respectively, compared to an average of 11.7 mm at age 7 [1].
- The average anterior chamber depth is 2.1 mm in full-term newborns compared to 3.0–3.2 mm in adults [2]. Other studies report the newborn anterior chamber is approximately 75–80% the depth of the adult chamber [1, 2].
- The premature eye has a steeper corneal curvature and shallower anterior chamber compared to the full-term eye.
- The newborn lens is spherical and relatively thicker than the adult lens. The lens axial length is 3.8 mm in full-term newborns and 3.9–4.0 mm in adults [2].
- The pediatric lens is soft and attached to the anterior vitreous. Anterior lensectomy can lead to retinal traction and breaks if caution is not exercised.

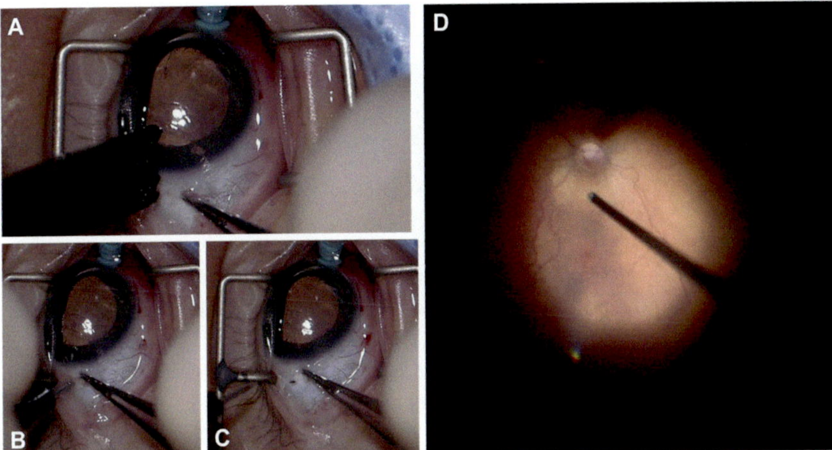

Fig. 2.1 Intraoperative Views of Vitrectomy for Stage 4A Retinopathy of Prematurity. Lens-sparing vitrectomy was performed for worsening vitreoretinal traction temporally several weeks post peripheral laser ablation. **A** Sclerotomies were planned 1 mm posterior to the limbus to clear the ora serrata by at least 1 mm. **B** An MVR blade was used to create sclerotomies since trocars should be avoided in infants. Note that the angle of entry for sclerotomy creation was parallel to the visual axis to avoid iatrogenic lens touch. **C** Sclerotomies were used for direct insertion of vitrectomy instrumentation. Note the blue sewn in infusion cannula inferonasally. **D** Surgeon's view with temporal positioning of instruments to safely remove traction along the temporal ridge

Additionally, children do not tolerate intraocular surgery, especially corneal transplantation, as well as adults given their propensity to mount significant immune responses; this can often lead to graft failure from neovascularization [1]. Surgeons should be cautious in placing intraocular lenses in young children given the heightened intraocular fibrin reaction that may occur; the approach to pediatric cataract surgery and lens placement is discussed further in Sect. 2.8.

Pars Plana Development

One of the most important distinctions between pediatric and adult eyes is the pars plana width. This measurement determines the surgical landmark for sclerotomy entry, and a 1 mm error can lead to inadvertent injury to the lens or retina. In full-term neonates, the pars plana is not fully developed and measures less than 2 mm in width [2]. This fully develops in the early childhood years, reaching an average of 3.28 mm at 1–2 years [3]. Hairston, et al. reported a 95% chance of the pars plana width being at least 3 mm at 64.4 weeks gestational age (GA) [4]. Sclerotomies can be performed without adjusting for age after 6 years, as the pars plana is then comparable to the adult [5]. Lemley and Han in 2007 published an

Table 2.1 Recommendations for Sclerotomy Placement in Children. The age-based sclerotomy distances posterior to the limbus are provided to obtain at least 1 mm clearance from the ora serrata

	Distance posterior to limbus (mm)						References
	1.0	1.5	2.0	2.5	3.0	3.5	
Age of child	n/a	0–6 months	6–12 months	1–2 years	2–3 years	3 + years	Lemley and Han [5]
	1–3 months	4–7 months	8–12 months	18 months–2 years	3–5 years	6–12 years	Wright et al. [6]

age-based method for planning sclerotomy placement during pediatric vitrectomy [5]. A similar, optimized nomogram was subsequently published by Wright et al. [6]. These are summarized in Table 2.1.

These surgical landmarks should *not* be used on premature infants; instead, instruments and/or injections should enter the pars plicata, no more than 0.5–1.0 mm posterior to the limbus, in these neonates. Additionally, the indication for surgery should be taken into consideration when planning sclerotomy placement. For instance, in cases of familial exudative vitreoretinopathy (FEVR) and/or persistent fetal vasculature (PFV), the pars plana should be visualized by transillumination prior to sclerotomy placement (Fig. 2.2). Trans-scleral illumination can be performed using the light pipe directly on the sclera with visualization of the ora serrata, pars plana, and any aberrant retinal tissue through a non-contact viewing system.

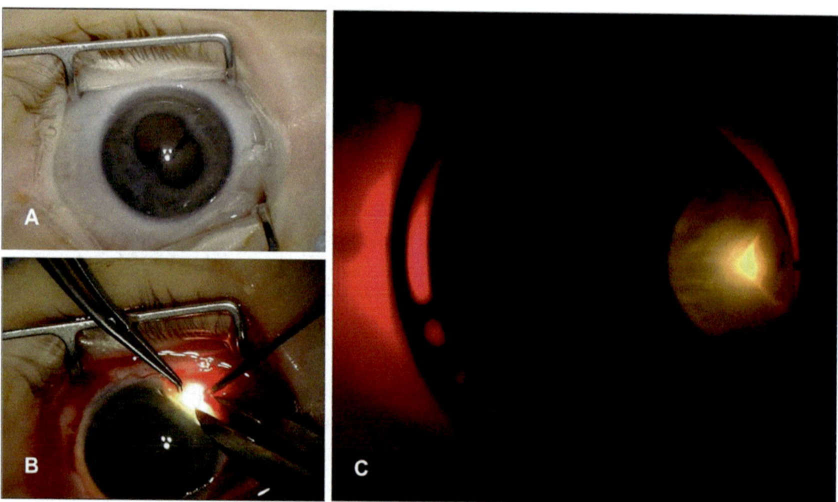

Fig. 2.2 Transillumination for Pars Plana and Ora Serrata Visualization. **A** A case of pediatric uveitis with vitreous debris required pars plana vitrectomy and synechiolysis. **B** Calipers were used to measure 1.5 mm posterior to the limbus. The light pipe on full brightness was placed at the planned sclerotomy site. **C** While the light pipe was directly on the sclera, a non-contact viewing system allowed trans-scleral illumination to verify safe entry through the pars plana with no aberrant retinal tissue. Photos used with permission by Dr. Emmanuel Chang

Axial Eye Length

The eye at birth has an average axial length of 16.8–17.7 mm and is approximately 70% the size of the adult eye, which averages 23.5 mm [1, 2, 4]. A morphometric analysis of over 200 human eyes demonstrated that the eye is at least 19 mm by 62 weeks GA [4]. The axial length often increases by 3.5 mm within the first year of life [1]. However, this growth slows considerably to an estimated rate of 0.1 mm per year between ages 3–14 [1]. The process of emmetropization requires visual input, and visual form deprivation can lead to axial myopia. For this reason, neonatal vitreous opacities should be cleared promptly, especially when unilateral [1].

The standard 25-gauge adult vitrectomy set is equipped with a 23 mm light pipe and 27 mm vitrector [2]. Given the neonatal eye is often under 17 mm with a vitreous chamber depth of 10.5 mm, there are dedicated pediatric vitrectomy sets designed with shorter and more rigid instruments [2]. Figure 2.3 demonstrates use of a cut buckle element to create shorter trocars; this is one way to improve safety during pediatric vitrectomies. Chapter 7 of this section highlights the differences between pediatric and adult vitreoretinal surgical instrumentation.

Despite a smaller eye and orbit, administration of a weight-based retrobulbar block (e.g., 0.1 mL/kg of 0.5% ropivacaine) has been shown to be safe [7]. General anesthesia with retrobulbar block is effective at reducing pain and the stress response during pediatric vitreoretinal surgery; this combination decreases the need for systemic opioids [7]. A similar block can be administered into the subtenon's

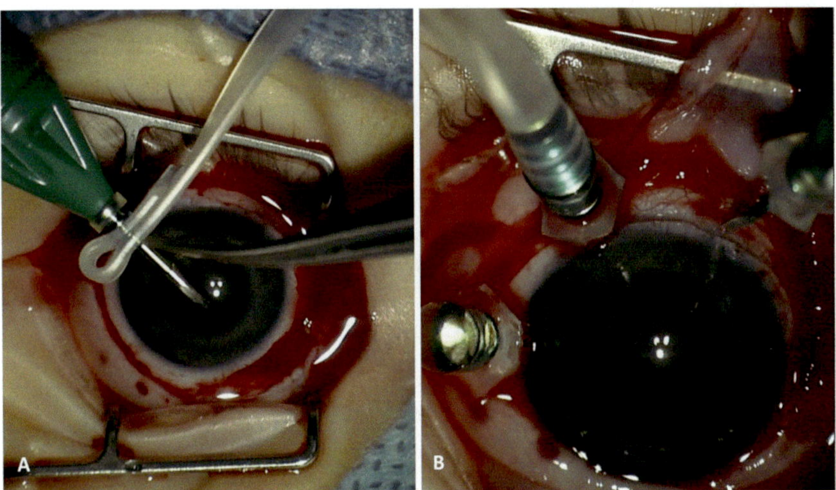

Fig. 2.3 Trocar Modification and Placement for Pediatric Vitrectomy. **A** A buckle element was secured on trocar cannulas for shortening effect for this pediatric case. **B** Trocar insertion shows entry parallel to the visual axis for avoidance of crystalline lens. Note the location of the cannulas approximately 1.5 mm posterior to the limbus. Photos used with permission by Dr. Emmanuel Chang

space in young children; many prefer this approach to decrease the risk of globe perforation, retrobulbar hemorrhage, or chemosis [7]. Chapter 6 of this section further discusses general anesthesia in children.

Pediatric Lens

Given the posterior segment at birth is less than half the adult volume [2], the lens to globe ratio is greater for children than for adults. The infant lens is also thicker and more spherical, further limiting the space to safely operate. When lens-sparing vitrectomy is performed, the instruments should be placed and positioned appropriately to avoid lens touch; lens trauma often leads to visually significant cataracts in children. Specifically, trocars and instruments should be inserted parallel to the visual axis during pediatric vitrectomy (Fig. 2.3). Adhering to the sclerotomy placement nomogram (Table 2.1) should further decrease risk of iatrogenic lens or retinal trauma.

In children with retinal vascular disorders (Sect. 2.3) or developmental disorders (Sect. 2.4) requiring vitrectomy, the risk of retinal anteriorization and/or dysplasia may necessitate crystalline lens removal using a limbal-based approach. The surgical approach to the crystalline lens in pediatric retinal surgery is discussed in Sect. 2.8.

Intraoperative Pressure Control During Pediatric Vitrectomy

Children have lower systolic blood pressure, which puts the pediatric eye at risk of iatrogenic occlusion of the central retinal artery [8]. Surgeons must be cautious to avoid excessive scleral depression or elevated intra-operative pressure levels [8]. Reduction in infusion pressures throughout the case helps prevent corneal clouding, which occurs more commonly children [8]. The infusion pressure should be decreased even further during the removal of instruments to prevent retinal or vitreous incarceration [8].

Pediatric Sclera: Implications for Sclerotomies and Scleral Buckling in Children

The pediatric sclera has increased elasticity and decreased stiffness compared to the adult sclera [8]. These differences change how vitreoretinal surgery is performed in children. For older children undergoing vitrectomy, port placement is often difficult due to the sclera composition. Often, a surgeon must twist the trocar with consistent pressure while using a second instrument to provide counter-traction. Younger age has been associated with thinner sclera [9]; the sclera of infants averages 0.4 mm and increases significantly until age 2 [1]. The thin nature of the sclera makes the use of the trocar blade to insert cannulas fully dangerous, because of the risk of inadvertent posterior touch. For younger children, sclerotomies, rather than the use of trocars, may be preferred for direct insertion of instruments (Fig. 2.1). The short path through the pediatric sclera increases the risk of intra-operative cannula dislodgement; thus, pediatric vitrectomy kits often include sutured infusion lines.

Given most pediatric vitrectomies are incomplete, there is risk of vitreous incarceration with resultant traction if the sclerotomies are not sutured. Thus, it is preferable, when possible, to perform air-fluid exchange at the end of surgery and to strongly consider suturing sclerotomies. The task of suturing on the pediatric eye may seem slightly more challenging than the adult case since the pediatric sclera is less rigid. This decreased rigidity relative to the adult also leads to eye collapse more easily; a Flieringa scleral fixation ring is necessary for combination pediatric cases requiring corneal transplantation [1].

The pediatric sclera introduces additional challenges for scleral buckling. First, the thin sclera should be considered. Second, the relative size of the buckle to the eye is much larger, and therefore care should be taken in choosing and placing buckle elements on young eyes, to minimize risk of exposure, strabismus, and post-operative discomfort. Third, since the eye continues to grow over time while the buckle remains fixed, younger children may require a buckle revision. While there is no hard and fast rule, buckles placed in younger children should be monitored for impact on the shape and contour of the growing eye, especially in children under 2 or 3 at the time of buckle placement. In these cases, the buckle may be cut, but not necessarily removed, approximately 3–6 months after the buckling surgery when the retina appears stable. The retained element continues to support the pathology, while the eye continues to grow appropriately. Removal of the buckle element, if attempted, is often difficult since the pediatric eye forms capsular tissue rapidly around the scleral buckle [10]. Finally, anisometropia resulting from an encircling procedure may be greater in pediatric populations [1].

Pediatric Hyaloid and Vitreous

The pediatric vitreous is well-formed with strong vitreoretinal adhesions throughout the pediatric eye [8]. In most pediatric retinal detachment cases, scleral buckling should be considered over vitrectomy, at least as an initial option, to relieve traction, to redirect forces, and to avoid interacting with an adherent hyaloid. With primary scleral buckling, the formed vitreous tamponades the retinal breaks and secondary surgeries (e.g., cataract extraction, silicone oil removal) are avoided [2]. Vitrectomy is sometimes necessary, and a posterior vitreous detachment must be induced in children with rhegmatogenous retinal detachments. Use of an intraocular steroid (e.g., triamcinolone) improves vitreous visualization, which is especially helpful in pediatric eyes with significant vitreoschisis. However, it is inadvisable to routinely lift the hyaloid in cases of heightened interface adhesion, such as in ROP and hereditary vitreoretinopathies. Iatrogenic retinal breaks should especially be avoided in pediatric cases; thus, in all cases the surgeon must use discretion in the level of aggression for membrane removal and vitreous shaving, balancing what is necessary to achieve the goals of the surgery, with the risk of iatrogenic breaks.

The pediatric eye is at risk of proliferative vitreoretinopathy (PVR) and membrane proliferation in the setting of iatrogenic injury, including lens touch, retinal break, or even retinotomy creation. If a retinotomy is necessary, an anterior location should be considered to decrease PVR risk. The heightened intraocular fibrin reaction and immune response with associated membrane proliferation should be considered with all pediatric cases, especially those in which the lens is removed.

Pediatric Retinal Vasculature

The choroid meets the metabolic needs of the retina in early fetal life with vascularization by six weeks GA. As the retina becomes increasingly complex and metabolically active, this single circulation becomes insufficient, which leads to a state of physiological retinal hypoxia [11]. The developing retina responds to excessive or insufficient oxygen by trimming or inducing growth in the microvasculature, respectively, to match the retina's metabolic requirements [12]. In normal development, the retinal vessels reach the ora serrata nasally at 36 weeks GA and temporally soon after birth at approximately 40 weeks GA. The likelihood of developing severe retinopathy is closely related to the state of retinal vascularization [13]. ROP and hereditary vitreoretinopathies are discussed later in this chapter.

Retina and Retinal Pigment Epithelium Adherence in the Pediatric Eye

Subretinal injections of novel therapeutics (e.g., gene augmentation, oligonucleotide therapy, stem cell-derived therapy, etc.) are being tested in pre-clinical and clinical trials for treatment of pediatric retinal diseases primarily affecting the photoreceptors and retinal pigment epithelium (RPE); such emerging therapies are discussed in Sect. 2.10. Anatomic differences in the retina-RPE adherence of children have implications for subretinal bleb formation in pediatric eyes. To create a subretinal bleb, the abnormally adherent retina must be detached. Multiple blebs may be needed to achieve detachment of the target zone and/or to avoid overstretching the retina where the bleb stopped propagating [14].

Patients between the ages of 5 and 20 (average 11.6 years) have experienced perifoveal chorioretinal atrophy following subretinal injection of voretigene neparvovec-rzyl, the first prescription gene therapy [15, 16]. Younger patients have been shown to require higher injection pressures for bleb propagation, which may lead to development of atrophy within the bleb region [14]. Thus, pediatric vitre-oretinal surgeons should perform subretinal injections using a foot-pedal control system with a maximum injection pressure limit to prevent photoreceptor or RPE shearing, solution egress that may stimulate intraocular inflammation, and/or retinal thinning that could lead to secondary macular hole formation [14].

Pediatric Anatomical Anomalies

In addition to the structural differences between pediatric and adult eyes, specific pediatric vitreoretinal pathologies should also be considered in surgical planning. A few common pediatric retinal diseases and the surgical implications of their unique abnormalities are discussed below.

Retinopathy of Prematurity

ROP is a vasoproliferative disease of extremely preterm infants. Children who are preterm have an increased prevalence of all refractive errors, especially myopia [17–19]. The myopia is low and has the following characteristics: steep corneal curvature, shallow anterior chamber, thick lens, and an axial length shorter than expected for the degree of myopia due to because of the arrest of anterior chamber development [17, 19, 20]. Advanced ROP may be associated with anterior vitreous causing further anterior displacement of the iris–lens diaphragm, shallowing of the anterior chamber and, if severe, corneal opacity and cataract [21]. The extent of laser-treated areas may have an influence on structures of the anterior chamber angle in these patients [20].

The proliferative phase of ROP can lead to arteriovenous shunts, retinal neo-vascularization, vitreoretinal traction, retinal detachments, and blindness. Severing transvitreal traction vectors should guide surgical management of extrafoveal retinal detachments (stage 4A), sub-total foveal-involving retinal detachments (stage 4B), and total retinal detachments (Stage 5); techniques for these complex surgeries are discussed in Sect. 2.3. Anatomic differences to consider when performing surgery on ROP eyes include:

- The premature eye does not have a pars plana; entry into the vitreous cavity should be performed through the pars plicata, approximately 0.5 mm posterior to the limbus [10].
- Shallow anterior chambers increase the risk of angle-closure glaucoma after scleral buckling.
- When scleral buckling is performed for ROP, the ridge should be supported on the anterior aspect of the band.
- Limbal-based approach to vitrectomy should be considered for nearly all advanced ROP detachments to avoid iatrogenic breaks.

- Extensive anterior contraction is common in Stage 5 ROP cases. Removal of the lens and capsule should be performed to remove scaffold for anterior proliferation [22].
- Total capsulectomy should be approached cautiously to prevent retinal breaks from aberrant attachments of zonular fibers [1].
- Patients with ROP are at high risk of anesthesia complications. Consider supplementing with an ophthalmic block to decrease use of intraoperative opioids [7] and performing immediate sequential bilateral surgery, when appropriate [23].

Persistent Fetal Vasculature

Patients with persistent fetal vasculature (PFV) often have microphthalmos and anterior segment dysgenesis. The hallmark of these cases is failure of the primary vascular vitreous to regress. A stalk of tissue persists, often between the posterior lens and/or anterior retina and the optic nerve. Echography can be helpful to detect blood flow within the stalk and to rule out retinoblastoma. The pediatric surgeon must carefully differentiate the stalk from the retinal fold as cutting the retinal tissue posteriorly can lead to PVR and/or retinal detachment [22]. Further complicating vitreoretinal surgery for PFV, the vitreous base and the pars plana may be displaced or dystrophic with abnormal adhesions and/or location of retinal tissue [22]. Progressive glaucoma can complicate post-operative care due to incomplete angle development.

In some PFV cases, the pars plana may be entirely absent or circumferential retinal folds may be pulled anteriorly to the lens or to the elongated ciliary processes [22]. Dense retrolental plaques necessitate careful lens removal, and nearly all advanced PFV cases should be approached by trans-limbal entry due to these abnormal anatomic findings (Fig. 2.4). A PFV case is highlighted later in this chapter (Figs. 2.4 and 2.5), and the surgical management of PFV cases can be reviewed in Sect. 2.4. As is common with all pediatric cases, iatrogenic retinal breaks can lead to a massive PVR response.

Vitreoretinopathies

FEVR may be misdiagnosed as PFV due to related retinal folds that can resemble stalks. Like PFV and ROP, FEVR eyes often have associated anterior segment abnormalities involving the pars plana, vitreous base, and anterior retinal tissue. Temporal dragging of the macula in FEVR may result in positive angle kappa or strabismus. Fibrovascular scarring and neovascularization are hallmarks of this disease, and fluorescein angiography is invaluable in detecting areas of peripheral retinal nonperfusion that are difficult to appreciate clinically. Imaging in pediatric eyes is discussed further in Sect. 2.2.

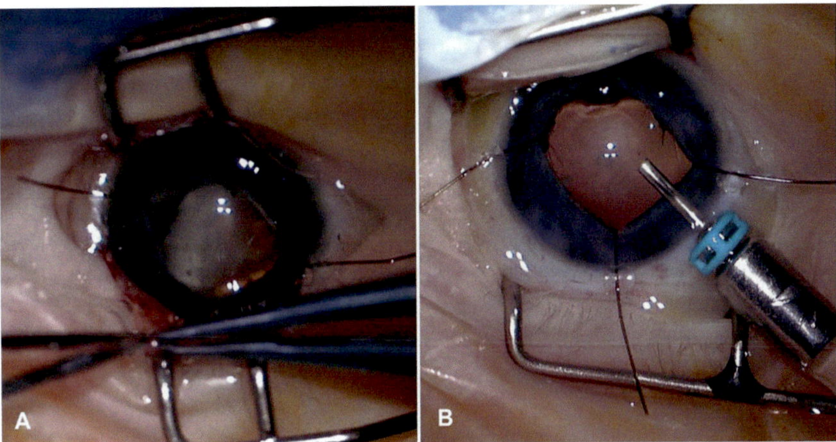

Fig. 2.4 Anterior Intraoperative Views of Limbal-based Vitrectomy for Persistent Fetal Vasculature. **A** A dense central opacity on the posterior lens is noted. Prior B-scan ultrasonography demonstrated a stalk, consistent with PFV. Note the elongated ciliary body processes and the small pupil with need for iris hooks to improve visualization. **B** Post-vitrectomy image demonstrates placement of infusion cannula in paracentesis and clear visual axis. A total capsulectomy was also performed during this case

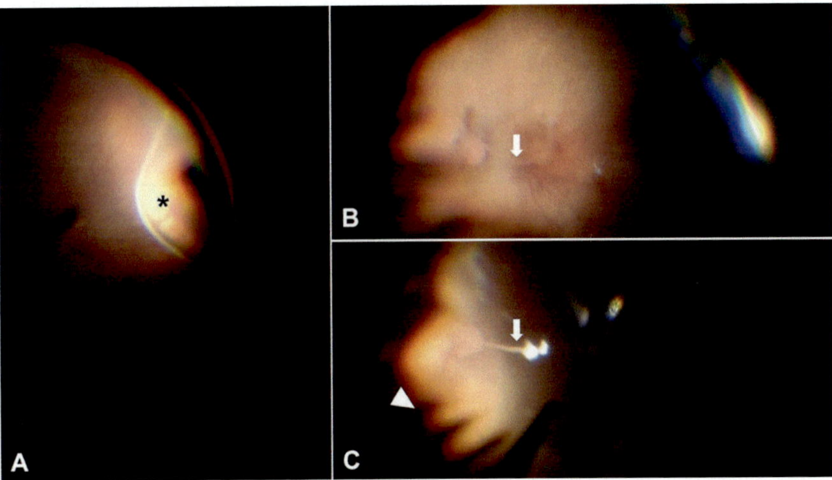

Fig. 2.5 Posterior Intraoperative Views of Limbal-based Vitrectomy for Persistent Fetal Vasculature. **A** Scleral depression (*) demonstrates normal anterior retina and no retinal breaks. **B–C** Remaining PFV stalk (white arrows) is shown after limited core vitrectomy. The ciliary body processes were elongated (white arrowhead). The vitrector was used to relieve vitreous traction from stalk and to carefully remove the capsular remnants

In some cases of advanced vitreoretinopathy with significant retinal dysplasia (e.g., Norrie Disease), the anatomic anomalies may be too severe to merit surgical intervention. Often the goals in these complex cases are (1) to maintain the eye size and/or appearance or (2) to preserve any visual function, even if only light perception [24]. Management of FEVR and Norrie Disease is discussed in Sect. 2.3, whereas management of the deformed blind eye is discussed in Sect. 2.10.

Stickler syndrome, which is the most common hereditary vitreoretinopathy, is secondary to a procollagen mutation. High myopia, frequent retinal detachments, and systemic features (e.g., facial dysgenesis, debilitating arthritis) cause increased morbidity in these patients. Section 2.5 highlights management of these cases. A few anatomic abnormalities are highlighted to guide one's surgical approach for vitreoretinopathies:

- Patients with Stickler syndrome have vitreous liquefaction and equatorial and perivascular lattice. These anatomical changes lead to retinal detachments in over half of cases and retinal tears in approximately 90% of cases. Patient counseling should include discussion of prophylactic laser and/or scleral buckling to support the pathology.
- Vitreoretinopathies, especially Stickler syndrome, are associated with multiple, large, posterior breaks and PVR. Vitrectomy in these cases can be challenging since areas of lattice can unzip and cause more retinal breaks.
- Increased retinal friability and vitreoretinal traction exist in all vitreoretinopathies. Surgeons should use extreme caution to avoid aggressive maneuvers and to avoid intraoperative traction [22].

Clinical Case

A 1-month-old child presented with leukocoria in the right eye. Anterior segment examination showed a shallow anterior chamber and a minimally reactive pupil secondary to superotemporal synechiae. There was a dense lens opacity affecting the entire central visual axis. Ultrasonography showed a thin stalk connecting the optic nerve to the posterior capsule, consistent with PFV. The retina remained attached. Given the centrally located opacity, decision was made to proceed with limbal-based lensectomy and capsulectomy with core vitrectomy.

Figure 2.4 demonstrates the limited exposure in these pediatric cases. Viscoelastic was used to deepen the anterior chamber to ensure adequate room for the infusion cannula. A 25-gauge trocar cannula was inserted into the anterior chamber through a paracentesis and connected to the infusion line. Note the long, oblique course of the paracentesis to secure the cannula in a position away from the cornea and iris (Fig. 2.4). The pupil was enlarged with iris hooks and elongated ciliary body processes were noted nasally.

Corneal paracenteses were created superiorly for entry of the vitrectomy cutter, which was used to remove the lens and capsule. The stalk was noted to retract posteriorly once severed from the posterior capsule. A limited vitrectomy without hyaloid removal was performed to relieve traction around the stalk and to remove residual capsular remnants (Fig. 2.5). The stalk was left intact to ensure no injury to the retinal tissue. The eye was inspected for retinal breaks and left aphakic with a partial air fill. All corneal wounds were closed with 10–0 absorbable suture.

Since the surgical plan involved lensectomy, the safest approach in this case was a trans-limbal entry of instruments. Although pars plana lensectomy and vitrectomy can be performed, pediatric surgeons should remember that PFV eyes often have abnormal pars plana sizes and locations with aberrant and anteriorly located retinal tissue. Thus, in cases with attached retina, lens opacity, and a central stalk, a pars plana approach may put the eye in an unnecessarily dangerous situation. This case also highlights the importance of good visualization of the lens, capsule, ciliary processes, and anterior retina; iris hooks should be considered for similar cases with inadequate dilation. Lastly, it may be tempting to completely truncate the stalk, but surgeons should bear in mind that the posterior retina can be drawn up into the stalk.

The patient in this case did well with a clear visual axis and attached retina. Vision rehabilitation with an aphakic contact lens and pediatric ophthalmology management of amblyopia were promptly initiated. The patient maintains good fixation with the operative eye.

Review Questions

1. Which disease state can present with elongated ciliary processes, microphthalmos, and a malformed anterior chamber?

A. Advanced retinopathy of prematurity (ROP)
B. Persistent Fetal Vasculature (PFV)
C. Familial Exudative Vitreoretinopathy (FEVR)
D. Stickler Syndrome

2. You are operating on a 4-month-old child with shaken baby syndrome to clear a visually significant vitreous hemorrhage by pars plana vitrectomy. What distance posterior to the limbus is safest to avoid lens touch and iatrogenic trocar-related retinal breaks?

A. 0.5 mm
B. 1.5 mm
C. 2 mm
D. 3 mm

3. Compared to adults, children have _____ sclera with _______ elasticity and _______ stiffness?

A. Thinner, increased, decreased
B. Thinner, decreased, increased
C. Thicker, increased, decreased
D. Thicker, decreased, increased

4. A 4-year-old patient with anterior dysgenesis has a normal appearing lens and a macula-sparing retinal detachment. Pars plana abnormalities may complicate lens-sparing vitrectomy. How might this be assessed intra-operatively?

A. Intraoperative optical coherence tomography
B. B-scan ultrasonography
C. Trans-scleral illumination
D. Measurement of corneal diameter

5. The pars plicata can be used for entry to the vitreous cavity in a full-term infant.

A. True
B. False

Answers

1. B
2. B
3. A
4. C
5. A

References

1. Meier P, Wiedemann P, Surgery for pediatric vitreoretinal disorders. In: Ryan S, ed. Surgical Retina Surgical considerations and techniques—Posterior segment surgical techniques 5th ed. ed. 2013:1936–1939: chap Chapter 115 vol. Part 1.
2. Leung EH, Berrocal AM. Pediatric Microincision vitreoretinal surgery. Int Ophthalmol Clin. 2016;56(4):203–8.
3. Aiello AL, Tran VT, Rao NA. Postnatal development of the ciliary body and pars plana. A morphometric study in childhood. Arch Ophthalmol 1992;110(6):802–5. https://doi.org/10.1001/archopht.1992.01080180074031.
4. Hairston RJ, Maguire AM, Vitale S, Green WR. Morphometric analysis of pars plana development in humans. Retina. 1997;17(2):135–8. https://doi.org/10.1097/00006982-199703000-00009.
5. Lemley CA, Han DP. An age-based method for planning sclerotomy placement during pediatric vitrectomy: a 12-year experience. Trans Am Ophthalmol Soc. 2007;105:86–89; discussion 89–91.
6. Wright LM, Harper CA, Chang EY. Management of infantile and childhood retinopathies: optimized pediatric pars Plana vitrectomy Sclerotomy Nomogram. Ophthalmol Retina. 2018;2(12):1227–1234. https://doi.org/10.1016/j.oret.2018.06.008.

7. Yao L, Zhao H, Jiang B, Feng Y. Retrobulbar block in pediatric vitreoretinal surgery eliminates the need for intraoperative fentanyl and postoperative analgesia: a randomized controlled study. Reg Anesth Pain Med. 2017;42(4):521–526. https://doi.org/10.1097/AAP.0000000000000610.

8. Gan NY, Lam WC. Special considerations for pediatric vitreoretinal surgery. Taiwan J Ophthalmol. 2018;8(4):237–242. https://doi.org/10.4103/tjo.tjo_83_18.

9. Read SA, Alonso-Caneiro D, Vincent SJ et al. Anterior eye tissue morphology: scleral and conjunctival thickness in children and young adults. Sci Rep. 2016;6:33796. https://doi.org/10.1038/srep33796.

10. Trese M, Capone A. Surgical approaches to infant and childhood retinal diseases: Invasive methods. In: ME H, ed. Pediatric Retina. Lippincott Williams & Wilkins; 2005.

11. Smith LE, Hard AL, Hellström A. The biology of retinopathy of prematurity: how knowledge of pathogenesis guides treatment. Clin Perinatol. 2013;40(2):201–14. https://doi.org/10.1016/j.clp.2013.02.002.

12. Provis JM. Development of the primate retinal vasculature. Prog Retin Eye Res. 2001;20(6):799–821. https://doi.org/10.1016/s1350-9462(01)00012-x.

13. Palmer EA, Flynn JT, Hardy RJ, et al. Incidence and early course of retinopathy of prematurity. The cryotherapy for retinopathy of prematurity cooperative group. Ophthalmology 1991;98(11):1628–40. https://doi.org/10.1016/s0161-6420(91)32074-8.

14. Scruggs BA, Vasconcelos HM, Matioli da Palma M, et al. Injection pressure levels for creating blebs during subretinal gene therapy. Gene Ther. 2021. https://doi.org/10.1038/s41434-021-00294-2.

15. Russell S, Bennett J, Wellman JA, et al. Efficacy and safety of voretigene neparvovec (AAV2-hRPE65v2) in patients with RPE65-mediated inherited retinal dystrophy: a randomised, controlled, open-label, phase 3 trial. Lancet. 2017;390(10097):849–60. https://doi.org/10.1016/S0140-6736(17)31868-8.

16. Gange WS, Sisk RA, Besirli CG, et al. Perifoveal Chorioretinal Atrophy after Subretinal Voretigene Neparvovec-rzyl for RPE65-Mediated Leber Congenital Amaurosis. Ophthalmol Retina. 2021. https://doi.org/10.1016/j.oret.2021.03.016.

17. O'Connor AR, Stephenson T, Johnson A, et al. Long-term ophthalmic outcome of low birth weight children with and without retinopathy of prematurity. Pediatrics. 2002;109(1):12–8. https://doi.org/10.1542/peds.109.1.12.

18. Quinn GE, Dobson V, Repka MX, et al. Development of myopia in infants with birth weights less than 1251 grams. The cryotherapy for retinopathy of prematurity cooperative group. Ophthalmology 1992;99(3):329–40. https://doi.org/10.1016/s0161-6420(92)31968-2.

19. Fledelius HC. Pre-term delivery and subsequent ocular development. A 7–10 year follow-up of children screened 1982–84 for ROP. 3) Refraction. Myopia of prematurity. Acta Ophthalmol Scand. 1996;74(3):297–300. https://doi.org/10.1111/j.1600-0420.1996.tb00096.x.

20. Chang SHL, Lee YS, Wu SC, et al. Anterior chamber angle and anterior segment structure of eyes in children with early stages of Retinopathy of prematurity. Am J Ophthalmol. 2017;179:46–54. https://doi.org/10.1016/j.ajo.2017.04.010.

21. Multicenter trial of cryotherapy for retinopathy of prematurity. Preliminary results. Cryotherapy for retinopathy of prematurity cooperative group. Arch Ophthalmol. 1988;106(4):471–9. https://doi.org/10.1001/archopht.1988.01060130517027.

22. Ranchod TM, Capone A. Tips and tricks in pediatric vitreoretinal surgery. Int Ophthalmol Clin. 2011;51(1):173–83. https://doi.org/10.1097/IIO.0b013e3182009b73.

23. Yonekawa Y, Wu WC, Kusaka S, et al. Immediate sequential Bilateral pediatric vitreoretinal surgery: an international multicenter study. Ophthalmology. 2016;123(8):1802–1808. https://doi.org/10.1016/j.ophtha.2016.04.033.

24. Trese M, Ferrone P. Pediatric vitreoretinal surgery. Duane's Ophthalmology: Lippincott Williams and Wilkins; 2006.

Preoperative Visual Assessment in Neonates and Preverbal Children

3

H. Tuba Atalay

Abstract

Preoperative visual assessment in neonates and preverbal children is crucial but challenging as well. It should include inspection of the baby-overall appearance, history taking and visual acuity testing. Obtaining a reliable and reproducible response is difficult. Different methods may be used according to patient's age. Here in this chapter we are explaining the visual assessment techniques in preverbal children.

Keywords

Visual acuity · Preverbal children · Fixation · Preferential looking

Introduction

Visual acuity, in preverbal infants, is defined as a motor or sensory response to a threshold stimulus of known size at known testing distance. In preliterate but verbal children, visual acuity is defined as the smallest target of known size at known testing distance correctly verbally identified by a child.

Supplementary Information The online version contains supplementary material available at https://doi.org/10.1007/978-3-031-14506-3_3.

H. T. Atalay (✉)
School of Medicine, Ophthalmology Department, Gazi University, Ankara, Turkey
e-mail: htatalay@yahoo.com

Ş. Özdek et al. (eds.), *Pediatric Vitreoretinal Surgery*,
https://doi.org/10.1007/978-3-031-14506-3_3

In order for a visual system to develop normally, several components are required. To receive visual stimulation the anatomical structures must be present, the two eyes must be positioned correctly and have clear media. The neurological connections of the visual pathway to the visual cortex must also be functional. Compared with the relatively dark environment within the uterus, the newborn is bombarded with visual stimuli of differing light intensity and contours within the first few months of life. This encourages the development of the lateral geniculate nucleus and striate cortex. Structural development is largely complete by 2–3 years of life but functional changes continues throughout life.

Visual acuity improves rapidly during the first year of life and then matures more gradually to adult levels at approximately 5–6 years of age. Although the central cones function by term birth, acuity as measured by the different techniques does not approach 20/20 (6/6) until from 6 to 30 months (depending upon the examination technique used). Reasons for this delay include the incomplete development and specialization of photoreceptors, maturation of synapses in the inner retinal layers, and myelination of the upper visual pathways. Foveal cones do not attain adult appearance until 4 months after term birth, and visual pathway myelination continues until 2 years of age.

Vision testing in neonates and preverbal children is often the most challenging part of a comprehensive eye examination, in fact it is an art. The examination should begin as the child enters the examination room. The child's overall appearance and level of alertness can be evaluated during the history taking. Specifically, the examiner should be aware of head position, nystagmus, photophobia, or strabismus.

Parents often are aware of a vision problem before it is readily apparent to the clinician. It is important to ask the parents specific questions about the child's vision, including whether the child has eye-to-face contact, holds things close, or squints; the eyes appear to cross or wander; the eyelids droop; or disturbed by bright light.

Visual Acuity Assessment

The acuity of the newborn infant is close to 6/240, and at 7 weeks of age the infant has eye-to-face contact. Visual acuity rapidly increases to 6/180–6/90 at 2–3 months. At 6 months visual acuity is between 6/18 and 6/9. The assessment of visual acuity, however, depends on the testing method used; here visual acuities are given as Snellen equivalents. Table 3.1 summarizes pooled information of visual development, indicating the difficulties in examining infant vision [1].

To evaluate vision in the preverbal child, we should use the smallest age-appropriate target that will hold attention and observe the difference between the two eyes. An appropriate target for a 1-year-old child may be a small figure (Fig. 3.1); but a 1-month-old may fixate only on a human face. Infants are unable to pursue targets smoothly until 6 to 8 weeks of age [2].

Table 3.1 Visual acuity according to different methods, given as Snellen equivalents

Technique	Newborn	2 months	4 months	6 months	1 year
Optokinetic nystagmus	20/400	20/400	20/200	20/100	20/60
Preferential looking	20/400	20/200	20/200	20/150	20/50
Visual evoked potential	20/100–20/200	20/80	20/80	20/20–20/40	20/20–20/40

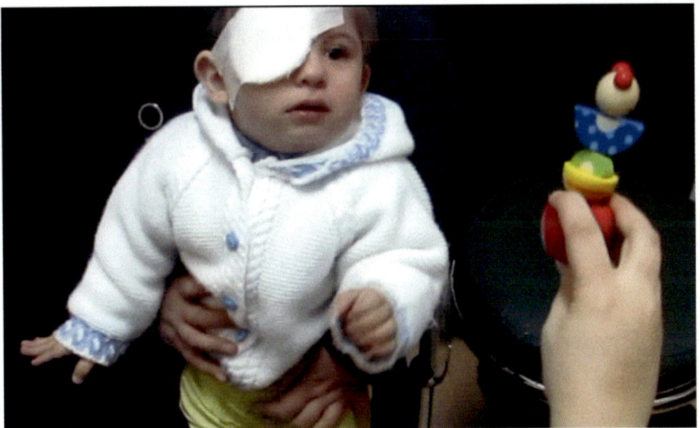

Fig. 3.1 Evaluation of the fixation pattern by using a small toy

Video 1: *Evaluation of the fixation pattern on right and left eye covered in turn.*

Cover Test can detect the amblyopic eye in a pre-verbal child. Such children resist or cry when the better eye is covered or occluded.

Fixation

In the first few weeks of life, infants sleep frequently, and it can be difficult to sufficiently assess her vision. It can be helpful to see the child when she is more alert.

There are two types of fixation testing; monocular and binocular. In monocular fixation testing each eye is occluded in turn. CSM for central, steady, and maintained, or FF for fix and follow are used to describe fixation behavior. The neonate with normal visual functions should respond to lights and to faces. The baby's gaze should fixate on and follow the face of the examiner as the examiner moves in different directions or the smallest possible target that elicits a fixation response. The ability to fix and follow an object should be present by 2 to 3 months of age. Yet it can be present at birth in a very healthy, alert infant [3].

When no fixation or following movements can be elicited, room lights can be turned on and off. A consistent reaction to the change in room illumination is a gross measure of visual response. Avoidance reactions to light of the indirect ophthalmoscope are also useful [3].

> **CSM Classification**
> C = Central: Is the visual axis central in each eye, in contrast with eccentric (recorded as nC) fixation? If so, the macula is fixating.
> S = Steady: Is the monocular fixation without movement, or does the eye wander? If not steady (recorded as nS), the type of movement must be described.
> M = Maintainsed: Can the fixation be maintained with each eye individually under binocular viewing? In strabismus, the amblyopic eye may not maintain fixation under binocular conditions, and the patient will preferentially fixate with the dominant or sound eye.

The Induced Tropia Test (ITT)

The induced tropia test (ITT) test was developed to assist practitioners in diagnosing possible amblyopia, or other vision deficits. To perform, a loose prism, either 10 prism diopter base down or 20 prism diopter base in, is placed in front of one eye at a time, while asking the child to look at a toy or a light source. Symmetric fixation behavior indicates there is no fixation preference, and asymmetric fixation behavior indicates a fixation preference is present. The fixation preference may indicate a relative difference in acuity, possibly due to amblyopia [4].

The benefits of using the ITT are that it requires minimal time and cooperation from the patient, but due to the contradictory results regarding its specificity, using it alone may not be advisable [5].

There are three basic methods for estimating visual acuity in the preverbal or impaired child: optokinetic nystagmus (OKN), preferential looking (PL), and visually evoked potentials (VEP).

Optokinetic Nystagmus (OKN)

In this test, nystagmus is elicited by passing a series of black and white stripes in front of the infant. Gross vision (ie, 20/400) is present if the child responds to the optokinetic drum (Fig. 3.2) with thick stripes. Visual acuity can be estimated by using drums with thinner and thinner stripes until the response is no longer detected. False-positive results, presumably caused by the presence of other

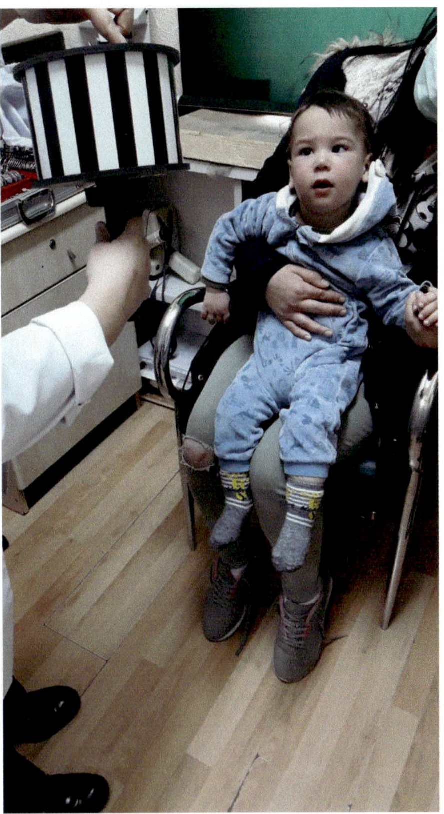

Fig. 3.2 Optokinetic nystagmus testing using a OKN drum

vision-related neural pathways, can occur in children who do not have a normal visual cortex. The absence of an OKN response to a moving stripe may represent nothing more than a lack of interest or attention [6].

It is important to note that the use of optokinetic nystagmus to assess visual acuity may lead to errors of interpretation, because one is evaluating a motor response in an attempt to assess sensory function. The absence of optokinetic nystagmus may be due to some alteration in the ocular motor systems necessary to generate this eye movement and not to the patient's failure to "see" the stimuli.

Preferential Looking Test (PLT)

This test is based on the fact that when an infant is presented with 2 visual stimuli, one striped and the other plain, the infant looks at the striped pattern for a greater amount of time. Lea cards (Fig. 3.3), Teller acuity cards II and Cardiff acuity test utilize this method.

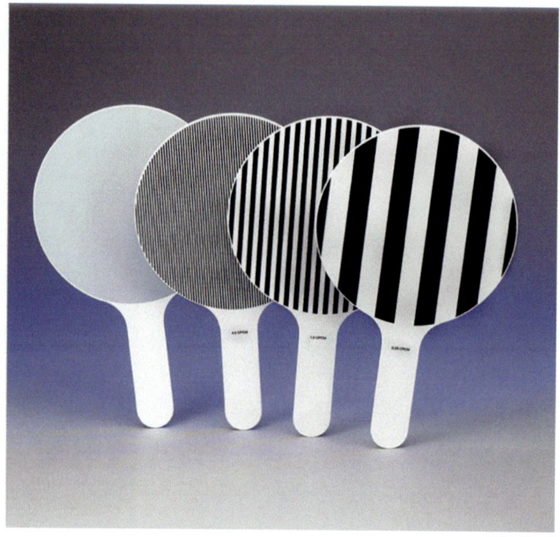

Fig. 3.3 LEA grating paddles

There are several advantages of using the acuity card procedure for measurement of visual acuity in infants. Measurements can be made quickly and easy to learn, the procedure allows the tester to interact with the infant visually between card presentations, the procedure relies on the infant's natural eye movement responses to a patterned stimulus, the cost of the equipment is relatively low, the procedure can be used with infants of all ages, as well as with children whose developmental age is that of an infant, data are available on the distribution of acuity results in normal infants of different ages, making it possible to interpret an infant's visual acuity score in terms of number of standard deviations below normal [6].

Visual Evoked Potential (VEP)

If the etiology of a severe visual impairment is not clinically obvious, the child requires electrodiagnostic investigations (electroretinography (ERG) and visual evoked potential (VEP) as well as imaging of the brain and orbits with magnetic resonance imaging (MRI)). Electrodiagnostic tests in the first year of life are often unreliable, therefore clinical examination is of superior importance.

The visual evoked potential (VEP, also called the visual evoked response or VER) is an electrical signal generated by the occipital cortex of the brain in response to visual stimulation. It is recorded through one or more electrodes placed on the scalp over the visual cortex. Visual acuity can be estimated by recording VEP responses to patterned stimuli, such as phase-alternating, black and white gratings, in which the overall luminance of the target remains constant but the spatial configuration of the pattern changes [7].

Normative data are available for VEP acuity for infants between birth and age 1 year [8, 9]. The use of the VEP for measurement of visual acuity in infants has been limited, due to the expense of the equipment and the technical expertise required to conduct the test.

Conclusion

There are many methods of assessing visual acuity in the preverbal child depending on the child's age. The examiner familiar with all techniques will be able to use the best method for obtaining the most accurate result.

Review Questions

1. Which test is not useful in visual assessment in preverbal children?

a. Teller acuity cards
b. CSM evaluation
c. ETDRS chart
d. Visual Evoked Potential
e. The induced tropia test (ITT)

2. Which one is wrong about visual assessment of a neonate?

a. Child's overall appearance and level of alertness should be evaluated
b. The examiner should be aware of head position, nystagmus
c. Presence of photophobia and strabismus are not clinically significant symptoms
d. History taking is an important part of evaluation
e. Parents should be asked whether the child has eye-to-face contact

3. Which one is not one of the basic methods for estimating visual acuity in the preverbal or impaired child?

a. Optokinetic nystagmus (OKN)
b. Preferential looking (PL)
c. Visually evoked potentials (VEP)
d. Fixation behavior (FF or CSM)
e. Teller Acuity Cards

Answers

1. C
2. C
3. D

References

1. Day SH, Sami DA. History, examination, and further investigation. In: Taylor D, ed. Paediatric Ophthalmology, 3rd ed. Philadelphia: Elsevier; 2005:66–77.
2. Hoyt CS, Nickel BL, Billson FA. Ophthalmological examination of the infant. Dev Aspects Surv Ophthalmol. 1982;26:177.
3. Ellis GS Jr, Prichard C. Visual assessment. In: Gallin PF, editor. Pediatric Ophthalmology, A Clinical Guide. New York: Thieme; 2000. p. 14–23.
4. Wright KW, Walonker F, Edelman P. 10-diopter fixation test for amblyopia. Arch Ophthalmol. 1981;99(7):1242–1246.
5. Nanda KD, Blaha B, Churchfield WT, Fulwylie CR, Medsinge A, Nischal KK. Induced Tropia test and visual acuity testing in nonverbal children. J Binocul Vis Ocul Motil. 2018;68(4): 134–136.
6. National Research Council (US) Committee on Disability Determination for Individuals with Visual Impairments; Lennie P, Van Hemel SB, editors. Visual Impairments: Determining Eligibility for Social Security Benefits. Washington (DC): National Academies Press (US); 2002. 4, ASSESSMENT OF VISION IN INFANTS AND CHILDREN. Available from: https://www.ncbi.nlm.nih.gov/books/NBK207548/
7. Lamkin JC. Can this baby see?: estimation of visual acuity in the preverbal child. Int Ophthalmol Clin. 1992 Winter;32(1):1–23.
8. McCulloch, DL, Orbach H, Skarf B. Maturation of the pattern- reversal VEP in human infants: a theoretical framework. Vis Res. 39(22):3673–3680.
9. Norcia AM, Tyler CW. Spatial frequency sweep VEP: Visual acuity during the first year of life. Vis Res. 25(10):1399–1408.

Surgical Decision Making in Pediatric Retinal Diseases

4

Matthew G. J. Trese, Michael T. Trese, and Antonio Capone Jr.

Abstract

This chapter aims to prime the reader by describing the salient points of pediatric vitreoretinal surgical decision making. Recognizing that pediatric vitreoretinal surgery does not exist in a vacuum, we start this chapter by describing the importance of establishing a multidisciplinary pediatric vitreoretinal surgery team. In the later portions of the chapter, we focus specifically on general principles of pediatric scleral buckling and vitrectomy which can be applied broadly to nearly any pediatric vitreoretinal disease.

Keywords

Surgical decision · Retinal detachment · Scleral buckling · Membrane dissection technique · Lens sparing vitrectomy · Intraocular tamponades

M. G. J. Trese · M. T. Trese · A. Capone Jr. (✉)
Department of Ophthalmology, Oakland University William Beaumont School of Medicine, Royal Oak, MI Rochester, USA
e-mail: acaponejr@arcpc.net

M. G. J. Trese
e-mail: matttrese@arcpc.net

M. T. Trese
e-mail: mtrese@arcpc.net

Ş. Özdek et al. (eds.), *Pediatric Vitreoretinal Surgery*,
https://doi.org/10.1007/978-3-031-14506-3_4

45

Introduction

Many of the principles which guide pediatric vitreoretinal surgery differ from adult vitreoretinal surgery. A thorough understanding of these differences provide a framework for surgical decision making in pediatric patients. This chapter focuses on general guidelines for incisional pediatric vitreoretinal surgery which can be applied broadly. However, a more nuanced discussion regarding the management of specific disease entities will be described in their respective chapters.

General Considerations

Although this chapter focuses on surgical decision making, it is first necessary to address that surgical intervention in a child evokes unique psychological issues for both the patient and the parents. To provide the patient with the highest quality of care and allay any parental concerns, it is necessary to construct a pediatric vitreoretinal surgery team. Key members of this team may include pediatric vitreoretinal surgeons, pediatric ophthalmologists, neonatologists, pediatric anesthesiologists, pediatricians, Neonatal Intensive Care Unit (NICU) nurses, vision/social services, school system contacts and parents. Although the members of this team may vary depending on the patient's age, the vitreoretinal surgeon, patient and parents are constants.

Therefore, it is essential to develop a rapport with the parents (and if age permitting, the patient) that is based on candor and trust. Important first steps toward establishing this relationship are to open a dialog regarding the disease process, describe the surgical goals in terms that are understandable, define realistic expectations for vision, express the mutual goal of preserving and/or restoring all levels of vision and discuss the potential need for multiple procedures and long-term follow up care. Interventions which preserve even low levels of Snellen visual acuity can be deeply meaningful for pediatric patients. By taking these steps, surgical intervention can be approached in a way that mitigates apprehensions for the both the patient and family and aligns the core members of the care team.

Rhegmatogenous retinal detachments in children require careful consideration as the mechanism of retinal detachment in this age group is often different than in the adult population. Trauma should be at the forefront of the ophthalmologist's mind when confronted with a pediatric rhegmatogenous retinal detachment. Further, trauma that is unexplained or inconsistent with the exam findings should alert the physician to the potential for abuse. Such concerns should be reported to child protective services to ensure the safety and well-being of the patient. It is also important to consider prematurity and vitreoretinal dystrophies (such as Stickler syndrome) which is a prime consideration for spontaneous rhegmatogenous retinal detachment in pediatric patients. A thorough history and examination with particular attention to the patient's birth history, family history of retinal detachments, stature, facial features and joint extensibility may provide valuable clues suggesting an underlying unifying diagnosis. The importance of this thorough history and examination cannot be overstated because children presenting with rhegmatogenous retinal detachments will often present with advanced proliferative vitreoretinopathy. Thus surgically addressing not only the involved eye, but also prophylactically treating the companion eye (prophylactic peripheral retinopexy or scleral buckle) is arguably the most important aspect of their care plan.

Scleral Buckling

Scleral buckling can be a valuable therapeutic treatment modality for pediatric patients with retinal detachments. Scleral buckling in infants and small children carries some unique considerations. First, amblyopia is an ever-present concern when operating on pediatric patients. Scleral buckling induces a refractive shift which has the potential to induce anisometropic amblyopia. In fact, scleral buckling in retinopathy of prematurity (ROP) has been shown to induce up to 12 diopters of refractive shift [1]. Mitigating the amblyogenic impact of scleral buckling requires a collaborative effort between the vitreoretinal surgeon, the parents and the pediatric ophthalmologist to manage the amblyopia factors. Second, scleral buckling in children whose eyes who are still growing should always be presented as a potentially staged surgery [2]. The first stage being the placement of the scleral buckle and the second stage being the division of scleral buckle, if needed.

In recent years, scleral buckles have been used less frequently for tractional retinal detachments, such as those in Retinopathy Of Prematurity (ROP). In these detachments it is unusual that the tractional vectors responsible for the retinal detachment can be completely addressed with scleral buckling alone. Therefore, there has been a shift towards vitreous surgery and when possible, lens sparing vitrectomy. Scleral buckle procedures remain an essential therapeutic tool in children with rhegmatogenous retinal detachments and it can be performed as either a primary procedure or in combination with vitreous surgery.

The scleral buckle that we use in children is a tire and an encircling element. We advocate for a proportionally larger scleral buckle than we might use in the adult eye because of the aggressive nature of the PVR seen in children following rhegmatogenous detachments. For example, we use a 2.5-mm solid silicone band (such as a 240-style) to encircle the eye. Then we will use a large sponge (2.5-mm; such as a 5,025-style) or a large asymmetric silicone tire (7.0-mm; such as a 276-style) for the buckling elements. Nylon sutures are used for scleral fixation of the sponge/tire and the silicone band. Treatment around the dialysis or retinal break(s) is often performed with cryotherapy, however laser may also be used. Breaks are localized on the sclera, and the buckle is chosen to support the breaks adequately ($\sim$2 mm beyond the anterior and posterior extents of the break localized on sclera). Intrascleral mattress sutures are placed approximately 2 mm farther apart than the width of the buckling element to optimize buckle height. If drainage of subretinal fluid is considered, we prefer a scleral cutdown and use diathermy to cause the sclera fibers to retract and expose the choroid. Diathermy is placed onto the choroid once it is exposed and prior to release of subretinal fluid. Transillumination may be performed to locate, so as to avoid perforating large choroidal vessels. A preplaced mattress suture of 7–0 silk is placed into the lips of the scleral cutdown if it is not supported by the buckle. Tension on the rectus muscle sutures is lessened. Then, subretinal fluid is released with a cold thin perforating electrode. In cases with thick subretinal fluid that is difficult to drain, a 5–0 polyglactin suture with a S-14 needle can be used to create a small opening in the choroid. When perforating, care is taken not to stick the needle into the eye but rather to pierce and lift up on the knuckle of choroid protruding from the scleral cutdown site.

It often is difficult to ascertain symptoms in the younger, especially preverbal, child. Therefore, the child often already has some PVR on the presenting examination. We believe larger buckles can be helpful in overcoming the tractional forces caused by the PVR.

Customarily, children are evaluated approximately 3 months after scleral buckling to determine if division of the buckle is possible. We usually leave the large buckling element in place and divide the encircling band in an area where the retina is flat without any clinical evidence of traction. In children, capsular tissue can form rapidly around the scleral buckle, even after a relatively short period of time. This is noted on attempted division of the encircling band. The band can be located by tapping gently in the area where it is suspected with a closed pair of forceps. Once the band's location is determined, a blade can be used to make a 2–3-mm incision through the capsule on the anterior buckle edge along the length of the band. The band then can often be lifted from the sclera and divided with scissors. After longer periods of time, even 6 to 12 months, the band might rarely erode into or through the sclera. In that situation, it is important to avoid any deep tissue dissection. Sometimes division of the band over the larger buckling element can be performed. In the author's experience, it is extremely rare that redetachment results after division of the encircling elements, particularly in eyes where buckling has been performed for a predominantly nonrhegmatogenous retinal detachment.

Drainage of subretinal fluid is always an important consideration. If the retina is stretched and all traction is not removed, drainage of subretinal fluid can be dangerous and lead to retinal breaks. Therefore, drainage is rarely performed in ROP and Familial Exudative Vitreo Retinopathy (FEVR). However, drainage might be considered in these cases if there is a total retinal detachment with extensive amounts of subretinal fluid; then, often only partial drainage is performed to reduce the risk of iatrogenic retinal tears. In addition, unless there is an existing retinal break, which makes subretinal fluid drainage possible in vitreous surgery, external drainage is more desirable. This is true because it is unlikely that the posterior hyaloid can be mechanically removed in a child during standard vitreous surgery.

Vitreous Surgery

Over the last 2 decades, advances both in our understanding of the pathophysiology of pediatric retinal diseases and the instrumentation that we use to approach these complex retinal detachments has allowed vitrectomy to become a leading therapeutic option for pediatric retinal detachments. From an instrumentation standpoint, two and three-port vitrectomy as well as open-sky vitrectomy, can be used for pediatric indications. Although open sky vitrectomy is rarely used today, it is a viable approach when corneal opacity prevents visualization of the posterior segment and can be used with or without a temporary keratoprosthetics. More commonly, both two and three-port vitrectomy allow for two-handed dissection in a pressurized eye with a variety of instruments. The authors employ 20-, 23- and 25-gauge instrumentation when approaching pediatric retinal detachments. Smaller instrumentation offers some potential benefits in terms of smaller wounds, less post-operative inflammation and the potential for the procedure being sutureless. However, instrument flex of the finer gauges limits the ability to access proliferation in the far periphery—as is often the case in eyes with ROP and FEVR. This combined with a smaller range of instruments available in 25-gauge results in the authors favoring 20- and 23-gauge vitrectomy surgery. Essential instruments include the wide-angle high-flow light pipe, the infusion spatula, the infusion forceps, the retractable-lighted pick and the irrigating illuminated pick. These, in addition to the vitreous cutter and Membrane Peeler Cutter (MPC) scissors, make up the instrumentation customarily used by the authors for vitreous surgery in infants and children. The viewing system used is an operating microscope with adjustable horizontal and vertical movement (X–Y) and a wide-angle noncontact viewing system.

The location of the sclerotomies often is determined by the anatomic configuration of the pathology and the age of the child. The premature eye does not have a fully developed pars plana; therefore, entry into the vitreous cavity of the premature infant eye should be performed near or through the pars plicata, approximately 0.5 mm posterior to the limbus. A developed pars plana is not present until 8–9 months post-term [3]. Even at that age, sclerotomy placement is significantly more anterior than in the average adult.

In retinal detachments with vitreoretinal membranes that contact the posterior lens capsule, a lensectomy–vitrectomy often is required to relieve the vitreous traction and permit the retina to reattach. The entry for the lensectomy–vitrectomy in the premature eye is located immediately posterior to the limbus through the iris root directed into the lens anterior to the equator of the lens. This entry avoids the possibility of injuring the retina which has been pulled anteriorly into the posterior chamber. A bent 23-gauge butterfly needle attached to lactated ringers solution or anterior chamber infusion cannula (Lewicky anterior chamber maintainer, right-angled 20-gauge infusion cannula or valved 23-gauge vitrectomy cannula) allow for infusion into the anterior chamber without contacting the corneal endothelium. Once an infusion has been established, the vitreous cutter is used to remove the lens within the capsule. Once the lens material is aspirated, the remaining capsule can be removed using a broad flat Sutherland or Max Grip forceps. The forceps grasps the capsule approximately one-third of the distance from the equator to the posterior pole of the lens; in that fashion, all of the capsule (i.e. anterior and posterior leaflets) can frequently be removed *in toto*. Complete removal of the capsule is essential to reduce the risk of retinal-iridal adhesions postoperatively—a common mode of surgical failure in children. When lensectomy is performed in the absence of a fibrous proliferative sheet immediately behind the lens, a posterior approach can be used to remove the capsule using a vitrector.

In many pediatric eyes with ROP, opaque retrolental/preretinal tissue is in contact with retinal tissue. It is important to open this retrolenticular tissue without damaging the retina beneath or peripheral to it. This opening can be created with the sharp point of the 23-gauge infusion butterfly needle, the tip of a 26-gauge needle or a microvitreoretinal (MVR) blade. When encountered with an anteriorly closed funnel retinal detachments, for example in a stage 5 ROP eye, a cross-action dissection technique allows one to create an opening in the retrolental tissue without creating traction on the peripheral retina. Traction on the peripheral retina can cause a retinal dialysis, which almost uniformly results in surgical failure. Once opened, the retrolenticular tissue then can be dissected using two-hand dissection with the infusion spatula and forceps, either Grieshaber-Sutherland forceps or other positive action forceps that can grasp and fixate tissue using one hand and allow tissue to be spread or cut using the other hand. This technique is termed lamellar dissection. Particularly in ROP, FEVR, and other vitreoretinal dystrophies where the vitreous is formed in solid and liquid sheets, it is possible to perform lamellar dissection, peeling off one layer of preretinal membrane or vitreous at a time. This allows the surgeon to approach the retina safely, taking advantage of the collapsed layers of vitreous collagen. The MPC scissors also can be used to divide, in a sharp fashion, this tissue from the retinal surface. This vitreous pattern is present in many retinal dystrophies and the surgical approach described above can be used in many scenarios.

Another technique involves using the retractable lighted pick with the pick extended in one hand and the infusion spatula beneath tissue adherent to, but not part of the retina, in the other hand. The instruments are pulled away from each other, thus avoiding inducing traction on the peripheral or other areas of the retina. This frequently permits large areas of tissue to be stripped from the retinal surface, which can exert both circumferential and radial traction on the retina.

The goals of vitreous surgery in the pediatric eye must be considered differently from those in adult eyes. It is not necessary, and is dangerous, to try to remove all vitreous or preretinal membranous tissue from the inner retinal surface. Particularly in diseases such as ROP, much of the preretinal tissue is attached and sometimes is intrinsic to the retinal surface from whence it arose. Often preretinal membranes can be segmented and left in place after the main vectors of vitreoretinal traction have been relieved. This technique minimizes the risk of damage to the extremely thin peripheral retina.

Unlike in adult vitreoretinal surgery where iatrogenic breaks can be managed by removal of preretinal membranes, retinotomies, and endophotocoagulation, iatrogenic retinal breaks in most pediatric retinal diseases result in inoperable retinal detachments. This statement holds true despite the use of laser, perfluorocarbon, and silicone oil, because of the inability to completely dissect the vitreous from the inner retinal surface which limits retinal reattachment and therefore the ability to perform effective retinopexy. Thus the guiding tenet of pediatric vitreous surgery should be to use extreme caution and avoid creating a retinal break. This is often difficult because of the convoluted nature of the retinal anatomy and the fact that the retina can be stretched into an appearance unfamiliar to most surgeons. This is particularly true in ROP, FEVR, congenital retinoschisis, and persistent fetal vasculature syndrome.

Modification of the lens-sparing vitrectomy may be required in some cases. The entry must be made where there is adequate space between the lens and the neurosensory retina. As the surgeon becomes more familiar with this technique, a larger number of eyes can be operated upon by adapting to anatomic differences. Very often there are spaces between circumferential or radial folds of retina and the posterior lens capsule. The surgeon can create entry wounds at sites other than the customary 3 and 9 o'clock positions. It may be necessary to enter through the sclera with an MVR blade and make an incision between the retinal fold and posterior lens by what we have described as an ab interno incision. This ab interno incision is made by placing the MVR blade through the sheet of tissue between the circumferential retinal fold and the posterior lens capsule and drawing back, extending the internal incision by cutting parallel to the lens capsule. The opening between the preretinal tissue or retinal fold and the posterior lens capsule can be extended from 90–120 degrees of arc. Entry into these eyes also requires care to avoid the lens equator. This is accomplished by pointing the MVR blade posteriorly, parallel to the visual axis. As the point of the blade comes into view, the blade is angled toward the center of the eye, avoiding contact with the clear lens material. The same angle of entry is used with all other surgical instruments such as the MPC scissors, intraocular forceps, and light pipe.

Vitreous Infusion

The infusion fluids used for vitreous surgery are Balanced Salt Solution (BSS) Plus and lactated Ringer solution. We customarily use BSS Plus as our main infusion; this can be delivered via the wide-angle high-flow infusion light pipe or irrigating pic when performing 2-port vitrectomy. In certain scenarios, a manifold system can provide infusion from a single source of lactated Ringer solution. This single source can supply the infusion spatula, the infusion forceps, and the 23-gauge irrigating butterfly needle. As the surgery progresses the infusion supporting the butterfly needle can be swapped for an infusion contact lens which may be needed for higher-magnification dissection in the posterior pole. Finally, an infusion cannula with BSS Plus may be used when performing 3-port vitrectomy as is customarily done in adult vitreoretinal surgery. Placement of the cannula must be done with caution to avoid injuring the retina or intraocular structures as the cannula is proportionally larger in the pediatric eye as compared to the adult eye.

In scenarios where the retina is bullously detached (Coats disease with total exudative retinal detachment, for example), the infusion cannula can be placed in the anterior segment via a clear corneal wound. This wound is created by grasping the limbus with toothed forceps adjacent to the planned infusion site, normally inferotemporal. The trocar is inserted to the widest point of the blade. Next, the toothed forceps releases and then holds the limbus at 6 o'clock and the cannula is gently introduced through the corneal wound using a twisting motion. With this technique one can safely enter a very narrow anterior chamber without injuring the retina or any anterior segment structures. Further, this technique provides trans-zonular infusion to the posterior segment which can be moved to a more traditional location once adequate space can be surgically obtained.

Vitreous Tamponades and Replacements

As in adults, vitreous tamponades and replacements such as sodium hyaluronate (Healon), perfluorocarbon liquids, long-acting gases, and silicone oil are required in pediatric vitreoretinal surgery. However, there use carries higher risks because accurate intraocular pressure measurements are often difficult to obtain and post operative positioning is difficult to ensure. For these reasons, we tend not to use expanding gases in young children. If, however, it is necessary to use a long-acting gas bubble, we use 10% octafluoropropane (C3F8). Families are cautioned that until the air/gas is gone from the eye, nitrous oxide anesthesia, air travel, and high altitudes should be avoided to prevent expansion and contraction of the bubble and, thus, dangerously high or low intraocular pressures. We place a bracelet on the child to caution against using nitric oxide anesthesia while air or other gases are in the vitreous cavity. Our preference is to use air which can be used at the end of the case to facilitate closure of the sclerotomy wounds. If submacular blood is present, the child can be placed face down in the parent's arms overnight using an air bubble to displace the blood.

The use of silicone oil has proven to be a helpful tamponade in complex pediatric retinal detachments. We have found silicone oil to be a great help in eyes with long-standing hypotony from ciliary body destruction or detachment. Although generally well tolerated, complications associated with its use include uncontrolled intraocular pressure, silicone oil emulsification, cataract and band keratopathy. Barring these issues, pediatric patients may maintain the intraocular oil for extended periods of time, often for years. Leading some to suggest that 5000-centistoke silicone oil may be a preferable alternative to 1000-centistoke silicone oil. Regardless of the oil used, children with intraocular silicone oil will need to be monitored closely for as long as the oil remains in the eye.

Ophthalmic viscoelastic devices, such as sodium hyaluronate, can be used as a surgical adjunct and ca be left within the vitreous cavity much like a short acting vitreous substitute [4]. For example, sodium hyaluronate injections can be used to separate tight retinal folds and facilitate dissection of proliferative tissue. Care must be taken not to inject the sodium hyaluronate under such force that either a peripheral dialysis or posterior retinal break is created.

Perfluorocarbon liquids can also be useful in pediatric vitreoretinal surgery. However, they should be used cautiously as the weight of perfluorocarbon can tear the very thin peripheral retina. Therefore, it is safest to use perfluorocarbons once all traction has been relieved. Perfluorocarbon liquids in conjunction with silicone oil, have also been reported to displace blood from the posterior pole [5]. In some circumstances, perfluorocarbon and silicone oil can be used together and left in the eye temporarily facilitating retinal reattachment. Post operative positioning represents a challenge as the child must remain on his or her back for up to 1 week. The perfluorocarbon liquid is then removed and the silicone oil replaced.

Pharmacologic Adjuncts

The use of intraocular agents, such as ocriplasmin, a truncated recombinant form of plasmin, have been studied in children [6, 7]. This recombinant enzyme or autologous plasmin enzyme have been successfully used when the vitreous needs to be completely removed from the retinal surface. The authors feel enzyme-assisted vitrectomy in children offers value although several questions remain regarding the timing of injection relative to surgery. In addition, intravitreal antimetabolites, such as 5-fluorouracil and methotrexate, have gained popularity in recent years. They are believed to suppress intraocular proliferation, particularly in traumatized eyes with epithelial downgrowth or fibrous ingrowth. Both 5-fluorouracil (combined with low-molecular weight heparin) and methotrexate have antiproliferation and anti-inflammatory properties. While the available evidence for 5-FU is conflicting [8], the data for methotrexate are more promising [9]. These agents often require frequent follow up visits and retreatment with intravitreal injections, which in the pediatric population may mean frequent general anesthesia. Further, their use requires human subject's approval if they are to be used for research data collection.

Conclusion

Pediatric vitreoretinal surgery is far more than adult surgery in a smaller eye. There are unique considerations ranging from philosophical considerations, family interactions, and developmental issues, as well as surgical anatomy, strategies, techniques, and instrumentation. Those aspiring to provide surgical care for children with vitreoretinal pathology should seek to master all aspects of this field.

References

1. Maguire AM, Trese MT. Lens-sparing vitreoretinal surgery in infants. Arch Ophthalmol. 1992;110:284–6.
2. Trese MT. Scleral buckling for retinopathy of prematurity. Ophthalmology. 1994;101:23–6.
3. Hairston RJ, Maguire AM, Vitale S, et al. Morphometric analysis of pars plana development in humans. Invest Ophthalmol Vis Sci. 1992;33:1197.
4. Stirpe M, Michels RG. Sodium hyaluronate in anterior and posterior segment surgery. Padova: Fidia Spa, Abano Terme Publishers; 1989.
5. Shaikh S, Trese M. Retinal reattachment facilitated by short term perfluorocarbon liquid tamponade in a case of FEVR and rhegmatogenous retinal detachment. Retina. 2002;22:674–6.
6. Trese MT, Williams GA, Hartzer MK. A new approach to stage 3 macular holes. Ophthalmology. 2000;107:1607–11.
7. Verstraeten TC, Chapman C, Hartzer M, et al. Pharmacologic induction of posterior vitreous detachment in the rabbit. Arch Ophthalmol. 1993;111:849–54.
8. Khan MA, Brady CJ, Kaiser RS. Clinical management of proliferative vitreoretinopathy: an update. Retina. 2015 Feb;35(2):165–75.
9. Amarnani D, Machuca-Parra AI, Wong LL, et al. Effect of methotrexate on an in vitro patient-derived model of proliferative vitreoretinopathy. Invest Ophthalmol Vis Sci. 2017 Aug 1;58(10):3940–9.

Preparation for the Surgery: Preoperative Measures

Linda A. Cernichiaro-Espinosa and Luis Gilberto Pérez-Chimal

Abstract

Preoperative management constitutes a cornerstone in the treatment of pediatric retina patients. The complete plan includes a checklist with integral management, discussion with the parents or the caregivers, explaining the realistic results, potential complications, and all the follow-up needed to avoid amblyopic problems, rehabilitation, and quality of life. Having informed consent for each surgical and non-surgical procedure, special pediatric instrumentations, and ancillary tests.

Keywords

Preoperative · Pediatric surgery · Vitreoretinal surgery · Presurgical · Examination under anesthesia

Introduction

Checklists are a must when the picture is tough. Many aspects need to be put at ease just before entering the operating room to perform an interventional procedure on a baby. Having a complete plan for the comprehensive management of the pediatric retinal patient includes extensive discussion with parents or caregivers, explaining realistic results, possible complications, and follow-up. Sometimes, in the pediatric retina, gaining function is generally better than quantifying vision. If a procedure does not offer the possibility of improving the functional status of a child, it should

L. A. Cernichiaro-Espinosa (✉) · L. G. Pérez-Chimal
Asociación Para Evitar La Ceguera en México IAP, CDMX, Mexico
e-mail: linda.cernichiaro@retinakids.org

© The Author(s), under exclusive license to Springer Nature Switzerland AG 2023
Ş. Özdek et al. (eds.), *Pediatric Vitreoretinal Surgery*,
https://doi.org/10.1007/978-3-031-14506-3_5

55

be considered whether this is necessary. As this is one of the many reasons why the pediatric retina is not an easy task, having a clear presurgical plan is mandatory for everyone who will face pre, trans and postoperative complications as intrinsic traits of pediatric retinal pathologies [1–3].

The entire first section of this book includes specific topics that range from embryological aspects that lead to decisions on how to approach a pars plana by age, when to operate or not, anesthetic characteristics, equipment and pediatric instrumentation. This chapter is intended to provide the reader with an easy way to keep many relevant aspects together.

Informed Consent in Pediatric Patients

In pediatrics, patients are not legally allowed to consent to medical procedures and treatments. Parents or caregivers are often the main decision-makers for their children. In some cases, when children are old enough to understand medical procedures, they may be asked to consent to care. The ophthalmologist should involve pediatric patients in making decisions about their medical care, providing information about their disease and options for diagnosis and treatment in a developmentally appropriate manner and seeking consent for medical care when appropriate [3, 5]. Before any procedure, the ophthalmologist will maintain a broad and careful conversation with parents or caregivers about the procedure to be performed, the risks involved, and the necessary follow-up for their children. Parents should recognize those who make the appropriate legal and ethical deci- sions for the treatment of their children. If a surgical decision is to be made during EUA, it should be clearly stated that there is the possibility of surgery or an interventional procedure if the current status of the examination requires it [5, 6].

In addition to the need for a pediatric retinal specialist, these patients tend to be challenging preoperatively, perioperatively, and postoperatively, as more than half of patients with low vision will have at least one other disability, so we need an anesthesiologist and an anesthesiologist. pediatrician who is comfortable working with challenging pediatric patients, especially those with very low birth weight [7, 8, 15].

Types of Interventions in an Operating Room

First, there are two major types of interventions that are done in the operating room: *non surgical* and *surgical* procedures.

Non-surgical interventions

Exam under anesthesia (EUA)

An EUA serves both for an initial diagnosis in an uncooperative child and for the follow up where treatment can be given based on the current status of the eye. It is advised that even when scheduling an EUA there is a pre-interventional plan to maximize the duration of the anesthesia, especially in kids that require multiple EUAs (i.e. retinoblastoma). Refraction, intraocular pressure, biomicroscopic exam, and dilated fundus exam with or without pictures are mandatory [7, 8] (Fig. 5.1).

Ablative therapies

Different types of lasers are used for various purposes. As a general rule, an 810 nm laser is useful for developmental vascular disease (ie, FEVR), retinopathy of prematurity, vascular tumors, and retinoblastoma. Some 810 nm and 577 nm lasers have micropulse configurations. The 810 nm laser allows the pediatric glaucoma specialist to perform external cyclophotocoagulation. In some cases, it is helpful to have a 532 nm laser available in the operating room. Cryotherapy is the second frequently used ablative tool in pediatric pathologies [3, 7].

Intravitreal or periocular medications

Whether the drug is readily available upon request or must be requested ahead of time will depend on local regulations and this should be prepared in advance.

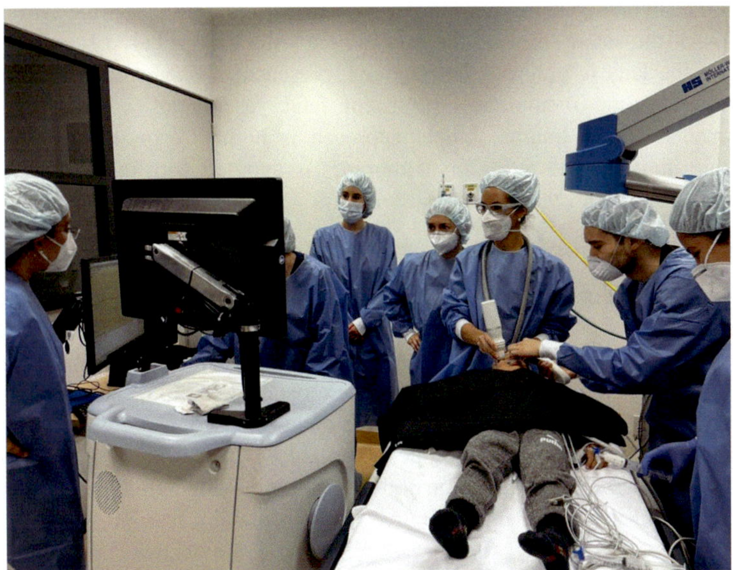

Fig. 5.1 Examination under anesthesia. (*Note*: The fundus camera with FA, and electroretinogram displayed on the picture)

Ancillary testing

Equipment availability is often a limitation for many centers. However, if most tests can be performed on a child who does not otherwise allow an in-office examination, it is recommended [9]. Fluorescein Angiography [FA] requires knowledge of the infant's current weight, the recommended dose by our group is 8 mg/kg, however, different doses can be consulted elsewhere since they all seem to work in different ways. FA protocols are discussed in a different book chapter. Other tests that can be done are: OCT, OCT-A, B-scan, A-scan, UBM, AS-OCT, autofluorescence (AF), electroretinogram (ffERG, EOG), VEP and autorefraction keratometer. B-scan, A-scan and keratometries are useful when planning intraocular lens implantation in a child [9, 10].

It should be noted that most of the ideal equipment is not available in all operating rooms, however it is recommended to build a fully equipped operating room for best results in children.

Surgical interventions

Vitrectomy

After an examination has been performed in the office or under anesthesia, the best approach to a vitrectomy should be clearly defined in the mind of the surgeon just prior to entering the eye. In general, Pars Plana Vitrectomy (PPV) or pars plicata should be performed in children where preservation of the lens is preferred (most cases) and where there is little evidence of anterior retinal pathology. For the latter purpose, the preoperative B-scan and UBM guide is the best area to insert the trocars (i.e. avoiding the cyclitic membrane in pars planitis), as well as transillumination of the sclera to place the trocars below the limbus [11, 12].

When the lens is going to be removed, presence of extensive anterior retinal pathology, cyclitic membranes, persistent fetal vasculature, anterior choroidal detachments, and/or trauma, limbal approach is highly recommended. Usually, iatrogenic injury to the retina or membranes is avoided with this maneuver and moving backwards to the pars plana is always a secondary option [11, 13].

Scleral buckle

Even in the presence of extensive proliferative vitreoretinopathy (PVR), scleral buckling is an excellent first step in the repair of retinal pathologies in children. Therefore, a good understanding of the forces and dynamics of the vitreous by a skilled surgeon, coupled with a good preoperative examination, can lead to a good justification for a buckle. Ideally, the type of buckle should be decided prior to surgery in order to have the instrument available. Also, some surgeons advocate sutures and others for tunnels. For both scenarios, having sutures and the scleral blade is helpful in making intraoperative decision making feasible [12, 13].

<u>Combined procedures</u>

Most pediatric retinal surgeons will agree with combined surgeries: scleral buckle and vitrectomy. Importantly, there is a subset of patients who require combined glaucoma-retina or glaucoma-cornea procedures. The multidisciplinary preoperative approach has improved our results as a center [3, 12, 13].

<u>Phacoemulsification with or without IOL implant</u>

As mentioned earlier, in young children sometimes the IOL calculation in the operating room is more accurate. There is a subset of older children or adolescents who will also allow this calculation in the office so that the precise IOL is available before surgery. Otherwise, whoever makes the IOL available in the operating room must be notified in advance that a possible special IOL will be required at the time of surgery [13].

<u>Tamponade</u>

SF6, C3F8 and silicone oil (1000cs, 5000cs or heavy silicone oil) should be available ahead of time in the OR.

Planning the Follow-Up

Once a patient is discharged from the hospital, it is essential to have a clearly defined plan for follow-up care in these complex cases. Integrated management starts from the preoperative plan with a multidisciplinary approach. From the outset, a pediatric retinal patient in need of surgical treatment, the findings, prognosis, and management plan should be discussed extensively with the parents/caregivers. Ideally explained by a pediatric ophthalmologist or pediatric retina specialist trained to describe the problems associated with visual impairment, the approach to treatment, amblyopia management, drop instillation, and the support system that parents can trust [3, 6, 13].

Once a patient is discharged from the hospital, it is essential to have a clearly defined plan for follow-up care in these complex cases. Integrated management starts from the preoperative plan with a multidisciplinary approach. From the outset, a pediatric retinal patient in need of surgical treatment, the findings, prognosis, and management plan should be discussed extensively with the parents/caregivers. Ideally explained by a pediatric ophthalmologist or pediatric retina specialist trained to describe the problems associated with visual impairment, the approach to treatment, and the support system that parents can trust [3, 6, 13].

The low vision support centers and the visual rehabilitator, supported by the pediatric ophthalmologist, are essential to prevent the factors that generate amblyopia and provide stimulation to promote maximum visual development. The window of time to acquire good vision can be short and therefore it is important to start training without wasting time, usually starting earlier and continuing immediately after the surgical procedure [15].

Finally, parents play an important role in every moment of our treatment and rehabilitation process, they will support us with postural compliance, treatment application, transportation to the rehabilitation centers and, put into practice the therapy every day [6] (Fig. 5.2).

Clinical case scenario

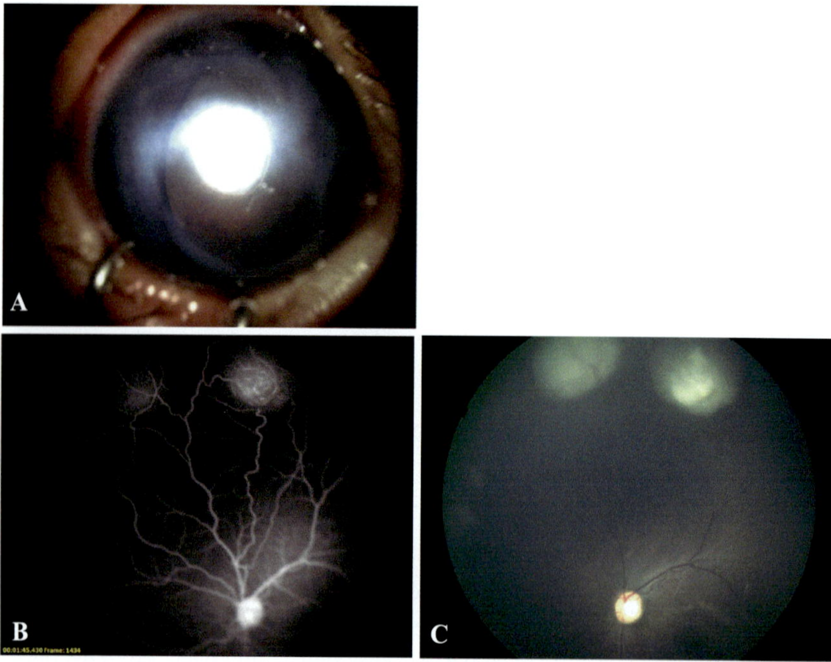

Fig. 5.2 11 month old male with OD leukocoria since 6 months of age noted by the mother. OD showed a buphthalmic eye with a vitreous hemorrhage and a possible mass touching the lens **A**. On the office exam it was not clear if the OS was normal or not. The following day an EUA with a B-scan confirmed bilateral retinoblastoma with peripheral OS tumors **B** and **C**. MRI was performed and treatment was discussed with the retinoblastoma multidisciplinary team. On a second EUA, TTT was placed on the left eye to the peripheral masses and primary enucleation was done OD before systemic chemotherapy. This exemplifies the importance of informed consent and multiple modalities of treatment within the same anesthetic event

CHECKLISTS

Complete EUA instruments

1	Tonometer	
2	Caliper	
3	Portable slit lamp	
4	Indirect ophthalmoscope	
5	Lenses (28D, 30D, 20D)	
6	Speculum	
7	Scleral depressor	
8	Dilating drops	
9	Anesthetic drops	
10	Fluorescein strips	
11	Retinoscope and test box or plates	

Ancillary testing

1	Fluorescein angiogram [FA] and IV fluorescein 10–20%	
2	Optical coherence tomography [OCT]	
3	OCT Angiography [OCT-A]	
4	B-scan	
5	UBM	
6	Anterior segment OCT [AS-OCT]	
7	Electroretinogram (ffERG, EOG) and visual evoked potentials (VEP)	

Ablative therapies

1	Laser	
	•532 nm	
	•810 nm	
	▪Indirect ophthalmoscope	
	▪Glaucoma cyclophotocoagulation probe	
	•577 nm	
2	Cryotherapy	

Intravitreal injections

1	Anti-VEGF	
2	Steroids	
3	Immunomodulators	
4	Implants	
5	Antibiotics	
6	Chemotherapy	

Surgical Procedures

1	Vitrectomy	
	Pars plana vitrectomy	
	Pars plicata vitrectomy	
	Limbal vitrectomy	
2	Scleral buckle	
3	Phacoemulsification $\pm$ Intraocular lens implant	
4	Combined procedures	
5	Tamponades	

Conclusion

There are many complex factors that play a star role in the management of pediatric patients with retina pathology. Checklists are offered in this chapter to the reader. Although there are many considerations in the management of pediatric retinal patients, including management during surgery and follow-up, preparing for surgery with a detailed plan increases the chance of a positive outcome after surgery and improves quality of life of these patients.

Review Question

1. What is the most important feature of an EUA:

a. The informed consent stating the possibility of surgical or non-surgical interventions at the time of anesthesia
b. Refraction
c. VEP
d. None

Answer

1. (**A**) If a surgical decision is to be made during EUA, it should be clearly stated that there is the possibility of surgery or an interventional procedure if the current status of the examination requires it.

References

1. Beck KD, Rahman EZ, Chang EY, Gunn ML, Harper CA. A Practical approach to pediatric retinal surgery. Int Ophthalmol Clin. 2020;60(3):115–34. https://doi.org/10.1097/IIO.0000000000000321.
2. Ranchod TM, Capone A Jr. Tips and tricks in pediatric vitreoretinal surgery. Int Ophthalmol Clin. 2011;51(1):173–83.
3. Baumal CR, Berrocal AM. Pearls for pediatric retinal surgery. Retin Today. 2018; SE.
4. Grajewski AL, Bitrian E, Papadopoulos M, et al. Surgical management of childhood glaucoma: clinical considerations and techniques. Cham, Switzerland: Springer; 2018.
5. Committee AAP, Bioethics ON. Informed consent in decision-making in pediatric practice. Pediatrics. 2016;138(2): e20161484.
6. Denham EJ, Nelson RM. Selfdetermination is not an appropriate model for understanding parental permission and child assent. Anesth Analg. 2002;94(5):1049–51.
7. Chang TC, Cavuoto KM. Anesthesia considerations in pediatric glaucoma management. Curr Opin Ophthalmol. 2014;25(2):118–21.
8. Sun LS, et al. Association between a single general anesthesia exposure before age 36 months and neurocognitive outcomes in later childhood. JAMA. 2016;315(21):2312–20.
9. Agarwal K, Vinekar A, Chandra P, Padhi TR, Nayak S, Jayanna S, et al. Imaging the pediatric retina: an overview. Indian J Ophthalmol. 2021;69:812–23.
10. GoyalP, PadhiTR, DasT, PradhanL, SutarS, ButolaS.Outcome of universal newborn eye screening with wide-field digital retinal image acquisition system: a pilot study. Eye (Lond) 2018; 32:67–73.
11. Wenick AS, Barañano DE. Evaluation and management of pediatric rhegmatogenous retinal detachment. Saudi J Ophthalmol. 2012;26(3):255–63.
12. Wright LM, Harper CA, Chang EY. Management of infantile and childhoode retinopathies: optimized pediatric pars plana vitrectomy sclerotomy nomogram. Ophthalmol Retin. 2018;2 (12):1227–34.
13. Cai S, Therattil A, Vajzovic L. Recent developments in pediatric retina. Curr Opin Ophthalmol. 2020;31(3):155–60. https://doi.org/10.1097/ICU.0000000000000650.
14. Kashani AH, Brown KT, Chang E, Drenser KA, Capone A, Trese MT. Diversity of retinal vascular anomalies in patients with familial exudative vitreoretinopathy. Ophthalmology. 2014;121(11):2220–7.
15. Hartnett ME. Pediatric retina. Chapter 58 early intervention and rehabilitation. 2nd edition. Lippincott Williams & Wilkins; 2013.

Vitreoretinal Surgical Equipment and Instruments Why and How Are They Different in Children?

6

Janani Sreenivasan, Pramod S. Bhende, and Muna Bhende

Abstract

This chapter deals with the special considerations in vitreoretinal instrumentation that a retinal surgeon should know while planning a pediatric retinal surgery. The instrumentation is designed to address the important anatomical differences such as the small size of the eye, reduced scleral rigidity, the relatively large size of the lens, immature pars plana, and a densely adherent formed vitreous. Starting from eye speculum to the short 25-G vitrectomy packs to the eye shield, all these are designed specifically for children. 25G short instruments occupy less space in already narrow pars plana and allow for better visualization compared with 20-gauge instrumentation. In addition to instrument design, the surgical steps also need modification which may be a slight variation from the normal technique like more perpendicular sclerotomy entry or need for additional steps like suturing. Knowing these variations between adult and pediatric retina surgery can play a major role in reducing the complications and improving the outcomes of pediatric retinal surgery.

Keywords

Pediatric vitreoretinal surgery · Anatomical differences in pediatric eyes · 25G short vitrectomy instruments · Pediatric eye speculum · Instruments in pediatric retinal surgery · Pediatric eye shield

J. Sreenivasan · P. S. Bhende · M. Bhende (✉)
Medical Research Foundation, Shri Bhagwan Mahavir Vitreoretinal Services, Sankara Nethralaya, Chennai 600006, India
e-mail: drmuna@snmail.org

© The Author(s), under exclusive license to Springer Nature Switzerland AG 2023   65
Ş. Özdek et al. (eds.), *Pediatric Vitreoretinal Surgery*,
https://doi.org/10.1007/978-3-031-14506-3_6

Introduction

"Children are not small adults" is a famous adage among pediatricians. Similarly, children's eyes are not merely small adult eyes. The anatomy and physiology of the child's eye as well as the pathophysiology of pediatric vitreoretinal disorders are very different from adults posing unique challenges in the diagnosis and management [1–6]. Knowing how the rulebooks differ between adult and pediatric retina surgery can go a long way in improving the outcomes of pediatric retinal surgery [1–6]. In this chapter, we briefly discuss how pediatric vitreoretinal surgical instrumentation varies from its adult counterpart.

Anatomical and Physiological Differences in Children

1. Narrow palpebral fissure and small orbits in children can lead to difficulties in accommodating buckle elements.
2. Small eyes with a relatively large lens [1–6].
3. The pars plana through which vitreoretinal surgical instruments are usually safely introduced in adults, is not fully formed until approximately the age of 8–9 months [1–6].
4. Children have thick conjunctiva and thick tenon's capsule, which is white, sticky, and glistening, becoming thinner in adulthood [7]. This may pose difficulties in dissection and requires separate layered closure at the end.
5. Children have thinner anterior sclera (0.4 mm at 6 months of age and well developed by 2 years of age), which is less rigid, especially in babies less than two years of age [1–8]. With age, the anterior scleral thickness increases. The posterior scleral thickness is influenced by factors like muscle insertion and axial length [8]. Since the sclera is thin, care must be taken during cryopexy, passage of anchor sutures, and while making scleral tunnels. Also, two-step or angled incision for sclerotomies may not be possible.
6. Children tend to have thin extraocular muscles and the thickness increases with age [9]. Careful handling of extraocular muscles is needed while tagging them and rotating the globe as the muscles are thin.
7. The vitreous is well-formed, sticky, and densely adherent to the retina [1–6].
8. The newborn eye has varying levels of vascular endothelial growth factor (VEGF), insulin-like growth factor-1, tumor growth factor-b, and other cytokines, which may affect the progression or stabilization of pediatric vitreoretinopathies [4].

Preoperative Considerations

Preoperative assessment, including visual acuity, intraocular pressure, and clinical findings is difficult, may be inaccurate, and sometimes insufficient for diagnosis and further management [1–5]. Ultrasonography plays an important role in such cases. If there is a doubt, there must be a low threshold for planning examination under anaesthesia (EUA) with or without fluorescein angiography, especially if there is a vascular pathology necessitating treatment in both eyes [3, 4]. It can help the surgeon to decide on which eye to be operated first if both eyes need surgery and assess the location of sclerotomies. It also allows discussion with the parents regarding further management and possible outcomes. However, if the child's systemic condition is not conducive for frequent general anaesthesia, one might plan the assessment in the same sitting of the planned surgery. During preoperative counselling of the parents, the outcomes of pediatric vitreoretinal surgeries, risk of amblyopia, risks of general anaesthesia, need for a multidisciplinary approach (pediatrician, retinal specialist, pediatric ophthalmologist) and regular postoperative follow-up needs to be clearly explained. Except for older children requiring short procedures, most pediatric vitreoretinal surgeries are done under general anaesthesia with a team skilled in handling premature babies and infants with significant co-morbid conditions.

Draping

Care must be taken while draping a child under general anaesthesia and while removing the drape, which can get stuck to the airway tubes. It is a good idea to place sterile gauze over the tubes at the likely contact area with the drape, to prevent this. Commercially available sterile drapes come in smaller sizes (40 × 40 cm, 50 × 50 cm), pre-cut/non-pre-cut usually with pouches.

Speculum

An appropriately sized speculum should be used which retracts the eyelids sufficiently without tearing the tissues and interfering with the instruments, especially the infusion cannula. The Barraquer wire speculum (Fig. 6.1A) of the pediatric age group can be used which has fenestrated blades of 11 mm size with a blade spread of 12 mm. The Alfonso eye speculum (Fig. 6.1B), specially designed for newborn babies has an overall length of 45 mm. It has finger grips and interlacing fenestrated blades (5 mm) to facilitate insertion in eyes with narrow palpebral fissure.

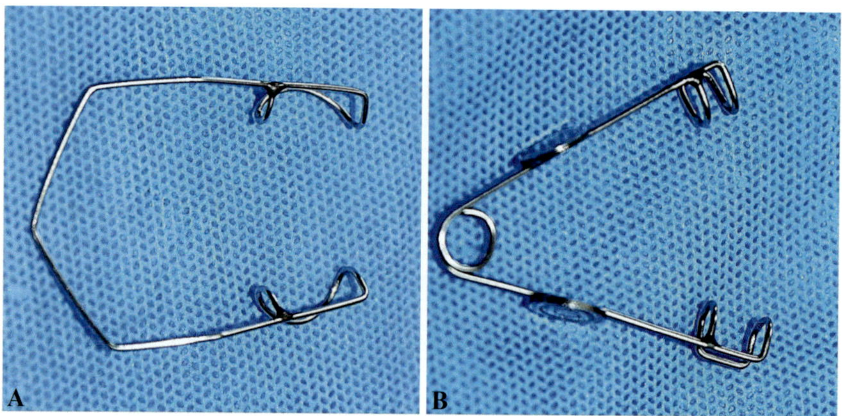

Fig. 6.1 **A** shows the photographic image of the Barraquer pediatric eye speculum and **B** shows the Alfonso eye speculum. One can appreciate the finger grips in the Alfonso speculum which enables easier handling in smaller eyes

Buckle Elements

In older children with rhegmatogenous retinal detachment, buckle elements used are not different from adults. The segmental element is chosen based on the extent of the posterior most break and an encircling band is placed along with segmental element to support the vitreous base [10]. In peripheral TRDs due to ROP/FEVR, broad buckle elements like 2.5 mm band (240 style) (Fig. 6.2A) or a 41 or 42 band (3.5 mm wide by 0.75 mm thick) (Fig. 6.2B) are preferred [11]. When encircling bands are used in children less than 2 years of age, they need to be removed at a later date to allow for the growth of the eye [11].

Sclerotomies

Before starting sclerotomies, one has to decide whether to enter via pars plana or pars plicata or limbus, which in turn depends mainly on age and the extent of pathology. Entering at more perpendicular angles and using shorter cannulas may decrease the risk of damage to the lens and surrounding retina. As a rule of thumb, the sclerotomies are placed at 4 mm from the limbus only in children aged 4 years and older [1]. Although the distance of the sclerotomies from the limbus varies widely based on age and pathology, it can be easily remembered as adding 1 mm to the distance from the limbus with each year of age after the 1st year of life [1]. For eyes with stage 5 ROP and unusual anatomy such as microphthalmos in persistent fetal vasculature (PFV)/severe anterior segment abnormalities, **trans-scleral illumination** is another useful method to determine the location of safe sclerotomy

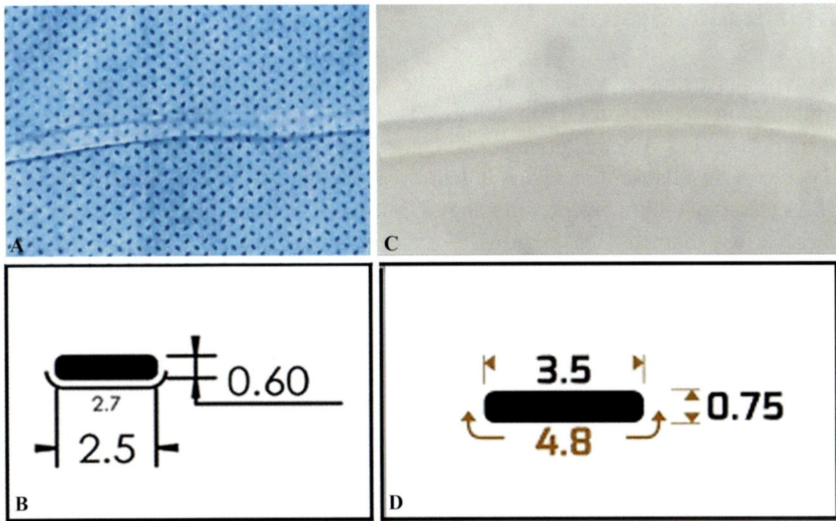

Fig. 6.2 **A** shows the photographic image of the #240 encircling silicone band with dimensions shown in **B**. **C** and **D** depict the image and dimensions of band 41 respectively

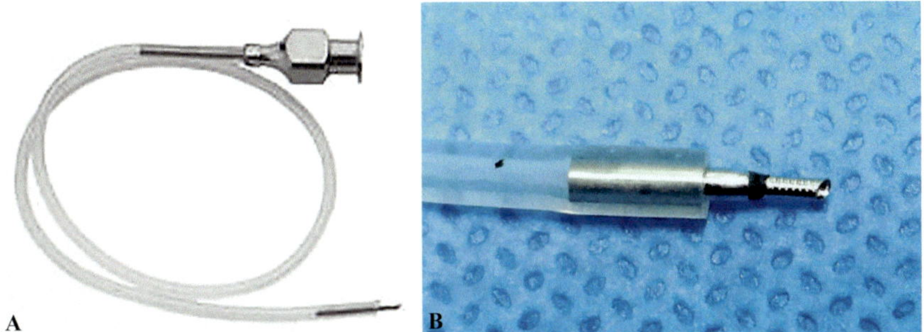

Fig. 6.3 It shows the photographic image of the AC maintainer **A** used to maintain anterior chamber infusion in cases of limbal entry for pediatric vitrectomy. The grooves **B** at the tip helps in retaining the AC maintainer in the corneal wound.

entry[2]. When there is no space in the pars plicata/plana, **corneal limbal or iris root entry** is the preferred entry site [1–6]. Infusion is accomplished by an anterior chamber maintainer or a small gauge infusion cannula [1–6]. The infusion in the anterior chamber (AC) could be an irrigating one which does not easily permit bimanual dissection or can be via an AC maintainer which allows bimanual dissection. A shelving corneal wound is made with a 20G MVR blade, and the anterior chamber maintainer is anchored in the corneal wound via grooves [Fig. 6.3] on its side [1].

Visualization System

Most of the pediatric vitrectomies can be managed with the routine wide-angle visualization systems used for adults. There are some commercially available pediatric viewing systems (contact and non-contact) for use mainly in infant's eyes. The Ocular Pediatric Landers Vitrectomy Lens Set (Ocular® instruments, inc. USA) (Fig. 6.4) is a contact wide-angle viewing system designed for infant eyes. These 8 mm diameter lenses provide a clear view of the entire retina and optic nerve while avoiding the difficulties caused by size mismatch with large adult lenses. A groove on the side of the lens allows securing with the lens ring. The set includes three lenses, a lens ring, forceps, and an autoclavable case. Ocular Peyman Pediatric Wide Field Vitrectomy Lens (Fig. 6.5) is a two-piece lens system that comes with a contact diameter of 7 mm [12]. It is excellent for panoramic viewing of the far peripheral retina for both premature infants and adult patients, and autoclavable. Designed to reduce image cropping from lens tilt on the eye, it produces an indirect image, and requires an image inverter.

MIVS (Microincision Vitrectomy Systems)

The routine 23G Microincision vitrectomy systems (MIVS) are widely used by surgeons for pediatric vitreoretinal surgery, the main advantage being stiffness and its ability to handle formed vitreous and dense membranes at the periphery. Although scleral buckling is the procedure of choice in children with

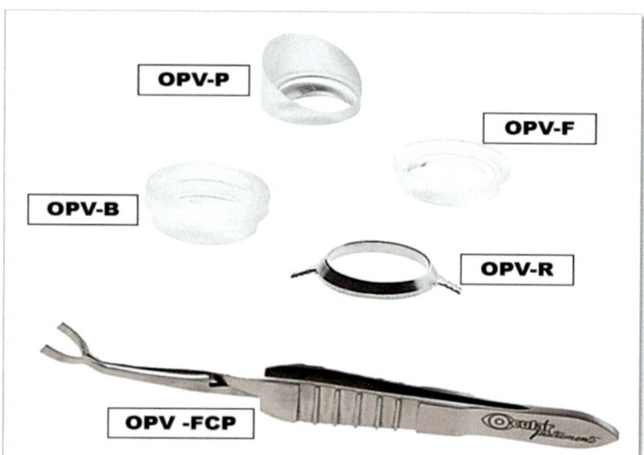

Fig. 6.4 It shows the ocular pediatric vitrectomy lens set, which is a contact type wide-angle viewsing system designed for infant's eyes. The biconcave lens (OPV-B) allows a clear view of fundus in an air-filled vitreous cavity in phakic eyes; the flat lens (OPV-F) helps in visualizing the central retina and 30 degrees prism (OPV-P) allows peripheral viewing beyond the equator with minimal distortion. The ring (OPV-R) helps to hold the lenses and the forceps (OPV-FCP) is used for handling the lenses. Image source: Ocular instruments catalogue, oscular instruments inc., USA

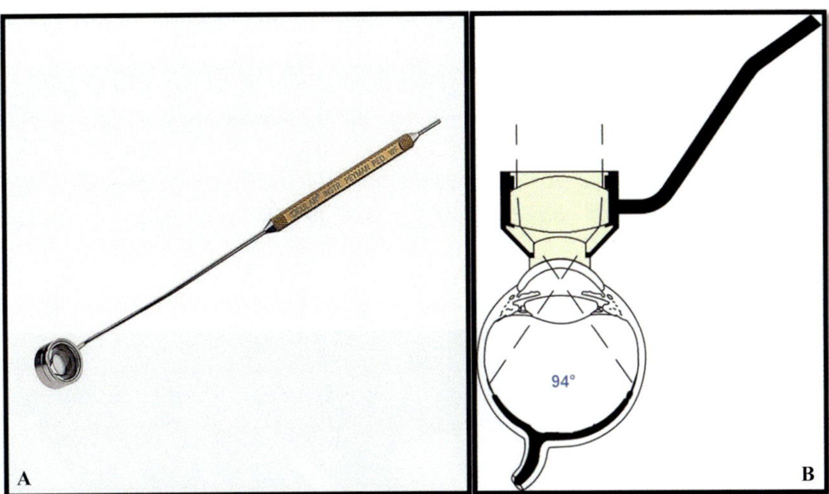

Fig. 6.5 Ocular Peyman pediatric wide field vitrectomy lens. It is again a contact type wide-angle viewing system which is excellent for panoramic viewing of the far peripheral retina in both infant and adults eyes. Its wide field of view and low magnification makes it particularly useful during fluids-gas exchange. Image souce: Ocular instruments catalogue, Ocular instruments inc., USA

rhegmatogenous retinal detachment, vitrectomy is needed in cases of complex detachments like a giant retinal tear, closed funnel retinal detachment, those associated with vitreous hemorrhage/endophthalmitis/posterior scleral dehiscence, Grade C PVR, and re-detachment after scleral buckling [2–5, 10, 11]. In addition, retinal detachments secondary to retinopathy of prematurity, Familial exudative vitreoretinopathy, Persistent fetal vasculature, and other complications of vascular retinopathies also require vitrectomy [11].

23G instruments are long, making it difficult for the surgeon to operate in a small infant's eye with a relatively large lens. While making sclerotomies using a normal adult trocar- cannula system, there is increased risk of damaging the retina if it is anteriorly pulled. Hence it is preferable to use short 25G/27G MIVS systems in pediatric retinal surgeries, in an attempt to reduce lens damage and iatrogenic retinal breaks [13–16]. Differences in dimensions among the 23G, 25G, 23G short, and 27G instruments are elaborated in Table 6.1.

The short 25-G vitrectomy packs (Fig. 6.6) designed specifically for children are commercially available (Alcon/DORC). The vitrectors and light pipes are 9 mm shorter and 50–90% more rigid than standard 25-G instruments (Fig. 6.7), allowing for easier manipulation of the globe with less instrument warpage [2]. The effective length of the cutter is 18 mm, while that of endolaser and endoilluminator is 14–15 mm. The length of the infusion cannula is 3.2 mm, which needs to be anchored with a suture. The entry is directly through the sclera without the cannula.

Table 6.1 Comparison of dimensions between 23G/25G/27G MIVS instruments. *Source* Leung et al. [2]

Instrument	23G (mm)	25G + (mm)	25G + short (mm)	27G + (mm)
Intraocular length of cannula	4	4	3.2 infusion line	4
Sclerotomy size	0.6	0.5	0.5	0.4
Effective length of light pipe	30	23	14	23
Effective length of vitrector	32	27	18	26

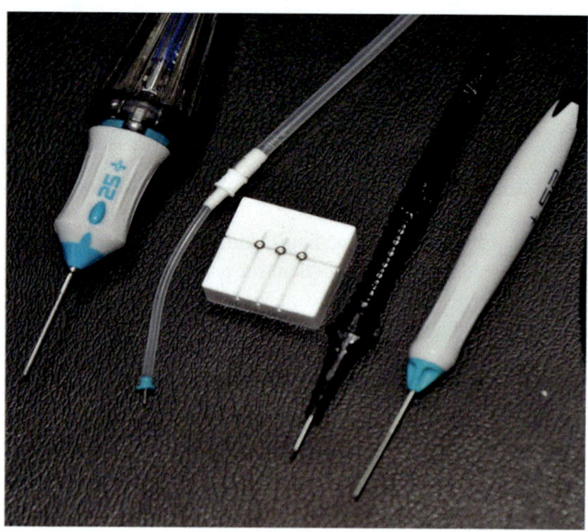

Fig. 6.6 A photograph of the complete set of the short 25G MIVS instruments which consist of vitrector, Infusion tubing, sclerotomy plugs, sclerotomy trocar and endoilluminator from left to right

The slender profile of the 25-gauge instrumentation has a distinct advantage within the small confines of an infant's eye [13–16]. 25-gauge instrument occupies less space in already narrow pars plana and allows for better visualization compared with 20-gauge instrumentation [14]. The advent of a newer generation 25-gauge endoilluminator has also improved visualization, and stiffer instrumentation allows for better instrument maneuverability while dealing with peripheral and anterior retinal pathology [14, 15]. The disadvantages of the 25-G short packs are the lack of small cannulas and the need to suture the infusion lines and sclerotomies, which can be challenging in the less rigid sclera of children [2].

Difficulties in using 25G system [14]

– Any finding that precludes adequate visualization of the retinal periphery, such as vitreous hemorrhage or extraretinal fibrous proliferation, could preclude the use of the 25-gauge system and safe positioning of the intraocular portion of the trocar and instrument insertion.

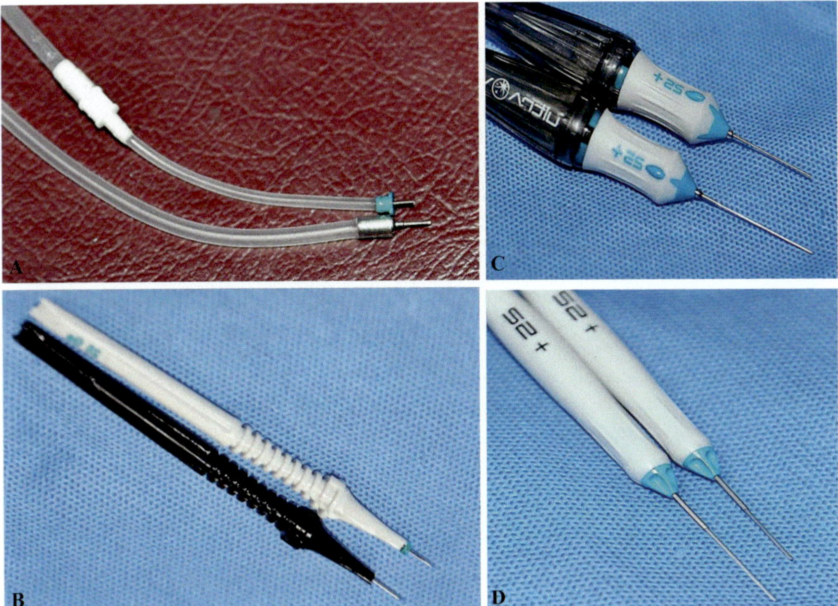

Fig. 6.7 **A–D** shows the differences in the length of the instruments between the routine 25G and the short 25G MIVS instruments, which include infusion tubing, sclerotomy plugs, sclerotomy trocar and endoilluminator from left to right

– In cases where there is significant anterior and peripheral traction because the flexibility of the instrumentation may not permit reliable ability to remove the peripheral and dense fibrous membranes due to lack of control at the tip and tendency of the instrument to bend.

The advantages and disadvantages of 25G MIVS in pediatric retinal surgery are summarized in Table 6.2.

The 27-G instruments are less than half the size of the 20-G instruments and 0.1 mm smaller than the 25-G [2]. The 27-G instruments, therefore have tighter spheres of influence, allowing for more controlled fluidics, allow closer shaving of the vitreous, and more precise dissections of preretinal membranes [2]. The 0.4 mm self-sealing sclerotomies may decrease the risk of postoperative hypotony, postoperative bleeding, and endophthalmitis [2]. The disadvantages of 27-G vitrectors include decreased flow rates and increased instrument flexibility [2]. New pediatric-sized 27-G vitrectomy sets are being developed. The effective lengths of the vitrectors are 19.8 mm, the light pipes are 16 mm, and the cannulas are 3 mm (Dutch Ophthalmic Research Center, Exeter, NH) [2].

Table 6.2 Advantages and disadvantages of the 25G instruments in pediatric vitreoretinal surgery

Advantages	Disadvantages
1. Smaller instrumentation—access smaller spaces within the eye	1. Possibility of lens damage during trocar insertion
2. Allows a three-port vitrectomy with the advantage of a constant infusion and thus good intraoperative IOP control (as opposed to two-port vitrectomy using an irrigating light pipe for infusion, done in neonatal VR sx)	2. Subretinal entry can occur if the site is not properly chosen
	3. Short light pipe may not be a very good helping second hand for membrane dissection as compared to adult counterparts
3. For older children with a mature pars plana, the sclerotomies can be placed more posteriorly, and the transconjunctival sutureless technique can be employed without postoperative hypotony	4. Flexible instruments—difficult for anterior/peripheral dense membranes
	5. In neonates, due to pars plicata entry which is usually perpendicular, sclerotomies are leaky, need suturing

Modifications

Few surgeons use **trocar-cannula systems** only at $\geq$ 2 years of age due to thin sclera in children less than 2 years [1]. Some prefer relatively larger gauge sclerotomies for smooth entry of instruments. For 23 G or 25 G instruments, 20 or 23 G sclerotomies respectively allow safe and snug entry [13, 14]. It is possible that the absence of the trocar sleeve and a shorter fulcrum at the wound allows for better instrument maneuverability and control that may be helpful for cases involving anterior traction [14]. Inserting cannulas through stacked silicone bands can decrease the intraocular lengths [5]. Babu et al. devised a simple technique to shorten the intraocular length of the 25-gauge trocar and the cannula by inserting a small piece (2 × 2 mm) of 42 silicon band, which is pushed till the hub of the cannula [17]. This can help reduce the chances of the lens and retinal injury during vitrectomy in infant's eyes. One complication reported was that the cannula had come out along with the cutter, which could be minimized by withdrawing the instruments slowly [17]. Few commercially available chandelier systems have the option of simultaneous infusion, thereby avoiding the clutter of another sclerotomy and the cable of an independent chandelier. In this device, the optical fiber which runs parallel to the infusion line is connected to a separate console and the infusion tubing is connected to the MIVS system as usual. 20G illuminated infusion comes in two forms, conventional sew-in infusion line, and the trocar cannula system. 25G illuminated infusion (Fig. 6.8) requires a special transconjunctival cannula to accommodate the optical fiber without limiting infusion flow. The optical fibers are partly shielded by the infusion line, thereby reducing glare in air-filled eye, but provide less illumination (when compared to independent Chandelier) due to the small diameter of the optical fibers.

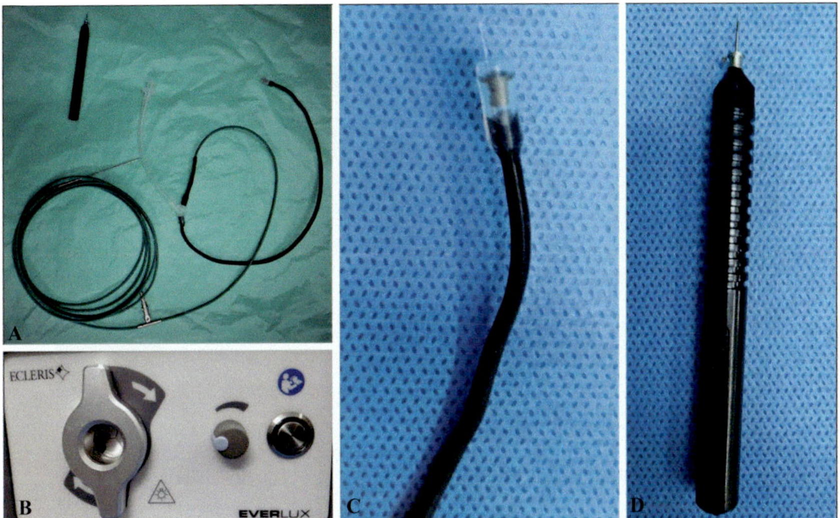

Fig. 6.8 25G illuminated infusion system. The entire tubing with optical fiber is shown in (**A**), the console in (**B**), the trip of tubing is shown in (**C**), and the transconjunctival trocar in (**D**)

Suture Materials

The suturing of sclerotomies in children is recommended to ensure a water-tight closure for three reasons:

1. The pediatric sclera has decreased scleral stiffness and increased elasticity [1–6].
2. The sclerotomies are inserted more perpendicularly to avoid lens damage, they may not be self-sealing [1–6, 13–16].
3. Postoperative hypotony due to frequent rubbing may be a concern in children. Additionally, in pediatric vasoproliferative disorders, hypotony in the immediate postoperative period may result in an increased risk of bleeding from the vascular ridge [16].

Closure of the sclera and conjunctiva may be done with absorbable 8–0 vicryl sutures [13–16]. To reduce the likelihood of wound leakage, at the conclusion of the surgery, **a partial fluid–air exchange** can be performed before trocar removal [15]. For limbal or corneal wounds, 10–0 vicryl is widely used in the pediatric age group as it is associated with less suture-related complications and obviates the need for general anaesthesia for suture removal [18].

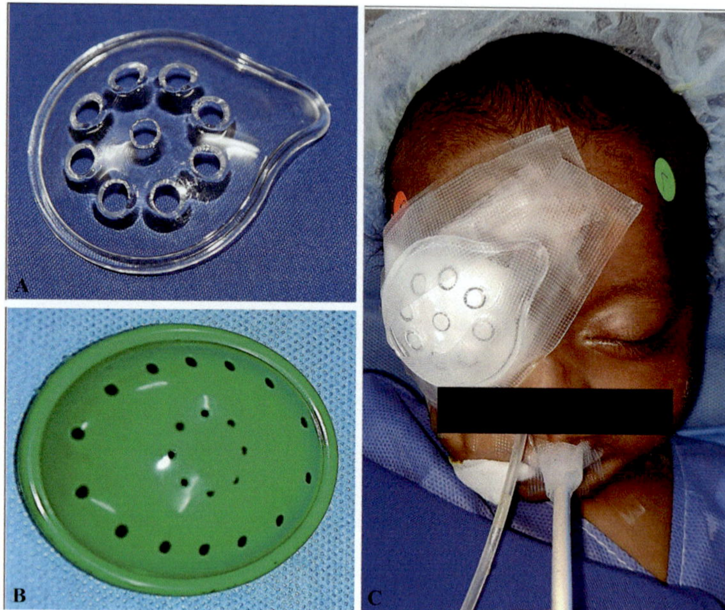

Fig. 6.9 It shows the photographic image of the pediatric eye shield which is available in two form (**A** and **B**). **C** shows the image of the eye shield after being applied at the end of the surgery over the dressing

Eye Shield

Eye shields are used to protect the eye after surgery and to hold dressings in place. It is more important in the pediatric age group due to concerns of frequent rubbing. They are made of clear Polycarbonate shatterproof plastic in a universal shape for use over either eye (Fig. 6.9). Holes in the eye shield provide ventilation as well as allows the child to see, thereby minimising the chances of amblyopia.

Conclusion

To summarize, the instrumentation of pediatric retinal surgery is designed to address the important anatomical differences such as small size of the eye, reduced scleral rigidity, relatively large size of the lens, immature pars plana and a densely adherent formed vitreous. Variations may be in the form of size of instruments, modification of the current technique and need for additional steps like suturing. It is important for the surgeon to remember the anatomy as well as the differences in the instrumentation to avoid complications and achieve the maximal surgical outcomes.

Review Questions

1. The pars plana is fully formed at

A. At birth
B. At 6 months of age
C. Between 8–9 months of age
D. At 1 year of age

2. Children have

A. Thin tenon's capsule, thin sclera and thick extraocular muscles
B. Thick tenon's capsule, thin sclera and thin extraocular muscles
C. Thin tenon's capsule, thick sclera and thin extraocular muscles
D. Thick tenon's capsule, thick sclera and thick extraocular muscle

3. All are true regarding Alfonso speculum except

A. Specifically designed for infant eyes
B. Interlacing blades of 11 mm
C. Finger grips
D. Overall length of 45 mm

4. When encirclage is used in infants, it needs to be removed at 1 year of age

A. To allow growth of the eye
B. To avoid amblyopia
C. To avoid anterior segment ischemia
D. To avoid buckle infection

5. All are true regarding sclerotomies in infants except

A. Biplanar entry is better
B. Suturing is preferred
C. More perpendicular entry
D. Location depends on age and extent of pathology

6. Difference between the length of adult 25G and short 25G cutter is

A. 10 mm
B. 8 mm
C. 7 mm
D. 9 mm

7. Advantages of the short 25G MIVS instruments include all except

A. Shorter, so less damage to lens
B. Allows a three-port vitrectomy with the advantage of a constant infusion and thus good IOP control
C. Stiffer and suited for dissection of severe peripheral traction
D. Self-sealing sclerotomies in older children

8. The advantage of 23G over 25G/27G in pediatric vitreoretinal surgeries is

A. Shorter
B. Stiffer
C. Flexible
D. Self-sealing

9. Modifications to reduce the intraocular length of MIVS instruments include all except

A. Avoiding trocar cannula systems and direct MVR entry
B. Stacked silicone bands
C. Using large gauge sclerotomies
D. Increasing intrascleral length of sclerotomies

10. The purpose of eye shield in children include all except

A. To hold the dressing in place in immediate post op period
B. Protection against rubbing
C. Has holes for ventilation and also permit the child to see
D. Prevention of hypotony

Answers

1. C
2. B
3. B
4. A
5. A
6. D
7. C
8. B
9. C
10. D

References

1. Gan NY, Lam WC. Special considerations for pediatric vitreoretinal surgery. Taiwan J Ophthalmol. 2018;8(4):237–242. https://doi.org/10.4103/tjo.tjo_83_18. PMID: 30637195; PMCID: PMC6302561.
2. Leung EH, Berrocal AM. Pediatric microincision vitreoretinal surgery. Int Ophthalmol Clin. 2016;56(4):203–8. https://doi.org/10.1097/IIO.0000000000000143. PMID: 27575768.
3. Yonekawa Y, Fine HF. Practical pearls in pediatric vitreoretinal surgery. Ophthalmic Surg Lasers Imaging Retin. 2018 Aug 1;49(8):561–5. https://doi.org/10.3928/23258160-20180803-02 PMID: 30114299.
4. Ranchod TM, Capone A Jr. Tips and tricks in pediatric vitreoretinal surgery. Int Ophthalmol Clin. 2011;51(1):173–83. https://doi.org/10.1097/IIO.0b013e3182009b73. PMID: 21139483.
5. Turgut B, Demir T, Çatak O. The recommendations for pediatric vitreoretinal surgery. Adv Ophthalmol Vis Syst. 2019;9(6):142–5. https://doi.org/10.15406/aovs.2019.09.00366.
6. Bhende PS. Commentary: Entry sites and access in retinopathy of prematurity surgery: How important are they? Indian J Ophthalmol. 2020 Oct;68(10):2211–2. https://doi.org/10.4103/ijo.IJO_766_20.PMID:32971645;PMCID:PMC7727963.
7. Fernández-Vigo JI, Shi H, Burgos-Blasco B, De-Pablo-Gómez-de-Liaño L, Almorín-Fernández-Vigo I, Kudsieh B, Fernández-Vigo JÁ. Impact of age, sex and refractive error on conjunctival and tenon's capsule thickness dimensions by swept-source optical coherence tomography in a large population. Int Ophthalmol. 2021 Nov;41(11):3687–98. https://doi.org/10.1007/s10792-021-01928-5 Epub 2021 Jun 28 PMID: 34181192.
8. Read SA, Alonso-Caneiro D, Vincent SJ, Bremner A, Fothergill A, Ismail B, McGraw R, Quirk CJ, Wrigley E. Anterior eye tissue morphology: scleral and conjunctival thickness in children and young adults. Sci Rep. 2016 Sep;20(6):33796. https://doi.org/10.1038/srep33796.PMID:27646956;PMCID:PMC5028711.
9. Saccà S, Polizzi A, Macrì A, Patrone G, Rolando M. Echographic study of extraocular muscle thickness in children and adults. Eye (Lond). 2000 Oct;14(Pt 5):765–9. https://doi.org/10.1038/eye.2000.200 PMID: 11116701.
10. Errera MH, Liyanage SE, Moya R, Wong SC, Ezra E. PRIMARY SCLERAL BUCKLING FOR PEDIATRIC RHEGMATOGENOUS RETINAL DETACHMENT. Retina. 2015 Jul;35(7):1441–9. https://doi.org/10.1097/IAE.0000000000000480 PMID: 25741811.
11. Hansen ED, Hartnett ME. A review of treatment for retinopathy of prematurity. Expert Rev Ophthalmol. 2019;14(2):73–87. https://doi.org/10.1080/17469899.2019.1596026. Epub 2019 Mar 29. PMID: 31762784; PMCID: PMC6874220.
12. Peyman GA, Canakis C, Livir-Rallatos C, Whalen P. Small-size pediatric vitrectomy wide-angle contact lens. Am J Ophthalmol. 2003 Feb;135(2):236–7. https://doi.org/10.1016/s0002-9394(02)01911-6 PMID: 12566036.
13. Gonzales CR, Boshra J, Schwartz SD. 25-Gauge pars plicata vitrectomy for stage 4 and 5 retinopathy of prematurity. Retina. 2006 Sep;26(7 Suppl):S42–6. https://doi.org/10.1097/01.iae.0000244288.63757.be PMID: 16946678.
14. Chan-Kai BT, Lauer AK. Transconjunctival, sutureless 25-gauge lens sparing vitrectomy for stage 4 retinopathy of prematurity-related retinal detachments. Retina. 2009 Jun;29(6):854–9. https://doi.org/10.1097/IAE.0b013e3181a3b7b1 PMID: 19516123.
15. Gadkari S, Kamdar R, Kulkarni S, Kakade N, Taras S, Deshpande M. Vitreoretinal surgery for advanced retinopathy of prematurity: presentation and outcomes from a developing country. Can J Ophthalmol. 2015 Feb;50(1):54–60. https://doi.org/10.1016/j.jcjo.2014.08.017 PMID: 25677284.
16. Gonzales CR, Singh S, Schwartz SD. 25-Gauge vitrectomy for paediatric vitreoretinal conditions. Br J Ophthalmol. 2009 Jun;93(6):787–90. https://doi.org/10.1136/bjo.2008.155655 Epub 2009 Feb 11 PMID: 19211601.

17. Babu N, Shah PK, Narendran V, Kalpana N, Kim R. An easy method to raise the 25-gauge trocar and cannula system for retinopathy of prematurity-related lens-sparing vitrectomy. Retina. 2014 May;34(5):1014–5. https://doi.org/10.1097/IAE.0000000000000128 PMID: 24695066.

18. Matalia J, Panmand P, Ghalla P. Comparative analysis of non-absorbable 10–0 nylon sutures with absorbable 10–0 vicryl sutures in pediatric cataract surgery. Indian J Ophthalmol. 2018 May;66(5):661–4. https://doi.org/10.4103/ijo.IJO_654_17.PMID:29676310;PMCID: PMC5939158.

Philosophical Considerations in Pediatric Vitreoretinal Surgery

7

Antonio Capone Jr.

Abstract

This chapter addresses philosophical considerations relevant to Pediatric Vitreoretinal Surgery (PVS) ranging from interactions with the parents/caregivers and children, philosophical orientation toward surgical goals and surgical approach, aftercare requirements, outcome considerations and more. This chapter differs from others in this text in that it draws less from the scientific literature than from over three decades of personal clinical experience.

Keywords

Pediatric vitreoretinal surgery · Philosophy · *Primum non nocere* · Rapport · Interaction with the patient/family · Anatomical variability · Surgical judgement

Introduction

The courage to cut. The heart of what it means to be a surgeon, and what makes surgeons a breed apart. Innately intrusive, the therapeutic trauma that is surgery invokes unique moral and philosophical demands, particularly for those who operate on children. The differences between adult and pediatric vitreoretinal sur-

A. Capone, Jr. (✉)
Oakland University William Beaumont Hospital School of Medicine, 2000 N Squirrel Road, Auburn Hills, MI, USA
e-mail: acaponejr@arcpc.net

Associated Retinal Consultants PC, Neuroscience Center Building, 3555 W 13 Mile Rd, Ste LL-20, Royal Oak, MI, USA

© The Author(s), under exclusive license to Springer Nature Switzerland AG 2023
Ş. Özdek et al. (eds.), *Pediatric Vitreoretinal Surgery*,
https://doi.org/10.1007/978-3-031-14506-3_7

gery span the entire "therapeutic arc" from the initial clinical encounter to post-operative considerations.

As detailed in Chaps. 2 and 4, PVS is far more than surgery in smaller eyes—a reality which extends beyond anatomical considerations. Projections suggest that the lifespan of many infants born today is 100 years [1], and thus the potential impact of our interventions.

Training

The paths to a career as a pediatric vitreoretinal surgeon are varied. Many vitreoretinal surgeons gain scant experience in pediatric vitreoretinal diseases and surgery in their training. Consequently, most with an interest in this career path are self-taught to meaningful degree and travel to centers with high surgical volume to gain experience. Some abandon the path within the first five years following the completion of their retina fellowships due to low surgical volume or other challenges to acquiring skills. For those who persevere, those first five years are critical for acquiring both clinical judgement and surgical skills. When possible, a senior surgeon-junior surgeon relationship has great value in accelerating the journey up the learning curve. While we all continue to accrue expertise over the course of our careers, the pediatric vitreoretinal surgeon's training after residency is long—the two years of fellowship and the five or so years thereafter.

Expectations and Rapport—the Physician: Parent + Patient Interaction

Some aspects of the physician patient relationship that are unique to PVS are obvious. One is interacting with a child not an adult—consequently one needs to be aware of and know how to manage issues unique to both the parents and their child.

Setting and managing expectations

Expectations of the parents (and children old enough to understand) regarding PVS are likely guided by their experience with "one and done" surgeries such as an appendectomy, tonsillectomy, or repair of a laceration. It is important to address the unique aspects of PVS early in the course of the therapeutic relationship:

- **PVS is a team sport**. In some regards, the surgical intervention—while technically complex and the reason the parents have entrusted their child to you—is the most straightforward aspect of the child's care. The surgeon is part of the team comprising the child (when old enough to interact), the parents, the referring physician, and other consultants—neonatal intensive care unit staff for infant in-patients through pediatric ophthalmologists, and low vision therapists—all working together on the child's behalf. In common parlance, we pediatric vitreoretinal surgeons put the anatomy back together as best we can—often in a procedure that transpires over an hour or two—then the other members of the team are critical to optimizing visual outcome.

- **PVS is often more of a journey than an event**. As compared to the procedures above, or adult vitreoretinal surgery, the likelihood is high that there will be a need for multiple surgeries for both the index eye and in light of the fact that pediatric vitreoretinal diseases are commonly bilateral.
- **Broken and fixed is not the same as normal.** Unlike adult surgery where the goal is normalizing anatomy, in PVS often the best than can be achieved is to render vitreoretinal anatomy less abnormal or to mitigate progression to worse disease. By way of example, anything less than complete reattachment in an adult with rhegmatogenous retinal detachment is a failure, at least in part. In surgery for advanced retinopathy of prematurity (ROP) or familial exudative vitreoretinopathy (FEVR), partial reattachment is considered a success. Anatomic and functional outcomes are generally better than the untreated course of disease, but often short of normal.

Rapport

In a typical interaction the physician greets the parents on entering the exam room, acknowledges the child, gathers information from the parents, examines the child, then explains the findings and plan. Parents of children with pediatric vitreoretinal pathologies are often anxious to the point of desperation. How you interact with their child in front of them communicates to them how you seriously you consider their concerns, and how you will treat their child when they are absent: in the operating room. On initial encounter with a child and caregivers, to address the adults and ignore the child may seem practical as it is time-efficient but is wrong in virtually every other way.

After infancy and certainly by the time a child is four or five years of age, it's important to relate to the child in the interest of building a therapeutic relationship. It is the child whom you will be examining and who will undergo the surgical procedure(s). Exams and procedures will on occasion be uncomfortable or painful. You are the source of the demand that they submit to eyedrops, or that they wear a patch or protective eyewear. Building a relationship enhances trust and compliance. Developing a rapport with older children and adolescents is important regarding the procedure and outcome considerations described just above.

The steps for gaining the confidence of a child and building a relationship may seem obvious: speak in a calm and reassuring voice, after explaining the findings and the plan to the parents turn to the child and explain at a level they can comprehend, tell them what you are going to do to them to examine them or perform an office-procedure before you do it, and if something will be uncomfortable do all you can to mitigate the discomfort then be honest about what they will experience.

Surgical Considerations

A nuanced discussion on the surgical management of specific disease entities is found in their respective chapters. General surgical considerations are discussed below.

Size of the Globe

The smaller size of the pediatric eye, while not unimportant, is the least important difference between adult and pediatric vitreoretinal surgery. There is a learning curve to adjusting to the difference in dimensions, of the eye as well as of the dimensions of one's hands and the instrument relative to the size of the eye. That small instrument excursions in an adult eye are far greater in an infant eye are logical differences, and their impact predictable.

Anatomic Variability

By far the greatest challenges relate to the unique anatomy of eyes impacted by pediatric vitreoretinal diseases, as many of these are rare diseases with rare and varied clinical manifestations. This variability is perhaps the most daunting aspect of PVS. Simply put, anatomic variability is the rule and not the exception, such that things are often not as you expect them to be. Gaining experience with these variations requires years of experience, facilitated by an experienced surgeon/junior surgeon practice relationship when possible.

Developmental Considerations: Lensectomy and Chronic Retinal Detachment

The decisions as to whether to perform lensectomy or operate on longstanding retinal detachment are best considered in a developmental context.

Lensectomy is commonly considered when leukocoria is present in advanced ROP, FEVR, Norrie Disease, Persistent Fetal Vascular Syndrome (PFVS), and other conditions. The notion is that if the pupil is leukocoric then the lens must be cataractous. For all of these conditions save PFVS, leukocoria is due to retrolental fibrovascular proliferation (FVP) present just posterior to the Anterior Hyaloidal Face (AHF) and the lens and lens capsule are often intact and transparent. Nevertheless, lensectomy may be necessary in cases where there is no other way to access the proliferation which must be removed to reattach the retina.

Removing the lens places the eye at developmental disadvantage. The lens should be left in place unless the anatomic advantage outweighs the developmental downside. Two examples are PFVS with a stalk to an otherwise clear lens, and FEVR with a retinal fold and FVP to the temporal AHF with an otherwise clear lens. In the case of PFVS, relieving traction from the stalk as the eye grows forestalls both posterior lenticonus and epipapillary traction retinal detachment. However, removing the lens often results in severe anisometropic amblyopia and poor visual development. These typically small eyes are fitted with a contact lens with difficulty, and the required amblyopia therapy beyond what some parents are able or willing to provide. Similarly, in the eye with a fold due to FEVR, if the FVP is densely consolidated temporally at the pars plana/pars plicata, lensectomy will provide little or no retinal relaxation. In an eye with PFVS the stalk can be transected and crystalline lens left in place. In the FEVR eye the disadvantages of aphakia outweigh the meager anatomic gain from lensectomy, and such eyes are also best served by leaving the crystalline lens in place.

Chronic retinal detachments may be tempting to operate on when they are in a wide-open or other configuration which seems amenable to repair. Detachments up to a year old can have surprising improvement in vision—generally not in Snellen acuity but ambulatory vision. However, repair of longstanding retinal detachment typically yields an unrewarding functional outcome despite anatomic success.

Presumed Visual Potential

Children and infants with markedly abnormal ocular anatomy, particularly when asymmetrically so, are often referred with a notion that "this eye will never see" or that the visual prognosis is so dismal as to preclude surgery. Those judgements, predicated on experience with adult eyes, are so often wrong that they should rarely guide the decision to perform surgery. Surgical intervention is routinely offered to adults with conditions which have a decidedly poor visual prognosis, such as endophthalmitis, trauma, severe alkali injuries, advanced glaucoma, and more. Our smallest patients deserve no less.

The neural plasticity of children is such that they derive far more function from an anatomically abnormal eye than an adult eye abruptly reduced to the same level of anatomic abnormality. Further, the value of low vision to a visually impaired child is significantly underestimated—even by their own parents [2]. Only form vision is required for ambulation using visual cues, not 5/200 visual acuity as is widely held. Even children with only LP objected strenuously to bilateral occlusion, suggesting that they value any residual vision [3]. Light perception is beneficial for the maintenance of normal circadian rhythms and sleep–wake cycles, important in maximizing the potential for attention and learning in children with limited vision [4]. Presumed visual potential is a poor surgical determinant.

The future holds promise for the development of technologies for vision restoration. It is reasonable to assume that a child with at least LP is likely to be in a better position to benefit from these technologies than a child with no ability to perceive light.

Clinical judgement

In making surgical decisions, one relies on established rules for routine procedures and clinical experience/intuition to guide decisions that involve higher levels of uncertainty. This is particularly true for PVS given the variable anatomy and clinical presentations discussed above.

When clinicians encounter a child with vision loss due to a complicated vitreoretinal disease, there are two paths at the extreme: do nothing given versus aggressive. Newly minted surgeons are often more aggressive than experienced ones. Fresh out of training, predicated on experience with adult vitreoretinal surgery, the goal is often to render every eye anatomically perfect. This temperament generally serves the adult vitreoretinal surgeon well, but not always. A notable exception is the complicated diabetic traction retinal detachment (TRD) with dense nasal fibrous proliferation. Such eyes are often better left with an island of circumscribed residual nasal proliferation than subjected to an attempt to "clean" the retina of proliferation to near perfection at the expense of a retinal break and detachment, intractable bleeding or subsequent proliferative vitreoretinopathy. Dicta such as "perfection is expensive in terms of risk", "sometimes less is more", "perfect is the enemy of good" and "don't risk an eye over nasal retina" all come to mind.

As a surgeon gains in experience, complications and their consequences contribute to surgical judgement and temper the quest for anatomic perfection. In PVS perfection is frequently unattainable or impractical to pursue. Unlike adult vitreoretinal surgery where iatrogenic breaks can be managed by removal of preretinal membranes and application of endophotocoagulation once the retina is re-attached, intraoperative retinal breaks in some pediatric conditions may result in inoperable retinal detachments. Residual proliferation precludes bringing the retina in contact with the retinal pigment epithelium, and retinopexy cannot be applied to seal the break.

Knowing when to stop is one of the hardest things to teach—and learn—for a vitreoretinal surgeon. "Stop just before you make the first break" isn't practical advice. Successful pediatric retinal surgeons perform a running risk–benefit analysis during challenging procedures as to whether to remove all proliferation or leave some behind to minimize the risk of a retinal break. What has worked best for me as a surgeon and teacher is to tilt away from the frame of mind that dictates that all that needs to be done must be done in a single surgery. The goal is to influence the eye to move in a more correct direction, not to bend it to one's absolute will. *Primum non nocere.* As with the example of the complex diabetic TRD, many times the goal is better instead of perfect as the quest for perfection may come at too high a cost.

Skill Acquisition and Transfer

How does one go about gaining expertise considering the "rare manifestations of rare diseases" reality? I spoke above about the advantages of a surgeon/junior surgeon practice relationship. Whether one has such an opportunity or not, it is incumbent on all surgeons to prepare for uncertainty by being an avid student of the universe of pediatric vitreoretinal diseases. Learn the most common permutations by reading voraciously and visiting colleagues. Once armed with all the experience and knowledge you can acquire, be systematic, creative, adaptable. The nature of the work will ensure that you remain humble.

Implicit in the paragraph just above is the role of the teacher. "To teach is to learn twice" is a quote attributed to the nineteenth century French writer Joseph Joubert. One benefits from being the teacher as does the one being taught. I have benefitted immensely from the intellectual and personal generosity of my mentors and strive to follow their example. The pediatric vitreoretinal community is characterized by its deep commitment to the children and its intellectual generosity. Collaborate with more capable peers. You will both benefit. Welcome visiting scholars who ask to learn from you. Everything we know belongs to the children who have taught us and is ours only to share.

Aftercare Considerations

Given the rarity of the diseases within our purview and the high level of training and skill required, pediatric vitreoretinal surgeons tend to work in major metropolitan centers, generally within academically oriented private practices or universities. Consequently, it is common to see children who hail from remote locations. There are obvious follow-up care issues as the children return home. Developing a relationship with treating physicians close to the home of the patient is critical to post-operative management success. Many times, the retina is only partially attached after surgery, slowly reattaching in the ensuing weeks and months. Absent communication with the home physicians, after the first post-operative visit the parents will relate that the referring doctor informed them that the retina remained detached. The solution is obvious—detailed communication of the pre-operative findings, the therapeutic rationale and anatomic goal, the procedure performed, intra-operative and post-operative findings and the anticipated post-operative clinical course. Typically, on-week and one-month visits are routine, and the next important clinical decision-making visit is at three months post-operatively.

Conclusion

PVS is a challenging, richly rewarding, and often stressful career sub-specialty. Success impacts a child born today for their projected potential life-span of a century. The consequences of small errors may lead to lifelong visual disability. A thorough understanding of principles unique to PVS informs decision-making in pediatric patients. The path to mastery of PVS is unique in many ways. The learning curve is long and steep. It takes time to put miles on your eyes as a clinician and surgeon. Acquiring diagnostic expertise, experience with disease progression, clinical decision-making skills as to intervention opportunity and timing inclusive of the impact of developmental factors on visual rehabilitation and visual potential, a deep sensibility as to risk/reward considerations, and of course surgical expertise—all require long dedication to the task. These are the necessary prerequisites to an informed philosophy of pediatric retinal surgery, which guide one's ability to practice our art with confidence.

References

1. Christensen K, Doblhammer G, Rau R, Vaupel JW. Ageing populations: the challenges ahead. Lancet. 2009 Oct 3;374(9696):1196–208. https://doi.org/10.1016/S0140-6736(09)61460-4.
2. Tadić V, Cumberland PM, Lewando-Hundt G, et al. Do visually impaired children and their parents agree on the child's vision-related quality of life and functional vision? Br J Ophthalmol. 2017;101:244–250. https://doi.org/10.1136/bjophthalmol-2016-30858
3. Seaber JH, Machemer R, Eliott D, Buckley EG, deJuan E, Martin DF. Long-term visual results of children after initially successful vitrectomy for stage V retinopathy of prematurity. Ophthalmology. 1995;102(2):199–204.
4. Davitt BV, Morgan C, Cruz OA. Sleep disorders in children with congenital anophthalmia and microphthalmia. J AAPOS. 1997;1(3):151–3.

Part II

Conservative Interventions for Pediatric Retinal Diseases

Examination Under General Anesthesia in Children

8

Abhishek Das and Parag K. Shah

Abstract

A thorough eye examination is extremely important in children suspected to have any congenital or genetic or acquired ocular disorders. Apart from examining anterior segment using a portable slitlamp, it is extremely important to examine posterior segment using indirect ophthalmoscopy with scleral indentation to view the retina till the ora serrata. Investigations like measurement of intra ocular pressure, fundus digital imaging, ultrasound biomicroscopy, B scan ultrasound, optical coherence tomography and even fundus fluorescein angiography need to be performed on a case-to-case basis. Unlike adults, children cannot cooperate and hence they need to be examined under anesthesia (EUA). Children with retinoblastoma require serial examinations not only to monitor the regression after every chemotherapy cycle, but also to give laser or cryotherapy. This chapter gives the nuances of performing a successful EUA and also tips to give a smooth experience to the anxious child and their families especially in cases require serial examinations.

Keywords

Examination under anesthesia · Children · Serial examinations · Retinoblastoma

Supplementary Information The online version contains supplementary material available at https://doi.org/10.1007/978-3-031-14506-3_8.

A. Das · P. K. Shah (✉)
Department of Pediatric Retina and Ocular Oncology, Aravind Eye Hospital and Post Graduate Institute of Ophthalmology, Coimbatore, Tamilnadu 641014, India
e-mail: parag@aravind.org

Introduction

Examination under anesthesia (EUA) is very important for the complete evaluation of posterior segment especially far periphery of retina or even posterior pole which includes optic disc and macula in a child who cannot be examined adequately in outdoor setting as most of the times these children are not cooperative for examination. It is ideal to perform EUAs in the hospital or in an ambulatory center having pediatric anesthesiologist.

General Anesthetic Drugs

For short examinations, inhalation anesthetics such as sevoflurane, are less stressful for the patients as it avoids the intravenous route, has a well scented odor, causing less airway irritation with smooth and quick induction and recovery. It is most helpful in the management of retinoblastoma since these children require several repeated EUAs within a short duration, which can be quite stressful to both the patients and the parents. Hence, sevoflurane based EUA with a face mask by an experienced pediatric anesthesiologist is the preferred choice in most of our patients. We have observed that children become so comfortable that they even hold the mask on their own with the parent or guardian at their side (Fig. 8.1 left panel). Some children prefer their parents holding the mask (Fig. 8.1 right panel). Fragrant masks can be used but are of single use and quite expensive. Desflurane is an another inhalational drug which has a rapid uptake and elimination from the body, which results in a fast onset of anesthesia and fast recovery also making it as an ideal agent for ambulatory anesthesia. However its major disadvantage over sevoflurane is that it has a pungent odor which causes irritation to the upper airway

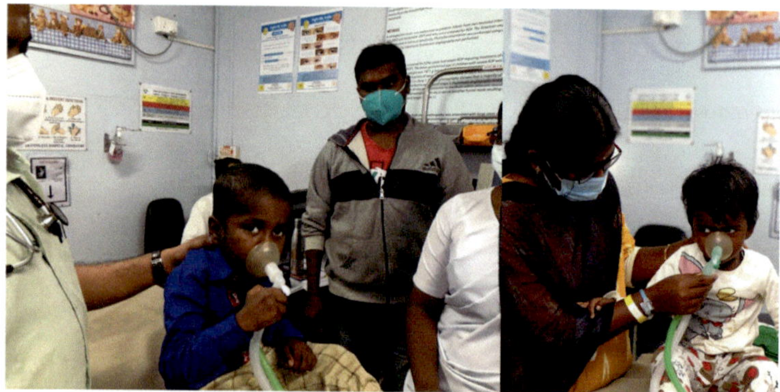

Fig. 8.1 Retinoblastoma child holding the inhalational anesthesia mask with the help of the anesthetist and accompanied by child's father (left panel). Inhalational anesthetic mask held by the mother (right panel) (Consent: Informed consent and parental consent has been taken from the families to publish the photographs.)

and may cause significant respiratory complications [1–3]. Laryngeal Mask Airway (LMA) can also be used. It is especially helpful in an extended eye examination under anesthesia and laser procedures [4]. LMA has shown to provide a satisfactory airway in infants during minor surgical procedures and results in less respiratory problems compared to an endotracheal tube. Most anesthetic drugs lower the intra ocular pressure with the exceptions of ketamine and chloral hydrate.

During long procedures, infants may not tolerate more than moderate to low inspired concentrations of sevoflurane or isoflurane. In these conditions, low concentrations of these agents can be used augmented with propofol infusion beginning at 100 µg/kg/min and titrating up or down as and when required. Pulse and O_2 saturation is monitored throughout the procedure. For recording electro retinogram (ERG) propofol infusion is preferred.

Age-appropriate fasting carried out for the patients is very important. Fasting guidelines and recommendations have been published, with the majority advocating a 6 h fast for solids, 4 h for juice, milk or breast milk and 2 h for clear fluids for elective surgery in both adults and children, the so-called 6–4–2 rule [5, 6]. However whatever fasting protocol the anesthesiologist is comfortable with, should be followed. Before EUA, a written consent form should be signed by the parents. Dilatation of pupils should be checked. All the necessary equipment and personnel for a complete ocular examination should be kept ready before induction of the anesthesia. Pre-anesthetic medications can also be tried like oral triclofos sodium syrup or midazolam syrup, but requires constant monitoring and it delays recovery from anesthesia. Complete recovery either by an appropriately trained nurse under supervision of an anesthesiologist or by the anesthesiologist himself should be ensured before the child is handed over to the parents. Typically feeding can begin couple of hours after the procedure starting with clear liquids.

While the patient is under anesthesia, a general physical examination can be performed and blood can be collected for various investigations such as baseline haemogram, genetic analysis etc.

Components of Anterior Segment Examination

Intraocular Pressure Measurement

Intraocular pressure (IOP) measurement in infants and children is often challenging. The importance of measuring IOP lies in the fact that most of the infants or child with retinal diseases like retinoblastoma, Coats disease or syndromes like Sturge Weber syndrome may present with high intraocular pressure. The gold standard to assess the intraocular pressure while the child is under anesthesia is the Perkins hand held tonometer with a blue filter after installation of fluorescein dye. Both the eyes should be in the primary position and motionless as position can be altered by the effect of the anesthetic drugs. Alternatively, a Tono-pen can be used for assessment of IOP after calibrating the device. It should be noted that the IOP should be measured multiple times in both the eyes. Tonometry under anesthesia provides only with approximation of the true tension and not an accurate one.

Corneal Diameter Measurement

The normal horizontal corneal diameter is approximately 10.5 mm increasing by about 1 mm in the first year of life. If the measurement of corneal diameter is greater than 13 mm in child of any age or asymmetrically enlarged or reduced then it is abnormal. During EUA, both vertical and horizontal corneal diameter is measured with calipers from limbus to limbus. An increasing corneal diameter in a vulnerable eye suggests high IOP requiring further treatment. For example, an advanced case of coats disease may present with enlarged corneal dimensions. Similarly infants with persistent fetal vasculature may present with microphthalmos and micro cornea.

Corneal Thickness

Pachymetry to measure corneal thickness may be indicated in certain cases where patients present with glaucomatous changes. An increase in corneal thickness as seen in infants with aphakia, there may be an over-reading of IOP and Pachymetry may have a role in it.

Anterior Segment Examination

Any child undergoing examination under anesthesia, which may fall under any pediatric retinal disease spectrum, anterior segment examination is an important aspect. The cornea is examined for the presence of any opacities, edema or Haab's striae. Under anesthesia, a portable slit-lamp is the ideal instrument to examine the anterior segment. Slit-lamp can be adjusted to magnify and produce oblique illu-mination as the signs can be subtle. Any anterior chamber anomalies like anterior chamber seeding due to retinoblastoma, hyphema or hypopyon can be ruled out. Detecting iris, pupil abnormalities or lens opacities is also important.

Gonioscopy

Gonioscopy plays an important role especially in congenital glaucoma or to look for involvement of the angles in case of a ciliary mass. Under anesthesia, direct gonioscopy can be performed with a variety of lens including a Koeppe lens (direct gonioscopy) or the 4 mirror lens.

Refraction

In case where satisfactory cycloplegic refraction is not possible in the outpatient setting, retinoscopy will need to be performed during the EUA.

Posterior Segment Examination

Examination of posterior segment in both the eyes is performed following anterior segment examination. Indirect ophthalmoscope with + 20 or + 28 diopter lens with scleral indentation is the gold standard for assessing the posterior segment. It is mandatory to check the retinal periphery till ora serrata not only to assess the peripheral avascular retina in cases of regressed retinopathy of prematurity (ROP) post anti vascular endothelial growth factor injections or in proliferative disorders like Familial Exudative Vitreo Retinopathy (FEVR) or incontinentia pigmentii but also to look for tumors in malignant conditions like retinoblastoma where new tumors usually appears anteriorly as the child grows older. Also, the optic disc and nerve fiber layer should be examined. A cup disc ratio of > 0.3 in an infant less than 1 year or > 0.5 in a caucasian child and disc asymmetry should increase suspicion of glaucoma. In Coats disease, we can look for subretinal exudates with telangiectatic vessels which may be associated with exudative retinal detachment. We can diagnose other associated abnormalities such as foveal hypoplasia associated with aniridia, choroidal hemangiomas in Sturge-Weber syndrome, and pigmentary retinopathy associated with rubella. All the retinal findings should be carefully recorded and documented with a drawing or photograph. Retcam or similar wide field fundus photography can be used to document the pathology and on serial follow-ups to see the progression or regression of the disease. Ultrasound b-scan can be carried out during EUA and document certain characteristic features like calcification in case of retinoblastoma or even a thin stalk from optic disk where there is no visibility because of corneal clouding. Ultrasound biomicroscopy (UBM) can also be done when ciliary body tumors like medulloepithelioma are suspected. Cryotherapy or laser treatment in the form of transpupillary thermo therapy (TTT) or pan retinal photocoagulation (PRP) can be also be performed in cases of retinoblastoma, ROP or FEVR. Fundus fluorescein angiography (FFA), optical coherence tomography (OCT) and ERG can also be performed during EUA.

Checklist for EUA

- Informed consent form regarding EUA signed by parents or legal guardians
- Age-appropriate visual assessment is required
- Age-appropriate fasting
- Inhalation based anesthesia using agents like Sevoflurane or Isoflurane
- Monitoring is performed using monitors

- Calipers for corneal diameter and Perkins hand held tonometer or Tonopen for IOP measurement
- Eye speculum and scleral depressor for indenting the globe
- Instrumentation like Indirect ophthalmoscope with 28 or 20 diopter lens, hand-held slit lamp, wide field fundus photography using Retcam or alternative photography for documentation, B scan, A scan, cryotherapy machine with retinal cryotherapy probe, TTT/Green laser with indirect ophthalmoscope delivery, UBM (optional)
- Fundus fluorescein angiography (optional).

Commonly Used Agents in EUA

- Preferred choice is inhalational agents like Sevoflurane, isoflurane, desflurane.

Advantages of EUA

- Complete fundus examination is carried out till the periphery
- Staging and grouping of various pediatric retinal disorders like Retinoblastoma, Coat's disease, FEVR, etc.
- Local treatment in the form of laser or cryotherapy can be performed
- Documentation and reviewing at each visit to look for progression or regression patterns
- Investigations like FFA or OCT or ERG can be done.

Case Scenario Which Needs Frequent EUA

Retinoblastoma is one case scenario which requires frequent EUA. The usual age of presentation of these children is from 3 months to 3 years and they may require periodic EUA till 7 years of age. As soon as a child is diagnosed of retinoblastoma, they tend to undergo frequent sessions of general anesthesia not only by the treating ophthalmologist for the ocular exams in-between the chemotherapy cycles but also by the radiologist for taking MRI scans and the interventional radiologist, if intra-arterial chemotherapy (IAC) is planned. On an average a child requires 3 cycles of IAC once a month. Even a child who has undergone enucleation as the primary treatment for unilateral retinoblastoma, requires frequent sessions of EUA every 3–4 months, as most clinicians prefer to examine the other eye thoroughly to look out for new tumors till 4 years of age (even if genetic testing has come negative for germinal mutation). If intra-venous chemotherapy is planned, the child is also exposed to multiple needle sticks every 3 weeks for at least six cycles (unless chemo port is inserted, which is quite costly). This frequent needle pricks also increases the anxiety of the child and the parents.

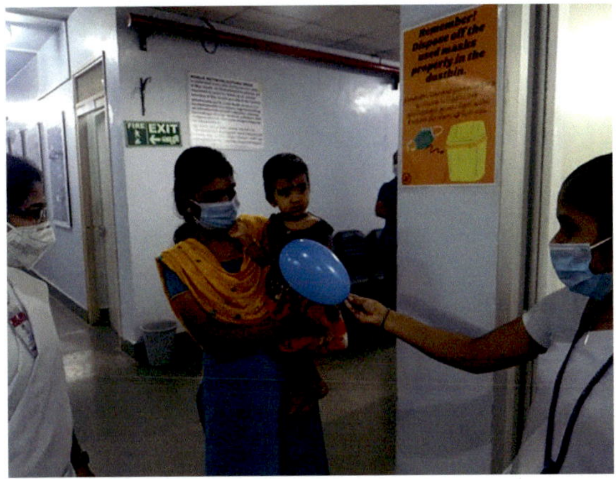

Fig. 8.2 Balloon given to the child to keep them occupied before the procedure

Since these patients tend to come in and out of the various hospitals quite often during the entire treatment, we prefer doing EUA as a daycare procedure where we encourage the family to get the child fasting early in the morning by 7 am, do the procedure by 9 am and get discharged by noon on the same day. To keep the children occupied before the procedure, we usually give them balloons to play with, which is a cheap and an all-time favorite toy (Fig. 8.2).

We perform the sevoflurane mask anesthesia technique where we encourage the children to blow themselves into the mask as if they are blowing a balloon while keeping one of the parents to hold their hands, thus making them comfortable (**see the video**). This makes a smooth induction and even recovery is quick.

We usually avoid doing routine pre anesthetic blood work before every EUA session, as far as possible (in order to avoid needle pricks), as most would have done a blood work up two weeks after their chemotherapy session. Thus, we try to follow the 'no needle prick' short anesthesia technique using just the sevoflurane mask. If a longer duration is required, then an intravenous line can be secured under anesthesia with switching from face mask to laryngeal mask airway (LMA). With over 15 years of using this technique, under the guidance of an experienced pediatric anesthesiologist, we have not faced any major complications and found this technique to be quite comfortable and acceptable amongst the families.

Video: *A short video showing a retinoblastoma child self-inducing the anesthesia under the supervision of an experienced pediatric anesthesiologist in the presence of the child's mother.*

Review Questions

1. Fasting duration for children before general anesthesia

a. 6 h for solids
b. 4 h for milk

c. 2 h for water
d. All of the above
e. None of the above

2. Which anesthetic drug does not lower the intra ocular pressure

a. Sevoflorane
b. Desflurane
c. Propofol
d. Ketamine

Answers

1. D
2. D

References

1. Kim EH, Song IK, Lee JH, Kim HS, Kim HC, Yoon SH, Jang YE, Kim JT. Desflurane versus sevoflurane in pediatric anesthesia with a laryngeal mask airway: A randomized controlled trial. Medicine (Baltimore). 2017;96(35): e7977.
2. He J, Zhang Y, Xue R, Lv J, Ding X, Zhang Z. Effect of Desflurane versus sevoflurane in pediatric anesthesia: a meta-analysis. J Pharm Pharm Sci. 2015;18(2):199–206.
3. Gupta A, Stierer T, Zuckerman R, Sakima N, Parker SD, Fleisher LA. Comparison of recovery profile after ambulatory anesthesia with propofol, isoflurane, sevoflurane and desflurane: a systematic review. Anesth Analg. 2004;98(3):632–41.
4. Ferrari LR, Goudsouzian NG. The use of the laryngeal mask airway in children with bronchopulmonary dysplasia. Anesth Analg. 1995;81(2):310–3.
5. Lambert E, Carey S. Practice guideline recommendations on perioperative fasting: a systematic review. JPEN J Parenter Enteral Nutr. 2016;40:1158–65.
6. Brady M, Kinn S, Ness V, O'Rourke K, Randhawa N, Stuart P. Preoperative fasting for preventing perioperative complications in children. Cochrane Database Syst Rev 2009; 7: CD005285.

Imaging in Pediatric Eyes

9

Nita Valikodath, S. Tammy Hsu, Cynthia A. Toth, and Lejla Vajzovic

Abstract

Multimodal imaging in pediatric eyes is useful for the diagnosis, treatment, and monitoring of several disease processes. Imaging in pediatric patients can be challenging to perform in clinic and an exam under anesthesia (EUA) may be required. Coordination with the anesthesiologist and entire operating room team are necessary to ensure efficient acquisition of images to limit the time the patient is under general anesthesia. The most common imaging modalities obtained during surgery or EUA include fundus photography, optical coherence tomography, fluorescein angiography, and ultrasound.

Keywords

Imaging · Fundus photography · Widefield fundus photography · Optical coherence tomography · Optical coherence tomography angiography · Fluorescein angiography · Indocyanine green angiography · Ultrasound · Exam under anesthesia · Intraoperative imaging

N. Valikodath · S. Tammy Hsu · C. A. Toth · L. Vajzovic (✉)
Department of Ophthalmology, Duke University, Durham, NC, USA
e-mail: lejla.vajzovic@duke.edu

N. Valikodath
e-mail: nita.valikodath@duke.edu

S. Tammy Hsu
e-mail: s.tammyhsu@duke.edu

C. A. Toth
e-mail: cynthia.toth@duke.edu

© The Author(s), under exclusive license to Springer Nature Switzerland AG 2023
Ş. Özdek et al. (eds.), *Pediatric Vitreoretinal Surgery*,
https://doi.org/10.1007/978-3-031-14506-3_9

Introduction

Imaging in pediatric retinal diseases can be a valuable adjunct to the clinical exam and in the operating room. The utility of multimodal imaging in pediatric retina is evolving. Advantages of imaging include accurate documentation and means for additional information when clinical exam is not possible.

This chapter will focus on imaging and its role in pediatric retina for exams under anesthesia (EUA) and vitreoretinal surgery. It is important to discuss the imaging plan with the parents/guardian of the patient and obtain informed consent. In addition, the entire surgical team including the nursing staff and anesthesiologists should be aware of the imaging plan to coordinate image acquisition safely and efficiently to minimize the patient's time under anesthesia. Visualization is important and the status of the ocular surface, amount of dilation and exposure are factors that affect image quality.

We will discuss the use of fundus photography, autofluorescence, fundus fluorescein angiography (FFA), indocyanine green angiography, optical coherence tomography (OCT), optical coherence tomography angiography (OCTA), B-scan ultrasonography, and ultrasound biomicroscopy. These imaging modalities can be used for general screening, diagnosis, management, and monitoring of various pediatric retinal diseases. See Table 9.1 for general indications of each imaging

Table 9.1 General indications by imaging modality in pediatric retina

Imaging modality	Indications
A scan ultrasonography	Axial length measurements
B scan ultrasonography	Poor view to retina secondary to media opacity; retinal or choroidal detachments, intraocular tumors, vitritis, congenital anomalies, inflammation, trauma
Ultrasound biomicroscopy	Intraocular tumors, uveitis, trauma
Color fundus photography	Documentation and monitoring of vitreoretinal diseases (retinal detachment, retinal tears/holes, intraocular tumors, vascular disorders, congenital anomalies, inflammation, trauma, retinal dystrophy)
Autofluorescence	Retinal dystrophies, retinal pigment epithelium
Fluorescein angiography	Documentation and monitoring of vitreoretinal diseases (vascular disorders, intraocular tumors, inflammation, retinal dystrophy)
Indocyanine green angiography	Choroidal pathology
Optical coherence tomography	Vascular disorders, inherited retinal diseases, uveitis and infectious diseases, trauma and retinal detachment, intraocular tumors, drug toxicity, or congenital diseases
Optical coherence tomography angiography	Vascular disorders

modality. Although the focus of this chapter is mainly on imaging modalities that are currently used in clinical practice, we do mention a few investigational devices.

Types of Imaging Modalities

Fundus Photography

Color fundus photography is one of the most common imaging tests performed during exams under anesthesia (EUA) for pediatric retina. It is an excellent tool to capture the posterior pole and periphery for disease monitoring and documentation purposes for a variety of pediatric retinal diseases, such as retinal detachment, retinal tears/holes, intraocular tumors, vascular disorders, congenital anomalies, inflammation, trauma, retinal dystrophy [1]. Typically, five standard fields are obtained: posterior pole, superior periphery, temporal periphery, inferior periphery, and nasal periphery.

There are many types of fundus cameras including RetCam (Clarity Medical System, Pleasanton, CA, USA), Forus 3Nethra (3Nethra Neo™, Forus Health, Bangalore, India), PanoCam LT (Visunex Medical Systems) and Phoenix ICON (NeoLight LLC., Scottsdale, AZ, USA). Camera systems may be mydriatic or non-mydriatic, contact or non-contact and have variable fields of view. Cameras with larger fields of view are especially useful in the management of pediatric retinal diseases such as retinopathy of prematurity (ROP) or familial exudative vitreoretinopathy (FEVR). Ultra-widefield systems are available with a 200-degree field of view. See Table 9.2 for types of fundus cameras and their features. Other features that differ among camera systems are probe weight, portability, light source, and cost [1, 2].

For EUAs, a contact fundus camera is more commonly used. A wire speculum and coupling medium are required. The focus and illumination can be modified to highlight pathology in the retina or vitreous, and more peripheral views can be obtained via scleral depression. Image quality can be affected by fundus pigmentation, resolution, and illumination.

Clinical scenario: 8-year-old female (gestational age 22 weeks and birth weight 400 grams) with a history of ROP status post bevacizumab in both eyes (OU), pathologic myopia, amblyopia in the right eye (OD), and cerebral palsy was noted to have a retinal detachment OD on routine eye exam. She was referred to our institution for further evaluation. Optos imaging was obtained and showed an inferior macula-off detachment and area of extrafoveal neovascularization inferotemporally with dragged retina (see Fig. 9.1).

An EUA was performed and showed a total retinal detachment with a dragged retinal fold inferotemporally, hemorrhages and pigmentation in this area. Lattice degeneration was noted superiorly with retinal breaks at 12 and 5 o'clock positions. Two circumferential rows of whitening were visualized which likely represented an irregular vitreoretinal interface in areas of prior and current avascular-vascular retina border (ridge) (see Fig. 9.2).

Table 9.2 Examples of digital fundus cameras

Name	Field of view	Handheld versus tabletop	Contact versus non-contact	Mydriatic versus non-mydriatic	Other
RetCam	Widefield and ultra-widefield; 130	Handheld and tabletop	Contact	Mydriatic	
3Nethra Neo	Widefield and ultra-widefield; 120	Handheld and tabletop	Contact	Mydriatic	
PanoCam LT	Widefield; 130	Handheld	Contact	Non-mydriatic	
Optos ™ panoramic 200Tx	Widefield and ultra-widefield; 200	Handheld and tabletop	Non-contact	Non-mydriatric	
The heidelberg spectralis	Widefield and ultra-widefield; 102	Handheld and tabletop	Non-contact	Mydriatic	
Topcon TRC NW400	50	Tabletop	Non-contact	Mydriatic	
ICON	100	Handheld	contact	Mydriatic	
NIDEK	30	Tabletop	Non-contact	Non-mydriatic	
PEEK	55	Handheld	Non-contact	Not specified	Direct ophthalmoscopy: mobile phone camera
D-Eye	20	Handheld	Non-contact	Non-mydriatic	Direct ophthalmoscopy: mobile phone camera
Arclight					Direct ophthalmoscopy: mobile phone camera

The patient underwent retinal detachment repair with a 4050 scleral buckle and scleral buckle segment augmentation inferotemporally, 25-gauge pars plana vitrectomy, membrane peeling, 532 nm endolaser, fluid air exchange and silicone oil OD.

At the post-operative month 1 visit, an Optos image showed that the retina was attached, and both the encircling scleral buckle and inferotemporal scleral buckle segment were in good position with adequate height (see Fig. 9.1). OCT showed improvement of subretinal fluid in the macula with residual intraretinal cysts (see Fig. 9.1).

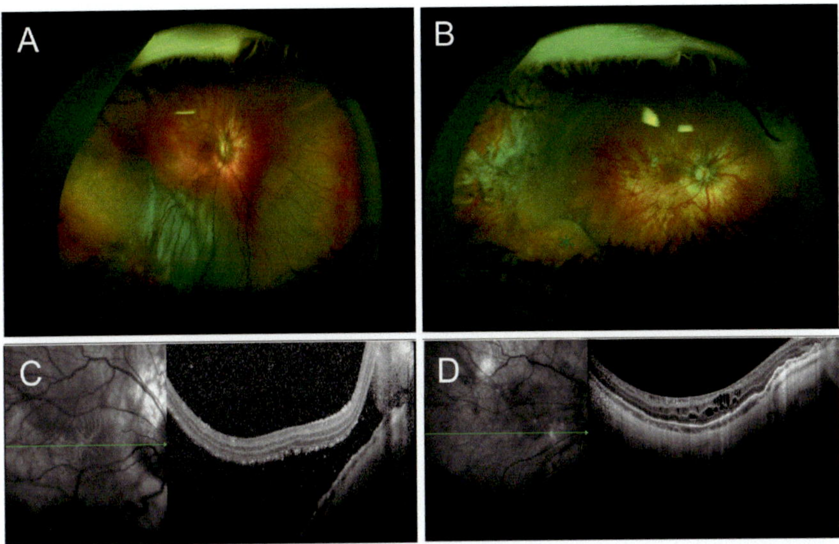

Fig. 9.1 Preoperative and post-operative widefield fundus photos and OCT images. Pre-operative Optos widefield fundus image OD showed an inferior macula-off detachment and area of extrafoveal neovascularization inferotemporally with dragged retina (**A**). Optos widefield fundus image 1 month after surgery showed that the retina was attached, and both the encircling scleral buckle and inferotemporal scleral buckle segment (*) were in good position with adequate height (**B**). Preoperative OCT images of the right eye showed subretinal fluid in the macula (**C**). OCT 1 month after surgery showed significant improvement in subretinal fluid in the macula with mild cystic changes (**D**)

Autofluorescence

Fundus autofluorescence can be used to document changes in the retinal pigment epithelium (RPE) and photoreceptors and is especially useful for retinal dystrophies. It is a non-invasive imaging tool. The mechanism involves blue-light excitation of lipofuscin and emission of light of a longer wavelength [3]. Currently available fundus autofluorescence systems require an upright position and thus are not used during EUAs.

Fluorescein Angiography

Fundus fluorescein angiography (FFA) can be utilized in the operating room with RetCam, ICON and Heidelberg Spectralis camera/OCT systems. Fluorescein dye is administered through an intravenous cannula followed by a saline flush. It is important to work together with the anesthesiologist to administer an accurate dose of fluorescein (5–7.5 mg/kg, max dose 500 mg) and to ensure accurate timing of image acquisition once fluorescein has been injected [4]. The transit eye should be identified beforehand for the initial image acquisition, and then the camera can be alternated between the two eyes.

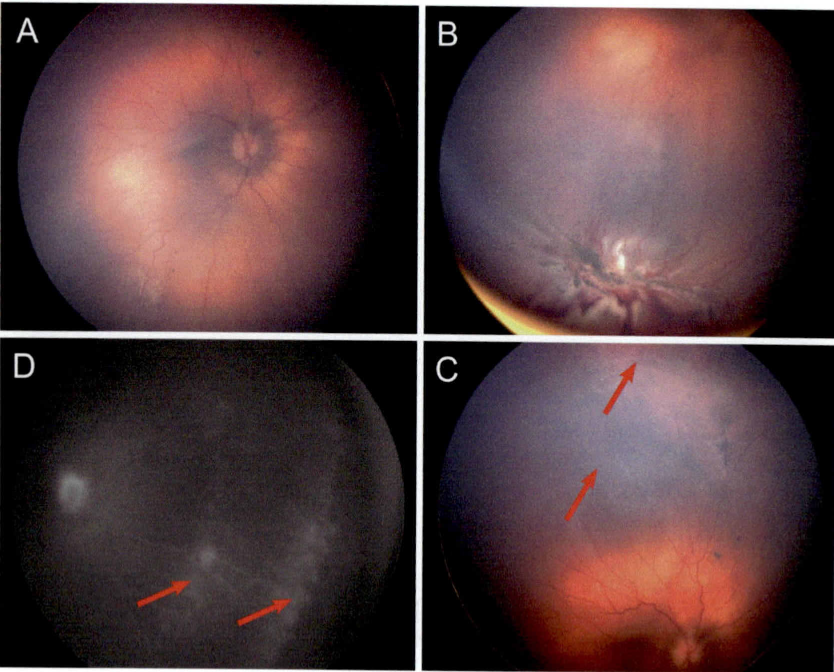

Fig. 9.2 Intraoperative Retcam photos with fundus fluorescein angiography. RetCam images (**A** and **B**) showed a total retinal detachment with a dragged retinal fold inferotemporally and associated hemorrhage and pigmentation. Two circumferential rows of whitening (red arrows) were visualized which represented an irregular vitreoretinal interface in areas of prior and current avascular-vascular retina border (ridge) (**C**) and is more prominent on fluorescein angiography (**D**)

FFA is useful in several pediatric vascular disorders, such as ROP or FEVR. It can be used to document and monitor the avascular retina or areas of new neovascularization. For Coats' disease or other exudative retinopathies, it can help identify telangiectasias and leakage as well as non-perfused retina to guide laser treatment. FFA can be useful in sickle cell disease, diabetic retinopathy, inflammatory or infectious conditions, and inherited retinal diseases.

Clinical scenario: 5-year-old male with history of Coat's disease of the left eye (OS) with macular exudates and visual acuity of counting fingers OS had been undergoing serial EUAs status post multiple intravitreal bevacizumab injections, laser therapy, and posterior subtenon kenalog injections. At a follow up visit patient was noted to have areas of active leakage on fluorescein angiography. Repeat EUA was performed.

Retcam OS showed a subfoveal nodule and fibrosis with exudates in the temporal, superior and inferior macula, as well as exudates, telangiectatic vessels and lightbulb aneurysms in the temporal periphery (see Fig. 9.3). Scattered laser scars were also present. OCT OS showed a subretinal nodule with increased cystoid macular edema. FFA OS showed temporal peripheral leakage that was more prominent in the superotemporal region (see Fig. 9.4A–F). Laser photocoagulation and intravitreal off-label bevacizumab were performed.

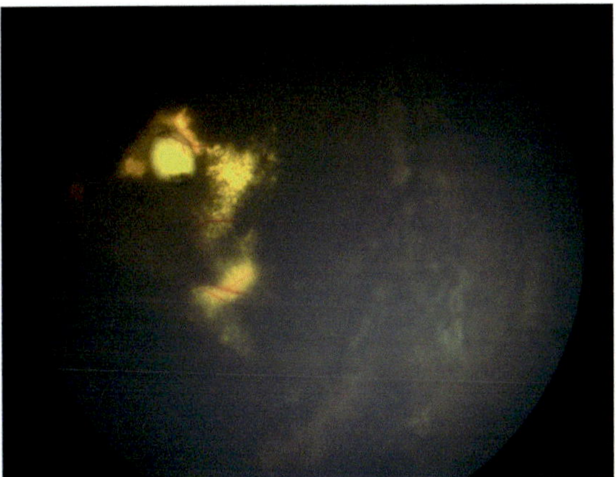

Fig. 9.3 Retcam image of the left eye. Retcam images OS showed a subfoveal nodule and fibrosis with exudates in the temporal, superior and inferior macula, and temporal telangiectatic vessels with terminal lightbulb aneurysms

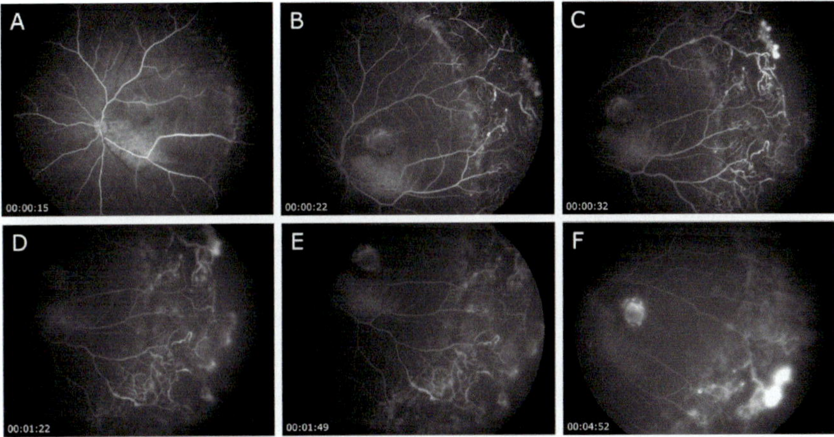

Fig. 9.4 Fundus fluorescein angiography of the left eye. Fundus fluorescein angiography OS showed telangiectasias, lightbulb aneurysms, and areas of non-perfusion. There was peripheral leakage temporally and staining of the macular fibrosis/nodule (**A–F**)

Indocyanine Green Angiography

Indocyanine green angiography (ICGA) can be used to monitor choroidal pathology such as choroidal neovascularization or to assess choroidal thickness. The dye fluoresces in the infrared range and is largely protein bound. ICGA is not commonly used in the OR setting due to limited availability with current intraoperative imaging systems.

Optical Coherence Tomography

Optical coherence tomography (OCT) has been quickly evolving in the field of pediatric retina. It is used for several diseases including vascular disorders, inherited retinal diseases, uveitis and infectious diseases, trauma, retinal detachment, intraocular tumors, drug toxicity, and congenital diseases [1]. It can be used to evaluate foveal architecture, vitreoretinal interface disorders, macular edema, neovascularization, loss of retinal tissue or subretinal fluid [5, 6]. In diseases such as Coats or diabetic macular edema, OCT can identify if treatment is warranted with intravitreal anti-vascular endothelial growth factor.

Ivue/Istand from Optovue and Heidelberg Spectralis are tabletop spectral domain OCT devices that are available for commercial use. The Bioptigen/Leica Envisu c2300 is a handheld portable OCT that can be used to image pediatric patients in the supine position. The patient's age and axial length should be considered when setting imaging parameters as this will affect image quality. Scans can be obtained at the macula, the periphery or optic nerve.

Intraoperative OCT (iOCT) can be very beneficial in pediatric retina surgery. Handheld portable iOCT can be used to distinguish different anatomical planes, identify abnormalities in the vitreoretinal interface, or locate subtle retinal breaks. Ultra-widefield handheld OCT prototypes are available and can assist in imaging the periphery to identify vitreoretinal pathology in a variety of pediatric diseases, such as ROP or familial exudative vitreoretinopathy (FEVR). However, handheld portable iOCT require longer operating times because the surgeon must stop the surgical procedure to obtain images without contaminating the surgical field. Microscope-integrated OCT (MIOCT) allows real time visualization and has many uses in pediatric vitreoretinal surgery. It can provide guidance in retinal detachment repair, macular surgery, or gene therapy for inherited retinal diseases.

> **Clinical scenario**: 4-year-old boy with history of ruptured globe OD status post repair who presented to our institution for worsening vision OS and was diagnosed with sympathetic ophthalmia. In the left eye, he was noted to have optic disc edema and elevation in the macula. Preoperative and intraoperative OCT showed bacillary layer detachments (see Fig. 9.5A and B). FA showed late leakage. The patient underwent laboratory workup which was negative, and he was started on prednisone. 1 week later, OCT during clinic visit showed improvement in subretinal fluid OS (see Fig. 9.5C). EUA was performed again 1 month later, and OCT demonstrated resolution of subretinal fluid at the fovea (see Fig. 9.5D–F). The patient was transitioned off prednisone and started on infliximab and methotrexate.

Optical Coherence Tomography Angiography

Optical coherence tomography angiography (OCTA) is used to better understand the retinal microvasculature [7]. It is a functional extension of OCT that evaluates vascular flow and identifies superficial, penetrating and deep vascular complexes. Currently, there are a few portable investigational OCTA systems that has been

Fig. 9.5 Preoperative, intraoperative and follow up OCT images. Preoperative OCT demonstrated bacillary retinal detachments with subretinal fluid (**A**). Intraoperative OCT at initial EUA also demonstrated bacillary retinal detachments with subretinal fluid (**B**). Repeat OCT showed improving subretinal fluid 1 week later after starting treatment with prednisone (**C**). OCT with B-scan (**D**) and 3D views (**E–F**) showed resolution of subretinal fluid at the fovea 1 month later

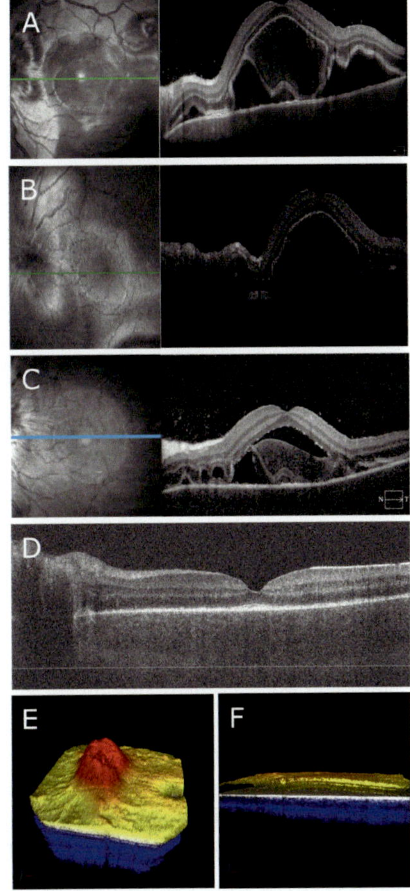

used in the pediatric population -Heidelberg Spectralis with Flex Module [7, 8], Axsun Technologies [9], and Avanti RTVue XR (Optovue Inc, Fremont, CA) [10]. A study by Hsu et al. in 2019 evaluated OCTA in healthy pediatric eyes and showed that factors such as age, race and axial length should be considered in quantitative measures [11]. OCTA has also been studied in diseases such as retinoblastoma [12, 13] and retinal vascular diseases including ROP [14] and FEVR [15]. Chen et al. is investigating a microscope-integrated OCTA device for retinal vascular diseases in the pediatric population [16].

> **Clinical scenario**: An 18-month-old female with retinoblastoma treated with intra-arterial chemotherapy and transpupillary thermotherapy returned for a scheduled EUA. She had a stable calcified, treated retinoblastoma tumor OD as seen on Retcam fundus photo (see Fig. 9.6A). OCT with OCTA were also obtained, and OCTA showed a tortuous network of capillaries in the tumor (see Fig. 9.6B).

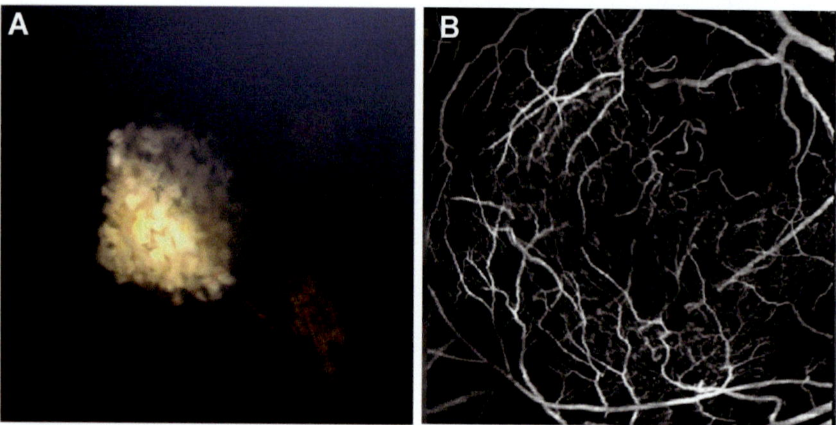

Fig. 9.6 Retcam and OCTA image of the right eye. Retcam OD showed a stable calcified, treated retinoblastoma tumor (**A**). En face OCTA image of all the retinal blood flow is demonstrated (**B**). The superficial and deep vascular complexes were difficult to segment properly due to the irregular retinal layers and calcifications of the tumor

Ultrasonography

A scan biometry is useful in obtaining axial length measurements. In patients with pathologic myopia, nanophthalmos, or posterior microphthalmos, it may be useful to determine the axial length [1]. In other cases, A-scan ultrasound can be used for IOL power calculations.

There are contact or immersion-based methods for A-scan ultrasonography. Pediatric patients have low corneal and scleral rigidity which leads to greater likelihood of corneal compression in the contact method. The immersion method uses a coupling fluid between the cornea and probe and has been shown to be more accurate than contact biometry. However, in the operating room, a trained technician may not be available to perform immersion A-scan and the surgeon more commonly uses the contact technique [17].

B-scan ultrasonography is commonly used when there is a media opacity in the cornea or lens, poorly dilated pupil, or vitreous hemorrhage, precluding a clear view to the retina. It can be used to identify and characterize retinal or choroidal detachments, intraocular tumors, vitritis, congenital anomalies, inflammation, intraocular foreign bodies, or trauma [1]. In addition, it can help guide operative planning. For example, B-scan can help guide one's surgical approach in patients with persistent fetal vasculature with anterior and posterior involvement. In patients with a retinal detachment, trocar placement may be modified depending on the configuration of the detachment. B-scans can also be used to evaluate anterior segment structures and optic nerve.

A coupling medium is required for B-scan ultrasonography. The probe can be placed over the lids or over the cornea taking caution to avoid corneal damage. It can be oriented in the axial, transverse and longitudinal positions and moved to

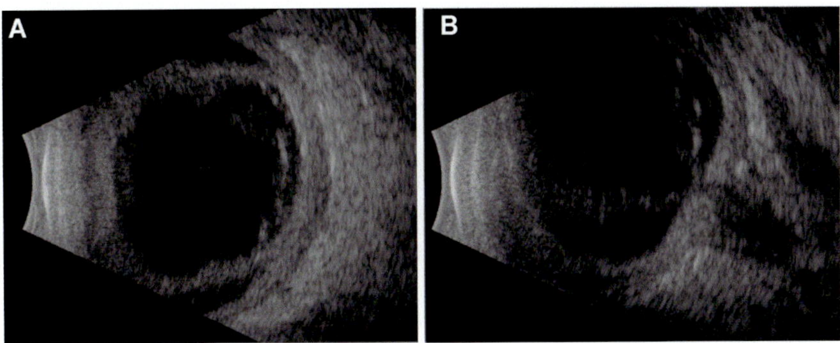

Fig. 9.7 B-scan of both eyes. B-scan OD showed a total retinal detachment and vitreous hemorrhage (**A**). Bscan OS showed a funnel shaped retinal detachment and vitreous hemorrhage OS (**B**)

obtain more anterior or posterior views. The gain can be adjusted for optimal viewing, especially to identify subtle vitritis. Dynamic ultrasonography can be useful and can help distinguish hyaloid from retina.

> **Clinical scenario**: 10-year-old boy with history of West syndrome and self-injurious behavior was noted to have worsening vision by his parents and referred to our clinic for evaluation of retinal detachment. He was noted to have bilateral traumatic white cataracts with no view to the posterior pole. B-scan showed bilateral retinal detachments (see Fig. 9.7).

> **Clinical scenario**: 3-month-old female with combined persistent fetal vasculature (PFV) in the right eye status post cataract extraction OD and no view to the posterior pole due to a dense pupillary plaque across visual axis. Retcam photo of the right eye demonstrated an anterior vascular stalk obscuring the visual axis (see Fig. 9.8A) and B-scan ultrasonography showed an anterior membrane (asterisk) with traction to the ciliary processes and retina near the pars plana (see Fig. 9.8B). A broadened attachment where the stalk extended from the optic nerve (arrow) was consistent with limited central posterior involvement with a tractional retinal detachment involving the posterior one-third of the stalk. Vitreous hemorrhage was also seen.

Ultrasound Biomicroscopy

Ultrasound biomicroscopy (UBM) is a high-resolution and non-invasive way to evaluate cases of uveitis, intraocular tumors especially ciliary body tumors, or trauma [1]. UBM can identify involvement of the anterior retina or ciliary body in retinoblastoma and anterior hyaloidal fibrovascular proliferation in ROP. It requires a coupling medium, uses high frequency transducers, and can image structures up to 4 mm from the surface [18].

Multimodal Imaging

Fundus photography, FFA, OCT, and B-scan are the most common imaging modalities used during EUAs or surgery. A combination of these can help guide diagnosis, management, and treatment of various pediatric retinal diseases.

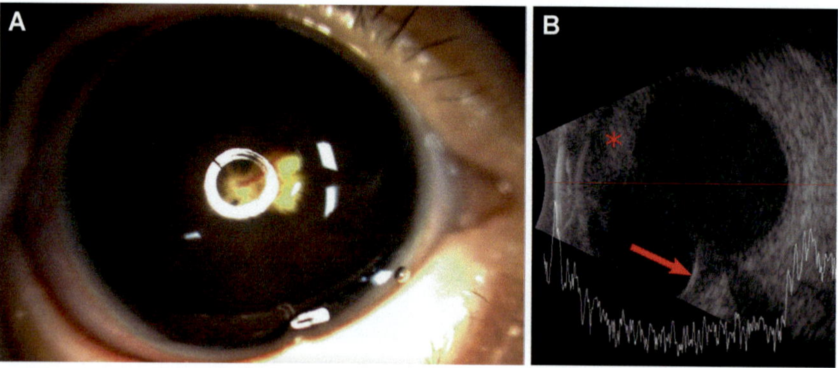

Fig. 9.8 Retcam photo and B-scan ultrasonography of the right eye. Retcam image OD demonstrated an anterior vascular stalk obscuring the visual axis (**A**). B-scan ultrasonography showed an anterior membrane (asterisk) with traction to the ciliary processes and retina near the pars plana. There was also a broadened attachment where the stalk extended from the optic nerve (arrow) with a tractional retinal detachment to the posterior one-third of the stalk. Vitreous hemorrhage was also visualized by static and dynamic ultrasound (**B**)

Clinical scenario: 5-year-old boy (born 31 weeks and 1397 g) with history of ROP with bilateral retinal detachment status post vitrectomy and laser OU in Mexico 5 years prior to presentation. The patient was seen for a routine exam by his ophthalmologist and noted to have a "tube of retina" emanating from the optic disc OU and referred to our institution for further evaluation. However, examination in clinic was difficult in this 5-year-old boy. The patient was closing his eyes frequently and limited views of the periphery were seen on clinical examination or on Optos imaging. An EUA was performed.

Retcam images demonstrated macular dragging with retinal folds OU (see Fig. 9.9A and F). The left eye had a peripheral tractional retinal detachment temporally, ischemic retina and sclerotic vessels. FA in the right eye showed a retinal fold, no leakage, and peripheral laser

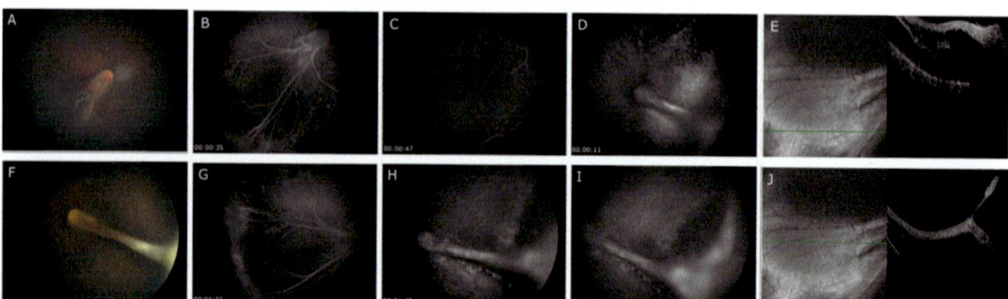

Fig. 9.9 Multimodal imaging with Retcam, FFA, and OCT. Retcam images of the right (**A**) and left eye (**F**) demonstrated macular dragging with retinal folds OU. There was a peripheral tractional retinal detachment temporally in the left eye as well as ischemic retina and sclerotic vessels. FA in the right eye (**B–D**) showed a retinal fold, no leakage, and peripheral laser scars. FA in the left eye (transit) (**G–I**) confirmed the diffusely ischemic retina and showed mostly choroidal vasculature and peripheral laser scars. Retinal vessels were visible within the fold and were dragged temporally. Hand-held OCT showed tractional schisis and retinal fold in the right eye (**E**) and left eye (**J**).

scars (see Fig. 9.9B–D). FA in the left eye confirmed the diffusely ischemic retina and showed mostly choroidal vasculature and peripheral laser scars (see Fig. 9.9G–I). Retinal vessels were visible within the fold and were dragged temporally.

Review Question

1. Which of these steps should be performed first during an exam under anesthesia?

A. Obtain OCT images
B. Communicate imaging and surgical plan with the OR team, including anesthesiology and nursing staff
C. Administer fluorescein dye with help from the anesthesiology team.
D. Obtain Retcam images

Answer

1. B

References

1. Agarwal K, Vinekar A, Chandra P, et al. Imaging the pediatric retina: An overview. Indian J Ophthalmol. 2021;69(4):812–23. https://doi.org/10.4103/ijo.IJO_1917_20.
2. Valikodath N, Cole E, Chiang MF, Campbell JP, Chan RVP. Imaging in retinopathy of prematurity. Asia-Pac J Ophthalmol Phila PA. 2019;8(2):178–86. https://doi.org/10.22608/APO.201963.
3. Salcedo-Villanueva G, Lopez-Contreras Y, Gonzalez-H. Leon A, et al. Fundus autofluorescence in premature infants. Sci Rep. 2021;11(1):8823. https://doi.org/10.1038/s41598-021-88262-z.
4. Marmoy OR, Henderson RH, Ooi K. Recommended protocol for performing oral fundus fluorescein angiography (FFA) in children. Eye. 2022;36(1):234–6. https://doi.org/10.1038/s41433-020-01328-6.
5. Toth, CA, Ong SS. Handbook of pediatric retinal OCT and the eye-brain connection. Elsevier Inc.; 2020.
6. Hartnett ME, et al. Pediatric retina, 3rd ed. Wolters Kluwer; 2020.
7. Hsu ST, Chen X, Ngo HT, et al. Imaging infant retinal vasculature with OCT angiography. Ophthalmol Retina. 2019;3(1):95–6. https://doi.org/10.1016/j.oret.2018.06.017.
8. Viehland C, Chen X, Tran-Viet D, et al. Handheld OCT angiography probe for imaging of infants in the clinic or nursery. Invest Ophthalmol Vis Sci. 2019;60(9):3094.
9. Campbell JP, Nudleman E, Yang J, et al. Handheld optical coherence tomography angiography and ultra–wide-field optical coherence tomography in retinopathy of prematurity. JAMA Ophthalmol. 2017;135(9):977–81. https://doi.org/10.1001/jamaophthalmol.2017.2481.
10. Vinekar A, Chidambara L, Jayadev C, Sivakumar M, Webers CAB, Shetty B. Monitoring neovascularization in aggressive posterior retinopathy of prematurity using optical coherence tomography angiography. J AAPOS Off Publ Am Assoc Pediatr Ophthalmol Strabismus. 2016;20(3):271–4. https://doi.org/10.1016/j.jaapos.2016.01.013.

11. Hsu ST, Ngo HT, Stinnett SS, et al. Assessment of macular microvasculature in healthy eyes of infants and children using OCT angiography. Ophthalmology. 2019;126(12):1703–11. https://doi.org/10.1016/j.ophtha.2019.06.028.

12. House RJ, Hsu ST, Thomas AS, et al. Vascular findings in a small retinoblastoma tumor using OCT angiography. Ophthalmol Retin. 2019;3(2):194–5. https://doi.org/10.1016/j.oret.2018.09.018.

13. Thomas AS, Hsu ST, House RJ, et al. Microvascular features of treated retinoblastoma tumors in children assessed using OCTA. Ophthalmic Surg Lasers Imaging Retin. 2019;51(1):43–9. https://doi.org/10.3928/23258160-20191211-06.

14. Hsu ST, Chen X, House RJ, Kelly MP, Toth CA, Vajzovic L. Visualizing macular microvasculature anomalies in 2 infants with treated retinopathy of prematurity. JAMA Ophthalmol. 2018;136(12):1422–4. https://doi.org/10.1001/jamaophthalmol.2018.3926.

15. Hsu ST, Finn AP, Chen X, et al. Macular microvascular findings in familial exudative vitreoretinopathy on optical coherence tomography angiography. Ophthalmic Surg Lasers Imaging Retin. 2019;50(5):322–9. https://doi.org/10.3928/23258160-20190503-11.

16. Chen X, Viehland C, Carrasco-Zevallos OM, et al. Microscope-integrated optical coherence tomography angiography in the operating room in young children with retinal vascular disease. JAMA Ophthalmol. 2017;135(5):483–6. https://doi.org/10.1001/jamaophthalmol.2017.0422.

17. Wilson ME, Trivedi RH. Axial length measurement techniques in pediatric eyes with cataract. Saudi J Ophthalmol. 2012;26(1):13–7. https://doi.org/10.1016/j.sjopt.2011.11.002.

18. Guthoff RF, Labriola LT, Stachs O. Diagnostic ophthalmic ultrasound. In: Schachat AP, editor. Ryan's Retina. 6th ed. Amsterdam, Netherlands: Elseiver; 2018. p. 273–374.

Laser Photocoagulation of the Retina in Babies and Children

10

Ulrich Spandau

Abstract

Indirect laser photocoagulation of the nonvascular retina is a major tool in preventing blindness. This chapter shows step-by-step the technique of lasercoagulation of children.

Keywords

Indirect laser photocoagulation · Laser · Argon · Diode · ROP · FEVR · Coats

Introduction

Indirect laser photocoagulation of the nonvascular retina is a major tool in preventing blindness. Confluent photocoagulation burns are applied to the nonvascularized retina. The most common pediatric retinopathy is ROP; less common is FEVR, Coats, Sickle cell retinopathy and Incontinentia pigmenti. Two laser types are used for treatment of the retina: Argon laser with a wave length of 510 nm and diode laser with 810 nm wave length.

U. Spandau (✉)
St Eriks Eye Hospital, University of Stockholm, Stockholm, Sweden
e-mail: ulrich_spandau@yahoo.de

© The Author(s), under exclusive license to Springer Nature Switzerland AG 2023
Ş. Özdek et al. (eds.), *Pediatric Vitreoretinal Surgery*,
https://doi.org/10.1007/978-3-031-14506-3_10

113

Our Experience

In our experience laser coagulation is always successful for ROP 3+ in zone II. A failure or recurrence is seldom. Successful laser coagulation is "normal" for clinical centers which treat many ROP newborns per year. The success rate in the ETROP study is 90% for zone II [1]. But the failure and recurrence rate for laser coagulation is much higher (30%) for clinics which treat only a handful newborn per year [2]. The most common reason for failure after laser coagulation is an incomplete laser treatment [3, 4].

This is not the case for zone I. In zone I a recurrence may occur after a complete laser photocoagulation. It is therefore essential to distinguish between zone I and zone II eyes. This is only possible with an imaging device such as Retcam (Clarity Medical System Inc, USA).

The technique of lasercoagulation is difficult and requires much training. An eye with ROP 3+ requires a COMPLETE laser coagulation within ONE session. This is different to diabetes. Here a laser coagulation in many sessions is possible.

First you must learn to examine adults with the binocular indirect ophthalmoscope. If you master this technique fluently, then examine newborns on the weekly ROP examinations. This training requires at least 12 months. Then you can start with laser coagulation. You laser one eye and your mentor lasers the fellow eye. After approximately five laser treatments with your teacher you can start to treat alone.

One eye or both eyes? Sometimes ROP 3+ is not present in both eyes. One eye may have ROP 3+ and the other eye may have ROP 3 preplus. We laser treat always both eyes. Why? In the most cases the preplus eye will progress later on to a plus disease. Furthermore, an asymmetric treatment results in a grave anisometropia. The treated eye will become highly myopic and the fellow eye not. Finally, the newborn avoids a second general anaesthesia.

Instruments for Laser Coagulation

(1) Diode laser device (Fig. 10.1)
(2) Binocular indirect ophthalmoscope (Fig. 10.2)
(3) Volk 25D lens (Fig. 10.3)
(4) Scleral depressor (Fig. 10.4)
(5) Lid speculum (Fig. 10.5)

Laser device (Fig. 10.1): We use always a diode laser (Iridex, CA). An alternative is an Argon laser. The initial settings of the laser device are 100/100/300: Power: 100 ms, Duration: 100 ms, Interval: 300 ms.

Laser indirect ophthalmoscope (LIO) (Fig. 10.2): The laser indirect ophthalmoscope is a helmet which contains a light source and a laser device. The laser indirect ophthalmoscope is connected to the diode laser (Iridex, CA).

Fig. 10.1 A diode laser (Iridex) and two attached cables from binocular laser ophthalmoscope for laser and light

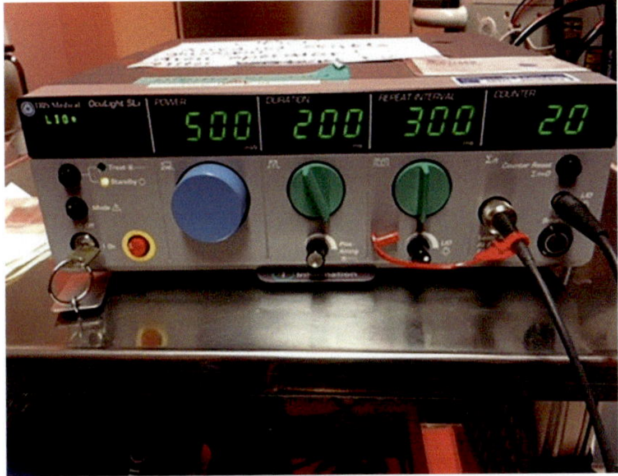

Fig. 10.2 A binocular indirect laser ophthalmoscope (LIO) (Iridex, Iridex). The two cables are attached to the laser device (Fig. 10.1)

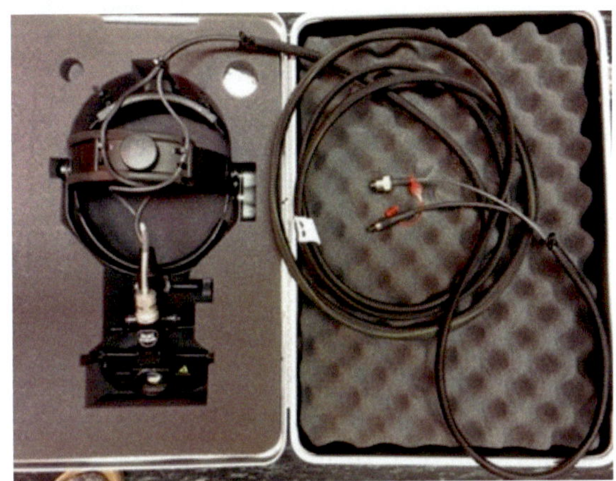

Fig. 10.3 20D and 25D lens from Volk. Both lenses are suitable for laser. We use preferably the 25D lens

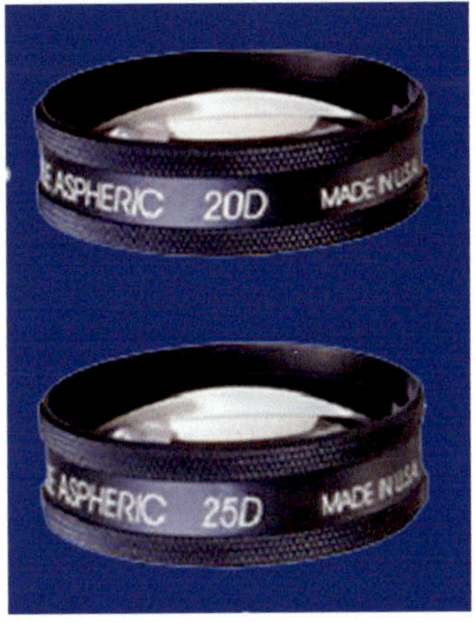

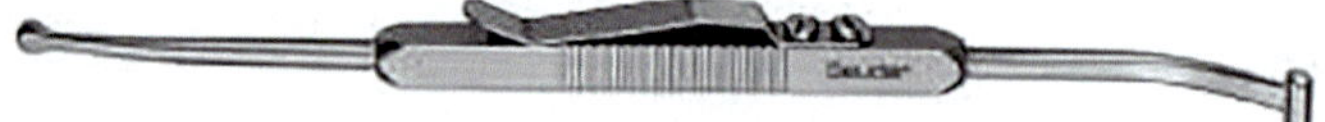

Fig. 10.4 Sclera depressor with small and large indentor (Geuder, Germany)

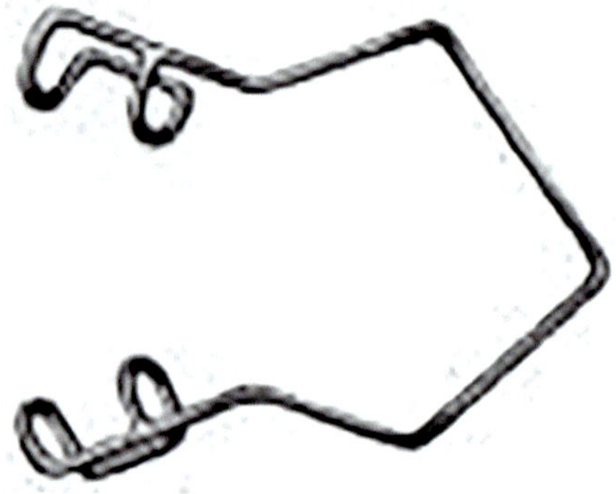

Fig. 10.5 Lid speculum for ROP newborns (Geuder No. 17023, Germany)

Volk 25D lens (Fig. 10.3): We use usually the 25D lens from Volk. An alternative is the 20D lens which is better for the ridge but not so good for ora serrata. Another alternative is the 30D lens which may give a too small image.

Scleral depressor (Fig. 10.4): A scleral depressor is very important for laser coagulation. You can only reach the ora serrata with a scleral depressor. If possible, we laser with the big indentor because it enables treating more tissue at once. At the ora serrata we prefer the small indentor. Alternatively, you can use a cotton wool swab or a strabismus hook.

Lid speculum (Fig. 10.5): We recommend a small lid speculum for newborns.

The laser treatment of newborn with ROP is very different because the eyes are very small and because the pathology is located in the periphery of the eye. If you laser treat the temporal periphery and the central ridge it is best to laser in a standing position (Fig. 10.6). If you laser treat the nasal, superior and inferior retina you may need to laser in a sitting position (Fig. 10.7).

We use usually a diode laser. Alternatively, you can use an Argon laser. The *normal amount* of laser effects is 1200–1800 laser spots (minimum: 1000 laser spots, maximum: 2500 laser spots).

The start settings for a diode laser are: 300 ms (power), 100 ms (duration) and 300 ms (interval) (Fig. 10.8). Remark: Be careful with duration. Too high duration may result in vitreous haemorrhage and detachment. Start always with 100 ms. Increase first power to maximal settings before you increase duration to 200 ms.

Fig. 10.6 A standing position is fine for the temporal ischemic retina. Note the sclera depressor

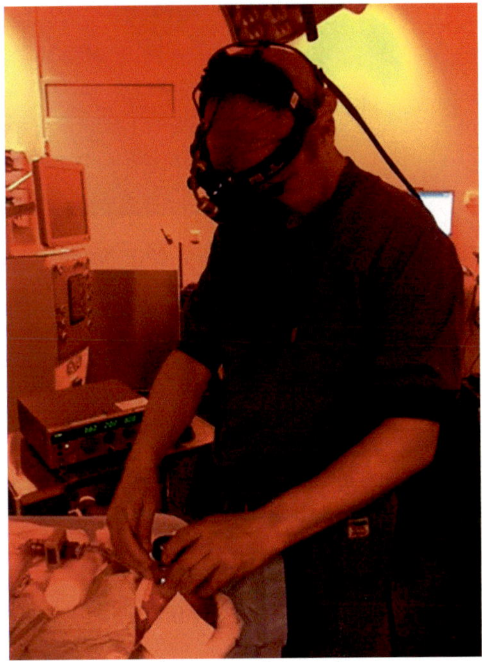

Fig. 10.7 A sitting position is sometimes required to reach the nasal, superior and inferior ischemic retina

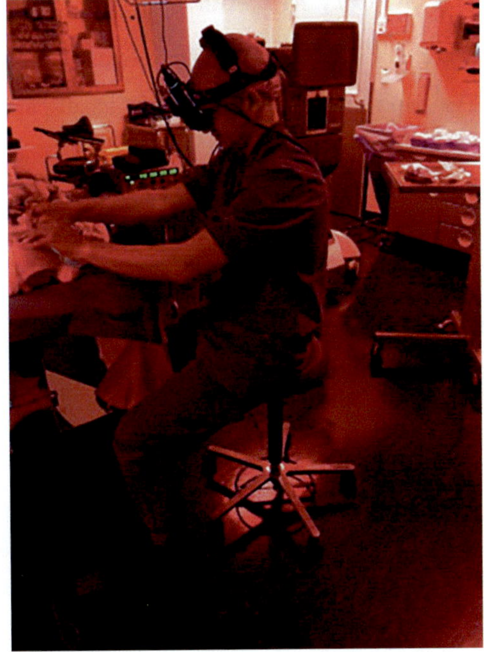

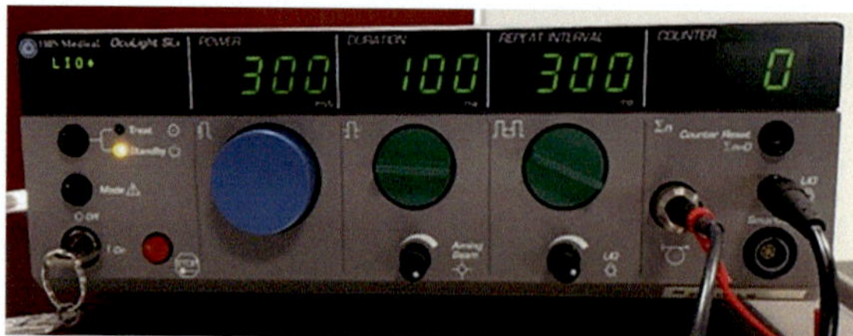

Fig. 10.8 A diode laser (Iridex, CA). Normal laser settings for laser coagulation of a ROP newborn

Laser Treatment Step-By-Step: (Figs. 10.9, 10.10, 10.11, 10.12, 10.13, 10.14, 10.15, 10.16, 10.17, 10.18 and 10.19)

(1) Start with the temporal retina. Find the correct laser power.
(2) Laser treat the temporal retina from ora serrata almost to the ridge.
(3) Laser treat the superior, nasal and inferior retina.
(4) Treat the ridge.
(5) Inspect the retina for skip lesions and incomplete laser.

The Surgery in Detail

(1) Start with the temporal retina. Find the correct laser power

The pupil must be well dilated, a small pupil is not sufficient for laser photocoagulation. See chapter pupil dilatation.

Laser coagulation of the newborns eye is best performed in two 360° rounds. The first round treats the ischemic retina from the ora serrata almost to the ridge. In the second round the ridge is laser treated.

We start always with the temporal retina. Why? The temporal retina has the biggest ischemic area. Therefore, the visualization of the temporal ischemic retina is the best of all quadrants and the ridge is well visible.

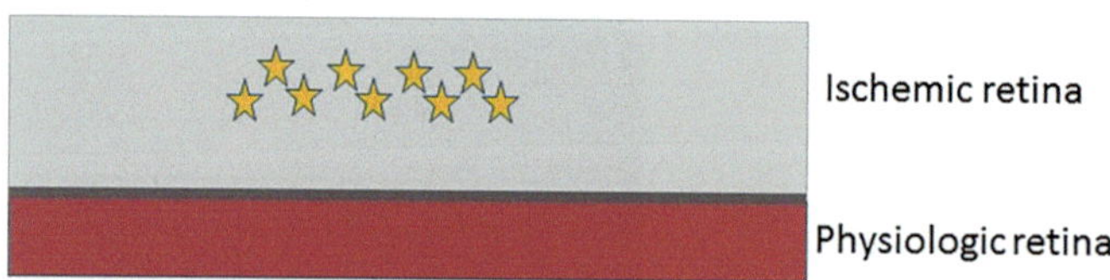

Fig. 10.9 Start at the temporal quadrant and find the appropriate laser settings

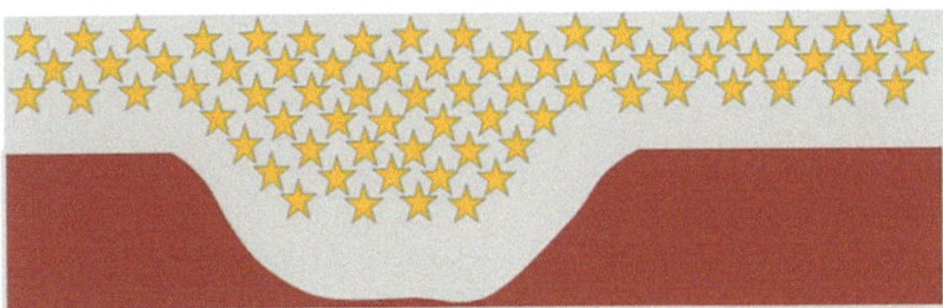

Fig. 10.10 Laser photocoagulation of the temporal pole from ora serrata almost to the ridge

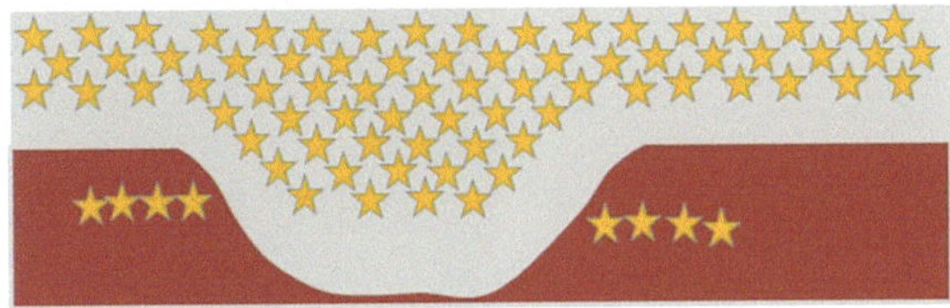

Fig. 10.11 Avoid overtreatment when moving from temporal to inferior and superior retina

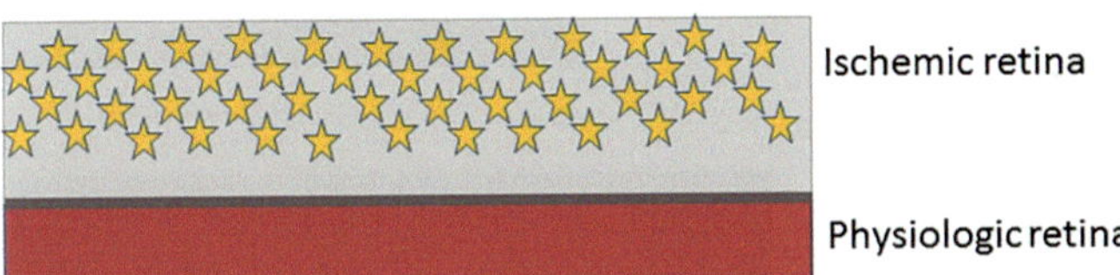

Fig. 10.12 Treat from the ora serrata until close to the ridge

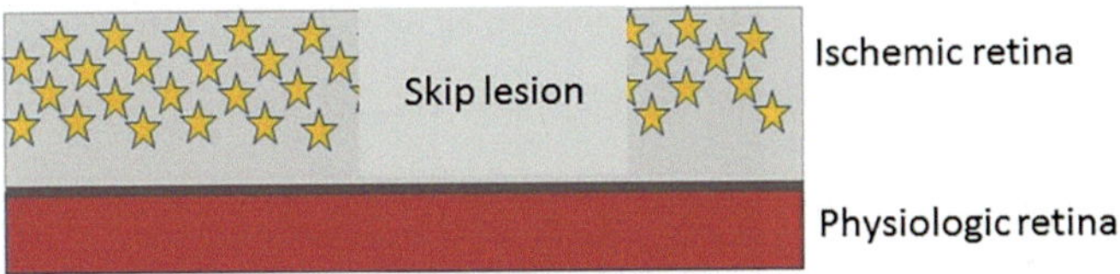

Fig. 10.13 When moving from one treated area to the next avoid creating a skip lesion

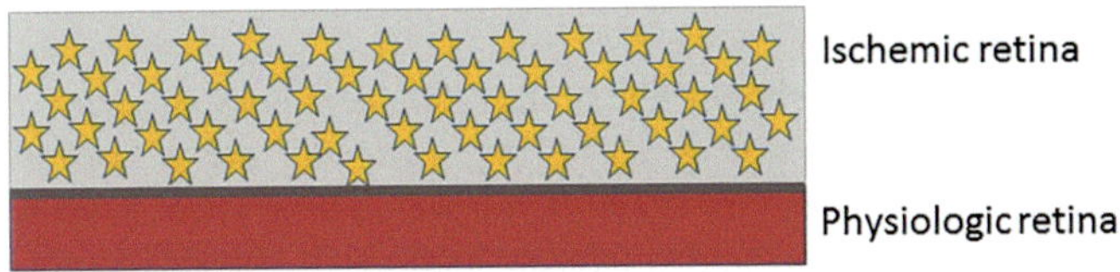

Fig. 10.14 Now treat the ridge. Increase power and work without scleral depressor

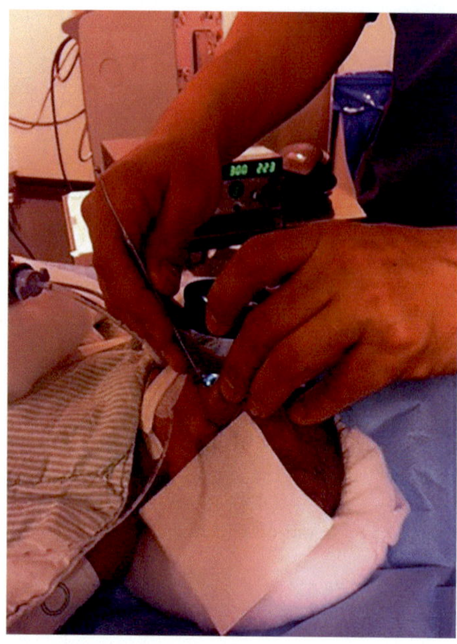

Fig. 10.15 For peripheral laser coagulation use the scleral depressor to indent the ora serrata

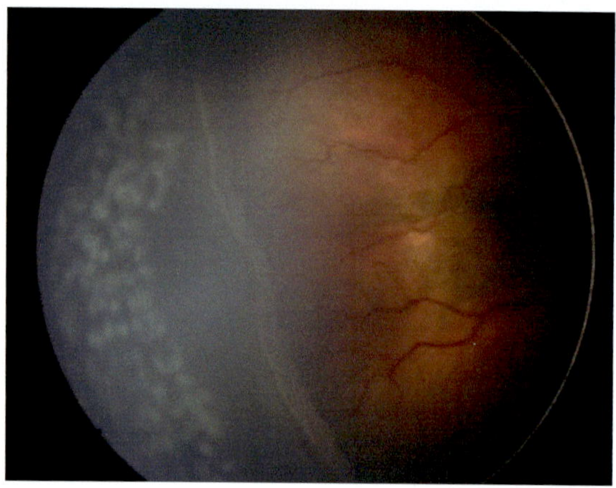

Fig. 10.16 Laser treat from the ora serrata almost to the ridge

Indent the retina with the broad side of the sclera depressor and place a few laser spots on the indented retina (Fig. 10.9). If you do not see a laser effect, then increase **power** to 200 ms and try again. If you see no laser effect increase power to 300 ms and continue like this until you reach 1000 ms. If you still do not see a laser effect, then increase **duration** to 200 ms and reduce power to 100 ms. Then increase power again in 100 ms steps to 1000 ms.

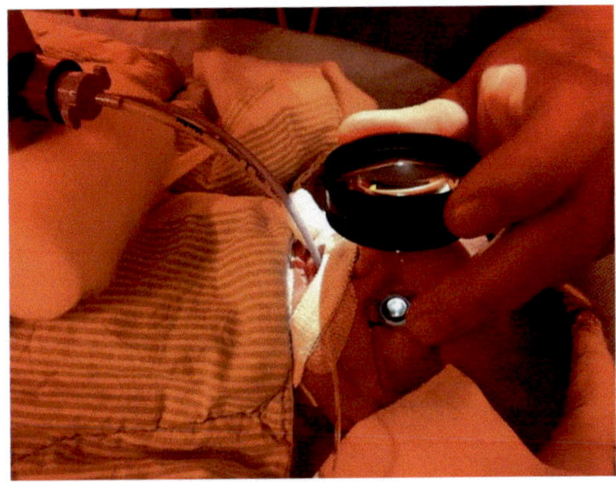

Fig. 10.17 For central laser treatment of the ridge work without scleral depressor

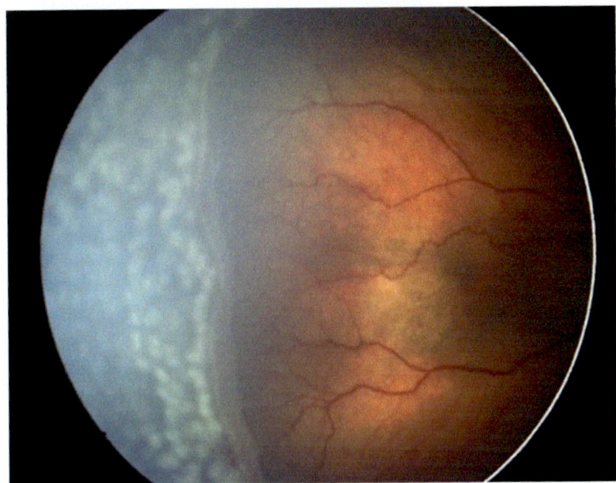

Fig. 10.18 Laser treat the ridge. Usually a higher laser power is required

You should achieve a laser effect with approximately 300–600 ms power and 200 ms duration. A laser duration of 300 ms is too high and never necessary in our experience. A normal laser setting with our (old) laser device (Iridex, CA) is power: 400–700 ms, duration: 200 ms and interval: 300 ms.

If the retina bleaches very much or you see a burst in the retina with a bleeding, then the laser power is too high. Reduce power by 100 ms and try again.

Important: If you laser the eye with too high laser energy it may happen that within 1 week the ROP progresses so much that the "eye tilts". Too aggressive laser coagulation aggravates the intraocular VEGF expression. This may happen if you use a duration of 300 ms for laser. Use a maximal duration of 200 ms. Otherwise, a rubeotic iris and finally a retinal detachment develops.

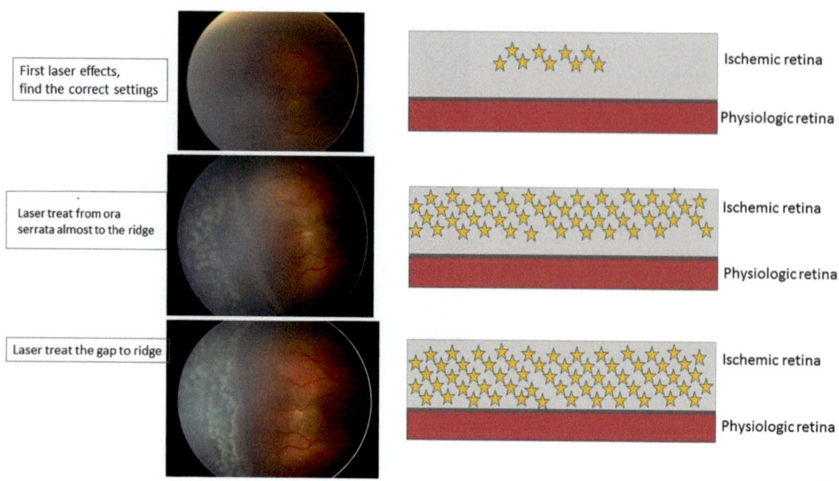

Fig. 10.19 A brief overview of the laser coagulation of ROP newborn

(2) **Laser treat the temporal retina from ora serrata almost to the ridge** (Figs. 10.10, 10.11, 10.16)

If you achieve laser spots on the retina then the first difficult step is achieved. Continue now with laser coagulation of the temporal ischemic retina. Treat with a density of a distance of maximal one laser spot between two spots (Fig. 10.10). Use the scleral depressor to reach the ora serrata (Figs. 10.15 and 10.16). Do not treat the ridge yet.

By moving the 25D or 20D lens forwards or backwards you can increase or decrease the size of the laser spots. Large laser spots save time. Large laser spots are advisable for the periphery and small laser spots for the ridge.

(3) **Laser treat the superior, nasal and inferior retina** (Figs. 10.12, 10.13, 10.14)

If you continue from the temporal to the superior or inferior retina be aware that the size of ischemic retina reduces very much. The ischemic retina becomes a thin strip inferior and superior and a bit broader nasally. This circumstance may easily lead to overtreatment into the physiologic retina (Fig. 10.11).

If you treat the inferior, superior and nasal retina it is easier to start with the small indentor of the scleral depressor. Place the scleral depressor at the limbus and move it slowly towards the equator. As soon as you see the ora serrata, start with laser treatment. Continue with laser treatment almost to the ridge (Fig. 10.12).

If you are done with one area, then place the depressor again at the limbus and continue with the next area. But do not lose contact to the old treatment area in order to prevent a skip lesion (Fig. 10.13). The inferior and superior retina is difficult to assess. You often have to move like a monkey to find a suitable position for laser coagulation. Remember that the ischemic retina decreases substantially in size outside the temporal pole. It is a thin strip of ischemic retina.

(4) **Treat the ridge** (Figs. 10.14, 10.17, 10.18)

In the second round you treat the ridge (Fig. 10.14). The lasercoagulation is easier without scleral depressor. Here you need an increased laser power because the retina is thicker. You need approximately 200 ms extra power. The duration remains unchanged at 200 ms.

(5) **Inspect the retina for skip lesions and incomplete laser**

If you have completed laser, double check that the complete retina 360 deg from the ora serrata to the ridge is treated. You can do this with:

(1) 25D Volk lens
(2) Retcam

Look for untreated areas, examine the retina up to the ora serrata and ascertain yourself that the complete ridge is treated. Do not close the case before you are really certain that you treated the complete ischemic retina because undertreatment may result in a progression of the disease and finally end in a retinal detachment.

Pits and pearls:

Visualization of the ischemic retina is difficult: The ischemic retina is a thin strip superior and inferior, a broader strip nasal and a broad tongue temporal. The ischemic retina is grey and has no vessels. The demarcation line is the border between ischemic and physiologic retina. The physiologic retina is light red and has vessels.

Follow-up: We prescribe the eye drops Dexamethasone 1 mg/ml 2×d and Atropine 0,1% 2×/d for 2 weeks. The eyes require a weekly follow-up. On the first follow-up the retinopathy should be stable or less but not worse. If the retinopathy is worse, then perform a thorough examination in order to exclude an undertreatment. If you do not find an undertreatment then examine the newborn again after three days. If the retinopathy has worsened, we recommend an immediate examination in general anaesthesia to exclude skip lesions. We recommend also an immediate anti-VEGF injection.

On the second week follow-up, the retinopathy should have further regressed. After 4 weeks laser scars have formed, and the retinopathy has resolved.

In Conclusion

Laser coagulation of a newborn is technically a very difficult procedure which requires much training. See Fig. 10.19. An optimal laser coagulation within ONE session is however required to achieve a regression of the retinopathy. An undertreatment results within a few weeks in progression of the retinopathy.

If a progression occurs, we recommend an immediate intravitreal anti-VEGF injection.

Angiography Assisted Laser Photocoagulation for Newborn and Children

Laser photocoagulation of a ROP newborn may be difficult due to poor visualization. Especially the border between physiologic and ischemic retina is sometimes difficult to determine.

In other pediatric retinal diseases such as familial exudative vitreoretinopathy (FEVR) or incontinentia pigmenti (IP) the border between ischemic and physiologic retina cannot be discerned with ophthalmoscopy. Only angiography can tell us where exactly the border between physiologic and ischemic retina is localized. In these cases, an angiography is required before laser coagulation.

We developed therefore an angiography assisted laser photocoagulation (Fig. 10.20). Within one session, several laser coagulations and Retcam angiographies are performed until the complete ischemic retina is laser treated.

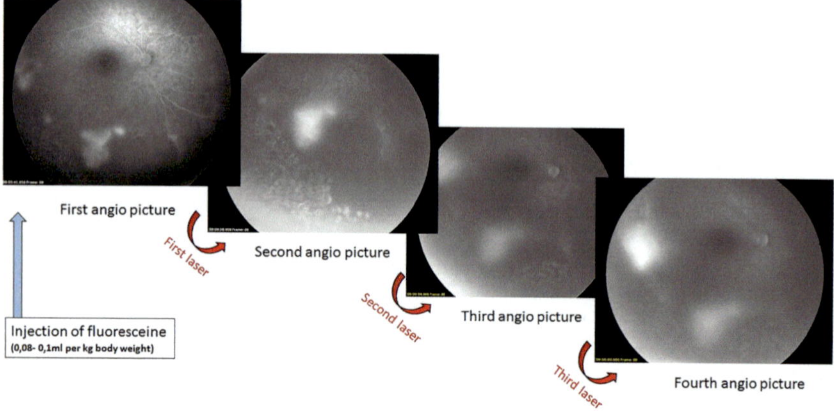

Fig. 10.20 Fluorescein is injected once. After the first angiography pictures a laser photocoagulation is performed. Then the second angiography picture is taken and so on

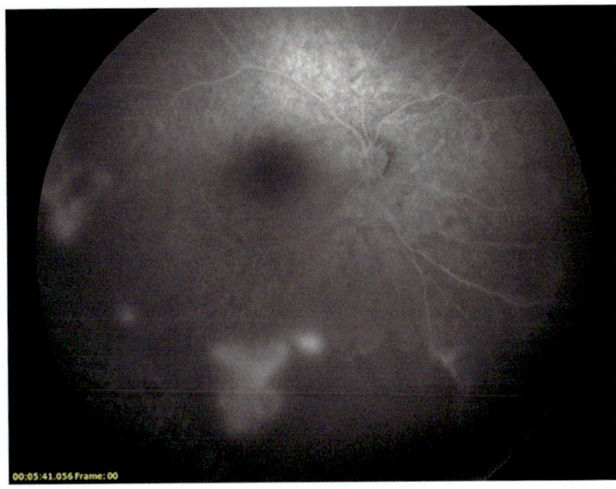

Fig. 10.21 First angiography: Note the inferior ischemia

The Technique Step-by-Step (Fig. 10.20):

(1) Fluorescein is injected, and the first angiography is performed. The border between physiologic and ischemic retina is determined (Figs. 10.20 and 10.21).

(2) The first laser photocoagulation is performed.

(3) No fluorescein is reinjected. The second first angiography is performed. The skip lesions are determined.

(4) A second laser photocoagulation is performed.

(5) No fluorescein is reinjected. The third angiography is performed. The skip lesions are determined.

(6) A third laser photocoagulation is performed.

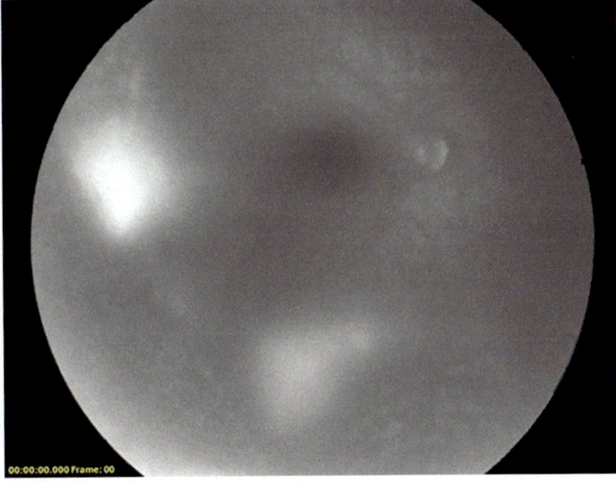

Fig. 10.22 Last angiography: After 3 laser photocoagulations the inferior ischemia is filled up with laser

Fig. 10.23 The first angiography. A newborn with Incontinentia pigmenti. Note the irregular vascular sprouting, vascular pruning and the ischemic retina. In the periphery old laser effects are visible

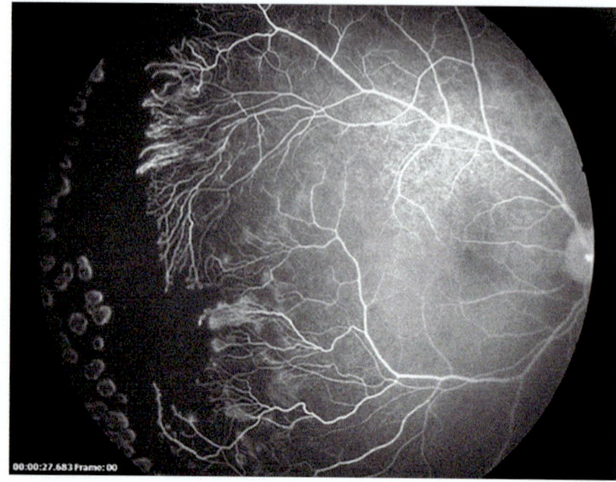

Fig. 10.24 New laser effects have been added. A visualization of the ischemic retina is not possible

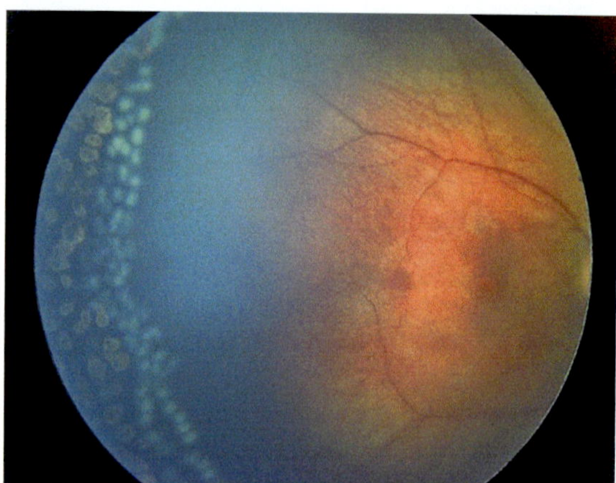

Fig. 10.25 The third angiography. Note the old and fresh laser effects

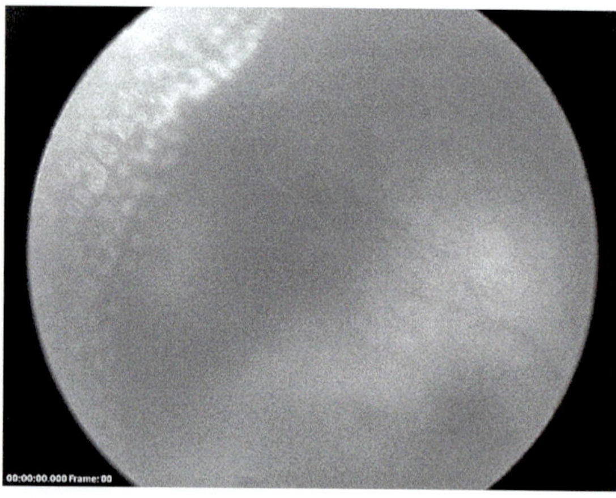

(7) No fluorescein is reinjected. The fourth angiography is performed. Now, laser coagulation is usually completed (Fig. 10.22).

We demonstrate the technique with a case report. A full-term newborn with incontinentia pigmenti was laser treated before due to a peripheral ischemia. In this session the old laser coagulation is assessed with angiography and an additional laser coagulation planned if necessary. The Retcam angiography shows a residual ischemia which has not yet been laser treated (Fig. 10.23). A laser photocoagulation with binocular ophthalmoscope is performed. Then a second angiography is performed. A small residual ischemia is still visible (Fig. 10.24). Two additional rows of laser are added. The ischemia is now filled up with laser (Fig. 10.25).

Review Questions

Q1: A laser photocoagulation in a newborn (one correct answer):

(A) Can be done in several sessions
(B) Can be done in two sessions
(C) Must be done in one session

Q2: How many degrees of retina in case of ischemic retinopathy in a newborn or child need to be laser photocoagulated? (One correct answer).

(A) 90°
(B) 180°
(C) 270°
(D) 360°

Q3: Skip lesions in a 360° must be avoided because (One correct answer).

(A) They are aesthetically a sign of poor surgery
(B) They increase the risk for progression of the ischemic retinopathy
(C) They cause visual field defects

Q4: The negative side effects of a laser photocoagulation are: (several answers are correct):

(A) Visual field defects
(B) Increased risk for myopia
(C) Increased risk for hyperopia
(D) Increased risk for retinal detachment

Q5: What is the most critical laser parameter? (one answer is correct):

(A) Power
(B) Duration
(C) Repeat interval

Answers

Q1: C

Q2: D

Q3: B

Q4: A, B

Q5: B

References

1. Repka MX, Tung B, Good WV, Capone A Jr, Shapiro MJ. Outcome of eyes developing retinal detachment during the early treatment for retinopathy of prematurity study. Arch Ophthalmol. 2011;129(9):1175–9.
2. Holmström G, Tornqvist K, Al-Hawasi A, Nilsson Å, Wallin A, Hellström A. Increased frequency of retinopathy of prematurity over the last decade and significant regional differences. Acta Ophthalmol. 2018;96(2):142–8.
3. Austeng D, Källen KB, Ewald UW, Wallin A, Holmström GE. Treatment for retinopathy of prematurity in infants born before 27 weeks of gestation in Sweden. Br J Ophthalmol. 2010;94 (9):1136–9.
4. Spandau U, Larsson E, Holmström G. Inadequate laser coagulation is an important cause of treatment failure in type 1 retinopathy of prematurity. Acta Ophthalmol. 2020;98(8):795–9. https://doi.org/10.1111/aos.14406. Epub 2020 Apr 6. PMID: 32250547.

Intravitreal Injections for Pediatric Retinal Diseases

Christa Soekamto, Luca Rosignoli, and Clio Armitage Harper III

Abstract

The advent of anti-vascular endothelial growth factor (VEGF) agents has allowed for a new treatment option in pediatric diseases, most specifically retinopathy of prematurity (ROP). In this chapter, the authors discuss indications for anti-VEGF use in pediatric ocular diseases. Special considerations and appropriate injection technique are explained, given the unique anatomy and health issues specific to the pediatric population. Additionally, a protocol for anti-VEGF injections in ROP patients called the SAFER protocol is described, which stands for: (S)hort needle, (A)ntiseptic/antibiotic, (F)ollow-up, (E)xtra attention to detail, and (R)echeck. Lastly, monitoring for vascularization with a fluorescein angiogram is an important part of follow up in ROP management.

Keywords

Anti-VEGF · Intravitreal injection · Retinopathy of prematurity · SAFER protocol

C. Soekamto · L. Rosignoli · C. A. Harper III (✉)
University of Texas Health San Antonio, San Antonio, TX, USA
e-mail: armieharper3@gmail.com

L. Rosignoli
e-mail: rosignoli@uthscsa.edu

C. A. Harper III
Austin Retina Associates, Austin, TX, USA

University of Texas at Austin, Austin, TX, USA

© The Author(s), under exclusive license to Springer Nature Switzerland AG 2023
Ş. Özdek et al. (eds.), *Pediatric Vitreoretinal Surgery*,
https://doi.org/10.1007/978-3-031-14506-3_11

Introduction

Indications for Anti-VEGF in ROP

Retinopathy of prematurity (ROP) is the leading cause of treatable blindness in children in the world, and it is the leading cause of ocular morbidity of premature infants [1]. If left untreated, severe ROP can lead to retinal detachment and blindness. Historically, conventional treatment options included laser photocoagulation and cryotherapy. The advent of anti-vascular endothelial growth factor (VEGF) agents, which is commonly used in adult eyes, has allowed for a new therapy in the armamentarium of ROP treatment. Anti-VEGF medications are used worldwide for treatment-requiring ROP. Even though they are not FDA approved for ROP treatment in the United States, the intravitreal anti-VEGF drug, ranibizumab, has been approved for the treatment of ROP by the European Medical Agency July 20, 2019. Currently, ranibizumab is the only medication approved for ROP treatment whereas bevacizumab is used off-label.

The pathogenesis of ROP involves increased local VEGF response secreted by ischemic tissue after the infant is born. Treatment is aimed at decreasing VEGF response, which has conventionally been achieved through confluent laser [2]. Of the currently available anti-VEGF agents, the most widely studied in the management of ROP are bevacizumab and ranibizumab. In rabbit models, ranibizumab has shown faster retinal diffusion and decreased systemic half-life compared to bevacizumab [3]. Intravitreal bevacizumab has been reported to lower systemic VEGF levels for up to 8 weeks following injection for ROP treatment [2]. These findings have led to a hypothesized decreased risk of adverse events with ranibizumab compared to bevacizumab that has not been formally established.

Based on current available evidence, anti-VEGF therapy in management of type 1 ROP seems to carry no increased risk compared to its use in the adult population. Despite concerns of neurodevelopmental delay in infants receiving anti-VEGF therapy, a true cause-effect relationship has not been established, with no difference found in Bayley-III scores for neurodevelopmental outcomes in infants who received intravitreal bevacizumab compared to primary laser therapy for the treatment of type 1 ROP [4]. Bevacizumab use has been associated with decreased refractive error compared to laser therapy alone in the management of type 1 ROP [5].

The landmark BEAT-ROP study published in 2011 was the first randomized controlled trial comparing intravitreal bevacizumab (0.625 mg/0.025 ml) to laser in infants with zone I or zone II posterior stage 3+ disease [6]. This study demonstrated a significant benefit in using intravitreal bevacizumab in infants with zone I disease when compared to laser. Commonly cited limitations of the trial include lack of long-term follow-up and higher-than-predicted laser treatment failure rate. The RAINBOW study published in 2019 was a randomized controlled superiority trial which showed intravitreal ranibizumab (0.2 mg/0.02 mL) may be superior to laser therapy in the treatment of type 1 ROP [7]. Aflibercept has been used for ROP in multiple reports and is currently being studied against laser therapy in the

BUTTERFLEYE trial. Patients that should be considered for anti-VEGF treatment are those with type 1 ROP, defined as: zone I, any stage with plus; zone I, stage 3 without plus disease; or zone II, stage 2 or 3 with plus disease [8]. Infants with aggressive posterior ROP (AP-ROP) disease may also benefit. Anti-VEGF medications can be used as monotherapy or in combination with laser photocoagulation.

There is currently no unified protocol directing the ideal dosage and frequency of anti-VEGF injections in the management of type 1 ROP, which relies on close monitoring (every 1–2 weeks) to assess for disease reactivation. Similarly, there is currently no established protocol in the implementation of delayed laser therapy in the management of residual retinal avascularity following anti-VEGF injections. One recommended strategy is to perform angiography-guided laser photocoagulation approximately 60 weeks post-menstrual age (PMA) in all infants with residual avascular retina following anti-VEGF therapy or with persistent mild or type 2 ROP without previous treatment, with assessment of fluorescein angiogram at the time of treatment [9].

Indications for Anti-VEGF in FEVR

Anti-VEGF agents have also been used in the management of familial exudative vitreoretinopathy, although the evidence addressing this treatment option is limited, partly due to the rarity of this disease. The long-term effects of anti-VEGF use in FEVR remain unclear.

Ranibizumab, bevacizumab and pegaptanib have been used to manage FEVR stage 2 or greater, resulting in regression of retinal neovascularization and leakage noted on fluorescein angiography [10–12]. Subsequent vitreous hemorrhage and tractional retinal detachment following pegaptanib therapy have been reported, but the relationship between these complications and the anti-VEGF injection remains unclear. Although anti-VEGF therapy may help in delaying progression of FEVR, there is not enough evidence of support management with anti-VEGF therapy alone.

Indications for Anti-VEGF in Coats' Disease

The use of Anti-VEGF therapy in Coats' disease remains controversial. A case series shows improvement in retinal exudations through 1 year follow-up in Coats' disease stages 2B-3B treated with monthly (n = 1–3) bevacizumab 2.5 mg/0.1 ml injections followed by laser photocoagulation or cryotherapy [13]. However, new-onset vitreoretinal fibrosis and tractional retinal detachments following bevacizumab 1.25 mg/0.05 ml injection combined with laser/cryotherapy have also been reported [14].

Considerations in Anti-VEGF Injections in ROP

When treating a preterm infant, several considerations must be made given the unique anatomy. These include the following: a smaller size globe, the crystalline lens in relation to the globe is wider in the anterior–posterior dimension, the ciliary body is located more anteriorly, and the pars plana is either absent or incompletely developed [15]. These anatomic findings can predispose the preterm infant to iatrogenic trauma, such as anterior or contralateral retinal breaks and injury to the lens, especially with the use of a standard ½ inch needle [17]. The RAINBOW study employed the use of a 30-gauge ½ inch (12.7 mm) needle, which may allow for complications due to its large size in relation to the infant globe. Wright et al. reported histopathologic evidence of damage to the posterior pole and lens with a standard 30-gauge 12.7 mm needle fully introduced into the globe of a postmortem enucleated 56-week old infant eye [16]. Additionally, the study demonstrated that the short 32-gauge 4 mm needle inserted into its hub enters the vitreous cavity completely without threatening the lens or retina [16]. A small volume syringe (0.5–1.0 ml) is preferred to allow for precise hand control throughout the procedure, which is important when patient cooperation is unpredictable. In terms of needle placement, Wright et al. described an age-based nomogram for sclerotomy placement for pediatric vitrectomies [17]. This data can be applied to proper location of needle placement in intravitreal injections as it includes a range of pediatric ages and variety of ocular diseases, including ROP, based on in vivo ora-limbus measurements of eyes. Another consideration is the higher risk of infection in these infants due to an underdeveloped immunity and other medical comorbidities. Exclusion of risk factors for infection is a crucial part of evaluation prior to intravitreal injection. The ophthalmologist must also ensure there is no congenital nasolacrimal duct obstruction, which can be simply be evaluated by applying digital pressure to the nasolacrimal sac to confirm there is no reflux of mucus material. Being informed of the past medical history and other current infections also helps one assess the risk factors for endophthalmitis.

Technique for Anti-VEGF Injection in ROP

There is no standardized protocol describing the use and technique of intravitreal injection in pediatric patients for the treatment of ROP. There are, however, published protocols for intravitreal injection in adults [18, 19]. The authors propose a protocol described by Wright et al. which accounts for the unique considerations that should be made for infants with premature eyes and systemic comorbidities [16, 17]. The acronym SAFER is used to describe the authors' protocol of anti-VEGF injections for ROP, which stands for:

- (S)hort needle
- (A)ntiseptic/antibiotic
- (F)ollow-up
- (E)xtra attention to detail
- (R)echeck

The "short needle" is a single-use 32-gauge thin-walled stainless steel, hypodermic 4 mm needle (TSK STERiJECT, TSK Laboratory, Japan). The "antiseptic/antibiotic" includes either 5 or 10% betadine, instilled before and after the injection. The "follow up" should be 48–72 hours following the injection to rule out endophthalmitis. The "extra attention to detail" involves referencing the ora nomogram to determine the safest distance from the limbus for injection [17]. It also includes the use of sterile instruments, gloves and masks for all team members involved in the injection. "Recheck" entails following the patient every 1 to 2 weeks following the injection until complete vascularization has occurred or laser has been applied to avascular retina. The precise technique is outlined as below.

If injections are performed on awake infants they should have cardiorespiratory monitoring and a pulse oximeter. A registered nurse should be present throughout the entire procedure. Gloves and masks should be worn by all involved in the procedure, including nurses or respiratory therapists holding the baby. Patients on continuous positive airway pressure (CPAP) ventilation are at increased risk of dispersed flora from the nasopharynx contaminating the injection field. This can be avoided by replacing the CPAP with long nasal prongs for the duration of the injection procedure. Additional sedation or anesthesia can be given depending on the ophthalmologist's preference in consultation with the neonatologist, but it has not been found to affect adverse outcomes [15].

Topical tetracaine or proparacaine hydrochloride 0.5% is applied for anesthesia and a sterile speculum is placed in the eye. Drops of either 5% or 10% betadine are placed in the eye. The eye is then marked with calipers 0.75–1 mm posterior to the temporal limbus based on the ora nomogram described by Wright et al. [17]. The medication is then prepared by pushing the plunger of the syringe until the rubber stopper aligns with the desired dose mark, so the drug completely fills the needle shaft and syringe [17]. The medications include bevacizumab (0.625 mg/ 0.025 mL) or ranibizumab (0.2 mg/0.02 ml) in a prefilled syringe with a single-use 32-gauge thin-walled stainless steel, hypodermic 4 mm needle (TSK STERiJECT, TSK Laboratory, Japan). The needle tip is directed into the central of the vitreous cavity and completely inserted in the eye until it reaches the hub, and the plunger pushed slowly until it reaches the end of the syringe (Fig. 11.1). A sterile calcium alginate tipped applicator or lens loop can be used to stabilize the eye prior to injection but is not necessary. When initially performing this procedure or when teaching trainees, the authors recommend a two-hand approach with one hand stabilizing the syringe and the other hand pushing down on the plunger to avoid unintentional change in needle direction while injecting the medicine. An additional drop of 5 or 10% betadine is instilled into the eye. The fundus is

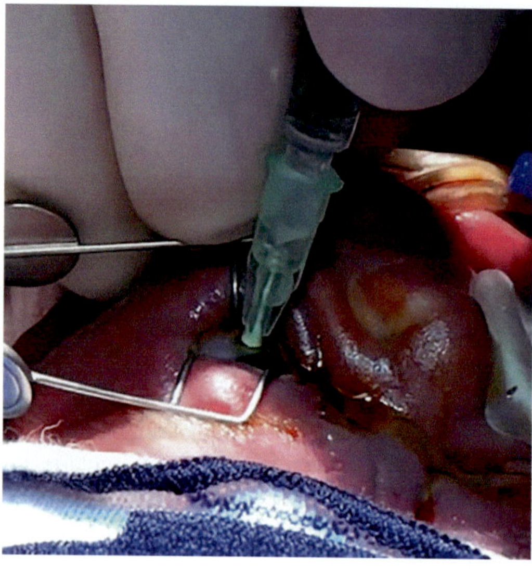

Fig. 11.1 Intravitreal injection of an infant with a 4 mm needle completely inserted until it reaches the hub

examined for a central retinal artery occlusion and the speculum is removed. A retrospective 2018 multicenter study demonstrates the safety of the proposed technique. Two hundred and twenty eyes were treated without complications, including endophthalmitis, vitreous hemorrhage, cataract and corneal ulcer [15].

Follow up for Anti-VEGF Injection in ROP

Patients should be followed 48–72 h after the injection and at 1 week to ensure there is no initial infection, as well as to confirm vascularization. The authors recommend performing a fluorescein angiogram for treated patients 60–65 weeks postmenstrual age. Additional laser photocoagulation should be given if they are not vascularized into zone III. Studies show that a substantial number of neonates remain incompletely vascularized with anti-VEGF treatment, with reports ranging from 39 to 50% [20, 21]. Furthermore, treatment failure must be differentiated from recurrence of ROP, with recurrence typically occurring 4–16 weeks' post-injection [22]. Findings of the RAINBOW trial demonstrated that approximately 20% of patients showed recurrence of ROP with ranibizumab [23].

Conclusion

In conclusion, the increasing use of anti-vascular endothelial growth factor drugs in clinical trials and daily practice for ROP treatment warrants the need for a standardized protocol for safety of preterm infants. The use of a shorter needle has been proven to avoid inadvertent damage to intraocular structures, and a sterile environment protects against infection. Close follow up to monitor for vascularization with a dilated exam and fluorescein angiogram is as important as the procedure itself, and additional laser photocoagulation should be performed if vascularization is incomplete.

Case Discussion

A former 25-week old 790 g male twin presents with type 1 ROP. At 37 5/7 weeks he was treated with 0.15 mg/0.025 mL ranibizumab OU (the authors used this dose prior to the publication of the RAINBOW trial which recommends a dose of 0.2 mg/0.02 mL). Fluorescein angiogram (FA) was performed at 60 weeks to identify vascular changes, recurrence or detachment (Fig. 11.2). FA showed leakage in the periphery and growth to the anterior edge of zone II. The patient was subsequently treated with laser photocoagulation to the areas of avascular retina.

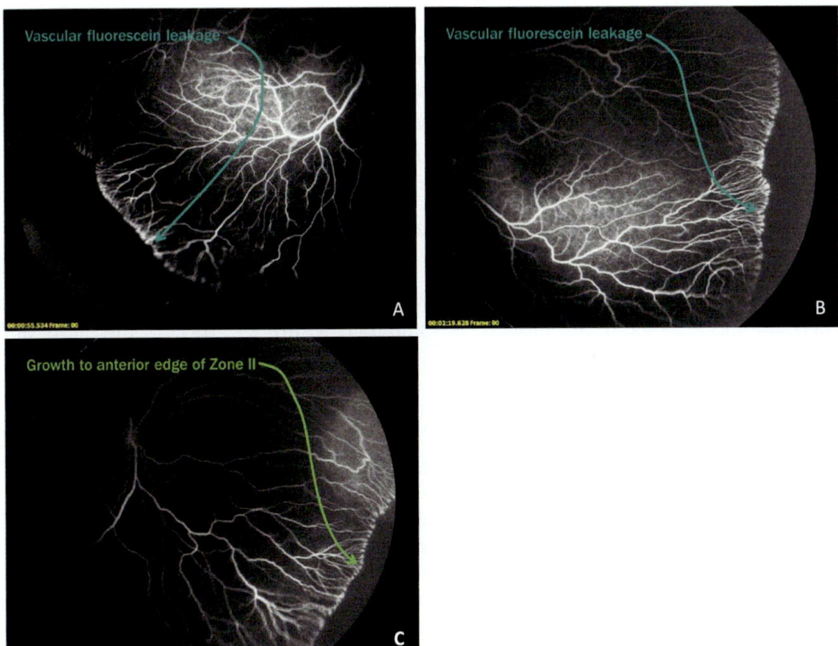

Fig. 11.2 Fluorescein angiogram performed at 60 weeks of an infant with type 1 ROP treated with intravitreal ranibizumab with temporal leakage of the right eye **A** and the left eye **B**. FA also showed vascular growth to the anterior edge of Zone II **C**

Review Questions

1. Which is true regarding the anatomy of an infant with ROP?

a. The ciliary body is located more posteriorly
b. The lens size is proportionally smaller in relation to the globe than in an adult eye
c. The pars plana is absent or incompletely developed
d. The sclera is tougher to penetrate with a needle for intravitreal injections

2. Which of the following is NOT true regarding follow up for anti-vegf injection in ROP?

a. First follow-up should be 1–2 weeks after the injection
b. Treatment failure and recurrence of ROP must be differentiated
c. Fluorescein angiogram should be performed at 60–65 weeks postmenstrual age for treated patients
d. Laser photocoagulation should be performed if vascularization does not reach zone III

Answers

1. (**C**) The pars plana is absent or incompletely developed, which can predispose the infant to retinal breaks during intravitreal injections due to improper needle placement. Additionally, the ciliary body is located more anteriorly, and the lens has a proportionally wider anterior-posterior dimension in comparison to an adult eye.

2. (**A**) Initial follow-up should occur 48–72 hours after injection to rule out endophthalmitis. Unlike adult patients, neonates are unable to inform us of symptoms such as eye pain, redness or decreased vision. Endophthalmitis must be ruled out and thus the infant must be re-examined within 2–3 days of injection, and again at 1 week.

References

1. Solebo AL, Teoh L, Rahi J. Epidemiology of blindness in children. Arch Dis Child. 2017;102 (9):853–857. doi: https://doi.org/10.1136/archdischild-2016-310532. Epub 2017 May 2. Erratum in: Arch Dis Child. 2017;102(10):995. PMID: 28465303.
2. Hong YR, Kim YH, Kim SY, Nam GY, Cheon HJ, Lee SJ. Plasms concentrations of vascular endothelial growth factor in retinopathy of prematurity after intravitreal rescizumab injection. Retina. 2015;35(9):1772–7. https://doi.org/10.1097/IAE.0000000000000535.
3. Bakri SJ, Snyder MR, Reid JM, Pulido JS, Ezzat MK, Singh RJ. Pharmacokinetics of intravitreal ranibizumab (Lucentis). Ophthalmology. 2007;114(12):2179–82. https://doi.org/10.1016/j.ophtha.2007.09.012.
4. Ahmed K, Ali AS, Delwadia N, Greven MA. Neurodevelopmental outcomes following intravitreal bevacizumab with laser versus laser photocoagulation alone for retinopathy of

prematurity. Ophthalmic Surg Lasers Imaging Retina. 2020;51(4):220–4. https://doi.org/10. 3928/23258160-20200326-03.

5. Geloneck MM, Chuang AZ, Clark WL, et al. Refractive outcomes following bevacizumab monotherapy compared with conventional laser treatment: a randomized clinical trial. JAMA Ophthalmol. 2014;132(11):1327–33. https://doi.org/10.1001/jamaophthalmol.2014.2772.

6. Mintz-Hittner HA, Kennedy KA, Chuang AZ. Efficacy of intravitreal bevacizumab for stage 3 + retinopathy of prematurity. N Engl J Med. 2011;364(7):603–15. https://doi.org/10.1056/ NEJMoa1007374.

7. Stahl A, Lepore D, Fielder A, et al. Ranibizumab versus laser therapy for the treatment of very low birthweight infants with retinopathy of prematurity (RAINBOW): an open-label randomised controlled trial. Lancet. 2019;394(10208):1551–9. https://doi.org/10.1016/ S0140-6736(19)31344-3.

8. Early Treatment For Retinopathy Of Prematurity Cooperative Group. Revised indications for the treatment of retinopathy of prematurity: results of the early treatment for retinopathy of prematurity randomized trial. Arch Ophthalmol. 2003;121(12):1684–94. https://doi.org/10. 1001/archopht.121.12.1684. PMID: 14662586

9. Wood EH, Chang EY, Beck K, Hadfield BR, Quinn AR, Harper CA 3rd. 80 Years of vision: preventing blindness from retinopathy of prematurity. J Perinatol. 2021;41(6):1216–24. https://doi.org/10.1038/s41372-021-01015-8.

10. Lu Y-Z, Deng G-D, Liu J-H, Yan H. The role of intravitreal ranubizumab in the treatment of familial exudative vitreoretinopathy of stage 2 or greater. Int J Ophthalmol. 2018;11(6):976– 80. https://doi.org/10.18240/ijo.2018.06.13.

11. Tagami M, Kusuhara S, Honda S, Tsukahara Y, Negi A. Rapid regression of retinal hemorrhage and neovascularization in a case of familial exudative vitreoretinopathy treated with intravitreal bevacizumab. Graefe's Arch Clin Exp Ophthalmol. 2008;246(12):1787–9. doi:https://doi.org/10.1007/s00417-008-0949-6

12. Quiram PA, Drenser KA, Lai MM, Capone AJ, Trese MT. Treatment of vascularly active familial exudative vitreoretinopathy with pegaptanib sodium (Macugen) Retina 2008;28(3 Suppl):S8–12. https://doi.org/10.1097/IAE.0b013e3181679bf6

13. Lin C-J, Hwang J-F, Chen Y-T, Chen S-N. The effect of intravitreal bevacizumab in the treatment of Coats disease in children. Retina. 2010;30(4):617–22. https://doi.org/10.1097/ IAE.0b013e3181c2e0b7.

14. Ramasubramanian A, Shields CL. Bevacizumab for Coats' disease with exudative retinal detachment and risk of vitreoretinal traction. Br J Ophthalmol. 2012;96(3):356–9. https://doi. org/10.1136/bjophthalmol-2011-300141.

15. Cernichiaro LA, Harper CA 3rd, Read SP, Wright LM, Scribbick FW 3rd, Young R, Negron CI, Rodríguez A, Berrocal AM. Report of safety of the use of a short 32G needle for intravitreal anti-vascular endothelial growth factor injections for retinopathy of prematurity: a multicenter study. Retina. 2018;38(6):1251–5. https://doi.org/10.1097/IAE.00000000000 02172 PMID: 29689029.

16. Wright LM, Vrcek IM, Scribbick FW, 3rd, Chang EY, Harper CA, 3rd. Technique for infant intravitreal injection in treatment of retinopathy of prematurity. Retina 2017.

17. Wright LM, Harper CA 3rd, Chang EY. Management of infantile and childhood retinopathies: optimized pediatric pars plana vitrectomy sclerotomy nomogram. Ophthalmol Retina. 2018;2(12):1227–34. https://doi.org/10.1016/j.oret.2018.06.008 Epub.

18. Avery RL, Bakri SJ, Blumenkranz MS, Brucker AJ, Cunningham ET Jr, D'Amico DJ, Dugel PU, Flynn HW Jr, Freund KB, Haller JA, Jumper JM, Liebmann JM, McCannel CA, Mieler WF, Ta CN, Williams GA. Intravitreal injection technique and monitoring: updated guidelines of an expert panel. Retina 2014;34(Suppl 12):S1–18. doi: https://doi.org/10.1097/ IAE.0000000000000399. PMID: 25489719.

19. Grzybowski A, Told R, Sacu S, Bandello F, Moisseiev E, Loewenstein A, Schmidt-Erfurth U. Euretina board. 2018 update on intravitreal injections: euretina expert consensus

recommendations. Ophthalmologica 2018;239(4):181–93. doi: https://doi.org/10.1159/000486145. Epub 2018 Feb 1. PMID: 29393226.
20. Harper CA 3rd, Wright LM, Young RC, Read SP, Chang EY. Fluorescein angiographic evaluation of peripheral retinal vasculature after primary intravitreal ranibizumab for retinopathy of prematurity. Retina. 2019;39(4):700–5. https://doi.org/10.1097/IAE.0000000000001996 PMID: 29300248.
21. Isaac M, Tehrani N, Mireskandari K. Medscape. Involution patterns of retinopathy of prematurity after treatment with intravitreal bevacizumab: implications for follow-up. Eye 2016;30(3):333–41. doi: https://doi.org/10.1038/eye.2015.289. Epub 2016 Feb 12. PMID: 26869159; PMCID: PMC4791711.
22. Martínez MA, González-H León A, Romo-Aguas JC, Gonzalez-Gonzalez LA. A proposal of an algorithm for the diagnosis and treatment of recurrence or treatment failure of retinopathy of prematurity after anti-VEGF therapy based on a large case series. Graefes Arch Clin Exp Ophthalmol. 2020;258(4):767–72. https://doi.org/10.1007/s00417-020-04605-y Epub.
23. Stahl A, Lepore D, Fielder A, Fleck B, Reynolds JD, Chiang MF, Li J, Liew M, Maier R, Zhu Q, Marlow N. Ranibizumab versus laser therapy for the treatment of very low birthweight infants with retinopathy of prematurity (RAINBOW): an open-label randomised controlled trial. Lancet. 2019;394(10208):1551–9. https://doi.org/10.1016/S0140-6736(19)31344-3 Epub.

Cryotherapy for Pediatric Vitreoretinal Diseases

12

Hussain Ahmad Khaqan

Abstract

The word cryotherapy comes from Greek word cryo—cold and therapy—to cure. With the advent of liquefied gases in 1899, it was used for skin and inoperable brain tumors. Introduction to ophthalmology was pioneered by Bietti in 1933 to seal a retinal hole. Since then, cryotherapy was used for intracapsular cataract extraction, retinal detachment and benign and malignant tumors of the eye. Based on Joule-Thompson effect, it causes ischemia, ice crystal formation, lipid protein complexes denaturation, osmotic stress leading to tissue necrosis and cellular apoptosis. The ophthalmic use of cryotherapy is indicated both for the ocular surface diseases and for intraocular use with a few contraindications and complications. This chapter describes in detail the medical background of the cryotherapy with the principle, mechanism of action, indications, contraindications, equipment, technique with complications and the important diseases for which cryotherapy is done with result outcomes.

Keywords

Cryotherapy · Joule-Thompson effect · Retinopathy of prematurity · Coats disease · Retinoblastoma · Toxoplasmosis · Rhegmatogenous retinal detachment

H. A. Khaqan (✉)
Post-Graduate Medical Institute, Ameer-Ul-Din Medical College, Lahore, Pakistan
e-mail: drkhaqan@hotmail.com

Introduction

Background

Medical cryotherapy's fascinating history (also known as cryocautery, cryogenic surgery, and cryosurgery) has been thoroughly recorded by Lubritz [1], Cooper and Dawber [2], and Freiman and Bouganim [3], among others. The advantages of cryotherapy have been documented dating all the way back to 2500 B.C., when the ancient Egyptians utilised cold to ease injuries [1, 4]. Hippocrates advocated for the use of cold to alleviate swelling, bleeding, and discomfort [5]. Arnott made the earliest report on freezing biologic tissue, in which he described freezing tissue locally in the presence of malignancies [6]. Arnott employed cryotherapy to relieve pain in patients with breast cancer, uterine malignancies, and certain skin cancers by using a salt and crushed ice combination. He also utilised his cold therapy to cure acne, neuralgia, and migraines, achieving temperatures of $-24°C$.

With the introduction of liquefied gases, it was discovered that rapidly freezing tumours with a colder cryogen was an efficient treatment method. White [7, 8] pioneered the use of commercially accessible refrigerants (liquefied gases) in medical treatment in 1899. He produced articles describing the use of liquid air to treat lupus, herpes zoster, nevi, warts, chancroid, varicose leg ulcers, carbuncles, and epitheliomas. Irvine and Turnacliffe extended the indications for liquid air therapy to include seborrheic keratosis, senile keratosis, lichen simplex, and poison ivy dermatitis [9].

Allington pioneered the use of liquid nitrogen to treat skin lesions [10]. Cooper developed a liquid nitrogen probe capable of reaching a temperature of $-195.6°C$ [11]. Torre and Zacarian took the field further by constructing one-handed cryospray and cryoprobe devices [12].

In the early and mid-1930s, Bietti [13] and Deutschmann [14] pioneered the use of cryotherapy to treat retinal detachments. They employed cryotherapy in place of diathermy in a retinopexy operation that focused on treating the choroid and retina and draining subretinal fluid.

Cryotherapy was first employed in ophthalmic surgery in 1961, when Krwawicz [15] developed an intracapsular cataract extraction probe made of metal. The probe was chilled using an alcohol/solid carbon dioxide combination, but lacked a means for quick defrosting. Following that, other cryotherapy devices were created, the most significant of which being the Cooper-Linde unit, which was initially intended to treat parkinsonism. The instrument's design comprised an insulated probe through which liquid nitrogen flowed, resulting in a temperature control of up to $-196 °C$. The temperature at the probe's tip may be adjusted manually. Kelman and Coopers first described the use of this instrument to remove cataracts in 1963. Additionally, they documented the formation of a chorioretinal scar in a cat after transscleral freezing.

The original Cooper-Linde equipment was large, and Lincoff and McLean designed a smaller one for treating retinal detachments. Lincoff et al. had previously conducted cryotherapy experiments with solid carbon dioxide applicators, but preferred the Cooper-Linde device due to its ability to generate lower temperatures. Their original study reported the clinical and histopathologic examination of rabbit, dog, and cat transscleral cryotherapy lesions. They decided that a temperature range of −35 to −40° C should be utilised therapeutically after studying the effects of different temperatures.

Lincoff performed the first cryotherapy treatment on patients in 1963. The early patients had acute retinal tears coupled with regions of vitreoretinal degeneration, with or without accompanying minor detachments; a silicone sponge was sometimes sutured to the episcleral surface.

Amoils invented a cryoprobe in 1965 that used carbon dioxide gas and was first used for cataract surgery. Amoils described a retinal cryoprobe in 1968 that could be adjusted to a temperature range of −40 to −70° C by altering the pressure valve. Due to its simplicity, this kind of carbon dioxide-based cryosurgical tool became the instrument of choice for retinal surgery.

Principle

The fundamental physical principle is the Joule–Thomson effect, which states that when a gas such as compressed carbon dioxide or nitrous oxide gas is quickly expanded to atmospheric pressure, a rapid reduction in temperature occurs.

The tip is often made up of two tubes: an inner delivery tube and an outer exhaust tube. Compressed nitrous oxide (N_2O) gas with a pressure range of 400–625 psi flows via the inner delivery tube and out through a tiny hole at the probe tip. The gas then expands as the pressure in the huge exhaust tube decreases. The expanding gas cools the tip as it expands. The same gas is also used to thaw the cryoprobe tip.

Defrosting is accomplished in certain probes by passing a warm, lower-pressure gas at 85–90 psi via a wider aperture that is not affected by the Joule-Thompson effect. In some probes, high-pressure gas travels through a tiny aperture to cool the tip, but the exhaust tube is occluded, compressing the gas again and heating the probe.

The Joule-Thompson principle, which regulates the cooling of a cryoprobe, may be described using simple physical and thermodynamic ideas, and its mathematical derivation yields a complicated formula. The Joule-Thompson effect may be reduced to $\Delta T = \mu_{JT}\Delta p$, however the simplified formula is neither accurate or rigors mathematically or thermodynamically. The change in temperature ΔT is equal to the product of the Joule-Thompson coefficient μ_{JT} and the change in pressure Δp, according to the simplified formula. The difference between the effort needed to force gas through the cryoprobe's aperture and the work created by the expanding gas controls the temperature change's direction and amplitude. For the majority of gases, μ_{JT} has a positive value, which means that the temperature of the gas falls as the pressure of the gas reduces as it passes through the cryoprobe's narrow aperture.

For an ideal gas, μ_{JT} equals zero, and the temperature does not vary in response to pressure reduction. As a result, if a perfect gas were available, the cryoprobe's temperature would remain constant. At ambient temperature, a few gases, such as helium, have a negative μ_{JT} value. These gases would, ironically, cause the probe's tip to heat up.

Gases having a big, positive Joule-Thompson coefficient experience a significant temperature reduction when the pressure is decreased. Nitrous oxide and carbon dioxide both have a positive μ_{JT} value, which makes them good refrigerants. Although both nitrous oxide and carbon dioxide have been employed in cryoprobe units, nitrous oxide is the more efficient refrigerant. Nitrous oxide has a boiling point of −88.5 °C, which is lower than carbon dioxide's triple point of −56.6 °C. Thus, nitrous oxide has a stronger cooling capacity than carbon dioxide. Allowing pressurised carbon dioxide to expand to a pressure of one atmosphere results in the formation of a solid, dry ice, at −56.6 °C without passing through a liquid phase. Carbon dioxide's transformation from a gas to a solid restricts its usefulness to temperatures below −56.6 °C, but nitrous oxide operates at all pressures down to its freezing point.

Mechanism of Action

Cryotherapy's medical use is based on the changes in tissue caused by subfreezing temperatures. When exposed to very low temperatures, living tissue reacts by forming ice, both inside cells and in the extracellular fluid that surrounds them. Additionally, subfreezing temperatures result in the production of ice inside tiny blood vessels, cutting off blood flow to neighbouring cells. Through ischemia and necrosis, a combination of these factors damages live tissue and induces inflammation in reaction to cell death [16].

When the choroid and retinal pigment epithelium are exposed to cold, cell death and scarring occur, resulting in the closing of the borders of retinal breaks.

Cryotherapy has the following effects:

- Ischemia caused by vascular stasis and the destruction of small calibre blood vessels
- Ice crystal formation within cells, resulting in cell wall rupture
- Denaturation of lipid-protein complexes
- Osmotic stress
- Tissue necrosis
- Cellular apoptosis following freezing injury caused by the accumulation of toxic solute concentrations inside cells.

Indications

Cryotherapy for Surface Eye Pathology

Benign Pathology

- Advancing wavelike epitheliopathy
- Conjunctival amyloidosis
- Conjunctival lymphangiectasia
- Conjunctival sarcoidosis
- Conjunctival vascular tumors
- Pterygia
- Superior limbic keratoconjunctivitis
- Trichiasis: Freezing of lash roots for recurrent trichiasis
- Vernal keratoconjunctivitis.

Pre-Malignancy and Malignancy

- Primary acquired melanosis and melanoma of the conjunctiva
- Conjunctival intraepithelial neoplasia
- Squamous cell carcinoma
- Basal cell carcinomas
- Reactive lymphoid hyperplasia and conjunctival lymphoma
- Cryoablation of malignant peripheral melanomas of the choroid or ciliary body—This allows salvage of vision and the eye in selected cases
- Cryoablation of retinoblastomas—Peripheral retinoblastomas can be successfully treated with transconjunctival or transscleral cryopexy
- Cryoablation of metastatic lesions to the choroid. These secondary malignancies (most commonly from the breast or lung) can be destroyed with cryosurgery if their location is peripheral enough.

Cryotherapy for Intraocular Pathology

- Used to repair retinal breaks (holes or tears)
- Used during scleral buckling procedures and pneumatic retinopexies for retinal detachment [17].
- Utilised during pars plana vitrectomy to create chorioretinal adhesions, albeit it has been mostly supplanted in this situation by endolaser methods.
- Cyclocryopexy for advanced glaucoma—In patients with severe intractable glaucoma who are not candidates for standard glaucoma medication or surgery,

ocular cryopexy given transscleral to the ciliary body may inhibit aqueous production, therefore decreasing intraocular pressure.

- Cryoablation of the peripheral retina for neovascular glaucoma—Cryotherapy may induce the iris neovascularization to shrink in neovascular glaucoma.
- Cryoablation of the peripheral retina in premature infants with retinopathy of prematurity (ROP)—In multicenter prospective clinical trials, destruction of the peripheral retina slows disease progression and increases the likelihood of maintaining vision in premature infants with ROP; ocular cryotherapy has significantly improved the prognosis of ROP.
- Retinal cryoablation for peripheral uveitis (intermediate uveitis or pars planitis) —Destruction of the far peripheral retina can alleviate peripheral uveitis and improve macular edoema secondary to peripheral uveitis.
- Transconjunctival cryotherapy for retinal toxoplasmosis—Active Toxoplasma gondii lesions in the peripheral retina can be treated with transconjunctival cryotheraphy.
- Cryoablation of the retina for Coats disease—The most probable reason for its application is a reduction in vascular endothelial growth factor (VEGF) synthesis by the peripheral retina, which results in a decrease in vascular proliferation [18].
- Cryoablation of the peripheral retina to promote regression of proliferative diabetic retinopathy—Although this technique has been effectively employed in the past, it has been completely superseded by panretinal photocoagulation with an argon laser, which is more effective [19–21].
- Transconjunctival cryopexy for ocular larva migrans—If the intraocular nematode (Toxocara canis or Toxocara cati) is located away from the posterior retina, transconjunctival cryopexy can be used to destroy it.
- Peripheral cryoablation of the retina and choroid for retinal vasculitis of various etiologies
- Retinal capillary hemangiomas

Contraindications

Contraindications are:

- Active infection of the ocular surface or eyelids (bacterial, viral, or fungal)
- The patient's reluctance to cooperate.

Technical Consideration

Cryotherapy needs a very cold material (i.e., a cryogen). Cryogens that are often utilised include the following:

- Liquid nitrogen, which has a boiling point of –196°C.
- Carbon dioxide snow, with a melting point of –79°C.
- Argon or Freon liquid, which has a boiling point of –35°C.

These compounds may be sprayed or probed into tissue using an aerosol spray or a cryoprobe.

Today, liquid nitrogen is the most often used cryogen in medicine. Carbon dioxide (melting point = $-79°C$) is still widely utilised around the globe due to its relative ease of storage. Carbon dioxide, on the other hand, is often only useful for treating benign illnesses because to its higher boiling point.

A cryoprobe is a closed system that circulates cryogen inside a metal probe and applies the cold probe to the tissue. Specifically, a cryogen (e.g., liquid nitrogen) is delivered to the probe through a pressurised source. Within the probe, liquid nitrogen turns to gaseous nitrogen, chilling it to very low temperatures.

The probe is constructed from three long concentric tubes. The inner tube acts as a conduit for the liquid nitrogen to reach the probe's tip. The gap between the inner and middle tubes provides a conduit for gaseous nitrogen to be returned from the tip. The probe's tip is a chamber into which liquid nitrogen enters from the inner tube and out of which gaseous nitrogen returns through the gap between the inner and middle tubes. Freezing occurs in the tissue around the chamber on the probe's tip.

The quantity and pace of tissue death are dependent on the cryogen's temperature, the cryoprobe's size, the circulation to the treated tissue, the kind of tissue treated, and the length of the cryogen application. On tissue, cryotherapy has both immediate and delayed effects.

Equipment

Cryotherapy equipment comprises the following:

- Cryoconsole
- Appropriately sized cryoprobe for the procedure—The cryoprobe is connected to the cryoconsole via insulated tubing that is integrated into the probe; probes with varying tip sizes and angulations have been developed for various applications; generally, the larger the probe tip is, the colder it will become.
- Power source for the cryoconsole.
- Tank of gas, typically carbon dioxide, that is connected to the cryoconsole via valves and tubing to the cryoconsole.
- In all situations involving the retina, an indirect ophthalmoscope and condensing lens are used (Figs. 12.1 and 12.2).

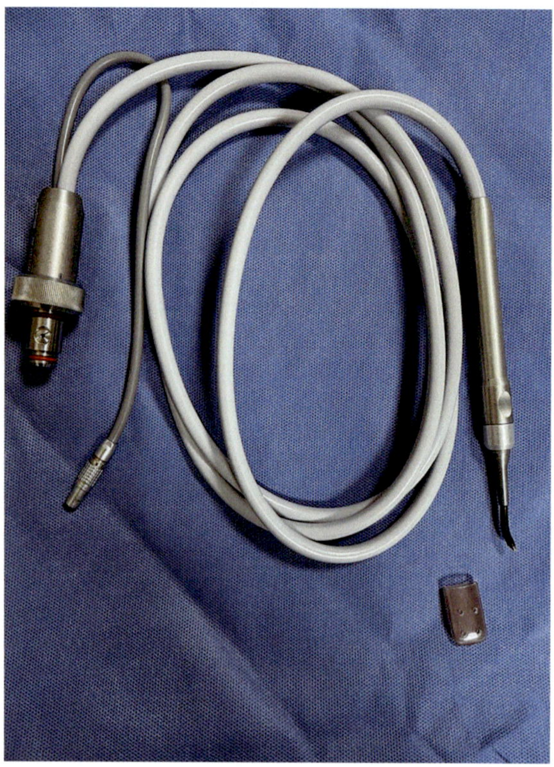

Fig. 12.1 Cryoprobe with insulated tubing

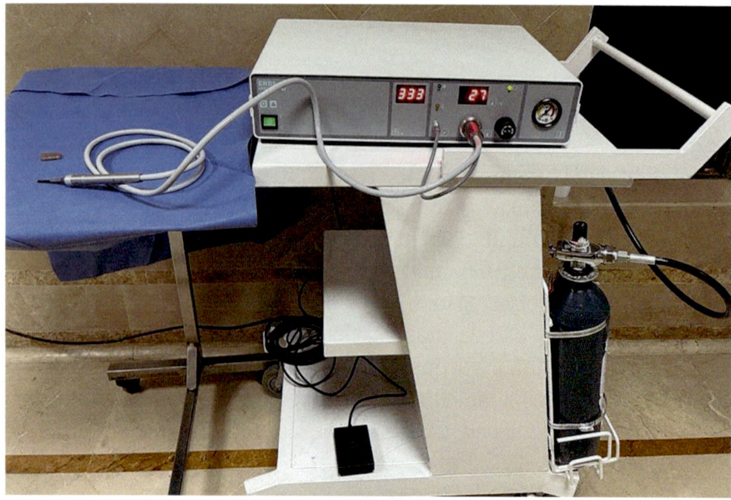

Fig. 12.2 Cryoconsole with cryoprobe and gas cylinder

Cryotherapy Probes

- **Freezing Temperature** (°C)-89
- **Probe Type:** CE-2000™ Straight Hammerhead Retinal Probe
- **Probe Specs:** Dimensions: shaft 40 mm long × 2.5 mm dia.; tip 6.5 mm long × 4.5 mm dia.
- **Probe # 145**

- **Probe Type:** CE-2000™ Super Cool Curved Retinal
- **Probe Specs:** Completely non-electric and autoclavable for safety and ease of use the super cool probes achieve their operating temperature 30% faster than standard probes. Dimensions: shaft 38 mm long × 2.5 mm dia.; tip 2.5 mm dia.
- **Probe # 161**

- **Probe Type:** CE-2000™ Super Cool 3.2 mm Straight Retinal
- **Probe Specs:** Completely non-electric and autoclavable for safety and ease of use the super cool probes achieve their operating temperature 30% faster than standard probes. Dimensions: shaft 38 mm long × 3.2 mm dia.; tip 3.2 mm dia.
- **Probe # 166**

- **Probe Type:** CE-2000™ Straight Retinal Probe
- **Probe Specs:** Dimensions: shaft 40 mm long × 4.0 mm dia.; tip 3.2 mm dia. Precise freeze location with fibre optic illumination.
- **Probe # 708–4**

- **Probe Type:** CE-2000™ Vitreous Intraocular Probe 20 Gauge
- **Probe Specs:** Dimensions: shaft 35 mm long × 0.89 mm dia.; tip 0.89 mm dia. Thermocouple absent.
- **Probe # 134**

- **Probe Type:** CE-2000™ Straight Retinal Probe
- **Probe Specs:** Dimensions: shaft 38 mm long × 2.5 mm dia.; tip 2.5 mm dia.
- **Probe # 124**

- **Probe Type:** CE-2000™ 3 mm Disc Pediatric Retinal Probe
- **Probe Specs:** Dimensions: shaft 35 mm long × 1.5 mm dia.; tip 3 mm long × 15 mm dia. Thermocouple absent.
- **Probe # 123**

- **Probe Type:** CE-2000™ 6 mm Pediatric Hammerhead Retinal Probe without thermocouple
- **Probe Specs:** Dimensions: shaft 34 mm long × 1.5 mm dia.; tip 6 mm long × 1.5 mm dia. Thermocouple absent.
- **Probe # 149**

- **Probe Type:** CE-2000™ 1.88 mm Curved Pediatric Retinal Probe
- **Probe Specs:** Dimensions: shaft 26 mm long × 2.5 mm dia.; tip 1 mm long × 1.88 mm dia.
- **Probe #** 120

Patient Preparation

Anaesthesia

- For the majority of instances of retinal cryopexy, topical anaesthetic with proparacaine drops is sufficient.
- Lidocaine is used locally in cryotherapy to treat conjunctival neoplasms, lid neoplasms, and trichiasis.
- Retrobulbar or peribulbar anaesthesia is used to perform cryoablation of choroidal cancers (melanoma or metastatic tumours), peripheral cryoablation of the retina or choroid, cryotherapy for ocular toxoplasmosis or Coats disease, and cyclocryotherapy for neovascular glaucoma.
- Cryotherapy for retinopathy of prematurity and retinoblastoma is performed under general anaesthesia.

Positioning

The majority of ocular cryotherapy treatments are conducted with the patient recumbent on a narrow table, allowing the surgeon to approach the patient from either side or from the head of the table.

Application of Cryoprobe

Ascertain that there is sufficient gas in the tank and that all connections have been made and fastened properly. The appropriate cryoprobe must be used for the job. Before beginning, check that the cryotherapy equipment is operating properly by depressing the foot switch and noting that the tip is properly cooled.

After administering the required anaesthetic, the cryoprobe is introduced to the tissue receiving treatment while it is still warm. After that, the footswitch is depressed to initiate coolant flow to the tip. At the tip, an ice ball should develop. After tissue begins to adhere to the tip, the probe should not be moved to avoid ripping or breaking the tissue.

The probe is put to the conjunctiva for retinal cryopexy while the surgeon examines the eye with an indirect ophthalmoscope and gently pushes on the probe. The probe's pressure may be seen as an indentation in the retina. When the probe is positioned properly in relation to the retinal break, cryogen is released into the probe, and the retina whitens as it freezes. After the probe is withdrawn, swelling of the retina may be noticed, and scarring occurs within approximately a week.

Complications

Cryotherapy complications include the following:

- Over freezing—Because cryotherapy destroys tissue, extremely low temperatures or prolonged cryotherapy may cause harm to normal tissue; the quantity and duration of cryotherapy must be acceptable for the intended goal.
- Under-freezing—Cryotherapy will not provide the intended outcomes if the tissue temperature is not sufficiently low.
- Freezing nearby tissue that was not intended to be treated—This may occur if the cryoprobe is applied accidently to adjacent tissue that was not intended to be treated.
- Tissue breaking—This may occur if the probe is moved after adhering to the tissue; the probe should be allowed to fully thaw before attempting to remove it.
- Additional complications include visual loss, lid notching, corneal ulceration, accelerated symblepharon formation, xerosis, trichiasis, cellulitis, herpes zoster activation, skin depigmentation, severe soft-tissue reaction, intravitreal dispersion of viable retinal pigment epithelial cells, and retinal tear extension through the cryosurgical scar.
- New retinal tears have been documented as a late consequence of cryotherapy for retinopathy of prematurity and more recently as an early complication of retinal detachment surgery and retinal necrosis in the Japanese literature

Indications of Cryotherapy in Retinopathy of Prematurity

- Ablative surgery should be done within 72 h if threshold disease is present, defined as five contiguous clock hours of stage III illness with plus disease or eight non-contiguous clock hours of stage III disease with plus disease.

Outcome

- Cryotherapy for Retinopathy of Prematurity (CRYO-ROP), a prospective randomised study of cryotherapy for threshold ROP, demonstrated a 50% decrease in unfavourable outcome for zone 2 and 3 disease [22].

- Early treatment of high-risk pre-threshold ROP substantially decreased adverse ROP outcomes at 9 months and 2 years, according to the Early Treatment for Retinopathy of Prematurity (ET-ROP) Trial [23, 24].
- Although therapy was beneficial in newborns with threshold disease, infants with ROP in zone 1 had a poor result despite treatment.

Indications of Cryotherapy in Coats Disease

- For exudation with subretinal fluid of such thickness that cryo reaction can reach the retina
- Exudative detachment
- Peripheral lesions, stage 3A and 3B.

Indications of Cryotherapy in Retinoblastoma

- Pre-equatorial lesions without either deep invasion or vitreous seedings
- Lesions up to 3.5 mm in diameter and 2.0 mm in thickness.

Outcome

- Abramson concluded that overall, 70% of tumors were cured with cryotherapy and 93% of patients treated with cryotherapy survived [25].

Indications of Cryotherapy in Toxoplasmosis

- Transconjunctival cryotherapy for active lesions in the peripheral retina.

Outcome

- It decreases the number of recurrences.

Indications of Cryotherapy in Rhegmatogenous Retinal Detachment

- Far anterior retinal breaks
- If retinal visibility is difficult due to hazy media, not amenable to laser application
- Pneumatic retinopexy
- Scleral buckling
- Pars plana vitrectomy.

Review Questions

1. Cryotherapy is indicated in which stage of Coats disease?

(a) Stage 2
(b) Stage 3A
(c) Stage 3A and 3B
(d) Stage 3B

2. Which cryogen(s) is used in cryotherapy?

(a) Liquid nitrogen
(b) Carbon dioxide snow
(c) Argon or Freon liquid
(d) All of the above

3. Which of the following is NOT an indication for cryotherapy.

(a) Pneumatic retinopexy
(b) Scleral buckling
(c) A large posterior break
(d) Pars plana vitrectomy

4. All of the followings are the effects of cryotherapy EXCEPT:

(a) Ischemia caused by vascular stasis
(b) Decrease retinal demand of oxygen
(c) Cell wall rupture
(d) Osmotic stress

5. Nitrous oxide is more efficient refrigerant than carbon oxide because:

(a) It operates at all pressures down its freezing point
(b) It has a positive Joule-Thompson coefficient value
(c) Its boiling point is higher than that of carbon dioxide
(d) Its transformation from a gas to solid state.

Answers

1. C
2. D
3. C
4. B
5. A

References

1. Lubritz RR. Cryosurgery. Clin Dermatol. 1987;5(4):120–7. https://doi.org/10.1016/0738-081X(87)90033-2.
2. Cooper SM, Dawber RP. The history of cryosurgery. J R Soc Med. 2001;94(4):196–201.
3. Freiman A, Bouganim N. History of cryotherapy. Dermatol Online J. 2005;11(2):9.
4. Squazzi A, Bracco D. A historical account of the technical means used in cryotherapy. Minerva Med. 1974;65(70):3718–22.
5. Brock A. Greek medicine, being extracts illustrative of medical writers from Hippocrates to Galen. 2nd ed. New York: Dutton; 1972.
6. Arnott J. On the treatment of cancer by the regulated application of an anaesthetic temperature. London: Churchill; 1851.
7. White A. Liquid air: its application in medicine and surgery. Med Rec. 1899;56:109–12.
8. White A. Possibilities of liquid air to the physcian. JAMA. 1901;36(7):426–9. https://doi.org/10.1001/jama.1901.52470070012001d.
9. Irvine HG, Turnacliff DD. Liquid oxygen in dermatology. Arch Dermatol Syphilol. 1929;19(2):270–80. https://doi.org/10.1001/archderm.1929.02380200098007.
10. Allington H. Liquid nitrogen in the treatment of skin disease. Calif Med. 1950;72(3):153.
11. Cooper IS, Hirose T. Application of cryogenic surgery to resection of parenchymal organs. N Engl J Med. 1966;274(1):15–8. https://doi.org/10.1056/NEJM196601062740103.
12. Zacarian S. Cryogenics: the cryolesion and the pathogenesis of cryonecrosis, in cryosurgery for skin cancer and cutaneous disorders. St. Louis: Mosby; 1985. p. 1–30.
13. Bietti GB. Research on the variation of temperatures of some areas of the eyeball for episcleral diathermocoagulation, thermocauterization and cryocoustication. Boll Ocul. 1933;12:1427–57.
14. Deutschmann R. The treatment of detachment of the retina with tincture of iodine and carbonic acid snow. Klin Montasbl Augenh. 1935;94:349.
15. Krwawicz T. Intracapsular extraction of intumescent cataract by application of low temperature. Br J Ophthalmol. 1961;45(4):279–83. https://doi.org/10.1136/bjo.45.4.279.
16. Prohaska J, Bermudez R. Cryotherapy. Treasure Island;2018
17. Stewart S, Chan W. Pneumatic retinopexy: patient selection and specific factors. Clin Ophthalmol. 2018;12:493–502.
18. Bhat V, D'Souza P, Shah PK, Narendran V. Risk of tractional retinal detachment following intravitreal bevacizumab along with subretinal fluid drainage and cryotherapy for stage 3b coats' disease. Middle East Afr J Ophthalmol. 2016;23(2):208–11.
19. Veckeneer M, Van Overdam K, Bouwens D, Feron E, Mertens D, Peperkamp E. Randomized clinical trial of cryotherapy versus laser photocoagulation for retinopexy in conventional retinal detachment surgery. Am J Ophthalmol. 2001;132(3):343–7.
20. Shalev B, Farr AK, Repka MX. Randomized comparison of diode laser photocoagulation versus cryotherapy for threshold retinopathy of prematurity: seven-year outcome. Am J Ophthalmol. 2001;132(1):76–80.

21. Margo C, Hidayat AA, Marshall CF, Renaldo DP. Cryotherapy and photocoagulation in the management of retinoblastoma: treatment failure and unusual complication. Ophthalmic Surg. 1983;14(4):336–42.
22. Cryotherapy for Retinopathy of Prematurity Cooperative Group. Multicenter Trial of Cryotherapy for Retinopathy of Prematurity: ophthalmological outcomes at 10 years. Arch Ophthalmol. 2001;119(8):1110–8.
23. VanderVeen DK, Coats DK, Dobson V, et al. Prevalence and course of strabismus in the first year of life for infants with prethreshold retinopathy of prematurity: findings from the Early Treatment for Retinopathy of Prematurity study. Arch Ophthalmol. 2006;124(6):766–73.
24. Good WV, Hardy RJ, Dobson V, et al., for the Early Treatment for Retinopathy of Prematurity Cooperative Group. The incidence and course of retinopathy of prematurity: findings from the early treatment for retinopathy of prematurity study. Pediatrics 2005;116 (1):15–23.
25. Abramson DH, Ellsworth RM, Rozakis GW. Cryotherapy for retinoblastoma. Arch Ophthalmol. 1982;100(8):1253–6.

Taku Wakabayashi and Yoshihiro Yonekawa

Abstract

Patients with Stickler syndrome and related collagen disorders, traumatic retinal detachment resulting from self-injurious behavior, and giant retinal tear (GRT) in the initial eye, are at high risk of visual loss from bilateral retinal detachment. Therefore, prophylactic treatment for fellow eyes is recommended for these patients depending on the clinical scenarios. Although there are no prospective randomized clinical trials, several studies have shown the potential benefits of prophylaxis with laser photocoagulation, cryotherapy, and scleral buckling, to prevent future detachment. In this chapter, we review the current status of prophylactic treatments in fellow eyes with high risk of retinal detachment, as well as reviewing other pediatric vitreoretinopathies where treatment of the fellow eye is important.

Keywords

Bilateral retinal detachment · Cryotherapy · Ehlers-Danlos syndrome · Fellow eyes · Giant retinal tears · Laser photocoagulation · Marfan syndrome · Prophylaxis · Scleral buckle · Self-injurious behavior · Stickler syndrome · Wagner syndrome

T. Wakabayashi · Y. Yonekawa (✉)
Wills Eye Hospital, Mid Atlantic Retina, Thomas Jefferson University School of Medicine, Philadelphia, PA, USA
e-mail: yyonekawa@midatlanticretina.com

© The Author(s), under exclusive license to Springer Nature Switzerland AG 2023
Ş. Özdek et al. (eds.), *Pediatric Vitreoretinal Surgery*,
https://doi.org/10.1007/978-3-031-14506-3_13

Introduction

Prophylactic treatment of unaffected fellow eyes can be considered for some pediatric vitreoretinopathies that pose a very high risk of bilateral retinal detachment, such as Stickler syndrome and related collagen disorders, traumatic retinal detachment resulting from self-injurious behavior, and history of giant retinal tear (GRT) in the initial eye. The risk of bilateral retinal detachment has been reported to be as high as 48% in patients with Stickler syndrome [1], 54–57% in patients with self-injurious behavior [2, 3], and 11–18% in patients with contralateral GRT [4–6].

Anatomical retinal reattachment can be achieved through surgery in most cases of routine pediatric rhegmatogenous retinal detachment. However, there is a substantial risk of surgical failure in patients with complex retinal detachment accompanied by proliferative vitreoretinopathy, particularly in the setting of systemic and ophthalmic co-morbidities [7–11]. Surgical failure often results in eventual phthisis and blindness. Therefore, effective prophylactic treatment for fellow eyes at high risk of retinal detachment has been explored to prevent future retinal detachment, in order to protect what is often the better-seeing eye. To date, no randomized clinical trials have been conducted on this topic. Therefore, there is no definitive consensus on the indication or standardized methods of treatments. However, several studies have shown the potential benefits of prophylaxis (such as with laser retinopexy, cryopexy, and scleral buckling). Herein, we provide an overview of prophylactic treatments in fellow eyes at high risk of retinal detachment.

Stickler Syndrome

Stickler syndrome, first described in 1965, is a hereditary connective tissue disorder affecting 1 in 7500–9000 births [12, 13] (see Sect. 6, Chap. 1 for more details). Gene mutations affecting the formation of types II and XI collagen may result in a wide variety of symptoms, such as distinctive facial features, hearing loss, joint problems, and ocular abnormalities [14, 15]. Ocular manifestations include severe myopia, vitreous liquefaction, and perivascular retinal degeneration with strong vitreoretinal adhesions [16]. Degenerative vitreoretinal changes predispose patients to retinal breaks and GRTs, resulting in rhegmatogenous retinal detachment (RRD) often occurring in younger ages. The anatomical success rate has been reported to be between 67 and 84% after scleral buckle (SB), pars plana vitrectomy (PPV), or combined SB/PPV [17]. Primary surgical failure and redetachments are frequent. One study reported that the mean number of vitreoretinal surgeries required for retinal reattachment was 3.1 [18]. After an awerage of 3.1 surgeries, visual acuity only improved from 20/914 to 20/796; this improvement was not statistically significant. The higher chance of recurrence and poor visual outcomes are due to the high incidence (approximately 75%) of proliferative vitreoretinopathy [18]. Based on the younger age of presentation and the challenges of surgical repair, prophylaxes such as 360-degree laser photocoagulation, cryotherapy, and encircling SB have been performed as treatments to prevent subsequent retinal detachment [1, 19–22]. Although there is no evidence-based consensus regarding prophylactic treatment in patients with Stickler syndrome, several studies have shown the potential benefit of prophylactic treatment [23].

Indication of Prophylaxis

Some studies have investigated the use of bilateral prophylaxis for attached retinas of patients with Stickler syndrome [20], but prophylactic treatment may be especially indicated in fellow eyes of patients with retinal detachment in one eye.

Methods of Prophylaxis

Prophylactic methods include 360-degree laser photocoagulation [19, 22], 360-degree cryotherapy [1, 20], and encircling SB with or without cryotherapy [21]. Each method has been reported to reduce the risk of subsequent retinal detachment in patients with Stickler syndrome compared with observation. However, no studies have compared the differences between treatments or the superiority of a specific treatment. The geographic area of treatment (far anterior retina only vs to the equator, lattice degeneration only vs. 360°) also remains controversial.

Outcomes After Prophylaxis

A summary of studies on prophylactic treatment in patients with Stickler syndrome is shown in Table 13.1. All studies are retrospective in nature without randomization.

Laser

Leiba et al. [19] compared the results of 360-degree and focal prophylactic lasers applied at the border between the pathological and normal peripheral retina to observation. During the 1- to 15-year follow-up, 10% (1/10) of the patients with laser treatment and 44% (15/34) of the observed patients developed RRD. Thus, the incidence of subsequent retinal detachment was significantly lower in laser-treated eyes (P < 0.025). One eye developed retinal detachment despite laser prophylaxis (5 years after the laser prophylaxis).

Khanna et al. [22] reported the efficacy of using 360-degree laser from the ora serrata to the equator with laser burn spacing between ½ and 1 spot size, which they termed "extended vitreous base laser" (EVBL). The results of 129 eyes with EVBL were compared with those of 92 eyes without prophylaxis and 9 eyes with non-protocol laser that did not follow the pattern of EVBL. Retinal detachment

Table 13.1 Summary of studies of prophylactic treatment in Stickler syndrome

Year	Author	No. of patients/eyes	Age at prophylaxis	Disease	Prophylactic treatment	Follow-up	Outcomes
1996	Leiba et al.	Laser treated (10 eyes) vs. non-treated (34 eyes)	N/A	Type 1 Stickler syndrome	Argon laser photocoagulation (focal or 360° depending on the extent of pathological changes)	1–15 years	10% (1/10 eyes) of laser-treated patients vs. 44% (15/34 eyes) of non-treated patients developed RD (unilateral or bilateral) ($P < 0.025$)
2008	Ang et al.	111 patients (222 eyes) without prophylaxis, 62 patients (124 eyes) with bilateral prophylaxis, 31 patients (31 eyes) with unilateral prophylaxis	2–92 years	Type 1 Stickler syndrome	360° cryotherapy applied just posterior to the ora serrata	11.5 (1–27) years	73% (81/111), 8% (5/62), and 10% (3/31) developed RD in no prophylaxis, bilateral prophylaxis, and unilateral prophylaxis group, respectively ($P < 0.001$)
2014	Fincham et al.	293 patients with prophylaxis (229 with bilateral and 64 with unilateral prophylaxis) and 194 untreated control patients	N/A	Type 1 Stickler syndrome	360° cryopexy including the ora serrata	Up to 36.1 years	7.4-fold and 10.3-fold reduction in the risk of RD in bilateral and unilateral prophylaxis group compared with bilateral and unilateral untreated patients

(continued)

Table 13.1 (continued)

Year	Author	No. of patients/eyes	Age at prophylaxis	Disease	Prophylactic treatment	Follow-up	Outcomes
2021	Ripandelli et al.	52 patients (52 eyes)	10.7 ± 2.3 years	Type 1 Stickler syndrome	360° encircling SB with (n = 39) or without (n = 13) cryopexy	15.6 ± 2.4 years	RD developed in 0% (0/39) that received cryo and 38% (5/13) that did not have cryo (P < 0.001). Thus, encircling SB with cryo significantly reduced the risk of RD
2021	Khanna et al.	92 eyes with no laser, 9 eyes with non-protocol laser, and 129 eyes with EVBL	9.5 (6–13) years	Stickler syndrome (type not specified)	Observe/Non-protocol laser or EVBL	1–7 years	RD developed in 3% (4/129 eyes) after EVBL, compared to 73% (74/101 eyes) after no laser or non-protocol laser (P < 0.001)

EVBL = extended vitreous base laser; SB = scleral buckle; RD = retinal detachment developed in 3% (4/129) eyes after EVBL, compared to 73% (74/101) after no laser or non-protocol laser, during 1 to 7 years of follow-up (P < 0.001). EVBL was significantly associated with better final visual acuity also. The cohort size of non-EVBL was likely too small to directly compare to EVBL, but the study does nicely show the benefit of laser prophylaxis in general.

Cryotherapy

In 2008, Ang et al. [1] reported the results of a large cohort study comparing 111 patients without prophylaxis, 62 patients with bilateral prophylaxis, and 31 patients with unilateral prophylaxis with cryotherapy. The transconjunctival 360-degree cryotherapy was performed just posterior to the ora serrata. Retinal detachment developed in 73% (81/111), 8% (5/62), and 10% (3/31) of patients in the no-prophylaxis, bilateral prophylaxis, and unilateral prophylaxis groups, respectively (P < 0.001). The time from prophylaxis to failure (RRD) was 7.7 years (0.2–15 years) after bilateral prophylaxis and 11.6 years (4.1–15 years) after unilateral prophylaxis.

In 2014, the same group of researchers further increased the sample size and reported the results of the same prophylaxis procedure (360-degree cryotherapy), which they termed the Cambridge prophylactic cryotherapy protocol [20]. In this study, the investigators compared the results of 229 patients who received bilateral prophylaxis and 194 who did not receive any prophylaxis. During the mean follow-up period of 6.3 years, RRD developed in 8% (19/229) and 54% (104/194) of patients, respectively, suggesting that bilateral prophylaxis led to a 7.4-fold reduction in the risk of retinal detachment. They also compared 64 patients with Stickler syndrome who received unilateral prophylaxis after retinal detachment in their fellow eyes and 104 control patients with previous retinal detachment in one eye but who did not receive prophylactic treatment in the fellow eye. During the mean follow-up period of 10.1 years, retinal detachment developed in 13% (8/64) of those who received unilateral prophylaxis, compared with 81% (84/104) of unilateral controls, suggesting that unilateral prophylaxis in eyes with a history of fellow eye retinal detachment can provide a 10.3-fold reduction in the risk of subsequent retinal detachment.

Scleral Buckling

Ripandelli et al. [21] compared the outcomes of 360-degree encircling SB with cryotherapy (39 patients) and without cryotherapy (13 patients). RRD developed in 0% (0/39) of patients who received cryotherapy and 38% (5/13) of those who did not receive cryotherapy during the mean follow-up period of 15.6 years (P < 0.001). Therefore in this particular study, prophylactic encircling SB with cryotherapy reduced the risk of RRD.

Prophylaxis Failure

Although the efficacy of prophylactic treatment in reducing the risk of subsequent retinal detachment has been reported as described above, the failure of prophylaxis (retinal detachment despite prophylaxis) has been reported in approximately 10% of patients. According to the Cambridge prophylactic cryotherapy study, the average time from prophylaxis to failure was 5.6 (0.1–22.4) years, indicating that late retinal detachment may still develop [20].

Follow-Up

Patients who have undergone prophylactic treatment still remain with lifelong risk of retinal detachment, albeit at a reduced rate. Therefore, patients should be monitored regularly on a long-term basis.

Case Presentation

A 7-year-old boy with Stickler syndrome, genetically confirmed with a COL2A1 mutation, presented for fundus examination. He had a strong family history of RRD. Given the high risk of future retinal detachment in this patient, 360-degree laser photocoagulation from the ora serrata to the equator was performed in both eyes under anesthesia. The patient has been subsequently stable without retinal detachment (Fig. 13.1).

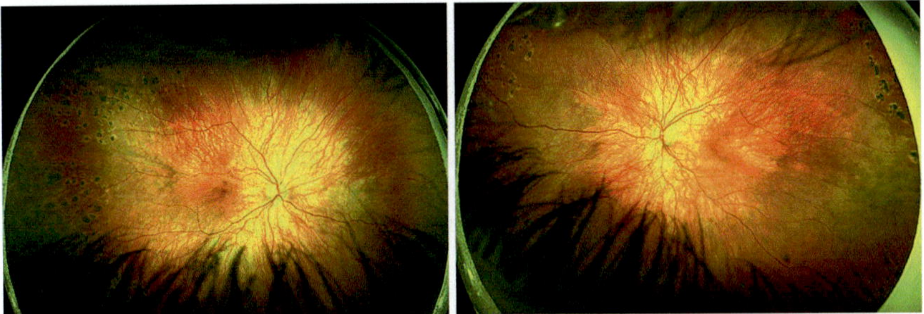

Fig. 13.1 Widefield fundus images of a child with Stickler syndrome who had undergone prophylactic 360-degree laser photocoagulation

Traumatic Retinal Detachment Associated with Self-Injurious Behavior

Traumatic retinal detachment from self-injurious behavior in patients with cognitive impairment is a surgical challenge because of delayed and advanced presentation, limited patient cooperation, and recurrent retinal detachment due to ongoing ocular trauma. According to an international multicenter study, anatomical success was only 23% without tamponade (37% including silicone oil) after a single surgery and 36% after multiple surgeries [3]. The fellow eye is at risk of developing retinal detachment also. Fifty-four percent of patients had bilateral retinal detachment or phthisis bulbi in their fellow eyes. Another study also showed an anatomical success rate of 55% (also not favorable) [2]. Given the challenges of surgery and the high rate of bilaterality, prophylactic treatment seems to be a reasonable approach to prevent retinal detachment. Although no dedicated studies have investigated the efficacy of prophylaxis in the fellow eyes of patients with retinal detachment associated with self-injurious behavior, the aforementioned international multicenter study showed that 4 eyes that were attached on presentation and underwent prophylactic encircling SB did not experience retinal detachment (0%), whereas 19% of the initially attached eyes without SB developed retinal detachment (although this was not statistically significant because of the small sample size) [3]. In addition, none of the 3 attached eyes that underwent prophylactic laser treatment developed retinal detachment.

Giant Retinal Tears

Giant retinal tears (GRTs)—full-thickness circumferential retinal breaks that involve more than 3 clock hours (90 degrees)—have been reported in 5–25% of pediatric cases of retinal detachment [7–9, 11]. (see Sect. 6 Chap. 7 for more details). The risk factors for GRTs include trauma, high myopia, and connective tissue disorders, such as Stickler, Marfan, Wagner, and Ehlers-Danlos syndromes [5]. The fellow eyes of patients with GRTs are at elevated risk for developing retinal breaks detachment. In 1962, Schepens et al. [24] reported that the fellow eyes of 122 patients with GRTs developed GRTs (2.5%), retinal detachment (28.0%), and retinal breaks (16.0%). In 1978, Freeman et al. [25] also reported the high incidence of GRTs (12.8%), retinal detachment (15.9%), and retinal breaks (22.5%) in 226 fellow eyes during 44 months of follow-up. The British Giant Retinal Tear Epidemiology Eye Study prospectively showed that fellow eyes developed GRTs (9.7%), retinal detachment (4.8%), and breaks (3.2%) [26].

Currently, there is no consensus on the need for prophylaxis or the type of prophylactic treatment for the fellow eyes of patients with GRTs, particularly in non-syndromic patients. However, several studies have retrospectively shown the potential benefits of fellow-eye prophylaxis [6, 27, 28]. Ripandelli et al. [6] compared the results of 62 patients without prophylaxis and 98 patients who had undergone 360-degree prophylactic laser photocoagulation and found that 14.5% (9/62) of patients without prophylaxis developed GRTs, while only 2% (2/98) of patients with prophylaxis developed GRTs, a difference that was statistically significant. Patients with prophylaxis experienced a higher number of small tears resulting in localized retinal detachment (3.2% vs. 11.2%), but there was significantly few cases of macula-off RRDs (0% vs. 14.5%). Verhoekx et al. [28] also reported the results of 51 patients without prophylaxis and 78 patients who had undergone 360-degree prophylactic laser photocoagulation. Prophylactic laser significantly reduced the incidence of fellow-eye GRT (23.5% vs. 2.6%) and retinal detachment (19.6% vs. 10.5%). The incidence of retinal breaks without retinal detachment was comparable between those with no prophylaxis and those with prophylactic laser treatment (7.8% vs. 7.7%). Those studies showed that prophylactic laser may reduce the risk of GRTs but may not decrease the incidence of retinal breaks, indicating that regular follow-up is required even after prophylactic treatment.

Adult Retinopathy of Prematurity and other Pediatric Vitreoretinopathies

Older children or adults with a history of retinopathy of prematurity (ROP) often have persistent avascular retina (PAR) and other peripheral lesions such as lattice degeneration and atrophic retinal holes. These patients are categorized currently as "adult ROP," and are at elevated risk for retinal detachment. Prophylactic laser treatment can be treated in such eyes, especially if there are peripheral lesions in addition to PAR. A recent study has shown that patients with PAR had concomitant lattice degeneration (54%), retinal tears (31%), atrophic holes (35%), and retinal detachment (39%) [29]. However, there is little data about the long-term outcomes of prophylactic laser for PAR, the precise indications, and the number needed to treat, so therefore future studies are needed to evaluate the efficacy of prophylaxis (see Sect. 6, Chap. 3 for more details).

Many other pediatric vitreoretinopathies are also associated with retinal detachment, including familial exudative vitreoretinopathy (FEVR) and sickle cell retinopathy, usually in the form of traction retinal detachment. Therefore, when the patients develop retinal detachment in one eye, the fellow eye should be examined well and treated accordingly before the fellow eye develops complications. For example in FEVR, eyes with neovascularization and/or peripheral vascular leakage are often treated with laser photocoagulation. Similarly for proliferative sickle cell retinopathy, the avascular retina should be treated in eyes with active seafan fronds. Norrie disease, incontinentia pigmenti, and dyskeratosis congenita are also some systemic disease where both eyes should be examined well for pathology.

Some systemic pediatric diseases cause retinal tumors such as retinal capillary hemangiomas in the setting of von Hippel-Lindau disease. This is also a bilateral condition, so the fellow eye must be examined well, and tumors treated accordingly, usually with laser photocoagulation.

Conclusion

The role of prophylactic treatment in fellow eyes of high-risk patients remains relatively controversial in many clinical scenarios, and further studies are needed to clarify the indications. However, the results of fellow-eye prophylaxis in the literature are encouraging when compared with observation. 360-degree laser photocoagulation, cryotherapy, or encircling scleral buckling may indeed be considered for patients with Stickler syndrome and related conditions, GRTs, and patients with traumatic retinal detachment associated with self-injurious behavior. Because of the highly variable nature of retinal detachment in these populations, the approach to prophylaxis can be considered on an individual basis. In addition, even with prophylactic treatment, lifelong, regular follow-up is recommended to preserve vision. Future studies are needed to determine the indication, modality, and area of treatment for preventing fellow-eye retinal detachment in the high-risk patients that we care for.

Review Questions

1. Which of the following is true:

A. Prophylactic laser will always prevent retinal detachment in fellow eyes of patients with giant retinal tears.
B. Pars plana vitrectomy is a preferred approach for prophylaxis in patients with Stickler syndrome.
C. There is level 1 evidence to support that scleral buckling is required in fellow eyes of patients with traumatic retinal detachment associated with self-injurious behavior.
D. Even with prophylactic laser treatment in Stickler syndrome and other high-risk clinical scenarios, lifelong, regular follow-up is recommended due to the ongoing, albeit lower, risk to develop retinal detachment.

Answer

1. D

References

1. Ang A, Poulson AV, Goodburn SF, Richards AJ, Scott JD, Snead MP. Retinal detachment and prophylaxis in type 1 stickler syndrome. Ophthalmology. 2008;115(1):164–8. https://doi.org/10.1016/j.ophtha.2007.03.059.
2. Liu Q, Campomanes AG de A, Stewart JM. Outcomes after retinal detachment resulting from self-inflicted injury. Ophthalmol Retina. 2019;3(8):690–3. https://doi.org/10.1016/j.oret.2019.03.021.
3. Rossin EJ, Tsui I, Wong SC, et al. Traumatic retinal detachment in patients with self-injurious behavior an international multicenter study. Ophthalmol Retina. 2021;5(8):805–14. https://doi.org/10.1016/j.oret.2020.11.012.
4. Sharma T, Gopal L, Shanmugam MP, et al. Retinal detachment in Marfan Syndrome. Retina. 2022;22(4):423–8. https://doi.org/10.1097/00006982-200208000-00005.
5. Hasan N, Azad SV, Kaginalkar A, et al. Demography, clinical profile and surgical outcomes of paediatric giant retinal tear related retinal detachments. Eye. 2021;35(11):3041–8. https://doi.org/10.1038/s41433-021-01621-y.
6. Ripandelli G, Rossi T, Cacciamani A, Scarinci F, Piaggi P, Stirpe M. Laser prophylactic treatment of the fellow eye in giant retinal tears. Retina. 2016;36(5):962–6. https://doi.org/10.1097/iae.0000000000000805.
7. Read SP, Aziz HA, Kuriyan A, et al. Retinal detachment surgery in a pediatric population. Retina. 2018;38(7):1393–402. https://doi.org/10.1097/iae.0000000000001725.
8. Gonzales CR, Singh S, Yu F, Kreiger AE, Gupta A, Schwartz SD. Pediatric rhegmatogenous retinal detachment. Retina. 2008;28(6):847–52. https://doi.org/10.1097/iae.0b013e3181679f79.
9. Weinberg DV, Lyon AT, Greenwald MJ, Mets MB. Rhegmatogenous retinal detachments in children Risk factors and surgical outcomes. Ophthalmology. 2003;110(9):1708–13. https://doi.org/10.1016/s0161-6420(03)00569-4.
10. Chang PY, Yang CM, Yang CH, et al. Clinical characteristics and surgical outcomes of pediatric rhegmatogenous retinal detachment in Taiwan. Am J Ophthalmol. 2005;139(6):1067–72. https://doi.org/10.1016/j.ajo.2005.01.027.
11. Wang NK, Tsai CH, Chen YP, et al. Pediatric rhegmatogenous retinal detachment in East Asians. Ophthalmology. 2005;112(11):1890–5. https://doi.org/10.1016/j.ophtha.2005.06.019.
12. Stickler GB, Belau PG, Farrell FJ, et al. Hereditary progressive arthro-ophthalmopathy. Mayo Clin Proc. 1965;40:433–55.
13. Stickler GB, Hughes W, Houchin P. Clinical features of hereditary progressive arthro-ophthalmopathy (Stickler syndrome): a survey. Genet Med. 2001;3(3):192–6. https://doi.org/10.1097/00125817-200105000-00008.
14. Snead MP, McNinch AM, Poulson AV, et al. Stickler syndrome, ocular-only variants and a key diagnostic role for the ophthalmologist. Eye. 2011;25(11):1389–400. https://doi.org/10.1038/eye.2011.201.
15. Snead MP, Richards AJ, McNinch AM, et al. Stickler syndrome–lessons from a national cohort. *Eye*. Published online 2021:1–7. https://doi.org/10.1038/s41433-021-01776-8.
16. Parma ES, Körkkö J, Hagler WS, Ala-Kokko L. Radial perivascular retinal degeneration: a key to the clinical diagnosis of an ocular variant of Stickler syndrome with minimal or no systemic manifestations. Am J Ophthalmol. 2002;134(5):728–34. https://doi.org/10.1016/s0002-9394(02)01646-x.
17. Abeysiri P, Bunce C, da Cruz L. Outcomes of surgery for retinal detachment in patients with Stickler syndrome: a comparison of two sequential 20-year cohorts. Graefe's Archive Clin Exp Ophthalmol. 2007;245(11):1633–8. https://doi.org/10.1007/s00417-007-0609-2.
18. Yonekawa Y, Reddy D, Thomas B, Nudleman E, Williams G. Long-term surgical outcomes of retinal detachment in patients with Stickler syndrome. Clin Ophthalmol. 2016;10:1531–4. https://doi.org/10.2147/opth.s111526.

19. Leiba H, Oliver M, Pollack A. Prophylactic laser photocoagulation in stickler syndrome. Eye. 1996;10(6):701–8. https://doi.org/10.1038/eye.1996.164.
20. Fincham GS, Pasea L, Carroll C, et al. Prevention of retinal detachment in Stickler syndrome the Cambridge prophylactic cryotherapy protocol. Ophthalmology. 2014;121(8):1588–97. https://doi.org/10.1016/j.ophtha.2014.02.022.
21. Ripandelli G, Rossi T, Pesci FR, Cecere M, Stirpe M. The prophylaxis of fellow-eye retinal detachment in Stickler syndrome. A retrospective series. Retina. 2021;Publish Ahead of Print. https://doi.org/10.1097/iae.0000000000003304.
22. Khanna S, Rodriguez SH, Blair MA, Wroblewski K, Shapiro MJ, Blair MP. Laser prophylaxis in patients with stickler syndrome. Ophthalmol Retina. 2021. Published online2021. https://doi.org/10.1016/j.oret.2021.11.001.
23. Coussa RG, Sears J, Traboulsi EI. Stickler syndrome: exploring prophylaxis for retinal detachment. Curr Opin Ophthalmol. 2019;30(5):306–13. https://doi.org/10.1097/icu.0000000000000599.
24. Schepens CL, Dobble JG, McMEEL JW. Retinal detachments with giant breaks: preliminary report. Trans Am Acad Ophthalmol Otolaryngol Am Acad Ophthalmol Otolaryngol. 1962;66:471–9.
25. Freeman HM. Fellow eyes of giant retinal breaks. T Am Ophthal Soc. 1978;76:343–82.
26. Ang GS, Townend J, Lois N. Epidemiology of giant retinal tears in the United Kingdom: The British Giant Retinal Tear Epidemiology Eye Study (BGEES). Invest Ophth Vis Sci. 2010;51(9):4781–7. https://doi.org/10.1167/iovs.09-5036.
27. Wolfensberger TJ, Aylward GW, Leaver PK. Prophylactic 360° cryotherapy in fellow eyes of patients with spontaneous giant retinal tears. Ophthalmology. 2003;110(6):1175–7. https://doi.org/10.1016/s0161-6420(03)00256-2.
28. Verhoekx JSN, van Etten PG, Wubbels RJ, van Meurs JC, van Overdam KA. Prophylactic laser treatment to decrease the incidence of retinal detachment in fellow eyes of idiopathic giant retinal tears. Retina. 2020;40(6):1094–7. https://doi.org/10.1097/iae.0000000000002494.
29. Hamad AE, Moinuddin O, Blair MP, et al. Late-onset retinal findings and complications in untreated retinopathy of prematurity. Ophthalmol Retina. 2020;4(6):602–12. https://doi.org/10.1016/j.oret.2019.12.015.

Part III

Retinopathy of Prematurity (ROP)

Classification of Retinopathy of Prematurity

14

Graham E. Quinn and Alistair R. Fielder

Abstract

ICROP3 is the third iteration of classification of retinopathy of prematurity (ROP) and it further expands the descriptions of this potentially blinding disorder of premature infants. It is organized several categories in terms of: (1) location of vascularization (zone) including a segmenting of the middle zone 2, (2) plus disease, pre-plus disease, and normal posterior retinal vessels (3) stages 1–3 of acute phase disease including A-ROP, (4) retinal detachment (stages 4 and 5), (5) extent of vascularization, and (6) regression, reactivation, and long-term sequelae. Importantly, each eye needs to be classified in terms of zone, plus disease, stage, and extent of disease, along with additional notation if A-ROP is present. This classification will facilitate more detailed descriptions of ROP for improvements in clinical care and research.

Keywords

Classification of retinopathy of prematurity · Regression · Reactivation · Aggressive ROP · Subclassification of stage 5 ROP

G. E. Quinn (✉)
Children's Hospital of Philadelphia, University of Pennsylvania, Philadelphia, PA, USA
e-mail: QUINN@chop.edu

A. R. Fielder
FRCP, Department of Optometry and Visual Science, City, University of London, London, UK
e-mail: A.Fielder@city.ac.uk

Classification of Retinopathy of Prematurity

Classification of any disease evolves for use in clinical practice and research provide further insight into the causation and manifestations of the disorder. This is true for the description of the clinical findings associated with retinopathy of prematurity (ROP) noted over the past three-quarters of a century since its first description largely in countries with high levels of human development. With improving neonatal care of premature infants throughout the world, this potentially blinding disorder has become increasingly prevalent and further development of the classification would enhance both communication about and management of this disorder. The first international classification of acute phase ROP (ICROP) was published in 1984 [1] with the collaboration of 23 ophthalmologists and vision scientists from 12 countries with a further expansion in 1987 [2] to include classification of retinal detachment and a description of retinal sequelae. Four basic parameters of the clinical appearance of the retinopathy were used to describe the severity by stage, location by zone, circumferential extent of disease, and the appearance of the posterior pole vessels, i.e., plus disease. The classification was revisited in 2005 [3] and additional concepts included then were pre-plus disease as an intermediate form between normal posterior pole vessels and plus disease, and a description of aggressive posterior ROP (AP-ROP) to indicate a rapidly developing severe form of the retinopathy that was being observed with increasing frequency in some regions of the world.

In the years since the 2005 classification, there has been a dramatic increase in the technology to detect and describe abnormalities of ROP during the initiation and later manifestations of the disease. This led to the recognition of the need to develop a subsequent classification called ICROP3 that was recently published [4]. A number of important advances were made that begin to address a series of current issues. The subjectivity of an ROP classification based on clinical appearance can now be supplemented and clarified using innovations in ophthalmic imaging that is increasingly available in the neonatal intensive care unit. In addition, there are a number of novel pharmacologic interventions for serious disease (e.g. anti-vascular endothelial growth factor agents) that present different post-treatment patterns of regression and reactivation compared to retinal ablation using laser photocoagulation or cryotherapy. Further the patterns of developing serious ROP have been found to vary in some regions of the world and the 2005 ICROP term "aggressive posterior ROP" has been changed to "aggressive ROP", A-ROP.

ICROP3 is organized in terms of: (1) location of vascularization (zone), (2) plus and pre-plus disease, (3) stage of acute phase disease including A-ROP, (4) retinal detachment (stages 4 and 5), (5) extent of vascularization, and (6) regression, reactivation, and long-term sequelae. Importantly, ICROP3 recommends that each eye be classified in terms of zone, plus disease, stage, and extent of disease, along with additional notation if A-ROP is present. This latest classification will facilitate more detailed descriptions of ROP for improvements in clinical care and research.

Location of Vascularization

The vascularization of the inner retina begins in the peripapillary region at about week 13 of gestation and proceeds centrifugally, reaching the far peripheral retina at approximately full term. Though developing retinal vascularization proceeds in a lobular pattern and displays nasal-temporal asymmetry, ICROP 3 recommends at this time the continued use of describing the stage of vascularization in terms of 3 circles that are arrayed concentrically around to the optic disc (Fig. 14.1).

Zone I, the most posterior zone, consists of a circle with a radius that is twice the estimated distance from the center of the optic disc to the center of the fovea. The extent of zone I can be judged clinically using a 28-diopter lens by viewing the nasal edge of the optic disc and estimating the limit of zone I temporally.

Zone II consists of a ring-shaped area that extends nasally from the outer extent of zone I to the nasal ora serrata with similar estimated distances in the remaining retina. One region of zone II that extends 2-disc diameters posterior to zone I is highlighted as "posterior zone II" that the ICROP3 committee considered more worrisome disease than disease that occurs in more peripheral zone II.

ICROP3 also introduces a new term, "notch," to indicate a frequently observed feature in which the ROP lesion makes an incursion of 1–2 clock hours along a horizontal meridian and intrudes into a more posterior zone than the rest of the ROP. When a notch is present and most of the retinopathy is in a more peripheral zone, the ROP should be noted as occurring in the most posterior zone with the notation of "secondary to a notch" (ie Zone I, secondary to notch).

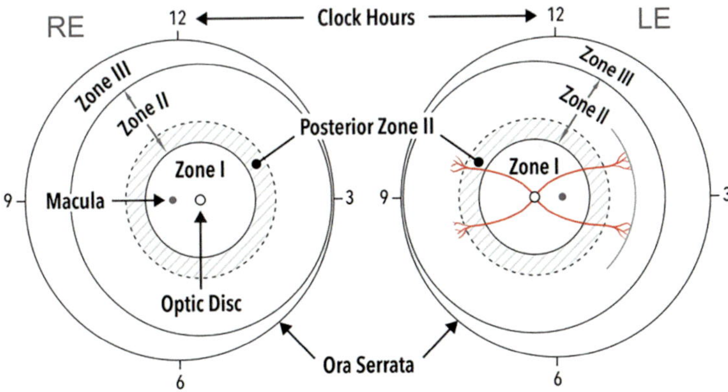

Fig. 14.1 Schema of right eye (RE) and left eye (LE) showing zone borders and clock hour sectors used to describe the location of vascularization and extent of retinopathy. Solid circles represent borders of zones I-III, and dotted circles represent borders of posterior zone II (two disc diameters beyond zone I). A hypothetical example of examination findings is shown in the left eye, representing approximately three clock hours of stage 1 disease in zone II (note single line on drawing to document presence of stage 1 disease). (This text and figure were published as Fig. 1 in Ophthalmology, Vol 128, Chiang MF, Quinn GE, Fielder AR et al. e51–e68, International Classification of Retinopathy of Prematurity, 3rd edition. Copyright Elsevier, 2021.)

Zone III is that region of the retina beyond zone II and ROP in zone III requires that the nasal portion of the retina is vascularized completely to the ora serrata in at least 2 clock hours.

The Plus Disease Spectrum

Plus disease, defined as a marked increased tortuosity and/or engorgement of posterior inner retinal vessels (Fig. 14.2A, B, C), is the current major indication for treatment. However, inter-expert agreement on grading across the range of vascular changes from normal to preplus to plus is low, though with better agreement if normal or severe.

To improve agreement, increase grading granularity, and provide a more consistent approach in clinical diagnosis, the ICROP3 Committee has presented the vascular changes within zone I associated with ROP as a spectrum (see traffic-light figure). This clinical diagnosis is made by comparing the appearance of the posterior vessels with a range of reference photographs (Fig. 14.3) in the ICROP3 classification [5]. The term "pre-plus" disease [5] indicates posterior vascular which is insufficient to be termed plus disease (Fig. 14.2D, E, F). It alerts to the likelihood of impending severe retinopathy.

Engorgement of the iris vessels and poor pupillary dilatation and vitreous haze are late signs and generally indicate advanced disease. Such changes are not required for the diagnosis of plus disease. Importantly, the term plus disease does not refer to vascular changes in the retinal periphery.

Stage of Disease

Peripheral retinal vascular changes in the premature infant range from incomplete vascularization to changes associated with ROP and, in ICROP 3, these changes are categorized in terms of acute retinopathy and retinal detachment. In the absence of peripheral changes of ROP, the term "incomplete vascularization" is used and accompanied with a designation of the most posterior zone of vascularization, e.g. incomplete vascularization in zone II.

Acute Phase Disease

Stage 1–Demarcation Line

A relatively flat and gray-white demarcation line separates the vascularized from non-vascularized retina. This line appears to lie within the plane of the retina and often has abnormal vessel branching posterior to the line (Fig. 14.4A).

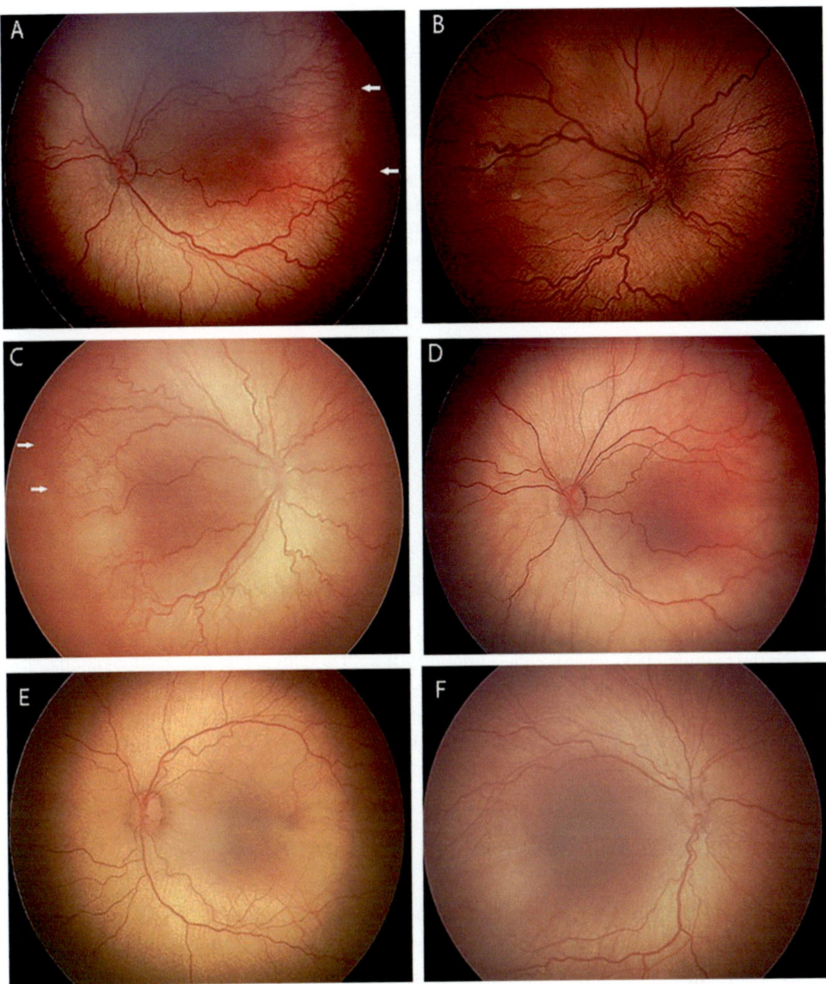

Fig. 14.2 Wide-angle fundus photographs demonstrating examples of plus disease and preplus disease. In Figures **A**, **B**, and **C** there is marked dilations and tortuosity of the posterior pole vessels while in Figures **C**, **D**, and **E**, there is an increase in tortuosity and dilation of vessels beyond normal, but insufficient for plus disease. (This figure was published as Fig. 2 in Ophthalmology, Vol 128, Chiang MF, Quinn GE, Fielder AR et al. e51–e68, International Classification of Retinopathy of Prematurity, 3rd edition. Copyright Elsevier, 2021.)

Stage 2–Ridge

A white or pink ridge with width and height develops in the region of the demarcation line and extends out of the plane of the retina (Fig. 14.4B). Small neovascular tufts, termed "popcorn," occur posterior to the ridge, but are not sufficient to upgrade the eye to a more serious stage.

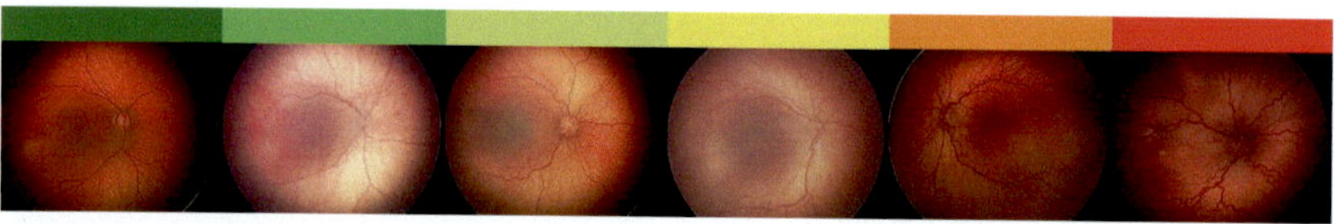

Fig. 14.3 Continuous vessel severity spectrum seen in ROP from normal to plus disease. The 34 members of ICROP3 of rated a series of 30 images ranging from normal, preplus, to plus. The average gradings are presented from normal (green) to plus disease (red) demonstrating the continuous spectrum of posterior vascular abnormalities in ROP. (This figure was published as Fig. 3a in Ophthalmology, Vol 128, Chiang MF, Quinn GE, Fielder AR et al. e51–e68, International Classification of Retinopathy of Prematurity, 3rd edition. Copyright Elsevier, 2021.)

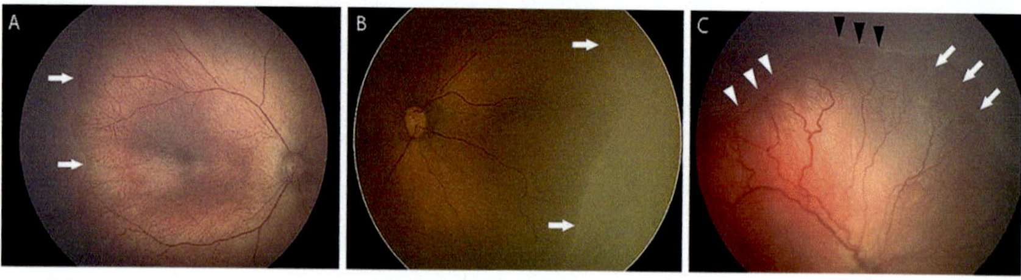

Fig. 14.4 Images documenting stages of acute ROP. 14.4**A** a grey-white line of demarcation between the vascularized and avascular retina. 14.4**B** a ridge with height and depth extending from the retinal surface in the region of the demarcation line. 14.4**C** extraretinal neovascularization extending into the vitreous. (This figure was published as Fig. 5a, c and f in Ophthalmology, Vol 128, Chiang MF, Quinn GE, Fielder AR et al. e51–e68, International Classification of Retinopathy of Prematurity, 3rd edition. Copyright Elsevier, 2021.)

Stage 3–Extraretinal Neovascular Proliferation

In stage 3, extraretinal neovascularization (Fig. 14.4C) extends from the ridge into the vitreous cavity. As the neovascularization progresses, a "ragged" pattern of the vessel abnormality appears. In more posterior ROP, the neovascularization may appear to lie flat on the retinal surface.

Aggressive ROP (A-ROP)

Aggressive-posterior ROP (AP-ROP) was added to ICROP in 2005 to describe a severe, rapidly-progressive form of ROP located in zone I or posterior zone II that occurred in the smallest premature infants [5]. However, aggressive ROP is increasingly recognized to also occur in larger preterm infants and in more peripheral retina, particularly in regions of the world with limited resources and experience in caring for premature infants. Therefore, in ICROP 3, the new term Aggressive ROP (A-ROP) is recommended to replace AP-ROP since the key diagnostic features of A-ROP are the tempo of disease and the appearance of the vascular abnormalities, but not the location of disease.

In A-ROP, pathologic neovascularization and severe plus disease without noting earlier stages of ROP constitute hallmark findings. Early on, capillary abnormalities posterior to the original border of vascularized retina may be noted including arterio-venous shunting resembling dilated vascular loops surrounding areas of vascular injury (Fig. 14.5A, B), sometimes with apparent loss of vessels of the entire retina (Fig. 14.5C). Eyes with A-ROP often develop a form of stage 3 which may appear as deceptively featureless networks of "flat" neovascularization (Fig. 14.5C–D), which are difficult to visualize on ophthalmoscopy using a 28-diopter lens and the use of greater magnification (e.g., 20-diopter lens) or fluorescein angiography may be helpful. It is important to note that A-ROP and classic stage 3 disease are not mutually exclusive but can coexist in a single eye.

Of interest, A-ROP may have been the florid ROP type seen in the 1940s and 50s as shown in the drawing included in the very first classification of retrolental fibroplasia by Reese King and Owens [5] (Fig. 14.6).

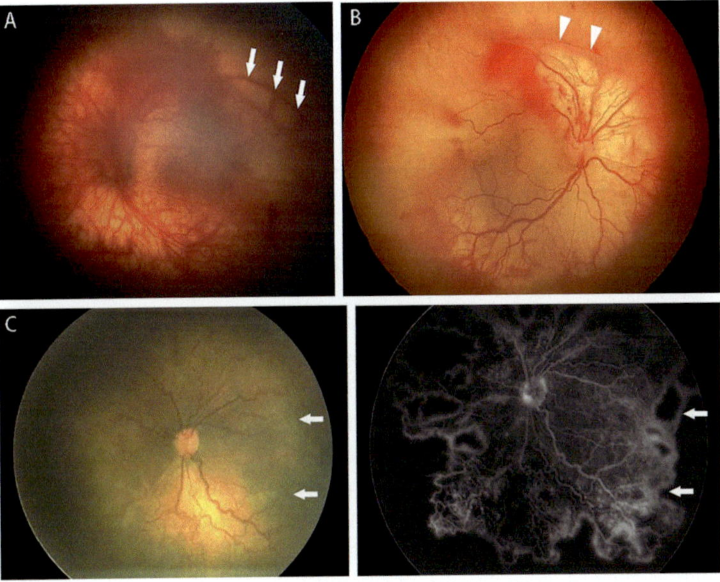

Fig. 14.5 Images showing aggressive ROP (A-ROP) with arteriolar-venular loops (14.5**A**–**B**), loss of retinal vessels (14.5**C**), and flat neovascularization (14.5**C**–**D**). (This figure was published as Fig. 7b–d in Ophthalmology, Vol 128, Chiang MF, Quinn GE, Fielder AR et al. e51–e68, International Classification of Retinopathy of Prematurity, 3rd edition. Copyright Elsevier, 2021.)

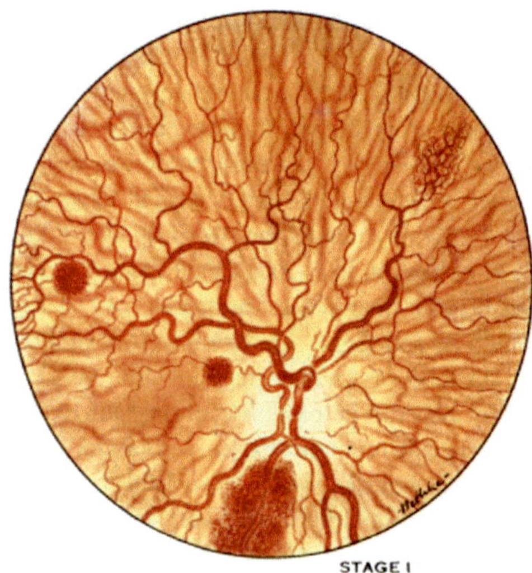

Fig. 14.6 An image from Reese, King, and Owens 1952 article documenting "florid" ROP. [This image was used with permission of the American Journal of Ophthalmology, "A classification of retrolental fibroplasia," Volume 36 (10), Fig. 1for Stage 1, copyright Elsevier (1952)]. *This figure was published in Am J Ophthalmol. 36(10), Reese AB, King MJ, Owens WC, Classification of retrolental fibroplasia, pp. 1333–35, Figure stage 1 in Volume 36, plate 8, Copyright Elsevier (1953)

Retinal Detachment (Stages 4–5)

Stage 4: Partial Retinal Detachment

A partial retinal detachment in ROP is defined as stage 4 ROP, which can be foveal sparing (stage 4A, Fig. 14.7A) or foveal involving (stage 4B, Fig. 14.7B). Features on examination suggesting retinal detachment include loss of fine detail of the choroidal vasculature or granular pigment epithelium, and/or a "ground glass" appearance relative to adjacent attached retina. Subtle foveal involvement may be most effectively discerned using optical coherence tomography (OCT) imaging. Stage 4 ROP may be exudative or tractional, occur in treated or untreated eyes, and vary in appearance depending on the tractional vectors and presence of exudation.

Exudative stage 4 detachments occur most commonly within days following laser treatment. They are typically convex in appearance, sometimes localized, and self-limited. Tractional detachments are associated with progressive fibrovascular organization and vitreous haze and may be associated with lipid and/or subretinal hemorrhage. Distinction by clinical examination between retinoschisis and detachment can be difficult. Eyes with A-ROP can develop a unique posterior "volcano" tractional detachment generally involving the fovea, in which the peripheral retina remains attached While the clinical appearance is reminiscent of a

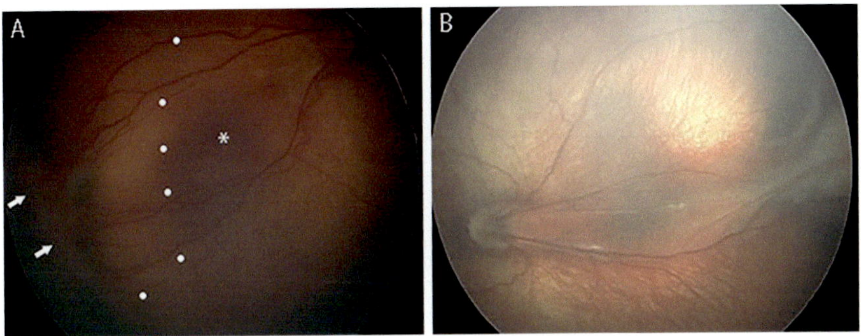

Fig. 14.7 Partial retinal detachment in ROP. Stage 4A represents a partial detachment with foveal spared while Stage 4B partial detachment with foveal involvement. (This figure was published as Fig. 8a, c in Ophthalmology, Vol 128, Chiang MF, Quinn GE, Fielder AR et al. e51–e68, International Classification of Retinopathy of Prematurity, 3rd edition. Copyright Elsevier, 2021.)

stage 5 funnel shaped detachment, these are more correctly considered stage 4B since the treated peripheral retina remains attached and thus the detachment is not total.

Stage 5: Total Retinal Detachment

Stage 5 ROP is defined by the presence of a total retinal detachment. When fibrosis precludes visualization of the posterior pole, the extent of detachment can be examined by B-scan ultrasonography. ICROP 3 subcategorizes total detachment into three configurations: stage 5A, in which the optic disc is visible by ophthalmoscopy (Fig. 14.8A), suggesting open-funnel detachment); stage 5B, in which the optic disc is not visible secondary to retrolental fibrovascular tissue or closed-funnel detachment (Fig. 14.8B); and stage 5C, in which findings of stage 5B are accompanied by anterior segment abnormalities (e.g., anterior lens displacement, marked anterior chamber shallowing, irido-capsular adhesions, and/or capsule-endothelial

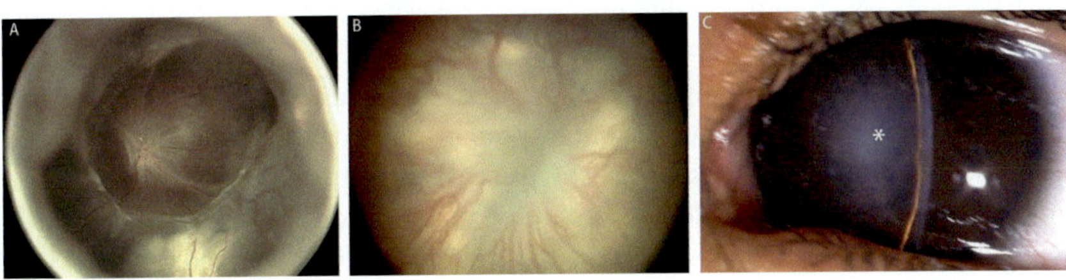

Fig. 14.8 Complete retinal detachment. In Stage 5A (Fig. 8a), the optic disc is visible while in Stage 5B, the optic disc is not visible. In Stage 5C, severe anterior segment abnormalities are noted along with findings of Stage 5B. (This figure was published as Fig. 10a, b, d in Ophthalmology, Vol 128, Chiang MF, Quinn GE, Fielder AR et al. e51–e68, International Classification of Retinopathy of Prematurity, 3rd edition. Copyright Elsevier, 2021.)

adhesion with central corneal opacification) (Fig. 14.8C, suggesting a closed-funnel configuration) [4].

Extent of Disease

The extent of disease along the junction between the vascularized and avascular retina is described in clock hours or by 30° sectors.

Regression, Reactivation, and Long-term Sequelae

To date regression, whether spontaneous or following treatment, has received relatively little attention. The advent of anti-VEGF treatment has increased the need for retreatment, thus detailed understanding of the events following acute phase disease is critical and as yet incompletely documented.

When describing later phases of ROP, two terms are recommended: first, "regression," to include both disease involution and resolution, and second, "reactivation," which refers to recurrence of acute phase features. Regression may be complete or incomplete. Neither regression nor reactivation should be regarded as the acute ROP process in reverse.

Regression

The first indication that regression has commenced is failure of acute signs to increase. Vascular features regress (plus) more rapidly than the peripheral lesion and also more rapidly following anti-VEGF therapy compared to laser (1–3 days vs around 7–14 days) or spontaneous regression. The vascular features regress before changes in the peripheral retina. Of note, while vessel dilatation is reduced tortuosity may persist. During regression there is involution of tunica vasculosa lentis, improvement of: pupillary dilation media clarity, and resolution of retinal hemorrhages.

In the peripheral retina, signs of regression are thinning and whitening of neovascular tissue. Vascularization of the avascular retina can be complete or incomplete, the latter resulting in the persistent avascular retina (PAR). PAR may occur in either the peripheral or posterior retina and may be seen following anti-VEGF treatment and also spontaneous regression. Ophthalmologists should describe PAR by its location by zone and extent. The risk of retinal detachment with PAR remains to be clarified and an important topic for future research.

Reactivation

The Committee recognized the importance of including reactivation into ICROP3. It is seen most frequently after anti-VEGF treatment and considered by some ophthalmologists as an indication for treatment, despite a lack of an agreed description of its features, natural history, and treatment criteria.

Reactivation may occur after incomplete or complete regression of the original ROP lesion. The time interval between anti-VEGF administration and reactivation is not fully understood, but evidence to date suggests it occurs most commonly between 37–60 weeks postmenstrual age (PMA) but this may be influenced by choice and dosage of anti-VEGF agent.

Signs of reactivation range from development of a new demarcation line to stage 3 with plus disease (Fig. 14.9A, B) Critically, reactivation may not progress and if it does, it may not proceed, through the usual sequence of stages of acute phase disease. Vascular changes in ROP reactivation include vascular dilation and/or tortuosity, similar to the plus disease spectrum. Extraretinal new vessels may develop which can be fine or appears as a fibrovascular ridge. Reactivation may progress to fibrosis, contraction, and tractional detachment.

Notation of reactivation should include zone and stage be preceded by reactivated, eg "reactivated stage 3, zone II'. Reactivation may occur at the site of the original ridge or elsewhere within the vascularized retina. Signs of reactivation may

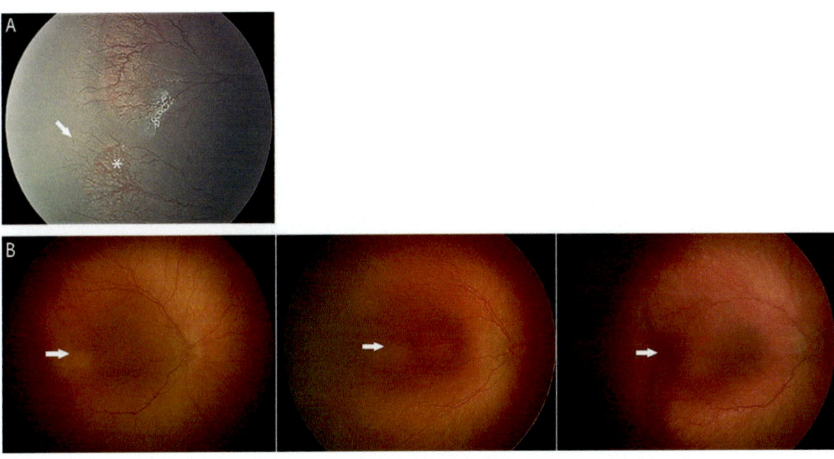

Fig. 14.9 ROP Reactivation. **A** Image showing reactivation at 67 weeks PMA in an eye that had received an injection of intravitreal anti-VEGF at 33 weeks PMA and again at 52 weeks PMA. **B** Image showing an eye with zone I ROP treated at 34 weeks PMA, appeared regressed on examination at 38 weeks PMA and showing reactivated stage 3 ROP at 51 weeks PMA. (This figure was published as Fig. 13d, g in Ophthalmology, Vol 128, Chiang MF, Quinn GE, Fielder AR et al. e51–e68, International Classification of Retinopathy of Prematurity, 3rd edition. Copyright Elsevier, 2021.)

be relatively subtle but with progression to stages 4 and 5 ROP is associated with vitreous condensation, haze, fibrotic contraction, and/or retinal breaks.

The Committee acknowledges that our understanding of reactivation is currently incomplete and is another topic for future study.

Long-Term Sequelae

Patients with a history of premature birth, even without history of ROP, exhibit a spectrum of ocular abnormalities that may lead to permanent sequelae.

- Late tractional, rhegmatogenous, or rarely exudative retinal detachments. The Committee stressed retinal detachment occurring in the absence of signs of ROP activity should not be designated as being due to reactivation, but rather as a sequela
- Retinoschisis from chronic traction of involuted Stage 3 may progress without retinal detachment into the macula and threaten visual field and acuity.
- PAR. Avascular retina is prone to retinal thinning, holes, lattice-like changes, and may be associated with retinal detachments later in life (Fig. 14.10A and B). PAR was observed over 30 years ago following spontaneous regression, so it is not a new problem. However, as mentioned above, following anti-VGEF therapy the area of avascular retina may be extensive. As yet, the clinical significance of PAR has yet to be clarified.
- Macular anomalies including smaller foveal avascular zone and blunting or absence of the foveal depression. These may be related to the degree of acute phase ROP and may be more apparent with fluorescein angiography or OCT imaging. More research is required to elucidate the clinical significance of these findings.
- Retinal vascular changes. These may include persistent tortuosity, straightening of the vascular arcades with macular dragging, and falciform retinal fold. Abnormal non-dichotomous retinal vessel branching, circumferential interconnecting vascular arcades, and telangiectatic vessels frequently occur. Vitreous hemorrhage may occur.
- Glaucoma. Eyes with history of ROP can develop secondary angle closure glaucoma later in life – usually in eyes with end-stage ROP.

Conclusion

There have been tremendous advances in the detection and management of ROP over the past 30–40 years—from no widely accepted treatment in the 1970s and 1980s, to cryotherapy, laser and now, in the new millennium, anti-VEGF treatment. These advances have been made possible and, in effect, were kicked started by the

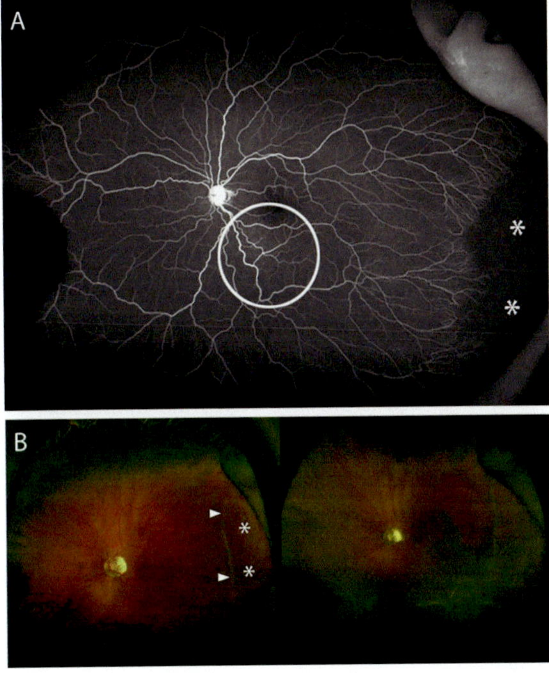

Fig. 14.10 PAR. Examples of persistent avascular retina (PAR). **A** Fluorescein angiogram demonstrating in a 7-year-old with a history of regressed ROP. **B** Fundus image showing incompletely regressed redige with PAR in a 15-year-old with extreme prematurity and no prior ROP treatment. (This figure was published as Fig. 12b, d in Ophthalmology, Vol 128, Chiang MF, Quinn GE, Fielder AR et al. e51–e68, International Classification of Retinopathy of Prematurity, 3rd edition. Copyright Elsevier, 2021.)

first ICROP of 1984. This, for first time, enabled robust comparison of findings between ophthalmologists and across centers and countries. ICROP Revisited (2005) incorporated advances in knowledge resulting from the Cryotherapy for ROP (CRYO-ROP) trial (REF) and, also the introduction of digital imaging and so increased granularity/sensitivity in the grading of acute phase ROP. ICROP 3 takes us on a step by hopefully eliminating a number of ambiguities, and further increasing detail by which ROP is graded. Of particular relevance in this anti-VEGF therapy era, ICROP 3 includes the phases of regression and reactivation in detail. There is still much to learn and we can anticipate that the addition of fluorescein angiography, OCT and artificial Intelligence in ROP will contribute greatly to a 4th version of ICROP in the future. However, this is an opportune moment to remind the reader that ICROP 3 has been largely devised so that it is accessible to anyone in any country and for this reason it is based on the ophthalmoscopic appearances of this potentially blinding condition.

Review Questions

1. A temporal notch is observed impinging on zone I compared to zone II in which most of the ROP lesion is observed. How is this noted in ICROP3?

a. zone II with notch
b. zone I with secondary notch
c. zone I secondary to notch
d. zone II with anterior notch

2. Why was AP-ROP changed to AROP?

a. Characteristics of this form of ROP occurs more rapidly than most ROP
b. In some eyes with serious aggressive ROP, the retinopathy is noted only in zone II
c. To make the distinction that this form of ROP occurs without any findings of classic ROP regardless of location
d. In some regions, serious aggressive ROP is noted in more peripheral regions

3. Are eyes with preplus progress more or less likely to progress to plus disease than eyes with no preplus disease?

a. More than 80%
b. Progression to plus disease is noted to be variable from 7 to > 70% in several small studies.
c. Always less than 40%

Answer

1. C
2. D
3. B

References

1. An international classification of retinopathy of prematurity. The Committee for the Classification of Retinopathy of Prematurity. Arch Ophthalmol. 1984;102:1130–4.
2. An international classification of retinopathy of prematurity. II. The classification of retinal detachment. The International Committee for the Classification of the Late Stages of Retinopathy of Prematurity. Arch Ophthalmol. 1987;105:906–12.
3. International Committee for the Classification of Retinopathy of Prematurity. The International classification of retinopathy of prematurity revisited. Arch Ophthalmol. 2005;123:991–9.
4. Chiang MF, Quinn GE, Fielder AR, Ostmo SR, Chan RVP, Berrocal A, Binenbaum G, Blair M, Campbell JP, Capone Jr. A, Chen Y, Dai S, Ells A, Fleck BW, Good WV, Hartnett ME, Holmstrom G, Kusaka S, Kychenthal A, Lepore D, Lorenz B,

Martinez-Castellanos MA, Özdek S, Ademola-Popoola D, Reynolds JR, Shah PK, Shapiro M, Stahl A, Toth C, Vinekar A, Visser L, Wallace DK, Wu W-C, Zhao P, Zin A. International classification of retinopathy of prematurity, 3rd ed. Ophthalmology 2021; 128: e51–e68.
5. Reese AB, King MJ, Owens WC. Classification of retrolental fibroplasia. Am J Ophthalmol. 1953;36(10):1333–5.

Major Clinical Trials in ROP

15

Johanna Madeleine Pfeil, Milena Grundel, Sonja Katharina Eilts, Marie-Christine Bruender, and Andreas Stahl

Abstract

First described about 80 years ago, the management of retinopathy of prematurity (ROP) has changed tremendously since. This development was only possible due to the conduction of a number of clinical trials in the field of ROP. The following chapter will summarize the most important interventional clinical trials on ROP treatment. The chapter will describe the journey from cryocoagulation to laser coagulation and anti-VEGF treatment. In addition, it will describe trials aimed not on treatment but prevention of severe ROP by targeting exposure to oxygen, light or nutrition. And finally, the chapter will introduce some of the current non-interventional registry studies SWEDROP, Retina.net ROP registry and EU-ROP that aim to improve ROP care beyond clinical trials by collecting and analyzing real-world data.

Keywords

Retinopathy of prematurity · Interventional clinical trials · Non-interventional clinical trials · Registry · Cryocoagulation · Laser coagulation · Anti-VEGF treatment · Prevention

J. M. Pfeil · M. Grundel · S. K. Eilts · M.-C. Bruender · A. Stahl (✉)
Department of Ophthalmology, University Medicine Greifswald, Greifswald, Germany
e-mail: andreas.stahl@med.uni-greifswald.de

J. M. Pfeil
e-mail: johanna.Pfeil@med.uni-greifswald.de

M. Grundel
e-mail: milena.Grundel@med.uni-greifswald.de

S. K. Eilts
e-mail: sonja.eilts@stud.uni-greifswald.de

M.-C. Bruender
e-mail: marie-Christine.Bruender@med.uni-greifswald.de

© The Author(s), under exclusive license to Springer Nature Switzerland AG 2023   185
Ş. Özdek et al. (eds.), *Pediatric Vitreoretinal Surgery*,
https://doi.org/10.1007/978-3-031-14506-3_15

Abbreviations

AA	Arachidonic Acid
BPD	Bronchopulmonary Dysplasia
DHA	Docosahexaenoic Acid
GA	Gestational Age
IGF-1	Insulin like Growth Factor 1
IGFBP	IGF Binding Protein
IVH	Intraventricular Hemorrhage
PAR	Persistent Avascular Retina
PMA	Postmenstrual Age
rhIGF-1	Recombinant human Insulin-like Growth Factor 1
rhIGFBP-3	Recombinant human Insulin-like Grow Factor 1 Binding Protein 3
ROP	Retinopathy of Prematurity
VEGF	Vascular Endothelial Growth Factor

Introduction

Since the first description of retinopathy of prematurity (short ROP) about 80 years ago, the management of the disease including prevention, detection and treatment has changed tremendously [1]. The following chapter will summarize some of the most important interventional as well as non-interventional clinical trials on treatment and prevention of ROP. Clinical trials on these topics are challenging, due to several reasons. One reason is the relative rareness of ROP requiring treatment, another reason is the relatively high number of neonatal clinical trials and the fact that patients often cannot be included in multiple clinical trials, and lastly, it is often a difficult decision for parents to consent to trial participation on behalf of their children.

When looking at the results of clinical trials in ROP, one needs to keep in mind that the first trials were conducted in the late 1980s, which means that the patients included in these first trials are not even 40 years old. Longer-term data on ROP sequelae into adulthood do not exist. In addition, treatment options as well as neonatal care have changed tremendously since the 1980s making long-term data from these early trials difficult to adapt for today's patients. Long-term data, however, are extremely important in ROP since the disease affects the whole life of a patient with some sequelae only becoming apparent years after active ROP and treatment.

Interventional Clinical Trials on Treatment of ROP

- After several reports had been published on cryotherapy for ROP, the prospective clinical trial **CRYO-ROP** started in 1986 as the first prospective randomized clinical trial on the treatment of ROP. The main inclusion criterion in this study was the presence of threshold disease, which was defined as stage 3 ROP in zone I or II in at least 5 contiguous or 8 cumulative clock-hours with plus disease. When a child had bilateral disease, one eye was randomized to receive cryocoagulation, the other eye was left without treatment. In unilaterally affected children, the child was randomized to one of the two study arms [2]. The preliminary study results after the inclusion and follow-up for three months of 172 infants revealed a reduction of unfavourable outcomes (defined as retinal detachment, macular fold or retrolental mass) from 43% in the untreated eyes to 21.8% in the eyes treated by cryocoagulation [3]. These results led to the termination of randomization in the study (by then a total of 279 infants had been randomized) because the benefit of cryotherapy was so evident that it would have been unethical to bar infants access to treatment. The complete study results confirmed the preliminary results showing a risk reduction of unfavorable outcome from 51.4% in the untreated eyes to 31.3% in the treated eyes [4]. Following the publication of the final results in 1990, cryocoagulation became the first evidence-based treatment option for threshold ROP [5]. The children enrolled in the CRYO-ROP trial were followed-up for up to 15 years with regular examinations of ocular findings and visual acuity. These long-term results further supported the efficacy and safety of cryocoagulation for the treatment of ROP [2, 6, 7].

The CRYO-ROP trial was followed by a number of small randomized controlled clinical trials, in which laser coagulation and cryocoagulation were directly compared, showing that **laser coagulation** was at least as effective as cryocoagulation for the management of ROP if not advantageous [8–10].

- One of the next milestone studies in the field of ROP, the **ETROP (Early Treatment for Retinopathy of Prematurity) trial,** started in 2000. The study used the earlier definition of threshold disease as defined in the CRYO-ROP trial: At least five contiguous or eight cumulative clock hours of stage 3 ROP in zone I or II in the presence of plus disease [11].

In addition to threshold disease, the term prethreshold ROP was used. Prethreshold ROP was defined as any ROP in zone I that was less than threshold; or in zone II stage 2 with plus disease; or zone II, stage 3 disease without plus disease; or zone II, stage 3 with plus disease but fewer than five contiguous or eight cumulative clock hours. The ETROP study randomized children with prethreshold ROP that had a high risk of developing an unfavorable outcome (assessed by a risk model based on the CRYO-ROP study) to receive either early treatment by laser coagulation or conventional management of the disease. The conventional management consisted of regular eye exams until ROP either progressed to threshold disease (then followed by treatment) or regressed without intervention. The results of the ETROP trial favored the earlier treatment option leading to both a significant reduction in rates of unfavorable visual acuity (19.8% in the conventional group vs. 14.3% in the early treatment group) as well as less unfavorable structural outcomes (15.6% vs 9.0% respectively). Following the ETROP trial, **type I ROP** was defined as any stage of ROP with plus disease in zone I, or zone I stage 3 without plus disease, or zone II stage 2 or 3 with plus disease, and laser treatment was recommended for these stages. **Type II ROP** was defined as stage 1 or 2 without plus disease in zone I or stage 3 without plus disease in zone II, and continued observation was recommended for these stages [11].

Definition of prethreshold disease: any ROP in zone I that was less than threshold; or in zone II stage 2 with plus disease; or zone II, stage 3 disease without plus disease; or zone II, stage 3 with plus disease but fewer than five contiguous or eight cumulative clock hours.

Definition of threshold disease: at least five contiguous or eight cumulative clock hours of stage 3 ROP in zone I or II in the presence of plus disease.

Long-term follow-up assessments of the children in the trial found significantly better visual acuity for children in the early treatment arm but no difference regarding (high) myopia at 4 and 6 years of age [12]. Although these results favor an early treatment at times of prethreshold disease, one needs to keep in mind that a substantial part of infants with prethreshold ROP never progress to threshold disease, but regress without intervention. The benefits of early treatment have therefore to be weighed against the risks and stress associated with an intervention. This is particularly true for stage 2+ in zone II where the rate of spontaneous regression is relatively high without treatment. Today, some national treatment guidelines have adopted the ETROP recommendations (for example in the USA, Australia, Poland) while others have only adopted parts of the ETROP recommendations (for example Germany, where ROP stage 2+ in zone II is currently not a treatment indication) [13–16].

Type 1 ROP:

Zone I: any stage of ROP with plus disease or stage 3 without plus disease
Zone II stage 2 or 3 with plus disease

Type 2 ROP:

Zone I: stage 1 or 2 without plus disease
Zone II: stage 3 without plus disease

Combined, the CRYO-ROP and ETROP trials laid the foundation for today's standard laser treatment for ROP.

- The next milestone study was the **BEAT-ROP (Bevacizumab Eliminates the Angiogenic Threat of ROP) trial**, which started in 2008. The study enrolled 150 infants born with a birthweight ≤ 1500 g or a gestational age < 30 weeks who developed bilateral stage 3 ROP with plus disease in zone I or in posterior zone II. Children were randomized to either laser therapy (75 children) or intravitreal bevacizumab (0.625 mg in 0.025 ml, corresponding to 50% of the bevacizumab dose regularly used in adults; 75 children). Infants were stratified based on zone of ROP (67 infants with ROP in zone I and 83 infants in posterior zone II). The primary endpoint (treatment failure defined as recurrence of neovascularization in any eye requiring retreatment) was assessed up to 54 weeks postmenstrual age. Despite the fact that laser for skip lesions within the first week after initial treatment was not considered as retreatment but as part of the original treatment, the rate of ROP reactivation was relatively high in the laser arm (22%), and considerably lower in the bevacizumab arm (4%). A sub-analysis looking at the treatment effect by zone found a statistically significant difference between the two arms in favor of bevacizumab for zone I but not for posterior zone II eyes. A positive finding after treatment with bevacizumab was that physiologic vessel growth into the periphery continued while laser coagulation permanently destroyed the peripheral part of the retina [17] (Fig. 15.1).

Follow-up results of retinoscopic refraction at 2.5 years of age favored bevacizumab over laser coagulation, as significantly higher rates of high myopia were found after laser than after bevacizumab treatment, both in eyes with zone I and zone II ROP. Also the mean spherical equivalent was considerably lower in bevacizumab treated eyes independent of zone [18]. Neurological and developmental assessments at around 2 years of age found no significant differences between bevacizumab and laser [19].

Following the publication of the BEAT-ROP study, the use of anti-VEGF drugs, especially bevacizumab, for ROP increased considerably [20]. In parallel with the increase in anti-VEGF use, the number of articles reporting late reactivation of ROP increased [21–23], stressing the importance of frequent and long-term follow-up exams for months after anti-VEGF treatment for ROP. Low grade reactivation (stage 1 or 2) may be observed, as it often disappears spontaneously. If, however, reactivation reaches stages requiring treatment, either re-injection with anti-VEGF or laser treatment must be performed in a timely manner, usually within days.

Another concern regarding the increasing use of bevacizumab for ROP is its potential for systemic side effects. Different to laser therapy, anti-VEGF drugs injected into the eye leak out into the systemic circulation. In the case of bevacizumab, the systemic drug exposure after a single bilateral ROP treatment suppresses VEGF levels in the circulation for weeks [24–26]. Since organ development is still in full progress at that early developmental age, it is unknown whether

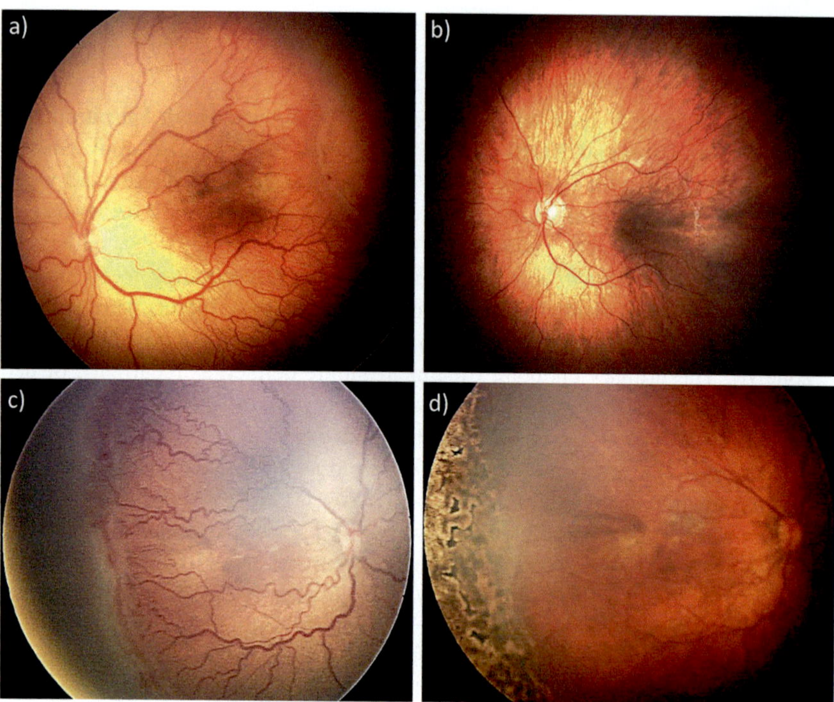

Fig. 15.1 Top row: Retinal images before (**a**) and after (**b**) bevacizumab treatment. Bottom row: Retinal images before (**c**) and after (**d**) laser treatment. Note that after laser therapy, the retinal periphery is scarred (**d**). (Images courtesy of Prof. Dr. Şengül Özdek)

systemic VEGF suppression has the potential to harm other organs. In the BEAT-ROP trial, neither VEGF levels nor bevacizumab blood levels were measured [17]. In addition to safety, the ideal bevacizumab dose has been the focus of scientific debate ever since publication of the BEAT-ROP trial. BEAT-ROP used half the adult dose (0.625 mg in 0.025 ml).

- The first dose de-escalation study for bevacizumab was conducted between 2015 and 2016 on 61 infants with type 1 ROP (see ETROP definition above) in the **PEDIG (pediatric eye disease investigator group) trial**. The trial started with a dose of 0.25 mg of bevacizumab (corresponding to 40% of the dose used in the BEAT-ROP trial, or 20% of the regular adult dose). If treatment was successful in at least 80% of the infants treated with that dose, the dose was halved for the next 10 to 14 patients. The criteria for treatment success were regression of ROP activity by 4 days post injection and the absence of a recurrence of type 1 ROP or severe neovascularizations over 4 weeks. Dose de-escalation was continued until the predefined lowest dose of 0.031 mg was reached. Even the lowest dose, which corresponds to only 2.5% of the adult dose, was still effective in treating acute ROP in 9 of 9 infants [27]. It has to be acknowledged, however, that re-treatments due to either treatment failure within four weeks after treatment, or due to "late" recurrences after > four weeks, or due to persistent avascular retina were frequent in all treatment arms (total of 41%) and one study eye even progressed to stage 5 ROP [28]. From a practical point of view, the use of these very low doses of any anti-VEGF drug is complicated by the fact that bevacizumab needs to be diluted to achieve the low doses described in the PEDIG trials. From a scientific point of view, however, the study demonstrates that the ideal concentration for anti-VEGF in ROP may yet to be defined and may well differ from patient to patient depending on the individual area of avascular retina and the individual VEGF levels present.

- In order to respond to concerns regarding systemic anti-VEGF exposure and dosing, the **CARE-ROP (Comparing Alternative Ranibizumab dosages for safety and efficacy in ROP) trial** (starting in 2014) investigated two lower anti-VEGF doses (24% and 40%) and with ranibizumab a molecule with significantly lower risk for systemic VEGF suppression [29, 30]. A total of 19 infants with stage 1+, 2+, 3+ or 3− or AP-ROP in zone I or stage 3+ or AP-ROP in posterior zone II were randomized to receive either 0.12 mg or 0.20 mg of ranibizumab at 6 centers in Germany. This was the first clinical trial, in which a re-injection of the same dose of ranibizumab was allowed after at least 28 days in case of treatment requiring reactivation of ROP if it had initially responded well to ranibizumab. Both doses of ranibizumab were found to be effective in controlling acute ROP while they did not suppress systemic VEGF-levels [30]. The CARE-ROP core study was followed by a follow-up period, which consisted of ophthalmological assessments at 1 and 5 years as well as pediatric assessments at 2 and 5 years of age. The 1- and 2-year results from CARE-ROP found no indications for negative effects of ranibizumab on neurodevelopmental or ophthalmic outcomes [23]. The follow-up period did, however, report one case of late reactivation of ROP after the end of the core study that had been missed due to cancelled ophthalmologic follow-up exams by the parents. This case of missed late reactivation led to stage 5 ROP in both eyes and once again highlights the importance of frequent and long-term follow-up examinations after anti-VEGF treatment for ROP [23]. As a lesson learned from this case and similar ones reported in the literature [21, 22], the German Ophthalmologic and Neonatal Societies have developed with the **ROP ID card**, a tool that helps reminding patients and physicians of scheduled ophthalmologic follow-ups. The ROP ID card (in German) can be downloaded from this website: https://t1p. de/lmu4.

- With only 19 patients randomized, CARE-ROP was a pilot study. Starting in 2015 the use of ranibizumab for ROP was examined further and in a much larger cohort by the **RAINBOW (Ranibizumab versus laser therapy for the treatment of very low birthweight infants with retinopathy of prematurity) trial** [31]. RAINBOW investigated two doses of ranibizumab (0.1 mg vs. 0.2 mg, corresponding to 20 and 40% of the adult dose) and compared them directly to laser therapy in infants with a stage 1+, 2+, 3+ or 3− or AP-ROP in zone I or stage 3+ or AP-ROP in zone II. Similar to CARE-ROP, re-treatment after a minimum of 28 days with the same dosage of ranibizumab was allowed if treatment-requiring ROP recurred after the eye had initially responded well to ranibizumab. With a total of 225 infants from 26 countries, RAINBOW was one of the largest prospective, interventional clinical trials in the field of ROP conducted to date. Participants were randomized to the three treatment arms (77 infants to 0.1 mg ranibizumab, 74 to 0.2 mg ranibizumab and 74 to laser coagulation). According to the study results, 0.2 mg ranibizumab appeared likely to be more effective than laser coagulation in the treatment of ROP, although statistical significance to demonstrate superiority was marginally missed (p = 0.051). Numerically, treatment success occurred more often in the 0.2 mg arm than in the laser arm (80% vs. 66%) and the odds ratio for treatment success was 2.19 in favor of ranibizumab 0.2 mg vs. laser. In addition, the number of infants with unfavorable structural outcome was lower in the 0.2 mg ranibizumab arm compared to laser (one infant vs. 7 infants). The difference between 0.2 mg ranibizumab and laser was observed both in zone I and zone II eyes. The results for 0.2 mg ranibizumab were superior to 0.1 mg ranibizumab (80% vs. 75% treatment success) [31]. Confirming the results from CARE-ROP, the study did not identify any impact of ranibizumab on free VEGF levels in the circulation [31, 32]. The 2-year results from RAINBOW found less structural abnormalities and fewer cases of high myopia (-5 diopters or worse) after ranibizumab compared to laser. Pediatric and ophthalmic development was comparable between the two treatment arms adding no new safety concerns for ranibizumab in ROP [33].

The results of the RAINBOW trial lead to the approval of 0.20 mg ranibizumab for the treatment of ROP zone I stage 1+, 2+, 3+ or 3− as well as zone II stage 3+ and aggressive posterior ROP (AP-ROP) in Europe [34]. The 5-year results from both CARE-ROP and RAINBOW are expected for 2023.

- In 2021, the global phase III **FIREFLEYE trial** was concluded and first results were presented at the EURETINA meeting in September 2021 [35]. FIRE-FLEYE compared the anti-VEGF drug aflibercept to laser and found treatment success rates of 85.5% for aflibercept and 82.1% for laser. FIREFLEYE enrolled a total of 113 participants from 27 countries randomized 2:1 between aflibercept and laser. FIREFLEYE was the first randomized anti-VEGF study to include also unilateral cases of ROP and stage 2+ zone II eyes in addition to the stages enrolled in RAINBOW. In the study 0.4 mg aflibercept corresponding to 20% of the adult dose were injected in a volume of only 10 µl (as opposed to 20 µl in RAINBOW). The primary results missed the predefined endpoint of showing non-inferiority against laser, likely because of the relatively high success rates with laser in this trial (82.1%) compared to both RAINBOW (66%) and

BEAT ROP (78%). However, treatment success was still numerically higher with aflibercept (85.5%) compared to laser. Different to ranibizumab, aflibercept remains in the circulation for a longer period of time as shown in an adult population of AMD patients [36].

Summary table of interventional clinical trials on treatment of ROP

Study	Starting-year	Number of infants	Included stages of ROP	Intervention
CRYO-ROP [2]	1986	279	Threshold ROP (defined as stage 3 ROP in zone I or II in at least 5 contiguous or 8 cumulative clock-hours with plus disease)	Randomization to receive **cryocoagulation**, or no treatment
ETROP [11]	2000	317	Prethreshold ROP (defined as any ROP in zone I that was less than threshold; or in zone II stage 2 with plus disease; or zone II, stage 3 disease without plus disease; or zone II, stage 3 with plus disease but fewer than five contiguous or eight cumulative clock hours.)	Randomization to either early treatment by **laser coagulation** or conventional management of the disease (treatment when threshold ROP was reached)
BEAT-ROP [17]	2008	150	Stage 3 ROP with plus disease in zone I or in posterior zone II	Randomization to either laser coagulation or intravitreal **bevacizumab** (0.625 mg in 0.025 ml)
PEDIG [27]	2015	61	Type 1 ROP (any stage of ROP with plus disease in zone I, or zone I stage 3 without plus disease, or zone II stage 2 or 3 with plus disease)	Dose de-escalation study starting with 0.25 mg of **bevacizumab**; lowest dose used in the trial was 0.031 mg
CARE-ROP [30]	2014	19	Stage 1+, 2+, 3+ or 3 − or AP-ROP in zone I or stage 3+ or AP-ROP in posterior zone II	Randomization to either 0.12 mg or 0.20 mg **ranibizumab**

(continued)

(continued)

Study	Starting-year	Number of infants	Included stages of ROP	Intervention
RAINBOW [31]	2015	225	Stage 1+, 2+, 3+ or 3 − or AP-ROP in zone I or stage 3+ or AP-ROP in zone II	Randomization to either 0.1 mg or 0.2 mg **ranibizumab** or **laser coagulation**
FIREFLEYE [35]	2019	113	Stage 1+, 2+, 3+ or 3 − or AP-ROP in zone I or stage 2+, 3+ or AP-ROP in zone II	Randomization to either 0.4 mg **aflibercept** or **laser coagulation**

Interventional Clinical Trials on Prevention of ROP

Although treatment of ROP has evolved tremendously over the last years, each treatment option carries potential risks and side effects. Prevention of treatment requiring ROP could thus be a very interesting alternative. Preventive strategies in ROP have started long before any treatment option was available.

Oxygen

- The **Cooperative Study of Retrolental Fibroplasia and the Use of Oxygen trial** was conducted in the early 1950s allocating 786 infants to either the "routine-oxygen group", in which infants received more than 50% of oxygen for about 28 days, or to the "curtailed-oxygen group", in which infants received as little oxygen as compatible with the general condition of the child, while the concentration was not to exceed 50% and ranged between 40 and 50%. While mortality rates did not differ between the two study groups, the incidence of active ROP was higher in the routine-oxygen group than in the curtailed-oxygen group. The authors recommended that the period of times an infant received oxygen therapy as well as the oxygen concentration should be restricted to a minimum [37]. A few years later, Avery and Oppenheimer investigated retrospectively two cohorts, one before the introduction of curtailed oxygen levels and one after their introduction and discovered that while rates of ROP had actually decreased after the introduction of curtailed oxygen levels, infant mortality rates had increased [38]. Balancing the risk between increased rates of ROP and increased mortality and morbidity rates has since been the objective of many subsequent trials.

- Another big milestone trial exploring oxygen targets in ROP was the **STOP-ROP (Supplemental Therapeutic Oxygen for Prethreshold Retinopathy Of Prematurity) trial**, starting in 1994, which investigated if the progression of prethreshold ROP to threshold ROP could be prevented by the application of supplemental oxygen, once prethreshold ROP had been observed. A total of 649 infants were randomized to either the regular treatment arm (oxygen saturation targets of 89–94%) or the oxygen supplementation arm (oxygen saturation targets of 96–99%). In both study arms, oxygen was applied for at least two weeks and thereafter until either the study eye(s) progressed to threshold disease and received treatment or until regressing ROP in zone III was observed for at least two consecutive weeks or until complete vascularization of the retina was reached. Neither a reduction of progression to threshold disease in the higher saturation target group was observed, nor a further activation of the disease. In a subgroup analysis, a positive effect of oxygen supplementation was detected in infants who had threshold disease without plus disease. The higher oxygen saturation targets were on the other hand associated with higher rates of pulmonary events like pneumonia and exacerbation of chronic lung disease [39].

- In the **BOOST (Benefits of Oxygen Saturation Targeting) trial**, starting enrollment of patients in 2006, the effect of slightly different oxygen saturation targets on growth and neurodevelopmental outcomes were assessed. 358 infants born with a GA of less than 30 weeks were randomized to the standard saturation group (91–94%) or to a high saturation group (95–98%) if they were still dependent on oxygen supplementation at 32 weeks PMA. The treatment was maintained as long as the child needed oxygen supplementation. No differences between growth and neurodevelopmental abnormalities were observed between the two groups, but infants in the high saturation group needed oxygen for a longer period of time and a higher proportion of these infants was still dependent on oxygen at 36 weeks PMA [40]. Both trials helped to identify an upper level of oxygen saturation targets for preterm born babies, but lower levels were still open for discussion. Several case reports and smaller cohort studies were conducted with often contradicting results. In order to find an answer, the results of five prospective clinical trials (SUPPORT, the Canadian Oxygen Trial, BOOST, BOOST II in UK and BOOST II in Australia) conducted between 2005 and 2014 in different settings around the world were combined in the **NeOProM (Neonatal Oxygenation Prospective Meta-analysis) Collaboration**. All these studies used a similar study design comparing lower oxygen saturation targets of 85–89% with higher targets of 91–95% in a total of almost 5000 children (in all studies combined). The two BOOST II trials were stopped early based on an advice from their Data Monitoring Committee as higher survival rates in the group of infants receiving higher oxygen levels were identified in a joint safety analysis of the two studies [41]. Combining all available results from these trials found an increased risk of death and necrotizing enterocolitis in the lower oxygen saturation group while the risk for ROP was reduced [42].

Light

The **LIGHT-ROP trial** investigated from 1995 onwards if a reduction of ambient light in the neonatal intensive care units could reduce the risk for ROP. A total of 409 infants were randomized to either the control group (204 infants) or the group with reduced ambient light (205 infants). In the second group, ambient light was reduced by placing goggles on the eyes of the children within 24 hours after birth and was continued until four weeks after birth or until 31 weeks after conception, whichever was later. The control group was exposed to normal light in a neonatal intensive care unit. The study did not find any effect on the risk of developing ROP [43].

Nutrition

Arachidonic acid (AA) and docosahexaenoic acid (DHA) are important constituents of the retina as well as the brain, and are known to be lower in preterm born infants than in term born infants as the support by the mother during the third trimester is missing. Therefore, several trials to alter the systemic levels of these nutrients were conducted. Only very recently, the results of the **Mega Donna Mega trial** were published reporting that supplementation of AA and DHA in a ratio of 2:1 halved the risk for developing severe ROP. In this multicenter trial, 206 preterm infants born with a GA of less than 28 weeks were either randomized to the treatment arm (supplementation of enteral oil containing AA and DHA; n = 101) or to the control group (n = 105). Supplementation was started within 3 days after birth and was continued until 40 weeks PMA. Apart from the positive effect on ROP, no impact on other prematurity related comorbidities like BPD or IVH were observed. The authors concluded that in the future a supplementation of AA:DHA might be a useful strategy to prevent severe ROP in extremely preterm born infants [44].

Pharmacological Prevention of ROP

It is well established that low levels of IGF-1 are associated with an increased risk of ROP, and also other preterm associated complications [45, 46]. Therefore, an international, multicenter phase II trial investigated the effect of continuous application of rhIGF-1/rhIGFBP-3 from birth to 29 weeks PMA. A total of 61 infants with GA between 23 and 27 weeks were randomized to the intervention group (rhIGF-1/rhIGFBP-3) and 60 infants to standard of care group. The intervention did not reduce ROP severity nor the rate of ROP occurrence, but had a positive impact on the occurrence of severe bronchopulmonary dysplasia and intraventricular hemorrhage [47].

Non-interventional Clinical Trials on ROP

While clinical trials, with their strict inclusion and exclusion criteria and well-defined protocols lead to new insights into disease mechanisms and treatment options, they often do not reflect treatment reality in everyday life. Non-interventional trials, with their lack of predefined treatment protocols and lack of inclusion and exclusion criteria do just that: they capture everyday clinical routine and thus create access to extremely valuable data that has a very direct correlation to clinical practice. With treatment requiring ROP being a relatively rare disease, individual hospitals often treat only few patients per year. Real life studies must therefore be conducted in a joint effort and in a multicenter approach. Especially since the advent of new treatment options, the need for clinical routine data has increased in order to be able to evaluate how these new treatment options affect real world ROP outcomes.

Already in 2006, the Swedish national ROP registry, called **SWEDROP**, started as one of the first registries to collect ROP data from clinical routine settings. All infants in Sweden screened for ROP are included in SWEDROP [48]. Based on the SWEDROP results, the national screening guideline in Sweden has been reviewed and adapted several times over the recent years [49]. According to the latest publication from 2019, more than 8,473 patients are documented in SWEDROP, of which 440 were treated for ROP [49].

A few years later, in 2011, the German **Retina.net ROP registry** was launched with the goal to document exclusively cases of treated ROP [50]. Different from SWEDROP, the focus of this registry is thus on the treatment, not screening of ROP. Until the end of 2020, a total of 20 centers in Germany have contributed data of over 350 treated patients to the Retina.net ROP registry. It was estimated that this cohort represents about 10% of all patients treated for ROP in Germany during that time frame [51]. Apart from data on ROP treatment, demographic parameters and neonatal aspects of ROP, the registry also collects long-term follow-up data after treatment. In 2021, the Retina.net ROP registry was transferred from a national database addressing only centers in Germany to the EU-ROP registry which is now open for international participation.

The **EU-ROP registry** is an international, multicenter, non-interventional, observational registry intended to run open-ended in as many countries as possible. EU-ROP allows data entry for all infants treated for ROP, irrespective of the treatment modality. The parameters collected in the database were defined together with an international consortium consisting of ophthalmologists, neonatologists and parent representatives, putting the focus even more on ophthalmological aspects and on the follow-up after treatment. The EU-ROP registry represents a unique opportunity to jointly generate international comparable data that will help to improve ROP care. ROP centers interested in participating can contact contact@eu-rop.org or visit the www.eu-rop.org website.

Conclusion

Over the last years, treatment of ROP changed from no available treatment to cryocoagulation, laser coagulation and nowadays the choice between laser coagulation and several anti-VEGF drugs. Over these years, our understanding of the disease has improved dramatically and visual function outcomes are now in most cases much better than they would have been a few decades ago. However, long-term data, specifically on the new anti-VEGF treatment options, is still rare and late recurrences, which had been almost non-existent during the times of exclusive laser treatment, have become a new challenge with the use of anti-VEGF agents. The new treatment options thus require a completely new approach to the follow-up of ROP *after* treatment, with frequent and long-term follow-up examinations that can often be more challenging than the treatment itself. An important tool to increase our knowledge specifically regarding long-term outcomes and the required postinterventional follow-ups is the use of international, multicenter ROP registries.

Review Questions

1. Which statement about ROP is *incorrect*?

(a) The CRYO-ROP study was conducted in the 1980s.
(b) Cryocoagulation became the first evidence-based treatment option for ROP.
(c) The use of anti-VEGF drugs increased following publication of the BEAT-ROP study.
(d) CARE-ROP was the first clinical trial in which a re-injection of the same dose of ranibizumab was allowed.
(e) The RAINBOW study investigated the effect of oxygen supplementation on ROP.

2. Which study did *not* investigate at least one intravitreal anti-VEGF drug?

(a) FIREFLEYE
(b) BEAT-ROP
(c) ETROP
(d) CARE-ROP
(e) RAINBOW

3. Which statement about clinical ROP trials is *incorrect*?

(a) It is often a challenging decision for parents to consent to trial participation on behalf of their children.
(b) ROP requiring treatment occurs relatively rarely.

(c) Newborns are often already participating in other clinical trials, making participation in an ROP study difficult to achieve.

(d) Participation in a clinical trial for preterm born infants is only possible from a postmenstrual age of 30 weeks onwards.

(e) During the last years several clinical trials investigating the use of anti-VEGF drugs for the treatment of ROP were investigated.

Answers

1. (**E**) The RAINBOW trial compared the effect of ranibizumab 0.12 mg and 0.2 mg to laser therapy and led to the approval of ranibizumab 0.2 mg for the treatment of ROP by the European Medicines Agency (EMA) in 2019.

2. (**C**) In the FIREFLEYE trial the anti-VEGF drug aflibercept was compared to laser coagulation. The BEAT-ROP study compared the anti-VEGF drug bevacizumab to laser coagulation. The CARE-ROP study compared two different doses of ranibizumab for ROP treatment and in the RAINBOW trial ranibizumab was compared to laser coagulation. The ETROP trial, however, did not investigate the effect of anti-VEGF treatment on ROP but analyzed the effect of early laser treatment compared to conventional laser treatment.

3. (**D**) There is no general lower age limit for the inclusion of a child in clinical trials. Participation of a preterm born infant in a clinical trial depends on the inclusion and exclusion criteria of the respective trial and informed consent of the parents.

References

1. Hellström A, Hård A-L. Screening and novel therapies for retinopathy of prematurity–a review. Early Hum Dev. 2019;138: 104846.
2. Cryotherapy for Retinopathy of Prematurity Cooperative G. Multicenter trial of cryotherapy for retinopathy of prematurity. Snellen visual acuity and structural outcome at 5 1/2 years after randomization Arch Ophthalmol. 1996;114: 417–24.
3. Multicenter trial of cryotherapy for retinopathy of prematurity: preliminary results. Cryotherapy for Retinopathy of Prematurity Cooperative Group. Pediatrics. 1988; 81:697–706.
4. Multicenter trial of cryotherapy for retinopathy of prematurity. Three-month outcome. Cryotherapy for Retinopathy of Prematurity Cooperative Group. Arch Ophthalmol. 1990; 108:195–204.
5. Palmer EA. Results of U.S. randomized clinical trial of cryotherapy for ROP (CRYO-ROP). Doc Ophthalmol Adv Ophthalmol. 1990;74:245–51.
6. Cryotherapy for Retinopathy of Prematurity Cooperative Group. Multicenter trial of cryotherapy for retinopathy of prematurity: ophthalmological outcomes at 10 years. Arch Ophthalmol Chic Ill. 2001;1960(119):1110–8.
7. Palmer EA, Hardy RJ, Dobson V, Phelps DL, Quinn GE, Summers CG, Krom CP, Tung B, Cryotherapy for Retinopathy of Prematurity Cooperative G. 15-year outcomes following threshold retinopathy of prematurity: final results from the multicenter trial of cryotherapy for retinopathy of prematurity Arch Ophthalmol. 2005; 123: 311–18.

8. Algawi K, Goggin M, O'Keefe M. Refractive outcome following diode laser versus cryotherapy for eyes with retinopathy of prematurity. Br J Ophthalmol. 1994;78:612–4.

9. Connolly BP, McNamara JA, Sharma S, Regillo CD, Tasman W. A comparison of laser photocoagulation with trans-scleral cryotherapy in the treatment of threshold retinopathy of prematurity. Ophthalmology. 1998;105:1628–31.

10. White JE, Repka MX. Randomized comparison of diode laser photocoagulation versus cryotherapy for threshold retinopathy of prematurity: 3-year outcome. J Pediatr Ophthalmol Strabismus. 1997;34:83–7; quiz 121–122.

11. Good WV, Early Treatment for Retinopathy of Prematurity Cooperative Group. Final results of the Early Treatment for Retinopathy of Prematurity (ETROP) randomized trial. Trans Am Ophthalmol Soc. 2004; 102:233–48; discussion 248–250.

12. Quinn GE, Dobson V, Davitt BV, Wallace DK, Hardy RJ, Tung B, Lai D, Good WV, Early Treatment for Retinopathy of Prematurity Cooperative Group. Progression of myopia and high myopia in the Early Treatment for Retinopathy of Prematurity study: findings at 4 to 6 years of age J AAPOS Off Publ Am Assoc Pediatr Ophthalmol Strabismus. 2013; 17:124–8.

13. Fierson WM. American Academy of Pediatrics Section on Ophthalmology, American Academy of Ophthalmology, American Association for Pediatric Ophthalmology and Strabismus, American Association of Certified Orthoptists. Screening examination of premature infants for retinopathy of prematurity. Pediatrics. 2018; 142:e20183061.

14. Gotz-Więckowska A, Bakunowicz-Łazarczyk A, Hautz W, Filipek E, Niwald AM. Polish Ophthalmological Society revised guidelines for the management of retinopathy of prematurity. Klin Oczna. 2020;2020:14–6.

15. Maier RF, Hummler H, Kellner U, Krohne TU, Lawrenz B, Lorenz B, Mitschdörfer B, Roll C, Stahl A. Augenärztliche Screening-Untersuchung bei Frühgeborenen (S2k-Level, AWMF-Leitlinien-Register-Nr. 024/010, März 2020): Gemeinsame Empfehlung von Deutsche Ophthalmologische Gesellschaft (DOG), Retinologische Gesellschaft (RG), Berufsverband der Augenärzte Deutschlands (BVA), Deutsche Gesellschaft für Kinder-und Jugendmedizin (DGKJ), Berufsverband der Kinder-und Jugendärzte e. V. (BVKJ), Bundesverband „Das frühgeborene Kind" e. V., Gesellschaft für Neonatologie und Pädiatrische Intensivmedizin (GNPI). Ophthalmol. 2021. https://doi.org/10.1007/s00347-021-01353-0.

16. Sydney Local Health District. SLHD: Royal Prince Alfred Hospital Guideline: Women and Babies: Retinopathy of Prematurity 2018.

17. Mintz-Hittner HA, Kennedy KA, Chuang AZ, Group B-RC. Efficacy of intravitreal bevacizumab for stage 3+ retinopathy of prematurity N Engl J Med. 2011; 364:603–15.

18. Geloneck MM, Chuang AZ, Clark WL, Hunt MG, Norman AA, Packwood EA, Tawansy KA, Mintz-Hittner HA, Group B-RC 2014 Refractive outcomes following bevacizumab monotherapy compared with conventional laser treatment: a randomized clinical trial. JAMA Ophthalmol. 2014; 132:1327–33.

19. Kennedy KA, Mintz-Hittner HA, BEAT-ROP Cooperative Group. Medical and developmental outcomes of bevacizumab versus laser for retinopathy of prematurity J AAPOS Off Publ Am Assoc Pediatr Ophthalmol Strabismus. 2018; 22:61–65.e1.

20. Walz JM, Bemme S, Pielen A, et al. The German ROP registry: data from 90 infants treated for retinopathy of prematurity. Acta Ophthalmol. 2016. https://doi.org/10.1111/aos.13069.

21. Hu J, Blair MP, Shapiro MJ, Lichtenstein SJ, Galasso JM, Kapur R. Reactivation of retinopathy of prematurity after bevacizumab injection Arch Ophthalmol Chic Ill 1960. 2012; 130:1000–6.

22. Mintz-Hittner HA, Geloneck MM, Chuang AZ. Clinical management of recurrent retinopathy of prematurity after intravitreal bevacizumab monotherapy. Ophthalmology. 2016;123:1845–55.

23. Stahl A, Bründer M, Lagrèze WA, et al. Ranibizumab in retinopathy of prematurity–one-year follow-up of ophthalmic outcomes and two-year follow-up of neurodevelopmental outcomes from the CARE-ROP study. Acta Ophthalmol (Copenh). 2021; aos.14852.

24. Kong L, Bhatt AR, Demny AB, Coats DK, Li A, Rahman EZ, Smith OE, Steinkuller PG. Pharmacokinetics of bevacizumab and its effects on serum VEGF and IGF-1 in infants with retinopathy of prematurity. Invest Ophthalmol Vis Sci. 2015;56:956–61.
25. Sato T, Wada K, Arahori H, Kuno N, Imoto K, Iwahashi-Shima C, Kusaka S. Serum concentrations of bevacizumab (avastin) and vascular endothelial growth factor in infants with retinopathy of prematurity. Am J Ophthalmol. 2012;153(327–333): e1.
26. Wu WC, Lien R, Liao PJ, Wang NK, Chen YP, Chao AN, Chen KJ, Chen TL, Hwang YS, Lai CC. Serum levels of vascular endothelial growth factor and related factors after intravitreous bevacizumab injection for retinopathy of prematurity. JAMA Ophthalmol. 2015;133:391–7.
27. Wallace DK, Kraker RT, Freedman SF, et al. Assessment of lower doses of intravitreous bevacizumab for retinopathy of prematurity: a phase 1 dosing study. JAMA Ophthalmol. 2017. https://doi.org/10.1001/jamaophthalmol.2017.1055.
28. Wallace DK, Dean TW, Hartnett ME, et al. A dosing study of bevacizumab for retinopathy of prematurity: late recurrences and additional treatments. Ophthalmology. 2018;125:1961–6.
29. Krohne TU, Holz FG, Meyer CH. Pharmacokinetics of intravitreally administered VEGF inhibitors. Ophthalmologe. 2014;111:113–20.
30. Stahl A, Krohne TU, Eter N, et al. Comparing alternative ranibizumab dosages for safety and efficacy in retinopathy of prematurity: A randomized clinical trial. JAMA Pediatr. 2018. https://doi.org/10.1001/jamapediatrics.2017.4838.
31. Stahl A, Lepore D, Fielder A, et al. Ranibizumab versus laser therapy for the treatment of very low birthweight infants with retinopathy of prematurity (RAINBOW): an open-label randomised controlled trial. The Lancet. 2019;394:1551–9.
32. Fidler M, Fleck BW, Stahl A, et al. Ranibizumab population pharmacokinetics and free VEGF pharmacodynamics in preterm infants with retinopathy of prematurity in the RAINBOW trial. Transl Vis Sci Technol. 2020;9:43.
33. Marlow N, Stahl A, Lepore D, Fielder A, Reynolds JD, Zhu Q, Weisberger A, Stiehl DP, Fleck B. 2-year outcomes of ranibizumab versus laser therapy for the treatment of very low birthweight infants with retinopathy of prematurity (RAINBOW extension study): prospective follow-up of an open label, randomised controlled trial. Lancet Child Adolesc Health. 2021;5:698–707.
34. EMA.Europa.eu. 2020. Lucentis 10 mg/ml solution for injection SmPC.
35. Stahl A, Sukgen E, Wu W-C, Lepore D, Azuma N, Nakanishi H, Mazela J. Efficacy and safety of intravitreal aflibercept compared with laser photocoagulation for patients with retinopathy of prematurity: The FIREFLEYE study. 2021.
36. Avery RL, Castellarin AA, Steinle NC, et al. Systemic pharmacokinetics following intravitreal injections of ranibizumab, bevacizumab or aflibercept in patients with neovascular AMD. Br J Ophthalmol. 2014;98:1636–41.
37. Kinsey VE. Retrolental fibroplasia; cooperative study of retrolental fibroplasia and the use of oxygen. AMA Arch Ophthalmol. 1956;56:481–543.
38. Avery ME, Oppenheimer EH. Recent increase in mortality from byaline membrane disease. J Pediatr. 1960;57:553–9.
39. The STOP-ROP Multicenter Study Group. Supplemental Therapeutic Oxygen for Prethreshold Retinopathy Of Prematurity (STOP-ROP), a randomized, controlled trial. I: primary outcomes. Pediatrics. 2000;105:295–310.
40. Askie LM, Henderson-Smart DJ, Irwig L, Simpson JM. Oxygen-saturation targets and outcomes in extremely preterm infants. N Engl J Med. 2003;349:959–67.
41. Stenson B, Brocklehurst P, Tarnow-Mordi W. Increased 36-week survival with high oxygen saturation target in extremely preterm infants. N Engl J Med. 2011;364:1680–2.
42. Askie LM, Darlow BA, Finer N, et al. Association between oxygen saturation targeting and death or disability in extremely preterm infants in the neonatal oxygenation prospective meta-analysis collaboration. JAMA. 2018;319:2190–201.

43. Reynolds JD, Hardy RJ, Kennedy KA, Spencer R, van Heuven WAJ, Fielder AR. Lack of efficacy of light reduction in preventing retinopathy of prematurity. N Engl J Med. 1998;338:1572–6.
44. Hellström A, Nilsson AK, Wackernagel D, et al. Effect of enteral lipid supplement on severe retinopathy of prematurity: a randomized clinical trial. JAMA Pediatr. 2021. https://doi.org/10.1001/jamapediatrics.2020.5653.
45. Hellström A, Engström E, Hård A-L, et al. Postnatal serum insulin-like growth factor I deficiency is associated with retinopathy of prematurity and other complications of premature birth. Pediatrics. 2003;112:1016–20.
46. Löfqvist C, Engström E, Sigurdsson J, Hård A-L, Niklasson A, Ewald U, Holmström G, Smith LEH, Hellström A. Postnatal head growth deficit among premature infants parallels retinopathy of prematurity and insulin-like growth factor-1 deficit. Pediatrics. 2006;117:1930–8.
47. Ley D, Hallberg B, Hansen-Pupp I, et al. rhIGF-1/rhIGFBP-3 in preterm infants: a phase 2 randomized controlled trial. J Pediatr. 2019;206:56-65.e8.
48. Holmström GE, Hellström A, Jakobsson PG, Lundgren P, Tornqvist K, Wallin A. Swedish National Register for Retinopathy of Prematurity (SWEDROP) and the evaluation of screening in Sweden. Arch Ophthalmol. 2012;130:1418.
49. Holmström G, Hellström A, Gränse L, Saric M, Sunnqvist B, Wallin A, Tornqvist K, Larsson E. New modifications of Swedish ROP guidelines based on 10-year data from the SWEDROP register. Br J Ophthalmol. 2020;104:943–9.
50. Stahl A, Krohne T, Limburg E. Register zur Erfassung behandlungsbedürftiger Frühgeborenenretinopathie. Z Prakt Augenheilkd. 2012;500–4.
51. Walz JM, Bemme S, Reichl S, et al. Behandelte Frühgeborenenretinopathie in Deutschland: 5-Jahres-Daten des Retina.net ROP-Registers. Ophthalmol Z Dtsch Ophthalmol Ges. 2018;115:476–88.

Types of ROP: Threshold, Prethreshold, Type 1, 2, Aggressive-ROP

16

M. Margarita Parra, Melissa Chandler, and M. Elizabeth Hartnett

Abstract

Retinopathy of prematurity (ROP) is a disease that is associated with abnormal retinal vascular development followed by growth of blood vessels into the vitreous. Without early detection and treatment, abnormal intravitreal vascular growth can lead to complex retinal detachments and vision loss, making ROP a leading cause of childhood blindness worldwide. This chapter reviews definitions of levels of severity of ROP as well as new terms regression and reactivation from the International Classification of ROP third edition. Growing knowledge of the pathophysiology of ROP has led to the recognition that vascularization of the peripheral avascular retina can occur as a form of regression and is distinct from regression of adult forms of retinopathy. Clinical cases of ROP will be used as examples to clarify the terminology.

Keywords

Retinopathy of prematurity · Pathophysiology · Threshold · Regression · Vascularization into the peripheral avascular retina · Reactivation

M. M. Parra
Department of Ophthalmology and Visual Sciences, Moran Eye Center, University of Utah, Medellin, Antioquia, Colombia
e-mail: mparra.md@gmail.com

M. Chandler · M. E. Hartnett (✉)
Department of Ophthalmology and Visual Sciences, Moran Eye Center, University of Utah, Salt Lake City, Utah, USA
e-mail: me.hartnett@hsc.utah.edu; me.hartnett@stanford.edu

M. Chandler
e-mail: melissa.chandler@hsc.utah.edu

Introduction

Retinopathy of prematurity (ROP) is a vasoproliferative disease that affects developing retina in premature infants and is a leading cause of childhood blindness [1, 2]. The pathophysiology of ROP is complex and has evolved with changes in neonatal care [2]. Genetic factors as well as events that occur prenatally, perinatally and during the time the preterm infant spends in the neonatal nursery can be involved, some of which include maternal factors, nutritional status, oxygen supplementation, and oxidative stress [2–5]. Together the stresses involved in the preterm infant can trigger abnormal angiogenic and other signaling mechanisms in the retina [2–6].

Understanding the pathogenetic mechanisms is important as are effective screening, diagnosis and treatment [7]. In 2018, the American Academy of Ophthalmology, the American Association of Pediatrics, the American Association for Pediatric Ophthalmology and Strabismus, and the American Association of Certified Orthoptists established guidelines for screening premature infants for ROP in the US [7]. However, the parameters for screening premature infants, particularly birth weight and gestational age, vary geographically based on regional characteristics associated with developing severe ROP [8]. Therefore, screening criteria vary among different countries [8–11] (Table 16.1).

The classification of ROP has evolved over time also with advances in neonatal care, technology and treatments. The newest International Classification of ROP, third edition (ICROP3), proposed updates to the severity of ROP and defined the continuum of plus disease, as well as regression and reactivation [12]. Among other features, ICROP3 also included aggressive posterior ROP within a broader term, aggressive ROP (A–ROP), which has peripheral pathology with vascular loss [12].

The criteria for treatment-warranted ROP also differ throughout the world. It is helpful to put into context the evolution of definitions of treatment-warranted ROP based on major clinical trials performed over the years. The Cryotherapy for Retinopathy of Prematurity (CRYO-ROP) study addressed the risk of an unfavorable outcome of ROP and introduced the terms prethreshold ROP and threshold ROP [13–16]. The CRYO-ROP study defined treatment-warranted ROP as threshold disease, in which there was a 50% risk of an unfavorable outcome [13]. It was recognized that eyes in zone I had about an 80% risk of an unfavorable outcome [17, 18]. With this observation came the idea that earlier treatment might lead to improved outcomes. The technology to deliver laser through indirect delivery had also been developed since the CRYO-ROP study. The Early Treatment for Retinopathy of Prematurity (ETROP) study defined treatment-warranted ROP as a less severe form of prethreshold ROP, called type 1 ROP, in which the risk of an unfavorable outcome was ~15% [19].

Table 16.1 Different screening criteria for ROP worldwide

Study	Country	Criteria
Bas et al. Br J Ophthalmol. 2018[*]	Turkey	GA $\leq$ 34 weeks or a BW <1700 g
Rajvardhan et al. Asia–Pacific Journal of Opht. 2020[**]	India	GA <34 weeks or BW <2000 g
Carrion et al. Clin Ophthalmol. 2011[***]	Latin America	Inclusion criteria for patients in the studies ranged between birth weight $\leq$ 1500 g and $\leq$ 2000 g and gestational age $\leq$ 32 and <37 weeks
Mora et al., Br J Ophthalmol. 2018[****]	Dominican Republic	GA <35 weeks, BW <2500 g
	Egypt and Serbia	GA <37 weeks, BW <1500 g BW

GA: Gestational age, BW: Birth weight
* Bas AY, Demirel N, Koc E, Ulubas Isik D, Hirfanoglu İM, Tunc T; TR-ROP Study Group. Incidence, risk factors and severity of retinopathy of prematurity in Turkey (TR-ROP study): a prospective, multicentre study in 69 neonatal intensive care units. Br J Ophthalmol. 2018;102(12):1711–1716
** Azad R, Gilbert C, Gangwe AB, Zhao P, Wu WC, Sarbajna P, Vinekar A. Retinopathy of Prematurity: How to Prevent the Third Epidemics in Developing Countries. Asia Pac J Ophthalmol (Phila). 2020;9(5):440–448
*** Carrion JZ, Fortes Filho JB, Tartarella MB, Zin A, Jornada ID Jr. Prevalence of retinopathy of prematurity in Latin America. Clin Ophthalmol. 2011;5:1687–95
**** Mora JS, Waite C, Gilbert CE, Breidenstein B, Sloper JJ. A worldwide survey of retinopathy of prematurity screening. Br J Ophthalmol. 2018;102(1):9–13
The copyright holder of this content is M. Elizabeth Hartnett, MD and permission is required for reprint and reuse

Unlike threshold ROP that occurred on average at 37 weeks post-menstrual age (PMA), type 1 ROP peaked at approximately 35 weeks PMA [20–22] (PMA is the sum of gestational and chronologic ages in weeks). Type 2 ROP included other forms of prethreshold ROP that did not require treatment but that needed careful monitoring for the development of type 1 ROP [23, 24].

This chapter discusses pathophysiology and provides information regarding regression, progression of stage 4 ROP, and reactivation after treatment for ROP including the need to identify characteristics of physiologic versus pathologic angiogenic growth after anti-vascular endothelial growth factor (VEGF) agents.

Epidemiology

The incidence of ROP has changed over time and differs throughout the world [1]. In developing countries that previously experienced poor survival of preterm infants, advances in neonatal care have led to increased survival [1–3]. However, resources to optimize prenatal care and the regulation of supplemental oxygen were limited, and ROP resulted [3–5]. The time differences when advancements in neonatal care occurred aligns with the recognition of three different epidemics of ROP [25]. The second epidemic was described in the US and developed countries following the implementation of oxygen monitoring and regulation and the survival of extremely premature infants [26, 27]. The third epidemic was described in middle-income countries in Latin America and Eastern Europe and more recently is occurring in countries in East and South Asia, and in South Africa [25]. A review of studies from 10 Latin American countries reported the changes in prevalence of any stage of ROP to be from 6.6 to 82% and of severe ROP to be from 1.2 to 23.8% from 2000 to 2010 [10]. A study from the US reported an increase in ROP incidence from 14.70% in 2000 to 19.88% in 2012 [28]. While these increases in ROP were occurring, the number of trained ophthalmologists to screen and manage ROP has not kept up to meet the demand [2, 29, 30].

Since ROP is a common cause of childhood blindness worldwide, the unmet need for screening aligns with the concern of increases in blindness [2]. In 2010, it was estimated that globally 32,300 infants were becoming blind or visually impaired from ROP every year [2, 31–33]. Middle-income regions of Latin America and regions from East Asia/Pacific and North Africa/Middle East were estimated to account for 60% of ROP cases worldwide and 65% of visually impaired worldwide survivors [22]. In high-income countries, the estimated number of preterm births at risk of ROP was 149,000 with 1.1% risk of severe visual impairment or blindness [22, 34]. In low-income countries, the estimated number of preterm births at risk of ROP was 82,200 in North Africa and Middle East, and 31,200 in Sub-Saharian African, with 2.8% of visual impairment [22]. The use of telemedicine approaches to increase screening for referral-warranted ROP has been developed in countries worldwide [2, 29, 30, 35].

The prevalence of ROP severity and treatment-warranted ROP also vary depending on screening criteria and the definitions to diagnose ROP [2]. In the US, the 2018 guidelines for screening premature infants for ROP stated that infants with birth weights ≤ 1500 g or gestational ages ≤ 30 weeks should be screened [7] (see Diagram 1). Other countries have adopted their own screening criteria [24] (Table 16.1).

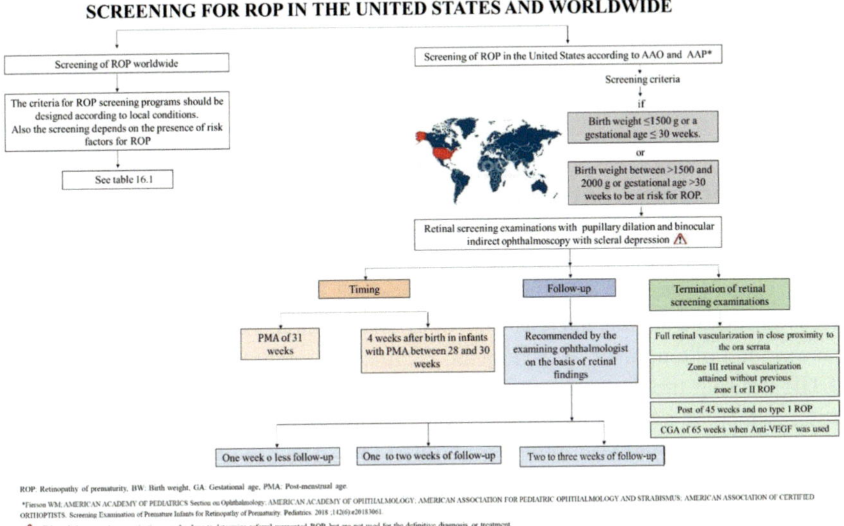

The copyright holder of this content is M. Elizabeth Hartnett, MD and permission is required for reprint and reuse.

Diagram 1 Screening criteria for ROP in the US

Pathophysiology of ROP

The understanding of the pathophysiology of ROP has evolved over time [2, 3]. This is due to increased knowledge and technical ability to delve into scientific processes and translate them to clinical care and because the ability to save and improve outcomes in preterm infants has improved.

When ROP was recognized in the US, it was prior to technology to monitor or regulate oxygen. The effect of oxygen on developing retinal vessels was analyzed in experimental studies [2–6]. A two-phase hypothesis of ROP was proposed based on studies in animal models [36]. Exposure of newborn (not premature) animals to 100% oxygen induced capillary attenuation or dropout, then known as vaso-obliteration of retinal vessels. When animals were returned to room air levels, the avascular retina became hypoxic, and this was postulated to lead to the release of pro-angiogenic factors that caused vaso-proliferation [2, 36]. As neonatal advances permitted extremely premature infants to survive, a new understanding of pathophysiologic mechanisms in ROP developed not only from clinical examinations, but also from studies using animal models that were more representative of the evolving ROP. It is now recognized that ROP involves not only capillary attenuation but also a delay in the development of the peripheral retinal vasculature [6, 22, 34, 37, 38].

The main risk factors for ROP are gestational age and low birth weight [1]. High oxygen at birth remains a risk factor. However, other factors such as extrauterine growth restriction, fluctuations in the oxygen tension and maternal factors have also been implicated [2–6].

Hypoxia-Inducible Factor (HIF)

Hypoxia inducible factors (HIF) are transcription factors that are degraded by prolyl hydroxylases in normal oxygen but are preserved in hypoxic conditions [39]. The HIFs translocate to the nucleus and bind DNA where they are involved in the transcription of a number of angiogenic factors. The suppression of the degradation of HIFs during the first phase of ROP when there is hyperoxia reduces avascular retina, which is a stimulus for the second phase of vaso-proliferation in animal models of oxygen-induced retinopathy (OIR) [39]. The use of a prolyl hydroxylase inhibitor during phase 1 to promote angiogenesis has been considered [39].

Maternal Factors, Nutrition and Extrauterine Growth Restriction

Several maternal factors important in infant health and development increase during the third trimester. When infants are born premature, they miss the benefit of such placentally-derived factors [40]. The interaction between insulin-like growth factor-1 (IGF-1) and VEGF play an important role in angiogenesis of developing retina [41–45]. Experimental studies in the mouse OIR model show that lack of IGF–1 is associated with reduced retinal vascularization even in presence of VEGF [41]. There has been a clinical trial to infuse IGF–1 to premature infants to reduce ROP (NCT01096784) [46].

IGF-I is required for maximum VEGF stimulation of angiogenic pathways through mitogen-activated protein kinase (MAPK) [43]. In preterm infants, the levels of IGF-1 are persistently low interfering with vascular growth in the developing retina. Once hypoxic retina stimulates the production of VEGF, there is enhanced angiogenesis that can lead to extraretinal vasoproliferation [43].

Another factor important in the pathophysiology of ROP are polyunsaturated fatty acids (PUFAs). Preterm infants lack maternal PUFAs [3]. It was been proposed that supplementation of omega-3 PUFAs during the first phase of ROP can provide protection from retinal neovascularization in animal models [3, 47–49]. A recent clinical trial evaluated the effect of enteral lipid supplements on severe ROP [50]. The study demonstrated that enteral supplementation of arachidonic acid and docosahexaenoic acid reduced the risk of severe ROP by 50% [50].

VEGF and Receptors

Animal models of OIR have provided a great deal of information on causes of extraretinal vasoproliferation, analogous to stage 3 ROP. The most commonly used model is in the mouse developed by Lois Smith and colleagues [51]. This model has several benefits including the ability to manipulate molecular pathways through gene modifications and to study angiogenesis, particularly in aggressive forms of ROP. The rat model of OIR, developed by John Penn [52], most closely represents ROP currently by demonstrating compromise of the newly developed vessels in the vascularized retina as well as delayed peripheral vascular development with regions of peripheral avascular retina in phase I and extraretinal vasoproliferation in phase II. The beagle model of OIR, developed by Jerry Lutty and colleagues, also represents ROP but uses extremely high oxygen similar to the mouse model [53].

From a number of experimental studies over the years, it is recognized that many different angiogenic factors and regulators are involved in retinal vascular development and extraretinal vasoproliferation. Of these, VEGF has become one of the most important angiogenic factors involved in adult retinovascular and choroidal neovascular diseases [54]. Since many of the preclinical models for anti-VEGF agents in adult diseases used models of OIR, it was relatively straight forward to postulate that anti-VEGF agents might reduce stage 3 ROP. Early case reports of anti-VEGF agents in infants with severe ROP and a later clinical trial showed encouraging effects with inhibition of stage 3 ROP and extension of peripheral retinal vascularization [54, 55]. However, understanding how an anti-angiogenic agent would reduce stage 3 disease and enhance angiogenesis into the peripheral retina came later using the representative model of ROP in the rat [56]. Inhibition and thereby regulation of a signaling pathway through VEGF receptor 2 (VEGFR2) in retinal endothelial cells not only inhibited abnormal intravitreal blood vessel growth, but also allowed extension of blood vessel growth into the retina [38]. The regulation of VEGFR2 in endothelial cells ordered endothelial cell divisions that permitted vessel extension to the ora serrata rather than growth of cells on top of one another [38, 53, 57, 58]. The use of an intravitreal neutralizing antibody to VEGF interferes with the binding to VEGFR2. However, it is not specific to that VEGF receptor nor to endothelial cells only. Too high of a concentrated intravitreal neutralizing antibody to the VEGF ligand damaged the developing retina [53, 59–63] and led to lower levels of VEGF in the blood stream [64]. These observations raised concerns as VEGF is important to other organ development in the premature infant.

The reason intravitreal anti-VEGF caused retinal damage was that other cells in the retina besides endothelial cells rely on VEGFR2 signaling for survival and neuroprotection [59]. These include neurons and glia [53, 62, 63]. Experimental studies in the beagle OIR model provided some insight that the dose of anti-VEGF could be adjusted to inhibit pathologic and extend physiologic angiogenesis [38, 55]. This led to several studies testing different agents and doses of anti-VEGF [60–63]. Ranibizumab has a shorter half-life in the eye and infant and does not significantly reduce VEGF in the bloodstream, whereas de-escalating doses of bevacizumab to 1/20th of the original BEAT-ROP dose have shown efficacy [40, 53, 62, 63, 65, 66]. Aflibercept is being tested at several doses in clinical trials and reflects the agent used in the beagle studies (NCT04101721, NCT04015180).

In premature infants treated with anti-VEGF agents now, recurrence of blood vessel growth occurs, but there is not consensus as to what patterns of blood vessel growth reflect "normal" extension into the peripheral avascular retina versus reactivated pathologic blood vessel growth into the vitreous. Therefore, it is unclear if all "reactivation" should be re-treated such as with additional anti-VEGF treatment. If treatment is performed erroneously for normal vascular growth into the peripheral avascular retina, there is risk of reducing vascular support, damaging the retina and reducing vision. However, if treatment is not done for new forming extraretinal neovascularization, blindness from progression of severe ROP could occur. This problem cannot be studied with the detail needed to ascertain blood vessel patterns in human infant retinas using current imaging methods. Therefore, additional experimental studies are needed.

Terminology

a. Threshold ROP

In the multicenter trial CRYO-ROP, threshold disease was defined as five or more contiguous or eight cumulative 30° sectors (clock hours) of stage 3 ROP in zone I or II in the presence of "plus disease" (defined as a certain degree of dilatation and tortuosity of the retinal blood vessels in the posterior pole of the eye). Threshold disease portended a 50% risk of an unfavorable outcome, which included posterior retinal detachment, retinal fold involving the macula, or retrolental tissue [13].

b. Prethreshold ROP

CRYO-ROP study defined prethreshold ROP as any stage of ROP in zone I, stage 2 in zone II with plus disease, or stage 3 in zone II without plus disease [13].

c. Types 1 and 2 ROP

In follow up studies, many of the failures of threshold disease were those in zone I, the most posterior zone with normal retinal vascular development. In zone I of eyes the risk of an unfavorable visual outcome, which was defined as a visual acuity of 20/200 or worse, was 95%, and the risk for an unfavorable structural outcome was

88% [18]. An unfavorable structural outcome was defined as stage 4 of ROP or worse [18]. Therefore, there appeared a need for earlier treatment. The ETROP study compared early treatment with laser to conventional treatment. The benefit of early treatment of eyes with type 1 ROP resulted in 30.8% of unfavorable visual outcomes versus 53.8% in the conventional treatment group [19]. The percentage of unfavorable structural outcomes was 29.6% versus 55.6% for early treatment with laser, and conventional treatment respectively [19]. Type 1 was defined as a form of prethreshold ROP that included: "Zone I, any stage with plus disease, Zone I, stage 3 without plus disease, or Zone II, stage 2 or 3 with plus disease," whereas type 2 included other forms of prethreshold ROP "Zone I, stage 1 or 2 without plus disease or Zone II, stage 3 without plus disease" (Fig. 16.1) [23].

d. Referral Warranted ROP: Telemedicine screening examinations can be done to determine referral-warranted ROP but are not used for the definitive diagnosis or treatment. The diagnosis of referral-warranted ROP is the presence of one of the following: Stage 3 ROP, ROP zone I, or Plus disease [32].

e. Regression: Regressed ROP is defined by the presence of signs such as decreased plus disease and thinning and whitening of neovascular tissue and can occur spontaneously (Fig. 16.2) or after treatment with laser (Fig. 16.3) or anti-VEGF agents (Fig. 16.4) [12]. Vascularization into peripheral avascular retina (VPAR) can occur with spontaneous regression or regression after anti-VEGF treatment but not after laser. However, persistent avascular retina (PAR) can occur in some eyes treated with anti-VEGF or in those that have had spontaneous regression. The signs of regression are typically visible earlier after anti-VEGF therapy compared to after treatment with laser; however, reactivation of ROP can occur after spontaneous regression or after regression following treatment with anti-VEGF [12]. Regression in the absence of VPAR occurs in type 1 ROP that has been fully treated with laser, although progressive stage 4 ROP can occur after laser in eyes with more advanced forms of type 1 ROP and occurred more often when treatment was withheld until threshold disease occurred in the era of the CRYO-ROP study.

These are examples demonstrating of ROP regression.

f. Reactivation: Reactivated ROP includes features such as a new stage (stage 1 [demarcation line], stage 2 [ridge] or stage 3 [extraretinal neovascularization]), or vascular changes of recurrent vascular dilation or tortuosity [12]. Reactivation can occur over a long period of time and infants are seen through 62 weeks PMA [7] (Figs. 16.5 and 16.6).

These are examples demonstrating of ROP reactivation.

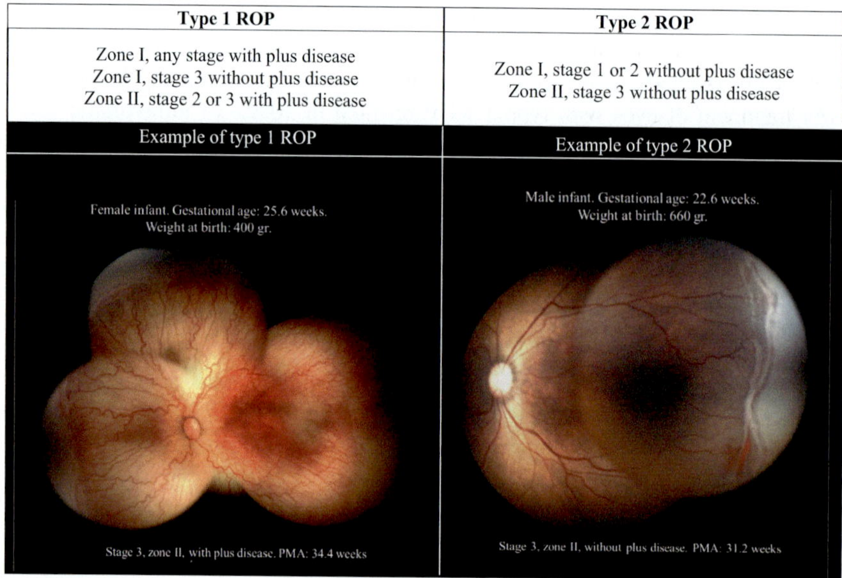

Fig. 16.1 Definitions and examples of type 1 and type 2 ROP. *The copyright holder of this content is M. Elizabeth Hartnett, MD and permission is required for reprint and reuse*

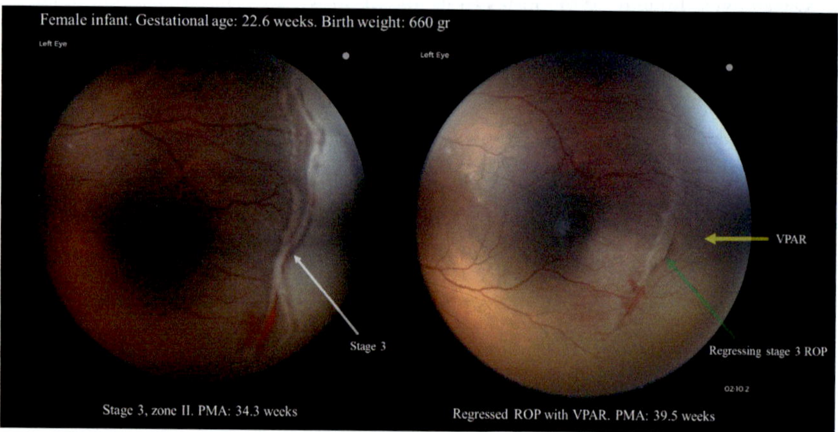

Fig. 16.2 Spontaneous regression. This patient presented with type 2 ROP (stage 3 in zone II without plus disease). Treatment was not performed. Note that ROP is regressing spontaneously, VPAR (yellow arrow) The green arrow shows a regressing stage 3 ROP. *The copyright holder of this content is M. Elizabeth Hartnett, MD and permission is required for reprint and reuse*

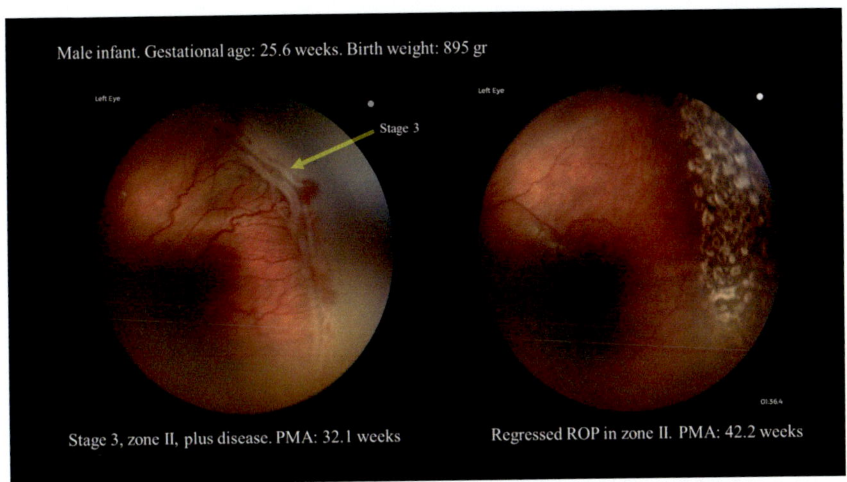

Fig. 16.3 Regression after laser treatment. Notice that the stage 3 ROP has regressed but there is no VPAR that is now ablated with laser. *The copyright holder of this content is M. Elizabeth Hartnett, MD and permission is required for reprint and reuse*

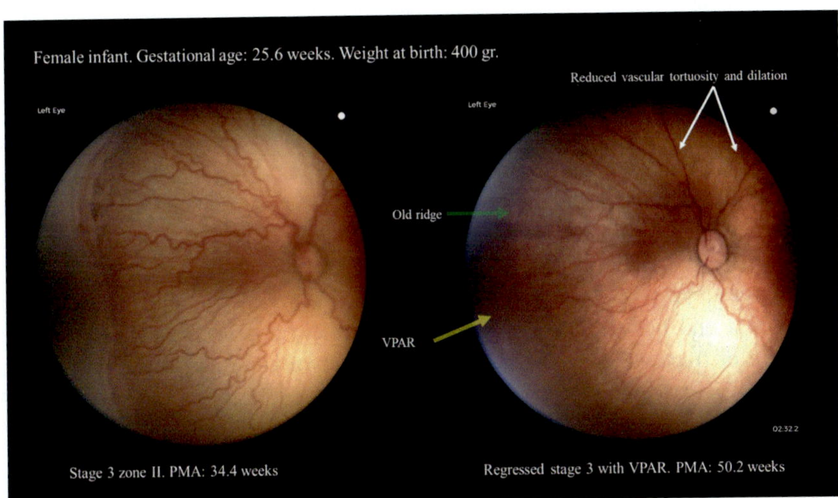

Fig. 16.4 Regression after anti-VEGF treatment. Note that regression of stage 3 ROP has occurred, and there is a faint line representing the old ridge (green arrow) and reduced vascular tortuosity and dilation. In addition, VPAR has occurred (yellow arrow). *The copyright holder of this content is M. Elizabeth Hartnett, MD and permission is required for reprint and reuse*

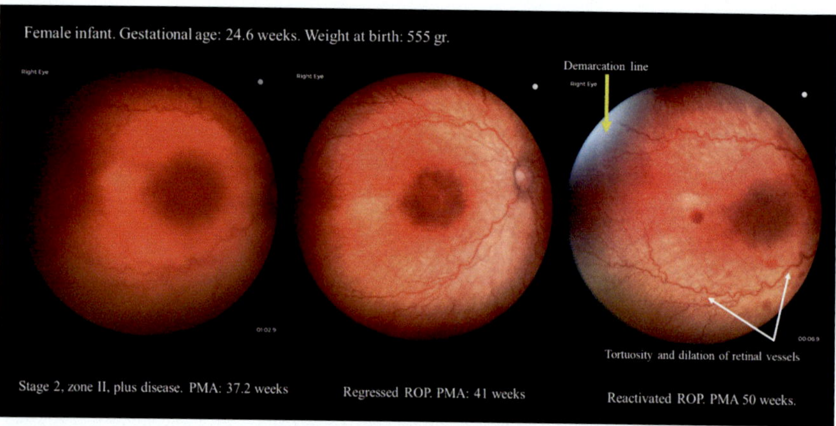

Fig. 16.5 Reactivation of stage 1, vascular dilation and tortuosity after anti-VEGF. In this case of treated type 1 ROP, there was regression of ROP with reduced vascular tortuosity and dilation (center). Nine weeks later, reactivation presented with increased dilation and tortuosity of retinal vessels (white arrows) and a new demarcation line temporally (yellow arrow). *The copyright holder of this content is M. Elizabeth Hartnett, MD and permission is required for reprint and reuse*

g. Progressive stage 4 ROP: Some patients can experience progressive stage 4 ROP (retinal detachment) following laser or anti-VEGF treatment, and the retinal elevation can be exudative or tractional or a combination of both [20, 22]. Progressive stage 4 ROP is seen less commonly since the adoption of early treatment with the ETROP study than when treatment was instituted at a more severe level for threshold disease based on the CRYO-ROP study. Features include ridge elevation, persistent or recurrent plus disease, vitreous hemorrhage and vitreous condensation or haze [67, 68]. After anti-VEGF, reactivation that is not treated can lead to progressive stage 4 ROP with elevation of the retina around the optic nerve and at the original and new ridges [69]. Other times, there can be the development of exudative or tractional stage 4 ROP that quiets down and does not progress. The presence of vitreous condensation, haze and fibrosis, plus disease and ridge elevation are concerning signs of progression.

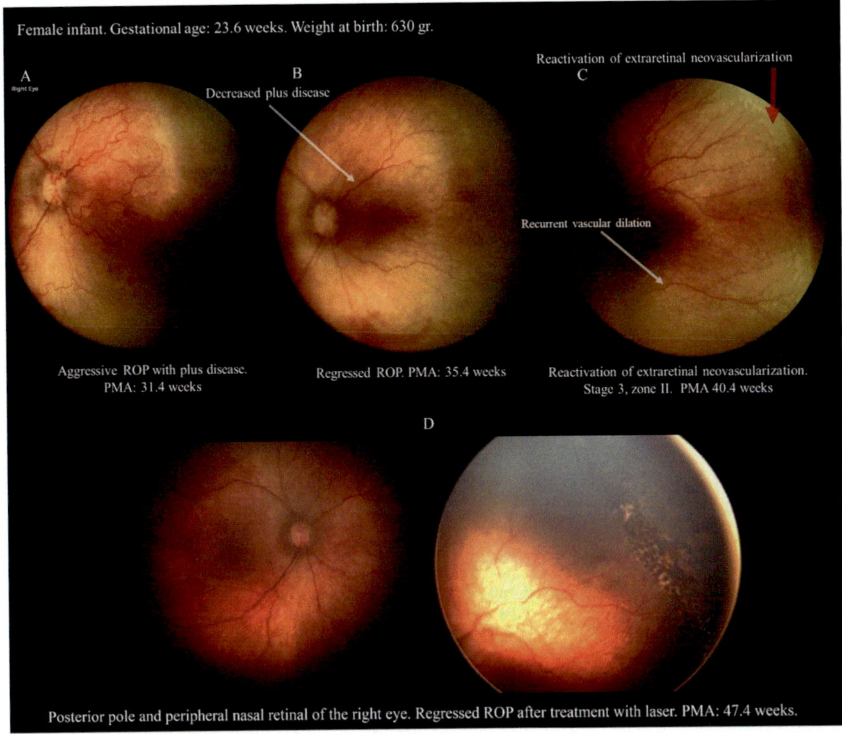

Fig. 16.6 Clinical case of reactivation of extraretinal neovascularization after anti-VEGF. A premature girl born at 23 6/7 weeks gestational age and 630 g birth weight presented at 31 4/7 weeks of PMA with aggressive ROP with dilated vascular loops and plus disease in zone I (Fig. 16.6a, right eye). Before developing ROP, she had a history of intraventricular hemorrhage grade I and severe bronchopulmonary dysplasia requiring supplementary oxygen. She received 0.25 mg Bevacizumab injection treatment at 32 5/7 weeks PMA. Three weeks after the injection, at 35 4/7 weeks PMA, reduced plus disease was evident with minimal vascularization into the peripheral avascular retina (VPAR, Fig. 16.6b). During the follow-up 8 weeks after injection, reactivation occurred with extraretinal neovascularization and retinal vascular dilation shown at PMA 40 4/7 weeks (Fig. 16.6c). At 42 3/7 weeks of PMA photocoagulation laser was delivered and regression recurred but without further VPAR (Fig. 16.6d) at 47 4/7 weeks of PMA. The copyright holder of this content is M. Elizabeth Hartnett, MD and permission is required for reprint and reuse

Review Questions

1. Which of the following statements is/are CORRECT

a. According to the CRYO-ROP study, threshold disease carries a 30% risk of an unfavorable outcome.

b. The ETROP study defined type 1 ROP as treatment-warranted ROP having a risk of an unfavorable outcome of ~ 15%.

c. Type 2 ROP is the most severe form of ROP and requires prompt treatment.

   d. Prethreshold ROP was defined by CRYO-ROP study as any stage of ROP in zone I, stage 2 in zone II with plus disease, or stage 3 in zone II without plus disease.

   e. b and d are correct

2. According to the epidemiology of ROP is CORRECT

   a. The third epidemic of ROP was described in Latin America, Eastern Europe and the US.

   b. The prevalence of ROP severity and treatment-warranted ROP do not vary worldwide.

   c. The recommended screening criteria for ROP are birth weights $\leq$ 1500 g or gestational ages $\leq$ 33 weeks, in the US.

   d. The screening criteria for ROP vary worldwide according to the local conditions and risk factors of each region.

   e. None of above is correct.

3. According to the pathophysiology of ROP which of the following questions is INCORRECT

   a. The main risk factors for ROP are gestational age and low birth weight.

   b. In animal models, the suppression of the degradation of HIFs during the first phase of ROP can prevent the progression to a vaso-proliferative phase.

   c. After birth, in preterm infants, the levels of IGF-1 are low and might interfere with vascular growth in the developing retina.

   d. Inhibition of VEGF signaling using drugs that neutralize VEGF can allow extension of vascular growth into the avascular peripheral retina.

   e. All above are correct.

4. According to regression and reactivation of ROP, which of the following is CORRECT

   a. Regression of ROP usually occurs earlier after laser treatment compared to anti-VEGF treatment.

   b. Vascularization into the peripheral retina (VPAR) is a common finding of regression of ROP after treatment with laser.

   c. Reactivation of ROP can occur after spontaneous regression, but never after treatment.

   d. Progressive stage 4 ROP seems less common since the adoption of early treatment with the ETROP study.

   e. A new stage, including a new demarcation line, ridge or stage 3, or recurrent vascular dilation or tortuosity, or VPAR are signs or reactivation of ROP.

Answers

1. (**E, B, D**) are correct.

2. (**D**) The screening criteria for ROP vary worldwide according to the local conditions and risk factors of each region.

3. (**E**)

4. (**D**) Progressive stage 4 ROP is seen less commonly since the adoption of early treatment with the ETROP study.

References

1. Gilbert CE, Lepvrier-Chomette N. In Pediatric retina. Hartnett ME, editor, 3rd ed. Philadelphia: Lippincott Williams & Wilkins. Worldwide Causes of Childhood Blindness, 2021. p. 763–84.
2. Al-Khaled T, Patel SN, Chan RVP. In Pediatric retina. Hartnett ME, editor. 3 rd ed. Philadelphia: Lippincott Williams & Wilkins. 2021. Education and Management of Retinopathy of Prematurity Worldwide, 2021. p. 784–95.
3. Hartnett ME, Penn JS. Mechanisms and management of retinopathy of prematurity. N Engl J Med. 2012;367(26):2515–26.
4. Hartnett ME. Advances in understanding and management of retinopathy of prematurity. Surv Ophthalmol. 2017;62(3):257–76.
5. Hartnett ME. Pathophysiology and mechanisms of severe retinopathy of prematurity. Ophthalmology. 2015;122(1):200–10.
6. Hartnett ME. Role of cytokines and treatment algorithms in retinopathy of prematurity. Curr Opin Ophthalmol. 2017;28(3):282–8.
7. Fierson WM. American Academy of Pediatrics Section on Ophthalmology; American Academy of Ophthalmology; American Association for Pediatric Opthalomlogy and Starbismus; American Association of Certified Orthoptists. Screening Examination of Premature Infants for Retinopathy of Prematurity. Pediatrics. 2018;142(6):e20183061.
8. Azad R, Gilbert C, Gangwe AB, Zhao P, Wu WC, Sarbajna P, Vinekar A. Retinopathy of prematurity: how to prevent the third epidemics in developing countries. Asia Pac J Ophthalmol (Phila). 2020;9(5):440–48.
9. Bas AY, Demirel N, Koc E, Ulubas Isik D, Hirfanoglu İM, Tunc T.TR-ROP Study Group. Incidence, risk factors and severity of retinopathy of prematurity in Turkey (TR-ROP study): a prospective, multicentre study in 69 neonatal intensive care units. Br J Ophthalmol. 2018;102(12):1711–16.
10. Carrion JZ, Fortes Filho JB, Tartarella MB, Zin A, Jornada ID Jr. Prevalence of retinopathy of prematurity in Latin America. Clin Ophthalmol. 2011;5:1687–95.
11. Mora JS, Waite C, Gilbert CE, Breidenstein B, Sloper JJ. A worldwide survey of retinopathy of prematurity screening. Br J Ophthalmol. 2018;102(1):9–13.
12. Chiang MF, Quinn GE, Fielder AR et al. International classification of retinopathy of prematurity, third edition. Ophthalmol. 2021;128(10):e51–68.
13. Cryotherapy for Retinopathy of Prematurity Cooperative Group. Multicentre trial of cryotherapy for retinopathy of prematurity Preliminary results. Arch Ophthalmol. 1988;106:471–9.
14. Cryotherapy for Retinopathy of Prematurity Cooperative Group. Multicenter trial of cryotherapy for retinopathy of prematurity: three month outcome. Arch Ophthalmol. 1990;108:195–204.
15. Cryotherapy for Retinopathy of Prematurity Cooperative Group. Multicenter trial of cryotherapy for retinopathy of prematurity: natural history ROP: ocular outcome at 5(1/2) years in premature infants with birth weights less than 1251g. Arch Ophthalmol. 2002;120:595–9.
16. Cryotherapy for Retinopathy of Prematurity Cooperative Group. Multicenter trial of cryotherapy for retinopathy of prematurity: ophthalmological outcomes at 10 years. Arch Ophthalmol. 2001;119(8):1110–8.
17. The Early Treatment for Retinopathy of Prematurity Cooperative Group. The early treatment for retinopathy of prematurity study: structural findings at age 2 years. Br J Ophthalmol. 2006;90(11):1378–82.
18. Vander JF, Handa J, McNamara JA, Trese M, Spencer R, Repka MX, Rubsamen P, Li H, Morse LS, Tasman WS. Early treatment of posterior retinopathy of prematurity: a controlled trial. Ophthalmol. 1997;104(11):1731–5; discussion 1735–6.

19. Good WV. Early treatment for retinopathy of prematurity cooperative. Final results of the early treatment for retinopathy of prematurity (ETROP) randomized trial. Trans Am Ophthalmol Soc. 2004;102:233–48; discussion 248–50.
20. Shulman JP, Hartnett ME. In Pediatric retina, Hartnett ME, editor. 3rd ed. Philadelphia: Lippincott Williams & Wilkins. Clinical Trials and Management of Retinopathy of Prematurity; 2021. p. 796–820.
21. Repka MX, et al. Outcome of eyes developing retinal detachment during the early treatment for retinopathy of prematurity study (ETROP). Arch Ophthalmol. 2006;124(1):24–30.
22. Blencowe H, et al. Preterm-associated visual impairment and estimates of retinopathy of prematurity at regional and global levels for 2010. Pediatr Res. 2013;74 Suppl 1:35-49.
23. Early Treatment For Retinopathy Of Prematurity Cooperative Group. Revised indications for the treatment of retinopathy of prematurity: results of the early treatment for retinopathy of prematurity randomized trial. Arch Ophthalmol. 2003;121(12):1684–94.
24. Good WV. Early Treatment for Retinopathy of Prematurity Cooperative Group. The incidence and course of retinopathy of prematurity: findings from the early treatment for retinopathy of prematurity study. Pediatrics. 2005;116(1):15–23.
25. Gilbert C, Malik ANJ, Nahar N, Das SK, Visser L, Sitati S, Ademola-Popoola DS. Epidemiology of ROP update - Africa is the new frontier. Semin Perinatol. 2019;43(6):317–22.
26. Reynolds JD, Hardy RJ, Kennedy KA, Spencer R, van Heuven WA, Fielder AR. Lack of efficacy of light reduction in preventing retinopathy of prematurity. Light Reduction in Retinopathy of Prematurity (LIGHT-ROP) Cooperative Group. N Engl J Med. 1998;338 (22):1572–6.
27. Gibson DL, Sheps SB, Schechter MT, Wiggins S, McCormick AQ. Retinopathy of prematurity: a new epidemic? Pediatrics. 1989;83(4):486–92.
28. Ludwig CA, Chen TA, Hernandez-Boussard T, Moshfeghi AA, Moshfeghi DM. The epidemiology of retinopathy of prematurity in the United States. Ophthalmic Surg Lasers Imaging Retina. 2017;48(7):553–62.
29. Paul Chan RV, Williams SL, Yonekawa Y, Weissgold DJ, Lee TC, Chiang MF. Accuracy of retinopathy of prematurity diagnosis by retinal fellows. Retina. 2010;30(6):958–65.
30. Chan RV, Patel SN, Ryan MC, Jonas KE, Ostmo S, Port AD, Sun GI, Lauer AK, Chiang MF. The global education network for retinopathy of prematurity (Gen-Rop): development, implementation, and evaluation of a novel tele-education system (an american ophthalmological society thesis). Trans Am Ophthalmol Soc. 2015;113:T2.
31. Blencowe H, Moxon S, Gilbert C. Update on blindness due to retinopathy of prematurity globally and in India. Indian Pediatr. 2016;53(Suppl 2):S89-s92.
32. Arnesen L, Durán P, Silva J, Brumana L. A multi-country, cross-sectional observational study of retinopathy of prematurity in Latin America and the Caribbean. Rev Panam Salud Publica. 2016;39(6):322–9.
33. Ells A, Hicks M, Fielden M, Ingram A. Severe retinopathy of prematurity: longitudinal observation of disease and screening implications. Eye (Lond). 2005;19(2):138–44.
34. Chan-Ling T, Gole GA, Quinn GE, Adamson SJ, Darlow BA. Pathophysiology, screening and treatment of ROP: A multi-disciplinary perspective. Prog Retin Eye Res. 2018;62:77–119.
35. Myung JS, Paul Chan RV, Espiritu MJ, et al. Accuracy of retinopathy of prematurity image-based diagnosis by pediatric ophthalmology fellows: implications for training. J AAPOS. 2011;15(6):573–8.
36. Ashton N, Ward B, Serpell G. Effect of oxygen on developing retinal vessels with particular reference to the problem of retrolental fibroplasia. Br J Ophthalmol. 1954;38(7):397–432.
37. Flynn JT, Bancalari E, Bachynski BN, Buckley EB, Bawol R, Goldberg R, Cassady J, Schiffman J, Feuer W, Gillings D, et al. Retinopathy of prematurity. Diagnosis, severity, and natural history. Ophthalmol. 1987;94(6):620–9.
38. Simmons AB, Bretz CA, Wang H, et al. Gene therapy knockdown of VEGFR2 in retinal endothelial cells to treat retinopathy. Angiogenesis. 2018;21(4):751–64.

39. Sears JE, Hoppe G, Ebrahem Q, Anand-Apte B. Prolyl hydroxylase inhibition during hyperoxia prevents oxygen-induced retinopathy. Proc Natl Acad Sci U S A. 2008;105 (50):19898–903.

40. Becker S, Wang H, Yu B, Brown R, Han X, Lane RH, Hartnett ME. Protective effect of maternal uteroplacental insufficiency on oxygen-induced retinopathy in offspring: removing bias of premature birth. Sci Rep. 2017;7:42301.

41. Hellstrom A, Perruzzi C, Ju M, Engstrom E, Hard AL, Liu JL, Albertsson-Wikland K, Carlsson B, Niklasson A, Sjodell L, LeRoith D, Senger DR, Smith LE. Low IGF-I suppresses VEGF-survival signaling in retinal endothelial cells: direct correlation with clinical retinopathy of prematurity. Proc Natl Acad Sci U S A. 2001;98(10):5804–8.

42. Smith LE, Shen W, Perruzzi C, Soker S, Kinose F, Xu X, Robinson G, Driver S, Bischoff J, Zhang B, Schaeffer JM, Senger DR. Regulation of vascular endothelial growth factor-dependent retinal neovascularization by insulin-like growth factor-1 receptor. Nat Med. 1999;5(12):1390–5.

43. Hellström A, Hård AL, Engström E, Niklasson A, Andersson E, Smith L, Löfqvist C. Early weight gain predicts retinopathy in preterm infants: new, simple, efficient approach to screening. Pediatrics. 2009;123(4):e638–45.

44. Löfqvist C, Andersson E, Sigurdsson J, Engström E, Hård AL, Niklasson A, Smith LE, Hellström A. Longitudinal postnatal weight and insulin-like growth factor I measurements in the prediction of retinopathy of prematurity. Arch Ophthalmol. 2006;124(12):1711–8.

45. Hellström A, Engström E, Hård AL, Albertsson-Wikland K, Carlsson B, Niklasson A, Löfqvist C, Svensson E, Holm S, Ewald U, Holmström G, Smith LE. Postnatal serum insulin-like growth factor I deficiency is associated with retinopathy of prematurity and other complications of premature birth. Pediatrics. 2003;112(5):1016–20.

46. Ley D, Hallberg B, Hansen-Pupp I, Dani C, et al. rhIGF-1/rhIGFBP-3 in preterm infants: a phase 2 randomized controlled trial. J Pediatr. 2019;206:56–65 e8.

47. Heidary G, Vanderveen D, Smith LE. Retinopathy of prematurity: current concepts in molecular pathogenesis. Semin Ophthalmol. 2009;24(2):77–81.

48. Mukherjee PK, Chawla A, Loayza NG, Bazan NG. Docosanoids are multifunctional regulators of neural cell integrity and fate: significance in aging and disease. Prostaglandins Leukot Essent Fatty Acids. 2007;77(5–6):233–8.

49. Connor KM, SanGiovanni JP, Lofqvist C, et al. Increased dietary intake of omega-3-polyunsaturated fatty acids reduces pathological retinal angiogenesis. Nat Med. 2007;13(7):868–73.

50. Hellström A, Nilsson AK, Wackernagel D, et al. Effect of enteral lipid supplement on severe retinopathy of prematurity: a randomized clinical trial. JAMA Pediatr. 2021;175(4):359–67.

51. Smith LE, Wesolowski E, McLellan A, Kostyk SK, D'Amato R, Sullivan R, D'Amore PA. Oxygen-induced retinopathy in the mouse. Invest Ophthalmol Vis Sci. 1994;35(1):101–11.

52. Penn JS, Henry MM, Tolman BL. Exposure to alternating hypoxia and hyperoxia causes severe proliferative retinopathy in the newborn rat. Pediatr Res. 1994;36(6):724–31.

53. Lutty GA, McLeod DS, Bhutto I, Wiegand SJ. Effect of VEGF trap on normal retinal vascular development and oxygen-induced retinopathy in the dog. Invest Ophthalmol Vis Sci. 2011;52 (7):4039–47.

54. Hartnett ME. Discovering mechanisms in the changing and diverse pathology of retinopathy of prematurity: the Weisenfeld award lecture. Invest Ophthalmol Vis Sci. 2019;60(5):1286–97.

55. Mintz-Hittner HA, Kennedy KA, Chuang AZ.BEAT-ROP Cooperative Group. Efficacy of intravitreal bevacizumab for stage 3+ retinopathy of prematurity. N Engl J Med. 2011;364 (7):603–715.

56. Penn JS, Tolman BL, Lowery LA. Lowery, Variable oxygen exposure causes preretinal neovascularization in the newborn rat. Invest Ophthalmol Vis Sci. 1993;34(3):576–85.

57. Hartnett ME, Martiniuk D, Byfield G, Geisen P, Zeng G, Bautch VL. Neutralizing VEGF decreases tortuosity and alters endothelial cell division orientation in arterioles and veins in a rat model of ROP: relevance to plus disease. Invest Ophthalmol Vis Sci. 2008;49(7):3107–14.

58. McLeod DS, Lutty GA. Targeting VEGF in canine oxygen-induced retinopathy - a model for human retinopathy of prematurity. Eye Brain. 2016;8:55–65.
59. Becker S, Wang H, Simmons AB, Suwanmanee T, Stoddard GJ, Kafri T, Hartnett ME. Targeted Knockdown of Overexpressed VEGFA or VEGF164 in Muller cells maintains retinal function by triggering different signaling mechanisms. Sci Rep. 2018;8(1):2003.
60. Wallace DK, Kraker RT, Freedman SF, et al. Assessment of lower doses of intravitreous bevacizumab for retinopathy of prematurity: a phase 1 dosing study. JAMA Ophthalmol. 2017;135(6):654–6.
61. Wallace DK, Dean TW, Hartnett ME, Kong L, Smith LE, Hubbard GB, McGregor ML, Jordan CO, Mantagos IS, Bell EF, Kraker. Pediatric Eye Disease Investigator Group. A dosing study of bevacizumab for retinopathy of prematurity: late recurrences and additional treatments. Ophthalmol. 2018;125(12): 1961–1966.
62. Wallace DK, Kraker RT, Freedman SF, et al. Short-term outcomes after very low-dose intravitreous bevacizumab for retinopathy of prematurity. JAMA Ophthalmol. 2020;138 (6):698–701.
63. Stahl A, Lepore D, Fielder A, Fleck B, Reynolds JD, Chiang MF, Li J, Liew M, Maier R, Zhu Q, Marlow N. Ranibizumab versus laser therapy for the treatment of very low birthweight infants with retinopathy of prematurity (RAINBOW): an open-label randomised controlled trial. Lancet. 2019;394(10208):1551–9.
64. Wang H, Yang Z, Jiang Y, Flannery J, Hammond S, Kafri T, Vemuri SK, Jones B, Hartnett ME. Quantitative analyses of retinal vascular area and density after different methods to reduce VEGF in a rat model of retinopathy of prematurity. Invest Ophthalmol Vis Sci. 2014;55(2):737–44.
65. Wang H, Han X, Gambhir D, Becker S, Kunz E, Liu AJ, Hartnett ME. Retinal inhibition of CCR3 induces retinal cell death in a murine model of choroidal neovascularization. PLoS ONE. 2016;11(6): e0157748.
66. Hartnett ME, Wallace DK, Dean TW, Li Z, Boente CS, Dosunmu EO, Freedman SF, Golden RP, Kong L, Prakalapakorn SG, Repka MX, Smith LE, Wang H, Kraker RT, Cotter SA, Holmes JM. For Writing Committee for the Pediatric Eye Disease Investigator Group. Plasma levels of bevacizumab and vascular endothelial growth factor after low-dose bevacizumab treatment for retinopathy of prematurity in infants. JAMA Ophthalmol. 2022 Apr 1;140(4):337–344. https://doi.org/10.1001/jamaophthalmol.2022.0030. Erratum in: JAMA Ophthalmol. 2022 Apr 1;140(4):441. PMID: 35446359; PMCID: PMC8895318.
67. Hartnett ME, McColm JR. Retinal features predictive of progressive stage 4 retinopathy of prematurity. Retina. 2004;24(2):237–41.
68. Hartnett ME, McColm JR. Fibrovascular organization in the vitreous following laser for ROP: implications for prognosis. Retina. 2006;26(7 Suppl):S24-31.
69. Yonekawa Y, Thomas BJ, Thanos A, Todorich B, Drenser KA, Trese MT, Capone A Jr. The cutting edge of retinopathy of prematurity care: expanding the boundaries of diagnosis and treatment. Retina. 2017;37(12):2208–25.

Type 1 ROP Management: Laser Versus Anti-VEGF Injection

17

María Ana Martínez-Castellanos, Alejandro Ortega-Desio, and Fernando Del Valle-Nava

Abstract

Laser retina ablation for ROP treatment remains as the standard treatment, however, due to the large number of side effects many ophthalmologists and retina specialist are encouraged to use anti-VEGF drugs. Many concerns exist about anti-VEGF therapy for ROP, most are due to lack of good quality trials and a different clinical definition. This chapter reviews the main advantages and disadvantages between two treatment modalities and some recommendations about injection technique.

Keywords

VEGF · Anti-VEGF · Ranibizumab · Bevacizumab · Aflibercept · ROP · Laser photocoagulation · Avascular retina · Intravitreal injection · Recurrence

Retinopathy of prematurity (ROP) remains as a leading cause of infant blindness worldwide, especially in developing countries because of frequently inappropriate access to adequate neonatal care and ROP screening programs. Due to VEGF role in ROP pathogenesis, leading to uncontrolled vasculogenesis and neovascularization, peripheral retinal laser photocoagulation remains the current standard of care for treatment-requiring ROP type 1 [1]. The aim of this modality is the destruction of avascular retina, in order to reduce vascular endothelial growth factor (VEGF) levels and induce regression of neovascularization. The theoretical mechanism is the destruction of the avascular retina producing increased levels of VEGF with laser photocoagulation. This eliminates the angiogenic signals by destroying distressed cells that produce VEGF-inducing cytokines and VEGF [2].

M. A. Martínez-Castellanos (✉) · A. Ortega-Desio · F. Del Valle-Nava
Hospital Luis Sanchez Bulnes, Asociación Para Evitar La Ceguera en Mexico,
46 Calle Vicente Garcia Torres, Coyoacan, Ciudad de Mexico, Mexico
e-mail: mamc@dr.com

© The Author(s), under exclusive license to Springer Nature Switzerland AG 2023   221
Ş. Özdek et al. (eds.), *Pediatric Vitreoretinal Surgery*,
https://doi.org/10.1007/978-3-031-14506-3_17

Being an ablative treatment, laser photocoagulation exerts several effects on the eye and retina specifically, that are subsequently evident during future development as unwanted effects.

Following the development of the anti-VEGF agents, controversy arose around laser being superior to anti-VEGF or vice versa, with advantages and disadvantages in both of them.

Advantages of Laser Treatment

- Less unfavorable outcomes as compared to cryotherapy.
- Less ROP recurrence and re-treatment as compared to anti-VEGFs (defined as recurrent plus disease, recurrent neovascularization, or reformation of ridge despite treatment) [2, 3].
- More effective in Zone II and III [3].
- Less need for follow-up after treatment [5, 8].
- Effectiveness with different wavelength lasers frequency-doubled Nd-YAG green laser (532 nm), Diode (810 nm).
- Portable and transferable.
- No risk of endophthalmitis.

Disadvantages of Laser Treatment

- Skipped areas (associated with recurrences and re-treatment) (Fig. 17.1) [3, 6].

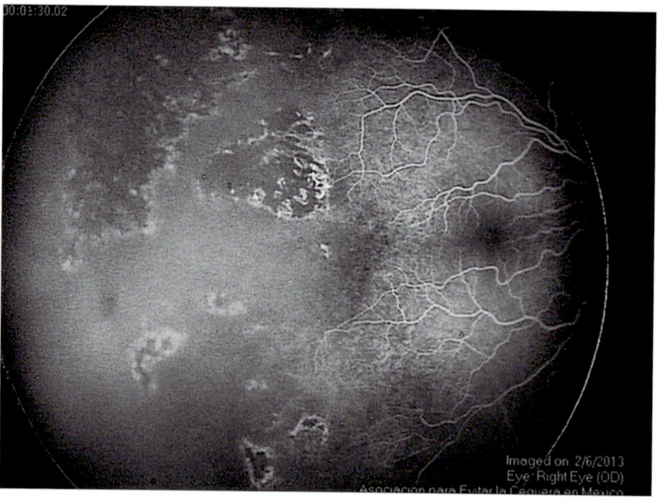

Fig. 17.1 Laser skipped areas in a zone 1 ROP case

- Experienced physician requirement.
- Blockage of emmetropization process and anterior segment development (presumably due to peripheral retina destruction) [3].
- Increased myopia rate (due to scleral wall weakness) and visual field loss [5, 7, 8].
- Less effective in Zone I disease [3].
- Sedation or general anaesthesia requirement at neonatal intensive care unit (NICU) or operating room (OR) [4].
- Increased adverse events rate and life-threatening events when applied under topical anaesthesia [4].
- More time is required for treatment as compared to anti-VEGF injection (1 or more sessions, requiring 30 or more minutes).
- Delayed anti-VEGF reduction [4].
- Anterior segment complications (corneal burn, iris burn, anterior synechiae, cataract formation, anterior segment ischemia and phthisis bulbi development) [8].
- Posterior segment complications (iatrogenic retinal tears, choroidal haemorrhage, exudative retinal detachment, vitreous haemorrhage) [10].

Despite several disadvantages, retinal photocoagulation remains as a very important treatment modality in ROP therapy, whereby specialists should be encouraged to improve their skills in laser application as it is proven useful and has relatively easy access to it.

In the case of patients who are unable to access to a proper follow up, laser is a fundamental tool, as its appropriate application allows an adequate disease stabilization with a permanent effect.

Anti-VEGF Treatment

Laser treatment has been shown to be associated with improved anatomical and visual outcome in the Early Treatment for Retinopathy of Prematurity (ETROP) Study. However, when ROP is present in the posterior retina that affects zone I or posterior zone II, the success of laser treatment is around 50% and has some disadvantages such as: the destruction of large areas of avascular retina that leads to a significant loss of the peripheral visual field and the development of high myopia. Furthermore, up to 50% of children with posterior aggressive disease progressed to tractional retinal detachment when treated with laser [11, 12].

At the beginning of the 2000s, the knowledge about retinopathy of premature (ROP) was improved; the role of VEGF as the main molecule involved in the development of ROP was demonstrated and the disadvantages of laser therapy in ROP motivated further research into new treatments. Consequently, the use of anti-VEGF drugs as an alternative to laser therapy was suggested with case reports [13–15].

With the publication of BEAT-ROP (Bevacizumab Eliminates the Angiogenic Threat for Retinopathy of Prematurity) study in 2011, clinical evidence was obtained for bevacizumab superiority in anatomical and recurrence results over laser, for the treatment of ROP [16]. Later, other clinical trials with different anti-VEGF drugs such as ranibizumab and aflibercept were conducted which enhanced available clinical evidence about anti-VEGF drugs in ROP [17–21, 23–26].

Advantages of Anti-VEGF Drugs

Recurrence Rate

BEAT-ROP study was a prospective, randomized laser-controlled clinical trial conducted in United States. A total of 286 eyes with zone I or posterior zone II, stage 3 + disease were randomized to 0.625 mg of intravitreal bevacizumab (IVB) versus conventional laser therapy in this study. A higher recurrence rate was found with laser therapy as compared to IVB for zone I and posterior zone II disease (26% vs. 6%. P = 0.002). The difference was even more remarkable for zone 1 ROP treatment, 6% in IVB group versus 42% in laser group (P = 0.003). Finally, the recurrence rate for zone II showed no significant difference compared to laser (5% vs. 12%; P = 0.27) [16].

The strongest clinical evidence for Ranibizumab monotherapy for the treatment of ROP was provided by the "ranibizumab compared with laser therapy for the treatment of infants born prematurely with retinopathy of prematurity (RAINBOW) study". The results have shown that ranibizumab 0.2 mg resulted in fewer eyes with unfavourable structural outcomes than did ranibizumab 0.1 mg or laser therapy. A higher proportion of infants treated with ranibizumab 0.2 mg reach success compared with laser therapy 80% versus 66% respectively (p = 0.051) [17].

The time and rate of recurrence were higher with ranibizumab compared with laser. Recurrence rate for laser treatment in the RAINBOW study were 18.9% and has shown-up at a mean of 16 days after baseline treatment. Conversely, recurrence among ranibizumab treatment groups was higher to be 31.1% and occurred later at a mean of 48 days.

The most recent anti-VEGF drug used in ROP is aflibercept. A few studies, mainly phase 2 studies, retrospective cohorts and large case series suggest that intravitreal aflibercept (IVA) was effective in achieving regression of all types of ROP with less need for both early and late re-treatment.

Salman et al. shows that IVA is an effective treatment for high-risk type 1 prethreshold ROP with a 7.7% recurrence rate [18]. Hovever, in a single-center retrospective cohort, Riazi-esfahani et al. found a higher recurrence rate of 58.3% (14 of 24 eyes) treated with aflibercept [19]. Ekinci et al., using two doses of IVA for ROP treatment, reported recurrence in 9 (28%) eyes in the low-dose group and 10 (24%) eyes in the standard-dose group after the complete regression of the disease with treatment (P = 0.845) [20]. Finally, Chen et al., found that a single

IVA injection resulted in total resolution of the disease in 15 eyes (88.2%), whereas 2 eyes (11.8%) needed retreatment [21].

It is to be noted that a wide discrepancy in ROP recurrence rates has been found in different studies. In a single center retrospective study comparing the recurrence rates of 3 anti-VEGFs for the treatment of ROP, there was no statistically significant difference between groups; recurrence rates were 25.9% for bevacizumab, 37.6% for ranibizumab and 23.2% for aflibercept (p = 0.15) [22]. These contradictory results may be due to the clinical definition of recurrence used, differences in dosing, treatment zones and follow-up. Therefore, although several clinical trials evaluate anti-VEGF agents, the comparison between them should be done carefully considering the differences between their protocols.

Regression

Anti-VEGF drugs induce a more rapid regression as compared to laser therapy (Fig. 17.2). Regression after laser treatment was found in 8%, 43%, 64%, 73%, and 86% of eyes at weeks 1, 2, 3, 4, and 9 respectively [22]. Following IVB, regression by at least one stage and absence of plus disease was observed in 29%, 82%, 88%, and 100% of eyes by weeks 1, 2, 3, and 4 post treatment, respectively. Mean number of days to regression was 11 ± 5.8 (median 8, range 3–23). Regression of

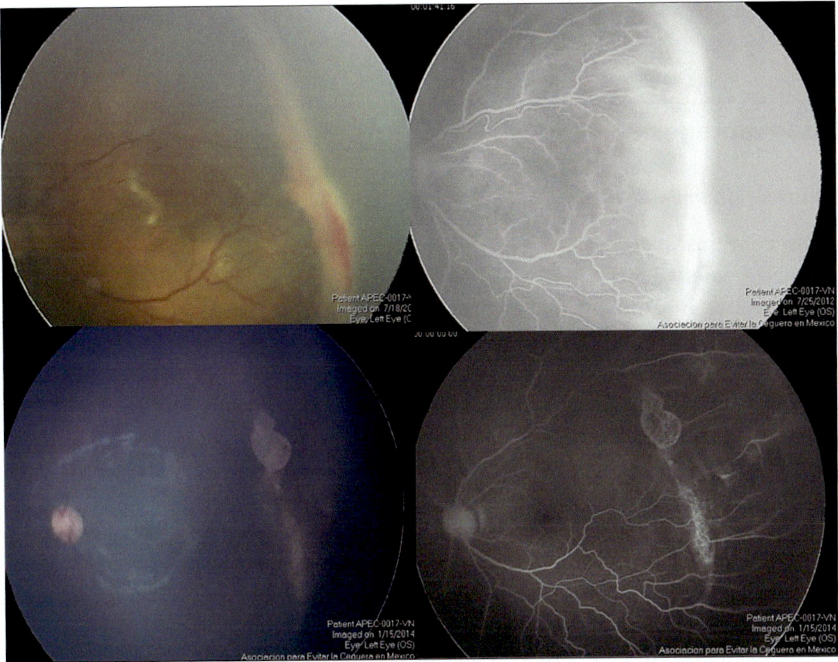

Fig. 17.2 Before and 3 years after anti-VEGF treatment for ROP type 1. Note that the previous avascular retina became vascularized during follow-up leaving some residual fibrotic tissue in the primary ridge area

plus disease was observed in 73.3%, 86.7%, and 100% of eyes by days 3, 5, and 8 post treatment, respectively [23]. The median days to regression after ranibizumab 0.2 mg versus laser were as follows: plus disease, 4 versus 16 days (P < 0.001); stage 3 ROP, 8 versus 16 days (P = 0.004); and AP-ROP, 7.3 versus 22 days (P = 0.03) [24].

Myopia

ROP eyes of children treated by laser generate a greater amount of myopia compared to those treated with anti-VEGF drugs. Chen et al. reported that the average refractive errors of patients were –0.98 ± 4.05 D (–15.6 to 5.5 D) in IVB group, –2.40 ± 3.13 D (–7.6 to 2.9 D) in IVB + laser group, and –14.38 ± 6.02 D (–21.8 to 8.1 D) in IVB + lens sparing vitrectomy group at 2 years follow up (P < 0.001) [25].

Additionally, RAINBOW study has shown that, high myopia (–5D or worse) in at least one eye was less frequent after ranibizumab 0.2 mg (7%) as compared to laser therapy (34%). (p = 0.0021) [26].

Accessibility

In comparison with laser treatment, anti-VEGF treatment can be applied in intensive care units, easy to transport and requires less physician training. Unfortunately, laser treatment may need general anesthesia, requires a longer training, and more difficult to transport.

Disadvantages

Neurodevelopmental Impair

Some concerns about anti-VEGF use in ROP remain, mainly due to the lack of long-term safety reports and the theoretical systemic VEGF suppression which could lead to impairment of newborn growth and development. Although at the time this text is written, there are only limited published evidence about growth and development impairment in children who received anti-VEGF drugs for ROP treatment, that evidence comes from biased studies. The majority of published studies did not found association of anti-VEGF drugs with neurodevelopmental impair. Finally, robust long term prospective studies are needed to assess the effects of anti-VEGF drugs on systemic biosecurity of infants [27, 28].

Endophthalmitis

The application of intravitreal injections poses a real risk of intraocular infection, fortunately, this risk is low. There are some published reports on cases of endophthalmitis associated with anti-VEGF drugs injection in infants with ROP [29, 30].

In both BEAT ROP and RAINBOW studies, the incidence of endophthalmitis was too low. In RAINBOW study only one infant in ranibizumab 0.1 mg group developed unilateral endophthalmitis and orbital infection 6 days after intravitreal injection. This infant was described as having bilateral conjunctivitis and left periocular staphylococcal infection 11 days before ranibizumab injection and treated with antibiotics. Another study found no cases of Endophthalmitis during folluw-up [31].

New initiatives have been carried out to inject children safely and with a defined protocol [32].

Cataract

Cataracts may develop as a complication of intravitreal injection of anti-VEGFs mainly due to poor intravitreal injection technique which occurs infrequently. In RAINBOW study, only one infant (ranibizumab 0.2 mg) had a moderate cataract in one eye noted on day 28, thought to be secondary to lens damage by the injecting needle. Cataract surgery was not done during the study. No cataract development was reported in bevacizumab group in BEAT ROP study.

To avoid trauma to the lens, we inject 1 mm posterior to the limbus, aiming the needle tip towards the optic nerve. We recommend inserting only half of the needle or use a short (4 mm) needle [33].

Persistent Avascular Retina (PAR)

PAR is a common finding in those eyes with ROP that does not require treatment, and those eyes who receive anti-VEGF therapy; moreover, laser treatment makes a permanent ablation in avascular retina that prevents peripheral vessel grow. Vural et al. found avascular retina in 23% of ROP type 1 eyes treated with bevacizumab, on the other hand in RAINBOW study, full vascularization of the retina was detected only in 59% of the eyes treated with ranibizumab during 2-years follow-up.

It seems that anti-VEGF treatment increase the frequency of PAR, and laser treatment reduce it.

Peripheral vascular anomalies other than PAR are also very common among ROP eyes treated with anti-VEGF drugs like anastomosing vessels forming loops, leakage in peripheral retina, rarely neovascularizations (Fig. 17.3).

Unfortunately, there are neither guidelines nor consensus about management of PAR in ROP. However, it is well known that PAR is prone to retinal thinning, development of holes, and lattice-like degenerations and may be associated with rhegmatogenous retinal detachments later in life (Fig. 17.4). Additionally, there are reports on the late recurrence of the ROP with neovascularizations and vitreous hemorrhage in these eyes. That is why many authors prefer to laser the persistent PAR in these eyes as a prophylaxis.

Currently there is no consensus about the timing and type of retreatment for ROP reactivation. Recently we proposed an algorithm based on the reactivation features. When reactivation presents with flat vessels, repeat intravitreal anti-VEGF injection

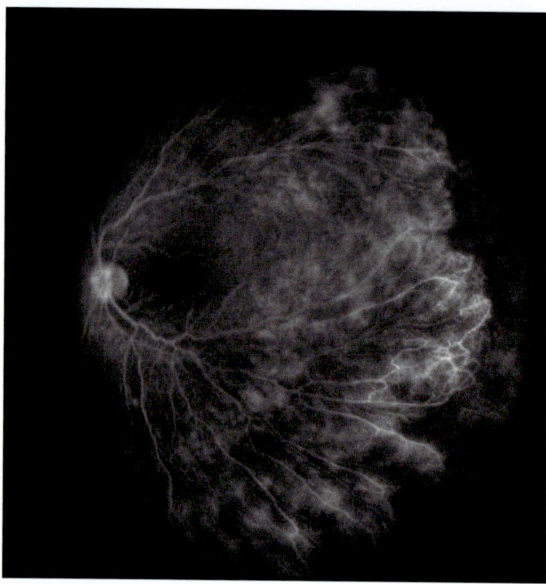

Fig. 17.3 FFA of a type 1 pretreshold ROP 4 years after treatment with anti-VEGF. Note the significant area of persistent peripheral avascular retina (PAR), late capillary leakage and peripheral anastomosing vessels forming loops

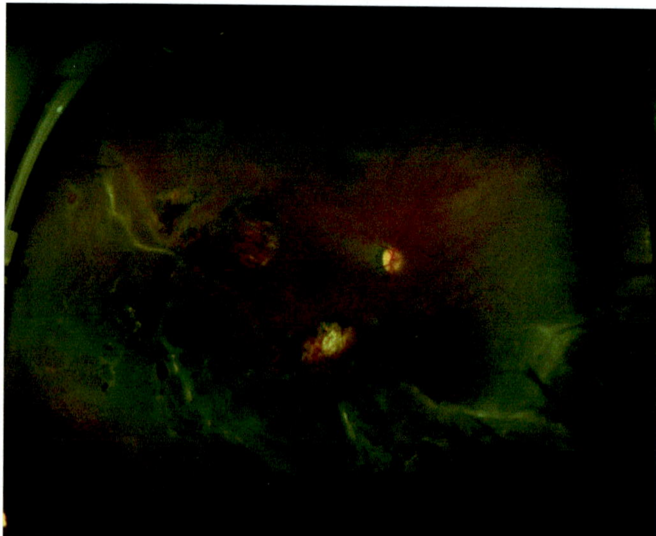

Fig. 17.4 28 years old female, born at 32 weeks never treated for ROP presented with sudden diminution of vision. Note that there are multiple retinal tears inferotemporally together with PAR and rhegmatogenous retinal detachment

is preferred; on the other hand, when neovascularization is present, a combination of anti-VEGF and laser is recommended. For fibrovascular proliferation causing retinal traction, vitrectomy is suggested.

Clinical Case Scenario (Fig. 17.5)

A premature female infant was born at 32 weeks' of gestation with a birth weight of 1,800 g in a rural hospital. She was diagnosed with respiratory distress syndrome and received continuous positive airway pressure treatment for 40 days. At 56 days after birth, the patient was transferred to our hospital for further evaluation and management. A comprehensive eye examination revealed a stage 3 ROP involving zone 2 in both eyes with vitreous traction with no retinal detachment. She underwent fluorescein angiography pre-treatment (Fig. 17.5 top). She received one injection of antiangiogenic therapy with bevacizumab 0.02 cc dose to both eyes. Three weeks after treatment we were able to assess regression of the pathological new vessels and growth of vascularization of the retina assessed with angiography, still with the mild vitreous traction with no detachment. Foveal avascular zone (FAZ) did not develop by then (Fig. 17.5 second row). Two months after treatment, we were able to see regression of the ridge and progression of the vessels towards periphery, by the time the vitreous was detached from the ridge, the FAZ is not detectable at the time (Fig. 17.5 third row). Two years after treatment we can see the growth of vessels in zone 3 and residual fibrosis in the primary ridge area. The FAZ looks fully developed. No laser was required (Fig. 17.5 bottom row).

Fig. 17.5 Look at the clinical case scenario

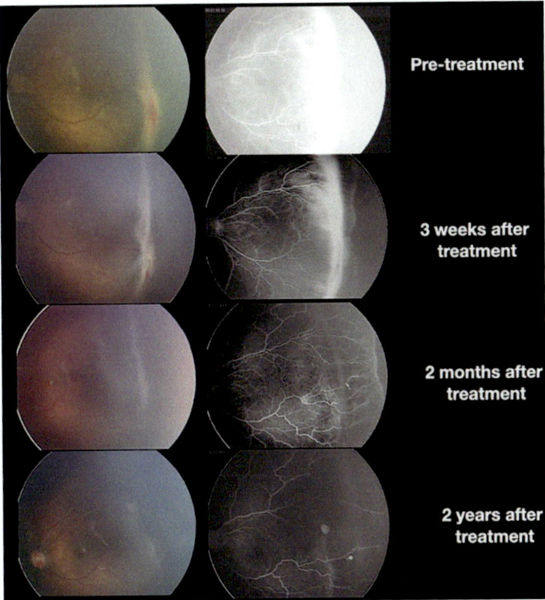

Conclusion

Laser remains as the golden standard for ROP treatment, however its lower rate of effectiveness for posterior ROP has led to the development of new treatments. There is an increase in the use of anti-VEGF therapy for ROP treatment, the advantages over laser treatment make it a very attractive treatment option. Compared with laser treatment, there is a low recurrence when posterior ROP is treated, induce a fast regression and the availability is better.

A considerable effort has been made for standardization of anti-VEGF treatment; nevertheless, the variety of protocols followed in each trial makes comparisons so difficult. When treating with anti-VEGF, it is important to consider an excellent injection protocol to avoid lens trauma and reduce endophthalmitis risk, close initial revision and then a longer follow-up to avoid late recurrences.

Injection technique suggested by SAFER-ROP report which describes an updated protocol for Anti-VEGF injections for ROP [33]:

- Injections are performed at the bedside in the neonatal intensive care unit on awake infants.
- Topical anesthetic is instilled into the eye followed by the placement of a sterile eyelid speculum.
- Betadine 5–10% drops are instilled.
- Calipers are used to measure and mark the location for the injection at 0.75 mm to 1.0 mm posterior to the temporal limbus.
- The medication is injected using the 4-mm, 32-gauge needle on a 1.0 cc syringe. The needle tip is kept parallel with the visual pupillary axis during the injection.
- Another drop of betadine is instilled, the retina is inspected for a central retinal artery occlusion, and the eyelid speculum is removed.

Technical Tips for Laser Photocoagulation [34]:

- The intensity must be grayish white rather than white and placement of spots must be nearly confluent.
- The laser power must be changed during the procedure; less energy must be used for the anterior and superior retina compared to the posterior and inferior retina or to the retina close to the ridge.
- Do not leave any untreated 'skip' areas near the posterior ridge of the avascular retina. It is safe to put 3000 – 4000 spots in each eye to cover the avascular retina to adequately treat zone I disease/ A-ROP eyes in one session. Make sure that the burns are not too intense to avoid complications like exudative retinal detachment.
- A scleral depressor is used to rotate and stabilize the globe, and to indent the anterior retina for laser. The depressor is held against the forniceal conjunctiva rather than pressing it against the globe. High pressure against the globe causes corneal haziness due to raised intraocular pressure and also hyphema and vitreous hemorrhage can occur.

- Do not depress too hard and release the pressure on the globe suddenly. This will lead to pupillary constriction and sometimes intraocular hemorrhage.
- Treat the easily accessible areas first and then proceed to the difficult areas. Start from a particular clock hour in temporal quadrant adjacent to the ridge (from posterior to anterior in the same clock hour) and do the same thing in the other areas.
- Avoid heavy confluent spots anteriorly in horizontal axis where long posterior ciliary vessels and nerves are present. Also avoid lasering beyond ora serrata to ciliary body. This may cause hypotony and cataract. Use milder intensity burns in these areas.

Review Questions

1. With which anti-VEGF drug has recurrence been found most often?

A. Bevacizumab
B. Ranibizumab
C. Aflibercept
D. Brolucizumab

2. If you decide to perform a ranibizumab injection in a patient with ROP type 1, how many weeks after initial ranibizumab injection do you expect reactivation?

A. 1 week.
B. 3 weeks
C. 7 weeks
D. 10 weeks

3. Two years after treating an infant with an injection of ranibizumab, what percentage would you expect to find an avascular peripheral retina?

A. 10%
B. 20%
C. 40%
D. 100%

Answers

1. (**B**) Despite larger differences in recurrence rates has been reported, an average of 25.9% for bevacizumab, 37.6% for ranibizumab and 23.2% for aflibercept. The difference is statistically not significant.

2. (**C**) It was reported to be 48 days with ranibizumab in the RAINBOW study.

3. (**C**) In RAINBOW study there were found a fully vascularization only in 59% of eyes treated with ranibizumab during 2-years follow-up.

References

1. Good WV; Early Treatment for Retinopathy of Prematurity Cooperative Group. Final results of the Early Treatment for Retinopathy of Prematurity (ETROP) randomized trial. Trans Am Ophthalmol Soc. 2004;102:233–48; discussion 248–50. PMID: 15747762; PMCID: PMC1280104.

2. Zhang G, Yang M, Zeng J, Vakros G, Su K, Chen M, Li H, Tian R, Li N, Tang S, He H, Tan W, Song X, Zhuang R. Shenzhen Screening for Retinopathy of Prematurity Cooperative Group. Comparison of intravitreal injection of Ranibizumab versus laser therapy for zone ii treatment-requiring retinopathy of prematurity. Retina. 2017;37(4):710–7. https://doi.org/10.1097/IAE.0000000000001241. PMID: 27529839; PMCID: PMC5388026.

3. Li Z, Zhang Y, Liao Y, Zeng R, Zeng P, Lan Y. Comparison of efficacy between anti-vascular endothelial growth factor (VEGF) and laser treatment in Type-1 and threshold retinopathy of prematurity (ROP). BMC Ophthalmol. 2018;18(1):19. https://doi.org/10.1186/s12886-018-0685-6.PMID:29378530;PMCID:PMC5789737.

4. Jiang JB, Strauss R, Luo XQ, Nie C, Wang YL, Zhang JW, Zhang ZW. Anaesthesia modalities during laser photocoagulation for retinopathy of prematurity: a retrospective, longitudinal study. BMJ Open. 2017;7(1): e013344. https://doi.org/10.1136/bmjopen-2016-013344.PMID:28119385;PMCID:PMC5278276.

5. Narnaware SH, Bawankule PK, Raje D. Aggressive posterior retinopathy of prematurity (APROP): LASER as the primary modality of treatment. J Ophthalmic Vis Res. 2021;16 (3):400–7. https://doi.org/10.18502/jovr.v16i3.9437.

6. Spandau U, Larsson E, Holmström G. Inadequate laser coagulation is an important cause of treatment failure in type 1 retinopathy of prematurity. Acta Ophthalmol. 2020;98(8):795–9. https://doi.org/10.1111/aos.14406 Epub 2020 PMID: 32250547.

7. Wang SD, Zhang GM. Shenzhen Screening for Retinopathy of Prematurity Cooperative Group. Laser therapy versus intravitreal injection of anti-VEGF agents in monotherapy of ROP: a Meta-analysis. Int J Ophthalmol. 2020;13(5):806–15. https://doi.org/10.18240/ijo.2020.05.17. PMID: 32420230; PMCID: PMC7201341.

8. Kong Q, Ming WK, Mi XS. Refractive outcomes after intravitreal injection of antivascular endothelial growth factor versus laser photocoagulation for retinopathy of prematurity: a meta-analysis. BMJ Open. 2021;11(2): e042384. https://doi.org/10.1136/bmjopen-2020-042384.PMID:33568373;PMCID:PMC7878142.

9. Nicoară SD, Ștefănuț AC, Nascutzy C, Zaharie GC, Toader LE, Drugan TC. Regression rates following the treatment of aggressive posterior retinopathy of prematurity with bevacizumab versus laser: 8-year retrospective analysis. Med Sci Monit. 2016;22:1192–209. https://doi.org/10.12659/msm.897095.PMID:27062023;PMCID:PMC4918525.

10. Houston SK, Wykoff CC, Berrocal AM, Hess DJ, Murray TG. Laser treatment for retinopathy of prematurity. Lasers Med Sci. 2013;28(2):683–92. https://doi.org/10.1007/s10103-011-1021-z Epub 2011 Dec 2 PMID: 22134790.

11. Repka MX, Tung B, Good WV, et al. Outcome of eyes developing retinal detachment during the early treatment for retinopathy of prematurity study (ETROP) Arch Ophthalmol. 2006;124:24–30.

12. Quinn GE, Dobson V, Barr CC, Davis BR, Palmer EA, Robertson J, Summers CG, Trese MT, Tung B. Visual acuity of eyes after vitrectomy for retinopathy of prematurity: follow-up at 5 1/2 years. The Cryotherapy for Retinopathy of Prematurity Cooperative Group. Ophthalmology. 1996;103(4):595–600.

13. Smith LEH. Through the eyes of a child: understanding retinopathy through ROP: the Friedenwald lecture. Invest Ophthalmol Vis Sci. 2008;49:5177–82 [PubMed: 18708611].

14. Quiroz-Mercado H, Ustariz-González O, Martinez-Castellanos MA, Covarrubias P, Dominguez F, Sanchez-Huerta V. Our experience after 1765 intravitreal injections of bevacizumab: the importance of being part of a developing story. Semin Ophthalmol. 2007;22 (2):109–25.

15. Quiroz-Mercado H, Martinez-Castellanos MA, Hernandez-Rojas ML, Salazar-Teran N, Chan RV. Antiangiogenic therapy with intravitreal bevacizumab for retinopathy of prematurity. Retina. 2008;28(Suppl):S19–25 [PubMed: 18317339].
16. Mintz-Hittner HA, Kennedy KA, Chuang AZ; BEAT-ROP Cooperative Group. Efficacy of intravitreal bevacizumab for stage 3+ retinopathy of prematurity. N Engl J Med. 201;364(7):603–15.
17. Stahl A, Lepore D, Fielder A, Fleck B, Reynolds JD, Chiang MF, Li J, Liew M, Maier R, Zhu Q, Marlow N. Ranibizumab versus laser therapy for the treatment of very low birthweight infants with retinopathy of prematurity (RAINBOW): an open-label randomised controlled trial. Lancet. 2019;394(10208):1551–9.
18. Salman AG, Said AM. Structural, visual and refractive outcomes of intravitreal Aflibercept injection in high-risk Prethreshold type 1 retinopathy of prematurity. Ophthalmic Res. 2015;53:15–20.
19. Riazi-Esfahani H, Mahmoudi A, Sanatkar M, Farahani AD, Bazvand F. Comparison of Aflibercept and bevacizumab in the treatment of type 1 retinopathy of prematurity. Int J Retina Vitreous. 2021;7(1):60.
20. Ekinci DY, Vural AD. Comparison of two different doses of intravitreal Aflibercept in the treatment of retinopathy of prematurity. J AAPOS. 2021;25(2):93.e1-93.e5.
21. Chen YT, Liu L, Lai CC, Chen KJ, Hwang YS, Wu WC. Anatomical and functional results of intravitreal Aflibercept monotherapy for type 1 retinopathy of prematurity: one-year outcomes. Retina. 2020;40(12):2366–72.
22. Süren E, Özkaya D, Çetinkaya E, Kalaycı M, Yiğit K, Kücük MF, Erol MK. Comparison of Bevacizumab, Ranibizumab and Aflibercept in retinopathy of prematurity treatment. Int Ophthalmol. 2022;42(6):1905–13.
23. Coats DK, Miller AM, Brady McCreery KM, Holz ER, Paysse EA. Involution of threshold retinopathy of prematurity after diode laser photocoagulation. Ophthalmology. 2004;111(10):1894–8.
24. Isaac M, Tehrani N, Mireskandari K. Medscape. Involution patterns of retinopathy of prematurity after treatment with intravitreal Bevacizumab: implications for follow-up. Eye (Lond). 2016;30(3):333–41.
25. Fleck BW, Reynolds JD, Zhu Q, Lepore D, Marlow N, Stahl A, Li J, Weisberger A, Fielder AR. RAINBOW Investigator Group. Time course of retinopathy of prematurity regression and reactivation after treatment with Ranibizumab or laser in the RAINBOW trial. Ophthalmol Retina. 2022:S2468–6530(22)00065–3.
26. Chen YH, Chen SN, Lien RI, Shih CP, Chao AN, Chen KJ, Hwang YS, Wang NK, Chen YP, Lee KH, Chuang CC, Chen TL, Lai CC, Wu WC. Refractive errors after the use of bevacizumab for the treatment of retinopathy of prematurity: 2-year outcomes. Eye (Lond). 2014;28(9):1080–6; quiz 1087.
27. Marlow N, Stahl A, Lepore D, Fielder A, Reynolds JD, Zhu Q, Weisberger A, Stiehl DP, Fleck B. RAINBOW investigators group. 2-year outcomes of Ranibizumab versus laser therapy for the treatment of very low birthweight infants with retinopathy of prematurity (RAINBOW extension study): prospective follow-up of an open label, randomized controlled trial. Lancet Child Adolesc Health. 2021;5(10):698–707.
28. Rodriguez SH, Blair MP, Shapiro MJ, Berrocal AM, Murray TG, Martinez-Castellanos MA, Baker Hubbard G. Neurodevelopmental outcomes of preterm infants with retinopathy of prematurity by treatment. Pediatrics. 2020;145(4):e20200056A.
29. Rodriguez SH, Blair MP, Shapiro MJ, et al. Neurodevelopmental outcomes following bevacizumab treatment for retinopathy of prematurity: a systematic review and meta-analysis. J Perinatol. 2021;41:2377–8.
30. Chandra P, Kumawat D, Tewari R, Azimeera S. Post-Ranibizumab injection endophthalmitis in aggressive posterior retinopathy of prematurity. Indian J Ophthalmol. 2019;67(6):967–9.

31. Suren E, Cetinkaya E, Kalayci M, Özyazıcı Özkan SE, Kucuk MF, Erol MK. Endophthalmitis in retinopathy of prematurity after intravitreal Aflibercept injection. Case Rep Ophthalmol Med. 2020;2020:Article ID 8861435:3.
32. Bazvand F, Riazi-Esfahani H, Mirshahi A, et al. Ocular complications following intravitreal bevacizumab injection for retinopathy of prematurity and assessment of risk factors. Int J Retin Vitr. 2021;7:5.
33. Beck KD, Rahman EZ, Ells A, Mireskandari K, Berrocal AM, Harper CA. 3rd SAFER-ROP: updated protocol for anti-VEGF injections for retinopathy of prematurity. Ophthalmic Surg Lasers Imaging Retina. 2020;51(7):402–6. https://doi.org/10.3928/23258160-20200702-05 PMID: 32706898.
34. Jalali S, Azad R, Trehan HS, Dogra MR, Gopal L, Narendran V. Technical aspects of laser treatment for acute retinopathy of prematurity under topical anesthesia. Indian J Ophthalmol. 2010;58(6):509–15. https://doi.org/10.4103/0301-4738.71689.

ROP Treatment in Complex Presentation

18

Michael J. Shapiro, Michael P. Blair, and Sarah Hilkert Rodriguez

Abstract

Randomized Clinical Trials (RCTs) have significantly improved outcomes for patients with retinopathy of prematurity (ROP). While these studies provide strong evidence for the management of most patients with ROP, inclusion and exclusion criteria limit the generalizability of some study conclusions in complex cases. Complexity can vary widely, from systemic fragility to ocular abnormalities, to socioeconomic barriers. Ophthalmologists must be prepared to adjust techniques with a variety of different approaches in the management of the complex patient. Overall, strict adherence to protocols from RCTs is important for patients who fit the study profile. Recognizing that each complex patient is unique, however, this chapter explores some general concepts as models that can be adapted to the care of individual complex patients with ROP.

Keywords

Retinopathy · Prematurity · Randomized Clinical Trials · Complex Presentation · Management

M. J. Shapiro (✉) · M. P. Blair
Retina Consultants, LTD, Des Plaines, Illinois, United States
e-mail: michaelj.shapiro@gmail.com

M. P. Blair
e-mail: michaelblairmd@gmail.com

M. J. Shapiro
Univerity of Illinois at Chicago, Chicago, Illinois, United States

Ann & Robert H. Lurie Children's Hospital, Chicago, Illinois, United States

M. P. Blair · S. H. Rodriguez
Department of Ophthalmology and Visual Science, University of Chicago, Chicago, Illinois, United States

Ş. Özdek et al. (eds.), *Pediatric Vitreoretinal Surgery*,
https://doi.org/10.1007/978-3-031-14506-3_18

Introduction: General Principles of Approaching Complexity

Complexity is an essential part of clinical practice. However, complex patients are usually excluded from randomized clinical trials (RCTs) in order to focus the particular question and limit the number of patients required. For example, infants with birth weights greater than 1251 g. were excluded from the CRYO-ROP and ET-ROP studies [1, 2], while infants with ocular or neurologic comorbidities were excluded from the RAINBOW study [3]. Data for these and other complex patients were either not collected or were diluted, such that there is no direct empiric evidence of treatment effect. In this situation, the RCT value is general. It describes the biologic response to the treatment. Therefore, to the extent that the complex case reflects the same pathogenesis, we can generalize that the response proven effective in RCTs remains valid. Although RCTs have powerful particular recommendations, there is no established best practice for complex cases. In clinical practice, all infants must be examined and treated as needed, and general biologic concepts, therapeutic principles and practical experience are the basis of clinical judgement. In this chapter, will share some aspects of our clinical judgement as applied to the problem of complex presentations of ROP.

A. The therapeutic principals for ROP from RCTs:

1. Mild-moderate disease (stage 1, stage 2 and ETROP-Type 2 ROP) is best allowed to regress [2].
2. Severe disease (ETROP-Type1 ROP) is nicely responsive to many interventions [1–4].
3. Extensive Severe disease: stage 3+, with increasing volume, circumferential extent, and active vascularity beyond baseline ETROP-Type 1 ROP increasingly fails primary intervention leading to retinal detachment. CRYO-ROP gives strong evidence for this effect when stage 3+disease extends beyond the minimal criterion for CRYO-ROP Threshold ROP.

B. The principles from non-randomized experience and reports with traction retinal detachment of ROP:

1. Mild stage 4A responds very well to vitrectomy.
2. Moderate stage 4 with increased circumferential extent and anterior traction and involvement of the macula often attaches but with low vision and less stability.
3. stage 5, even in mild configuration, often partially attaches but leads to low vision and poor stability

C. Zone. Conceptually, the zone of disease reflects the amount of avascular tissue that may become ischemic and fuels the progression of disease. Therefore, more posterior zones of disease have greater potential for severe and rapid progression.

D. Secondary Factors. Genetics, sepsis, and general health are occasionally major contributors to the progression of disease [5], especially among the complicated and surprising presentations.

E. Time Element. The time element cannot be overemphasized. The clinician must remember that late treatment results in blindness and an eye with minimal A-ROP may become untreatable in 2 weeks.

F. Uncertainty. The complex situation is outside the usual circumstance where we operate comfortably and confidently. The patients have increased uncertainty and the results are less predictable. The clinician should examine more often and more completely using additional tools and looking for clues outside the usual parameters of ICROP classification [6] and think ahead about the direction of changes over time. ROP colleagues should be enlisted and early consultation or referral to an expert may be the best in perplexing cases. Internationally, ROP experts are often happy to share their experiences and approaches. Retinal imaging may be helpful, and, although typically reliable in less complex ROP [7], may be challenging in the complex patient due to poor pupillary dilation, vitreous haze, and / or systemic instability.

G. General Protocols. As a rule, extraordinary situations do not reliably respond to ordinary management. We may need to adjust the routine treatment described in the RCT protocol. Needless to say, it is critical to remain calm and not respond fearfully because that limits the identification of options and estimation of relative risks in an unbiased and calculated manner.

H. Outcomes. In general, the outcomes are worse than the cases included in RCTs. Therefore, the team and family should be counseled accordingly.

Categories of Clinical Complexity.

There are different kinds of complexity: One dimension for dividing complex cases is between medical issues external to the eye (type 1) and pathologic features of the eye (type 2). These aspects of complexity may occur together or separately. In addition, family and socioeconomic issues (type 3) may present additional barriers to timely management and treatment.

Systemic Medical Barriers to Diagnosis and Treatment

The most common complex situation is the unstable or unwell infant with unstable oxygenation. These infants range from too unwell for safe examination to unstable for laser treatment. In the case of "too unstable for laser", we may have the option of anti-VEGF injection, which is a significantly less stressful than laser and has a later established moment for treatment based on timing in the BEAT-ROP study [3]. The infants that are "unsafe for an exam" arise from many causes including bronchopulmonary dysplasia and sepsis. For some infants that desaturate when moved, increasing the oxygen supplementation or in the case of intubation, a variety of medications, may be adequate, and some may be treated with a short course of methylprednisolone sodium succinate. Ultimately, the neonatologist is the expert here and will determine the potential remedies and the ultimate safety. If one is on a locally validated ROP examination schedule, a delay of less than a week is very low risk, and this may give the team enough time to treat the underlying cause. However, if the baby is too ill for the resources in the NICU, a transfer may be required and the sooner the better.

In order to maintain some control of the retina disease, the exam is critical. Often times, direct communication with the neonatologist regarding the potential for a modified exam is helpful. In such cases where a full exam cannot be safely performed, a brief exam of the posterior pole can determine the presence or absence of plus disease as well as zone I disease. This can be done very briefly, even without repositioning unstable patients requiring high-frequency oscillatory ventilation. If there is no plus, the risk of delay is low and the neontologist can take a full week to prepare the patient for a full exam. The limited exam ideally would be repeated at least once or twice weekly, depending on findings, until a full exam is possible. The low-risk period may last longer if the ROP is clearly in zone II.

In some unwell neonates the systemic effects of the dilating medication also require attention. Even a 1% solution drop dispenses a significant dose for a 3 kg neonate. For example, 1 drop of commercially packaged ophthalmic solution is around 40 µl or 400 µg in 1% solution. The pediatric IV dose of phenylephrine for Hypotension/Shock: Usual 0.1–0.5 mcg/kg/min titrated to effect. Clearly, an eye drop administered topically will not achieve serum concentrations as high as if it were administered intravenously, but can be absorbed through the nasal mucosa and avoid first pass metabolism, and, nonetheless in the unwell 3 kg infant, even lower doses of anticholinergics can be important. Cyclopentolate has been associated with decreased gastric acid secretion [8], while phenylephrine may raise blood pressure [9].

Although light dilation may be safer from a systemic perspective, inadequate dilation may compromise the quality of ophthalmoscopy and missing critical details may increase the chance of a poor ocular outcome. Rather than accepting poor dilation, placing drops over longer durations while monitoring blood pressure may help minimize systemic effects. Punctal occlusion may also help; it has been shown to effectively reduce systemic absorption of timolol in adult glaucoma patients [10] and may be considered in such cases. These options should be discussed with the neonatologist to balance systemic risks of topical eye drops with ocular risks associated with poor dilation.

If the unwell infant is found to have ETROP type 1 treatment criteria (such as stage 2 or 3, zone II with plus disease, or zone I, stage 3 or plus), antiVEGF offers a less stressful and potentially less dangerous alternative to laser. In such cases, delaying until stage 3+ROP is not unreasonable as improvements with antiVEGF are typically seen more quickly than laser, and the BEAT-ROP study waited until stage 3+for treatment [3]. In infants with known neurocognitive risk factors or microcephaly, the hypothetical concerns about adverse neurodevelopmental effects might be added to the equation. Although no study has been sufficiently powered to establish non-inferiority, a recent meta-analysis found no difference in risk of severe neurodevelopmental impairment or cerebral palsy comparing antiVEGF to laser [11]. Another important prospective study which compared infants treated with bevacizumab to infants with untreated ROP and found no difference in neurodevelopment [12]. As treatment bias would have made finding a difference more likely, yet none was found, this study provides reassurance. Nonetheless, this hypothesis is unlikely to be resolved adequately for all clinicians soon, and waiting for consensus will result in denial of an effective ROP treatment for many.

In classic ROP (in contrast to A–ROP), there are usually a few weeks between the first moment of ETROP type 1 and progression to stage 4. When extensive severe stage 3+is reached and the infant is too unstable for any treatment before stage 4, one needs to prepare for possible vitrectomy.

Local: Ophthalmic Complex Presentation of ROP

Another somewhat less common but not rare complex presentation is media opacity. This includes corneal opacity, engorged tunica vasculosa lentis (TVL), posterior synechia, cataract, pupillary membrane or vitreous hemorrhage. Vitreous haze is often present in extremely premature infants on early exams but may also be a sign of advanced disease. There is a range of severity, but any opacity that prevents the scheduled ROP examination is a problem. This includes not only complete opacity, but also partial opacity. In fact, mild opacity may be more deceptive because it may both prevent identification of subtle elements and leave the allusion of a good exam. This is a detection problem that is nicely explained by signal detection theory. Since ROP can be rapid moving and subtle, one must take appropriate and timely measures in order to reach a high level of certainty about the exam quality. In many cases, the second eye has a clear view and can be examined with ease. As ROP tends to present symmetrically [13], if the second eye has ETROP type 2 ROP or milder ROP, then the obscured eye is less likely to have severe ROP.

Again, as in the limited case of the unwell baby, if the exam allows determination of no plus and there is a sense that the view will improve, a week delay is well tolerated. Corneal edema can be treated with hyperosmotic saline solution or epithelial removal. Synechia may be broken with maximal topical dilating medication administration, with pledgets or with surgery. Pupillary membranes can be opened surgically. Engorged TVL can be treated with anti-VEGF. A dense cataract will need removal or endoscopy can be employed. Vitreous hemorrhage may require vitrectomy but may also clear spontaneously. Expectant management may be appropriate if recent treatment has been applied and posterior segment ultrasonography can reassure absence of retinal detachment [14]. Vitrectomy in an infant requires expertise and may require transfer. An injection of anti-VEGF may allow for a delay of the vitrectomy, and one can use indirect information from the iris and fellow eye to gauge the risk of the injection.

While waiting for the blood to clear, positioning may be helpful. Placing the infant in a vertical position either held up by parents or in a car seat may allow the blood to gravitate out of the posterior pole. This would allow adequate examination.

Within the category, local complexity, there is a second occasional barrier to treatment: local infectious disease, in particular conjunctivitis. Adenoviral conjunctivitis outbreaks have been reported [15] and small numbers of cases have been treated with laser and anti-VEGF; neither group has resulted in treatment failure or spread of infection into the vitreous cavity [16, 17]. Secondary bacterial infection is a true concern [18]. Of course, the clinical appearance is helpful. One can also reduce this concern for bacteria with a gram stain or conjunctival culture prior to injection. In the absence of bacteria, laser or anti-VEGF are safe. If bacteria are found, antibiotic treatment is indicated before injection or laser. A variety of solutions may be used in this situation.

A variety of congenital anomalies and diseases may also be present, and they will pose a variety of challenges. Some such examples are coloboma, microphthalmia, microcornea. In asymmetric microcornea, the smaller eye may be at higher risk. Although microphthalmos can be a feature of severe ROP, ocular growth may be abnormal even before late stage ROP, and ocular growth may be adversely affected by acute ROP itself [19].

Socioeconomic Complexity

Some of the most difficult situations are extrinsic to the eye and baby. The most common is a family unable to follow-up on the schedule. The disease after natural regression and standard laser is stable with very rare exceptions. However, after the use of anti-VEGF as monotherapy, some cases will recur and occasional retinal detachment will occur [20–23]. Therefore, the eye should be completely treated in a manner that the avascular zone which propels the pathology is minimal [24]. Ideally, treatment includes all abnormal avascular retina, greater than 2 disc diameters or more from the temporal ora serrata and 1 DD on the nasal side without stage 1 or greater disease. The avascular zone refers to the absence of normal retinal vessels and includes as part of the avascular zone areas of "flat" or fine vessel neovascularization near the junction [25]. As persistent avascular retina (PAR) may continue to produce VEGF leading to retinal detachment years to decades later, peripheral laser ablation should be considered in patients who are unlikely to maintain close follow-up regardless of prior treatment status [24, 26]. We hope the future literature will prove helpful and allow a more lenient recommendation for the infant without normal follow-up.

Another socioeconomic issue is inadequate equipment or expertise. In this case referral may be required and, given the tempo of some ROP eyes, the referral needs to be done in a timely manner. We have seen stage 4A evolve to stage 4B and stage 5 because of insurance and government bureaucratic barriers. Obviously, this is an unfortunate case for blindness.

In developing nations, as advances in NICU care lead to improved survival of premature infants, ROP is becoming an increasingly common cause of blindness [27]. Barriers to care include lack of standardized guidelines, equipment to regulate and monitor supplemental oxygen and treatment equipment [28].

Adjustment in Clinical Practice for the Complex Presentation

Adjustments are made in response to particular issues on a case-by-case basis. They must be monitored carefully because the adjusted protocol may stop working, and another approach may be needed. Generally, the greater the range of tools and expertise, the easier it is to adjust to unusual or even novel problems. It is a great advantage to have ROP vitrectomy equipment and expertise as a backup. However, the mindset to identify problems, figure out solutions and critique the results, is the most critical element.

Adjustments of observations. In the International Classification for ROP (ICROP), the essential descriptors of disease are included and graded [6]. There are associated findings that are correlated, but these features are de-emphasized to make ICROP widely useful. Since in the complex case, essential features may not be visible or may be ambiguous, the other features assume increased importance.

- Disease activity. The primary indication of disease requiring treatment rather than observation for regression, is plus disease. Plus disease is the widely accepted key indicator of activity and the gradation of this activity is now well documented in the ICROP3 [6]. However, in a complex case with the disc and posterior pole obscured, other observations can help determine disease activity. Severe disease activity is reflected throughout the eye including vascularity of the anterior segment (e.g.: iris and TVL engorgement) and at the junction between the vascularized and avascular retina (e.g. red color of the ridge and vascular proliferation). Most disease is symmetric because the eyes are genetically identical and environmentally similar [13]. This is particularly true at the extremes of the spectrum: for example, severe plus and normal without pre-plus. Therefore, if the second eye shows severe plus disease, the chance of activity in the obscured eye is significantly increased.
- Ultrasound, b-scan, seems like a standard approach to cases with poor media. The b-scan may help with identification of persistent fetal vasculature (PFV), retinoblastoma, and retina detachment. However, it has a significant rate of false negatives in stages 2, stage 3 and even stage 4a ROP. Consequently, this approach alone lacks sufficient sensitivity to eliminate progression of ROP beyond the point optimal intervention. The b-scan is likely to detect severe stage 4, rather than stage 3+or early stage 4a and therefore has limited usefulness in cases of risk for acute ROP. However, there may situations, after a high quality

treatment in which the b-scan in especially skilled operators may be somewhat reassuring [14].

- Wide-angle and ultra-wide-angle optical systems (eg Natus Retcam, Optos, Phoenix ICON and 3nethra Neo cameras), may allow useful imaging of the retina. In this situation central media opacity may be circumvented.
- Wide-angle imaging using fluorescein angiography is especially helpful because the filtering of the light reduces the ratio of noise to signal in addition to allowing emphasis on the periphery. The hyperfluorescence of stage 3 will have a particularly strong signal. These systems are strongest for vitreous opacities and are less helpful for cataract and vascularized pupillary membrane. The focus may be finicky, and using the fellow eye to set the focus may help improve the view. Knowing the relative axial length may also help in this effort.
- Correction of the media opacity should also be considered, especially if there is an experienced surgeon. Corneal edema may be treated with application of a hyperosmotic solution or epithelial removal. The pupil may be opened with nylon iris retractors, a cyclodialysis spatula and viscoelastic. Severe TVL may be cleared with anti-VEGF. Cataract has a range of extent and density. Ultimately it may be removed. However, aphakia is a very unfavorable situation for visual development with a high chance of amblyopia, particularly in unilateral cases, and alternatives must be considered first. If the cataract it is too dense for laser but not too dense for exam then anti-VEGF is the most efficient choice. If anti-VEGF is not optimal, cryotherapy can be performed through a mild cataract or to bridge areas of dense opacity. However, cryotherapy is technically demanding for the physician and can be stressful for the infant. Over treatment, in particular, multiple freeze thaws in the same location, can lead to necrosis, breaks and retinal detachment. It also causes more post-operative inflammation. If available, before deciding on cataract extraction, one might consider endoscopy as a viewing system for diagnoses. Additionally, it can be used for viewing with external anterior cryotherapy or with its own laser for posterior disease.
- Vitreous hemorrhage may block the view and makes the diagnosis less certain, but it does not reduce the effectiveness of anti-VEGF. Of course, the path of the needle needs to be safe. Vitreous hemorrhage may be allowed to gravitate. However, in most cases with moderate hemorrhage suspended in the vitreous matrix, the natural clearing process will take weeks to months, which is too long of a delay. Therefore, one must plan for vitrectomy, even as other measures are taken.

Adjustment is in the timeline. Delay is only reasonable if the reason for delay has potential for resolution. However, this requires a sense of the disease progression.

- ETROP Timeline. The ideal moment for laser treatment as determined by ETROP type 1 (approximately 15% risk pre-threshold) disease treatment is 48 h from diagnosis; this is the optimal moment and is the most likely to give a predictable mainly favorable outcome. Earlier treatment of type 2 ROP was not beneficial [2].

- The Beat ROP Timeline: In this study bevacizumab was used to treat zone I and posterior zone II at stage 3+, which is often a week later than ETROP Type 1 (ie: stage 2+or stage 3−), and this moment was very effective in the Beat ROP study [3]. This timeline may be more appropriate for anti-VEGF treatment and may represent one explanation for laser outcomes less than expected in this study.
- CRYO-ROP Timeline: In this study, cryotherapy of the avascular zone was used at extensive 3+ (5 continuous clock hours or 8 total clock hours) which was termed Threshold ROP [1]. In zone II it was very effective, but in zone I, more than 90% of eyes resulted in blindness. The plus disease in this study may have been well beyond the standard photo and, therefore, more severe than other RCTs. However, subsequent to CRYO-ROP, a large number of case series reported good results in laser cases of threshold ROP. Nonetheless, this extensive stage 3+is the group that most often progresses to retina detachment after laser treatment and "crunch" after anti-VEGF injection [29]. On occasion, the patients present with this severity, but our goal is to eliminate this late presentation. In these cases, one must also consider vigilant post-treatment observation for progression to stage 4a and vitrectomy.

Adjustments in treatment techniques is the second approach to the analysis of complex cases, emphasizing the range of interventions. The complex situation may require adjustments in tools. Including the full range of tools increases the potential for success.

Treatment tools:

- Anti-VEGF
- Green Laser
- Infrared Laser
- Cryotherapy
- Scleral Buckle
- Vitrectomy
- Anterior segment surgery
- Endoscope
- Laser requires visualization and is optimal at ETROP type 1 disease and less effective later. Infrared laser (rather than green laser) may be preferred in cases with TVL in order to reduce cataract as the green wavelength is uptaken by hemoglobin [30].
- AntiVEGF injection does not require any view and is effective at stage 3+, including A-ROP [31]. Often times repeat antiVEGF injections may quiet disease activity while other barriers can be overcome.
- Cryotherapy is an old technique that requires a minimal view and can be applied without a view in some cases; it is especially good near the ora when pupillary dilation is poor. It is less effective in posterior disease. It also causes

post-operative inflammation and can cause retina breaks especially if there are multiple freeze -thaw -freeze cycles to the same area.

- Scleral Buckle may reduce the development of stage 4. In situations where vitrectomy is not available or not feasible, antiVEGF and scleral buckle may be used to repair stage 4 detachments [32].
- Endoscope may resolve the cataract and anterior segment opacities, but requires a larger incision and safe entry is key.
- Staged procedures may be required to safely treat tractional elements without creating retinal breaks. This allows the RPE pump mechanism to open access to new surgical planes.
- Open-sky vitrectomy may be required for select eyes with severe anterior tractional elements.

Complex Presentations of ROP require a thoughtful and flexible approach. We have shared some of our thoughts as models rather than rules. It is obvious that each situation is particular and not relevant for all locations. We support strict adherence to protocols developed by RCTs when the patient fits the normative characteristics of the study patients. However, when the patient in clinical practice would have been excluded or is a statistical outlier in the study sample, we review the situation to determine if the RCT protocol can be generalized to the particular patient. If we find a complexity not well treated by the RCT, we support a thought process based on first principles in order to discover "out-of-the-box" solutions. Local experts as well as international experts are usually happy to consult in the hope of improving the infant's outcome.

Review Questions: (May Have More Than 1 Correct Response)

1. What are the high level types of complex presentation of ROP?

1. Conjunctival infection
2. Unstable oxygenation
3. Concurrent eye pathology
4. Socioeconomic issues

2. Which clinical trials only treated patients with stage 3+disease.

1. ETROP
2. CRYO-ROP
3. BEAT-ROP
4. STOP-ROP
5. RAINBOW

3. What is the ROP risk with patients that received anti-VEGF treatment who live far from an examination center.

1. Dehydration
2. Missed follow-up appointments
3. Poor oxygen supplementation
4. Lack of glasses

Answers

1. Correct answers are 3 and 4. There are three high-level types of complex presentation discussed in this chapter. They help conceptualize the topic. Many instances have been included from our experience, and different forms of complexity will be experienced in different locations at different times.

This chapter identifies three high-level types of complex presentation: medical issues external to the eye, concurrent eye pathology and socioeconomic issues. In each type there are many particular instances. 1. Conjunctival Infection is a particular instance under the category of concurrent eye pathology. 2. Unstable oxygenation is a example under the category of medical issues external to the eye. They are instances of complex presentation, but not high-level categories.

2. <u>Correct answers:</u> 2 CRYO-ROP and 3 BEAT-ROP: Both of these studies required stage 3 + before treatment, which is a later moment in the disease timeline than the ETROP criteria.

Incorrect.

4. STOP-ROP The STOP-ROP treatment was higher oxygen saturation endpoint of supplemental oxygen relative to the conventional management. Laser treatment or cryotherapy was done as part of routine care and was not determined by the trial.

1. ETROP the protocol compared treating at 15% risk prethreshold rather than at the conventional criterion for treatment which was the CRYO-ROP threshold. ETROP recommendation was simplified so that a computer risk model was not needed for clinical practice. The recommendation for treatment, which was called Type 1 ROP, which still stands for laser included treating stage 2 + as well as stage 3 + in zone II, and in zone I any stage with plus disease and stage 3 without plus disease.

5. RAINBOW in this study treated stage 1 and 2 with plus disease in zone I and only stage 3 + in zone II. They added AP-ROP as a separate criterion. It is certainly interesting that the studies have significant differences in the exact moment for treatment. It makes the comparisons more difficult.

3. <u>Correct answer:</u> Missed follow-up appointments.

This has always been an important problem, if the patient is not examined, then they might develop treatment warranted ROP. In this chapter we highlighted a second concern about occasional recurrences after antVEGF monotherapy. The exact risk is unknown, and it may vary from place to place. Certainly, the birth weights, NICU protocols and genetics varies by location. Late retinal detachment may not always be reported to the same physician that has treated. In our location we have seen a significant number of late stage 4 and 5, which results in blindness. Therefore, we have responded with laser treatments of the residual avascular zone before discharge if the patient may not return, or after 55–60, weeks in patients who will return. This late treatment allows the growth of blood vessels and treats the potential source of ischemic drive for the late disease.

Incorrect answers: 1. Dehydration, unrelated and fixable 3. Poor oxygen supplementation. Poor oxygen supplementation has a complex relationship with ROP and is a larger topic than this discussion. 4. Lack of glasses is important, and evaluation with refraction is recommended at 6 months.

References

1. Cryotherapy for Retinopathy of Prematurity Cooperative Group. Multicenter trial of cryotherapy for retinopathy of prematurity: preliminary results. Arch Ophthalmol. 1988;106:471–9.
2. Early Treatment for Retinopathy of Prematurity Cooperative Group. Revised indications for the treatment of retinopathy of prematurity: results of the Early Treatment for Retinopathy of Prematurity randomized trial. Arch Ophthalmol. 2003;121:1684–94.
3. Mintz-Hittner HA, Kennedy KA, Chuang AZ. BEAT-ROP Cooperative Group. Efficacy of intravitreal bevacizumab for stage 31 retinopathy of prematurity. N Engl J Med 2011;364:603–15.
4. Stahl A, Lepore D, Fielder A, Fleck B, Reynolds JD, Chiang MF, Li J, Liew M, Maier R, Zhu Q, Marlow N. Ranibizumab versus laser therapy for the treatment of very low birthweight infants with retinopathy of prematurity (RAINBOW): an open-label randomised controlled trial. Lancet. 2019;394(10208):1551–9.
5. Kim SJ, Port AD, Swan R, Campbell JP, Chan RVP, Chiang MF. Retinopathy of prematurity: a review of risk factors and their clinical significance. Surv Ophthalmol. 2018;63(5):618–37.
6. Chiang MF, Quinn GE, Fielder AR, Ostmo SR, Paul Chan RV, Berrocal A, Binenbaum G, Blair M, Peter Campbell J, Capone A Jr, Chen Y, Dai S, Ells A, Fleck BW, Good WV, Elizabeth Hartnett M, Holmstrom G, Kusaka S, Kychenthal A, Lepore D, Lorenz B, Martinez-Castellanos MA, Özdek Ş, Ademola-Popoola D, Reynolds JD, Shah PK, Shapiro M, Stahl A, Toth C, Vinekar A, Visser L, Wallace DK, Wu WC, Zhao P, Zin A. International Classification of Retinopathy of Prematurity. 3rd Edn Ophthalmology. 2021;128 (10):e51–68.
7. Biten H, Redd TK, Moleta C, Campbell JP, Ostmo S, Jonas K, Chan RVP, Chiang MF. Imaging & Informatics in Retinopathy of Prematurity (ROP) Research Consortium. Diagnostic Accuracy of Ophthalmoscopy vs Telemedicine in Examinations for Retinopathy of Prematurity. JAMA Ophthalmol 2018;136(5):498–504.
8. Isenberg SJ, Abrams C, Hyman PE. Effects of cyclopentolate eyedrops on gastric secretory function in pre-term infants. Ophthalmol. 1985;92(5):698–700.
9. Isenberg S, Everett S. Cardiovascular effects of mydriatics in low-birth-weight infants. J Pediatr. 1984;105(1):111–2.
10. Passo MS, Palmer EA, Van Buskirk EM. Plasma timolol in glaucoma patients. Ophthalmol. 1984;91(11):1361–3.
11. Tsai CY, Yeh PT, Tsao PN, Chung YE, Chang YS, Lai TT. Neurodevelopmental outcomes after Bevacizumab treatment for retinopathy of prematurity: a meta-analysis. Ophthalmol. 2021;128(6):877–88.

12. Fan YY, Huang YS, Huang CY, Hsu JF, Shih CP, Hwang YS, et al. Neurodevelopmental outcomes after intravitreal bevacizumab therapy for retinopathy of prematurity: a prospective case-control study. Ophthalmol. 2019;126(11):1567–77.

13. Lin LY, Jensen AK, Quinn GE, Spiller A, Tomlinson LA, Ying GS, Binenbaum G. Symmetry of disease in retinopathy of prematurity in the postnatal growth and retinopathy of prematurity (G-ROP) study. Ophthalmic Epidemiol. 2020;27(6):477–81.

14. Theophanous C, Schechet S, Rodriguez SH, Blair M. Bilateral vitreous hemorrhage following bilateral intravitreal injections of Bevacizumab in an infant with retinopathy of prematurity. Ophthalmic Surg Lasers Imaging Retina 2018;49(11):893–6.

15. Sammons JS, Graf EH, Townsend S, Hoegg CL, Smathers SA, Coffin SE, Williams K, Mitchell SL, Nawab U, Munson D, Quinn G, Binenbaum G. Outbreak of adenovirus in a neonatal intensive care unit: critical importance of equipment cleaning during inpatient ophthalmologic examinations. Ophthalmol. 2019;126(1):137–43.

16. Koçluk Y, Alyamaç SE. Intravitreal anti-VEGF treatment for retinopathy of prematurity in infants with active adenoviral keratoconjunctivitis. Cutan Ocul Toxicol. 2018;37(1):15–8.

17. Gunay M, Celik G, Con R. Treatment for retinopathy of prematurity in an infant with adenoviral conjunctivitis. Case Rep Pediatr. 2015;2015: 192717.

18. Buznach N, Dagan R, Greenberg D. Clinical and bacterial characteristics of acute bacterial conjunctivitis in children in the antibiotic resistance era. Pediatr Infect Dis J. 2005;24 (9):823–8.

19. Kelly SP, Fielder AR. Microcornea associated with retinopathy of prematurity. Br J Ophthalmol. 1987;71(3):201–3.

20. Snyder LL, Garcia-Gonzalez JM, Shapiro MJ, Blair MP. Very late reactivation of retinopathy of prematurity after monotherapy with intravitreal bevacizumab. Ophthalmic Surg Lasers Imaging Retina. 2016;47:280–3.

21. Hajrasouliha AR, Garcia-Gonzales JM, Shapiro MJ, Yoon H, Blair MP. Reactivation of retinopathy of prematurity three years after treatment with bevacizumab. Ophthalmic Surg Lasers Imaging Retina. 2017;48:255–9.

22. Hu J, Blair MP, Shapiro MJ, Lichtenstein SJ, Galasso JM, Kapur R. Reactivation of retinopathy of prematurity after Bevacizumab injection. Arch Ophthalmol. 2012;130:1000–6.

23. Ittiara S, Blair MP, Shapiro MJ, Lichtenstein SJ. Exudative retinopathy and detachment: a late reactivation of retinopathy of prematurity after intravitreal bevacizumab. J AAPOS. 2013;17:323–5.

24. Garcia Gonzalez JM, Snyder L, Blair M, Rohr A, Shapiro M, Greenwald M. Prophylactic peripheral laser and fluorescein angiograph after bevacizumab for retinopathy of prematurity. Retina. 2018;38:764–72.

25. Blair MP, Shapiro MJ, Hartnett ME. Fluorescein angiography to estimate normal peripheral retinal nonperfusion in children. JAAPOS. 2012;16:234–7.

26. Golas L, Shapiro MJ, Blair MP. Late ROP reactivation and retinal detachment in a teenager. Ophthalmic Surg Lasers Imaging Retina. 2018;49:625–8.

27. Herrod SK, Adio A, Isenberg SJ, Lambert SR. Blindness secondary to retinopathy of prematurity in Sub-Saharan Africa. Ophthalmic Epidemiol. 2021:1–8. Epub ahead of print. PMID: 33818253.

28. Lloyd T, Isenberg S, Lambert SR. Current management of retinopathy of prematurity in sub-Saharan Africa. J AAPOS. 2020;24(3):151.e1-151.e6.

29. Yonekawa Y, Wu WC, Nitulescu CE, et al. Progressive retinal detachment in infants with retinopathy of prematurity treated with intravitreal Bevacizumab or Ranibizumab. Retina. 2018;28(6):1079–83.

30. Shapiro MJ, Chow CC, Karth PA, Kiernan DF, Blair MP. Effects of green diode laser in the treatment of pediatric coats disease. Am J Ophthalmol. 2011;151(4):725-731.e2. https://doi.org/10.1016/j.ajo.2010.10.024 Epub 2011 Jan 22.

31. Blair M, Gonzalez JMG, Snyder L, Schechet S, Greenwald M, Shapiro M, Rodriguez SH. Bevacizumab or laser for aggressive posterior retinopathy of prematurity. Taiwan J Ophthalmol. 2018;8(4):243–8.
32. Shah RJ, Garcia-Gonzalez JM, Blair MP, Galasso J, Shapiro MJ. Concurrent scleral buckle and intravitreal bevacizumab for advanced retinopathy of prematurity-related retinal detachment. Retina Cases Brief Rep. 2016;10(2):183–6.

Vitreoretinal Surgery for Stage 4 ROP

19

Benjamin K. Young and Cagri G. Besirli

Abstract

Stage 4 retinopathy of prematurity can result in poor visual and anatomic outcomes, and requires urgent intervention. For most cases, lens-sparing pars plana vitrectomy is the preferred treatment strategy, with the key surgical goal of relieving transvitreal forces along the retinal ridges, while avoiding the creation of iatrogenic retinal breaks. Special considerations must be made in pediatric vitrectomy to optimize the odds for the best possible outcomes.

Keywords

Retinopathy of prematurity · Lens-sparing vitrectomy · Transvitreal forces · Retinal detachment · Surgical maneuvers

Supplementary Information The online version contains supplementary material available at https://doi.org/10.1007/978-3-031-14506-3_19.

B. K. Young · C. G. Besirli (✉)
Department of Ophthalmology and Visual Sciences, Kellogg Eye Center, University of Michigan, Ann Arbor, MI, USA
e-mail: cbesirli@med.umich.edu

B. K. Young
e-mail: youngbe@ohsu.edu

Case Presentation

A twin boy born at gestational age (GA) of 25 weeks 6 days and with a birth weight of 0.79 kg presents at 43-weeks post-menstrual age (PMA) weighing 3.115 kg. At the referring hospital, he was noted to have zone 2 stage 3 disease, and had undergone indirect laser ablation in both eyes, but was transferred for concern for retinal detachment. On our examination, the left eye has a stage 4A detachment in zone 2 from 1 o'clock to 5 o'clock with partial laser treatment in the avascular retina. The right eye had a regressed temporal ridge in zone 2 with partial laser treatment 360 degrees.

Introduction

Stage 4 retinopathy of prematurity (ROP) is the first stage where retinal detachment is noted, and is subdivided into two stages: 4A, with the fovea attached, and 4B, with the fovea detached. The goal of screening and ROP treatment with either laser therapy or intravitreal anti-VEGF agents is to prevent progression to stage 4 disease.

Stage 4A and 4B disease both require surgical intervention to prevent progression (ie from 4A to 4B, or 4B to stage 5), where outcomes become progressively worse or irrecoverable [1, 2]. Surgical outcomes worsen significantly with each stage. In lens-sparing vitrectomy, the reattachment rate after a single surgery was 82.1% for stage 4A, 69.5% for stage 4B, and 42.6% for stage 5 [3]. In one study, visual outcomes were 20/550 Snellen visual acuity equivalent for stage 4A, 20/1600 for stage 4B, and 20/4000 for stage 5 when excluding patients who were light perceptions or worse [4]. These findings highlight the importance of timing of intervention to maximize the odds of success.

It is valuable to always define the goals of surgery before planning any operative case. This is especially critical in pediatric retina surgery, where the stakes are high, and the margin of error is low. Steps that do not directly aid in achieving the goal of surgery should be minimized to lower the potential rate of complications.

Goals of Surgery in Stage 4 ROP

- Complete laser treatment of avascular retina to prevent disease progression and recurrence
- Avoid creating an iatrogenic retinal break at any cost
- Remove tractional forces on the retina which typically emanate from the ridge
- Stage surgical intervention to minimize risk of complications when necessary

The above goals are listed in priority order. We will note examples of possible objectives the adult retina surgeon may have that are NOT within the goals of ROP surgery in this scenario:

- Complete reattachment of the retina at the end of the surgery
- Dissecting or removing all membranes
- Performing shave vitrectomy, or removing the maximum amount of cortical vitreous
- Cauterizing all sources of intraoperative bleeding

Attempts at the above may increase the risk for an iatrogenic break being made. As others have reported, the eye may be considered lost with even a single iatrogenic break, with best case visual outcomes generally being light perception vision, even with the most aggressive surgical interventions.

Pre-operative Considerations

Timing

Timing to surgical intervention is critical once Stage 4A has been identified. Earlier surgical intervention is recommended to prevent foveal detachment and improve anatomic and functional outcomes. Even if the detachment appears peripheral, minimal or even questionable at time of identification, the following factors can cause the detachment to progress rapidly:

- Contraction of the ridge
- Pathologic vitreous organization and contraction
- Persistent vascular activity and exudation

Typical age for the patient is 38–42 weeks PMA. This is when Stage 4A may occur without prior treatment, and often neonates are better able to tolerate general anesthesia. Systemic health as it relates to toleration of extended time under general anesthesia should always be a team-based discussion between the neonatologist, pediatric anesthesiologist, the retina surgeon, and the patient's guardians.

We recommend a similar approach for surgical intervention in Stage 4B disease, as foveal re-attachment is critical for visual development and prevention of amblyopia. However, since the fovea is already detached, some surgeons may recommend a more flexible approach to urgency of surgical intervention, especially if the overall systemic status of the patient increases the risk of potential non-ocular complications during or after general anesthesia.

Laser Status

In general, patients who have progressed to Stage 4 disease have either inadequate or no laser therapy. As addressed in "Goals of Surgery", one of the primary goals is to ensure the avascular retina has been completely treated to prevent recurrence. Intravitreal anti-VEGF is useful for ROP treatment before Stage 4, but its role for treating Stage 4 disease is limited. Potential for "crunch" phenomenon of the fibrovascular ridge is concerning with anti-VEGF injection in late-stage disease. In addition, anti-VEGF treatment does not preclude the need for ablation of the peripheral retina to minimize the risk of early or late reactivation of disease [5].

If there is significant plus disease associated with iris neovascularization and no laser therapy has been performed, complete indirect laser therapy with or without anti-VEGF injection may be considered first, followed by vitrectomy approximately 1 week later. This staged approach may allow the plus disease to regress before surgery and optimize the intraoperative view (see below).

In essentially all other cases, laser therapy and vitrectomy can be performed on the same day. Attempting laser therapy using endolaser intraoperatively may be challenging in a premature eye, even with curved or articulating endolaser systems. It is difficult to obtain sufficient visualization to complete laser up to the ora serrata, position one's hands in the crowded pediatric surgical space, and still avoid lens-instrument touch. Therefore, we recommend starting these surgeries first with indirect laser photocoagulation, which can be done in a non-sterile fashion. Efficient, optimal technique is required for this indirect laser to avoid significant corneal edema and cataract via laser energy being applied to the tunica lentis, limiting intraoperative visualization.

If available, we recommend use of an 810 nm laser. While more widely available 532 nm green lasers are equally effective at treating the avascular retina, this wavelength is better absorbed by the common persistent tunica lentis which can promote corneal edema, which will be disadvantageous for intraoperative visualization.

Laterality

Often, patients will have stage 4 detachments in both eyes at the time for decision to surgery, except in circumstances where only one eye may have had insufficient prior therapy. Operating on both eyes at the same session may be considered to reduce the number of exposures to general anesthesia, given the risk of bilateral endophthalmitis is very low compared to anesthetic risks in this population [6–8].

If bilateral surgery is performed, each eye should be treated as if it were a completely fresh surgery, including completely finishing one surgery, patch and shielding, removal of previous instruments from the room to prevent accidental cross contamination, changing of intraocular fluid infusions, etc. Then, a completely new timeout is performed, followed by a sterile prep and drape, new instruments, freshly primed vitrectomy machine, etc.

Operating on the eye with better potential first is highly recommended, in case an intraoperative anesthetic risk or other concern prevent surgery on the fellow eye the same day or within a reasonable amount of time. An exam under anesthesia (EUA), including detailed anterior segment examination, fundus photography, and hand-held OCT if available, is recommended to determine which eye may have better potential.

Surgical Setup Considerations

Proper head positioning is critical for successful vitrectomy in a pediatric eye. The surgeon should ensure the tube, scope, IV lines, and child's head are all adequately positioned for ergonomic surgery. In addition to the standard superior entry into the eye, a temporal or even nasal approach may be considered, depending on where the patient's pathology is most severe, as determined by preoperative EUA as discussed above. As in adult vitreoretinal surgery, we suggest positioning the patient's head, so the cornea is parallel to the floor. The authors do not find routine use of a wrist rest to be helpful in neonatal surgery. Ensure that a properly sized speculum for a premature infant is available.

Intraoperative Considerations

Operative Strategy (See the Video)

Lens-sparing 25 g vitrectomy provides an effective surgical approach in most stage 4 detachments. Valved trocars improve intraocular pressure control and globe stability. 20G or 23G instrumentation are preferred by some surgeons.

- In general, we do not recommend scleral buckle for stage IV ROP detachment. A retrospective case series showed a lens sparing vitrectomy had a 72% success rate compared with a 34% success rate in scleral buckle [9]. The primary operative goal at this stage is to relieve transvitreal traction off the ridge from multiple vectors.
- While surgical planes may be too tight anteriorly in select cases with severe anteroposterior traction, which may require removal of the lens, lens-sparing surgery has the benefits of avoiding the problem of aphakic amblyopia management as well as aphakic glaucoma.
- Some surgeons may find advantages to using 27 g cutters to more easily dissect into tight surgical planes [10], though decreased stiffness of 27G instruments may limit globe manipulation.

Surgical Setup and Entry

Conjunctival Peritomy and Sutures

- For maximal control of post-operative wounds, we recommend a 180-degree conjunctival peritomy extending from the planned inferotemporal to superonasal trocar sites (Figure A). Given the difficulty of post-operative examinations, and possibility of self-induced trauma to the eyes, scleral closure ensures a sealed globe, and conjunctival closure may reduce the risk of endophthalmitis. We recommend pre-placing the suture for the infusion line in a figure-of-8 fashion to allow for immediate closure of that sclerotomy when the infusion line is removed (Fig. 19.1).
- Conjunctival cut down is simplest with a 180 peritomy, with care to excise Tenon's capsule to avoid incarceration while closing the sclera. Intraoperative subtenon's Marcaine after the conjunctival cut down may be beneficial for globe proptosis to improve surgical access. Discuss the maximum volume of anesthetic with your anesthesiologist before administering, as there are much more significant dose limitations in neonates compared to adults.

Trocar Placement

- Since the pars plana will either be undeveloped, or unpredictably developed, the recommended scleral entry is anterior, located 0.5–1.0 mm posterior to the limbus through pars plicata [11]. Though it may be safe to place trocars further

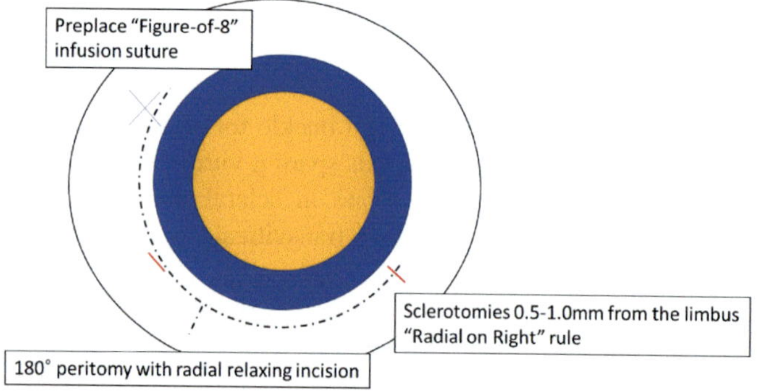

Fig. 19.1 Schematic of surgical strategy for sutured approach to ROP detachment repair. A peritomy (black dashed line) is made to ensure watertight closure of the sclera at the end of surgery. The radial relaxing incision allows for easy reapproximation at the end of surgery. The "Radial on Right" rule is to allow for ergonomic closure of the sclerotomies (red lines) at the end of surgery by a right-handed surgeon (reverse this for left-handed surgeons). The pre-placed "Figure of 8" suture (purple lines) is so that scleral closure can be complete immediately upon removal of the infusion trocar

posterior given modern nomograms of ora serrata location [12], we advise this slightly more anterior location given the experience that this does not typically result in lens strike, and the unpredictable development of the pars plana.

- Given how limited the surgical space is in the premature infant eye, tunneled or beveled cannulae may limit rotational freedom, and risk touching the lens or retina. Therefore, we recommend using a "straight in" trocar approach. Orient the trocar blades to be parallel, with the "Right side radial" rule (see Fig. 19.1). This will allow for ergonomic sutured closure for the right-handed surgeon.
- The path of the trocar cannulae should be straight posterior, visualizing that one is aiming through the lens zonules to avoid inadvertently striking the lens.
- Be mindful that in premature infants, the retina may have a larger surface area than the RPE, leading to retinal folds that may be attached to the lens, underscoring the importance of the preoperative EUA. If lensectomy is required, we recommend inserting the trocar into the anterior chamber to avoid these retinal folds in the posterior chamber.
- The standard 4 mm cannula may be too long for the neonatal eye to effectively maneuver vitrectomy instruments. We recommend using a silicone spacer to reduce the intraocular length of the cannula, unless specific pediatric trocars are available in your practice. A simple way to produce this is to cut segments of a 240 silicone scleral buckle band, and pierce these with the trocar (Fig. 19.2).
- Pediatric sclera is can be difficult to enter compared to adult sclera [13]. To create a controlled entry with the trocars, we recommend ensuring a firm grasp of the conjunctiva and episcleral at the limbus with a toothed forceps (ie a

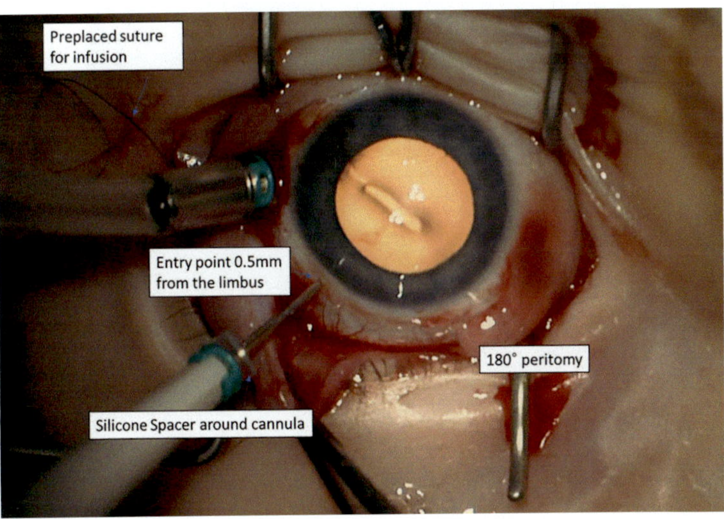

Fig. 19.2 Intraoperative photo of surgical opening during trocar insertion. The silicone spacer depicted is a piece of 240 band normally used for scleral buckle procedures. It is cut to the size of the cannula, then punctured before placement, reducing the length of cannula inside the neonatal eye

Thorpe or 0.12 forcep), tunneling straight into the sclera and twisting as needed to enter the eye. Inserting trocars slowly and smoothly is critical, as it is much easier for the trocar blade to pierce the opposing retina in the pediatric eye if there is a sudden, jerking motion.

- If most of the retinal pathology is temporal, a nasal approach may be considered. Although this surgical approach requires operating across the face, the smaller size of the patient makes it feasible. The use of a hard shield taped over the fellow eye is advised, so that undue pressure is not placed on this eye while the surgeon anchors their hands intraoperatively.

Operative Considerations

The goal is to address as many transvitreal forces as possible, which are focused on the ridges (Fig. 19.3).

- Ridge to ridge
- Ridge to periphery
- Ridge to lens or ciliary body
- Ridge to nerve

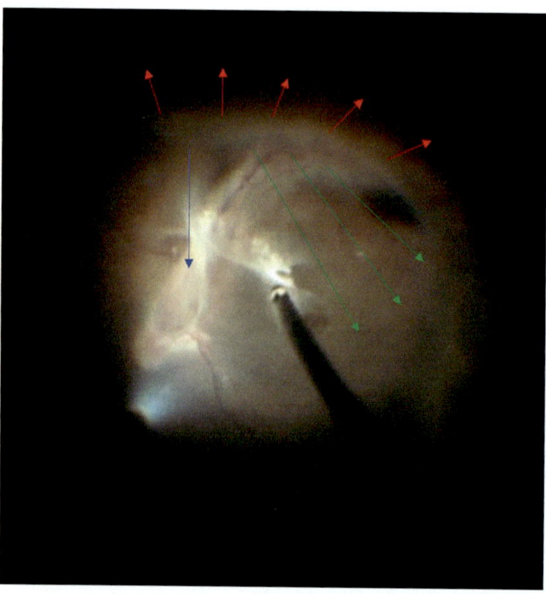

Fig. 19.3 Intraoperative posterior segment photo illustrating the transvitreal forces to address. Red = Ridge to Periphery. Blue = Ridge to Nerve. Green = Ridge to Ridge (forming a "drumhead). Further, anterior sources of traction that are not directly visualized here must also be relieved; ridge to lens and ridge to ciliary body. The primary goal of surgery is to sever these sources of traction to the ridge

The hyaloid will be extremely adherent; it tends to be organized into sheets, otherwise known as vitreoschisis. This frequently can fool the surgeon that they have removed the hyaloid. As a result, liberal use of triamcinolone throughout a surgery to highlight the vitreous may be helpful. If intraoperative OCT is available (Fig. 19.4), this can also be useful in identifying vitreous planes and retinal adhesion points.

In general, the authors' only instruments used during these surgeries are the vitreous cutter and endoilluminator. We do not routinely find instruments such as scissors, loops, picks or elevators useful in the goal of severing traction to the ridges.

The posterior hyaloid should be elevated carefully at the optic nerve to sever ridge to nerve transvitreal traction; others have shown this may improve functional and anatomic outcomes [14]. Hyaloid elevation is typically extended close to the ridge, stopping 1–2 disc diameters from the ridge to prevent any excess traction and retinal break at the ridge or within the detached retina. Elevation of the hyaloid is performed slowly to identify and observe focal areas of vitreoretinal adhesion, which may require trimming the vitreous around these areas to prevent creating full or partial-thickness retinal holes in attached retina.

While removing the maximal amount of cortical vitreous is often the goal in adult surgery, it is frequently necessary to leave significant amounts in ROP cases to avoid making retinal breaks. Always remember the number one goal is to avoid the creation of retinal breaks in ROP detachments. As such, we always advise using high cut rates with low aspiration, given the low margin for error.

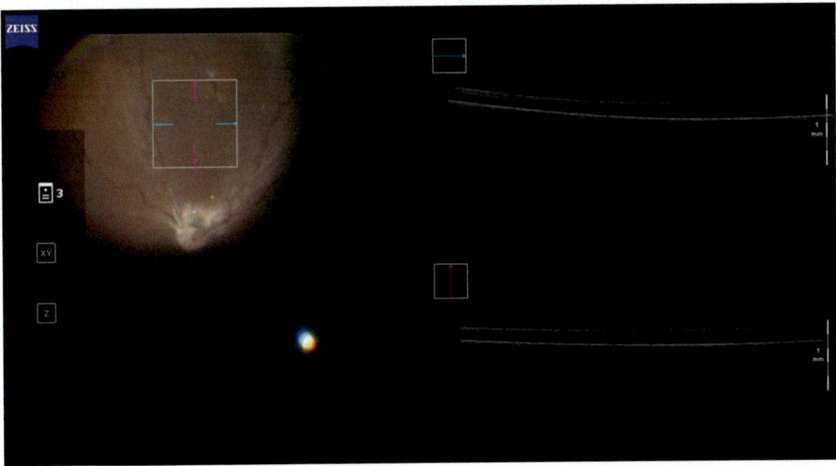

Fig. 19.4 Intraoperative optical coherence tomography (OCT) being used to demonstrate that the hyaloid has been elevated off the macula. During this case, there were several layers that appeared to be a hyaloid face which were elevated; these deceptive layers are caused by vitreoschisis. Also note the surgeon is sitting nasally in this case

Maneuvering in the Crowded Operative Field

Be exceedingly mindful of avoiding instrumentation crossing midline, as the lens is disproportionately thick in the neonatal eye compared to the size of the rest of the eye [13].

When using a standard indirect lighting system, such as the Resight or BIOM, the instruments will frequently bump the indirect lens due to the anterior placement of the trocars. One can consider using high magnification lenses (such as the green 60D lens in the Resight system), as the focal point is further from the eye, making lens bump easier to avoid, though this comes with limitation of field of view.

To further improve maneuverability issues, one can consider using a curved lighting system. While curved endoilluminators are not commonly available, a curved lighted endolaser can be used for such a purpose.

Some surgeons may prefer a chandelier lighting system to allow for bimanual techniques. While this is reasonable, recall that the goal of surgery is to sever traction, not to peel all membranes. The authors prefer to not add chandelier systems to the already crowded surgical field. In some cases, transcorneal (held by the assistant) or transscleral illumination can be helpful techniques for surgeons who prefer bimanual techniques [15]. Again, pre-planning the surgical approach based on the patient's pathology, such as approaching nasally for primarily temporal pathology, can help optimize the surgeon's ability to address tractional forces.

Closure

Begin closing when operative goals have been achieved. The retina will not be reattached at the end of these surgeries. Instead, once transvitreal traction has been relieved, the retina will reattach over the next weeks to months due to the underlying retinal pigment epithelial pump (Fig. 19.5).

If all transvitreal traction cannot be relieved safely without iatrogenic breaks, then we advise concluding the surgery for consideration of a stepwise approach to repair. Later surgeries may become more successful as some approximation of the retina to the RPE may better expose surgical planes that can be addressed in subsequent surgeries, and also improve margin for error to avoid iatrogenic breaks.

Be mindful of the position of the infusion canula as it can easily migrate in small eyes. The authors always recheck its positioning in the vitreous cavity before moving to fluid-air exchange. We routinely end cases with the vitreous cavity filled with air to aid with ensuring wound closure, and to theoretically debulk residual vascular endothelial growth factor.

We close all sclerotomies with 8–0 vicryl suture, and wounds are checked to be airtight. We then close conjunctiva with 8–0 vicryl suture, and place subconjunctival antibiotic and steroid. A drop of 1% atropine is placed, and a combination antibiotic + steroid ointment is placed on the eye, followed by a patch and shield which we leave until the post-operative day 1 evaluation.

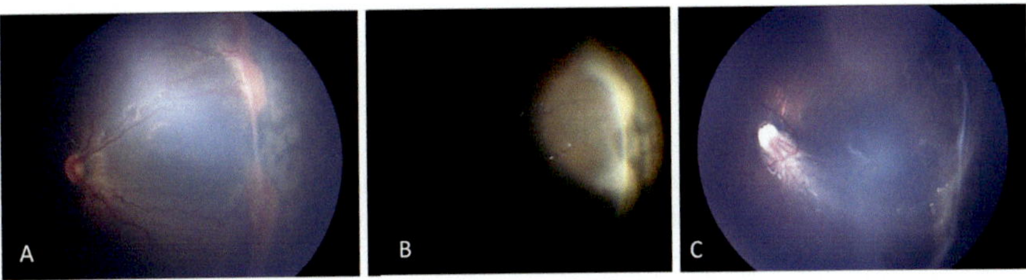

Fig. 19.5 25 6/7 wk GA, 790 g BW, twin premature baby now 43 wk PMA and 3115 g with a history of retinopathy of prematurity who was transferred from outside facility for recurrent ROP after laser treatment. **A.** Posterior Zone 2, Stage 4A ROP with plus disease in the left eye. **B.** Intraoperative photo showing the appearance of this ridge at the end of surgery; while it appeared somewhat relaxed, the temporal retinal fold is not completely attached, which is not an intraoperative goal of surgery. **C.** POM6, the retina is completely attached. There is a temporal prominent vitreous band which will be closely monitored. There is also inferior macular dragging

Ocriplasmin Assisted Vitrectomy

The use of intravitreal ocriplasmin to facilitate easier removal of the hyaloid, and facilitate dissection of vitreous planes was investigated in a small, prospective clinical trial, and it did not confer a benefit to retinal reattachment or ability to induce a posterior vitreous detachment [16, 17]. Given the lack of evidence for benefit, the authors do not currently recommend use of ocriplasmin in ROP detachment repair.

Intraoperative Hemorrhages

If intraoperative bleeding is noted emanating from a ridge, we encourage immediately increasing intraocular pressure, generally to around the neonate's mean arterial pressure, to attain hemostasis and prevent heme from possibly forming a scaffold for later membrane development. The authors typically set a timer of 60 s when increasing IOP to not lose track of how much time the eye may be ischemic. To achieve hemostasis, the authors encourage the use of endolaser for cautery instead of diathermy, to avoid full thickness retinal breaks, or later formation of atrophic holes.

Iatrogenic Breaks

If an iatrogenic break is formed, we advise aggressively removing all traction from this break, draining subretinal fluid through this break, using endolaser to achieve retinopexy, then performing a fluid-air exchange followed by instilling silicone oil into the vitreous cavity. Unfortunately, even with these measures, anatomic and functional outcomes are usually poor [1].

Postoperative Considerations

Care Instructions

If the patient is found to be manipulating the patch and shield, one can consider the use of "No-No" elbow restraints, however the authors do not find this is routinely needed in this age group. We advise a pediatric sized eye shield to be taped over the eye for the first week (without a patch) when eye drops are not being placed.

Our usual post-operative eye drop regiment is a combination neomycin-polymyxin-dexamethasone eye drop four times a day in the operated eye(s), and one drop of atropine 1% daily.

Follow-up Considerations

Our usual follow-up routine includes evaluation at 1 day, 1 week, then every 1–2 weeks depending on patient recovery. Patience is key in observing ROP detachment recovery; it may take months or even a year for the retina to flatten. As long as transvitreal traction was addressed, the retina should flatten. Handheld OCT and fundus photography can be helpful in monitoring improvement in subretinal fluid, if they are available.

When to reoperate

The primary reasons to re-operate is if the retinal detachment is not responding or worsening, or if neovascularization has worsened, with or without significant vitreous hemorrhage. We suggest intervention in a timely fashion, generally within 1 week of identification that the disease process is worsening to prevent progression to Stage 5 disease. Begin with an exam under anesthesia and consider a fluorescein angiogram to clearly demarcate avascular retina, and determine if further laser ablation is required, which may explain why the disease process has worsened.

Surgical Outcome and Prognosis

To reiterate, anatomic and functional success is most dependent on presenting stage of ROP detachment. Studies vary in outcomes, but a retrospective review from 2015 which included 496 eyes that had undergone vitrectomy for ROP detachment found a retinal reattachment rate of 82% for stage 4A, 69% for stage 4B, and 43% for stage 5 disease after a single surgery [3]. 20% of eyes required another surgery, of which 88% required lensectomy as well [3]. Another large study of 88 eyes in 2017 found similar results; 89% anatomic success in stage 4A, 63% in stage 4B, and 42% in stage 5 ROP [4].

Functional outcomes are variable depending on follow-up timing and type of visual acuity testing. Results range widely from a mean of 20/60 to 20/550 in stage 4A ROP, and 20/200 to 20/1600 for stage 4B, and 20/4000 or worse for stage 5 disease [4, 18]. In the original ETROP report, macular attachment was only attained in 5 of 16 stage 4A eyes, with only one patient having a visual acuity of 20/200 or better [19]. Only 2 of the stage 4B eyes had any measurable visual acuity, and no stage 5 patients had measurable visual acuity. Surgical results may be better in eyes with pre-operative laser or intravitreal anti-VEGF treatment, sparing the lens intraoperatively, and surgically inducing a posterior hyaloid detachment [14]. Note that neurologic injury may also limit vision in many extremely premature infants [19]. Other structural retinal problems may also limit vision, including foveal dragging, retinoschisis, and macular capillary injury from the initial oxygen insult [13]. Lastly, late retinal detachment may occur after childhood from the development of retinal breaks [5, 20].

Finally, anterior segment problems may complicate ROP patients after surgery. 17% may develop cataracts after lens-sparing pars plana vitrectomy [3]. Glaucoma is also more likely to occur in patients with ROP, though this may be associated with advanced ROP itself, and not necessarily ROP detachment surgery [21]. If a patient is left aphakic, their risk of glaucoma increases even more [21].

Conclusions

Recognition of progression to detachment in ROP and timing to surgical intervention are critical, as stage of ROP detachment at the time of surgery is the most important predictor of anatomic success and visual outcomes. In general, lens-sparing vitrectomy is the best surgical strategy to address stage 4 ROP detachments. To prevent further recurrence even after surgery, thorough completion of laser ablation of the avascular retina in both eyes is key. Then, the chief goal in surgery is to avoid creating retinal breaks. The second goal is to relieve traction by severing transvitreal forces on the ridge. We encourage staging surgeries when necessary if it appears there may be risk of creating a retinal break. We also encourage sutured closure of all sclerotomies for maximal control of wounds, the possibility of self-induced trauma post-operatively, and difficulty of post-operative examination.

Return to Case Presentation

This former 25 weeks 6 days GA twin boy, now 43-week PMA who had already undergone laser ablation therapy was taken to the operating room the day after transfer, where general anesthesia was induced. First, a thorough exam under anesthesia was performed, confirming the bedside examination; specifically, a stage 4A detachment was noted in the left eye. Then, indirect laser was performed in both eyes to thoroughly complete ablation of the avascular retina.

A sterile prep and drape were performed, and a 25G vitrectomy was performed using the principles described in the above text. Care was taken to sever all transvitreal traction to the ridge without causing retinal breaks. All sclerotomies were closed with 8–0 vicryl suture. The patient was followed the next day, then weekly until discharge. The Stage 4A detachment was noted to have improved by post-operative week 1, then nearly completely regressed by month 1 with a prominent residual vitreous band temporally. The retina remained attached with foveal dragging and ROP regression in both eyes, with the prominent residual vitreous band noted temporally in the left eye 6 months after surgery (Figure E).

Review Questions

1. **Which of the following are intraoperative goals of ROP detachment repair?**

   a. **Sever transvitreal forces**
   b. Completing a thorough shave vitrectomy
   c. **Avoid creation of any retinal breaks**
   d. Reattach the retina
   e. Peeling of all membranes, or as many membranes as possible
   f. Introduce silicone oil to compress the retina
   g. Introduce gas to tamponade the retina
   h. Cauterization of any source of intraoperative hemorrhage

2. **What technique is generally optimal for completing ablation of the avascular retina during or prior to ROP detachment repair?**

   a. Curved endolaser
   b. Cryotherapy
   c. **Indirect laser**
   d. Diathermy

3. **Where should one introduce trocars in the typical ROP detachment patient?**

   a. 0–0.5 mm posterior to the limbus
   b. **0.5–1 mm posterior to the limbus**
   c. 1–1.5 mm posterior to the limbus
   d. 5–3 mm posterior to the limbus

4. **Pre-operative intravitreal ocriplasmin has been shown to:**

   a. Improve retinal reattachment rate
   b. Improve ease of elevating the posterior hyaloid
   c. Improve visual outcomes
   d. **None of the above**

Answers

1. A and C
2. C
3. B
4. D

References

1. Asano MK, Papakostas TD, Palma CV, Skondra D. Visual outcomes of surgery for stage 4 and 5 retinopathy of prematurity. Int Ophthalmol Clin. 2014;54(2):225–37.
2. Capone A Jr, Trese MT. Lens-sparing vitreous surgery for tractional stage 4A retinopathy of prematurity retinal detachments. Ophthalmology. 2001;108(11):2068–70.
3. Nudleman E, Robinson J, Rao P, Drenser KA, Capone A, Trese MT. Long-term outcomes on lens clarity after lens-sparing vitrectomy for retinopathy of prematurity. Ophthalmology. 2015;122(4):755–9.
4. Karacorlu M, Hocaoglu M, Sayman Muslubas I, Arf S. Long-term functional results following vitrectomy for advanced retinopathy of prematurity. Br J Ophthalmol. 2017;101 (6):730–4.
5. Hamad AE, Moinuddin O, Blair MP, Schechet SA, Shapiro MJ, Quiram PA, et al. Late-onset retinal findings and complications in untreated retinopathy of prematurity. Ophthalmol Retina. 2020;4(6):602–12.
6. Steward DJ. Preterm infants are more prone to complications following minor surgery than are term infants. Anesthesiology. 1982;56(4):304–6.
7. Yonekawa Y, Wu WC, Kusaka S, Robinson J, Tsujioka D, Kang KB, et al. Immediate sequential bilateral pediatric vitreoretinal surgery: an international multicenter study. Ophthalmology. 2016;123(8):1802–8.
8. Yonekawa Y, Thomas BJ, Thanos A, Todorich B, Drenser KA, Trese MT, et al. The cutting edge of retinopathy of prematurity care: expanding the boundaries of diagnosis and treatment. Retina. 2017;37(12):2208–25.
9. Hartnett ME, Maguluri S, Thompson HW, McColm JR. Comparison of retinal outcomes after scleral buckle or lens-sparing vitrectomy for stage 4 retinopathy of prematurity. Retina. 2004;24(5):753–7.
10. Yonekawa Y, Thanos A, Abbey AM, Thomas BJ, Todorich B, Faia LJ, et al. Hybrid 25- and 27-gauge vitrectomy for complex vitreoretinal surgery. Ophthalmic Surg Lasers Imaging Retina. 2016;47(4):352–5.
11. Maguire AM, Trese MT. Lens-sparing vitreoretinal surgery in infants. Arch Ophthalmol. 1992;110(2):284–6.
12. Wright LM, Harper CA 3rd, Chang EY. Management of infantile and childhood retinopathies: optimized pediatric pars plana vitrectomy sclerotomy nomogram. Ophthalmol Retina. 2018;2(12):1227–34.
13. Hansen ED, Hartnett ME. A review of treatment for retinopathy of prematurity. Expert Rev Ophthalmol. 2019;14(2):73–87.
14. Özsaygili C, Ozdek S, Ozmen MC, Atalay HT, Yalinbas YD. Parameters affecting postoperative success of surgery for stage 4A/4B ROP. Br J Ophthalmol. 2019;103 (11):1624–32.
15. Wong SC, Capone A Jr. Illumination techniques for complex pediatric anterior retinal detachment and associated retrolental plaque. Retina. 2015;35(9):1905–7.
16. Wong SC, Capone A Jr. Microplasmin (ocriplasmin) in pediatric vitreoretinal surgery: update and review. Retina. 2013;33(2):339–48.

17. Drenser K, Girach A, Capone A Jr. A randomized, placebo-controlled study of intravitreal ocriplasmin in pediatric patients scheduled for vitrectomy. Retina. 2016;36(3):565–75.
18. Prenner JL, Capone A Jr, Trese MT. Visual outcomes after lens-sparing vitrectomy for stage 4A retinopathy of prematurity. Ophthalmology. 2004;111(12):2271–3.
19. Repka MX, Tung B, Good WV, Shapiro M, Capone A Jr, Baker JD, et al. Outcome of eyes developing retinal detachment during the Early Treatment for Retinopathy of Prematurity Study (ETROP). Arch Ophthalmol. 2006;124(1):24–30.
20. Smith JM, Ward LT, Townsend JH, Yan J, Hendrick AM, Cribbs BE, et al. Rhegmatogenous retinal detachment in children: clinical factors predictive of successful surgical repair. Ophthalmology. 2019;126(9):1263–70.
21. Nudleman E, Muftuoglu IK, Gaber R, Robinson J, Drenser K, Capone A, et al. Glaucoma after lens-sparing vitrectomy for advanced retinopathy of prematurity. Ophthalmology. 2018;125(5):671–5.

Vitreoretinal Surgery for Stage 5 ROP

20

Cemal Özsaygılı and Şengül Özdek

Abstract

Stage 5 retinopathy of prematurity (ROP) was considered an inoperable disease. Today, with the increasing experience of clinicians in ROP surgery, stage 5 ROP is no longer an incurable disease. The surgery is still very challenging with very limited functional outcomes. The preservation of the globe shape and appearance and even a light perception (LP) vision is a success in these eyes. The International ROP Classification (ICROP) committee recently recommended a subcategorization of stage 5 ROP into three and eyes in stage 5A ROP have the best chance to benefit from surgery. Since phthisis bulbi (PB) is the natural course of the disease in such eyes, vitreoretinal surgery can even be done for cosmetic purposes just to protect the globe shape and prevent the development of deformity and unacceptable appearance.

Keywords

Stage 5 ROP · Retinopathy of prematurity · Tractional retinal detachment · Leukocoria · Lens sparing vitrectomy · Limbal lensectomy-vitrectomy · Staged surgery · Cosmetic success

Supplementary Information The online version contains supplementary material available at https://doi.org/10.1007/978-3-031-14506-3_20.

C. Özsaygılı
Ophthalmology Department, Kayseri City Training and Research Hospital, Kayseri, Turkey

Ş. Özdek (✉)
School of Medicine, Gazi University, Ankara, Turkey
e-mail: sengulozdek@gmail.com

Introduction

Retinopathy of prematurity (ROP), a vasoproliferative disease, remains the main preventable cause of childhood blindness [1]. The International ROP Classification (ICROP) has provided a common staging among clinicians for this important disease [2, 3]. The CRYO-ROP study [4] showed that cryotherapy treatment of threshold disease and the ETROP study [5] showed that laser photocoagulation treatment of high-risk pre-threshold disease can prevent progression to retinal detachment (RD). However, despite timely screening, adequate laser ablation, and/or pharmacological treatment strategies (anti-VEGF), approximately 10% of eyes with ROP may develop total RD [6] and the treatment method of RD is undoubtedly surgical intervention.

Vitreoretinal surgery (VRS) has been applied for more than 30 years to prevent blindness for many vitreoretinal diseases with increasing success. The results of surgery for stage 4 ROP is very satisfactory and especially surgery for stage 4A eyes usually end up with very high anatomical and functional results. On the other hand, stage 5 ROP was used to be accepted as an inoperable disease. Today, with the increasing experience of clinicians in ROP surgery and the development of vitreoretinal surgical techniques and instruments, stage 5 ROP is no longer an incurable disease. The surgery for stage 5 ROP is still very challenging, and the anatomical and functional results are not always satisfactory [7–13]. The expectations are much different and lower than stage 4 ROP as expected, however, even the preservation of light perception (LP) is a success for such eyes. LP vision is very important in terms of maintaining the circadian rhythm of the baby for the secretions of hormones and for the general health [14]. Furthermore, preservation of the globe shape and cosmetic appearance is another goal for the surgery by preventing progression to phthisis bulbi (PB) which is the natural course of the disease in eyes with stage 5 ROP.

One of the major updates in the recent ICROP3 [15] was the subcategorization of stage 5 ROP. The ICROP committee recommends that the stage 5 ROP be subcategorized in three configurations. In stage 5A, the optic nerve head (ONH) can be seen by ophthalmoscopy and suggests open funnel RD. In stage 5B, the ONH is not seen secondary to retrolental fibrovascular tissue which is mostly associated with closed funnel RD. In stage 5C, on the other hand, stage 5B findings are accompanied by the abnormalities of the anterior segment (forward displacement of the crystallin lens, prominent shallowing of the anterior chamber, iridocapsular adhesions, corneal opacifications). It is widely accepted that eyes with stage 5A and B ROP may benefit from surgery to some extend either anatomically, functionally or at least cosmetically. Our group has recently reported an overall anatomical success of 57.5% in Group A and 16.5% in Group B [16]. Group C eyes with anterior segment abnormalities were not operated on, with the prediction that they would not benefit from the surgery [16].

VRS is still questionable, especially in unilateral cases. Some surgeons do not operate stage 5 eyes when the fellow eye is good. However, these eyes usually become deformed within time with development of phthisis bulbi and/or corneal opacification. We believe that, VRS may be done even for cosmetic purposes only to preserve the globe and to prevent development of deformed and unacceptable appearance.

Surgical Technique

Surgical intervention is advised in patients with open or closed funnel stage 5 ROP without corneal opacification. Surgical approaches include lens-sparing vitrectomy (LSV), and combined lensectomy-vitrectomy (LV) surgery. Scleral buckling may be added to the surgery in selected cases.

Scleral Buckling

Stage 5 ROP-related RDs are associated with fibrovascular membranes leading to tractional forces. SB supports the vitreous base, release circumferential cortical vitreous traction and has a very limited role in Stage 5A ROP [17]. In a study published in 1984 examining the anatomical and functional results of stage 5 ROP surgery, encircling band (240S) was used to support the posterior margin of the proliferation area in 40 eyes that underwent lensectomy and vitrectomy, and reported that 45% of the eyes were reattached at 6-month follow-up [10]. However, in another more recent study investigating the role of SB in reducing traction forces in stage 4 ROP detachments, it was stated that the use of SB with LSV did not provide any additional benefit [18]. Today, although VRS has replaced the SB in the surgical treatment of stage 5 ROP, SB may still be helpful as an auxiliary procedure for the treatment of holes caused by tractional forces in the thin retina, or in the treatment of iatrogenic retinal tears during surgery. It can be used to counteract the peripheral traction caused by residual membranes usually as an adjunct to pars plana vitrectomy (PPV). It supports the vitreous base and peripheral retina. The encircling buckle can cause high myopia close to -10 diopters, reduce ocular blood flow, and inhibit the growth of the globe. Therefore, the buckle should be removed after 6 months. When it is removed or loosened after 6 months, a reduction in myopia can be achieved by half [19].

Surgical Principles of Vitrectomy

The RD observed in stage 5 ROP is complex, but the surgical management of these eyes has evolved over time. A successful outcome depends on performing VRS after plus disease and neovascular activity has completely resolved. Surgery performed without regression of the undesirable vascular activity may result in failure associated with hemorrhage, exudation, proliferation, and contraction of vasoproliferative membranes after surgery. However, in early stage 5A cases, waiting will result in progression of the disease into stage 5B with a closed funnel RD where the prognosis is much poorer. So operating these eyes at the appropriate time and performing a successful surgery involve a decision-making process that is not easy to manage. Preoperative Anti-VEGF injection may be considered for these eyes 1–2 days before the surgery, but one should be cautious about the crunch phenomenon [15].

- LV surgery with a limbal entry is the preferred method for eyes with leukocoria (Fig. 20.1). However, LSV with pars plicata entry may still be used in eyes where the peripheral retina is not dragged to the back of the lens or ciliary body (Fig. 20.2).
- A "staged surgery" is a good option in leucocoric stage 5 cases. The main fibrotic bands causing tractions are usually removed during the first surgery and the retina is given time to settle down and go backwards to attach at least partially within a few months. Then, a second surgery can be planned to remove tinier membranes and to relieve the retinal tractions more. This kind of approach is called as "staged surgery" (Fig. 20.6).
- Late stage 5C cases usually come with anterior segment changes like very shallow anterior chamber and irido-corneo-lenticular adhesions leading to corneal opacification (Fig. 20.3). We do not prefer to do surgery after corneal opacification.
- Limbal versus Pars Plana/Plicata Approach: This is one of the most important and decisive steps of the surgery. The eye should be examined again just before the surgery to assess the peripheral retina to determine if there is any dragged retina anteriorly through the ciliary body towards the back of the lens. These parts should be avoided as an entry site for sclerotomy which may lead to retinal

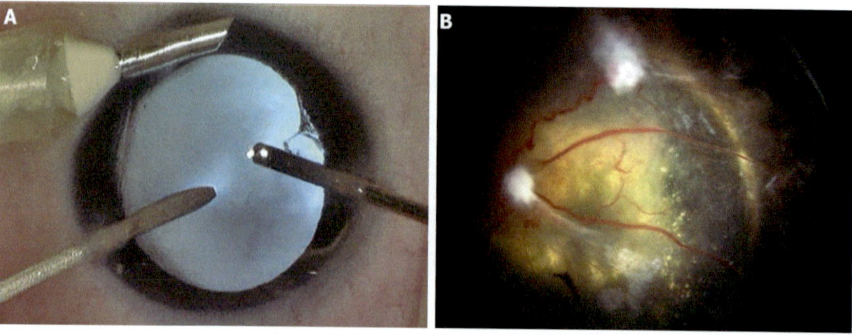

Fig. 20.1 **A** Leukocoric Stage 5B ROP treated with limbal LV. **B** Postoperative 4th year fundus picture with total shallow retinal detachment, subretinal exudates and some residual membranes over the disc and arcuate vessels. Visual acuity is hand motions. (See **video** 1 for stage 5B ROP surgery)

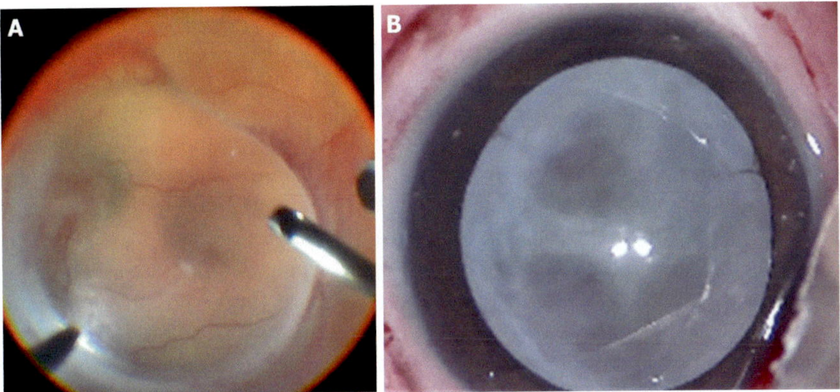

Fig. 20.2 Stage 5 ROP. **A** Stage 5A RD with open funnel where LSV is still possible. **B** Stage 5B with closed funnel RD and leukocoria presentation where a limbal LV is the preferred technique for surgery

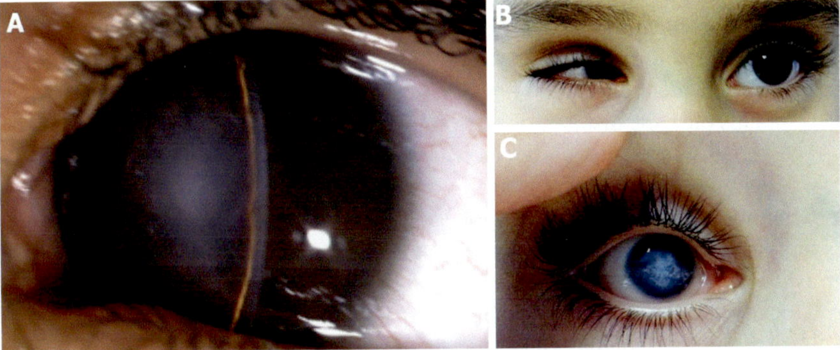

Fig. 20.3 **A** Corneal opacification with irido-corneo-lenticular adhesions in a late cicatricial stage 5C ROP. **B** Another bilateral stage 5 ROP. Right eye (RE) was unoperated, left eye (LE) was operated. Note that RE has bad cosmesis with phytisation and corneal opacification within years (**C**) while the operated LE is well-preserved in shape with good cosmesis

break formation at the beginning of the surgery. The safest place for the entry sites can be determined by using trans-scleral illumination which is another useful method to determine the location of the pars plana. At this point, the surgeon should decide if it is possible to enter the eye through pars plicata safely (to preserve the lens) or not. If the peripheral retina and pars plicata look safe, then sclerotomy through pars plicata/pars plana is the first choice. If not, a limbal approach with lensectomy has to be done.

- Limbal approach means that the surgeon has to sacrifice the lens which is the major disadvantage of this approach. The other disadvantages are risk of iris injury and induced miosis, endothelial damage & corneal edema induction, limited view of posterior segment because of the corneal distortion and edema caused by limbal entry sites and limited access of instruments to the posterior retina hitting the indirect viewing systems. Additionally, if 10/0 monofilament nylon sutures were used to close the limbal incisions they will need to be removed in another examination under general anesthesia (EUGA) session. There is no need for removal when 10/0 vicryl sutures are used. Additionally there may be a risk of fibrous ingrowth from the limbal entry sites postoperatively. The most important advantage of this approach is the avoidance of peripheral retinal damage during entry. Other advantages are; there is no need for canthotomy and conjunctiva is protected for future possible glaucoma surgeries by this approach.

- Trans-iris root approach where the trockars are entered just posterior to the limbus through the iris root to reach the back of the iris, is another alternative for the entry site. Lens has to be sacrified with this option but it is possible to avoid corneal distortion problems caused by limbal entry sites to some extend and still avoids peripheral retinal damage. However the complications of this option are bleeding from the iris root into the anterior chamber, iris root damage and iridodialysis.
- Sclerotomy Step: When we decide to do the pars plana/plicata approach the distance from the limbus for scleral entry should be arranged according to the age of the patient during the first 3 years of age. In prematures and neonates (till 6 months old), the distance of sclerotomy site from the limbus should be 1.5 mm and the distance should be increased accordingly with age, which reaches 3.5 mm after 3 years of age like in adults.
- Sclerotomy sites can even be moved from temporal to the nasal quadrant with the aid of preoperative comprehensive examination of the peripheral retina to avoid damage to the anteriorly dragged retinal folds.
- Trocars: Trocars should be entered perpendicularly without angulation in contrast to adults. Oblique entry may increase the risk of the lens or peripheral retinal damage. The length of the regular adult trocars is not appropriate for the babies and total insertion of the cannulas may cause damage to the structures like retinal folds within the vitreous cavity. Therefore, using a piece of silicone band or a tube at the bottom of the trocar to shorten the intraocular length of it may be a good solution (**see the Video** 2, Fig. 20.4). The tip of the infusion cannula should be secured and watched carefully throughout the surgery to prevent the lens and peripheral retinal damage with inadventant movement of the cannula.
- A peritomy at the sites of sclerotomies should be done at the beginning and all the sclerotomies should be sutured in pediatric cases. It is sometimes tricky to have watertight closure of the sclerotomies in pediatric cases. This is extremely important especially in eyes with active neovascularization, because leakage through the sclerotomies may end up with hypotonia causing postoperative hemorrhages and failure. A preplaced suture for infusion cannula may prevent such hypotonia during sclerotomy closure (Fig. 20.4).

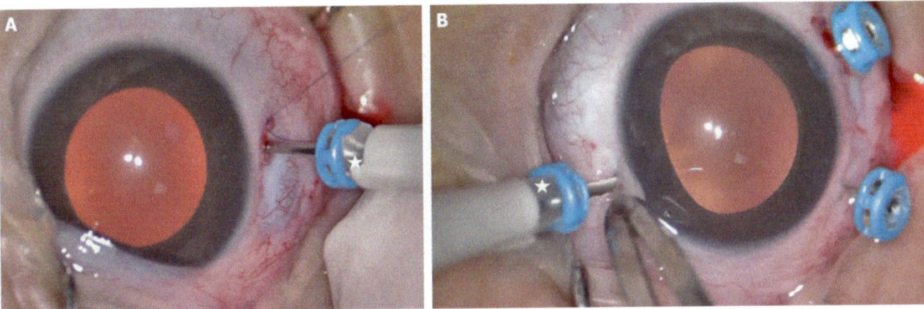

Fig. 20.4 **A** Insertion of the shortened 25-gauge trocar for the infusion cannula after placement of a piece of silicone band (white star) before the cannula, through the pre-placed 8/0 vicryl sutured sclerotomy area. **B** Pars plana insertion of other shortened-trocars after peritomy

- Vitreoretinal traction forces between the ridge to the lens/anterior hyaloid face, ridge to vitreous base, ridge to ridge, ridge to optic disc are released by excising the vitreous.
- Gauge: Any gauge (20G-23G-25G-27G) vitrectomy settings can be used during pediatric VRS. 23G and 25G are the most commonly used ones. Although there are vitrectomy settings with short vitrectomy and illumination probes, we do not believe that this has any advantage over regular adult probes since the surgeon can insert only the needed length of the instrument, unlike the trocars. However shorter trocars and cannulas would avoid peripheral retinal and lens problems during entry to some extent.
- Two versus 3 port entry: Two or 3 port entries can be used in pediatric VRS. Both have some advantages and disadvantages. Two-port vitrectomy needs different surgical instrumentation setup like infused forceps and scissors and endoillumination probes etc. since there is no separate infusion port in this setting. There are only superior 2 ports which give the advantage of enough space to move the eye during surgery which is normally limited with the third trocar in the inferotemporal quadrant, so that there is no need for canthotomy in neonates and prematures. However, one hand has to be within the eye all the time to avoid hypotony which may be tiring for the surgeon and there may be more risk of hypotony during the closure of sclerotomies. Three port vitrectomy, on the other hand, has the advantage of using the same instrumentation as in adults which all surgeons familiar with. There is no need for a different setup and instruments. Another advantage is less risk of hypotony because of the use of a separate infusion cannula. However, the third entry means additional risk for peripheral retina or lens damage and there is less space for maneuvers within the narrow interpalpebral rim especially in babies. This is also the reason why we do not prefer to use chandelier light for bimanual maneuvers in these small eyes which needs additional sclerotomy with additional sclerotomy associated risks.
- Use of Cannulas in entry sites: It is possible to do the surgery with or without cannula. Valved cannulas are useful to prevent vitreous herniation and leakage through the entry sites, however, it may prevent visualization and access to the

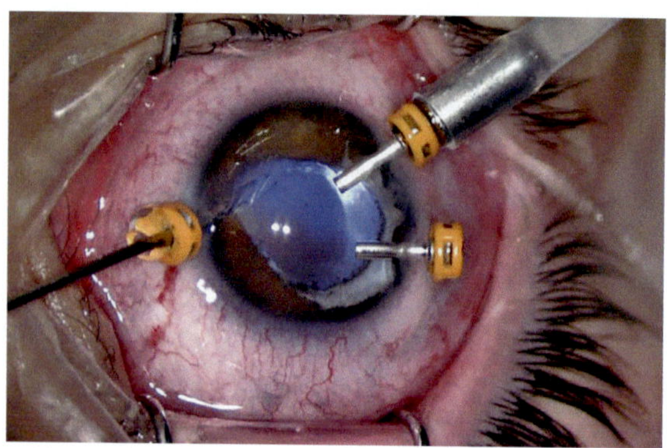

Fig. 20.5 Limbal entry with trocars

peripheral retina where you need to retract the cannula outwards. In eyes with predominantly anterior retinal pathologies, the risk of damage to the lens or peripheral retina with trocars & cannulas is higher and the cannulas may restrict the extent of maneuvers of microforceps and scissors in the peripheral retina by restricting the opening of the tips of the forcepses squeezed in the tight cannula. In such cases scleral or limbal entry can be done directly with a microblade without a cannula, however, this approach has the risk of vitreous herniation and leakage through the entry sites in pars plana/plicata approach and iris damage and herniation together with pupillary problems and increased incidence of corneal edema in limbal approach. (Fig. 20.1A, limbal entry without trocars, Fig. 20.5 limbal entry with trocars).

- Iris hooks can be used if there is significant posterior synechia preventing pupillary dilatation. Mechanical dilation of the pupil with iris retractors will be less traumatic, as incisions into the iris may cause reactive proliferation. However the surgeon may sacrifice the iris by performing a partial iridectomy when needed to perform effective membrane peeling. Diathermia can be applied to the pupillary border at the end of the surgery to stiffen the iris and pupil diaphragm.
- Lensectomy: When lensectomy is planned a total capsulectomy has to be performed since the residual capsule serves as a scaffold for membrane proliferation and secondary circumferential vitreoretinal contraction. This may result in ciliary body detachment and hypotony. It may be impossible to peel this membrane when it turns into a contractile anterior ring. In cases with lenticulo-retinal apposition, it is usually easy to dissect the capsular material with forceps without causing retinal breaks, however, one should be cautious for not causing retinal dialysis.

Major Principle: Always try to preserve the lens and do lens sparing vitrectomy (LSV) if possible! If there is a high risk of peripheral retinal damage during sclerotomy, do not hesitate to do limbal approach and do Lensectomy-Vitrectomy (LV) to avoid retinal break since retinal break may be catastrophic in such eyes.

- Perfusion pressure of the retina is lower in children since they have lower systolic blood pressure. The infusion pressure should be kept lower than the adults during surgery (15–20 mmHg) and prolonged scleral depression should be avoided to avoid central retinal artery occlusion.
- Posterior Hyaloid Removal: Although it is not essential for stage 5 ROP, we always attempt to remove the posterior hyaloid from a limited area in the posterior pole if possible. This will decrease the risk of future posterior hyaloid contractions leading to visual loss. Triamcinolone is a sine qua non for this purpose. (see **video** 3, LSV for stage 5A ROP) The posterior vitreous detachment (PVD) can be induced by using microforcepses to grasp the hyaloid at the edge of the disc together with a piece of inner limiting membrane (ILM) in some occasions. Vacuum is too dangerous over a totally detached retina which may cause engagement of retina into the vitrector. When a small opening is made, it is easy to detach the remaining hyaloid with hydrodissection of the circulating balanced salt solution (BSS) in the vitreous cavity. If it is not possible to detach it, one should not insist on it to avoid iatrogenic break and trim the vitreous as much as possible by using the triamcinolone again and again to see the remaining vitreous.
- The main aim of the surgery is to relieve the tractions as much as possible without inducing an iatrogenic break. Perioperative attachment of the retina should not be expected for these cases. Total peeling of all membranes or removal of all the hyaloid is never aimed. They may be left in place if the surgeon feels that further peeling is risky for a retinal break or hemorrhage. (**video** 1, LV for stage 5B ROP with leucocoria).
- Retina moves backwards after release of tractions even during the surgery. It is crucial to decide where and when to stop dissection of the peripheral membranes to avoid iatrogenic retinal breaks or dialysis. The fibrous stalk emerging from the ONH, which causes a funnel-shaped fixation of the retina, should be dissected as much as possible until the posterior funnel is opened (Fig. 20.5). Any bleeding can be stopped by increasing the bottle height and diathermi can be used to coagulate the bleeding vessels with caution. Care should be taken not to keep IOP elevated for a long time in these premature infants during the surgery. Schlieren's sign (serous fluid from the subretinal space) may warn the surgeon about presence of an iatrogenic retinal break.
- In cases with emerging corneal edema, ophthalmic viscoelastic devices (OVD) are used to fill the anterior chamber and vitreous space instead of infusion fluid to prevent further edema and the surgery may be completed under OVD support.
- There may be associated subretinal hemorrhage in some of the long-standing cases of stage 5 ROP which can be detected as hyperreflective material under the detached retina with ultrasonography before the surgery. Transscleral drainage of subretinal hemorrhage may be performed in those cases during vitrectomy.

- Tamponade & Iatrogenic Retinal Break: Air is our first choice in pediatric VRS if there is no retinal break. Air helps to seal the entry sites, to decrease the risk of postoperative hypotony and hemorrhage, and to decrease inflammation. If there is a retinal break, this will change the choice of the tamponade. If the retinal break is in a peripheral relatively silent membrane free area, try to clear the vitreous and any residual membrane at least locally around the break area, continue with argon laser photocoagulation (LPC) to the break and support the break with a local buckle. If it is in the most proliferative area where there is quite a lot membrane and fibrovascular tissue which has a very high contraction capacity, recurrent proliferative vitreoretinopathy (PVR) may be unavoidable and it may be logical to abandon the surgery. It is almost impossible to get rid of all the membranes in such conditions. Tamponade of choice is C3F8 gas in such situations. Although some surgeons advocate the use of standard or heavy silicone oil (SO) as a tamponade, we do not prefer use of SO since there are always residual membranes in these diseases which may contract and cause subretinal migration of SO.
- At the end of the surgery, air or OVD is used as a tamponade at the surgeon's discretion.

Adjuncts to Vitreoretinal Surgery

Improved outcomes have been reported with the combination of pharmacological adjuvants to VRS. In stage 5 ROP with vascular engorgement and neovascularization, it has been reported that intravitreal triamcinolone (2.0 mg/0.05 ml) applied at the end of the VRS, results in significantly higher anatomical success thanks to its ability to cause plus disease resolution and involution of neovascular activity [20].

It has also been reported that the use of plasmin in stage 5 ROP vitrectomy has a positive effect on the results. Plasmin releases laminin and fibronectin, helping to separate the cortical vitreous from the retinal surface. Thus, it is suggested that plasmin may facilitate the membrane peeling procedure in stage 5 ROP eyes by weakening the adhesion between the proliferative membranes and the retina [21].

Bilateral Sequential Surgery

In pediatric VRS, immediate sequential bilateral surgery reduces the risks associated with re-anaesthesia in infants and avoids the delay of surgery for advanced disease. If sequential bilateral surgery is planned, surgery should be started as a new case and the eye should be resterilized, new vitrectomy packs, new drapes, new instruments should be used, and the surgical team should be re-scrubbed before starting surgery on the fellow eye to reduce the risk of endophthalmitis. No endophthalmitis and anaesthesia-related complications were reported in studies that performed immediate sequential bilateral vitreoretinal surgery for pediatric vitreoretinal disorders and ROP [22, 23].

Complications of Vitreoretinal Surgery

The main intraoperative complications of vitrectomy surgery performed in stage 5 ROP eyes are retinal tear formation and vitreous hemorrhage, and postoperative complications include glaucoma, corneal decompensation in patients who underwent limbal access/surgery, cataract development in LSV patients, endophthalmitis, band keratopathy, PB, and conjunctival cyst [24–26].

Glaucoma is one of the most commonly reported complications after VRS for stage 5 ROP. It is reported that it occurs in 8–33% of eyes after VRS and is detected more frequently when lensectomy is performed [26, 27]. This is explained by degeneration of trabecular meshwork cells due to increased oxygen diffusion in patients undergoing lensectomy [28].

Complications of VRS for stage 4–5 ROP are mentioned in detail in Chap. 22.

Surgical Outcomes

Prospective studies of stage 5 ROP surgery are difficult, and our knowledge of the outcome of surgery is provided by retrospective studies. However, differences in experience of the surgeon and variations in the severity or extent of stage 5 ROP-related RDs make it difficult to do a one-to-one comparison between retrospective studies.

The success can be described in 3 categories: cosmetic, anatomical and functional. The natural course of stage 5 ROP is phytisation and bad cosmesis with corneal opacification (Fig. 20.3C). So preserving the cosmetic appearance by preventing progression to PB is very beneficial on children's social communication in their future lives. There is limited data in the literature on ocular cosmetic outcomes after VRS for stage 5 ROP. Our group has recently reported a good cosmesis in 62.5% of the stage 5 eyes who had undergone vitreoretinal surgery [16].

Anatomical results of VRS differ between 13–45% among the reported series of different surgeons, and the anatomical definition of success may also differ between studies. It should be noted that the severity of each series of stage 5 ROP is not the same. Different criteria has been used by each study to describe anatomical success like; attachment of the retina at least in the posterior pole, complete retinal reattachment, or partial reattachment posterior to the equator [12, 16, 24, 29–32].

Among the studies describing the anatomical success as the posterior pole reattached, the success rate was reported as 28% in a large series including 601 eyes [33], and as 29% [7] and 19% in other studies [34]. In the series of Lakhanpal et al. in which they analyzed 33 eyes of 21 patients with at least 6 months follow-up, the anatomical success rate was reported as 45%. In that study, most (63.6%) of the patients had stage 5A-like open anteriorly–open posteriorly configuration [35]. Our group reported an anatomical success rate over 50% in stage 5A ROP cases, which dropped to 15–18% in stage 5B cases where there is an apparent leukocoria and closed funnel RD in ultrasonography [16]. The new subdivision of stage 5 ROP as described recently in ICROP3 will enable authors to standardize and compare the results of surgery more accurately for stage 5 subclasses.

Similarly, functional outcomes reported after VRS for Stage 5 ROP are also variable and a common definition of functional success has not been established. Functional results were decribed according to light perception (LP), localization, ability to follow small objects, form identification with the help of Teller Acuity Card or Snellen chart in different studies [16, 22, 24–26, 30–34]. It is an obligation to make a functional evaluation according to the age groups. There is very limited data on functional results of VRS for stage 5 ROP [7, 10, 21, 35, 36–39]. Wu et al. reported that visual acuity in majority of eyes (73.8%) was between 20/600 and LP and 14% ended up with no LP (NLP) during 4 year follow-up of 80 eyes they operated [39]. Cusick et al. reported LP or better vision in 74% and, only 4% had better than 5/200 in 183 eyes operated for stage 5 ROP [33]. In our series, 35% of the operated eyes were able to fix and follow light and objects at the age of 1 year, 34.6% could follow small objects and move independently at the age of 2 years, and 18.2% had ambulatory vision at the age of 3 years [16]. In bilateral stage 5 patients who have undergone surgery, starting to walk without parental support is a valuable indicator of the ambulatory vision. Variables such as associated mental retardation and neurological disorders may complicate the assessment of functional outcomes in these children. Exposure of children to stimuli in environments enriched with light awareness will positively support their development, despite initial poor vision results.

Case Presentation

Staged Surgery in a Case with Stage 5B ROP (Fig. 20.6).

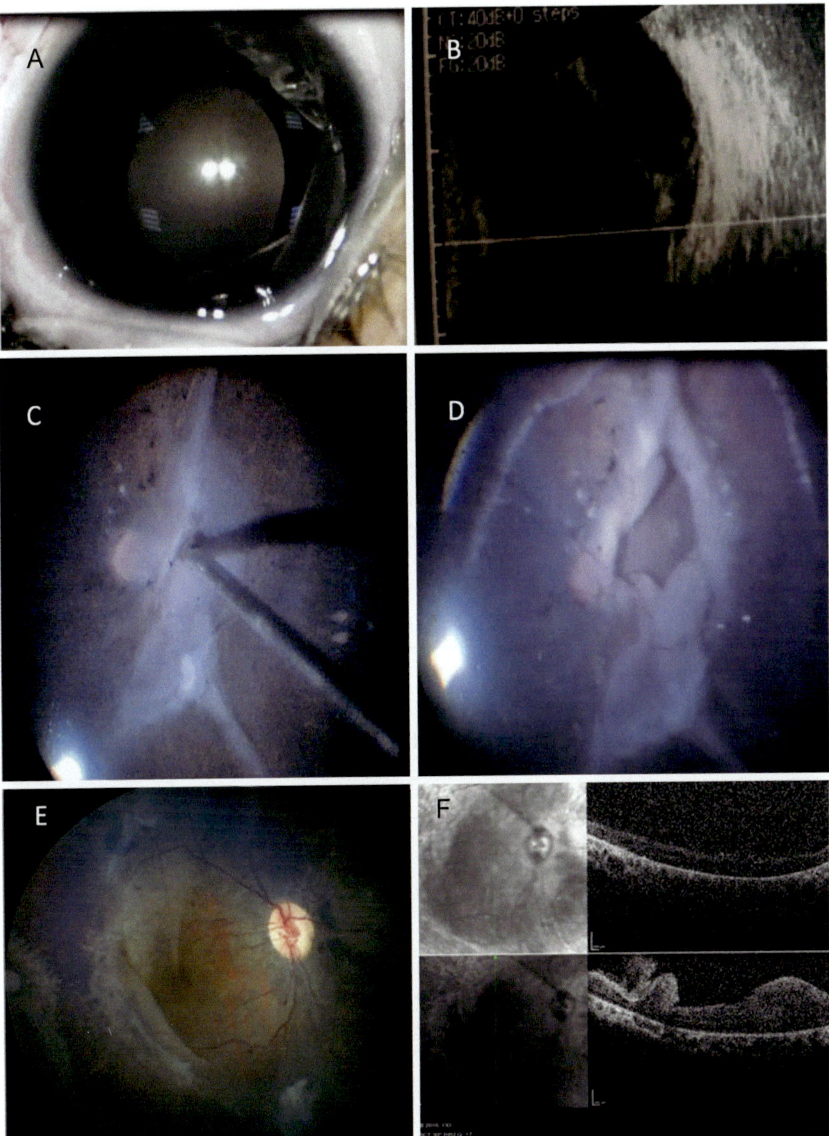

Fig. 20.6 This was a baby prematurely born at 29 postmestrual week with a birth weight of 950 gr who did not have any treatment before was referred to our clinic with leucocoria (**A**). B scan ultrasonography yielded tractional retinal detachment but not a closed funnel configuration (**B**). He had a limbal lensectomy, vitrectomy surgery which effectively released the anteroposterior tractions and ended up with attached retina with folds in the posterior pole. A second surgery is performed to open up these retinal folds 6 months after the first surgery (**C**) and the membranes causing macular folds could be peeled up extensively (**D**). **E** Shows the fundus picture at 5 years old; retina is attached with some minor folds in OCT (**F**) and vision was 20/100 with aphakic correction

Conclusions

- LSV or LV surgery may be preferred according to the configuration of the RD, the degree of peripheral anterior traction and retino-lenticular adhesions, and the preoperative or intraoperative clarity of the lens in stage 5 ROP.
- Intravitreal anti-VEGF injection 1–2 days before the surgery may reduce the risk of intraoperative hemorrhage in eyes with highly active plus disease.
- It is important to avoid any retinal break formation which may mandate the surgeon to abandon the surgery.
- It is usually not possible to reattach the retina in one surgery. A staged surgery principle is applied for these eyes.
- The results of surgery for stage 5 ROP is still far from satisfactory for the patients. The visual expectations should be kept very low, sometimes surgery may be planned just for anatomical and cosmetic reasons especially in stage 5B (closed funnel RD) cases.
- However, there is a trend for better anatomical and visual results in advanced ROP in the literature with the advances in vitreoretinal surgical techniques and equipments and increased experience.

Review Questions

1. Which one is correct for the natural course of the stage 5 ROP eyes?

a. Phytisation of the globe
b. Shallowing of anterior chamber followed by posterior synechia and irido-lenticulo-corneal adhesions.
c. Corneal opacification
d. Leucokoria
e. All of the above

2. Which of the following stage 5 ROP eyes has the best prognosis?

a. Stage 5A
b. Stage 5B
c. Stage 5C
d. Stage 5A associted with plus disease
e. Stage 5A associated with vitreous hemorrhage

3. A 39-week-old infant who was prematurely born at 27 weeks of PMA was referred to the clinic with bilateral leukocoria, and did not receive any treatment before. B-scan Ultrasonography yields a closed funnel RD. Which of the following statement is correct?

a. Parents should be informed that the patient will not benefit from surgery.
b. The patient's clinic is compatible with stage 5 B ROP, and bilateral lensectomy —vitrectomy surgery in the same session would be the right approach.
c. It would be an appropriate approach to inform the parents that the patient will benefit from the surgery and to perform a lens-sparing surgery to avoid amblyopia.
d. The patient should be given the chance of combined keratoplasty and open sky vitrectomy surgery.

4. Which of the following statement is correct about staged surgery for stage 5 ROP?

a. Surgery is graded according to subclassification of ROP
b. All membranes must be cleaned during the first surgery.
c. Complete reattachment of the retina is expected during the first surgery.
d. Major fibrotic membranes causing traction are usually removed during the first surgery, and a second surgery may be scheduled within a few months after the retina partly settles down to remove the tinier membranes to relieve more retinal traction.
e. Iatrogenic retinotomy can be done to achieve complete retinal reattachment during the second stage of the surgery.

Answers

1. **(E)**

2. **(A)** The prognosis is worst in stage 5C ROP which is associated with anterior segment abnormalities (shallow anterior chamber, iridocapsular adhesions, corneal opacifications). Stage 5B eyes are associated with frank leukocoria and closed funnel RD. The prognosis is best in stage 5A ROP cases characterized by open funnel retinal detachment. Hemorrhage in the vitreous cavity can act as a scaffold for proliferation and new membrane formation due to the growth factors it contains. The presence of plus disease may lead to bleeding during or after the surgery which adversely affects the prognosis.

3. **(B)** This is a typical stage 5B ROP. In stage 5 B ROP cases, performing LV surgery in the same session, if possible, would be the most appropriate option.

4. **(D)** The main fibrotic bands causing tractions are usually removed during the first surgery and the retina is given time to settle down and go backwards to attach at least partially within a few months. Then, a second surgery can be planned to remove tinier membranes and to relieve the retinal tractions more. This kind of approach is called as "staged surgery".

References

1. Reese AB, King MJ, Owens WC. Classification of retrolental fibroplasia. Am J Ophthalmol. 1953;36(10):1333e1335.
2. The Committee for the Classification of Retinopathy of Prematurity. An international classification of retinopathy of prematurity. Arch Ophthalmol. 1984;102(8):1130e1134.
3. International Classification of Retinopathy of Prematurity Committee for Classification of Late Stages of ROP. An international classification of retinopathy of prematurity: II. The classification of retinal detachment. Arch Ophthalmol. 1987;105:906e912.
4. Cryotherapy for Retinopathy of Prematurity Cooperative Group. Multicenter trial of cryotherapy for retinopathy of prematurity. Preliminary results. Arch Ophthalmol. 1988;106 (4):471e479.
5. Early Treatment of Retinopathy of Prematurity Cooperative Group. Revised indications for the treatment of retinopathy of prematurity. Arch Ophthalmol. 2003;121:1684–96.
6. Ng EYJ, Connolly BP, McNamara JA, Regillo CD, Vander JF, Tasman W. A comparison of laser photocoagulation with cryotherapy for threshold retinopathy of prematurity at 10 years: Part 1 Visual function and structural outcome. Ophthalmology. 2002;109:928–34.
7. Choi WC, Yu YS. Surgical management for stage 5 retinopathy of prematurity. Korean J Ophthalmol. 1994;8:37–41.
8. Tasman W, Borrone RN, Bolling J. Open sky vitrectomy for total retinal detachment in retinopathy of prematurity. Ophthalmology. 1987;94:449–52.
9. De Juan E, Jr MR, Charles ST, Hirose T, Tasman WS, Trese MT. Surgery for stage 5 retinopathy of prematurity. Arch Ophthalmol. 1987;105:21.
10. Trese MT. Surgical results of stage V retrolental fibroplasia and timing of surgical repair. Ophthalmology. 1984;91:461–6.
11. Fuchino Y, Hayashi H, Kono T, Ohshima K. Long-term follow up of visual acuity in eyes with stage 5 retinopathy of prematurity after closed vitrectomy. Am J Ophthalmol. 1995;120:308–16.
12. Gopal L, Sharma T, Shanmugam M, et al. Surgery for stage 5 retinopathy of prematurity: the learning curve and evolving technique. Ind J Ophthalmol. 2000;48:101–6.
13. Trese MT. Visual results and prognostic factors for vision following surgery for stage V retinopathy of prematurity. Ophthalmology. 1986;93:574–9.
14. Hartley S, Dauvilliers Y, Quera-Salva MA. Circadian rhythm disturbances in the blind. Curr Neurol Neurosci Rep. 2018;18:65.
15. Chiang MF, Quinn GE, Fielder AR, et al. International classification of retinopathy of prematurity, Third Edition. Ophthalmology. 2021;128(10):e51–68.
16. Ozsaygili C, Ozdek S, Ozmen MC, Atalay HT, Yeter DY. Preoperative anatomical features associated with improved surgical outcomes for stage 5 retinopathy of prematurity. Retina. 2021;41(4):718–25.
17. Trese MT. Scleral buckling for retinopathy of prematurity. Ophthalmology. 1994;101:23–6.
18. Sears JE, Sonnie C. Anatomic success of lens-sparing vitrectomy with and without scleral buckle for stage 4 retinopathy of prematurity. Am J Ophthalmol. 2007;143:810–3.
19. Lincoff H, Stopa M, Kreissig I, Madjarov B, Sarup V, Saxena S, Brodie S. Cutting the encircling band. Retina. 2006;26(6):650–4.
20. Lakhanpal RR, Fortun JA, Chan-Kai B, Holz ER. Lensectomy and vitrectomy with and without intravitreal triamcinolone acetonide for vascularly active stage 5 retinal detachments in retinopathy of prematurity. Retina. 2006;26(7):736–40.
21. Tsukahara Y, Honda S, Imai H, et al. Autologous plasmin-assisted vitrectomy for stage 5 retinopathy of prematurity: a preliminary trial. Am J Ophthalmol. 2007;144(1):139–41.
22. Özdek Ş, Özmen MC, Yalınbaş D, Atalay HT, Coşkun D. Immediate sequential bilateral vitrectomy surgery for retinopathy of prematurity: a single surgeon experience. Turk J Ophthalmol. 2021;51:225–30.

23. Yonekawa Y, Wu WC, Kusaka S, et al. Immediate sequential bilateral pediatric vitreoretinal surgery: an international multicenter study. Ophthalmology. 2016;123(8):1802–8.

24. Choi J, Kim JH, Kim SJ, Yu YS. Long-term results of lens-sparing vitrectomy for stages 4B and 5 retinopathy of prematurity. Korean J Ophthalmol. 2011;25:305–10.

25. Hartnett ME. Features associated with surgical outcome in patients with stages 4 and 5 retinopathy of prematurity. Retina. 2003;23:322–9.

26. Karacorlu M, Hocaoglu M, Sayman Muslubas I, Arf S. Long-term functional results following vitrectomy for advanced retinopathy of prematurity. Br J Ophthalmol. 101(6):730–734. https://doi.org/10.1136/bjophthalmol-2016-309198

27. Nudleman E, Muftuoglu IK, Gaber R, et al. Glaucoma after lens-sparing vitrectomy for advanced retinopathy of prematurity. Ophthalmology. 2018;125:671–5.

28. Cernichiaro-Espinosa LA, García-Huerta MM, Giordano VE, et al. Comparison of iridocorneal angle in infants with retinopathy of prematurity and healthy infants using spectral domain optical coherence tomography. J Aapos. 2014;18:344–6.

29. Machemer R. Closed vitrectomy for severe retrolental fibroplasias in the infant. Ophthalmology. 1983;90:436–41.

30. Kono T, Oshima K, Fuchino Y. Surgical results and visual outcomes of vitreous surgery for advanced stages of retinopathy of prematurity. Jpn J Ophthalmol. 2000;44:661–7.

31. Mintz-Hittner HA, O'Malley RE, Kretzer FL. Long-term form identification vision after early, closed, lensectomy- vitrectomy for stage 5 retinopathy of prematurity. Ophthalmology. 1997;104:454–9.

32. Yu YS, Kim SJ, Kim SY, et al. Lens-sparing vitrectomy for stage 4 and stage 5 retinopathy of prematurity. Korean J Ophthalmol. 2006;20:113–7.

33. Cusick M, Charles MK, Agrón E, Sangiovanni JP, Ferris FL 3rd, Charles S. Anatomical and visual results of vitreoretinal surgery for stage 5 retinopathy of prematurity. Retina. 2006;26(7):729–35.

34. Rajan RP, Kannan NB, Sen S, C L, Jena S, Kumar K, Vijayalakshmi P, Ramasamy K. Clinico-demographic profile and outcomes of 25-gauge vitrectomy in advanced stage 5 retinopathy of prematurity. Graefes Arch Clin Exp Ophthalmol. 2021;259(7):1695–1701.

35. Lakhanpal RR, Sun RL, Albini TA, et al. Anatomical success rate after primary three-port lens-sparing vitrectomy in stage 5 retinopathy of prematurity. Retina. 2006;26:724–8.

36. Seaber JH, Machemer R, Eliott D, Buckley EG, deJuan E, Martin DF. Long-term visual results of children after initially successful vitrectomy for stage V retinopathy of prematurity. Ophthalmology. 1995;102:199–204.

37. Shah PK, Narendran V, Kalpana N, Tawansy KA. Anatomical and visual outcome of stages 4 and 5 retinopathy of prematurity. Eye (Lond). 2009;23:176–80.

38. Gonzales CR, Boshra J, Schwartz SD. 25-Gauge pars plicata vitrectomy for stage 4 and 5 retinopathy of prematurity. Retina. 2006;26(7 Suppl):S42–6.

39. Wu WC, Drenser KA, Lai M, Capone A, Trese MT. Plasmin enzyme-assisted vitrectomy for primary and reoperated eyes with stage 5 retinopathy of prematurity. Retina. 2008;28(3 Suppl):S75-80.

Vitreoretinal Surgery for Cicatricial Retinopathy of Prematurity

21

Ehab N. El Rayes and Mahmoud Leila

Abstract

ROP is a blinding disease that affects premature infants. Though the child escapes the problems of active disease, yet he faces the problems of cicatricial ROP. Cicatricial stages of ROP pose significant morbidity due to the entailed irreversible visual loss and consequent adverse psychological and social impact on the infant and the caregivers. The magnitude of the problem is particularly large in developing countries due to lack of adequate screening programs for premature babies hence frequent late presentation with leucocoria and retinal detachment in a yet non-verbal baby, when the structural and functional outcomes of surgical intervention are already highly guarded. Nevertheless, surgical intervention using scleral buckle surgery, LSV, and non-lens sparing vitrectomy can still yield favorable outcomes providing proper preoperative evaluation and case selection are conducted. After successful surgery, it is important to follow-up these infants for long periods of time for early detection of amblyopia and other co-morbidities as glaucoma that can severely undermine the initial success.

Keywords

Cicatricial ROP · Surgery for ROP · Vitrectomy for ROP · Macular folds in ROP · Retinal detachment in ROP

Supplementary Information The online version contains supplementary material available at https://doi.org/10.1007/978-3-031-14506-3_21.

E. N. El Rayes (✉)
Chairman of Retina Department – Research Institute of Ophthalmology, Giza, Egypt
e-mail: erayes1@hotmail.com

M. Leila
Retina Department – Research Institute of Ophthalmology, Giza, Egypt

Ş. Özdek et al. (eds.), *Pediatric Vitreoretinal Surgery*,
https://doi.org/10.1007/978-3-031-14506-3_21

Introduction

Despite advances in screening programs and pre-emptive therapeutic interventions, late cicatricial stages of retinopathy of prematurity (ROP) still pose significant morbidity. In the cryotherapy for ROP (CRYO-ROP) study, the incidence of retinal detachment was 21.7% among eyes with threshold disease successfully treated with cryotherapy. The early treatment for ROP (ETROP) study protocol entailed earlier treatment for high-risk prethreshold ROP patients, namely type 1 ROP. The study succeeded in reducing progression to cicatricial stages to 9.1% of eyes [1, 2]. Infants progressing to cicatricial ROP are prone to develop a spectrum of disabling factors associated with low vision that could have profound effect on the quality of life of patients and their caregivers. These factors include stereotypic mannerism in the form of eye-poking or oculodigital phenomenon with consequent structural anomalies of the eye and behavioral changes secondary to social seclusion and stigma [3]. Cicatricial ROP includes myopia, pigmentary changes, macular folds and tractional retinal detachment. Surgical intervention in established cicatricial ROP must follow a carefully tailored approach. Firstly, it is mandatory for the treating physician to establish good rapport with the parents or caregivers through thorough discussion prior to intervention regarding the outcome of surgery to avoid unrealistic expectations and help educating them for integration in the postoperative plan of rehabilitation. Secondly, conducting meticulous preoperative evaluation for detection of criteria of disease severity, disease staging and pathogenetic factors associated with poor outcome for surgery. The goal of surgery is to provide the infant with at least navigational type of vision and to avoid phthisis bulbi or enucleation, which could have profound adverse psychological impact on the infant and parents [4, 5].

The International Classification for ROP (ICROP) Staging of Cicatricial ROP

Cicatricial ROP includes stages 4 and 5 and their respective sub-classification. Stage 4 represents partial retinal detachment. The nature of detachment is almost always tractional although exudative detachment might develop due to effusion from traction exerted on florid extraretinal fibrovascular proliferation in stage 3 ROP or in association with aggressive laser photocoagulation. The exudative variant could be identified by its smooth conspicuous convex anterior surface and absence of epiretinal proliferation or tented retina. The tractional variant is caused by contraction of fibrous membranes along the vitreoretinal interface complicating stage 3 ROP. Stage 4A describes partial retinal detachment confined to the periphery; whereas stage 4B is designated whenever the area of detachment extends to the macula or whenever the macula is involved by a fold of detached retina. Stage 5 describes total retinal detachment. In this stage the detachment has a funnel-shaped configuration, and the stage is sub-divided according to the morphology of the anterior and posterior parts of the funnel and the ability to visualize the optic disc. Accordingly, there are open-open, open-narrow, narrow-open and narrow-narrow configurations describing the anterior and posterior parts of the funnel. The most common configuration is the open-open and the least common is the narrow-open. More recently, The ICROP sub-categorized stage 5 into 3 configurations. Stage 5A, in which the optic disc is visible. Stage 5B, in which the optic disc cannot be visualized either due to closed-funnel retinal detachment or due to retrolental fibrovascular tissue. Stage 5C describes stage 5B plus anterior segment abnormalities [6].

Poor Prognostic Factors Related to Retinal Detachment

Thorough clinical examination could provide clues on the prognosis of surgical intervention if at all indicated. The presence of specific findings suggests a closed funnel retinal detachment and accordingly highly guarded visual prognosis. These findings include leucocoria caused by retrolental fibroplasia, which consists of whitish fibrous tissue with minimal vascularization occupying the retrolental space and obscuring visualization of the posterior segment. Anterior segment abnormalities including shallow or flat anterior chamber, iris atrophy, irido-corneal touch, posterior synechiae, and iris bombé. These abnormalities can progress to glaucoma or corneal decompensation thus further undermining the success of surgery. Subretinal fluid composed of blood, serum or cholesterol deposits is toxic to the retinal pigment epithelium (RPE) and the photoreceptors layer, hence causing poor visual results after surgery. Finally, ultrasound evidence of long length of the stalk of closed funnel from the optic disc indicates difficult unfolding of the funnel intraoperatively [7] (Fig. 21.1).

Pre-Operative Evaluation

Before deciding on surgical intervention, it is mandatory to examine the child to determine whether or not light perception is present. This could be performed clinically by eliciting the infant's reaction to bright light as well as the impression of the parents regarding the response of the infant to light. In addition, electrophysiology testing using awake visual evoked potential (VEP) or electrical evoked potential (EEP). Absence of response to light with recordable VEP still gives the infant a chance for surgery, while absence of infant's response to bright light and extinguished VEP preclude surgery. Anterior segment assessment could reveal hazy cornea, which might indicate high intraocular pressure (IOP). In absence of direct view of anterior segment structures ultra-sound biomicroscopy (UBM) using the modified immersion technique by a finger of latex glove is useful to identify anterior segment abnormalities. Ultrasound imaging is important in media opacities

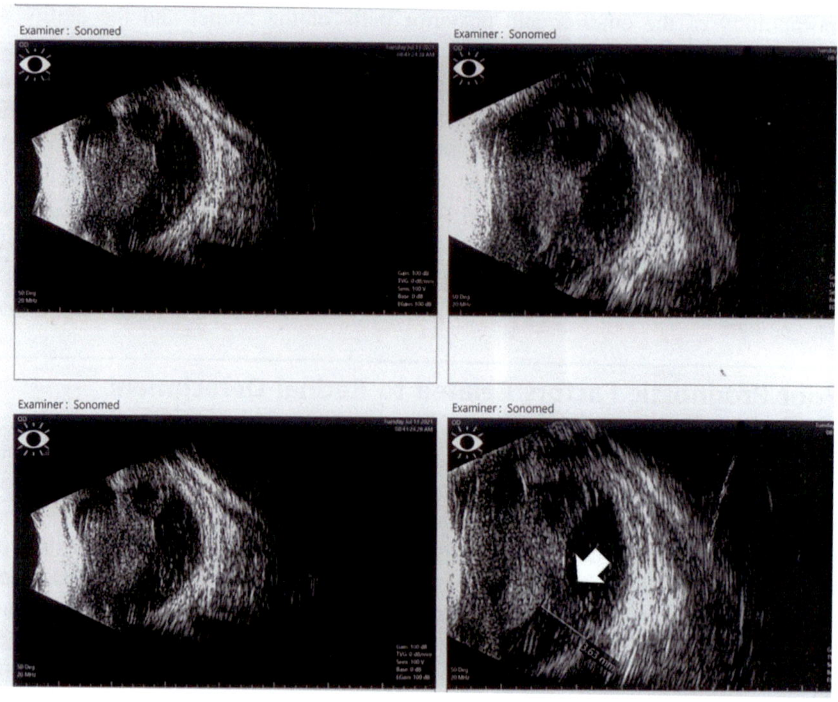

Fig. 21.1 B-scan ultrasound image of the right eye of an infant with stage 5 ROP demonstrates measurement of the length of the funnel stalk from the optic disc (white arrow)

of the anterior segment and in cases with retrolental fibroplasia in order to identify the configuration of the funnel, length of the stalk of the funnel from the optic disc, presence of blood in the sub-retinal space and the nature of subretinal fluid [5].

Surgery for Cicatricial ROP

Scleral Buckling

Scleral buckling could be performed in eyes with stages 4A and 4B with or without drainage of sub-retinal fluid. An encircling 2 mm buckle is placed over the area of highest ridge elevation and is combined with external cryotherapy to the avascular retina. The goal is to achieve re-attachment of the retina in zone 1. Greven and Tasman [8] reported 59% successful anatomical re-attachment of the retina using this technique in infants with stages 4 and 5 ROP. Final visual acuity was $\geq 20/400$ in 40% of eyes that achieved anatomical re-attachment at 18 months of follow-up. In case an encircling buckle is applied, division of the buckle must be performed in successful cases after the lapse of 3 months to allow for growth of the globe and to prevent anisometropia from unequal growth of both eyes [5, 8].

Lens-Sparing Vitrectomy (LSV)

LSV is indicated in infants with stages 4A and 4B ROP. Current advances in vitrectomy machine fluidics, bimanual techniques and wide-angle viewing systems facilitated adequate visualization and performing surgical maneuvers in the peripheral retina without the need for knocking-down the lens or scleral indentation intraoperatively, which could produce iatrogenic breaks during shaving the peripheral vitreous in presence of redundant retina. The advantage of preserving the crystalline lens is to avoid dealing with aphakia postoperatively and diminish the burden of amblyopia therapy on the ophthalmologist and the parents. LSV technique is sometimes difficult to execute due to tight retrolenticular space caused by organized vitreous or high retinal folds involving several clock hours. In this situation an ab interno incision technique could be performed to avoid inflicting iatrogenic injury to the lens or to the retina. First, the microvitreoretinal blade (MVR) is introduced through the pars plicata and then directed posteriorly towards the retrolental space. This is followed by inserting the trocar cannula with minimal resistance into the correct plane behind the lens anterior to the dragged retina. Once the anterior traction is released the retina falls back giving way to more room for safe introduction of vitrectomy instruments. Core vitrectomy is started followed by triamcinolone-assisted dissection of the posterior hyaloid. If the posterior hyaloid detaches easily from the posterior pole, detachment is not continued to the periphery and stops just anterior to the arcades to avoid inducing iatrogenic breaks. If the posterior hyaloid is tightly adherent at the posterior pole it is prudent to leave it in place and perform trimming of the peripheral vitreous. This is followed by peeling or trimming of vitreoretinal tractional membranes until the posterior pole is flattened. Finally fluid-air exchange is performed and the eye is left on air or sulfur hexafluoride gas (SF6) 20%. All sclerotomies are closed watertight [5, 9, 10].

Macular Folds

In patients with regressed ROP, organization and subsequent contraction of vitreous gel can cause the avascular elastic retina to form a retinal fold. These traction forces extend anteriorly from the ridge and also posteriorly from the disc. The resultant fold could involve the macula and manifests clinically as dragging and closing of the macula with shift of the nasal blood vessels towards the macula and straightening of temporal retinal blood vessels. Alternatively, contracture of remnants of the primary vitreous over the macular area could start the fold formation. A macular fold could take different forms and severity from just dragging an open macula to a totally closed macular fold obscuring the fovea with complete straightening of the temporal blood vessels like a napkin in a wine cup (Fig. 21.2). Surgical intervention to flatten the fold should be performed at the earliest possible to restore central fixation and to prevent permanent damage to the photoreceptors. Macular folds are particularly difficult to manage in cases with attached surrounding retina [5, 11].

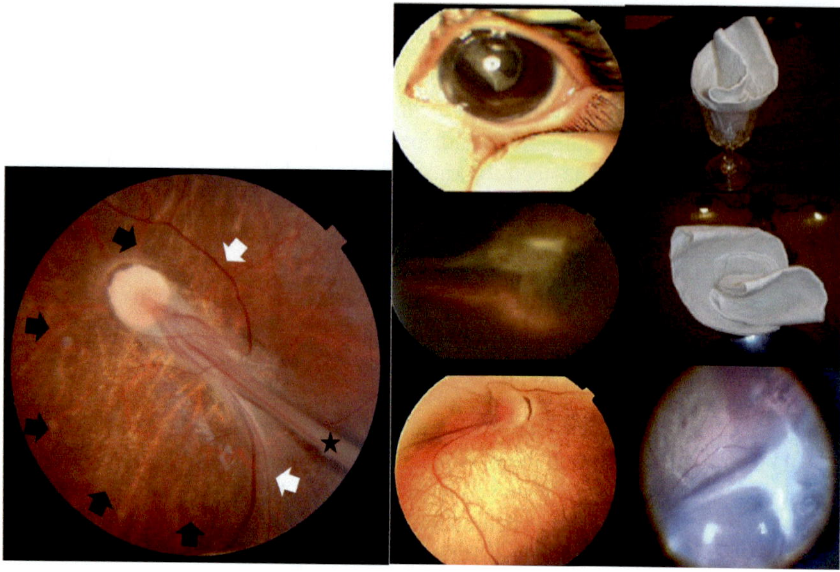

Fig. 21.2 **A** Color fundus photo of the left eye of an infant with stage 4B ROP and a full-thickness macular fold (asterisk). Note the extensive RPE mottling in the posterior pole (black arrows) and dragging and straightening of the temporal blood vessels (white arrows). **B** Color photos of different infants with macular folds reminiscent of a folded napkin in a wine cup

Surgical Technique for Management of Macular Folds

The surgical technique consists of LSV. After removing the core vitreous, we proceeded to release the peripheral point of fixation at the trough where the fold is drawn by the vitreous strand, representing the pillar of the detachment. This is aided by peripheral scleral indentation by the assistant to avoid lens damage during peripheral dissection. We then performed bimanual dissection of the sheet of condensed primary vitreous overlying the fold, which usually appears as glistening sheet coming off the retinal surface all the way to the periphery. The dissection of the stalk off the fold enables further manipulation to open the tissue in the fold and to undermine its edges and redistribute the macular tissue over the RPE using two diamond-dusted scrapers in a criss-cross manner under perfluorocarbon (PFC) liquid (Fig. 21.3).

The goal is to achieve anatomical repositioning of the fovea and displace the redundant tissue outside the arcades. The endpoint of surgery is flattening of the central foveal fold with visualization of the retinal vessels in the depth of the fold and formation of two extra-macular folds (Figs. 21.4 and 21.5). Care must be taken to avoid applying inadvertent mechanical pressure on the RPE while performing this maneuver. Finally air-fluid exchange is performed leaving the globe air-filled. Alternatively, non-expansile SF6 20% gas is placed to aid stretching of the macula area. **Supplemental digital content 1.**

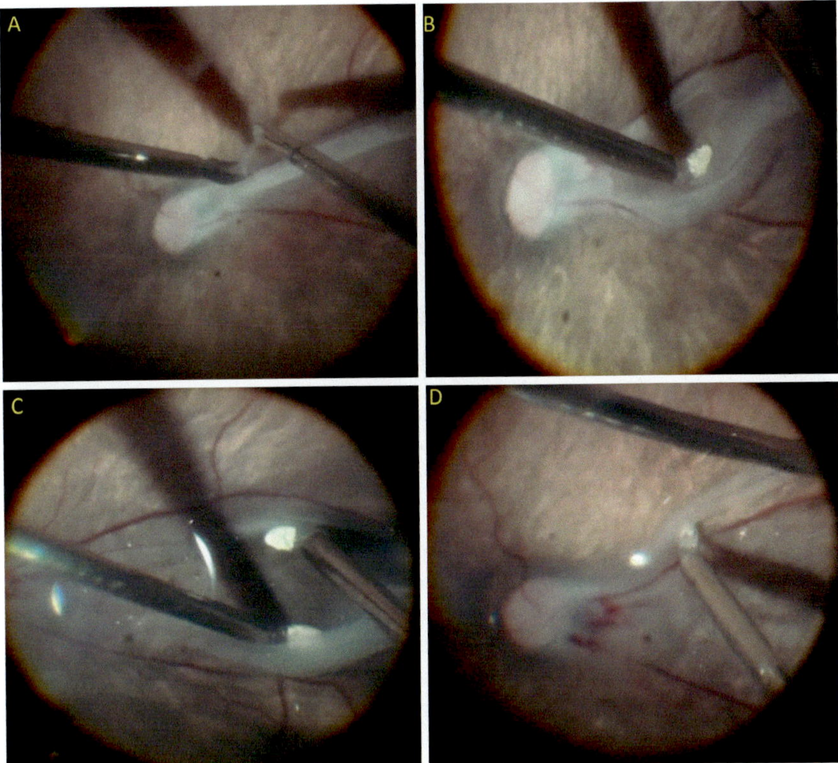

Fig. 21.3 Intraoperative photo demonstrating the surgical technique of unfolding a full-thickness macular fold using two diamond-dusted scrapers

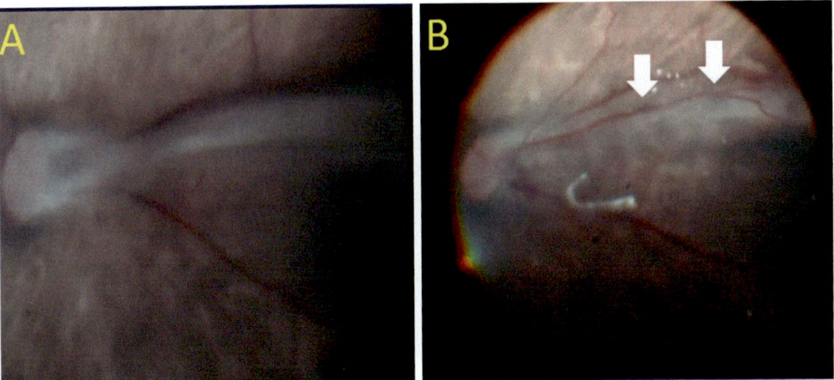

Fig. 21.4 A Intraoperative photo of the left eye of an infant with stage 4B ROP and a full-thickness macular fold at the start of surgery. **B** Intraoperative photo of the same eye at the conclusion of surgery and unfolding of the central foveal fold. Note the displacement of retinal tissue in the form of extramacular fold at the supero-temporal arcade (arrows)

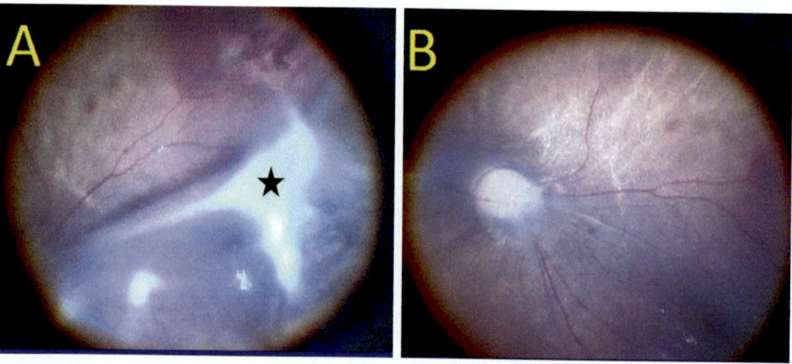

Fig. 21.5 A Intraoperative photo of the left eye of an infant with stage 4B ROP and a full-thickness macular fold at the start of surgery. Note the peripheral vitreous fibrous condensation causing dragging of the retina and perpetuating the macular fold (asterisk). **B** Postoperative fundus photo of the same eye shows successful complete flattening of the fold with clear visualization of the blood vessels in the depth of the fold

In successful cases, hypertrophy of the RPE can develop in the macular area at the site of the previous fold but this improves gradually with time [11] (Fig. 21.6).

We applied this technique in a series of 16 infants [11]. Follow-up period was at least 12 months. Eleven patients (68%) had complete flattening of the macular fold. Four patients had flattening of the central part of the fold with residual equatorial dragging. One patient (6%) had partial improvement in the height and thickness of the fold with incomplete central flattening. In 8 patients (50%) multifocal electroretinogram (mERG) showed improved pattern values in the macula relative to preoperative mERG at 3 months of follow-up and one more infant showed improvement at the fourth month. Four infants (25%) had no improvement up to 1 year after surgery. In 10 patients (62.5%), sweep visual evoked potential (VEP) improved during follow-up. The visual improvement is dependent on timing of intervention, height of the fold and possible RPE atrophy that ensues overtime (Fig. 21.7).

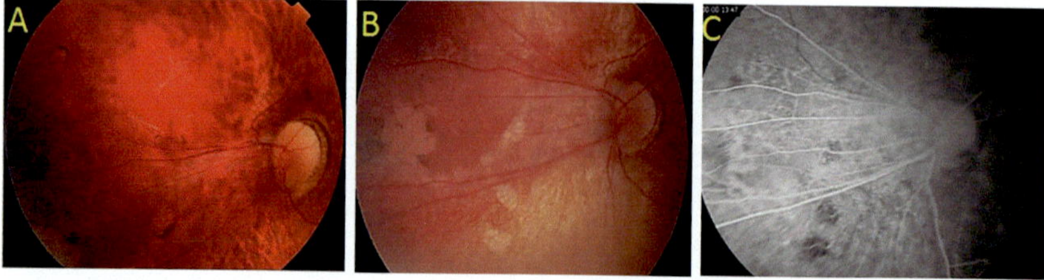

Fig. 21.6 Color fundus photo (**A-B**) and fluorescein angiography (**C**) of the right eye of an infant operated for stage 4B ROP. Note RPE mottling in the macular area at the site of previous macular fold

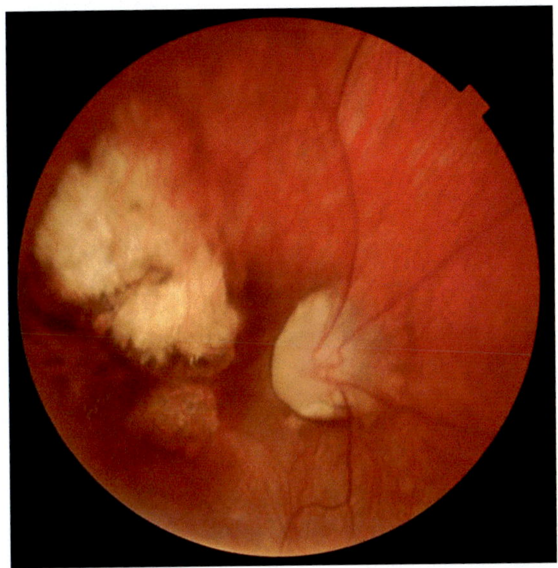

Fig. 21.7 Color fundus photo of the right eye of a child who had surgery for stage 4B ROP since 8 years. Note extensive RPE atrophy in the macular area at the site of previous macular fold

Lensectomy—Vitrectomy

Non-lens sparing vitrectomy is indicated in stage 5 ROP. Depending on corneal clarity, the surgical approach could be closed lensectomy and vitrectomy in clear corneas or open-sky intracapsular lensectomy followed by vitrectomy in cloudy corneas. The funnel-shaped retinal detachment extends from the ridge to the optic nerve head. Assessment of the configuration of the funnel is key to successful relieve of traction. Different configurations of the funnel could develop according to the vectors of traction along the ridge and the uniformity of depth of the residual peripheral trough of attached or shallow detached retina. Accordingly, the funnel could be closed centrally or eccentrically displaced in a crescent pattern or acquire a spiral configuration. The retina in the posterior pole could be dragged by tractional bands over the optic nerve head forming a triple-layered retinal fold [5] (Fig. 21.8).

Surgical Technique

The sclerotomy tract is better fashioned by the MVR blade prior to insertion of the trocar cannula to avoid unintentional lens damage or retinal breaks during trocar insertion. Non-lens sparing vitrectomy consists of an ab interno incision through the iris root or the limbus. Lensectomy is performed including removal of the entire lens capsule. A peripheral iridectomy is performed to prevent postoperative adhesions between the retina and the iris. The retrolenticular tissue is then dissected bimanually using two 27-gauge needles in a criss-cross pattern to create a slit in the retrolenticular membrane. The central slit could be enlarged using scissors or vitrectomy cutter to interrupt trans-vitreal vectors as much as possible and dissect the stalk which is the pillar of the cicatricial detachment. **Supplemental digital content**

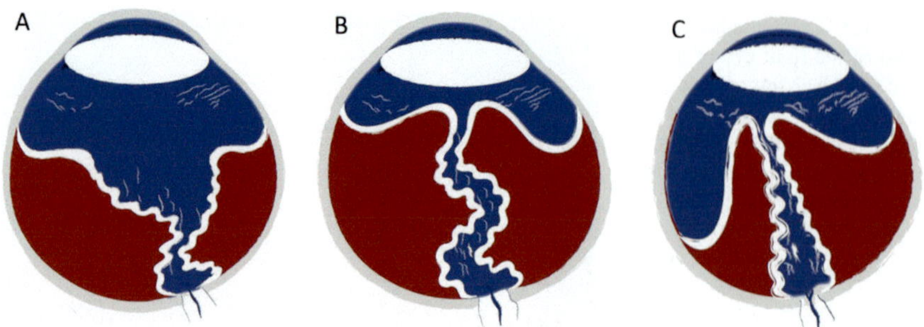

Fig. 21.8 Schematic diagram demonstrating different funnel configurations in stage 5 ROP. **A** Open-narrow configuration. **B** Narrow-narrow configuration. **C** Eccentrically displaced closed funnel

2. Aided with cohesive viscoelastic, the funnel is opened while dissecting the epiretinal tractional membranes until the posterior pole opens up. Afterwards, dissection is continued at the peripheral retinal trough. Viscoelastic is injected to open up the funnel and keep the retina open till posterior pole attachment is achieved. It is possible to use SF6 20% gas as well. Sclerotomies are closed watertight [5]. **Supplemental digital content 3**.

Results of LSV and Non-lens Sparing Vitrectomy for Cicatricial ROP

The author published a retrospective series of 56 eyes with stage 4B ROP [10]. Patients had either LSV (42.9%) or non-lens sparing vitrectomy (57.1%). Follow-up period was 36 months. Retinal re-attachment was achieved in 73.2% of the overall study subjects; 75% of patients who had LSV and 71.8% in patients with non-lens sparing vitrectomy. Postoperatively, visual acuity ranged between 20/300 and hand motion (<20/1900) at the last follow-up visit. Twenty-four eyes (42.8%) achieved visual acuity $\geq$ 20/800 at last follow-up. The remaining 32 eyes (57.2%) had visual acuity <20/800. Better anatomical and functional results were associated with LSV technique, prior ablation therapy and attached retina. In general, for Cicatricial stage 5 ROP our aim is at least partial posterior pole attachment which can give the infant navigational vision (Fig. 21.9).

Case Scenario

A female infant 4 months old presented at the retina clinic. Her parents mentioned that she was admitted to an incubator in the neonatal unit and received supplementary oxygen. Her gestational age was 30 weeks and she weighed 1200 g at time of birth. Examination of the right fundus revealed cicatricial macular fold obscuring

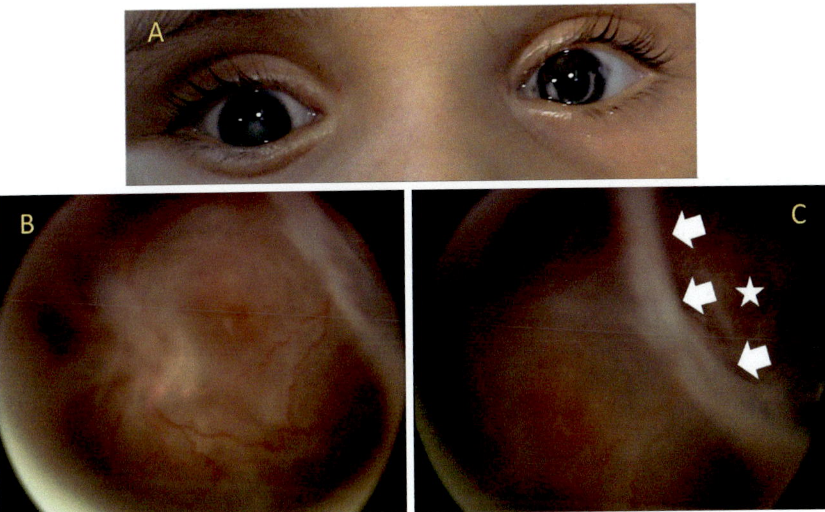

Fig. 21.9 **A** Postoperative photo of an infant with stage 5 ROP in the left eye. The patient had lensectomy-vitrectomy. Note restoration of normal reflex in the left eye compared to leucocoria of the right eye due to late cicatricial ROP. **B** Postoperative fundus photo of the left eye of the same patient 1 month after surgery. There is flattening of the retina in zone 1, with detached retina more peripherally. **C** Fundus photo of the same eye postoperatively showing the retinal periphery. The retina remained attached in zone 1. Note the ridge of fibrosis that formed during stage 3 disease (arrows) and the avascular atrophic retina peripheral to it (asterisk)

the temporal blood vessels and macular detachment. The left fundus showed regressed ROP with straightening and dragging of the temporal blood vessels and an attached macula. The patient was admitted for LSV in the right eye. After removal of epi-macular fibrous tissue, the fold was opened, and the redundant tissue was redistributed under PFC to open-up the foveal area and unveil the blood vessels and relocate the fovea. Finally, we did PFC/air exchange and applied SF6 20% gas tamponade. The infant was followed up for 6 months. Examination during follow-up visits revealed flattening of the fold and resolution of macular detachment and subretinal fluid. **Supplemental digital content 4.**

Supplemental digital contents (SDC)

SDC 1. Video shows surgical technique for management of macular fold.
SDC 2. Video shows stalk dissection in cicatricial tractional retinal detachment.
SDC 3. Video shows transvitreal dissection of membranes in cicatricial ROP.
SDC 4. Video shows LSV and flattening of a full-thickness macular fold in a 4 months old infant with cicatricial macular fold and macular detachment in the

right eye. Three still images in the video demonstrate: (a) intraoperative view before starting surgery, (b) intraoperative view after opening of the fold, (c) four months postoperatively with complete resolution of subretinal fluid.

Review Questions

1. Which of the following is considered an indication of an inoperable cicatricial ROP?

(a) Leucocoria
(b) Subretinal crystal deposits
(c) Narrow-open funnel configuration
(d) RPE mottling in the posterior pole
(e) Extinguished VEP

2. Which of the following ancillary tests is commonly used to determine surgical prognosis in cicatricial ROP?

(a) Ultrasound
(b) Magnetic Resonance Imaging
(c) Helical computed tomography scan of the orbit
(d) Vitreous sample
(e) Forced duction test

3. Which of the following is NOT considered a feature of cicatricial stage 5 ROP?

(a) Open funnel retinal detachment with readily visualization of the optic disc
(b) Full-thickness macular fold with subtotal retinal detachment
(c) Invisible optic disc due to closed-funnel retinal detachment with central corneal opacity
(d) Eccentrically displaced funnel
(e) Funnel-shaped retinal detachment with triple retinal fold overlying he optic disc

4. Which of the following surgical techniques is NOT used during surgery for cicatricial ROP?

(a) Lensectomy-vitrectomy
(b) Lens-sparing vitrectomy
(c) 2 mm encircling scleral silicone band + adjuvant cryotherapy
(d) Trans pars plicata ab-interno surgical approach
(e) Pars plana vitrectomy with episcleral macular buckle

5. Which of the following co-morbidities could develop in children with end-stage bilaterally inoperable ROP?

(a) Oedipus complex
(b) Pathological lying
(c) Obsessive compulsive disorder
(d) Stereotypic mannerism in the form of eye poking
(e) Attention deficit hyperactivity disorder

Answers

1. E
2. A
3. B
4. E
5. D

References

1. Cryotherapy for retinopathy of prematurity cooperative group. Multicenter trial of cryotherapy for retinopathy of prematurity. Arch Ophthalmol. 2001;119:1110–8.
2. Early treatment for retinopathy of prematurity cooperative group. Revised indications for the treatment of retinopathy of prematurity. Arch Ophthalmol. 2003;121:1684–96.
3. Kumawat D, Sahay P, Alam T, Bhari A, Chandra P. Ocular auto-stimulation and its morbidity in stage 5 retinopathy of prematurity. Indian J Ophthalmol. 2019;67:912–6.
4. Dogra MR, Katoch D, Dogra M. An update on retinopathy of prematurity (ROP). Indian J Pediatr. 2017;84:930–6.
5. Yonekawa Y, Faia LJ, Trese MT. Surgical management of retinopathy of prematurity. In: Schachat AP, editor. Ryan's Retina. 6th ed. China: Elsevier; 2018. p. 2155–69.
6. Chiang MF, Quinn GE, Fielder AR, Ostmo SR, Chan RVP, et al. International classification of retinopathy of prematurity, third edition. Ophthalmology. 2021;128:e51–e68.
7. Lee TC, Chiang MF. Pediatric retinal vascular diseases. In: Schachat AP, editor. Ryan's Retina. 6th ed. China: Elsevier; 2018. p. 1246–67.
8. Greven C, Tasman W. Scleral buckling in stages 4B and 5 retinopathy of prematurity. Ophthalmology. 1990;97:817–20.
9. Atalay HT, Özdek Ş, Yalinbaş D, Özsaygili C, Özmen MC. Results of surgery for late sequelae of cicatricial retinopathy of prematurity. Indian J Ophthalmol. 2019;67:908–11.
10. El Rayes EN, Vinekar A, Capone A Jr. Three-year anatomic and visual outcomes after vitrectomy for stage 4B retinopathy of prematurity. Retina. 2008;28:568–72.
11. El Rayes E. Macular unfolding for managing macular folds in infants with ROP. Retina Today 2011; May/June:78–80.

Complications of Vitreoretinal Surgery for ROP

22

Ihab Saad Othman

Abstract

Vitreoretinal surgery for stages 4 and 5 ROP carries a significant number of intraoperative complications. Surgery is not forgiving and bearing the responsibility of defining the visual future of a premature infant or child requires a great deal of expertise in understanding the anatomy of the eye, the severity of the disease with its different presentations and more importantly how to manage intra-operative complications. This is done by proper planning for surgery, using adequate surgical techniques and understanding the basics of intra-operative management of surgical complications and proper and swift management of such problems. In this chapter, the intraoperative surgical complications for stages 4 and 5 ROP are discussed in details, how to prevent and manage these complications to get the best outcome.

Keywords

ROP · Stages 4 and 5 · Pars plicata lensectomy · Pars plicata vitrectomy · Lens sparing vitrectomy · Preoperative assessment · Vascular activity management · Intraoperative bleeding · Sclerotomy complications · Posterior hyaloid detachment · Iatrogenic retinal breaks · Ciliary detachment · Semifluorinated silicone oil · Autologous plasmin · Trypan blue

Supplementary Information The online version contains supplementary material available at https://doi.org/10.1007/978-3-031-14506-3_22.

I. S. Othman (✉)
Cairo University, Giza, Egypt
e-mail: ihabsaad@hotmail.com

Eye World Hospital, 12 Mosaddak Street, Dokki, Giza, Egypt

Introduction

Before the nineties, cicatricial ROP in stages 5 and 4 were considered as inoperable with poor outcomes. Many of the cases were followed and many reports considered the natural history of stages 4 and 5 ROP with no surgical intervention, that included the following:

A. Microphthalmia, reported to be around 50% of cases and associated with shorter axial length and microcornea which is more severe the higher the stage of ROP. The presence of low-grade disruption in blood ocular barrier eventually results in band keratopathy and corneal scars [1–3].
B. Glaucoma, reported to be around 20% of case series. In stage 5 ROP with closed anterior funnel, the forward movement of the iris/lens diaphragm results in pupillary block, peripheral anterior synechiae formation and secondary angle-closure glaucoma. Chronic retinal detachment can also result in neovascular glaucoma [4, 5].
C. Lens opacities usually occurs in cicatricial ROP due to the extension of the fibrous tissue formed during contraction of the vitreous to the posterior pole of the lens or the posterior lens capsule in its periphery [6].

With the advancement in surgical techniques and better understanding of the patho-anatomy of cicatricial stages of ROP, anatomical success in stage 4 varies from 60 to 90% in different series, and decreasing from 13 to 40% for stage 5 ROP [7–10].

Results of surgery in stage 4 ROP with lens sparing vitrectomy (LSV) adequately preserves retinal stability and vision in children on long term basis, especially when the intervention is on a flat macula. Results of surgery in stage 5 ROP are less than optimal.

Operative complications seriously compromising anatomic success include retinal break creation, or dialysis, intra and postoperative vitreous hemorrhage, secondary glaucoma and cataract progression [7–13].

Other complications like endophthalmitis, postoperative hypotony, or atrophia are rare.

In this chapter, we will discuss the commonest operative complications in stages 4 and 5 with their management.

Taking the Decision for Surgery

Families presenting with a blind child during the first year of life are usually devastated when referred with strabismus, abnormal head posture, leukocoria and actual loss of facial recognition, social smiling and a clear oculo-digital reflex. Proper clinic evaluation of the child eyes should include proper anterior segment examination and posterior segment assessment. Anterior segment examination in the clinic would necessitate applying topical anesthesia and the use of a baby speculum. We prefer to use the 20 D/28 D Nikon lens as a magnifier along with the indirect ophthalmoscope to assess the following [14]:

a. Evaluation of the cornea:

   1. Presence of corneal clouding as an indicator of severe ischemia
   2. Presence of anterior synechiae
   3. Corneal diameter measurement as an indicator of secondary angle-closure glaucoma or severe microphthalmia.

b. Anterior chamber (AC) depth: A shallow AC reflects contraction of retro-lenticular fibrous tissue at 360° with the bulge of the iris/lens diaphragm forward, or a total retinal detachment in stage 5 ROP with excessive subretinal fluid.
c. Presence of posterior synechiae, poorly dilated or irregular pupil with an overlying membrane
d. Status of the lens clarity:

   1. A partially opaque lens periphery in stage 4 ROP reflects the direction of traction of the fibrovascular tissue on the retina with or without inducing a retinal fold.
   2. One should distinguish between a clear lens and the presence of a retro-lenticular fibrous membrane stretching onto the ciliary body. This membrane is usually a little further posterior to the posterior lens capsule and there is usually a potential space between them.

e. Status of the retrolental fibrous tissue:

   1. In stage 4 ROP, the peripheral fibrous tissue extends to the ora serrata, ciliary body and posterior lens capsule and is usually limited to one or two quadrants. Careful identification and annotation of the exact involved quadrants in the clinic chart is crucial in further sclerotomy design to avoid getting through an unnoticed retinal fold inducing an early retinal break that would compromise any planned surgery.
   2. In stage 5 ROP, the peripheral fibrous tissue bridges along the CB processes. It is important to identify a clear rim between the fibrous tissue and the CB processes as this may help the surgeon removing the fibrous tissue by cutting these frail adhesions in a centripetal fashion. Retcam photography may help determine that clear rim in presence of a narrow pupil.

Posterior segment evaluation is crucial in the clinic. Trying to dilate the pupil and examining the fundus is essential. Ultrasonography may be the only way in presence of corneal or retro-lenticular opacity. One should note the following [15]:

1. In stage 4 ROP:

   a. Direction and degree of the macular dragging or retinal fold or folds.
   b. Location and extent of the peripheral fibrous tissue and its ramification towards the retinal periphery, ciliary body and the lens
   c. Presence of retinal folding over the optic nerve and status of posterior fibrous tissue formation and extent.
   d. Presence of any associated retinal breaks

2. In stage 5 ROP, ultrasonography is imperative in posterior segment evaluation. It is difficult to discern retinal details from the vitreous and the lens. The following data are sought [16, 17]:

   a. Axial length of both eyes. The shorter the axial length the more severe the disease. The axial length of a newborn eye is 16 mm in the 34th gestational week and 17 mm in the 40th gestational week
   b. Status of stage 5 retinal detachment:

      i. Stage 5A, in which the optic disc is visible by ophthalmoscopy (suggesting open-funnel detachment);
      ii. Stage 5B, in which the optic disc is not visible because of retrolental fibrovascular tissue or closed-funnel detachment
      iii. Stage 5C, in which stage 5B is accompanied by anterior segment changes:

         1. Marked anterior chamber shallowing
         2. Iridocorneolenticular adhesions, corneal opacification, suggesting closed-funnel configuration
         3. Additional descriptors of funnel configuration (e.g., open-closed) may be applied if clinically useful.

      iv. By ultrasonography, the pattern of the funnel retinal detachment could be classified as follows:

         1. A closed both anterior and posterior funnel tractional retinal detachment
         2. An open anterior and closed posterior funnel retinal detachment
         3. An open anterior and posterior funnel retinal detachment
         4. A closed anterior and open posterior funnel retinal detachment

   c. Status of the subretinal fluid [17]:

      i. A clear echolucent subretinal fluid is a good prognostic sign

     ii. An echodense subretinal fluid indicates presence of hemorrhage or cholesterol crystals. Both findings indicate damaged RPE and if a desperate decision for surgery is taken, one should consider draining the dense subretinal fluid trans-sclerally

   d. Presence of peripheral retinal loops and cysts.

Once all the above data are clearly obtained and documented in the clinic, proper family counselling is carried out. One should never in these situations oversell optimistic expectations. Family members would always look to pinpoint the neonatologist, the NICU and the oxygen use as the cause of visual loss; in this matter, one should be very cautious in explaining that it is rather the prematurity and the low birth weight that are directly incriminated and should be very tactful in avoiding incriminating colleagues. A clear explanation of the advanced nature of stages 4 and 5 disease and the peculiarity of the tractional detachment and effect on vision should be elaborated upon. Also, one should mention that every effort will be done to preserve the lens in stages 4 and 5 disease with an open anterior funnel, however, the lens may be sacrificed if judged necessary. The recurrence of fibrosis or bleeding also should be mentioned with the necessity of a second or even a third intervention. Finally, one should stress upon the necessity of follow up and discuss briefly other potential long-term complications.

Vitrectomy for Stage 4 ROP

The variation noticed in the clinical presentation of stage 4 ROP warrants thorough clinical re-examination of the child's eyes under anesthesia to revise the surgical plan. Deep scleral indentation with indirect ophthalmoscopy or even the surgical microscope will highlight the extent and location of the anterior fibrovascular proliferation in relation to the retina, ciliary body and lens. This is primordial in further surgical planning.

Improving Outcomes in Stage 4 ROP Surgery

1. Manage vascular activity [18]:

   a. The presence of dilated congested vessels in stage 4 ROP is associated with worse prognosis.

   b. Anti-angiogenic factors should be considered for injection few days before surgery to minimize the risk of bleeding.

Fig. 22.1 Sclerotomy through pars plicata as seen from inside the eye (Arrow)

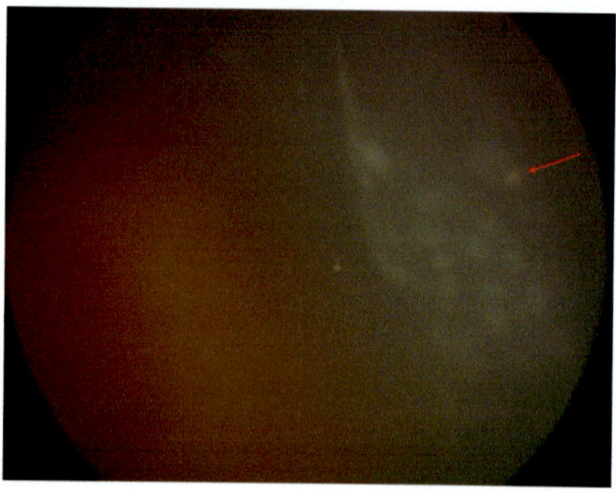

   c. Entry point of a 27/30 G needle should be 1–1.5 mm from the limbus away from the fibrous traction and the needle should be directed posteriorly towards the optic nerve in order not to injure the lens.

2. Possible complications at entry points [19] (Fig. 22.1):

   a. Surgeons should adapt a dynamic change from a comfortable position at the head of the surgical table to a temporal or sometimes a nasal approach. The child's head would need repositioning accordingly so that free access and mobilization of the surgeon's hand is warranted with no obstacles.

   b. Anesthetist should secure the airway so that the endotracheal tube or the laryngeal mask would not hinder the mobility of the surgeon's hands and at the same time would not be compromised if the head is manipulated or the eye indented.

   c. In infants a mature pars plana develops at 8–9 months post-term. The sclerotomies are placed at 1–1.5 mm from the limbus transconjunctivally through the pars plicata, after assuring that the entry point would not go through a peripheral fibrous tissue or a retinal fold resting on the pars plicata. The direction of entry should avoid the lens and be oriented towards the posterior pole taking care not to injure the retina. Trocars are inserted perpendicular on the sclera.

   d. Valved trocars are preferably used. A fourth trocar may be needed for chandelier light placement if bimanual dissection is planned and is preferably placed at 6 or 12 O'clock.

   e. If the eyelids are tight and the conjunctival sac becomes stretched to hinder free ocular motility or the surgeon's hands-free movement, one should consider a conjunctival periotomy or even a lateral canthotomy that would necessitate closure after completion of surgery.

   f. Sclerotomies should be closed after the completion of surgery using 8/0 vicryl sutures to avoid hypotony and possible hemorrhage.

3. Sharp entry into the vitreous: Sharp trocars should mark the entry point through the sclera into the vitreous. The formed vitreous in the infant eye and the presence of anterior fibrosis would make a blunt entry into the vitreous with the vitrectomy and light probes carry a risk of inducing traction on the retinal periphery or the ciliary body and eventually tears or dialysis. The entry of the instruments should be carefully watched with the surgical microscope and attention is given to the ease of insertion of the instruments while placing them very gently. Any presence of undue resistance would indicate dense vitreous condensation that may necessitate using a sharp MVR to clear a path for the instruments before insertion. Also, of note the direction of the instruments should be towards the optic nerve and away from the lens.

4. Detachment of the posterior hyaloid:

   a. Inducing a PVD in an infant eye is difficult and may carry the risk of inducing retinal breaks. Following a limited core vitrectomy, it is important to stain the vitreous with triamcinolone. This allows identifying the vitreous and fibrous traction direction and reveals its extent. We use a bent 23 G needle to engage the posterior hyaloid at the optic nerve margins. Gentle side to side manipulations of the needle will engage the hyaloid and minimal anterior traction would disengage the hyaloid from the retina.

   b. Care must be taken if the hyaloid is engaged near a retinal fold or an area of traction not to pull or engage the retina while inducing the posterior hyaloid detachment (PHD). Once detached from around the disc, it is much easier lifted off the macula or the retinal fold preferably till the vascular arcades. We believe that PHD is important in preventing late recurrences of the retinal detachment due to further PH contraction over time and also is primordial in further management of a retinal break [20].

5. Save the lens:

   a. Every effort should be done not to remove the lens. With the above techniques, a focal cataract or fibrous condensation at the lens periphery is preferably left if the central lens is clear.

   b. About a quarter of the eyes in stages 4a and 4b ROP will develop a significant cataract and required lensectomy to be performed within one year of the initial surgery [21].

6. Manage bleeding: Hemostasis is important during vitrectomy for stage 4 ROP. Bleeders develop while inducing a PHD, or during cutting the fibrous adhesions which are firmly adherent at vessels points. A simple way of hemostasis is to raise the IOP by increasing the infusion pressure. Care must be taken not to excessively elevate IOP to avoid inducing a ciliary body dialysis. Another method is to use cold sodium hyaluronate (healon) to fill the vitreous

cavity. Gentle indentation with the tip of the vitrectomy probe onto the bleeder while being on aspiration mode will prevent clot formation and assist in hemostasis. Light endodiathermy may be used with extreme caution not to induce a retinal break.

7. Managing retinal breaks (**Video** 1):

   a. Surgeons must make every effort to avoid retinal break formation. A retinal break is formed while separating the fibrous tissue from the retina specially in an area of a thinned or schitic retina. We believe that inducing a PHD using sharp bent needle is a safer technique in minimizing retinal break formation. Also the bimanual dissection techniques in dealing with the fibrous tissue at the posterior pole or the periphery markedly diminishes the risk.

   b. If a retinal break is formed, one should not panic. Although it has worse prognosis than regular iatrogenic retinal breaks in adult vitreoretinal surgery, this is an acceptable and manageable complication in most of the cases.

   c. Once a retinal break is created, the surgeon should resist the thoughts of inducing a retinotomy/retinectomy as in adult rhegmatogenous detachments. The presence of adherent posterior hyaloid will certainly prevent the retina from settling down against the posterior pole.

   d. The presence of a retinal break in the posterior pole would warrant sharp induction of a PHD beyond the break. Once the peripheral traction is released, a fluid/air exchange is performed, laser application and a tamponade agent is used.

   e. The presence of a retinal break at the periphery or at the retinal fold:

      i. This warrants thorough removal of the fibrous tissue and trying to bluntly relaxing the retina using a soft tip or bimanually using Tano scrapers.

      ii. If this technique doesn't work to flatten the retinal periphery, one should think about placing a segmental buckle to seal the peripheral retinal break, then endolaser application and use a tamponading agent.

      iii. If the tractional fold and fibrous tissue exert a significant centripetal elevation of the retina and a scleral buckle is not feasible or judged unnecessary, a last resort is to perform a limited retinectomy, and bimanually free and reposit the retina using Tano scrapers. Perfluorocarbons are used to flatten the retina and endolaser is applied with a long-term tamponade.

   f. Semifluorinated Silicone oil [22]:

      i. We used Semifluorinated ether or alkane silicone oil in management of stage 4 ROP with a retinal break due to their specific criteria:

1. Unique molecular design being heavier than water
2. Highly resistant against emulsification
3. Ideal for inferior and posterior pathologies
4. Can be injected through 23 G, and 25 G ports

ii. In presence of central or peripheral retinal break in stage 4 ROP, and after clearing of the vitreous and membranes, the semifluorinated silicone oils being heavier than water will tamponade the retina and allow the application of endolaser to the break(s). This increases the chances of success of the procedure.

iii. Semifluorinated silicone oil have a temporary tamponading effect and should be removed in 3 to 12 weeks' time.

Improving Outcome in Stage 5 ROP

1. Manage vascular activity [18]:

   a. The presence of dilated congested vessels in stage 5 ROP is associated with worse prognosis.
   b. Anti-angiogenic factors should be considered for injection before surgery.
   c. A firmly adherent retina to the fibrous tissue may warrant injecting anti-angiogenic factors few days before surgery into the anterior chamber through a paracentesis to minimize the risk of bleeding during surgery.

2. Possible complications at entry points:

   a. A conjunctival periotomy is performed at the planned site of AC infusion and sclerotomies
   b. As the retina is pushed onto the CB by the tractional membrane, the infusion is placed into the anterior chamber, preferably through a lamellar sclero-corneal penetrating wound using a 4–6 mm AC infusion cannula. The biplanar incision using a 20/23 G MVR will allow self-retention of the AC infusion cannula, otherwise it is secured in position by 7/0 vicryl sutures to the sclera. The sclero-corneal tunnel should not exceed 3 mm in length and the nozzle should be placed at ease into the AC to avoid stromal edema which can hinder success of surgery (Fig. 22.2).
   c. As an alternative to an AC infusion, a 23 G bent butterfly needle can be inserted in a similar fashion
   d. The sclerotomies are placed at the root of the iris which is 1–1.5 mm behind the limbus [19]. A 20 G MVR blade is used for the sclerotomies to allow the use of 23 G instruments without placing trocars and the wound is closed after surgery using 8/0 vicryl sutures. The site of the sclerotomy is preferably chosen where there is an adequate space between the lens and the retina. The

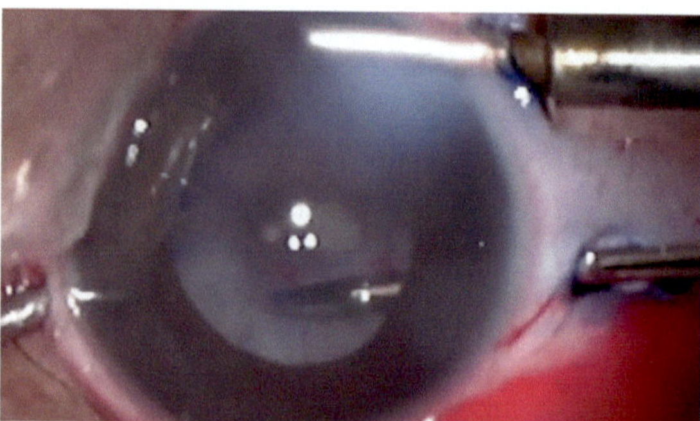

Fig. 22.2 Stromal corneal edema due to positioning of AC maintainer at the edge of stromal fibers due to a long track formation in the cornea

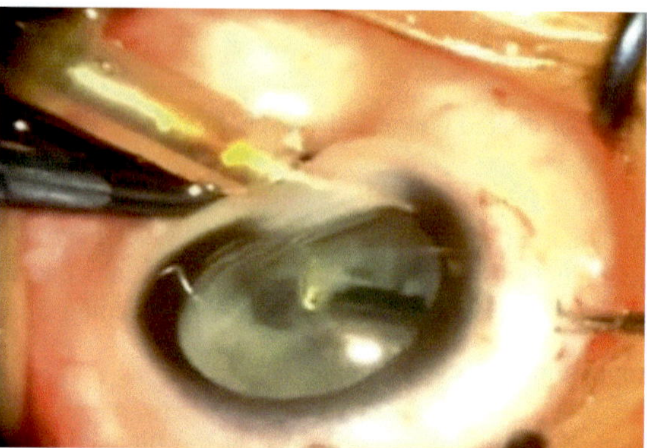

Fig. 22.3 Cutting of peripheral fibrous tissue behind the lens with deep scleral indentation to avoid its injury in an open anterior funnel retinal detachment in stage 5 ROP. Note the sclerocorneal tunnel with the anterior chamber maintainer in place

direction of the sclerotomy is parallel to the limbus at the iris root and parallel to the iris plane to avoid the possibility of perforating the retina dragged by the fibrous membranes onto the CB. The MVR may have to go through the lens before lensectomy.

3. Try to save the lens (Fig. 22.3):

  a. Despite the presence of a plane of cleavage between the posterior lens capsule and the fibrous membrane stretching to the CB, lensectomy has to be carried out in cases with closed anterior funnel detachment. The capsule has to be totally removed to avoid future retino-capsular or retino-iridal adhesions.

b. In rare cases of an open anterior funnel, the lens may be preserved. The direction of the instruments in this instance should be posterior parallel to the visual axis to avoid contact with the posterior capsule in case of LSV. This carries a better prognosis with a reattachment rate of about 43% compared to about 15% in closed funnel configurations [21]. Lens preservation decreases risk of late glaucoma development later [23].

4. Study the nature and behavior of the fibrous membrane:

   a. A thorough examination of the junction between the peripheral fibrous membrane and the pars plicata is done before surgery using the Retcam, and at surgery under the microscope by gentle deep indentation of the CB region.
   b. The presence of a peripheral clear rim between the fibrous membrane and the pars plicata may advocate a peripheral membrane dissection centripetally specially in presence of central corneal opacities.

5. Manage anterior synechiae: A separate paracentesis may be created in the presence of a very shallow/lost anterior chamber with anterior synechiae. Ocular viscoelastic device is injected into the AC, and a blunt spatula is used to separate delicately the anterior synechiae from the back of the corneal and AC angle.

6. Managing posterior synechiae and the pupil: During lensectomy, the iris adhesions to the anterior lens capsule can be separated bluntly or sharply. Additionally, the pupil can be stretched bimanually using two iris spatulas to induce mydriasis and the iris can be trimmed around the pupil for the same purpose. The use of adrenaline (1:1000 dilution in 0.1 ml or 1:1000,000 in 0.2 ml) in infusion line can help to keep the pupil well dilated. Iris hooks may also be useful (Fig. 22.4) [24].

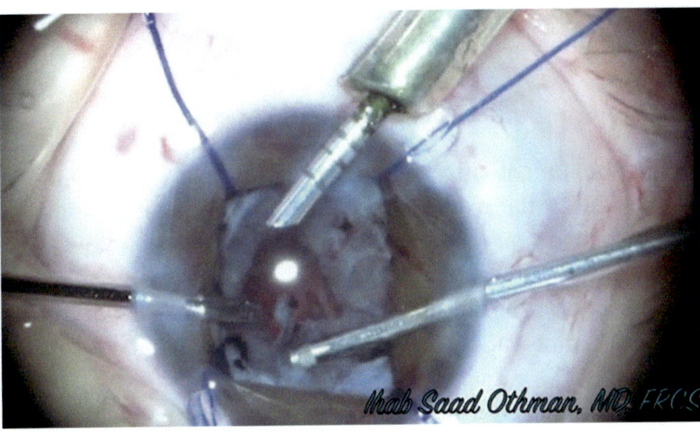

Fig. 22.4 Iris hooks used to dilate the pupil. Bimanual dissection with forceps and a vitrector is used to cut the fibrous membrane to the retinal periphery

7. Avoid retinal breaks during managing membranes: The fibrous membrane is best managed bimanually under good direct microscope illumination and keeping the area of dissection in sharp focus.

   a. Dissection may be initiated from the periphery separating the membrane from the retina and CB attachments and going centripetally. This method of dissection is particularly useful in presence of central corneal opacities.
   b. Care is taken to avoid inducing a retinal break specially towards the periphery as the retina is folded and extremely thinned and also to maintain good hemostasis. Healon is used to open the funnel as it is gradually released from the fibrous tissue.
   c. Membrane dissection should be carried out towards the periphery and if the membrane is firmly adherent to the CB region, radial cuts are performed to release that area.
   d. One should not try to remove all pre-retinal membranes from the inner retinal tissue as this is sometimes impossible due to the very firm adhesions to the retina which can even be anatomically part of the retinal surface. In this case scenario, segmentation of the membranes is done and the membrane is left in place after relieving the surrounding traction.
   e. Retinal breaks can be potentially created as dissection of the fibrous tissue is carried out to the periphery due to the lack of discrimination of the membranes from the retina specially at the retinal troughs. The author finds staining the fibrous membrane with trypan blue injected for 20–30 s in the potential space a great method of identifying the fibrous tissue from the thinned retina. Repeated staining may be indicated with further dissection [22] (Fig. 22.5A–C). Others used triamcinolone to better identify membranes and improve surgical dissection [25].
   f. Autologous plasmin or autologous plasminogen is prepared in a dose of 0.03–0.22 IU/0.15 ml and is injected into the vitreous cavity after removal of retrolenticular membranes to degrade glycoproteins assisting in separating the cortical vitreous from the internal limiting membrane [26].

8. Avoid retinal breaks during management of the stalk

   a. To open the funnel after removing the fibrous membrane, one should properly identify the extent of the fibrous stalk and its ramifications as it exerts the traction on the central retina around the optic disc. Using trypan blue helps tremendously (Fig. 22.5C) [22].
   b. Visco-dissection using healon to gently stretch and identify bridging membranes that can be cut by scissors or vitrector. Healon acts also as a hemostatic agent.
   c. Hemostasis is secured using endodiathermy, healon and gently elevating the infusion pressure.

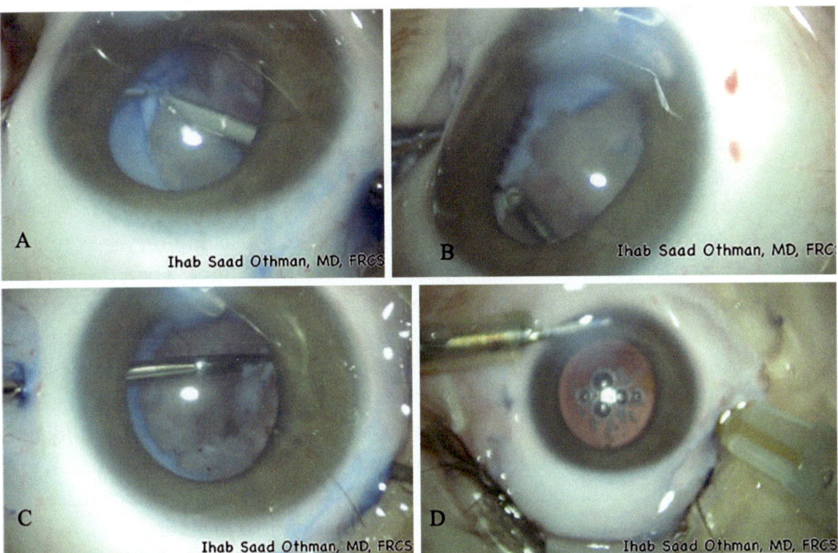

Fig. 22.5 **A** Staining of the fibrous membrane with Trypan blue allows better identification and discrimination of the plane between the retina and the fibrous tissue. **B** Dissection could be carried out to the ciliary processes. **C** identification and releasing of the fibrous stalk. **D** Semifluorinated silicone oil injection with a bright red reflex

9. Management of retinal breaks:

   a. CB dialysis:

      i. In severely ischemic eyes, the mere flow of fluid into the anterior chamber may precipitate ciliary body dialysis, with efflux of subretinal fluid (Schlieren sign) and the surgery is thus doomed to fail. Gentle start up infusion pressure of about 20 mmHg may be recommended initially to avoid such a drastic complication.

      ii. Another cause of inducing a CB dialysis is applying traction on the peripheral fibrous membranes on the ciliary processes. This is avoided by instructing a trained nurse to indent anteriorly deeply the CB region, and maintain maximum pupillary mydriasis to facilitate viewing of the membrane. Addition of Trypan blue would stain the membranes and discriminate them from the CB and peripheral retina [22].

      iii. If a minimal dialysis (1–2 clock hours) happen, with no fluid leak, an attempt at inserting an encircling element at the ora serrata may help in management and allow continuation of surgery.

      iv. One should think about unconventional ways of reversing such a drastic event, perhaps suturing the ciliary processes back to the eye wall, or applying a tissue adhesive (*n*-butyl or *n*-octyl cyanoacrylate) to the area of break or dialysis, would allow continuation of surgery [27].

  b. Retinal breaks:

     i. May occur while dissecting the peripheral fibrous tissue dragging the retina and not identifying a proper plane of cleavage between it and the retina. Sharp or blunt dissection may induce a break with sudden egress of subretinal fluid into the vitreous cavity. The same rules in 10 a apply to avoid such an event.

     ii. Another reason of inducing a retinal break is insisting on dissecting the posterior part of the stalk under the microscope light. The posterior part of the stalk do have many ramifications and is adherent to the retina at several points. An additional retinal bleeding while holding and gently pulling on the fibrous stalk increases the chances of such a posterior break. Avoiding such an event, would follow the same rules as 10a, with an additional use of healon to spread the retinal leaves open and identify the accurate extent of the fibrous stalk. Use of an illuminated pick with endovitreal curved scissors or MVR would allow bimanual dissection and proper removal of the stalk with minimal bleeding and minimal chance to create a break. Needless to say, that such a devastating event indicates a failure of surgery.

  c. Semifluorinated Silicone oil [22]:

     i. We used Semifluorinated ether or alkane silicone oil in management of stage 5 ROP with no breaks due to their specific criteria.

     ii. Being heavier than water, they allow tamponading the retina in an open funnel configuration, and may prevent recurrent fibrosis, thus enhancing retinal repositioning (Fig. 22.5D).

     iii. Semifluorinated silicone oil should be removed in 3–12 weeks time (Fig. 22.6).

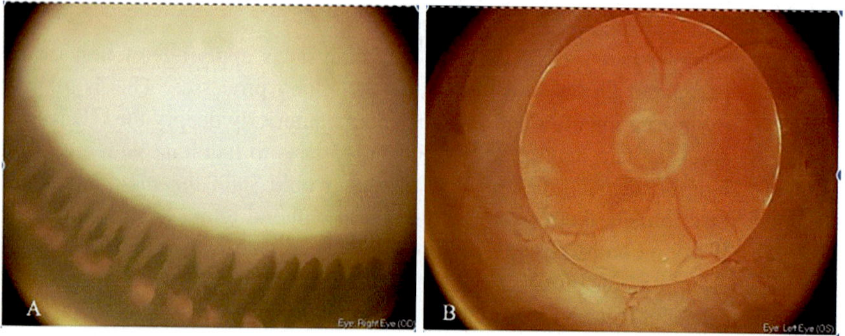

Fig. 22.6 **A** Stage 5 ROP OD with fibrous membrane stretching to the ciliary body. Note the clear rim towards the CB attachment allowing peripheral dissection of the fibrous tissue centripetally. **B** Same case OS at the time of Semifluorinated silicone oil removal. Note the flattening of the retina with appearance of the optic nerve and minimal recurrent fibrosis

Case Scenario

An 18-month-old premature boy presented with a history pars plicata lensectomy and vitrectomy OU with loss of the left eye and recurrent retinal detachment in his only right eye 8 months post-surgery OD due to late posterior hyaloid contraction.

On examination, the right eye was aphakic, fundus examination showed a total retinal detachment, with temporal fibrous ridge and wrinkling of the retina (Fig. 22.7A, B).

Decision: Surgery (**Video** 2)

Surgery with pars plicata vitrectomy was decided for the right eye. The posterior hyaloid face was found to be firmly attached to the detached retina and the fibrovascular ridge. Sharp dissection successfully detached the posterior hyaloid face, and the fibrous ridge. A temporal break was inevitably created. The surgery was completed with fluid/air exchange and semifluorinated silicone oil tamponade (Fig. 7C). Two months later, silicone oil was removed and the retina remained successfully reposited (Fig. 7D). Patient corrected vision allowed adequate ambulation.

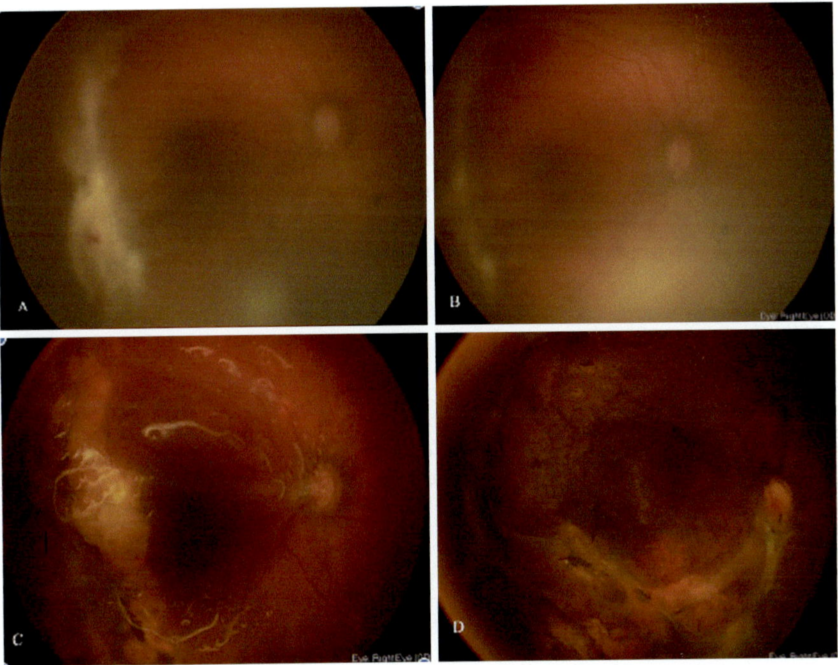

Fig. 22.7 **A, B** Retcam fundus photograph showing a recurrent retinal detachment in the right eye with a temporal fibrovascular ridge. **C** Retinal flattening post vitrectomy with removal of posterior hyaloid face and the fibrous ridge. A temporal break occurred during surgery necessitating semifluorinated silicone oil tamponade. **D** Retina is flat post silicone oil removal. New fibrous tissue formation is noted inferior to the optic nerve and at inferior retina. RPE shows pigmentary changes from the recurrent previous subretinal fluid

Review Questions

1. Select true or false for each sentence below:

a. Late recurrent retinal detachment in stage 4 or 5 ROP may not be rhegmatogenous.
b. An iatrogenic break during PPL/PPV in stages 4 and 5 ROP concludes the surgery as failure.
c. Late contraction of an attached posterior haloid face in stages 4/5 ROP can induce a late recurrent tractional retinal detachment.
d. Using semifluorinated silicone oil may assist in the success of ROP surgery in complicated stages 4/5 ROP.

2. Which of the following is true regrading complicated ROP surgery?

a. Unattended ROP in stages 4 and 5 are associated with microphthalmia and band keratopathy in over 50% of cases.
b. Surgical intervention in stage 5 ROP carries a 75% retinal reposition rate.
c. Lensectomy in stages 4 and 5 ROP carries a high retina reposition rate.
d. Post-operative phthisis bulbi is a common complication of vitrectomy for stages 4 and 5 ROP.

3. Which of the following regarding ROP surgery in stages 4 and 5 is false:

a. Surgery in stages 4a and 5a carries a better prognosis than stages 4b and 5b.
b. Thorough inspection of the retinal periphery before placing the sclerotomies is crucial to prevent iatrogenic peripheral retinal injury.
c. Anti-VEGF may be used 1 day before surgery to decrease vascular activity.
d. Vigorous dissection of all fibrous membranes is mandatory for success of surgery.

Answers

1. (**A**) True.
2. (**B**) False.
3. (**C**) True.
4. (**D**) True.

2. **A**

3. **D**

References

1. Pulido JS, Byrne SF, Clarkson JG, diBernardo CL, Howe CA. Evaluation of eyes with advanced stages of retinopathy of prematurity using standardized echography. Ophthalmology. 1991;98:1099–104.
2. Kelly SP, Fielder AR. Microcornea associated with retinopathy of prematurity. Br J Ophthalmol. 1987;71:201–3.
3. Laws DE, Haslett R, Ashby D, O'Brien C, Clark D. Axial length biometry in infants with retinopathy of prematurity. Eye. 1994;8:427–30.
4. Hittner HM, Rhodes LM, McPherson AR. Anterior segment abnormalities in cicatricial retinopathy of prematurity. Ophthalmology. 1979;86:803–16.
5. Pollard ZF. Lensectomy for secondary angle-closure glaucoma in advanced cicatricial retrolental fibroplasia. Ophthalmology. 1984;91:395–8.
6. Knight-Nanan DM, Algawi K, Bowell R, O'Keefe M. Advanced cicatricial retinopathy of prematurity-outcome and complications. Br J Ophthalmol. 1996;80:343–5.
7. Capone A Jr, Trese MT. Lens-sparing vitreous surgery for tractional stage 4A retinopathy of prematurity retinal detachments. Ophthalmology. 2001;108:2068–70.
8. Ozsaygili C, Ozdek S, Ozmen MC, et al. Preoperative anatomical features associated with improved surgical outcomes for stage 5 retinopathy of prematurity. Retina. 2021;41(4):718–25. https://doi.org/10.1097/IAE.0000000000002948 PMID: 32932381.
9. Shah PK, Narendran V, Kalpana N. Safety and efficacy of simultaneous bilateral 25-gauge lens-sparing vitrectomy for vascularly active stage 4 retinopathy of prematurity. Eye (Lond). 2015;29:1046–50.
10. Nudleman E, Robinson J, Rao P, Drenser KA, Capone A, Trese MT, et al. Long-term outcomes on lens clarity after lens-sparing vitrectomy for retinopathy of prematurity. Ophthalmology. 2015;122:755–9.
11. Lakhanpal RR, Davis GH, Sun RL, Albini TA, Holz ER. Lens clarity after 3-port lens-sparing vitrectomy in stage 4A and 4B retinal detachments secondary to retinopathy of prematurity. Arch Ophthalmol. 2006;124:20–3.
12. Shah PK, Narendran V, Kalpana N, Tawansy KA. Anatomical and visual outcome of stages 4 and 5 retinopathy of prematurity. Eye (Lond). 2009;23:176–80.
13. Gadkari S, Kamdar R, Kulkarni S, Kakade N, Taras S, Deshpande M, et al. Vitreoretinal surgery for advanced retinopathy of prematurity: presentation and outcomes from a developing country. Can J Ophthalmol. 2015;50:54–60.
14. Gadkari SS, Deshpande M, Kulkarni S. Minimally fibrotic stage 5 ROP: a clinical prognostic factor in eyes undergoing vitrectomy for stage 5 retinopathy of prematurity. Graefes Arch Clin Exp Ophthalmol. 2016;254:1303–9.
15. Muslubas IS, Karacorlu M, Hocaoglu M, Yamanel C, Arf S, Ozdemir H, et al. Ultrasonography findings in eyes with stage 5 retinopathy of prematurity. Ophthalmic Surg Lasers Imaging Retina. 2015;46:1035–40.
16. Chiang MF, Quinn GE, Fielder AR, et al. International classification of retinopathy of prematurity. Ophthalmology. 2021;128(10):e51-68. https://doi.org/10.1016/j.ophtha.2021.05.031 Epub 2021 Jul 8 PMID: 34247850.
17. Maidana EJ, Matieli LC, Allemann N, Melo LA Jr, Morales M, Moraes NS, et al. Ultrasonographic findings in eyes with retinal detachments secondary to retinopathy of prematurity. J Pediatr Ophthalmol Strabismus. 2007;44:39–42.
18. Yonekawa Y, Wu WC, Nitulescu CE, et al. Progressive retinal detachment in infants with retinopathy of prematurity treated with intravitreal bevacizumab or ranibizumab. Retina (Philadelphia, Pa). 2018;38(6):1079–83. https://doi.org/10.1097/iae.0000000000001685. PubMed PMID: 28471890.
19. Hairston RJ, Maguire AM, Vitale S, et al. Morphometric analysis of pars plana development in humans. Invest Ophthalmol Vis Sci. 1992;33:119.

20. Kondo H, Arita N, Osato M, Hayashi H, Oshima K, Uchio E. Late recurrence of retinal detachment following successful vitreous surgery for stages 4B and 5 retinopathy of prematurity. Am J Ophthalmol. 2009;147(4):661-666.e1.

21. Nudleman E, Robinson J, Rao P, et al. Long-term outcomes on lens clarity after lens-sparing vitrectomy for retinopathy of prematurity. Ophthalmology. 2015;122(4):755–9.

22. Othman IS. Retinopathy of prematurity: a major review and situation analysis in Egypt. J Med Sci Res. 2018;1:136–44.

23. Seaber JH, Machemer R, Eliott D, Buckley EG, deJuan E, Martin DF, et al. Long-term visual results of children after initially successful vitrectomy for stage V retinopathy of prematurity. Ophthalmology. 1995;102:199–204.

24. Gopal L, Sharma T, Shanmugam M, Badrinath SS, Sharma A, Agraharam SG, et al. Surgery for stage 5 retinopathy of prematurity: the learning curve and evolving technique. Indian J Ophthalmol. 2000;48:101–6.

25. Lakhanpal RR, Fortun JA, Chan-Kai B, et al. Lensectomy and vitrectomy with and without intravitreal triamcinolone acetonide for vascularly active stage 5 retinal detachments in retinopathy of prematurity. Retina. 2006;26(7):736–40.

26. Wu WC, Drenser KA, Lai M, Capone A, Trese MT. Plasmin enzyme-assisted vitrectomy for primary and reoperated eyes with stage 5 retinopathy of prematurity. Retina. 2008;28:S75-80.

27. Hartnett ME, Hirose T. Cyanoacrylate glue in the repair of retinal detachment associated with posterior retinal breaks in infants and children. Retina. 1998;18:125–9.

Genetics of Retinopathy of Prematurity from the Point of a Surgical Approach

Matthew G. J. Trese and Kimberly A. Drenser

Abstract

Retinopathy of prematurity is a leading cause of visual impairment for children globally. Currently, risk factor-based screening protocols have been successfully implemented and have dramatically reduced the incidence advanced ROP. Despite this success, we still are unable to accurately predict in whom advanced ROP will develop. This chapter aims to summarize our current understanding of the non-environmental risk factors which are known to influence ROP extent and severity.

Keywords

Retinopathy of prematurity · ROP · FEVR · Genetic predisposition · Wnt signaling · Familial exudative vitreoretinopathy · ROPER

M. G. J. Trese · K. A. Drenser (✉)
Department of Ophthalmology, Oakland University William Beaumont School of Medicine, Royal Oak, MI, USA
e-mail: kdrenser@arcpc.net

M. G. J. Trese
e-mail: matttrese@arcpc.net

K. A. Drenser
Pediatric Retinal Research Foundation, Birmingham, MI, USA

Eye Research Institute, Oakland University, Rochester, MI, USA

Ş. Özdek et al. (eds.), *Pediatric Vitreoretinal Surgery*,
https://doi.org/10.1007/978-3-031-14506-3_23

315

Introduction

Retinopathy of Prematurity (ROP) is a vasoproliferative retinal disease that occurs in premature infants. Decades of dedicated study have demonstrated that ROP is a common and largely predictable disease that progresses through various stages of severity. In fact, evidence from the Cryotherapy for Retinopathy of Prematurity (CRYO-ROP) study suggest that approximately 65% of preterm infants who met screening criteria developed some degree of ROP [1]. In most cases, acute signs of ROP regress without imparting significant long term visual consequences. However, a subset of patients will develop advanced ROP. In these infants, permanent vision loss occurs secondary to the development of pre-retinal neovascularization, vitreous hemorrhage, macular dragging, retinal folds and retinal detachments.

Since its original description, ROP has remained a significant source of childhood blindness. Early investigations aimed to identify environmental risk factors which would allow for adequate screening, timely intervention and hopefully visual preservation. These studies identified oxygen exposure, short gestational ages and low birth weights as significant risk factors for progression to advanced ROP. With timely and adequate treatment, the infants that progress represent a minority of patients, but the visual sequela for these infants can be severe and life-long. At present there are no clinically observable markers which allow physicians to predict in whom advanced ROP will occur. This has led some researchers to consider nonenvironmental factors which may contribute to advanced ROP pathogenesis. This chapter aims to summarize our current understanding of the genetic factors which drive advanced ROP.

Identifying a Genetic Predisposition

Although screening protocols which hinge upon the identification of environmental risk factors have proven largely successful, they inadequately characterize the risk of ROP progression within an individual. Anyone who cares for infants with ROP will undoubtably recall examples of high-risk infants with low birthweights and brief gestational ages who do not develop significant ROP. These same individuals will also recall low-risk infants who progress to advanced ROP. Risk based screening protocols cannot capture these outliers. In fact, a recent study demonstrated that the presence or absence of known risk factors in infants at phenotypic extremes does not correlate with ROP progression [2]. This combined with a retrospective twin study of premature monozygotic and dizygotic twins, found that genetic factors accounted for approximately 70% of the variance in liability for ROP [3]. Together these studies have provided support for the notion of that genetics play an important role in the pathophysiology which underlies ROP, but they did not define the culpable genes.

Given that ROP is a multifactorial disease, defining the genes which contribute to its pathogenesis is a difficult task. Thus, other heritable pediatric retinal diseases with similar clinical phenotypes to advanced ROP have been studied in hopes of elucidating a possible genetic connection. For example, Familial Exudative Vitreoretinopathy (FEVR), Norrie Disease (ND) and pseudoglioma osteoporosis syndrome (POS) have all been thoroughly evaluated through molecular genetic studies. All of these diseases are inherited vitreoretinal disorders that commonly occur in full term infants and have disease phenotypes that are reminiscent of advanced ROP. Specifically, these infants will develop abnormal pre-retinal neovascularization with varying degrees of compromised blood-retinal barrier function. Together, these pathologic features may result in both tractional and exudative retinal detachments. Mutations in FZD4, LRP5, TSPAN12, NDP, CTNNB1, KIF11 and ZNF408 are all known to cause FEVR; which can occur in an autosomal dominant (TSPAN12, FZD4, ZNF408), an autosomal recessive (LRP5) and an X-linked (NDP) manner. CTNNB1 and KIF11 mutations are associated with syndromes with microcephaly, chorioretinopathy, and/or cognitive delay [4, 5]. Regardless of the inheritance pattern, individuals affected with FEVR portray a spectrum of disease ranging from asymptomatic to severe vision loss. Norrie disease, on the other hand, is an X-linked condition associated with mutation in the NPD gene which effectively eliminates function of the protein product. In contrast to FEVR, whose disease findings are limited to the ocular structures, individuals affected with Norrie disease are almost universally blind by age 5 and often have sensorineural hearing loss and cognitive delay. Of the 5 previously mentioned genes which are known to cause FEVR and ND, all but KIF11 and ZNF408 are involved in the canonical Wnt signaling pathway.

Wnt Signaling

Wnt signaling is a highly evolutionarily conserved transduction signaling pathway that regulates many aspects of cellular survival, cellular differentiation, cellular migration and embryonic organogenesis (Fig. 23.1). Its role in retinal development is known to be crucial for angiogenesis and vascular maintenance [6]. Because the aforementioned Wnt-signaling vitreoretinopathies share an overlapping clinical phenotype with advanced ROP, a candidate gene approach was applied to better characterize the influence that genetic factors have on ROP progression.

Using this approach, mutations in the NDP, LRP5, TSPAN12 and FZD4, have all been described with variable frequencies in patients with advanced ROP. The NDP gene encodes a protein called norrin. Norrin, is a ligand that is capable of binding the Frizzled 4 receptor and its coreceptor low-density lipoprotein receptor-related protein 5. Once bound, norrin is capable of initiating wnt signaling cascades. Consequently, mutations in the NDP gene result in impaired wnt signaling. It has been suggested that NDP mutations account for approximately 3% of cases of advanced ROP [7–9]. Interestingly, this frequency was significantly higher

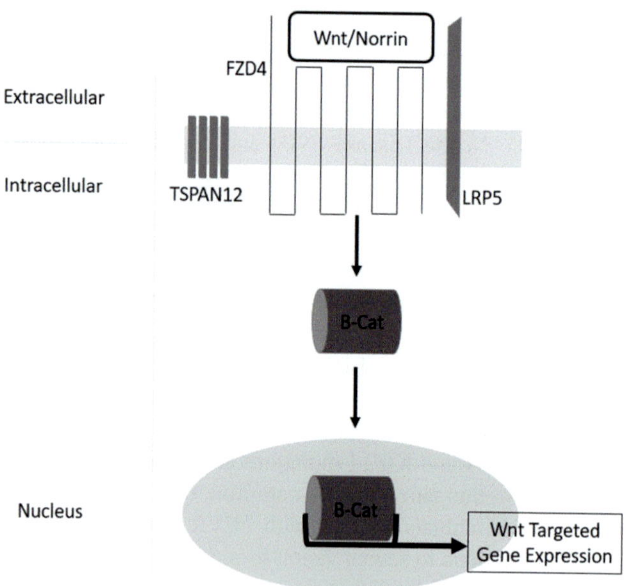

Fig. 23.1 Schematic of Canonical Wnt Signaling Pathway. Wnt and Norrin act as ligands which bind FZD4 receptor and its coreceptor LRP5. Once activated, β-catenin collects in the cytoplasm and is ultimately entering the nucleus where T-cell factor (TCF)/lymphoid enhancer factor family (Lef) interactions result in Wnt targeted gene transcription and ultimately gene expression. TSPAN 12 also interacts with the FZD4-LRP5 binding complex and acts to preferentially increase binding affinity for norrin. Abnormal Wnt signaling results in the failure of Wnt targeted gene activation and may give rise to clinical phenotypes such as Familial Exudative Vitreoretinopathy (FEVR), Norrie disease, pseudoglioma osteoporosis syndrome and a subset of patients with retinopathy o prematurity

in a Kuwaiti study which found a NDP597C > A polymorphism in 83% of patients with advanced ROP. Importantly, this polymorphism was not identified in patients whose ROP regressed spontaneously, and it was noted in 10% of the normal population [9].

The LRP5 gene encodes low-density lipoprotein receptor-related protein 5; which is the coreceptor for the frizzled 4 receptor. Mutations in this gene have the potential to result in altered wnt/norrin ligand binding affinity. Hiraoka et al. reported that sequencing of the 3'UTR region of the LRP5 gene resulted in the identification of a heterozygous polymorphism leading to the addition of a leucine amino acid in the signal peptide of a patient with advanced ROP. They postulated that this mutation could impair translocation function, protein processing and ultimately disrupt retinal development [8]. Kondo et al. also reported mutations in LRP5. They detected nonsynchronous mutations in the LRP5 gene in a small number of patients with advanced ROP (p.R1219H, p.H1383P, and p.T1540M). Although this study did not provide causality, it did use computational models which predicted that these mutations were likely pathologic [10].

The TSAPN12 gene encodes cell surface proteins that are members of the tetraspanin family. Tetraspanin family proteins can organize into tetraspanin enriched microdomains that are capable of acting as signal platforms within cellular membranes. Within the retina, TSPAN12 is required for successful norrin and LRP5 activity. Thus, TSPAN12 helps to regulates beta catenin mediated transcriptional activity by shifting receptor binding away from traditional wnt ligands and preferentially binding norrin. Mutations in TSPAN 12 have been reported in infants with advanced ROP in a Malaysian population [11]. However, their role in disease pathogenesis and its extrapolation to a more heterogenous patient population requires further investigations.

The FZD4 gene encodes the protein frizzled 4 receptors. The frizzled 4 receptor, together with its coreceptor low-density lipoprotein receptor-related protein 5, binds either the wnt or norrin ligand to initiate the wnt signaling cascades. Mutations in FDZ4 gene presumably result in misfolding of the frizzled 4 receptor and therefore hinders ligand affinity. Interestingly in evaluating patients with autosomal dominant FEVR and ROP, it was noted 10.6% of patients showed mutations in the FZD4 gene [12]. Four polymorphisms were identified in the autosomal dominant FEVR cohort (C117R, C181Y, Q505X and P33S/P168S), only one double missense mutation P33s/P168S was found in the ROP cohort. Importantly, no mutations of FZD4 were identified in infants without FEVR or ROP. Additionally, Elles et al. reported mutations in FZD4 (p.Ala370Gly (c.1109C > G), p.Lys203Asn (c.609G > T), and p.Arg466Trp (c.1396C > T) [13]. In their study, they concluded that roughly 3% of advanced ROP (i.e. treatment warranted) was related to these mutations. Thus, FZD4 mutations are noted to occur at a significantly higher frequency in individuals with FEVR and ROP than in the general population.

Wnt Signaling and Placental Insufficiency

In addition to a high prevalence of FZD4 mutations in patients with FEVR and ROP, it was noted that ROP infants with FZD4 mutation were born with lower birth weights than would be expected for their respective gestational ages. Consequently, our laboratory screened autosomal dominant FEVR and ROP children for FZD4 polymorphisms. Interestingly, a compound sequence variation P33S;P168 was found at a high frequency in patients with ROP.

Wnt signaling is a ubiquitous pathway that is not only important in retinal development but is also vital in the female reproductive system. In fact, animal studies have shown that there is impaired vascular development of the corpora lutea of FZD4 null mice and that NDP knock mice have defects in vascular development that result in embryonic loss [14, 15]. In humans, NDP expression has been reported in the placenta and localized to placental villous mesenchymal cells [15, 16]. These data suggest that FZD4 polymorphisms may play an important role in fetal and placental development. When juxtaposed with the notion that there is a higher frequency of FZD4 mutations in infants with ROP and that FZD4 mutations result in a predilection toward birth weight deficits, it seems convincing that FZD4 mutations are contributing to ROP severity in at least a subset of patients. In fact, our research has shown that infants with FZD4 mutations were generally older than expected (>26 weeks GA) but were small for gestational age. When considered in light of the weight, insulin like growth factor study (WINROP) study, which showed that infants with smaller birth weights were more likely to develop type 1 ROP, these results are quite compelling [17]. Thus implications of identifying this this genetic link, are potentially far reaching and suggest a potential role for genetic screening of at-risk infants.

Retinopathy of Prematurity or Familial Exudative Vitreoretinopathy

Prior to our understanding of the genetic factors which propagate FEVR, this rare proliferative vitreoretinopathy was often referred to as "ROP in a full-term infant." As our understanding of these two separate but related entities have expanded, it has become clear that the line that divides them is blurred. A good example of this diagnostic ambiguity comes from premature infants displaying significant proliferative retinopathy, but whose prematurity is a relatively underwhelming feature. When encountering these children, it is first important to consider the role of environmental factors, such as oxygen supplementation. In fact, the role of unregulated oxygen supplementation is inextricably linked to ROP progression and is commonly encountered in middle income countries who have a limited ability to supplement and monitor oxygen [18]. However in industrialized countries where the technology to regulate supplemental oxygen is readily available, it is imperative to consider alternative diagnoses, such as FEVR.

Those infants that do not clearly fit into archetypal disease categories and display features of both ROP and FEVR are often referred to as infants with FROP or ROPER [12, 19]. When considered in the background of wnt signaling, overlapping clinical features are almost expected. For example, an infant with a compound variation (P33S; P168) of the FZD4 gene may be born prematurely because of a relative placental insufficiency. Their mutation, which in the retina results in impaired wnt/norrin ligand binding affinity, may result in retinopathy which may be intensified due to environmental factors such as suboptimal oxygen supplementation. The history and clinical findings are consistent with ROP but they harbor a mutation closely associated with FEVR, creating a diagnostic dilemma. Consequently, when evaluating children with ROP it is essential to think about alternative diagnoses if the clinical course strays from the largely predictable and well-defined disease course of ROP.

Trophic Factors in Retinal Development

The trophic factors and molecular signaling pathways which govern normal retinal development as well as pathologic retinal neovascularization have also been carefully evaluated with the hopes of providing insight into the mechanisms which contribute to ROP extent and severity. The predominant focus of these investigations has been on signaling pathways which influence angiogenesis, inflammation and neural development. Signaling molecules that have been studied include but are not limited to vascular endothelial growth factor (VEGF), insulin like growth factor-1 (IGF-1), erythropoietin (EPO), endothelial nitric oxide synthase, brain derived neurotrophic factor, angiopoietins and a variety of inflammatory mediators [20]. Although a complete review of these signaling molecules is outside the scope of this chapter, special attention should be paid to VEGF and its critical role not only in normal retinal development, but also vasoproliferative retinal disease.

Our understanding of normal retinal development and the role of VEGF in part stems from rodent models [21–23]. These studies showed that developing retinal capillaries migrate anteriorly because of a wave of elevated VEGF expression. This process is thought to be driven by the presence of a zone of relative hypoxia in the avascular retina. Support for this notion is evidenced by the upregulation of hypoxia inducible factor 1 alpha (HIF1α), an upstream regulator of VEGF expression. As the immature retinal capillaries grow into the avascular retina and bring with them oxygenated blood, hypoxia is reduced and thus HIF1α and subsequently VEGF expression are down regulated. Although the above provides a helpful construct to study the role of VEGF in retinal development, it oversimplifies the myriad of carefully orchestrated events which culminate in retinal normal development and vascularization.

In and of itself premature birth, as well as the neonatal support required to sustain premature infants, likely alters the course of these carefully organized events. Given these changes it has been suggested the ROP progresses through 2 Phases [24]. In the first, supplemental oxygen provides a relative abundance of oxygen to the immature retinal tissues via diffusion from the choriocapillaris. This abundance of oxygen results in vaso-obliteration with the consequent development of retinal avascularity. In the second phase, retinal maturation results in a relative dearth of oxygen, leading to the over expression of trophic factors and cytokines, such as VEGF. This over expression ultimately results in pathologic pre-retinal neovascularization.

It is well established that VEGF, specifically VEGFA isoforms, play a critical role in ROP pathogenesis. In fact, treatment options such as peripheral retinal ablation and intravitreal anti-VEGF injections are predicated on VEGF suppression. Given this, numerous studies have employed a candidate gene approach to evaluate single nucleotide polymorphisms (SNP) in VEGFA expression. Of these, rs2010963 (−634G > C and +405G > C) has been the most widely investigated. Studies from the United Kingdom and Egypt showed that there was a higher frequency of the G allele in ROP patients [25, 26]. While others have shown a higher frequency of the C allele [27]. These conflicting results have made it difficult to infer the role of VEGFA polymorphisms in the pathogenesis of ROP. Despite several other investigations into a variety of SNPs, there are no known VEGF polymorphisms that are definitively associated with ROP.

Future Directions—Genome Sequencing for ROP

Linkage and SNP studies for the evaluation of multifactorial diseases, such as ROP, can be a daunting task. Therefore, high throughput assays have become powerful tools capable of evaluating the genome of patients with multifactorial disease. Genome-wide association studies (GWAS) use array technology to screen for common SNPs simultaneously. This approach has proven successful in glaucoma and age-related macular degeneration. On the other hand, next generation sequencing (NGS) utilizes massively parallel sequencing technology to evaluate regions of the whole genome. This approach can identify rare variants that may have phenotypic and functional correlations. Future studies employing this technology will require international collaboration not only to amass an adequate number of patients to identify significant variations, but also to define agreed upon disease phenotypes which may mitigate the intrusion of confounding clinical variables. Applying these techniques to ROP is an exciting next step that has the potential to promote our understanding of ROP pathophysiology and potentially provide new therapeutic targets.

Clinical Considerations

Despite the potential of exome and genome sequencing, current clinical care for preterm infants that meet screening criteria for ROP depends upon careful observation. Because a variety of diseases can have overlapping clinical phenotypes with ROP, which may be difficult to distinguish based on clinical exam alone, it is imperative to maintain a high level of suspicion for alternative diagnoses. This is particularly true in patients with presumed ROP who do not ascribe to its well-known and highly predictable disease course, or whose retinal disease is out of proportion with their risk factor profile or whose response to treatment is suboptimal. For example, we cared for a preterm infant who was referred for progression of ROP despite adequate laser treatment. The child was born at 23 weeks gestation with a birth weight of 730 g. An examination under anesthesia was performed and a blood sample was taken for genetic testing (Fig. 23.2A, B). Fundoscopic examination revealed adequate laser treatment, but there was extensive exudation bilaterally. The results of the genetic testing revealed a FZD4 mutation, which can be associated with persistent exudation. Unfortunately, the patient went on to develop bilateral retinal detachments despite multiple surgical interventions. Ultimately, we were unable to quell the patient's relentless exudation which resulted in severe

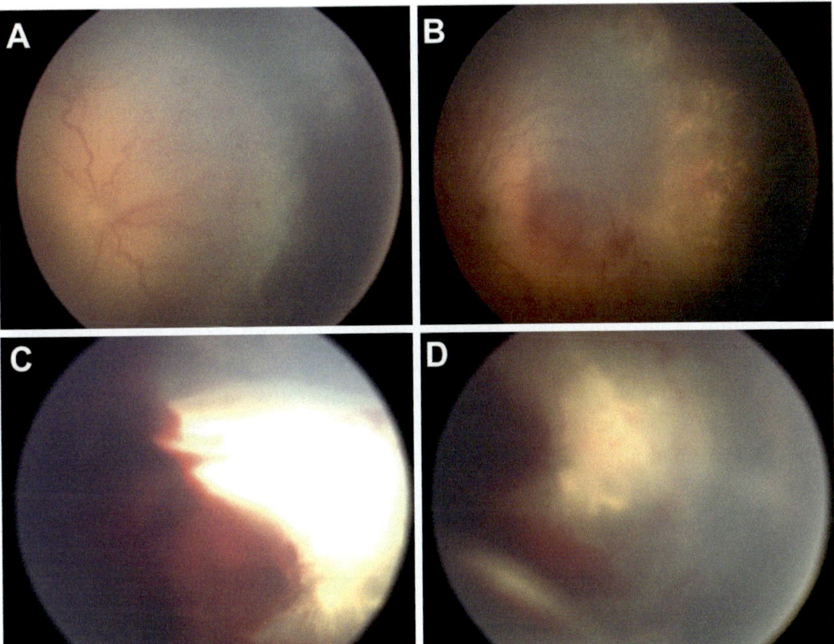

Fig. 23.2 A Diagnostic Dilemma—FEVR versus ROP. This child was referred for ROP progression despite peripheral retinal ablation with laser. The infant was born at 23 weeks with a birth weight of 730 g. Panel **A** and **B** shows the right and left eyes of this child at 36 weeks. These fundus images demonstrate dilated tortuous retinal vessels with near confluent laser treatment. Despite adequate laser treatment, and only two weeks later, this patient went on to develop extensive exudation, retinal and vitreous hemorrhage and retinal detachments of the right **C** and left **D** eyes. The patient was found to have a FZD4 mutation, which helped to explain their relentless exudation. In all patients with presumed ROP who stray from the well-defined clinical course, other diagnoses must be considered and widefield fluorescein angiography and genetic testing must be obtained

bilateral vision loss (Fig. 23.2C, D). Despite this poor visual outcome, the identification of this child's FEVR mutation provided clarity for why the patients clinical course was so complicated.

The importance of diagnostic accuracy cannot be overstated for this patient population. This is because the physician's treatment mentality shifts. This is in part because ROP can be thought of as a window disease, where the acute phase of the disease, and thus the period where optimal treatment can be applied, takes place within a pre-specified window. In contrast, FEVR is an inherited disease with the potential for life-long reactivation. Further, achieving disease control in ROP and FEVR is quite different. Although peripheral retinal ablation is a cornerstone treatment option for both diseases, control in treatment warranted ROP is often accomplished in a single session, while individuals with FEVR may require multiple laser session and/or multiple surgeries to quite the disease process.

Understanding these key differences is important in setting parental expectations regarding more aggressive life-long disease surveillance and surgical intervention. Taken together this underscores the importance of genetic screening for individuals with presumed ROP whose disease strays from what is expected. Finally, once an underlying genetic diagnosis has been identified, the screening of at-risk family members because an important feature of caring for patients with inherited vitre-oretinopathies. In fact, a review of our own patient records revealed that approximately 15% of newly diagnosed FEVR patients in the State of Michigan were the direct result of screening family members once a proband had been identified.

From a surgical standpoint, the identification of genetic factors which influence wnt signaling is also important. Because individuals with FZD4 and LRP5 mutations have an intrinsically compromised blood retinal barrier, premature infants that undergo vitrectomy are more likely to have post-operative inflammation, fibrin, and hemorrhage due to an intrinsically compromised blood retinal barrier. Awareness of these his information can inform intra and postoperative decision making such as the judicious use of intra and perioperative steroids.

Conclusions

Environmental risk-factor based screening protocols have dramatically improved outcomes for patients with ROP. The goal of these screening programs is to identify at-risk individuals prior to the development of macular distortion or retinal detachment. Through the evaluation of pediatric retinal diseases with similar clinical phenotypes we have identified genes which are in part responsible for ROP severity. However, these genetic variations represent a fraction of ROP cases, thus there is more work to be done. As technology evolves, we will be able to identify new genetic variations which influence ROP progression and offers the potential to better understand the disease pathophysiology, enhance our current screening paradigms and potentially identify new therapeutic targets.

Review Questions

1. A premature infant was born a 26 weeks gestational age and weighed 856 g. The child received no treatment for ROP and is currently 55 weeks post gestational age. The infant presents at the request of the pediatric ophthalmologist for persistent vascular tortuosity in both eyes with a mild peripheral preretinal hemorrhage in the left eye. What are the appropriate next steps?

a. Indirect ophthalmoscopy with detailed fundoscopic examination in the office
b. Examination under anesthesia with color photos and widefield fluoresceine angiography

c. Genetic Testing
d. All of the above

2. In approximately what percentage of patients suspected to have familial exudative vitreoretinopathy (FEVR) will genetic testing be positive?

a. 10%
b. 25%
c. 50%
d. 90%

3. All of the following genetic mutations have been consistently identified in infants with advanced retinopathy of prematurity, EXCEPT:

a. VEGF-A$_{165}$
b. NDP
c. FZD4
d. LRP5

Answers

1. (**D**) This child's clinical course is incongruent with the expected clinical course of a child with retinopathy of prematurity. Thus alternative diagnoses must be considered, despite the history of preterm birth. Indirect ophthalmoscopy is an essential component of the child's work up, but it can be challenging in the clinic. Thus examination under sedation or general anesthesia can be a valuable tool to better assess the peripheral retina in these children. At the same time, widefield fluoresceine angiography should be performed as it has been shown to enhance diagnostic accuracy for patients with familial exudative vitreoretinopathy (FEVR). Lastly, genetic testing plays an important role which can inform families and physicians about the expected clinical course, need for monitoring, the potential for surgery and the need to screen family members.

2. (**C**) In patients with clinically suspected FEVR, widfield fluoresceine angiography has been reported to enhance diagnostic accuracy. In these patients where widefield fluorescine angiography has been performed, the diagnosis of FEVR can be made approximately 90% of the time. Interestingly, only 50% of genetic testing will be positive for a FEVR mutation in patients with clinically suspected FEVR. Thus, widefield fluoresceine angiography remains the gold standard for the diagnosis and monitoring of patients with FEVR. This diagnostic discrepancy underscores the importance of continued research into the genetic factors which underly FEVR disease progression. As more genes are identified and genetic testing becomes more routine, this discrepancy is expected to narrow.

3. (**A**) Although the role of vascular endothelial growth factor (VEGF) has been proven to be critical in retinal vascular development in both the healthy and diseased states, no specific VEGF mutations have been unequivocally identified as being causative. Conversely, NDF, FZD4 and LRP5, members of the canonical wnt

signaling pathway, have been identified in several independent studies as being related to disease extent and severity in a significant minority of patients with advanced ROP.

References

1. Palmer EA, Flynn JT, Hardy RJ, Phelps DL, Phillips CL, Schaffer DB, Tung B. Incidence and early course of retinopathy of prematurity. The cryotherapy for retinopathy of prematurity cooperative group. Ophthalmology. 1991;98(11):1628–40.
2. Port AD, Chan RV, Ostmo S, Choi D, Chiang MF. Risk factors for retinopathy of prematurity: Insights from outlier infants. Graefes Arch Clin Exp Ophthalmol. 2014;252 (10):1669–77.
3. Bizzarro MJ, Hussain N, Jonsson B, Feng R, Ment LR, Gruen JR, Zhang H, Bhandari V. Genetic susceptibility to retinopathy of prematurity. Pediatrics. 2006;118(5):1858–63.
4. Coussa RG, Zhao Y, DeBenedictis MJ, Babiuch A, Sears J, Traboulsi EI. Novel mutation in CTNNB1 causes familial exudative vitreoretinopathy (FEVR) and microcephaly: case report and review of the literature. Ophthalmic Genet. 2020;41(1):63–8.
5. Rao FQ, Cai XB, Cheng FF, Cheng W, Fang XL, Li N, Huang XF, Li LH, Jin ZB. Mutations in LRP5,FZD4, TSPAN12, NDP, ZNF408, or KIF11 genes account for 38.7% of chinese patients with familial exudative vitreoretinopathy. Invest Ophthalmol Vis Sci. 2017;58 (5):2623–9.
6. Dejana E. The role of wnt signaling in physiological and pathological angiogenesis. Circ Res. 2010;107(8):943–52.
7. Shastry BS, Pendergast SD, Hartzer MK, Liu X, Trese MT. Identification of missense mutations in the norrie disease gene associated with advanced retinopathy of prematurity. Arch Ophthalmol. 1997;115(5):651–5.
8. Hiraoka M, Takahashi H, Orimo H, Hiraoka M, Ogata T, Azuma N. Genetic screening of wnt signaling factors in advanced retinopathy of prematurity. Mol Vis. 2010;05(16):2572–7.
9. Haider MZ, Devarajan LV, Al-Essa M, Kumar H. A C597–>A polymorphism in the norrie disease gene is associated with advanced retinopathy of prematurity in premature Kuwaiti infants. J Biomed Sci. 2002;9(4):365–70.
10. Kondo H, Kusaka S, Yoshinaga A, Uchio E, Tawara A, Tahira T. Genetic variants of FZD4 and LRP5 genes in patients with advanced retinopathy of prematurity. Mol Vis. 2013;19:476–85.
11. Mohd Khair SZN, Ismail AS, Embong Z, Mohamed Yusoff AA. Detection of FZD4, LRP5 and TSPAN12 genes variants in malay premature babies with retinopathy of prematurity. J Ophthalmic Vis Res. 2019;14(2):171–8.
12. Drenser KA, Dailey W, Vinekar A, Dalal K, Capone A, Trese MT. Clinical presentation and genetic correlation of patients with mutations affecting the FZD4 gene. Arch Ophthalmol. 2009;127(12):1649–54.
13. Ells A, Guernsey DL, Wallace K, Zheng B, Vincer M, Allen A, Ingram A, DaSilva O, Siebert L, Sheidow T, Beis J, Robitaille JM. Severe retinopathy of prematurity associated with FZD4 mutations. Ophthalmic Genet. 2010;31(1):37–43.
14. Hsieh M, Boerboom D, Shimada M, Lo Y, Parlow AF, Luhmann UF, Berger W, Richards JS. Mice null for Frizzled4 (Fzd4-/-) are infertile and exhibit impaired corpora lutea formation and function. Biol Reprod. 2005;73(6):1135–46.
15. Luhmann UF, Meunier D, Shi W, Luttges A, Pfarrer C, Fundele R, Berger W. Fetal loss in homozygous mutant Norrie disease mice: a new role of Norrin in reproduction. Genesis. 2005;42(4):253–62.
16. Knofler M, Pollheimer J. Human placental trophoblast invasion and differentiation: a particular focus on Wnt signaling. Front Genet. 2013;26(4):190.

17. Lofqvist C, Hansen-Pupp I, Andersson E, Holm K, Smith LE, Ley D, Hellstrom A. Validation of a new retinopathy of prematurity screening method monitoring longitudinal postnatal weight and insulinlike growth factor I. Arch Ophthalmol. 2009;127(5):622–7.
18. Bowe T, Nyamai L, Ademola-Popoola D, Amphornphruet A, Anzures R, Cernichiaro-Espinosa LA, Duke R, Duran F, Martinez-Castellanos MA, Multani PK, Nitulescu CE, Padhi TR, Tipsuriyaporn B, Chan RVP, Campbell JP, Yonekawa Y. The current state of retinopathy of prematurity in india, kenya, mexico, nigeria, philippines, romania, thailand, and venezuela. Digit J Ophthalmol. 2019;25(4):49–58.
19. Gologorsky D, Chang JS, Hess DJ, Berrocal AM. Familial exudative vitreoretinopathy in a premature child. Ophthalmic Surg Lasers Imaging Retina. 2013;44(6):603–5.
20. Swan R, Kim SJ, Campbell JP, Paul Chan RV, Sonmez K, Taylor KD, Li X, Chen YI, Rotter JI, Simmons C, Chiang MF, Imaging and Informatics in ROP Research Consortium. The genetics of retinopathy of prematurity: a model for neovascular retinal disease. Ophthalmol Retina. 2018;2(9):949–62.
21. Pierce EA, Avery RL, Foley ED, Aiello LP, Smith LE. Vascular endothelial growth factor/vascular permeability factor expression in a mouse model of retinal neovascularization. Proc Natl Acad Sci U S A. 1995;92(3):905–9.
22. Pierce EA, Foley ED, Smith LE. Regulation of vascular endothelial growth factor by oxygen in a model of retinopathy of prematurity. Arch Ophthalmol. 1996;114(10):1219–28.
23. Alon T, Hemo I, Itin A, Pe'er J, Stone J, Keshet E. Vascular endothelial growth factor acts as a survival factor for newly formed retinal vessels and has implications for retinopathy of prematurity. Nat Med. 1995;1(10):1024–8.
24. Smith LE. Pathogenesis of retinopathy of prematurity. Growth Horm IGF Res. 2004;14 Suppl A:140.
25. Cooke RW, Drury JA, Mountford R, Clark D. Genetic polymorphisms and retinopathy of prematurity. Invest Ophthalmol Vis Sci. 2004;45(6):1712–5.
26. Ali AA, Hussien NF, Samy RM, Husseiny KA. Polymorphisms of vascular endothelial growth factor and retinopathy of prematurity. J Pediatr Ophthalmol Strabismus. 2015;52(4):245–53.
27. Poggi C, Giusti B, Gozzini E, Sereni A, Romagnuolo I, Kura A, Pasquini E, Abbate R, Dani C. Genetic contributions to the development of complications in preterm newborns. PLoS One. 2015;10(7): e0131741.

Late Visual Prognosis in ROP Survivors

24

Lincoln T. Shaw, Saira Khanna, Sarah Hilkert Rodriguez, Michael J. Shapiro, and Michael P. Blair

Abstract

Retinopathy of prematurity (ROP) is a lifetime disease with the risk of late sequalae extending well into adulthood. Fortunately, careful screening and treatment when appropriate can lead to improved outcomes for ROP survivors, and a large majority achieve good visual function. This chapter discusses methods to prevent adverse structural outcomes that may result from ROP, as well as risk factors that affect visual function and long-term visual prognosis for ROP survivors.

Keywords

Retinopathy · Prematurity · Screening · Prognosis · Retinal detachment · Anti-VEGF · Laser photocoagulation

L. T. Shaw · S. Khanna · S. H. Rodriguez · M. P. Blair (✉)
Department of Ophthalmology and Visual Science, University of Chicago, Chicago, IL 60637, USA
e-mail: MichaelBlairMD@gmail.com

S. Khanna
e-mail: saira.khanna@uchospitals.edu

S. H. Rodriguez
e-mail: srodriguez5@bsd.uchicago.edu

M. J. Shapiro · M. P. Blair
Retina Consultants, Ltd., Des Plaines, IL, USA

© The Author(s), under exclusive license to Springer Nature Switzerland AG 2023   329
Ş. Özdek et al. (eds.), *Pediatric Vitreoretinal Surgery*,
https://doi.org/10.1007/978-3-031-14506-3_24

Late Visual Prognosis in ROP Survivors

In the age of advancing medical care for premature infants, survival rates of premature infants continue to rise, even in developing countries [1]. As a result, retinopathy of prematurity (ROP) has become a lifetime disease, with the risk of late sequelae (from 50 weeks and beyond) extending well into adulthood [2]. Fortunately, treatment for ROP can usually prevent significant adverse structural outcomes [3], although preventing adverse structural outcomes is necessary but not sufficient for good visual function. The long-term visual prognosis of ROP survivors depends on several factors, including the severity of disease, choice of treatment methods, early identification and treatment of amblyopia, and presence of comorbidities that may contribute to neurological visual impairment. With effective treatment, most ROP survivors are spared retinal detachment or macular folds [3, 4], but often there are secondary visual consequences as well such as myopia, amblyopia [5], glaucoma [6], cataracts [7], and strabismus [8] that can have a significant impact in the late visual prognosis of these infants. Comorbidities such as intracranial hemorrhage, hydrocephalus, and periventricular leukomalacia can also lead to cortical visual impairment in ROP survivors with structurally sound retinas.

Visual Acuity

While final visual acuity in ROP survivors depends on a variety of factors, less severe disease and early treatment of ROP when indicated improves visual acuity outcomes. The ET-ROP study showed that early treatment compared to conventional treatment improved visual outcomes for infants with Type 1 ROP but not Type 2 ROP [9]. In general eyes that underwent spontaneous regression of severe ROP, without reaching treatment criteria, had better vision than eyes that required treatment. As measured using optotypes at 36 months, the proportions of infants achieving 6/9 visual acuity or better in the untreated, laser, and cryotherapy groups were 68%, 40%, and 22.5%, respectively [10].

While highly successful at avoiding adverse outcomes (retinal detachment, macular fold, or retrolental mass), visual outcomes have remained suboptimal with cryotherapy and now laser therapy. Only approximately one third of early-treated eyes achieved normal vision (defined as 20/40 or better) at 6 years follow-up from the ET-ROP study [11]. Limited data exists for visual outcomes of Type 1 ROP treated with anti-vascular endothelial growth factor (VEGF) agents, but data from one retrospective study suggests potential for improved visual outcomes with anti-VEGF agents, as 85% of patients with Type 1 ROP in that study had normal vision (defined as >20/40) after treatment with bevacizumab [12].

Not surprisingly, eyes with more advanced disease (stage 4A, 4B, and 5) generally have poor visual outcomes. In the analysis of 70 eyes from the ET-ROP study at age 6 who experienced retinal detachment, favorable visual acuity (>20/200) was found in only 6 of the 70 eyes, and the majority of these eyes (5/6) were classified as stage 4A. Although most eyes with stage 4A had measurable vision, only one had normal vision (20/40 or better). All eyes with 4B detachment were worse than 20/200 and those with stage 5 had LP or NLP vision [13].

Reactivation

Reactivation of ROP is relatively uncommon but can occur months to years after initial ROP screening and treatment [14]. In fact, late ROP reactivation has even been reported as late as adulthood. Reactivation has been shown to occur not only in those ROP eyes that underwent spontaneous regression [2], but also those that were treated with cryotherapy, laser ablation, bevacizumab injection [15–18], scleral buckle, and vitrectomy [17, 19]. Treatment for reactivation must be tailored on a case-by-case basis, but generally involves similar techniques to initial ROP treatment, which may include repeat anti-VEGF injection or laser ablation, as well as surgical intervention when indicated. Although the number needed to treat to prevent detachment is unknown, delayed, prophylactic laser treatment completion should be considered after primary anti-VEGF treatment [14].

Retinal Detachment and Other Vitreoretinal Sequelae

Retinal detachments of all types are seen in ROP survivors. Cicatricial changes from ROP can cause tractional retinal detachments as well as predispose to retinal tears and subsequent rhegmatogenous retinal detachments. ROP-associated detachments are more likely to require multiple surgical procedures to achieve long-term reattachment, although many can maintain good long-term visual outcomes (Fig. 24.1) [20].

ROP eyes are at increased risk for:

- retinal detachment (Fig. 24.2)
- retinal tears
- residual traction
- tractional retinoschisis
- neovascularization
- atrophic holes
- lattice-like changes (Fig. 24.3)
- macular heterotopia (Fig. 24.4)
- peripheral avascular retina (PAR) (Fig. 24.3)
- abnormal vitreous condensation ridge-like interface
- premature vitreous syneresis [21].

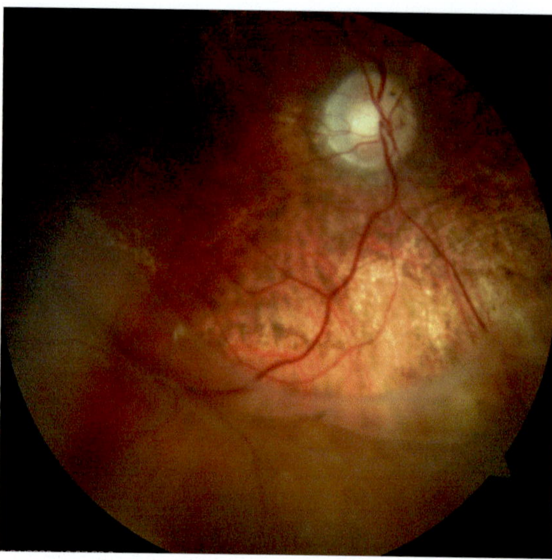

Fig. 24.1 40 year old with history of ROP and new onset tractional retinal detachment related to posterior stage 3 residual

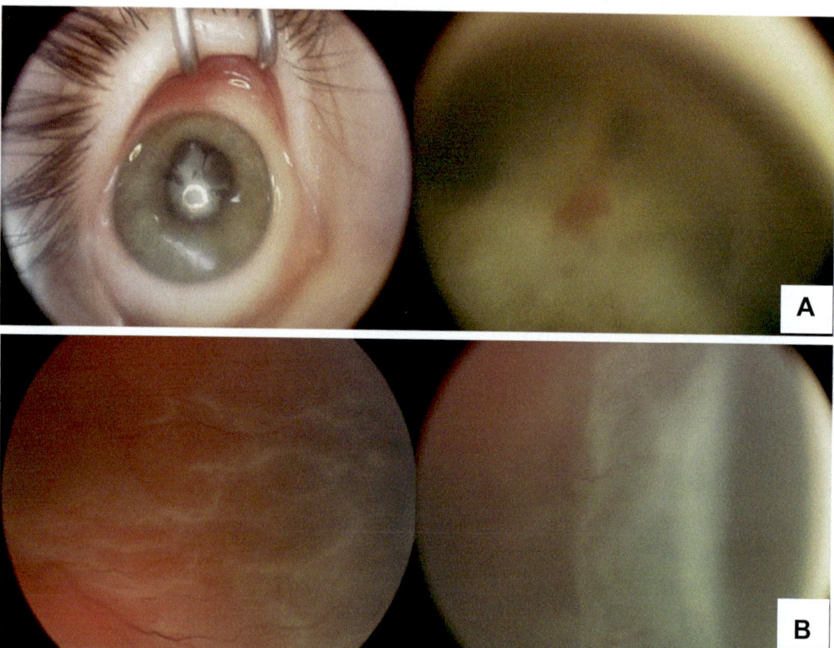

Fig. 24.2 5 year old boy with history of untreated ROP and developmental delay presented with new onset vision loss in the left eye. His visual acuity was NLP OD and 20/80 OS. **a** Right eye demonstrated a funnel retinal detachment. **b** Left eye had a combined tractional and rhegmatogenous retinal detachment related to the far temporal cicatrix. The chronic traction led to atrophic hole and vision loss from acute rhegmatogenous component

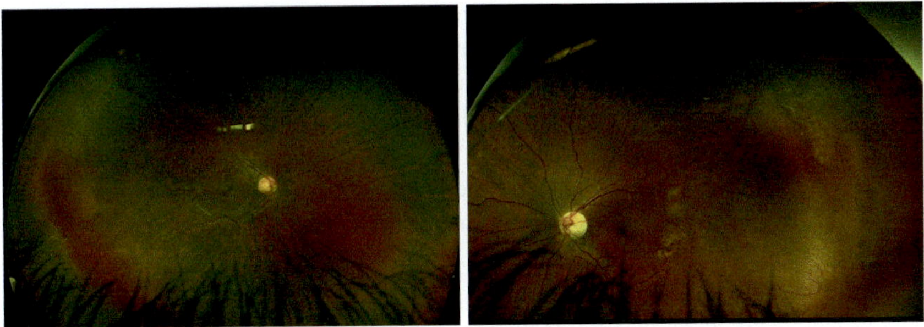

Fig. 24.3 16 year old female with spontaneously regressed ROP in both eyes. Lattice-like changes are noted in the PAR just anterior the vascular termination in both eyes

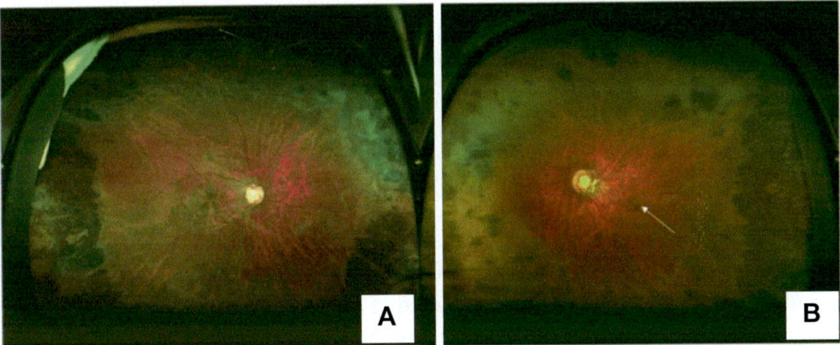

Fig. 24.4 27 year old female with history of ROP s/p laser, strabismic amblyopia s/p strabismus surgery, and myopia. Color fundus photo of right eye shows a healthy optic nerve, mild foveal dragging with chorioretinal scarring 360°. Color fundus photo of left eye fundus photos depicts slightly tilted optic nerve with fovea dragged temporally (arrow) with pigment mottling, straightened vessels, and 360° chorioretinal scarring from prior laser

Retinal detachment rates have been correlated to younger gestational age (<29 weeks) and larger area of peripheral avascular retina (PAR), with retinal vascularization only to zone 2 having higher risk of detachment than eyes with vascularized retina extending into zone 3 [21]. Additionally, adult eyes with a history of ROP that did not meet treatment criteria and that show no apparent persistent structural changes are still at increased risk for retinal tears and associated rhegmatogenous retinal detachments, and lack of apparent anatomical changes from ROP on fundus examination should not impede careful lifelong screening [20]. Frequent screening is particularly important in ROP survivors who are unlikely to report symptoms, which includes young children (5 or less) and those with cognitive impairment. Unfortunately, many times these patients present when the second eye has a detachment, with the first already with a chronic funnel-shaped retinal detachment (Fig. 24.2). Rhegmatogenous detachment may be due to residual stage 3 cicatrix exerting chronic traction on thin avascular retina, or development of atrophic holes in thin avascular retina. Circumferential pigmented patches similar to lattice degeneration may be seen in the atrophic PAR in some of the eyes.

PAR may be seen in ROP survivors who did not meet treatment criteria [19]. Although infrequent, this can lead to late exudative detachment, or combined exudative and tractional detachment [2, 19, 22–24]. As younger, smaller infants survive and have larger areas of PAR, whether untreated or treated with anti-VEGF, the incidence of detachment may increase [25].

Furthermore, exudative detachments are an uncommon complication of laser photocoagulation and bevacizumab injection for ROP. Unfortunately these detachments can leave lasting macular sequelae including macular pigmentary changes, macular atrophy, and photoreceptor loss, resulting in decreased visual potential in these eyes [26]. Exudative detachments reported after laser may be secondary to increased RPE permeability and inflammatory reactions to the laser therapy, and exudative detachments after bevacizumab treatment for ROP are thought to be related to telangiectasias, peripheral avascular retina, microaneurysms and lipid exudation similar to the pathophysiology of Coats disease and familial exudative vitreoretinopathy [18].

Myopia

Myopia is a common consequence of ROP and correlates to the degree to which the vascularization of peripheral retina is halted [27]. Furthermore, treatments for ROP such as laser photocoagulation (including endolaser during lens-sparing vitrectomy) can further increase the risk of myopia. Most eyes are myopic after laser photocoagulation treatment for ROP, and about half of eyes treated with laser have a long-term refraction greater than -4D [28, 29]. While myopia can be present in eyes that are treated with anti-VEGF agents, refractive data from the Bevacizumab Eliminates the Angiogenic Threat for Retinopathy of Prematurity (BEAT-ROP) study patients suggests this is significantly less likely [30]. When applied to reduce the risk of late reactivation after primary bevacizumab, delayed laser does not seem to increase myopia significantly [31].

Amblyopia

Survivors of ROP are at risk for all forms of amblyopia, including anisometropic, deprivational, and strabismic. Anisometropic amblyopia is a significant risk for patients with ROP, as these eyes often develop moderate to high myopia, and treatments for ROP such as laser photocoagulation can cause a further myopic shift. Deprivation amblyopia may occur from retinal detachment, vitreous hemorrhage associated with neovascularization of the posterior segment, or cataract formation as a sequela of lens-sparing vitrectomy [32] or laser photocoagulation [33].

Strabismus is more common among patients with ROP [8], and strabismic amblyopia typically can occur from either poor binocular fusion secondary to impaired vision early in life or after surgical repair of retinal detachment in cases where a scleral buckle is employed. As with amblyopia from other causes, careful screening as well as prompt diagnosis and treatment is key for improving long-term visual outcomes.

Cataract

Cataracts in infants with ROP are most commonly iatrogenically-induced by treatment methods. Cryoablative or laser treatment for ROP may induce an inflammatory response in the eye and cause lenticular changes such as milky lens vacuoles that may become increasingly opaque as the child progresses into early adulthood. Furthermore, if the tunica vasculosa lentis is still present at the time of laser treatment, the vascular tissue can absorb the laser and cause both anterior and posterior subcapsular cataracts [33, 34]. Lastly, while most lenses maintain clarity after lens-sparing vitrectomy for ROP-associated detachments, these eyes still are at increased risk for cataract formation, as with any vitrectomy procedure [32]. Cataracts early in visual development can lead to deprivation amblyopia, and therefore must be diagnosed promptly and removed if significantly blocking the visual axis.

Glaucoma

The anterior segment development of eyes with ROP is often abnormal, resulting in steeper corneal curvatures, shallow anterior chamber depths, and anterior effective lens position compared to normal eyes [34]. Data from the Cryotherapy for Retinopathy of Prematurity Study (CRYO-ROP) study demonstrated that 6.1% of control eyes with bilateral threshold ROP were diagnosed with glaucoma compared to 2.9% of treated eyes. In the ETROP study, 1.67% of pre-threshold patients were reported to have glaucoma in the first six years of life [35]. Glaucoma in infants with ROP may also be caused iatrogenically. Inflammatory reactions after cryoablation or laser therapy can lead to iris synechiae, as well as peripheral shallowing of the anterior chamber.

Cortical Visual Impairment and Other Neurologic Comorbidities

Unfortunately, ROP is a disease that commonly is associated with other comorbidities, including a high proportion of patients with concurrent neurologic disease. Given the association between cerebral palsy (CP) and severe ROP [36], and the association between CP and cortical visual impairment (CVI) [37], CVI also represents an important cause of vision loss among ROP survivors even when the ocular structures are functionally and structurally preserved.

In a 6-year follow up of the cohort of patients used in the Early Treatment for Retinopathy of Prematurity Study (ETROP) study, 11% of the cohort had poor vision ($\leq 20/200$) despite normal macular structure, and of these 77% had latent and/or manifest nystagmus, 46% had optic atrophy, and 8% had optic disc cupping. In addition, 7% of the ETROP patients that completed the 6-year examination had cortical visual impairment that was the primary cause for visual impairment [38].

Self-injurious behavior is another neurologic consequence present in some ROP survivors, and these patients can have a particularly poor visual prognosis as a result of delayed presentation, limited cooperation, proliferative vitreoretinopathy, bilateral involvement, and ongoing ocular trauma. Cases of self-injurious patients may particularly benefit from the use of scleral buckles during retinal detachment repair to provide ongoing retinal support [39].

Screening and Prevention Techniques

ROP survivors are a particularly high-risk group that should be monitored closely throughout their lifetime. After the acute phase of screening and treatment ends, infants treated for severe ROP should maintain frequent monitoring in infancy at least at 3–4 month intervals, or more frequently if clinical suspicion is high for early complications. Furthermore, the threshold for an exam under anesthesia should be low in uncooperative patients. Compared to adults, children are less likely to identify a problem in one eye, and behavioral changes are unlikely to indicate an obvious problem before the problem becomes bilateral. A careful discussion with the child's parents about changes in visual behavior that could indicate the child is developing a complication is important, and monthly unilateral patching checks at home can give further information to the parents and clinicians about changes in visual function. Special attention should be paid to eyes with residual traction, large PAR, residual cicatricial disease and monocular patients. Selected patients which have residual cicatricial changes that appear to be at high risk to develop detachment may benefit from early surgical intervention to avoid or reduce progression of the traction and reduce the risk for adverse outcomes in the future.

Conclusion

Retinopathy of prematurity is a life-long disease that can impair vision. While most treatment options are highly successful at preventing adverse structural outcomes, functional outcomes such as visual acuity have remained suboptimal. Although data are limited, treatment with anti-VEGF may be more likely to provide normal vision than treatment with laser. Regardless of treatment status, ROP survivors should be carefully and frequently monitored throughout their lifetime, as late sequelae have been reported even among eyes with spontaneously regressed ROP, and early intervention is critical.

Review Questions

1. For which of the following patients is termination of acute ROP evaluation with transition to chronic long-term follow-up appropriate?

a. Spontaneous regression of ROP with no type 1 ROP observed after 50 weeks postmenstrual age
b. Regression of Type 1 ROP after antiVEGF and no type 1 ROP observed after 50 weeks postmenstrual age
c. Regression of Type 1 ROP after laser treatment and no type 1 ROP observed after 50 weeks postmenstrual age

2. Which of the following is true regarding visual outcomes after treatment for Type 1 ROP?

a. Treatment in the CRYO-ROP study cut the rate of retinal detachment in half
b. Most patients in the ET-ROP study had normal vision at 6 years of age
c. Most patient in the BEAT-ROP study had normal vision at 6 years of age

3. Which of the following patients has a higher risk of high myopia?

a. Patient with Type 1 ROP s/p laser
b. Patient with Type 1 ROP s/p bevacizumab monotherapy
c. Patient with Type 1 ROP s/p bevacizumab and delayed laser prophylaxis

Answers

1. Correct answers are A and C. Traditionally, infants with regressed ROP have low risk of reactivation after 50 weeks postmenstrual age. Life-long follow-up is recommended even in cases of spontaneously regressed ROP, due to an increased risk of retinal detachments and other sequelae even into adult years.

Answer B is incorrect. After intravitreal bevacizumab treatment, complete retinal vascularization is rare with a high rate of peripheral avascular retina and/or leakage on fluorescein angiography (FA) with cases of reactivation leading to retinal detachment in toddlers, as described in this chapter. Although the number needed to treat is unknown, laser prophylaxis should be considered when there are more than 2 disc diameters of peripheral avascular retina or leakage on FA after 60 weeks postmenstrual age.

2. Answer A is correct. However, although the CRYO-ROP study reduced the rate of unfavorable structural outcomes (retinal detachment, retinal fold, retrolental tissue) from 44 to 22%, fewer than 20% of patients achieved normal vision at 5 years.

Answers B and C are incorrect. Although early-treated patients had improved visual outcomes compared to conventionally treated patients in ET-ROP, only 35% of patients achieved normal vision at 6 years (defined as 20/40 or better). Visual outcomes from BEAT-ROP are limited at this time, although a small single site study from the authors of this chapter found excellent visual acuity after 4 years of age among infants treated with bevacizumab, with most seeing 20/40 or better [12].

3. Answer A is correct. Laser has been shown to increase the risk of myopia compared to bevacizumab in the BEAT-ROP study. Delayed prophylactic laser, done to reduce the chance of late reactivation, is associated with near plano refractive state. Of note, prematurity itself increases the risk of myopia, and in a sense, all of the patients have an increased risk of myopia.

References

1. Chawla D, Suresh GK. Quality improvement in neonatal care-a new paradigm for developing countries. Indian J Pediatr. 2014;81(12):1367–72.
2. Golas L, Shapiro MJ, Blair MP. Late ROP reactivation and retinal detachment in a teenager. Ophthalmic Surg Lasers Imaging Retina. 2018;49(8):625–8.
3. Good WV, Early Treatment for Retinopathy of Prematurity Cooperative Group. Final results of the Early Treatment for Retinopathy of Prematurity (ETROP) randomized trial. Trans Am Ophthalmol Soc. 2004;102:233.
4. Cryotherapy for Retinopathy of Prematurity Cooperative Group. Multicenter trial of cryotherapy for retinopathy of prematurity: ophthalmological outcomes at 10 years. Arch Ophthalmol. 2001;119(8):1110–8.
5. Tolia VN, Ahmad KA, Jacob J, et al. Two-year outcomes of infants with stage 2 or higher retinopathy of prematurity: results from a large multicenter registry. Am J Perinatol. 2020;37 (2):196–203.
6. Bremer DL, Rogers DL, Good WV, et al. Glaucoma in the Early Treatment for Retinopathy of Prematurity (ETROP) study. J AAPOS. 2012;16(5):449–52.
7. O'Neil JW, Hutchinson AK, Saunders RA, et al. Acquired cataracts after argon laser photocoagulation for retinopathy of prematurity. J AAPOS. 1998;2(1):48–51.
8. VanderVeen DK, Bremer DL, Fellows RR, et al. Prevalence and course of strabismus through age 6 years in participants of the Early Treatment for Retinopathy of Prematurity randomized trial. J AAPOS. 2011;15(6):536–40.
9. Early Treatment for Retinopathy of Prematurity Cooperative Group. Revised indications for the treatment of retinopathy of prematurity: results of the early treatment for retinopathy of prematurity randomized trial. Arch Ophthalmol. 2003;121(12):1684–94.
10. Sahni J, Subhedar NV, Clark D. Treated threshold stage 3 versus spontaneously regressed subthreshold stage 3 retinopathy of prematurity: a study of motility, refractive, and anatomical outcomes at 6 months and 36 months. Br J Ophthalmol. 2005;89(2):154–9.
11. Early Treatment for Retinopathy of Prematurity Cooperative Group. Final visual acuity results in the early treatment for retinopathy of prematurity study. Arch Ophthalmol. 2010;128 (6):663–71.

12. Rodriguez SH, Schechet SA, Shapiro MJ, et al. Late visual outcomes in infants treated with primary bevacizumab for type 1 retinopathy of prematurity. J AAPOS. 2020;24(3):149.e1–e5.

13. Repka MX, Tung B, Good WV, et al. Outcome of eyes developing retinal detachment during the Early Treatment for Retinopathy of Prematurity study. Arch Ophthalmol. 2011;129 (9):1175–9.

14. Garcia Gonzalez JM, Snyder L, Blair M, et al. Prophylactic peripheral laser and fluorescein angiography after bevacizumab for retinopathy of prematurity. Retina. 2018;38(4):764–72.

15. Snyder LL, Garcia-Gonzalez JM, Shapiro MJ, et al. Very late reactivation of retinopathy of prematurity after monotherapy with intravitreal bevacizumab. Ophthalmic Surg Lasers Imaging Retina. 2016;47(3):280–3.

16. Hajrasouliha AR, Garcia-Gonzales JM, Shapiro MJ, et al. Reactivation of retinopathy of prematurity three years after treatment with bevacizumab. Ophthalmic Surg Lasers Imaging Retina. 2017;48(3):255–9.

17. Hu J, Blair MP, Shapiro MJ, et al. Reactivation of retinopathy of prematurity after bevacizumab injection. Arch Ophthalmol. 2012;130(8):1000–6.

18. Ittiara S, Blair MP, Shapiro MJ, et al. Exudative retinopathy and detachment: a late reactivation of retinopathy of prematurity after intravitreal bevacizumab. J AAPOS. 2013;17 (3):323–5.

19. Uner OE, Rao P, Hubbard GB. Reactivation of retinopathy of prematurity in adults and adolescents. Ophthalmol Retina. 2020;4(7):720–7.

20. Kaiser RS, Trese MT, Williams GA, et al. Adult retinopathy of prematurity: outcomes of rhegmatogenous retinal detachments and retinal tears. Ophthalmology. 2001;108(9):1647–53.

21. Hamad AE, Moinuddin O, Blair MP, et al. Late-onset retinal findings and complications in untreated retinopathy of prematurity. Ophthalmol Retina. 2020;4(6):602–12.

22. Brown MM, Brown GC, Duker JS, et al. Exudative retinopathy of adults: a late sequela of retinopathy of prematurity. Ophthalmic Lit. 1996;1(49):34.

23. Tasman W. Exudative retinal detachment in retrolental fibroplasia. Trans Sect Ophthalmol Am Acad Ophthalmol Otolaryngol. 1977;83(3 Pt 1):535–40.

24. Tasman W. Late complications of retrolental fibroplasia. Ophthalmology. 1979;86(10): 1724–40.

25. Hanif AM, Gensure RH, Scruggs BA, et al. Prevalence of peripheral avascular retina in spontaneously regressed retinopathy of prematurity. J AAPOS. 2021;25(4): e60.

26. Zhang DL, Shapiro MJ, Schechet SA, et al. Macular sequelae following exudative retinal detachment after laser photocoagulation for retinopathy of prematurity. Ophthalmic Surg Lasers Imaging Retina. 2020;51(12):698–705.

27. Dikopf MS, Machen LA, Hallak JA, et al. Zone of retinal vascularization and refractive error in premature eyes with and without spontaneously regressed retinopathy of prematurity. J AAPOS. 2019;23(4):211.e1-e6.

28. Ospina LH, Lyons CJ, Matsuba C, et al. Argon laser photocoagulation for retinopathy of prematurity: long-term outcome. Eye. 2005;19(11):1213–8.

29. Macor S, Pignatto S, Capone A Jr, et al. Lens-sparing vitrectomy for stage 4A retinopathy of prematurity in infants with aggressive-posterior ROP: anatomic and functional results. Eur J Ophthalmol. 2021;31(4):2020–6.

30. Geloneck MM, Chuang AZ, Clark WL, et al. Refractive outcomes following bevacizumab monotherapy compared with conventional laser treatment: a randomized clinical trial. JAMA Ophthalmol. 2014;132(11):1327–33.

31. Anand N, Blair MP, Greenwald MJ, et al. Refractive outcomes comparing primary laser to primary bevacizumab with delayed laser for type 1 ROP. J AAPOS. 2019;23(2):88.e1-e6.

32. Nudleman E, Robinson J, Rao P, et al. Long-term outcomes on lens clarity after lens-sparing vitrectomy for retinopathy of prematurity. Ophthalmology. 2015;122(4):755–9.

33. Lambert SR, Capone A Jr, Cingle KA, et al. Cataract and phthisis bulbi after laser photoablation for threshold retinopathy of prematurity. Am J Ophthalmol. 2000;129(5): 585–91.

34. Chang E, Rao P. Adult retinopathy of prematurity: treatment implications, long term sequelae, and management. Curr Opin Ophthalmol. 2021;32(5):489–93.
35. Hartnett ME, Gilbert MM, Hirose T, et al. Glaucoma as a cause of poor vision in severe retinopathy of prematurity. Graefes Arch Clin Exp Ophthalmol. 1993;231(8):433–8.
36. Schmidt B, Asztalos EV, Roberts RS, et al. Impact of bronchopulmonary dysplasia, brain injury, and severe retinopathy on the outcome of extremely low-birth-weight infants at 18 months: results from the trial of indomethacin prophylaxis in preterms. JAMA. 2003;289 (9):1124–9.
37. Ego A, Lidzba K, Brovedani P, et al. Visual-perceptual impairment in children with cerebral palsy: a systematic review. Dev Med Child Neurol. 2015;57(Suppl 2):46–51.
38. Siatkowski RM, Good WV, Summers CG, et al. Clinical characteristics of children with severe visual impairment but favorable retinal structural outcomes from the Early Treatment for Retinopathy of Prematurity (ETROP) study. J AAPOS. 2013;17(2):129–34.
39. Rossin EJ, Tsui I, Wong SC, et al. Traumatic retinal detachment in patients with self-injurious behavior: an international multicenter study. Ophthalmol Retina. 2021;5(8):805–14.

Part IV
Surgical Management of Pediatric Retinal Vascular Disorders

Familial Exudative Vitreo-Retinopathy

25

Komal Agarwal and Subhadra Jalali

Abstract

Familial exudative vitreoretinopathy is an autosomal dominant retinal disorder that starts at birth and manifests at various ages with a wide range of spectrum. The hallmark remains bilateral peripheral congenital avascular retina. Neonatal cases have more severe phenotypes including congenital bilateral leukocoria, than those that present later in life. The disease can follow a slow indolent course that can be asymmetric between the two eyes, or more progressive worsening especially when associated with exudative phenotypes. Neonatal screening and family screening especially using wide field imaging and retinal angiography, helps to detect early treatable stages. Laser photocoagulation and vitreoretinal surgery in early phases have better outcomes. FEVR can be a part of various syndromes. Genetic evaluation helps in clinical and family management.

Keywords

Autosomal dominant retinal disease · Combined retinal detachment · Exudative retinal detachment · FEVR · Familial exudative vitreoretinopathy · Family

Supplementary Information The online version contains supplementary material available at https://doi.org/10.1007/978-3-031-14506-3_25.

K. Agarwal
Srimati Kanuri Santhamma Centre for Vitreoretinal Diseases, and Jasti V. Ramanamma Childrens' Eye Care Centre, L V Prasad Eye Institute, Kallam Anji Reddy Campus, Hyderabad, India

S. Jalali (✉)
Network Director Newborn Eye Health Alliance (NEHA) and Consultant, Srimati Kanuri Santhamma Centre for Vitreoretinal Diseases, and Jasti V. Ramanamma Childrens' Eye Care Centre, L V Prasad Eye Institute, Kallam Anji Reddy Campus, Hyderabad, India
e-mail: subhadra@lvpei.org

retinal screening · Macular dragging · Macular fold · Neonatal leukocoria · Neonatal retinal screening · Peripheral avascular retina · Early vitrectomy · Pseudoglioma · Retinal photocoagulation · Tractional retinal detachment

Introduction

Familial exudative vitreo-retinopathy (FEVR, MIM # 133,780) are a group of bilateral, developmental retinal vascular disorders, primarily characterized by peripheral avascular retina and aberrant vascular differentiation [1]. Multiple mutations involving the Wnt (wingless related integration site) signaling pathways of retinal angiogenesis have been implicated in the disease process, the most important ones being in NDP, FZD4, LRP5, TSPAN12, ZN408, KIF11, CTNNB1, DOCK6, ATOH7, JAG1, RCBTB1 and ARHGAP31. These account for about 50% of FEVR cases [2, 3]. Variable inheritance patterns are reported, including autosomal dominant, autosomal recessive and X-linked recessive but is also seen in individuals with no family history. Both males and females are affected with equal severity, though due to X-linked families, overall, the number of males is more than the females. Some of these mutations have specific other organ involvement that needs appropriate management.

Peripheral primary avascular retina associated with vitreous abnormality is the clinical hallmark of the disease. Most patients have bilateral disease, but the phenotypic severity might differ in the two eyes and also between family members with the same mutation. Phenotypes show a variable proportion of retinopathy, vitreopathy and exudative components. Disease can range from asymptomatic disease to complete blindness from severely dysplastic retina with total closed funnel tractional retinal detachment (TRD) and from few hard exudates to massive exudation and from slow or no progression to severe fulminant course. While most clinical studies have focused on the abnormal vascularization, there is associated retinal neurodevelopmental lag also that results in subnormal vision and abnormal retinal neural function and architecture especially involving ganglion cells, which needs further elucidation [4]. Subnormal vision remains the presenting feature in many patients, even those with subtle retinal changes.

Classification: Pendergast and Trese [5] described the most widely used staging in FEVR (Table 25.1).

The same group of researchers further refined the classification to add features based on wide field Fundus fluorescein angiography and provided a new classification by Kashani et al. [6] (Table 25.2).

Table 25.1 Staging of FEVR by Pendergast and Trese [5]

Stage	Features
1	Peripheral avascular retina
2	A: Retinal neovascularization without exudates B: Retinal neovascularization with exudates
3	A: Extramacular Retinal Detachment without exudates B: Extramacular Retinal Detachment with exudates
4	A: Macula involving subtotal retinal detachment without exudates B: Macula involving subtotal retinal detachment with exudates
5	Total retinal detachment

Table 25.2 Revised FEVR staging using additional FFA by Kashani et al. [6]

Stage	Features
1	Avascular periphery or anomalous intraretinal vascularization 1A: without exudate or leakage 1B: With exudate or leakage
2	Avascular retinal periphery with extraretinal vascularization 2A: Without exudates or leakage 2B: With exudates or leakage
3	Extramacular Retinal detachment 3A: Without exudates or leakage 3B: With exudates or leakage
4	Macula involving subtotal retinal detachment 4A: Without exudates or leakage 4B: With exudates or leakage
5	Total retinal detachment 5A: Open funnel 5B: Closed Funnel

It is common to have different stages in two eyes of the same patient. This could probably suggest the involvement of additional local environment such as persistent fetal vasculature, or two-hit somatic mutations during the retinal vascular development, in addition to the primary genetic mutation. Further studies are awaited.

Clinical evaluation: Indirect Ophthalmoscopy alone in the clinic, may be inadequate to provide all clinical information that is needed to make management decisions in FEVR. Wide field fundus photography, wide field fundus fluorescein angiography, wide field Ocular coherence tomography, Gonioscopy, un-dilated slit lamp evaluation for iris new vessels and examination under anaesthesia help to get complete assessment of various changes in FEVR and make informed decisions about management.

Ocular signs of FEVR have a wide spectrum (Figs. 25.1, 25.2, 25.3, 25.4, 25.5, 25.6, 25.7, 25.8, 25.9, 25.10, 25.11, 25.12, 25.13, 25.14, 25.15, 25.16, 25.17 and 25.18). Patients can present at any age with variable symptoms and signs, depending on the severity of the disease [1, 6–8]. Mild cases of FEVR characteristically have only peripheral retinal avascularity with associated vitreous condensation at the 'V-shaped temporal ridge' and no ghost vessels, depicting vascular arrest (Figs. 25.1 and 25.2). These are asymptomatic and are diagnosed usually during familial retinal screening or screening for other disorders or fellow eyes of eyes that present with associated rhegmatogenous retinal detachment. Moderate cases present with retinal neovascularization and fibrovascular proliferation in localized areas. These can lead to vitreous haemorrhage (VH), TRD (Fig. 25.3) or combined with Rhegmatogenous retinal detachment and progress to neovascular glaucoma and hyphaema or phthisis bulbi.

Eyes that have severe phenotype in early infancy and were not treated at birth, show retinal drag and folds with or without macular ectopia as the infantile retina alone can develop such increase in retinal surface area from the abnormal vitreopathy that drags and stretches the tightly adherent retinal tissues. Extent and configuration of such folds is dictated by the presence or absence of the persistent fetal vasculature stalk and results in stage 3A and 4A tractional detachments. These evolve in a manner similar to ROP related retinal detachments.

The predominantly exudative types (type B) have more severe progression. Subretinal exudation can progress relentlessly towards the macular area. Peripheral avascular retina can later on develop one or more Vasoproliferative tumour (VPRT) like lesions that make the management difficult.

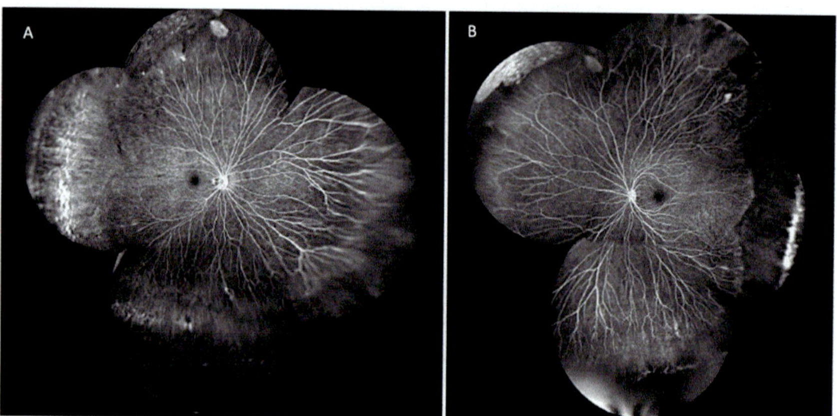

Fig. 25.1 Right **A** and left eye **B** of a 20 years female with bilateral stage 1 FEVR. The figures show arrested vascularization with no leaks on wide-field FFA. Note pruned and arborising vessel ends. Early vitreopathy is depicted by narrowed arcades left eye more than right eye leading to appearance of supernumerary macular vasculature. Annual review and family screening was advised

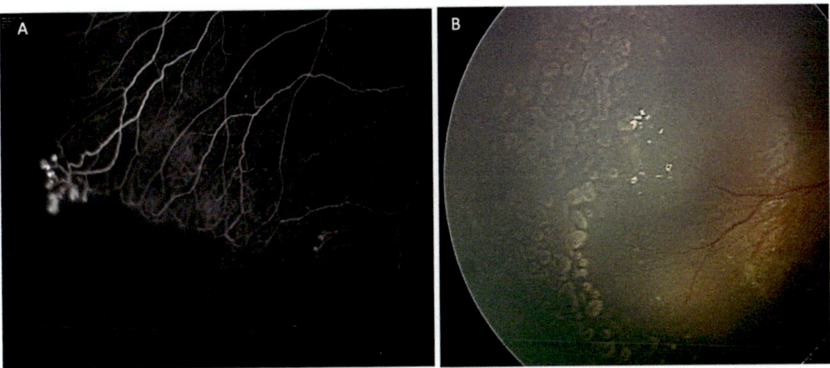

Fig. 25.2 Stage 1 FEVR early stages in two different patients. In Patient A, early leak was detected on annual FFA and was advised laser. In patient B, a clump of hard exudates was seen at the ridge at presentation and so laser was done. Early treatment reduces risk of severe stages

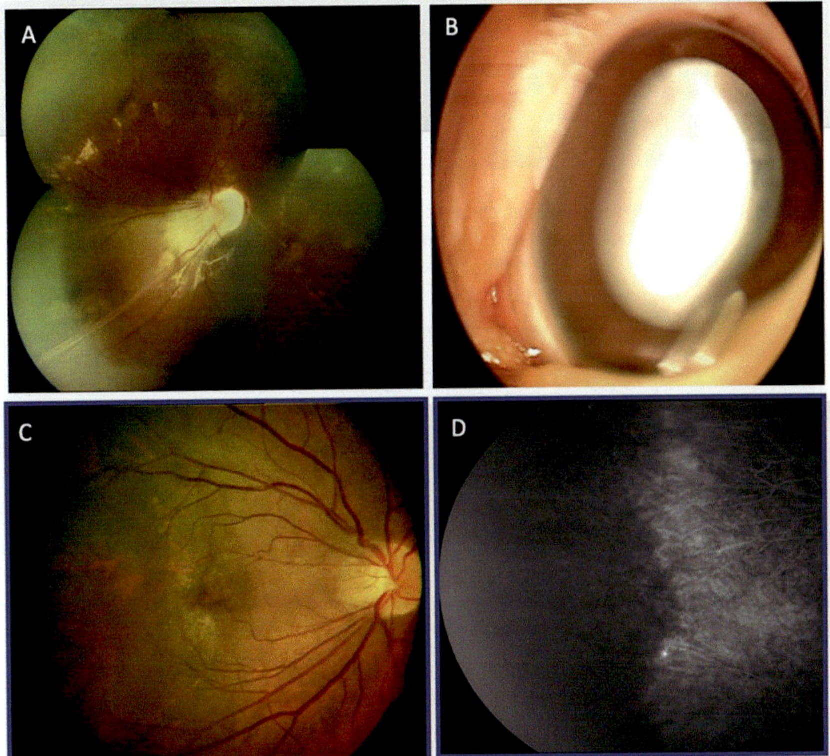

Fig. 25.3 A 4 year male child with right eye FEVR stage 3B (**A**) and leukocoria due to total retinal detachment and retrolental membrane in left eye (**B**). On family screening, father had peripheral avascular retina and dragging of vessels (**C**), more prominently seen on FFA with late stain due to vitreopathy (**D**)

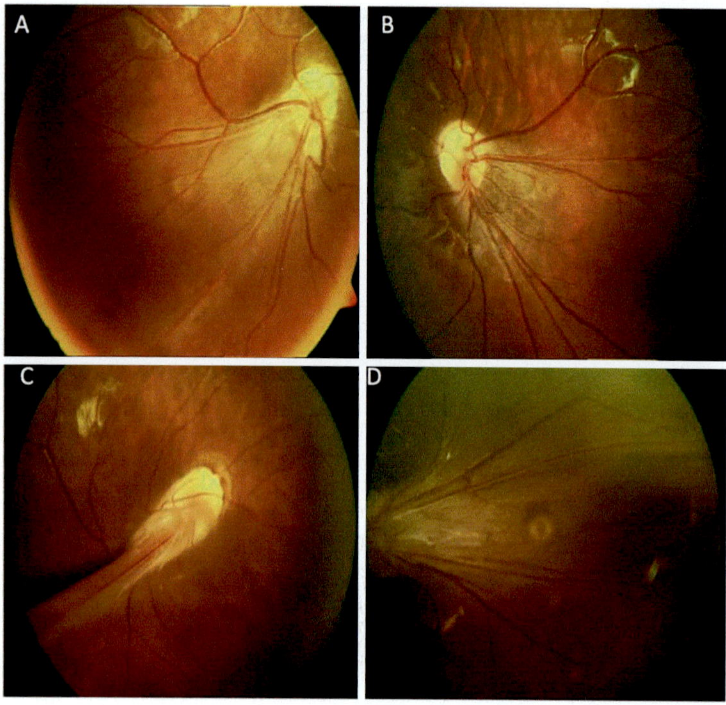

Fig. 25.4 FEVR stable fractional detachments in two sisters. One sister with retinal drag in both eyes (**A**, **B**). Other sister had retinal fold in right eye (**C**) and retinal drag in left eye (**D**). These are non-progressive, arrested stages of retinal detachments and need annual review

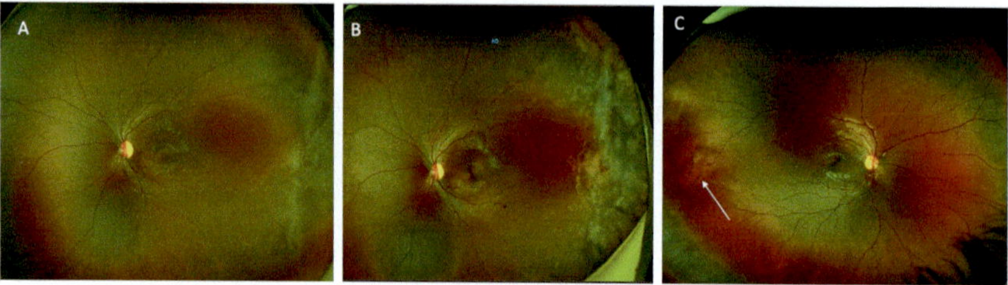

Fig. 25.5 Left eye of a 10 year old child whose mother was blind from FEVR. Retinal tear temporally with avascular temporal retina before (**A**) and after (**B**) barrage laser photocoagulation. At three months follow-up, similar area showing vitreous contraction and possible impending retinal tears in right eye (**C**) (arrow)

Any FEVR case detected needs thorough dilated retinal screening of all family members (parents/siblings/cousins) not only to help in the diagnosis but also to have an opportunity to detect and treat 'silent' vision threatening lesions in family members (Figs. 25.3, 25.4 and 25.5). Any newborns in the family must be screened immediately after birth (see neonatal FEVR later).

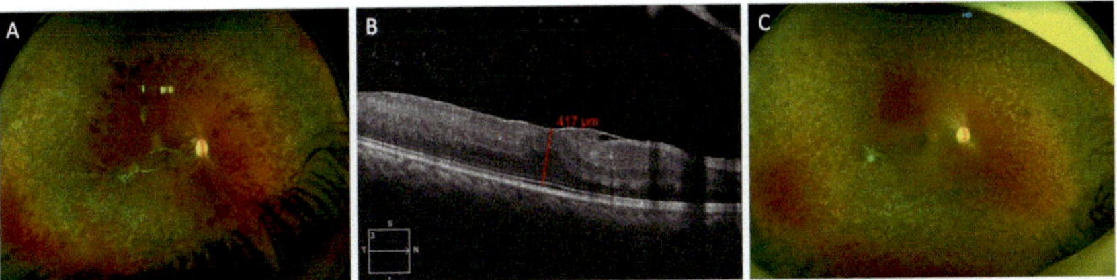

Fig. 25.6 **A** Preoperative epiretinal membrane with traction in Post Lasered FEVR in a 11 year old male with a visual acuity of 20/125. Preop OCT showing epiretinal membrane with foveal traction. **B** Post vitrectomy with judicious membrane removal with segmentation **c** with a visual acuity 20/60

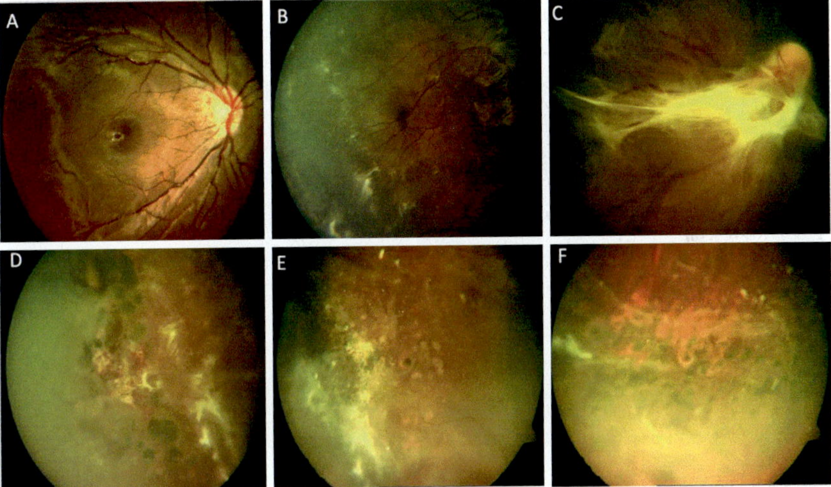

Fig. 25.7 Right eye (**A**, **B**) of 14 years female showing pre laser avascular temporal retina with hard exudates in a row. Note invisible vitreous condensation causing narrowed arcades. Visual acuity was 20/40. 8 months post incomplete laser, she developed dense fibrous proliferation and macular epiretinal membrane with traction (**C**, **D**). Visual acuity was 20/400. Post vitrectomy, stable retina with a visual acuity of 20/50 (**E**, **F**). Note inferior trimmed edge of posterior hyaloid at edge of vascularized retina beyond which vitreous left untouched with sparse laser ablation (**F**). Stable for over 15 years after oil removal

Genetic testing: We strongly encourage genetic testing wherever feasible which helps in diagnosing difficult cases, directs targeted screening for systemic associations, family counselling and identifying newborns for early treatment besides deeper understanding of pathogenesis and evolution of newer treatments. These genetic screening tests are becoming more and more available at reducing costs and

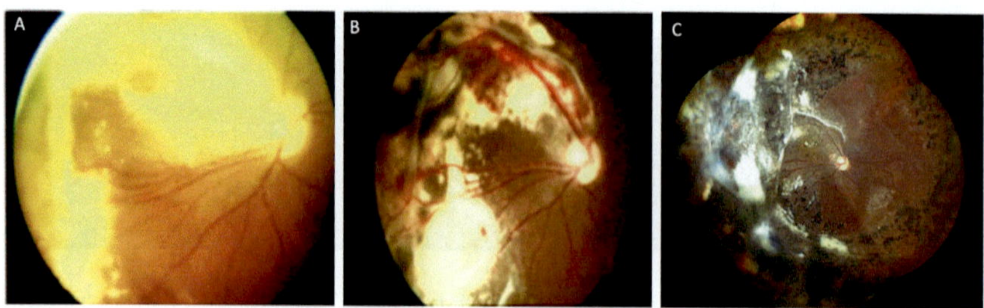

Fig. 25.8 **A** Right eye of a 22 years one-eyed male, showing dense confluent exudation, and mid-peripheral traction with macular dragging (BCVA CFCF) Multiple laser sessions did not halt progressive exudation. **B** Post vitrectomy and endolaser after one year: Note trimmed edge of uncut segmented thickened posterior hyaloid along superior arcade and temporally with reducing exudation. **C** Post Vitrectomy same eye after 15 years with no further treatment showing resolved exudates and BCVA of 20/100

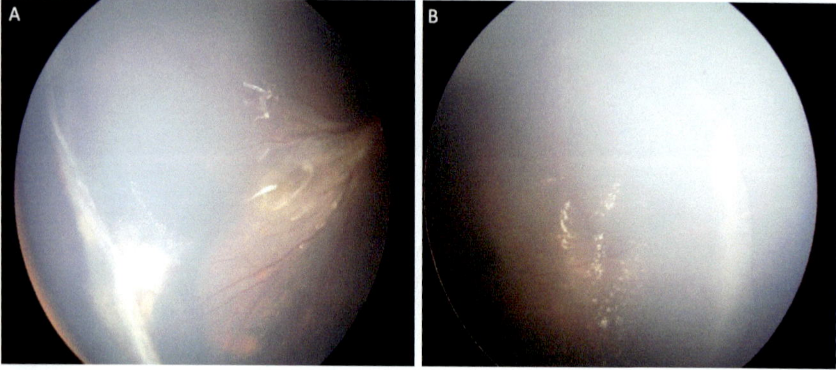

Fig. 25.9 FEVR Stage 3B right eye **A** needed vitrectomy and endolaser to take care of vitreopathy and retinopathy. The left eye **B** needed FFA based laser all around and close follow-up for development of any vitreopathy. Early definitive treatments based on interaction of the vitreous and retinal pathology may provide better outcomes

should be considered wherever possible. All children with FEVR should have a thorough review of systems by trained paediatrician to detect syndromic associations. Of course, as mentioned previously, all family members must be encouraged to have dilated fundus screening.

Follow-up and natural course: Unlike staging of disease in retinopathy of prematurity or retinoblastoma, the FEVR stages do not always progress from one stage to the next and are rather phenotypes with variable presentations and each presentation has its natural course. Understanding each phenotype and its likely course is what dictates surgical intervention versus observation. Retinal detachment (RD) can be seen in 21–64% of the cases in FEVR and constitute the most common indication for surgical intervention. It can be tractional, rhegmatogenous, exudative or combined. Other associations include secondary epiretinal membranes,

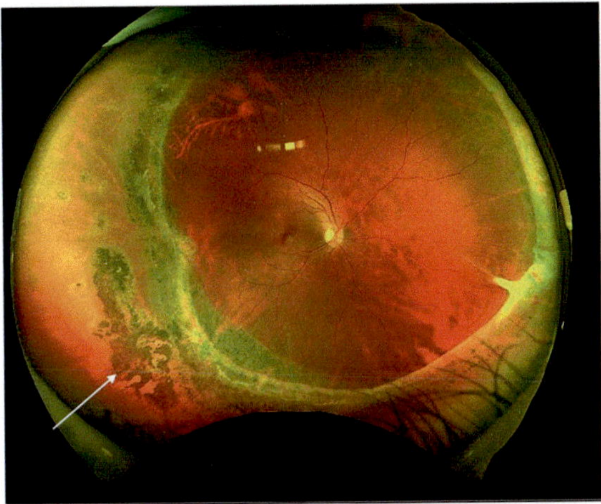

Fig. 25.10 Prophylactic buckle: FEVR stable over five years in a 12 years child with minimal laser to NVE (arrow), and 42 size encuxlageto counter vitreoretinal traction at temporal equator and beyond. Recent onset of exudation inferonasally would need focal laser. Note non-equatorial oblique placement of encirclage, more posterior temporally and more anterior nasally to counter area of maximum traction temporally. Extensive laser was avoided to prevent increase in vitreous traction. Other eye had been lost to giant retinal tear with severe vitreous abnormality

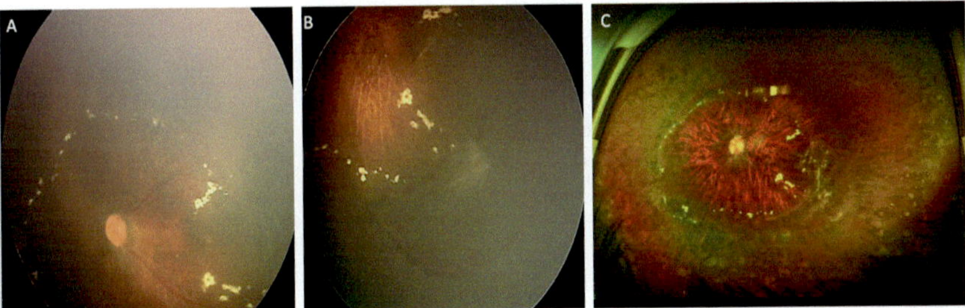

Fig. 25.11 **A** Composite photo: One-eyed FEVR female at 8 months of age. Left eye, Wreath pattern hard exudates and avascular retina beyond zone one encroaching near hypoplastic fovea seen. **B** New vessels and vitreous condensation at 4 O'clock, leading to vitreous haemorrhage inferiorly (lower segment of photo). This eye was lasercd at same visit. **C** Same eye at 17 years of age with no additional treatment. Note the arrested retinal vascularization never grows into laser scars, foveal hypoplasia and hard exudates persist with no increase. Fibrous proliferation at previous site of new vessels from 3 to 4 O'clock. Tiny new hard exudates and anomalous telangiectatic vessels at superior edge of fibrous proliferation (thin arrow) depicting possible reactivation effect of adolescence. Visual acuity 20/160

secondary retinoschisis, vasoproliferative retinal tumour (VPRT) lesions etc. When seen early enough, laser photocoagulation of the avascular retina helps to control disease progression, though advanced cases need additional vitrectomy with or without buckling procedures for treatment and also as prophylaxis against further progression.

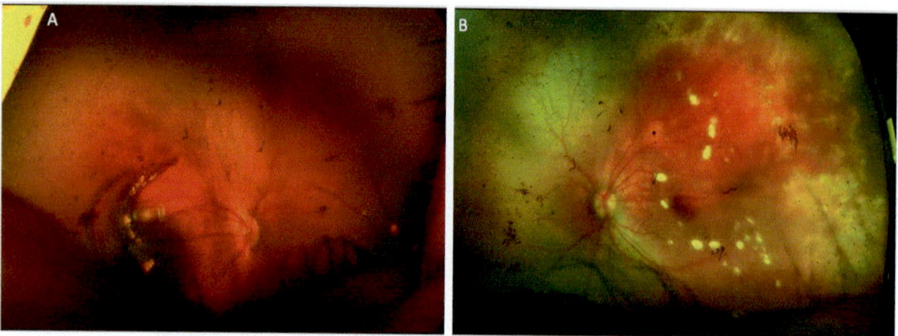

Fig. 25.12 Bilateral Neonatal FEVR. 28 days baby, 34 weeks gestational age and 2000 g birth weight. Note wreath like discrete hard exudates and zone one immature retinal vascularization both eyes. Associated vitreous haemorrhage and tractional detachment involving fovea in right eye and subfoveal haemorrhage in left eye. Left eye photo taken after starting laser therapy (OptosJFundus photos). Right eye underwent immediate surgery

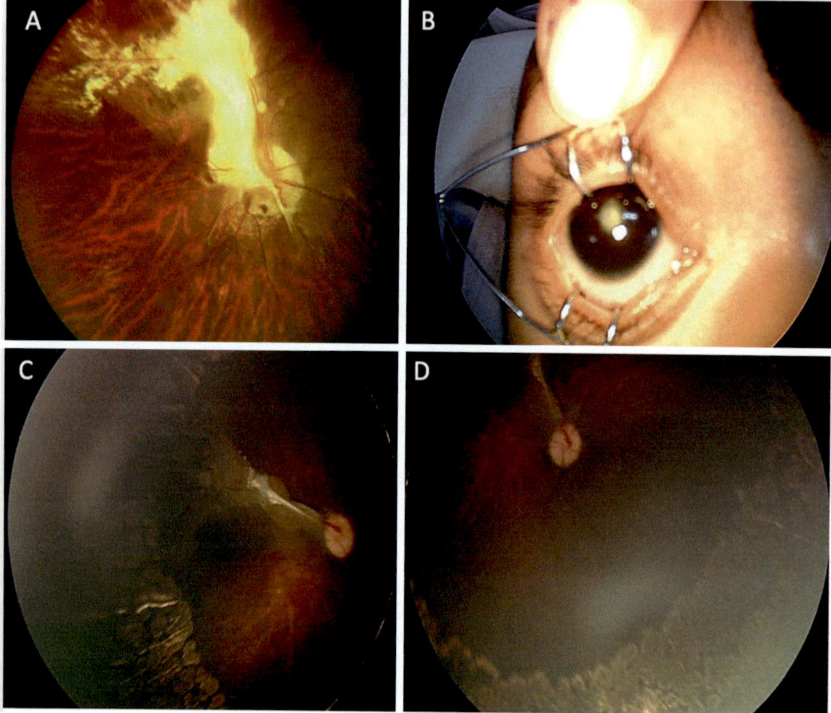

Fig. 25.13 One-year male child with congenital FEVR. **A** Right eye elevated retinal fold attached to centre of clear lens, with persistent fetal vasculature and exudates around the elevated fibrous stalk. **B** Stage 5 FEVR with leucocoria and phthisis in left eye. **C, D** 9 months after primary lens sparing vitrectomy, segmentation of adherent stalk from retinal fold and complete peripheral laser to the avascular retina seems to melt away the exudates and halt the progressive disease. Annual follow-up for any recurrence advised. Note associated hypoplasia of optic nerve

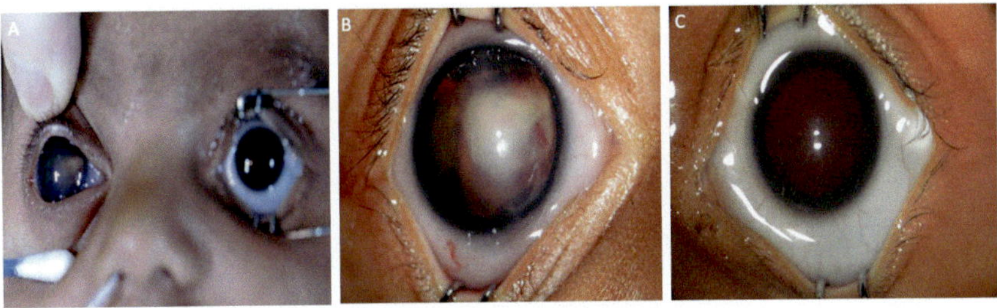

Fig. 25.14 **A** Neovascular glaucoma with ectropion uvea and total retinal dysplasia and detachment stage 5 FEVR in a one- day old male newborn referred as congenital retinoblastoma. **B** Right eye no treatment was done except topical eye drops for intraocular pressure control. **C** Left eye bright red glow of vitreous haemorrhage is seen that underwent vision salvage through lens sparing vitrectomy next day

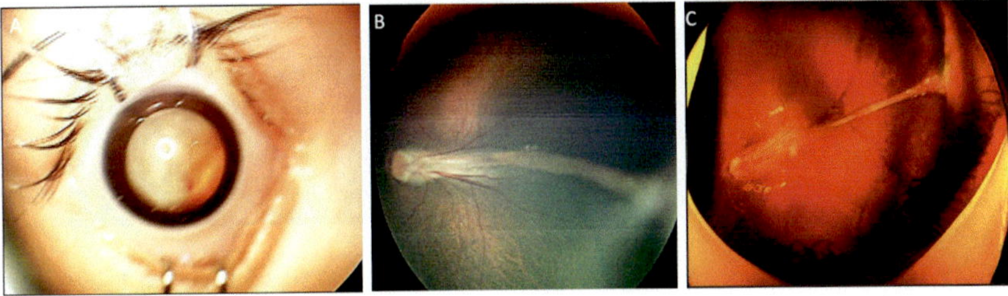

Fig. 25.15 Phenotype in a NDP gene mutation: **A** Newborn Boy at 6 weeks of age—Right eye "Nomes phenotype" with leukocoria, dyaglastic stage 5 retinal detachment. **B** Left eye "FEVR 4A phenotype" that underwent lens sparing vitrectomy and peripheral endolaser. **C** At 7 years of age stable retinopathy and visual acuity of 20/630

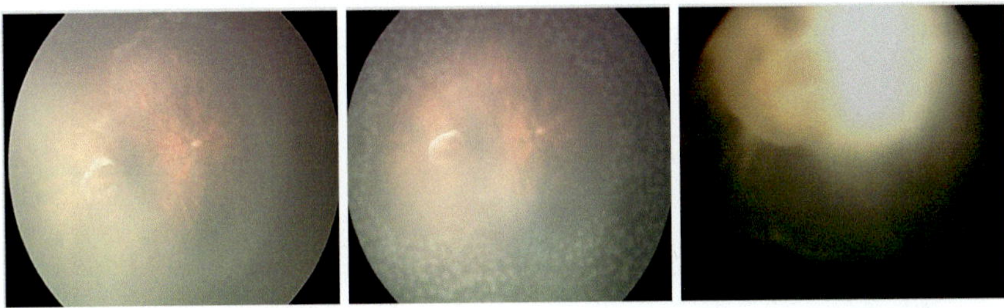

Fig. 25.16 Congenital FEVR in 2 days old term newborn. **A** Right eye Stage one FEVR with avascular periphery, subtle ridge, no vascular dilatation or tortuosity and no significant vitreopathy before (**A**) and after laser (**B**). **C** He presented with leucoooria stage 5 retinal detachment fractional and subretinal exudative components seen in left eye

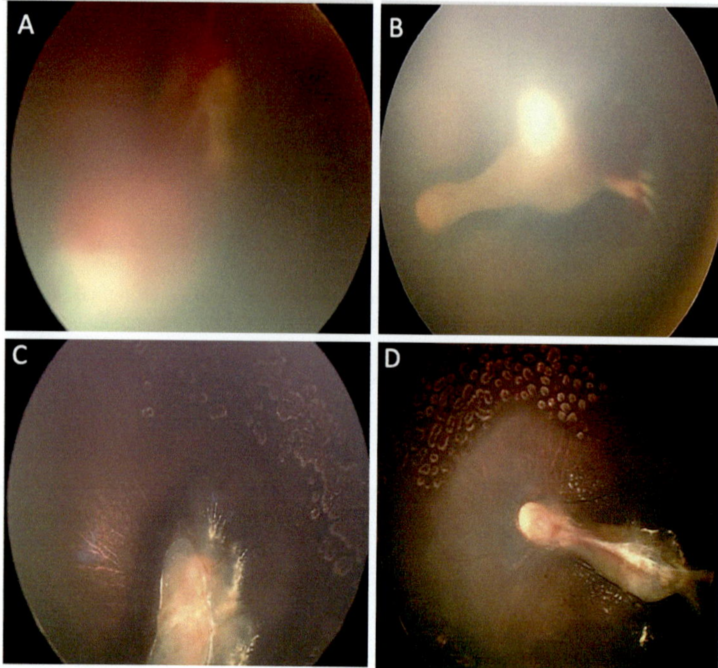

Fig. 25.17 Fulminant type of neonatal FEVR in full term 3000 g birth weight baby seen at 21 days of birth. **A, B** Severe active ncovascular process and Retinal dysplasia (upper panel, right and left eyes). Bilateral simultaneous lenscctomy with vitrectomy could salvage minimal ambulatory vision (**C, D**). At ten years of age, visual acuity 20/500 with + 15.00 D sphere glasses that improves to 20/160 with telescope lens. Near vision N24

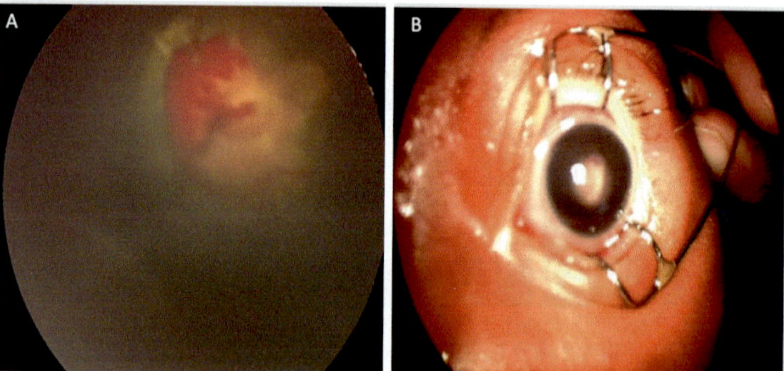

Fig. 25.18 Fulminant type of neonatal FEVR with severe active neovascular process and retinal dysplasia with retinal detachment at birth. **A** Stage 4B folded central retinal dysplastic tissue with overlying haemorrhage right eye and **B** stage 5 left eye. Even with AntiVegf injections and vitrectomy (right eye lens sparing and endolaser and left eye with lens removal) visual gain and anatomical outcome was poor

Management*:* Intervention might be required in following situations in FEVR cases.

a. Laser photocoagulation to prevent /treat new vessels, increasing exudation stage
b. Progressive Tractional retinal detachment—in Stages 3, 4 or 5
c. Rhegmatogenous retinal detachment
d. Exudative retinal detachment
e. Combined retinal detachment—combination of a retinal break with tractional retinal folds with or without exudative component
f. Vitreous haemorrhage
g. Secondary epiretinal membrane, vitreomacular traction, macular hole
h. Progressive exudation
i. Complicated cataract, secondary glaucoma, strabismus management
j. Management of amblyopia, anisometropia, low vision status
k. Systemic management of associations including but not limited to hearing loss, speech impairment, mental retardation, osteoporosis etc.

Based on our experience and literature review [5–11], we discuss in detail the choice of procedure and approach to surgery in FEVR in subsequent paragraphs, based on stage of the disease. Figures 25.1, 25.2, 25.3, 25.4, 25.5, 25.6, 25.7, 25.8, 25.9, 25.10, 25.11, 25.12, 25.13, 25.14, 25.15, 25.16, 25.17 and 25.18 and the videos provide further inputs to management approaches.

1. Stage 1: In most cases this is a stage of arrested vascular development with vitreous condensation at the 'ridge'. While most cases remain stable over decades, some show progression especially during adolescent/puberty years. These patients can be kept under observation and need annual retinal examination preferably with wide angle photos and wide- angle fundus fluorescein angiography (Figs. 25.1 and 25.3) to detect conversion to 1B (Fig. 25.2) or beyond. Any retinal breaks/lattice would need laser therapy and rarely additional cryopexy. Development of epiretinal membranes is rare in this stage but rhegmatogenous retinal detachments can occur. Scleral buckle for such detachments is the best option due to extreme difficulty in removing vitreous beyond the 'ridge'. If vitrectomy is needed due to break not visible, or posterior or large breaks, peripheral vitreous is supported on buckle, and limited careful vitrectomy is done. One can use segmentation techniques and 'shaving' of vitreous rather than trying to create a complete posterior vitreous detachment. Intravitreal triamcinolone left in for at least 10 min also helps. More recently, we have tried scleral imbrication with buckle in selected cases, with good outcomes. Stage 1B would need laser in most cases (Fig. 25.2).
2. Stage 2A and 2B: FFA may detect subtle new vessels or there could be obvious new vessels with associated fibrosis/haemorrhages or exudates. These eyes need judicious laser ablation of the avascular retina, that is sometimes done in a single sitting or preferably in 2–3 sittings to reduce vitreous contraction. Care should be taken to use low energy and keep an eye on the vitreopathy component.

While some eyes do well, others progress rapidly to epiretinal membranes, tractional detachments (Figs. 25.6 and 25.7) and sometimes combined tractional and rhegmatogenous retinal detachment.

Eyes with pre-existing exudation (2B) appear to be of two types. Those detected in neonatal period, have crystalline discrete or tiny cluster-based exudates that remain for ever but become non progressive after laser (Figs. 25.11 and 25.12). These appear to be more in the vitreoretinal interface rather than subretinal. Those exudates that are seen in adulthood are subretinal, confluent and often relentlessly progressive (Figs. 25.8 and 25.9) towards the posterior pole and may be associated with peripheral VPRT (vasoproliferative retinal tumours) lesions or schisis or both. They develop confluent progressive densely aggregated exudation and exudative retinal detachment often associated with vitreous traction. Repeated laser being ineffective seems to be due to inadequate laser from the overlying condensed abnormal vitreous over the avascular retina. Earlier our approach was to manage these complications with vitreous surgery with or without additional buckle as and when the tractional or rhegmatogenous or exudative retinal detachment developed. Literature shows that laser alone or with buckle can have a high 50–60% incidence of progression to stage 3 or 4 and same has been our experience.

In recent years we prefer to combine the primary laser ablation with primary vitrectomy in eyes with significant pre-existing vitreopathy or exudation. This allows good laser ablation and reduced likelihood of secondary complications or progression. The hard exudates seem to melt away with this approach (Figs. 25.8 and 25.13).

3. Stage 3A and 4A: Many of these eyes are detected due to strabismus or low vision in childhood beyond the neonatal period (Fig. 25.4). They remain stable and are characterised by retinal folds and macular heterotropia of varying degrees. These eyes seem to have reached a phase of arrested disease and remain so for prolonged period. Some eyes are treated with judicious laser and additional belt buckle to offset increasing traction (Fig. 25.10). Rarely they develop reactivation in form of new vessels/exudate (Fig. 25.10) or rhegmatogenous components. In quiescent adult stage we manage them similar to stage 1 disease. If seen in infancy, we carry out lens sparing vitrectomy especially in eyes with anteroposterior vitreous traction so as to protect from progressive traction during infantile and early childhood eye growth phase and provide peripheral laser ablation in adequate areas (Fig. 25.15).

4. Stage 3B and 4B retinal detachments in FEVR: The retinal changes in FEVR with new vessels or exudates are progressive and can worsen overtime (Fig. 25.7d). Development of retinal neovascularization and exudation when undiagnosed or left untreated (Fig. 25.7d) can lead to progressive fibrovascular proliferation (FVP). Worsening of FVP's can lead to combined exudative and tractional retinal detachment (TRD) and can also progress to a very complex association with rhegmatogenous retinal detachment. Studies have suggested that nearly 21% patients show worsening of FVP's and lead to TRD causing visual loss.

A. *Tractional Retinal Detachments in FEVR*: Surgical intervention in FEVR should include the management of avascular retina in all cases. Vitreal tractional forces are the major causative factor in many of the surgical indications and need to be meticulously judged and managed. These include antero-posterior, tangential and circumferential traction besides fine adhesions between disc and fovea sometimes with concomitant persistent fetal vasculature. The goal is to attain a complete retinal re-attachment with or without retinal folds, and control of exudation with adequately ablated avascular retina for long term success.

Choice of procedure

The choice of the procedure depends on the location and the extent of traction. Scleral buckling is effective in cases where the traction due to FVP is present in far periphery and where the circumferential traction is <2 clock hours. Scleral buckle can be tried in cases with circumferential traction more than 2 clock hours; however, it can be ineffective. Lens sparing vitrectomy is a safe and effective option to tackle antero-posterior traction, traction predominantly in the posterior retina or circumferential traction more than 2 clock hours. Vitrectomy combined with lensectomy might sometimes be required in cases with advanced TRD where the detached retina is reaching the lens, or total tractional retinal detachment with a retrolental membrane and no space between the retina and the lens. Fibrovascular proliferation and TRD can recur over the scaffold of posterior cortical vitreous when removed insufficiently or if the neovascularization is active. Laser photocoagulation to avascular areas can help reduce the chances of recurrence and further exudation.

Approach to surgery

1. Case selection and appropriate choice of procedure is very important for long term success.
2. Appropriate size of scleral buckle should be chosen preferably in the form of encirclage so as to cover the whole extent of peripheral FVP. It should be tightened with sutures till an extent to reverse the vitreo-retinal traction present. As the traction stabilizes over time with buckle in place, it can be cut (released) to prevent constriction of eyeball due to growth in small children. Any new areas of exudation should be watched for (Fig. 25.10).
3. While planning for vitrectomy, sclerotomy port placement should be planned prior. They should be placed away from the retinal folds or sites of lens-vitreous-retinal adhesion to prevent iatrogenic retinal breaks with the trocar.
4. Eyes with FEVR-TRD usually have a formed vitreous with minimal liquefaction. Careful and extensive vitrectomy to remove most vitreous is required for surgical success. All attempt should be made to remove as much of posterior cortical vitreous as possible to prevent re-proliferation. However, it should be moderated in a way to prevent retinal breaks. Intravitreal triamcinolone left inside for at least 10 min helps in this process.

5. Fibro-vascular proliferation tend to have multiple epicenters. These are also firmly attached to the underlying retina. Since the main aim of the surgery is to release traction, posterior vitreous detachment (PVD) is not necessary in all cases. If the FVP is predominantly vascular, the delamination and segmentation should be limited in order to prevent intra-operative retinal breaks and post-operative bleed.
6. Lens removal can have adverse effects on the visual development for the child. Amblyopia is common in such children. Hence, lens preservation should be attempted as far as possible. However, in cases with retrolental membrane or TRD close to the lens, lensectomy might be required for successful retinal re-attachment.
7. Add on endophotocoagulation should be done to peripheral avascular retina to prevent re-proliferation.

Tractional retinal detachments do not require a long-term tamponade with silicon oil. Vitreous cavity may be filled with air at the end of surgery to prevent bleeding from small neovascular twigs. Periodic follow up is required to assess for re-proliferation and development of myopia.

B. *Rhegmatogenous retinal detachment in FEVR*

Rhegmatogenous retinal detachment (RRD) is one of the most common indications for surgical intervention in FEVR. Patients with RRD tend to present in adolescence or early adulthood.

Anatomical considerations:

1. *Retinal breaks*: Retinal breaks in RRD due to FEVR include both atrophic holes and tears. Most of these breaks (>85%) are known to occur in the temporal retina. They are located either on the avascular retina (mostly atrophic holes; >96%) or the demarcation line (mostly tears). Atrophic holes are formed due the thinned atrophic avascular retina lacking the capillary bed; a mechanism similar to that described with lattice degeneration.
   Katagiri et al. have described the characteristics of retinal breaks in RRD associated with FEVR. Authors describe the presence of oval/almond shaped retinal tears at the demarcation line as opposed to the classical horseshoe tears in RRD. Abnormal vitreous adhesions at the ridge, at the junction of vascular and avascular retina, can be attributed to such oval tears (Fig. 25.5). The vitreo-retinal abnormalities are present all over the retina in FEVR, hence, atrophic holes and breaks can be found in other quadrants as well, although less common. Such a distribution should be kept in mind while managing RRD due to FEVR. Careful inspection of the retina near the ridge especially temporally will help to identify and manage all breaks intra-operatively.
2. *Vitreous adhesions:* Cases of FEVR have abnormal vitreal adhesions in the periphery. Such adhesions are seen preferentially at the edge of the vascular retina. Vitreous is also strongly attached to the avascular peripheral retina and difficult to remove completely with vitreous detachment induced posteriorly.

Hence, it is advisable to manage this by carefully shaving the peripheral vitreous. Avascular retina is also prone to intra-operative iatrogenic breaks while shaving. Operating surgeon should be cognizant of this fact while managing the vitreous. An encirclarge is of importance to manage peripheral uncut vitreous or anterior proliferative vitreo-retinopathy (PVR).

Choice of procedure

Scleral buckling (SB) is considered the first surgical choice for RRD associated with FEVR. It has the advantage of tackling the vitreous traction and supporting the retinal break after retinopexy, by changing the direction of vitreo-retinal tractional forces. A re-attachment rate of about 95% has been reported previously.

Pars plana vitrectomy (PPV) is considered in cases which are not amenable to SB. These include PVR Grade C or more, multiple breaks at different antero-posterior level, posterior breaks or substantial degenerated vitreous adherent at the retinal break. An encirclage should be preferred with PPV to support peripheral vitreous in view of tightly adherent vitreous over the avascular retina. Success rate of PPV with or without encirclage is reported to be around 55%, although the success rates might not be directly comparable due to selection bias of more severe cases undergoing PPV.

Approach to surgery:

1. Most of the cases for vitrectomy can be managed without lensectomy. Lensectomy can be considered in cases with very severe anterior PVR which would hinder posterior dissection or peeling of membranes and/or which cannot be managed with an encirclage.
2. Cases for scleral buckle should be chosen after a careful examination especially looking for breaks along the ridge. Additional encirclage may be of value in case of vitreous traction along the avascular retina.
3. Sclerotomy placement should be judged by thorough pre-operative examination. Anterior dragging of retina can predispose to inadvertent iatrogenic breaks which would complicate the surgery.
4. Posterior vitreous detachment (PVD) can be difficult in eyes with FEVR due to abnormal vitreous attachments especially in the periphery. Most of the patients with FEVR related RRD present at a young age. This can make the PVD induction difficult. Use of intravitreal triamcinolone after core vitrectomy to stain and loosen the posterior vitreous helps in complete PVD.
5. Identification of all breaks by careful intraoperative examination is of paramount importance. FEVR associated RRD can have multiple small breaks especially along the ridge. Thorough vitrectomy, release of traction from all retinal breaks and marking them is necessary to avoid subsequent recurrences.
6. Retinopexy of all breaks should be followed by laser photocoagulation of the avascular peripheral retina. This reduces the chances of recurrence. Fundus fluorescein angiography studies have shown that the avascular area extends posterior to the clinically perceived ridge. Hence, pre-operative FFA can

provide a guide to intra-operative laser. In a situation of unavailability of FFA, 3–4 rows of laser should also be done posterior to the ridge. Cryopexy can be done to the anterior retina if the access is limited.

7. Short acting gas like SF6 or C3F8 can used for tamponade after surgery in cases of no or minimal PVR. Most surgeons prefer silicon oil as it provides longer tamponade with a good view to the retina for post-operative examinations.

Patients with FEVR-RRD require a long follow up. FEVR is a life-long disease and even after surgical correction of RRD, exudative retinopathy can return and cause active subretinal exudation and exudative retinal detachment. These patients should hence, be periodically screened.

C. *Exudative retinal detachment in FEVR*

Aberrant vasculogenesis leading to abnormal angiogenesis is the main pathogenic factor leading to retinal vascular abnormalities in FEVR. Subretinal exudation is also a prominent feature in FEVR. Severe exudation can lead to exudative retinal detachment (ERD) which can be partial or total. Despite subretinal exudation being an important feature in FEVR, the incidence of ERD in FEVR is less as compared to rhegmatogenous or tractional RD.

Wnt-receptor: beta-catenin pathway has been implicated in the pathogenesis of FEVR. This is responsible for upregulation of VEGF levels which manifests as increased vascular activity and exudation. The role of anti-VEGF injections to reduce the exudation, has been sparingly described in the literature [12, 13]. Definitive treatments like laser photocoagulation or cryotherapy for treating the avascular retina is of utmost importance for prolonged effect and to prevent recurrences.

Choice of procedure:

1. Partial exudative retinal detachment: Partial ERD can be treated with laser photocoagulation and/or cryotherapy to treat the abnormal neovascularization and avascular areas in the periphery. In cases where these are not possible due to the subretinal fluid, intravitreal anti-VEGF can be used as an adjunct. As the ERD resolves, laser/cryo can be supplemented for sustained response. Worsening of tractional detachment has been reported with intravitreal anti-VEGF injections.

2. Total exudative retinal detachment: Subretinal external drainage can be planned for total ERD where the retina is seen just behind the lens. After adequate drainage, cryotherapy or laser with or without intravitreal anti-VEGF can be done to prevent recurrences.

Approach to surgery:

1. Case selection and appropriate choice of procedure is very important for surgical success. It would be absolutely detrimental to convert exudative RD to rhegmatogenous type iatrogenically.

2. Treatment of the avascular retina and exuding abnormal vasculature is the most important step determining the long-term success of the procedure.

3. Laser photocoagulation whenever needed, should be done to cover all the avascular retina and the avascular pockets posterior to the end of vessels. Fundus fluorescein angiography can be used as a guide whenever available (Fig. 25.1).

4. Infusion should be placed in the vitreous cavity in an area with maximum space near pars plana to avoid iatrogenic retinal breaks through the elevated retina. In cases, where placing an infusion is not possible, anterior chamber maintainer can be placed initially in a quadrant opposite to planned quadrant for external drainage.

5. Quadrant with maximum fluid should be chosen for external drainage.

6. External drainage can be done either by scleral cutdown or by needle drainage. Considering that the subretinal fluid might be thick and contain cholesterol crystals, a scleral cutdown might be preferred.

7. Intravitreal anti-VEGF can be considered after drainage to decrease the vascular activity.

An alternative approach of subretinal intravitreal anti-VEGF was tried by Peng et al. [14] in exudative vitreoretinopathies. The authors have described the procedure as an initial external drainage of the exudative fluid from one quadrant and then subretinal injection into the opposite quadrant. Although authors describe a good success rate, the procedure is still experimental and has not been tried widely.

Complications:

a. Re-proliferation: Ongoing disease and inadequately lasered peripheral avascular retina can lead to re-proliferation. This presents as subtle small NVE and exudates at the junction of vascular and avascular retina. Presence of exudates and NVE should alert the physician of ongoing activity. Fundus fluorescein angiography is used to delineate these proliferations better. Re-proliferation needs immediate attention and should be treated with additional laser photocoagulation or cryopexy to avascular retina.

b. Proliferative vitreo-retinopathy and re-detachment: Studies have reported a re-detachment rate of 15–20%. Re-detachment is more common with TRD. Development of advanced PVR and re-proliferation when left untreated can lead to re-detachment. A re-surgery can be undertaken in some cases however, the prognosis is usually guarded.

c. Cataract: Nuclear cataract can occur after vitrectomy and cataract surgery can be undertaken for them. Careful watch on any unablated avascular retina is needed. These eyes have a risk of neovascular glaucoma post-surgery especially when ablation was not thorough. In some eyes with advanced posterior disease, lensectomy with vitrectomy could be a better choice than intraocular lens placement especially where anterior camber is shallow (see below).

d. Glaucoma: Untreated or under-treated active disease with peripheral avascular retina leads to release of VEGF and other molecules which can lead to neovascular glaucoma. Neovascular glaucoma can be present at birth or be the presenting feature with or without hyphaema in young children or adults. Glaucoma can also be related to silicon oil emulsification in cases where it was used for tamponade. Shallow peripheral anterior chamber and progressive secondary angle closure, especially in temporal quadrants, are seen in eyes with peripheral vitreopathy/exudation as the fibrovascular tissues push the lens- iris diaphragm forwards. Intraocular pressure monitoring and periodic gonioscopy are an integral part of FEVR follow-up. Detection of glaucomatous cupping in dragged often small discs in FEVR is also a challenge.

  e. Amblyopia: Children are at risk of amblyopia after surgery for retinal detachment especially when lens has been removed. Proper refraction and patching should be recommended for these children in the post-operative period.

  f. Hypotony and phthisis bulbi: Ciliary membranes due to repeated surgery and long-standing ciliary inflammation can cause chronic hypotony and may lead to phthisis bulbi. Late adult untreated eyes or neonatal disease can also present with hypotony and phthisis bulbi.

Video 1: *This video is about a 2-month-old full term baby with bilateral asymmetric FEVR treated with immediate bilateral sequential vitrectomy.*

Video 2: *shows a lens sparing vitrectomy in a case of FEVR related macular fold.*

Neonatal FEVR spectrum (Figs. 25.11, 25.12, 25.13, 25.14, 25.15, 25.16, 25.17 **and** 25.18) is less frequently described in literature. Most babies are term babies with good birth weight and no NICU care. However, FEVR can be seen in preterm babies (called as ROPER) and needs to be differentiated from ROP [15]. While family retinal screening can help in few cases, differences on FFA and the temporal course of the disease is more likely to help to differentiate ROP and ROPER [15]. Genetic testing helps in some though not all cases since in many FEVR cases the molecular genetic defects are yet to be discovered and ROP cases also can have underlying FEVR associated genetic changes [16]. FEVR pathogenesis is mainly centered around failure of angiogenesis and is likely to become significantly aberrant beyond 34 weeks or so of gestational age. If one child is blind from FEVR, the next child can have an elective delivery by 37 weeks under monitoring by trained obstetrician and neonatologist. Examination of the newborn baby within a day or two of birth can detect FEVR early enough to be amenable to vision salvage treatment (personal unpublished data).

Neonatal FEVR can present as a slow smoldering disease with only a ridge (Fig. 25.16) or discrete, crystalline one (Fig. 25.2) or many wreath-shaped (Figs. 25.11 and 25.12) hard exudates. These hard exudates are mostly in the vitreoretinal interface to begin with and are not subretinal in neonatal period. They could also present as an evolving tractional fold or macular dragging (Figs. 25.9, 25.13 and 25.15). Neonatal FEVR can also be of a very fulminant aggressive vascular type (Figs. 25.14, 25.15, 25.17 and 25.18) even presenting with NVG and Buphthalmos (Fig. 25.14) at full-term birth, or bilateral stage 5 FEVR leukocoria. Strabismus, eye poking, nystagmus, corneal scarring with corneo-lenticular adhesion (resembling Peters' anomaly) are other presenting signs in non-verbal childhood ages. Selected few neonatal FEVR phenotypes and the management done are shown in the Figs. 25.11, 25.12, 25.13, 25.14, 25.15, 25.16, 25.17 and 25.18.

Conclusions: Most complications and advanced exudative or tractional drag/fold disease states of FEVR are seen due to lack of universal retinal screening in neonatal period. Detection of disease in neonatal period and its successful management with laser and early lens sparing vitrectomy change the natural course of the disease similar to that seen in ROP cases. Family awareness, intrauterine genetic testing and management of newborn eyes within 1–2 days of birth provides a window of opportunity. Screening of asymptomatic family members also provides this opportunity, though some already have advanced undetected stages when they are screened. Active FEVR may need one or more interventions to quieten the condition and stabilize visual function. Quiescent stages of disease should not give a false sense of security- life-long, periodic appropriate evaluation remains fundamental to have sustained visual function.

Review Questions

1. What are the various components to be watched for in FEVR?

a. Subretinal exudates and RD
b. Neovascular retinopathy and sequelae
c. Vitreopathy
d. All of the above

Variable proportions of Exudative process (subretinal exudates and exudative RD), Retinopathy (neovascular process and its sequalae), and vitreopathy (dragging/vitreous condensation, traction, membranes) need to be ascertained at presentation and follow-up.

2. What investigation is the best during follow-up of Quiescent disease?

a. Optical coherence tomography angiography
b. Wide-field fundus photography
c. Fundus fluorescein angiography
d. Autofluorescence

Annual Wide-field Fundus fluorescein angiography is the best; Annual Wide-field fundus photography is the second-best investigation for 'quiescent' stages, besides the usual comprehensive eye examination.

3. What precautions to be taken during Laser ablation of FEVR eyes?

a. Careful pre-op evaluation of avscular area and existing amount of votreopathy
b. Titrated power
c. Treat according to proper indications only
d. All of the above

Careful evaluation of vitreopathy component is absolutely essential before and after laser ablation. Avoid heavy confluent spots. Treat only progressive or active disease. Progression even after laser may need surgery sooner than later.

4. What Counselling to be given on detecting FEVR?

a. Life long follow up
b. Prenatal screening in subsequent pregnancies
c. Both a + b
d. None of the above

Being a genetic disorder, genetic counselling is very critical. Pre-natal genetic evaluation, early delivery and retinal screening of newborns immediately at birth and screening of other family members is counselled for. Need for long-term follow-up and various interventions that can help maintain visual function, need to be explained. The poor prognosis of advanced cases needs to be conveyed as appropriate.

5. Retinal breaks are most common in which part of the retina in RRD related to FEVR?

a. Junction of vascular and avascular area
b. In the vascularized retina
c. In the avascular area
d. Both a + b

Retinal breaks are most common as slit like breaks at the junction of vascular and avascular area where the neovascularization and traction develops. One should resort to segmentation/shaving and/ or external buckle support of the adherent peripheral vitreous rather than attempt complete vitreous removal that can result in iatrogenic breaks. Intravitreal triamcinolone usage during surgery is encouraged.

Answers

1. D
2. C
3. D
4. C
5. A

Funding/Support Hyderabad Eye Research Foundation.
The authors acknowledge that the institute has received support from Queen Elizabeth Diamond Jubilee Trust (UK), Miriam Hyman Memorial Trust (UK), Rashtriya Bal Swasthya Karyakram (RBSK) Government of India, Cognizant Foundation, India and Dalmia Holdings in India for its ongoing work in Newborn eye problems. None of the authors have any financial disclosures.

References

1. Gilmour DF. Familial exudative vitreoretinopathy and related retinopathies. Eye (Lond). 2015;29(1):1–14.
2. Kondo H. Complex genetics of familial exudative vitreoretinopathy and related pediatric retinal detachments. Taiwan Jl Ophthalmol. 2015;2(5):56–62.
3. Musada GR, Syed H, Jalali S, Chakrabarti S, Kaur I. Mutation spectrum of the FZD-4, TSPAN12 AND ZNF408 genes in Indian FEVR patients. BMC Ophthalmol. 2016;16:90.
4. Yaguchi Y, Katagiri S, Fukushima Y, et al. Electroretinographic effects of retinal dragging and retinal folds in eyes with familial exudative vitreoretinopathy. Sci Rep. 2016;6: 30523. Published 2016 Jul 26. https://doi.org/10.1038/srep30523.
5. Pendergast SD, Trese MT. Familial exudative vitreoretinopathy Results of surgical management. Ophthalmology. 1998;105(6):1015–23.
6. Kashani AH, Learned D, Nudleman E, Drenser KA, Capone A, Trese MT. High prevalence of peripheral retinal vascular anomalies in family members of patients with familial exudative vitreoretinopathy. Ophthalmology. 2014;121(1):262–8.
7. Shukla D, Singh J, Sudheer G, Soman M, John RK, Ramasamy K, Perumalsamy N. Familial exudative vitreoretinopathy (FEVR). Clinical profile and management. Indian J Ophthalmol. 2003;51(4):323–8. PMID: 14750620.
8. Nishina S, Suzuki Y, Yokoi T, Kobayashi Y, Noda E, Azuma N. Clinical features of congenital retinal folds. Am J Ophthalmol. 2012;153(1):81–7.
9. Yamane T, Yokoi T, Nakayama Y, Nishina S, Azuma N. Surgical outcomes of progressive tractional retinal detachment associated with familial exudative vitreoretinopathy. Am J Ophthalmol. 2014;158(5):1049–55.
10. Katagiri S, Yokoi T, Yoshida-Uemura T, Nishina S, Azuma N. Characteristics of retinal breaks and surgical outcomes in rhegmatogenous retinal detachment in familial exudative vitreoretinopathy. Ophthalmol Retina. 2018;2(7):720–5.
11. Ikeda T, Fujikado T, Tano Y, et al. Vitrectomy for rhegmatogenous or tractional retinal detachment with familial exudative vitreoretinopathy. Ophthalmology. 1999;106:1081–5.
12. Quiram PA, Drenser KA, Lai MM, Capone A Jr, Trese MT. Treatment of vascularly active familial exudative vitreoretinopathy with pegaptanib sodium (Macugen) [published correction appears in Retina. 2009;29(1): 127]. Retina. 2008;28(3 Suppl):S8–12
13. Lyu J, Zhang Q, Xu Y, Zhang X, Fei P, Zhao P. Intravitreal ranibizumab treatment for advanced familial exudative vitreoretinopathy with high vascular activity. Retina. 2021;41(9):1976–85.
14. Peng J, Liang T, Chen C, et al. Subretinal injection of ranibizumab in advanced pediatric vasoproliferative disorders with total retinal detachments. Graefes Arch Clin Exp Ophthalmol. 2020;258(5):1005–12.
15. John VJ, McClintic JI, Hess DJ, Berrocal AM. Retinopathy of prematurity versus familial exudative vitreoretinopathy: report on clinical and angiographic findings. Ophthalmic Surg Lasers Imaging Retina. 2016;47(1):14–9. https://doi.org/10.3928/23258160-20151214-02 PMID: 26731204.
16. Rathi S, Jalali S, Musada GR, Patnaik S, Balakrishnan D, Hussain A, Kaur I. Mutation spectrum of *NDP*, *FZD4* and *TSPAN12* genes in Indian patients with retinopathy of prematurity. Br J Ophthalmol. 2018;102(2):276–81. https://doi.org/10.1136/bjophthalmol-2017-310958 Epub 2017 Oct 5 PMID: 28982955.

Coats' Disease

Ahmet Yücel Üçgül and Şengül Özdek

Abstract

Coats' disease is one of the exudative retinopathies, commonly presented in childhood. Differentiation of Coats' disease from retinoblastoma is vital especially during the first years of life prior to commencing treatment. Early stages of the disease can be controlled with ablative therapies such as laser photocoagulation or cryotherapy; however, as the disease progresses to more advanced stage, transscleral drainage of subretinal fluid (SRF) may be needed to control the disease activity. Transscleral drainage of SRF increases the effectiveness of ablative therapies by attaching the retina. Recently, pars plana vitrectomy has been found useful in advanced Coats' disease. Removal of vitreous and concomitant vitreoretinal tractional membranes can reduce the need for further ablative treatment and prevent from the development of subsequent tractional retinal detachment. Anti-VEGF agents can be used as an adjunct to ablative therapies in cases where considerable leakage from abnormal vessels is present. Visual prognosis is mainly dependent on foveal involvement. Subfoveal exudation may transform into subfoveal nodule which indicates poor visual

Supplementary Information The online version contains supplementary material available at https://doi.org/10.1007/978-3-031-14506-3_26.

A. Y. Üçgül
Department of Ophthalmology, Training and Research Hospital, Ahi Evran University, Kırşehir, Turkey

Ş. Özdek (✉)
Department of Ophthalmology, School of Medicine, Gazi University, Ankara, Turkey
e-mail: sengulozdek@gmail.com

prognosis. In advanced disease, visual prognosis is unfortunately quite poor; therefore, the goal of the treatment is to preserve globe anatomically without causing any further disturbance to the patient in such advanced cases.

Keywords

Coats' disease · Anti-vascular endothelial growth factor · Cryotherapy · Laser photocoagulation · Pars plana vitrectomy · Transscleral drainage · Subfoveal nodule · Exudative retinal detachment · Tractional retinal detachment · Retinoblastoma

Introduction

Coats' disease, first described by George Coats in 1908, has been known as a clinical entity presenting with abnormal telangiectatic leaking vessels, subretinal and intraretinal exudation, and exudative retinal detachment [1]. Almost all clinical manifestations have been known to be unilateral; however, with increasingly using wide-field fluorescein angiography, it has been demonstrated that asymptomatic fellow eye may have peripheral retinal nonperfusion areas and subtle peripheral retinal capillary leakage (Fig. 26.1) [2]. Clinical picture can be highly variable, ranging from a few peripheral leaking retinal vessels and limited avascular area to total retinal detachment (RD), neovascular glaucoma, and even phthisis bulbi. Traditionally, the main purposes of the treatment include maintaining vision at early stages of the disease, and glob preservation in advanced disease. However, with recent improvements in the treatment modalities, favorable visual outcomes were reported even in some cases of advanced Coats' disease [3].

Epidemiology

Coats' disease is a rare exudative retinopathy, with an incidence of 1 in 100,000. It shows strong male predilection by approximately 90%, and mostly presents in first or second decade of life [4]. However, adults can be presented with similar clinical characteristics to those in children, but often milder [5]. Although rare cases of the disease such as Coats plus syndrome associated with other system abnormalities can be inherited in an autosomal recessive manner (STN1 gene) [6], isolated Coats' disease is considered as nonhereditary and purely sporadic. Moreover, no risk factors for developing the disease have been ascertained up to today.

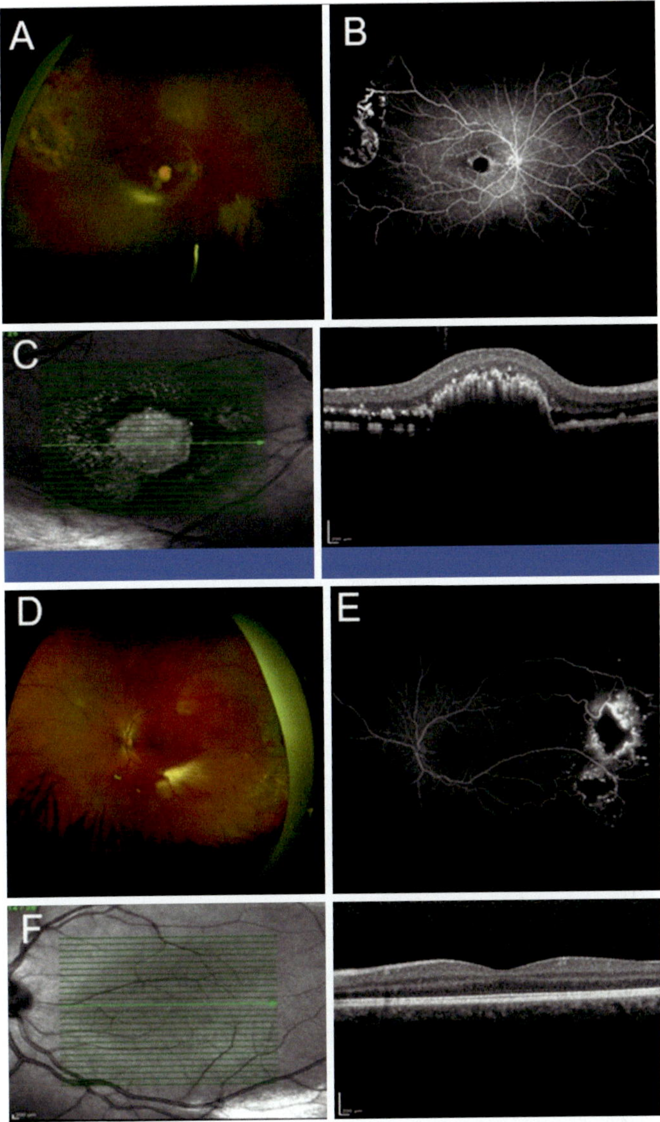

Fig. 26.1 Bilateral Coats' disease in a 17-year-old male. **A** RE has stage 2B1 Coats' disease which was successfully treated with cryotherapy, colored fundus imaging shows myelinated nerve fibers in the inferotemporal arcuate, a subfoveal hard exudate plaque and cryotherapy scar at the peripheral temporal retina. **B** FFA shows the ablated abnormal telangiectatic vessels located temporally. **C** OCT imaging of the right eye shows subfoveal accumulation of exudates. **D** Fundus picture of the left eye shows myelinated nerve fiber located on the inferotemporal macula, and telangiectatic vessels on temporal peripheral retina. **E** FFA shows the leaking telangiectatic vessels and associated capillary nonperfusion areas at the peripheral temporal retina of the same eye in **D**. **F** OCT was totally normal in the left eye

Clinical Characteristics and Stages

Infants and toddlers typically present with leukocoria/xanthocoria and strabismus at advanced stages of the disease, whereas less advanced cases, as in older patients, are usually detected during routine ophthalmic examination or eye screening [4]. Visual acuity can be affected at variable rates, depending on the stage of the disease. The longer and more advanced disease, the deeper vision loss. Patients may present with red and painful eye at the end stage of the disease due to iris neovascularization and neovascular glaucoma.

A classification system first described by Shields et al. [7] can be readily applied based on fundoscopic examination (Fig. 26.2). According to this classification system, stage 1 disease refers to the presence of retinal telangiectasia only, stage 2 disease to the presence of telangiectasia and exudation (2A, extrafoveal exudation; 2B, foveal exudation), stage 3 disease to the presence of exudative retinal detachment (RD) (3A, subtotal RD; 3B, total RD), stage 4 disease to the presence of total RD and neovascular glaucoma, and stage 5 disease to end-stage disease.

This classification system is of great importance in selecting therapeutic options and predicting visual prognosis. Recently, this classification system has been updated based on the presence of subfoveal nodule [9]. According to the updated classification system, stage 2B has been subdivided into two as stage 2B1 (without subfoveal nodule), and stage 2B2 (with subfoveal nodule) (Table 26.1).

On ophthalmic examination, anterior segment structures typically appear normal at early stages of disease; however, iris neovascularization, any types of cataracts, corneal haze, and cholesterolosis bulbi can be observed as the disease progresses to advanced stages. Vitreous usually remains clear until moderate to advanced stages in treatment-naïve patients [10]. However, patients with a history of cryotherapy, laser photocoagulation and intravitreal injection of anti-vascular endothelial growth factor (anti-VEGF) therapy or steroids may exhibit epiretinal membrane, vitreous bands, and vitreoretinal traction [11].

Retinal telangiectatic vessels are the main finding, found in all patients (Figs. 26.1 and 26.2). These vessels show bulbous terminal configuration and are associated with hard exudates, so are called as "light bulb telangiectasias" [12]. In most cases, retinal telangiectatic vessels are located in temporal and inferotemporal quadrants, and between equator and ora serrata [13]. In one-third cases, the area between equator and vascular arcades is involved; however, direct involvement of macula by telangiectatic vessels is rarely encountered [13].

As the disease progresses, intraretinal and subretinal exudates become prominent. Initially, peripherally located exudates tend to move towards the macula under the effect of gravity. In most advanced cases, longstanding submacular exudates give rise to the development of subfoveal nodule which is considered as a strong predictor for poor visual outcome (Figs. 26.3, 26.4 and 26.5) [9]. Subfoveal nodule develops secondary to the migration of retinal pigment epithelium (RPE) cells to subretinal space [9]. Some authors propose that subfoveal nodule result from a neovascular process in response to long-standing subfoveal exudates [14].

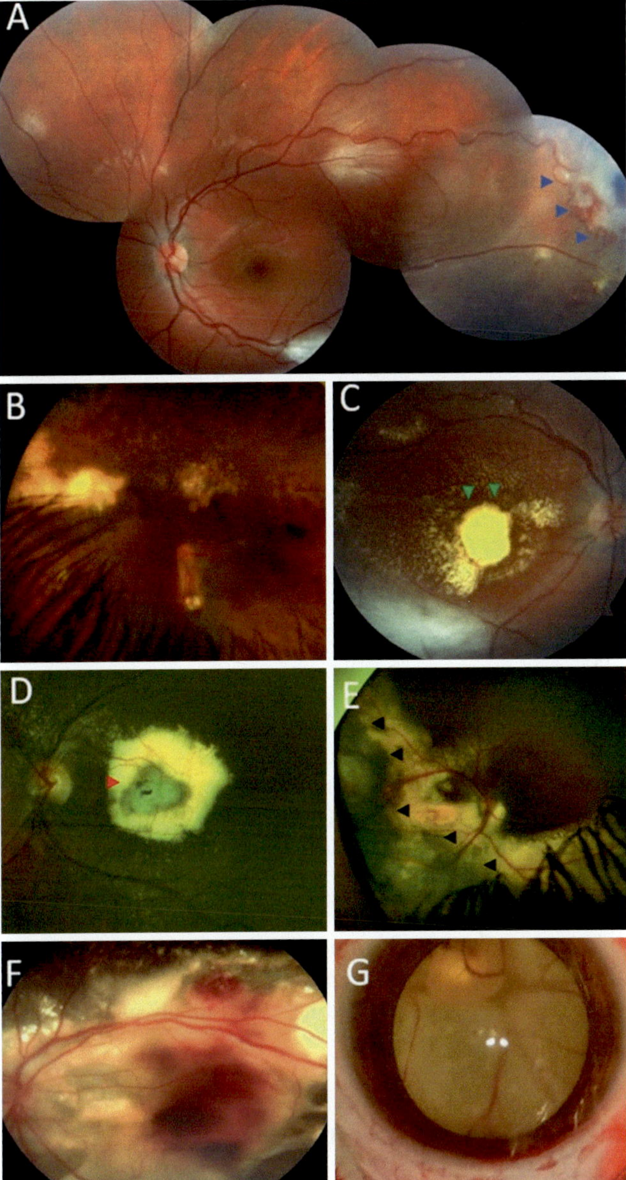

Fig. 26.2 The stages of Coats' disease. **A** stage 1, note the abnormal telangiectatic vessels (**blue arrowheads**) associated with mild exudation in the temporal periphery; **B** stage 2A, note the subretinal exudation not extending the fovea; **C** stage 2B1, note the subfoveal exudation without subfoveal nodule (**green arrowheads**); **D** stage 2B2, note the subfoveal exudation with subfoveal nodule (**red arrowhead**); **E** stage 3A1, note the serous RD inferotemporal to the macula (**black arrowheads**); **F** stage 3A2, note the serous RD extending into the entire macula; **G** stage 3B, note the total exudative RD

Table 26.1 Updated classification system for Coats' disease

Stage	Definition	Suggested treatment
1	Retinal telangiectasia only	Laser photocoagulation or observation
2A	Telangiectasia and extrafoveal exudation	Laser photocoagulation ± anti-VEGF therapy
2B	Telangiectasia and foveal exudation (2B1 without subfoveal nodule, 2B2 with subfoveal nodule)	Laser photocoagulation ± anti-VEGF therapy
3A	Subtotal exudative retinal detachment (3A1 with extrafoveal involvement, 3A2 with foveal involvement)	Laser photocoagulation or cryotherapy, external drainage of subretinal fluid ± anti-VEGF therapy
3B	Total exudative retinal detachment	Laser photocoagulation or cryotherapy, external drainage of subretinal fluid ± anti-VEGF therapy, vitreoretinal surgery
4	Total exudative retinal detachment and glaucoma	Laser photocoagulation or cryotherapy, external drainage of subretinal fluid ± anti-VEGF therapy, vitreoretinal surgery. Occasionally observation
5	End-stage disease	Observation if asymptomatic Enucleation if painful

From Daruich et al. [8]

However, none of those reports was able to answer whether neovascularization is the causative or resultant event in the exudation process. Other authors believed that retinal angiomatous proliferation-like foveal chorioretinal anastomosis might arise independently of peripheral exudation [15]. However, as there is no report showing subfoveal nodule in the absence of peripheral exudation, it is not possible to confirm this speculation.

In advanced Coats' disease, exudative retinal detachment occurs and may be complicated with tractional RD if left untreated. If the disease is not diagnosed at this stage, clinical picture may end up with neovascular glaucoma causing red painful eye with mature cataract, corneal haze, and finally phthisis bulbi in most of the cases of advanced disease.

Differential Diagnosis and Investigations

Patients with Coats' disease may be mistakenly diagnosed as retinoblastoma and familial exudative vitreoretinopathy [16]. Differentiating Coats' disease from retinoblastoma is of great importance, because an overlooked case of retinoblastoma can give rise to fatal consequences, moreover, a patient with Coats' disease misdiagnosed as having retinoblastoma will undergo enucleation inadvertently. The main clinical features that are helpful in differentiating Coats' disease from retinoblastoma are summarized in Table 26.2. Furthermore, telangiectatic vessels

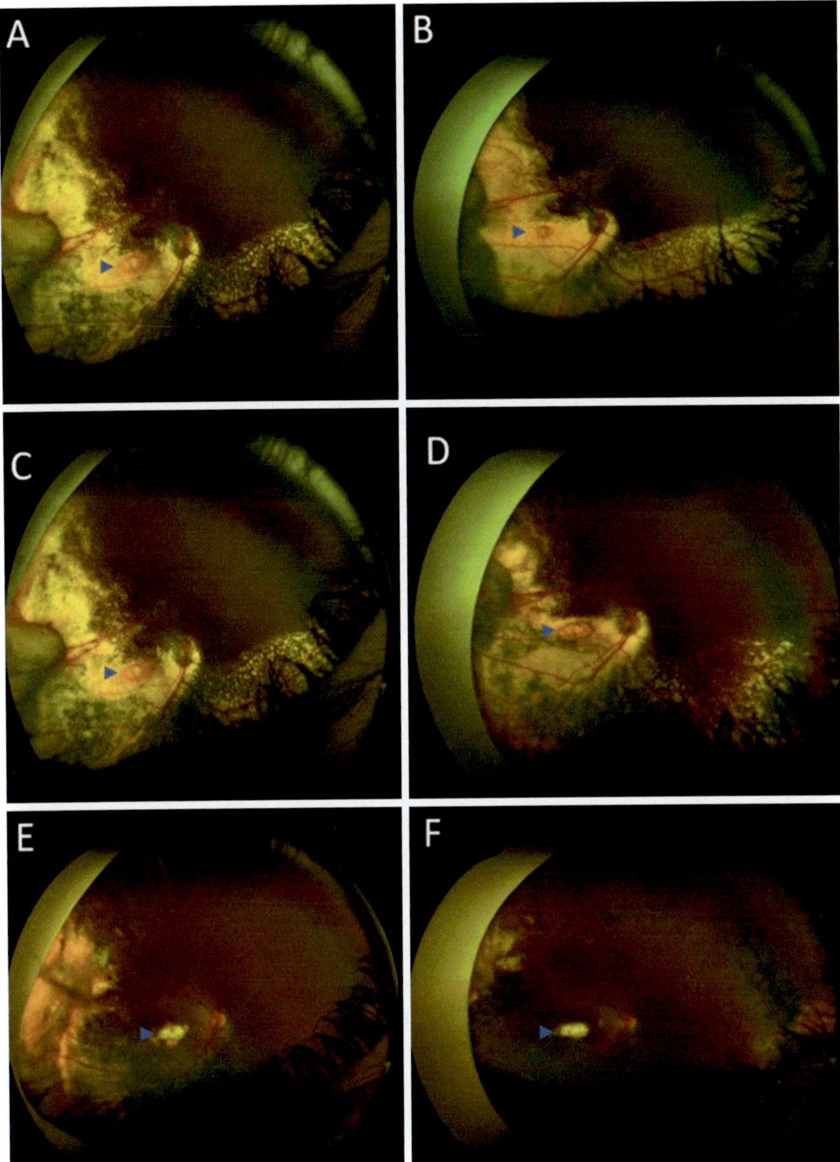

Fig. 26.3 Developmental stages of subfoveal nodule in a patient with Stage 2B Coats' disease who has been treated with multiple laser photocoagulation and intravitreal anti-VEGF injections. Note that long-lasting subfoveal exudates regress with the ablative therapies, leaving a subfoveal nodule (**blue arrowheads**), as going from **A** to **F**

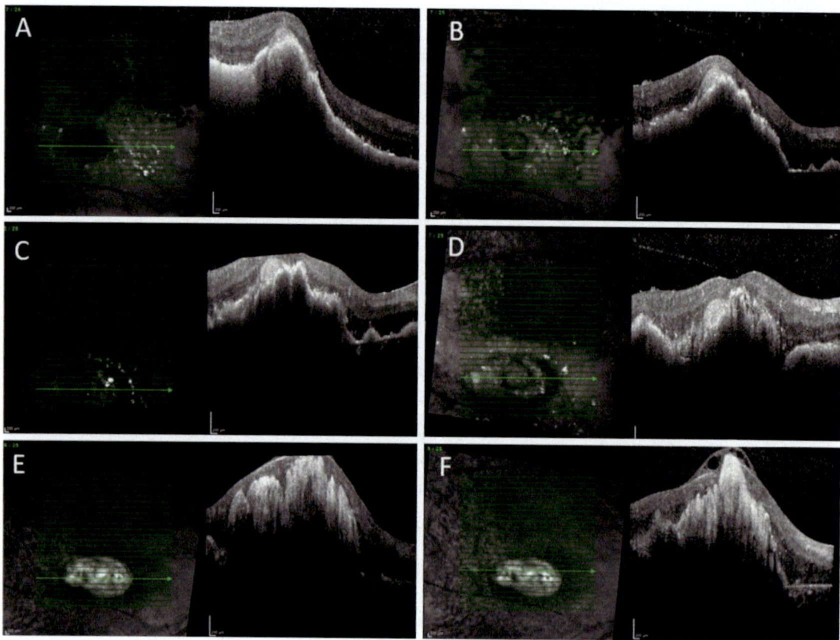

Fig. 26.4 OCT images show the transformation of subfoveal exudate to subfoveal nodule over time in the patient whose fundus images demonstrated in Fig. 26.3. Note the evolution of subretinal exudate with a relatively smooth interface and internal shadowing, into a subfoveal nodule with a more hyperreflective and multilobular interface with a thinning of the overlying sensorineural retinal layers, as going from **A** to **F**

are prominent in Coats' disease (Fig. 26.6), even if they can also be seen in retinoblastoma. Coats' disease can be differentiated from other exudative retinopathies such as familial exudative vitreoretinopathy or Norrie disease by the absence of a family history, retinal dragging, and vitreoretinal traction.

On fundus fluorescein angiography (FFA), abnormal retinal telangiectatic vessels exhibit hyperfluorescence in the venous phase and late leakage, nonperfused areas exhibit hypofluorescence in both arterial and venous phase, and exudation areas show late staining. FFA plays a pivotal role in evaluating the full extent of abnormal vessels and nonperfused areas, and thereby directing ablative therapies (Fig. 26.7). Recently, with coming into use of ultra-wide field FFA, the disease can be diagnosed earlier and the subtle changes in asymptomatic fellow eye can be documented (Fig. 26.1). Ultra-wide field fundus photography and FFA allows the imaging of 82% of the retina (200°) in a single capture without need for pupil dilatation or applanation. A recent ultra-wide field FFA study has shown that asymptomatic contralateral eyes of patients with Coats' disease have nonperfused peripheral retinal areas and retinal telangiectatic vessels by 77.8% [2]. In our case

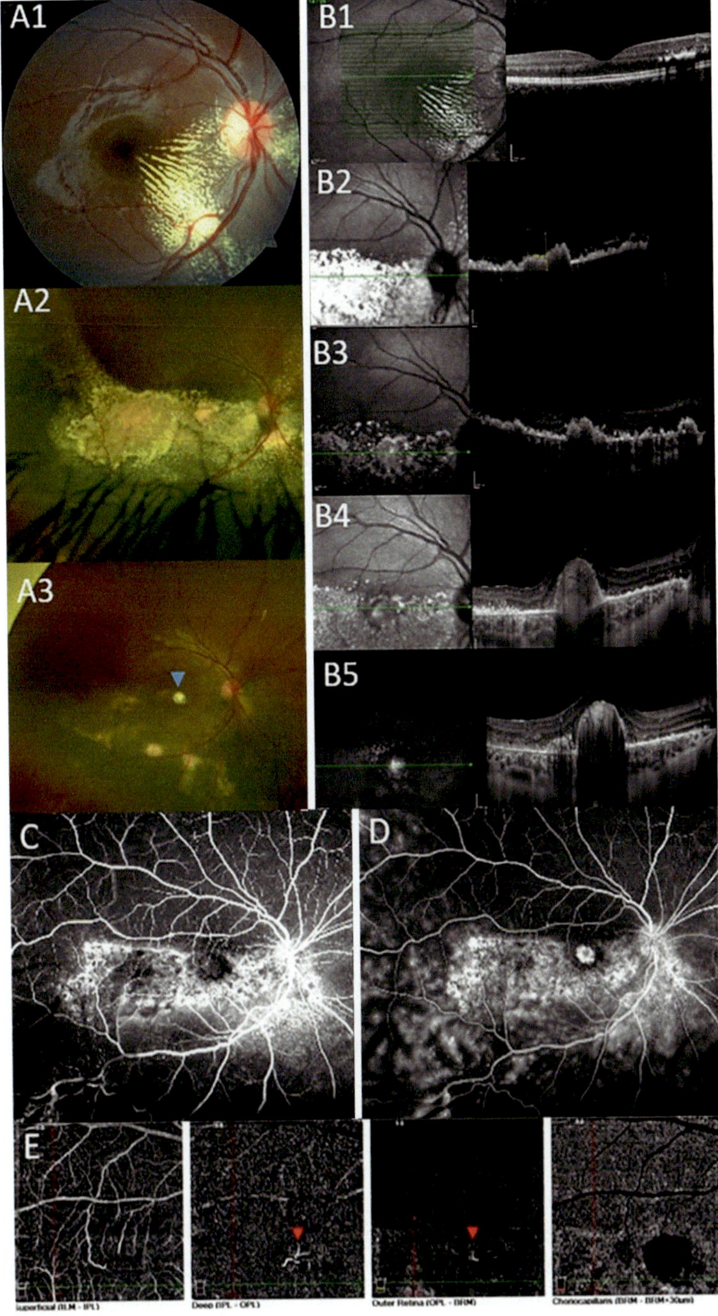
A1
A2
A3
B1
B2
B3
B4
B5
C
D
E
Superficial (ILM - IPL)
Deep (IPL - OPL)
Outer Retina (OPL - BRM)
Choriocapillaris (BRM - BRM+30um)

◀ **Fig. 26.5** Evolution of a subfoveal nodule. A 7-year-old patient with stage 2B Coats' disease had a vision of 20/50. Baseline fundus image shows submacular exudation threatening the fovea (**A1**). The exudates first migrated towards the fovea (**A2**) during treatments with multiple laser photocoagulation sessions and intravitreal dexamethasone implantation and then resolved leaving a subfoveal nodule (**A3-blue arrowhead**) at the first year of the follow-up. OCT images show the development of protruding subfoveal nodule while subretinal exudates vanishing over time (**B1–B5**). FA images demonstrate early hypofluorescence (**C**) and late hyperfluorescence (**D**) of the vascularized subfoveal nodule. (**E**) OCTA images show the diving retinal vessels in the superficial retinal plexus and abnormal vascular network at the level of deep retinal plexus and outer retinal layers (**E-red arrowheads**)

Table 26.2 Clinical clues in differentiating Coats' disease from retinoblastoma

	Coats' disease	Retinoblastoma
Fundus reflex	Yellow or bright yellow appearance (xanthocoria)	Grey-white appearance (leukocoria)
B-scan ultrasonography	– Acoustically clear subretinal fluid and diffuse medium reflective echoes of subretinal exudates – In advanced disease, osseous metaplasia of RPE appears as highly reflective echoes showing curvilinear pattern	– Solid mass with orbital shadowing – Highly reflective dense echoes of calcified substances showing diffuse distribution
Computed tomography	Calcification of subretinal nodule may be detected on CT in advanced cases (20%)	Intrinsic calcification of tumour
Magnetic resonance imaging (MRI)	Subretinal exudate appears as hyperintense on both T1 and T2	Tumour appears as hyperintense on T1, but hypointense on T2
Family history	Negative	Mostly positive in hereditary cases

series, 59% of patients with Coats' disease had telangiectatic vessels and capillary nonperfused areas in their asymptomatic fellow eyes (unpublished data). Cystoid macular oedema, subretinal fluid, ellipsoid zone and vitreomacular interface abnormalities can be documented on optical coherence tomography (OCT).

Treatment Options

The mainstay of treatment of Coats' disease is the ablation of all abnormal leaking vessels. In stage 1 disease, periodical monitorization without any intervention is generally advised; however, we consider that laser photocoagulation can be commenced in certain conditions in which very young patients with irregular follow-up. Once the progression to stage 2 disease is detected, ablative therapies should be initiated in order to prevent fovea from exudation. Laser photocoagulation and cryotherapy are commonly used for ablation of abnormal vessels.

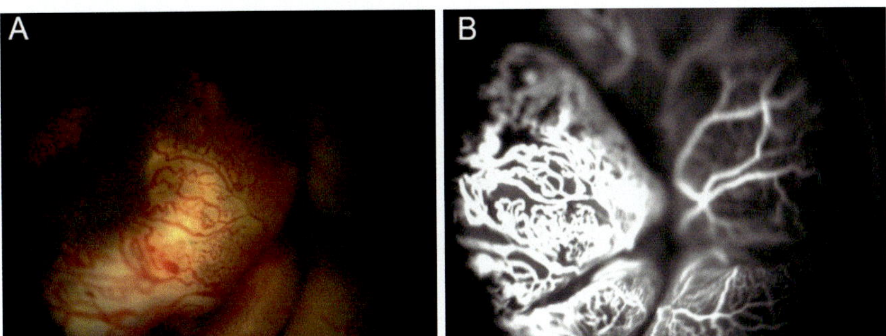

Fig. 26.6 A 10-month-old female patient with stage 3B Coats' disease. Colored fundus image (**A**) and FFA image (**B**) show marked telangiectatic vessels indicative of Coats' disease

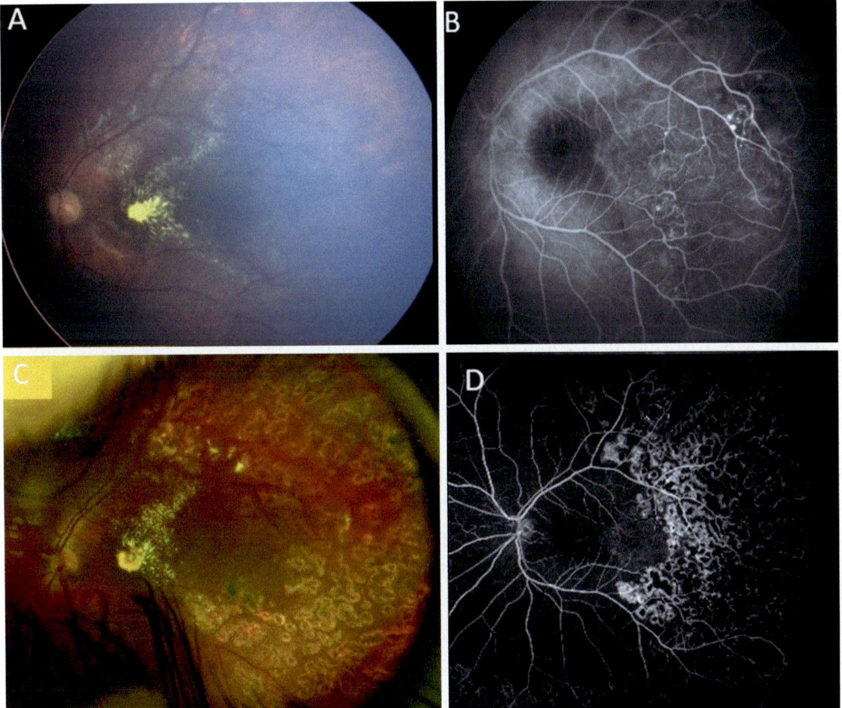

Fig. 26.7 A 6-year-old patient with stage 2B Coats' disease had a vision of 20/400. **A** Fundus picture shows subfoveal exudates. **B** late phase image of the fundus fluorescein angiography of the same patient. Note the leaky abnormal vessels at temporal retina, indicating the need for ablative treatment. **C** shows subfoveal newly formed nodule and laser photocoagulation scars in the temporal retina. **D** shows the effective ablation of the leaky vessels at temporal fundus with laser photocoagulation. Note the subfoveal nodule is hypofluorescent in this case. The final vision remained unchanged

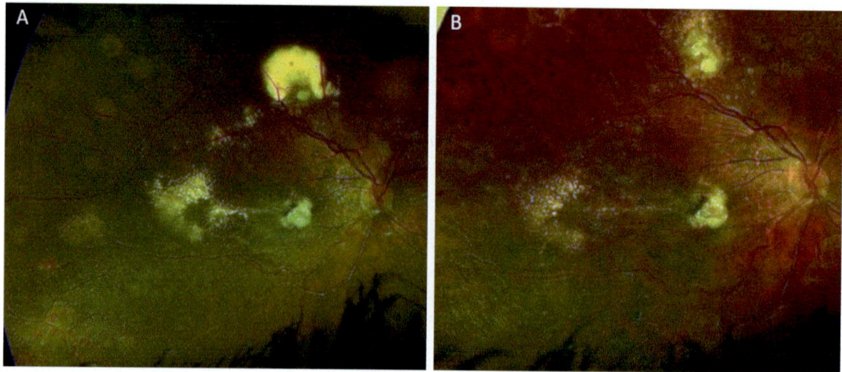

Fig. 26.8 A 7-year-old boy with stage 2 Coats disease. **A** abnormal telangiectatic vessels located temporally, subretinal exudates located on temporal and superior to macula, and fovea. **B** shrinking subretinal exudates six months after effective laser photocoagulation. Note the subfoveal nodule

Laser Photocoagulation (Stages 1, 2, 3a)

Laser photocoagulation offers obliterating leaking telangiectasias and abnormal vessels, and thereby, eliminating exudation (Fig. 26.8). A green or yellow laser in a setting of 0.1–0.5 s duration is preferred for effective vascular ablation [17, 18]. Most cases require multiple laser photocoagulation sessions to control vascular leakage and exudation. It is recommended that laser photocoagulation be performed at three- or six-monthly intervals if further treatment is needed, since resolution of exudate may take relatively long time [19]. However, some limitations come in sight with using laser photocoagulation. First, laser offers less effective vascular ablation when retina is detached. Second, abnormal retinal vessels located in far periphery may not be completely obliterated by laser.

Cryotherapy (Stages 1, 2, 3a)

In some cases where laser photocoagulation cannot be performed effectively, cryotherapy can be more beneficial because it works well even if retina is detached and provides satisfactory ablation of far peripheral abnormal vessels. Cryo-application consists of the steps of approximation of cryo probe externally, scleral indentation, and freezing of ocular tissues contacted by cryo probe. Cryotherapy is typically performed to a certain area two or three times during the same session (double or triple freeze–thaw technique) to produce satisfactory vascular obliteration. However, cryotherapy can cause severe blood-retinal barrier destruction which results in transient increase of subretinal fluid (ablatio fugax). Therefore, maximum two quadrant should be treated in one session and the treatment interval should be at least four weeks [7]. Moreover, cryotherapy can also cause the development of epiretinal membrane, vitreous bands, and even tractional retinal detachment which can cause the failure in controlling exudation process and visual impairment. Some authorities preferred performing cryotherapy after filling vitreous space with air to limit and localize adverse effects of cryotherapy [20].

When making a decision of retreatment of the same quadrant, there should be at least three months between initial and further treatments, like in laser photocoagulation cases, to respite for vanishing of exudates [7].

Anti-VEGF Agents (Stages 1, 2, 3a)

As a recent trend, anti-VEGF agents have been increasingly used as an adjuvant therapy in moderate to advanced Coats' disease. Anti-VEGF agents can ameliorate the effectiveness of ablative therapies by decreasing vascular permeability. Some studies demonstrated that a single dose of anti-VEGF agents alone decreased subretinal fluid markedly [21]. However, as they cannot produce a sustained therapeutic effect, use of anti-VEGFs remains limited to merely adjunct to ablative therapies.

External Drainage of Subretinal Fluid (Stages 3, 4)

In advanced Coats' disease (stages 3 and 4), controlling the disease requires more than laser photocoagulation, cryotherapy, and anti-VEGFs, because extensive subretinal exudates and fluid hinder performing vascular ablation effectively. External drainage of subretinal fluid and exudates in a transscleral way allows performing effective vascular ablation. A drainage sclerotomy should be located in the area corresponding to most massive subretinal fluid and exudate (Fig. 26.9,

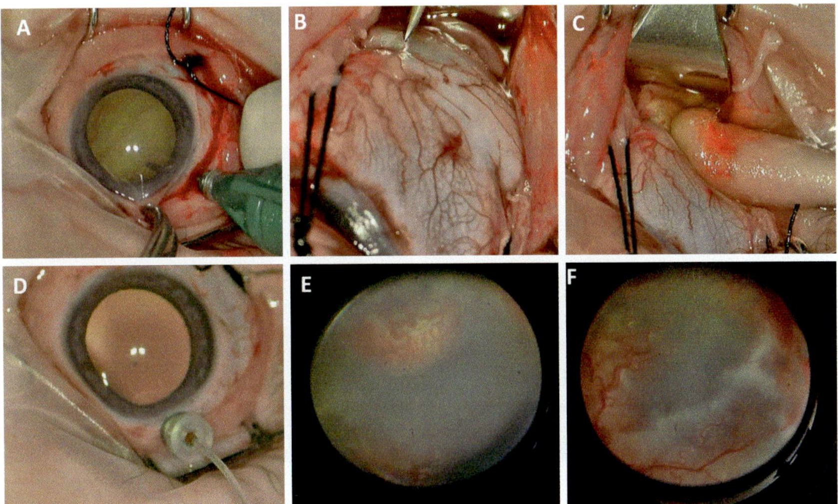

Fig. 26.9 Surgical steps of external drainage surgery. **A** the placement of trocar cannula superiorly. **B** transscleral drainage incision corresponding to most massive exudation area. **C** help of cotton bud for effective subretinal fluid drainage. **D** red fundus reflex obtained after the drainage. **E** Cryo-application by indenting sclera. **F** Attached retina at the end of the procedure

video 1). Meanwhile, maintaining ocular tonus with infusion fluid provides more effective transscleral subretinal fluid drainage and prevents the operated eye from the development of expulsive choroidal hemorrhage [3]. Internal drainage should be definitely avoided because it may be complicated with rhegmatogenous RD difficult to be treated.

Pars Plana Vitrectomy (Stages 3, 4)

Vitrectomy has been at clinicians' agenda for the treatment of advanced Coats' disease in recent years. Although external drainage appears to be sufficient adjunct to ablation therapies in order to accomplish retinal reattachment within early postoperative period, subsequent tractional RD may occur as a part of natural course of the advanced disease or an adverse effect of cryotherapy and anti-VEGFs in the long-term (Fig. 26.10) [22]. Vitrectomy may be needed to relieve vitreo-retinal tractions in such cases (**see the video** 1). A recent study of our group comparing external drainage alone with the combination of external drainage and vitrectomy in the advanced Coats' disease revealed that eyes having undergone the combination surgeries showed more favorable functional and anatomical outcomes and needed fewer further ablative therapies [3]. Furthermore, in advanced Coats' disease, we believe that the prophylactic removal of vitreous acting as a scaffold for tractional complications and housing all the VEGF molecules and other inflammatory cytokines can be protective against the development of subsequent vitreo-retinal traction and the recurrence of exudative RD in the long-term (Fig. 26.11) [3, 23] Other indications for vitrectomy include concomitant vitreous hemorrhage and opacity.

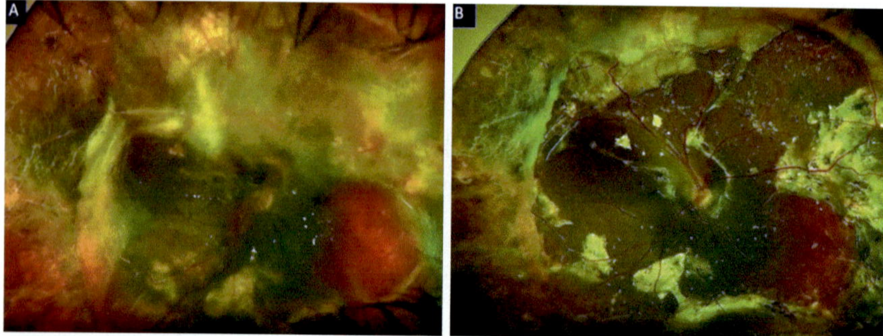

Fig. 26.10 The patient was referred to the eye clinic with the diagnosis of stage 3B Coats' disease on the right eye and underwent drainage of subretinal fluid and cryotherapy when he was 2 years old. He had multiple laser photocoagulation and cryotherapy sessions during following four years of the follow-up. **A** shows dense epiretinal and vitreous membranes causing tractional retinal detachment four years after initial surgery. The vision was questionable light perception. He underwent lens sparing vitrectomy with air tamponade as a second surgery at 6 years old. **B** shows completely attached posterior retina together with widespread peripheral subretinal fibrosis one year after the surgery. The final visual acuity improved slightly to hand hand motion level

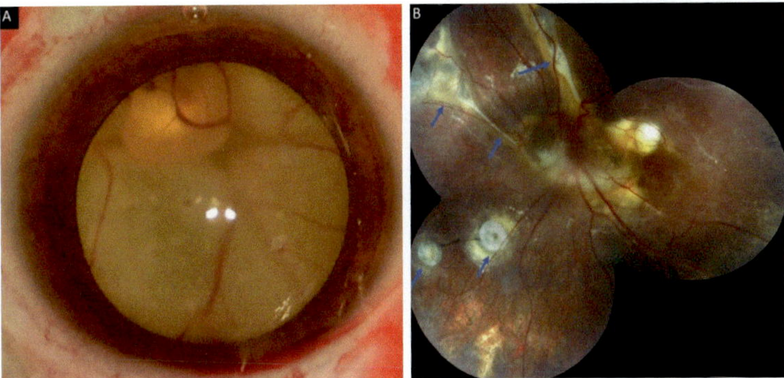

Fig. 26.11 **A** A preoperative image of 2-year-old girl with stage 3B Coats' disease, shows total exudative retinal detachment and widespread abnormal telangiectatic vessels. This patient underwent combined external drainage and vitrectomy surgery. **B** Retina was reattached completely six months after the surgery (Blue arrows indicate some of the subretinal fibrosis) (**see the video 1**)

Enucleation

Enucleation should be preferred in cases where the diagnosis of retinoblastoma cannot be excluded with clinical findings and available diagnostic tests [19]. Other indications for enucleation include the painful end-stage disease and stage 4 disease resistant to anti-glaucoma therapy [19].

Prognosis and Visual Outcomes

The most important prognostic factor in Coats' disease is the disease stage at presentation.

- Normal visual acuity levels can be maintained if the disease is diagnosed prior to foveal involvement. Therefore, advancements in the diagnostic scope are more important than those in the therapeutic scope.
- However, in stage 2B cases with foveal involvement, the disease can be controlled with ablative treatments, but a limited number of patients can achieve a visual acuity of 20/200 and above [16].
- The presence of a subfoveal nodule is another important poor prognostic factor [9]. In patients with subfoveal nodule and fibrosis, visual acuity remains poor at light perception to counting fingers levels despite the effective ablative therapies.
- Younger age at presentation is known to be poor prognostic factor for anatomical and functional successes [16]. The historical treatment goal in the advanced disease is to control the disease progression and protect the eye. However, visual improvement has been reported in a limited number of patients with the more aggressive approaches such as external drainage or vitrectomy

Table 26.3 Changing trends in the management of Coats' disease over the decades

Treatment and outcome	1970s	1980s	1990s	2000s	2010s	P
Observation	39%	21%	33%	21%	11%	0.002
Total number of treatments	2.9	2.0	1.8	3.6	4.5	0.001
Laser photocoagulation	55%	33%	38%	40%	72%	<0.001
Intravitreal anti-VEGF	0%	4%	2%	13%	18%	0.003
Primary enucleation	11%	16%	3%	4%	1%	0.001
Complete resolution	58%	45%	37%	55%	73%	0.002
Complete subretinal fluid resolution	64%	59%	38%	58%	72%	0.010

From Shields et al. [24]

preferred in the treatment of advanced disease in recent years. A recent comparative study of our group has reported that with the addition of vitrectomy to the treatment in the advanced Coats' disease, the need for ablative therapies is reduced, anatomical success is maintained for a longer time, and ambulatory vision is preserved in a limited number of patients [3].

- In a large series of 351 cases in which the change in trend of the treatment over last five decades was evaluated, from the 1970 to 2010s, less observation and enucleation, on the contrary, more anti-VEGF agents and laser photocoagulation were reported to be preferred in the treatment of Coats' disease (Table 26.3) [25].
- In conclusion, an appropriate screening method that can consistently detect the disease at an early stage is needed, as well as the treatment options mentioned above, to improve visual and anatomical outcomes in Coats' disease.

Review Questions

1. Which one of the followings is more valuable feature than others in differentiating advanced Coats' disease from retinoblastoma?

a. Telangiectatic vessels on fundoscopy
b. Intraocular calcification on CT imaging
c. Prominent serous retinal detachment
d. Intraocular hyperintense material on both T1 and T2 MRI

2. A toddler is referred for ophthalmic evaluation of leukocoria. Fundus examination shows stage 3A2 Coats' disease. Which management approach is more appropriate?

a. Pars plana vitrectomy
b. Anti-VEGF therapy

c. External drainage of subretinal fluid and exudate, combined with cryotherapy
d. Observation

3. An infant with Coats' disease, who progressed to the stage 3B disease despite previous multiple cryotherapy and anti-VEGF sessions, is referred for surgery. Fundus examination reveals total exudative retinal detachment and tractional preretinal membranes. What is the most recommended management approach?

a. Pars plana vitrectomy, membrane peeling and internal drainage of subretinal fluid
b. Transscleral drainage of subretinal fluid, combined with cryotherapy or laser photocoagulation
c. Transscleral drainage of subretinal fluid, combined with pars plana vitrectomy, membrane peeling and endolaser photocoagulation
d. Enucleation

Answers

1. **(D)** Telangiectatic vessels and prominent serous retinal detachment can be seen in both conditions. Although intraocular calcification is a well-known feature of retinoblastoma, calcification of subretinal nodule may be seen in advanced Coats' disease by 20%. However, subretinal exudate in Coats' disease appears as hyperintense on both T1 and T2 MRI, retinoblastoma appears as hyperintense on T1, but hypointense on T2.

2. **(C)** In the management of stage 3A disease, subretinal fluid and exudate should be drained in a transscleral way as much as possible to ablate telangiectatic vessels effectively. Stand-alone pars plana vitrectomy is unnecessary in lack of any tractional component in this stage.

3. **(C)** In stage 3B Coats disease, concomitant vitreoretinal tractions can contribute to recurrence of subretinal exudation and fluid after the transscleral drainage alone. Therefore, the transscleral drainage procedure should be combined with pars plana vitrectomy and membrane peeling to achieve better anatomical and visual outcomes. Internal drainage should be avoided as it markedly increases the risk of proliferative vitreoretinopathy and rhegmatogenous retinal detachment. Enucleation is an option for the management of stage 4 disease.

References

1. Coats G. Forms of retinal diseases with massive exudation. Roy lond ophthalmol hosp rep. 1908;17:440–525.
2. Rabiolo A, Marchese A, Sacconi R, et al. Refining Coats' disease by ultra-widefield imaging and optical coherence tomography angiography. Graefes Arch Clin Exp Ophthalmol. 2017;255(10):1881–90.
3. Ucgul AY, Ozdek S, Ertop M, Atalay HT. External drainage alone versus external drainage with vitrectomy in advanced coats disease. Am J Ophthalmol. 2021;222:6–14.

4. Morris B, Foot B, Mulvihill A. A population-based study of Coats disease in the United Kingdom I: epidemiology and clinical features at diagnosis. Eye (Lond). 2010;24(12): 1797–801.

5. Smithen LM, Brown GC, Brucker AJ, Yannuzzi LA, Klais CM, Spaide RF. Coats' disease diagnosed in adulthood. Ophthalmology. 2005;112(6):1072–8.

6. Simon AJ, Lev A, Zhang Y, et al. Mutations in STN1 cause Coats plus syndrome and are associated with genomic and telomere defects. J Exp Med. 2016;213(8):1429–40.

7. Shields JA, Shields CL, Honavar SG, Demirci H, Cater J. Classification and management of Coats disease: the 2000 Proctor Lecture. Am J Ophthalmol. 2001;131(5):572–83.

8. Daruich AL, Moulin AP, Tran HV, Matet A, Munier FL. Subfoveal nodule in Coats disease: toward an updated classification predicting visual prognosis. Retina (Philadelphia, PA) 2017;37:1591.

9. Daruich AL, Moulin AP, Tran HV, Matet A, Munier FL. Subfoveal Nodule in Coats' Disease: toward an updated classification predicting visual prognosis. Retina. 2017;37(8):1591–8.

10. Sigler EJ, Randolph JC, Calzada JI, Wilson MW, Haik BG. Current management of Coats disease. Surv Ophthalmol. 2014;59(1):30–46.

11. Glaser BM, Vidaurri-Leal J, Michels RG, Campochiaro PA. Cryotherapy during surgery for giant retinal tears and intravitreal dispersion of viable retinal pigment epithelial cells. Ophthalmology. 1993;100(4):466–70.

12. Adam RS, Kertes PJ, Lam WC. Observations on the management of Coats' disease: less is more. Br J Ophthalmol. 2007;91(3):303–6.

13. Shields JA, Shields CL, Honavar SG, Demirci H. Clinical variations and complications of Coats disease in 150 cases: the 2000 Sanford Gifford Memorial Lecture. Am J Ophthalmol. 2001;131(5):561–71.

14. Jumper JM, Pomerleau D, McDonald HR, Johnson RN, Fu AD, Cunningham ET Jr. Macular fibrosis in Coats disease. Retina. 2010;30(4 Suppl):S9-14.

15. Sigler EJ, Calzada JI. Retinal angiomatous proliferation with chorioretinal anastomosis in childhood Coats disease: a reappraisal of macular fibrosis using multimodal imaging. Retina. 2015;35(3):537–46.

16. Dalvin LA, Udyaver S, Lim LS, et al. Coats disease: clinical features and outcomes by age category in 351 cases. J Pediatr Ophthalmol Strabismus. 2019;56(5):288–96.

17. Shapiro MJ, Chow CC, Karth PA, Kiernan DF, Blair MP. Effects of green diode laser in the treatment of pediatric Coats disease. Am J Ophthalmol. 2011;151(4):725–31, e722.

18. Levinson JD, Hubbard GB 3rd. 577-Nm yellow laser photocoagulation for Coats disease. Retina. 2016;36(7):1388–94.

19. Sen M, Shields CL, Honavar SG, Shields JA. Coats disease: an overview of classification, management and outcomes. Indian J Ophthalmol. 2019;67(6):763–71.

20. Suesskind D, Altpeter E, Schrader M, Bartz-Schmidt KU, Aisenbrey S. Pars plana vitrectomy for treatment of advanced Coats' disease–presentation of a modified surgical technique and long-term follow-up. Graefes Arch Clin Exp Ophthalmol. 2014;252(6):873–9.

21. Zheng XX, Jiang YR. The effect of intravitreal bevacizumab injection as the initial treatment for Coats' disease. Graefes Arch Clin Exp Ophthalmol. 2014;252(1):35–42.

22. Ramasubramanian A, Shields CL. Bevacizumab for Coats' disease with exudative retinal detachment and risk of vitreoretinal traction. Br J Ophthalmol. 2012;96(3):356–9.

23. Li AS, Capone A Jr, Trese MT, et al. Long-term outcomes of total exudative retinal detachments in stage 3B coats disease. Ophthalmology. 2018;125(6):887–93.

24. Shields CL, Udyaver S, Dalvin LA, Lim LS, Atalay HT, L Khoo CT, Mazloumi M, Shields JA. Coats disease in 351 eyes: analysis of features and outcomes over 45 years (by decade) at a single center. Indian J Ophthalmol. 2019;67(6):772–83.

25. Shields CL, Udyaver S, Dalvin LA, et al. Coats disease in 351 eyes: analysis of features and outcomes over 45 years (by decade) at a single center. Indian J Ophthalmol. 2019;67(6): 772–83.

Incontinentia Pigmenti

James Kohler, Rusdeep Mundae, Ameay Naravane,
and Sandra R. Montezuma

Abstract

Incontinentia Pigmenti is a complex disease with both systemic and ocular findings. It requires early ophthalmological evaluation given risk of progressive retinal ischemia, neovascularization, and complex tractional and/or rhegmatogenous retinal detachments. Due to its rarity, there are no large-scale clinical trials to establish preferred practice patterns. Nevertheless, management guidelines can be adapted from other proliferative retinopathies that present in infancy. In particular, early identification of retinal ischemia through dilated fundus exams with fluorescein angiography is required to guide treatment course. Laser photocoagulation, cryotherapy, anti-vascular endothelial growth factor

Supplementary Information The online version contains supplementary material available at https://doi.org/10.1007/978-3-031-14506-3_27.

J. Kohler · R. Mundae · A. Naravane · S. R. Montezuma (✉)
University of Minnesota, Minneapolis, MN, USA
e-mail: smontezu@umn.edu

J. Kohler
e-mail: james.m.kohler@gmail.com

A. Naravane
e-mail: narav001@umn.edu

S. R. Montezuma
Department of Ophthalmology and Visual Neurosciences, 420 Delaware St SE, MMC 493, Minneapolis, MN 55455, USA

medications, scleral buckling, and vitrectomy are all used to curb disease progression. Despite advancements in care, outcomes in Incontinentia Pigmenti can be highly variable.

Keywords

Bloch-Sulzberger syndrome · Incontinentia pigmenti · Neovascularization · Proliferative retinopathy · Rhegmatogenous retinal detachment · Tractional retinal detachment

Introduction

Background

Incontinentia Pigmenti (IP), also known as Bloch-Sulzberger syndrome, is a rare X-linked autosomal dominant disorder that typically manifests at birth or early in childhood. It is a multiorgan syndrome that primarily affects the skin, eyes, central nervous system, and teeth. Initially described in 1906, it was further characterized by Bloch in 1926 and Sulzberger in 1928 [1–3].

Epidemiology

The incidence of IP has been reported to be 1 case per 40,000 births, with some estimating an incidence of 0.7 cases per 100,000 births [4, 5]. 90–97% of living patients with IP are female. Because IP is an X-linked dominant disorder, it is typically lethal in hemizygous male embryos. However, a total of at least 120 male patients with IP have been reported in the literature with a few additional case reports published every year since then [6, 7]. Survival in males is mediated through 47, XXY karyotype (Klinfelter syndrome) or somatic mosaicism [8]. Between 65 and 75% of cases are the result of sporadic mutations, while the remainder of the cases are familial [9].

Pathophysiology

In 80% of cases, IP is due to a loss of function, mutation in the *IKBKG* gene (inhibitor of the nuclear factor KB [NF-kB] kinase subunit gamma), also known as NF-kB Essential Modulator (*NEMO*), located on the X chromosome at position q28 [10]. NEMO plays a key role in the IK kinase complex; it works to cleave IKB, a protein that inhibits NF-kB.

NF-kB upregulates the immunogenic response and prevents cellular apoptosis. When the IK kinase complex (which includes NEMO) is activated, it cleaves IKB from NF-kB, allowing NF-kB to move to the nucleus to initiate transcription of proteins that prevent cellular apoptosis. Without NF-kB, cells in patients with IP are at an increased risk of apoptosis. These cells may upregulate production of chemotactic factors including eotaxin, a cytokine specific for eosinophils, and likely explains the eosinophilia seen in IP.

Currently, it is postulated that this inflammatory process is the common mechanism in IP. In the retina, the inflammation can result in vaso-occlusion and ischemia. The vaso-occlusion in the retinal arteries leads to areas of under perfused and avascular retina with resulting ischemia. Neovascularization (NV) can then occur as a damaging sequela [11, 12].

Clinical Features

Dermatological findings are typically the first manifestation of IP and are present in almost 100% of patients with IP. The most common dermatologic presentation is macular patches of hyperpigmentation in a swirling or whirling pattern, which are present in 98% of patients and typically fade by early adulthood. A vesicular rash can also be seen in 90% of patients and can be present at birth (Fig. 27.1). This is followed by a verrous rash, which can occur in the first few months of life in approximately 70% of patients (Fig. 27.2). Lastly, about 28% of patients are found to have hypopigmented lesions arranged in streaks or whorls [11].

While the dermatological findings aid in diagnosis of the disease, dermatologic manifestations are often benign. Patients with IP can also develop dental (54–80%) [11], central nervous system (40%) [13], and ophthalmic manifestations (36.5%) [7], the latter two of which have the most functional impact.

Ocular abnormalities include strabismus, microphthalmia, optic nerve atrophy, congenital cataracts, and retinal anomalies. Retinal anomalies are far more common and often occur in the first year of life [11]. They include incomplete vascularization leading to NV, retinal hemorrhage, and retinal detachment (RD). Foveal hypoplasia and foveal vascularization have also been reported, though there is some disagreement in the literature as to whether true "foveal hypoplasia" occurs [6, 7, 11]. An avascular peripheral retina is considered a classic retinal finding of IP (Fig. 27.3). Macular findings of IP are less obvious on exam but can include a blunted foveal pit and absence of a normal parafoveal vasculature pattern.

Fig. 27.1 Two-week-old baby girl with incontinentia pigmenti and typical vesicular rash noted on upper and lower extremities

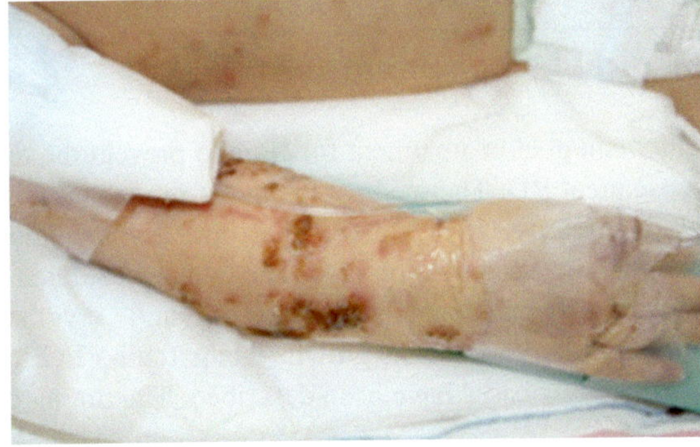

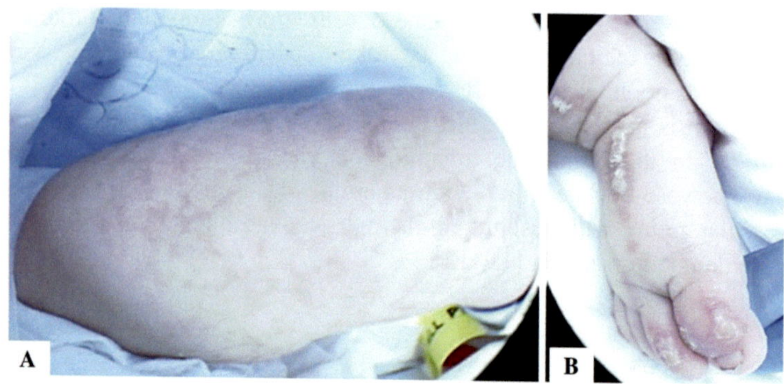

Fig. 27.2 Brownish pigmentation in a reticular pattern **A** and verrucous rash **B** noted on a 3-week-old baby with incontinentia pigmenti

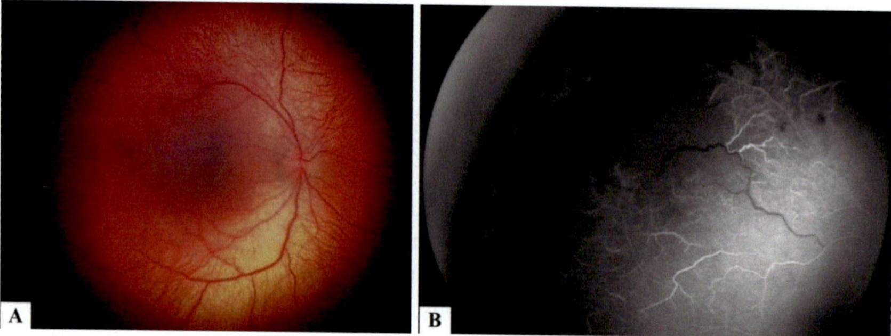

Fig. 27.3 Example of stage 1 disease with vessel tortuosity seen on color fundus photo **A** and incomplete peripheral vascularization without neovascularization on FA **B** on a 6-month-old female with incontinentia pigmenti

In describing the management of various stages of vitreoretinal disease in IP, we will refer to the staging scheme devised by Montezuma et al. in their systematic review (Table 27.1; Figs. 27.3, 27.4, 27.5 and 27.6) [12].

Medical Management

The main goal of treatment for IP is to prevent the development of retinal NV and subsequent RD. The medical treatment modalities are similar to that of retinopathy of prematurity (ROP), given that both retinopathies are a result of incomplete peripheral vascularization [14]. The two most studied non-surgical treatments for IP are laser photocoagulation therapy and cryotherapy. Recently, intravitreal anti-vascular endothelial growth factor (anti-VEGF) therapy has been employed, however few cases have been described. The timing of when to initiate treatment is

Table 27.1 Staging system of the retinal abnormalities seen in incontinentia pigmenti

Stage	Description
0	Complete vascularization of retina with no abnormal vessels
1	Incomplete peripheral vascularization, abnormal arteriovenous connections, tortuosity and/or engorgement of retinal vessels
2	Neovascularization of the retina or retinal hemorrhage
3	Retinal detachment with or without iris neovascularization
4	Chronic complete retinal detachment and development of retrolental fibrovascular membrane/mass
Sub-feature	
S	Foveal hypoplasia

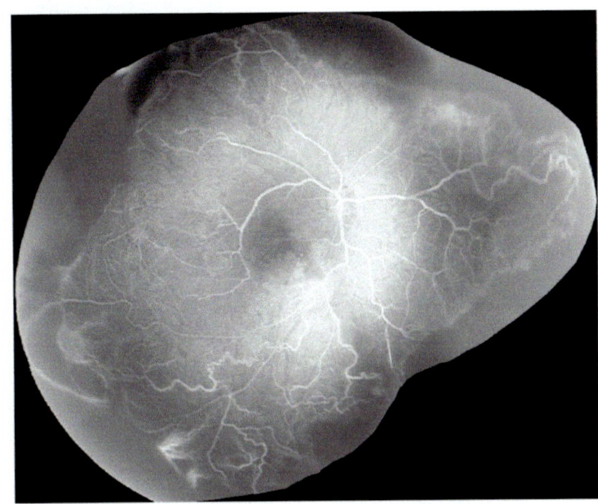

Fig. 27.4 Example of stage 2 disease with peripheral neovascularization noted on FA on a 2-week-old female with incontinentia pigmenti

debated [15], however many authors agree that early detection and treatment of IP can help prevent complications of retinal ischemia and progression to retinal detachment [12, 13, 16–18]. Non-surgical management is typically employed for stage 1 and stage 2 IP, while stage 3 IP and above would necessitate surgical intervention [12].

Laser Photocoagulation Therapy

Laser photocoagulation in treatment of IP has been described as early as the 1970s [19]. Most authors have suggested to start treatment at the first sign of incomplete peripheral vascularization (stage 1) [17, 20], while few have suggested to reserve treatment until fibrovascular proliferation develops (stage 2) [15]. Infants who are treated with laser photocoagulation should be re-evaluated in approximately 6–8 weeks at the office. If response is non-satisfactory, repeated laser photocoagulation should be performed [12].

Fig. 27.5 Example of stage 3 disease in a 50-year-old female with late diagnosis of incontinentia pigmenti. Peripheral neovascularization is noted on FA with OCT demonstrating a localized superonasal retinal detachment

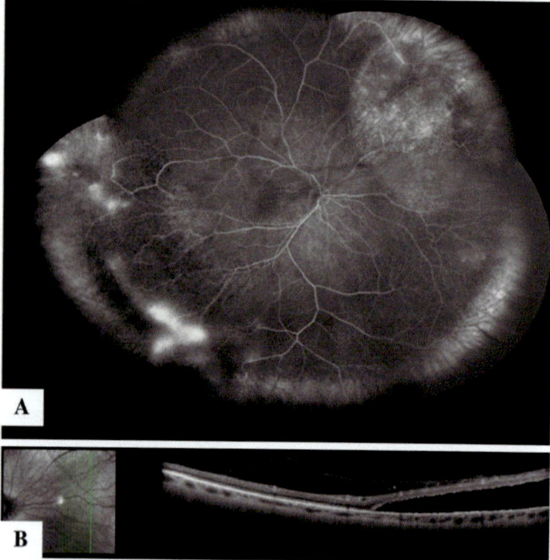

Fig. 27.6 Example of stage 4 disease in a 22-year-old female with wide-field photos demonstrating a chronic posterior tractional retinal detachment involving the optic nerve, extensive fibrosis, and abnormalities of the parafoveal vasculature

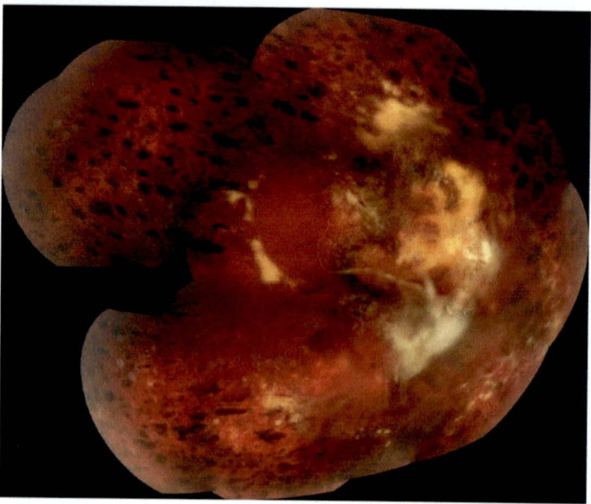

In general, retinal screening exams should be performed as early as possible with FA (either in the OR using RETeval or in-office examination with non-contact ultra-wide-field Optos imaging), to evaluate peripheral vascular changes and to guide surgeons on where to perform the retina photocoagulation treatment or cryotherapy. During the first year of life the patients should be followed approximately every 3 months at the office with repeated FA at least once a year, or earlier if concerns for persistent NV. Once stable, the recommendation is semiannually until 5 years of age and then annually for the rest of their life [12].

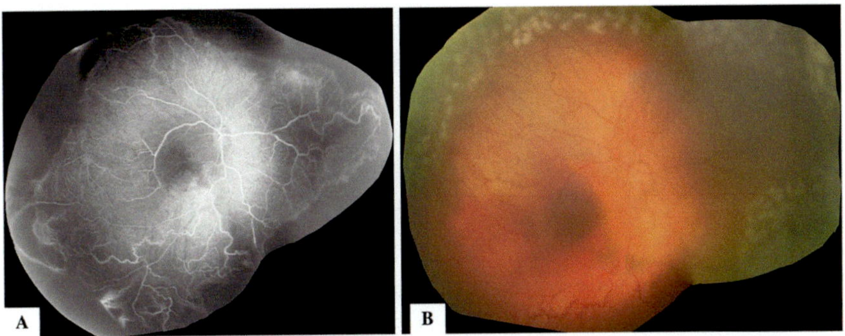

Fig. 27.7 **A** FA of right eye of 2-week-old female with peripheral neovascularization prior to photocoagulation treatment. **B** Fundus photo of right eye post-photocoagulation treatment

The laser treatment is similar to other lasers used in pediatrics with the Argon green laser as the most commonly used. The goal is to destroy the tissue that is producing VEGF and to treat the peripheral areas of avascularization and NV. We recommend FA guided laser photocoagulation as peripheral areas of retina avascularity and NV can often be difficult to identify on exam and FA can highlight areas that require treatment (Figs. 27.7 and 27.8). Similar to the laser recommendations for ROP [21], gray-white spots of near-confluent laser treatment are recommended. The laser parameters of laser power and duration should be adjusted for each patient based on the area being treated and the child's pigmentation.

Cryotherapy

Cryotherapy was a more common treatment option in the cases published prior to the late 1990s [22–24]. With increasing use of laser photocoagulation in the late 1990s, several studies were conducted comparing efficacy and visual outcomes in patients with threshold ROP. Cryotherapy was found to be associated with worse structural and functional outcomes [25], and leads to more inflammation compared to laser photocoagulation. Based on these studies, cryotherapy is now commonly regarded as the second line treatment for stage 2 IP. Moreover, cicatricial changes including epiretinal membranes or proliferative vitreoretinopathy can result from aggressive cryotherapy (and photocoagulation) [15], and have been associated with retinal tears at the edge of previously treated retina [26]. If cryotherapy is required, a similar follow up period to that of laser photocoagulation should be followed to assess treatment response.

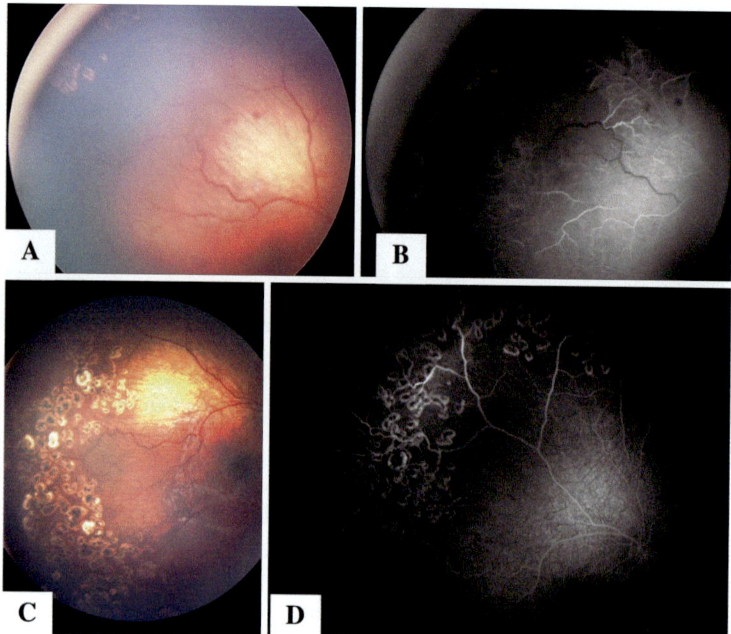

Fig. 27.8 **A** Fundus photo and **B** FA of a 6-month-old female with incontinentia pigmenti, demonstrating peripheral capillary dropout and panretinal photocoagulation scars in the far periphery prior to additional photocoagulation treatment. **C** Fundus photo and **D** FA post-additional photocoagulation treatment

Intravitreal Anti-vascular Endothelial Growth Factor

With the success of intravitreal anti-VEGF injections for retinopathy of prematurity, anti-VEGF therapy has recently been proposed as an additional treatment option of IP. It has been suggested that it could be used as sole first line therapy or as adjunct therapy after failed laser photocoagulation. However, the use of anti-VEGF injection has only been described in several case reports [27–29] with limited evidence on treatment outcomes. As such, it is the clinician's discretion to decide whether to use it based on the clinical context. It is important to note that patients with IP may develop cerebrovascular involvement, including occlusive arteriopathies and infarcts, which are theoretical contraindications for anti-VEGF injections [17, 30].

Surgical Management

When less invasive methods have failed to control retinal ischemia in infants and young children, retinal detachment (RD) may result (stages 3 or 4 IP) [12, 15, 31]. These primarily tractional detachments are complicated because retinal ischemia in

IP is not limited to developmental patterns of anterior avascularity and posterior vascularity. Due to the rarity of IP, no controlled trials exist evaluating treatments for retinal ischemia, and practice patterns vary based on physician preference [12]. Nevertheless, knowledge gained from late-stage ROP surgical management can guide surgical decision making in IP.

RD occurs in approximately 31% of patients with IP in a recent systematic review [12]. The RD pathophysiology appears to follow a bimodal age distribution, with tractional detachments occurring in children (median age 1.5 years) and rhegmatogenous detachments occurring in adults (age 31.5 years) [15]. This is not surprising as children are prone to retinal ischemia resulting in fibrovascular proliferations, whereas this ischemic process is more quiescent in adults. Neonates or young children with concurrent ocular pathology on initial examination, particularly ischemic optic neuropathy and/or retinal NV, must be identified because of greater odds of developing RDs [15]. These children should be followed closely due to the progressive nature of IP. The decision to pursue RD repair in IP is multifactorial. Care must be taken to weigh the visual potential of the patient. Coexisting eye disease is often present, including persistent fetal vasculature or macular ischemia, which may limit any visual potential and make repair futile [15, 32–34].

It is important to note that retinal detachment can occur late in life and early detection is critical because in some cases prophylactic laser demarcation can be performed in certain cases. This reinforces the concept that long life-term follow up is needed in patients diagnosed with IP (Fig. 27.9).

Tractional RD Repair (see the video, by courtesy of Şengül Özdek)

If repair of tractional RD is feasible, the surgical management in IP is similar to that used for late-stage ROP. The first decision is whether to pursue vitrectomy or scleral buckling (SB) or vitrectomy with SB. There is no consensus on the correct approach in IP. Due to similarities in pathophysiology to late-stage ROP, primary vitrectomy may lead to better outcomes in terms of anatomical and functional

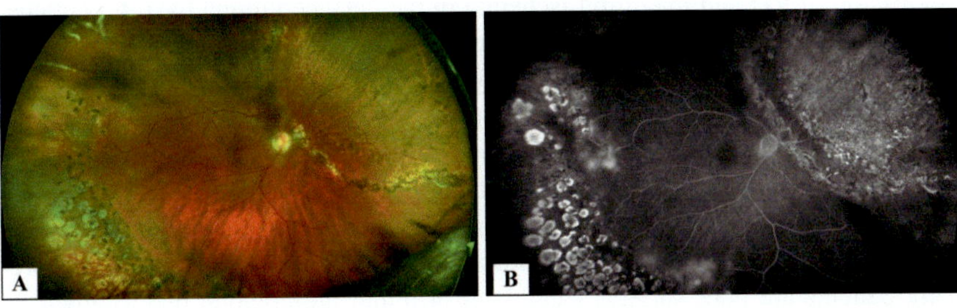

Fig. 27.9 **A** Wide-field fundus photo and **B** FA after FA-guided laser photocoagulation on the 50-year-old female from Fig. 27.5

success rates, particularly in lens-sparing vitrectomy [35]. Lens-sparing pars plicata vitrectomy is preferred if possible due to the risk of aphakic amblyopia. In this approach, a 3-port vitrectomy is performed through pars plicata rather than pars plana. Pars plicata sclerotomy can be approximated by 1 mm posterior to the limbus and adding 1 mm to the distance from the limbus with each year of age after the first year of life up to 4 years of age [36]. Instruments introduced through pars plana may penetrate the subretinal space or cause iatrogenic retinal tears [37]. Moreover, the trajectory of sclerotomy should be perpendicular rather than oblique to avoid lenticular injury and sutureless sclerotomies are not advised because pediatric sclera is thinner than adult which precludes a watertight seal [36]. Vitrectomy gauges typically used include 23G, 25G, and 27G [35]. Vitrectomy and membranectomy may then be performed taking care to avoid iatrogenic retinal breaks. For patients with retrolental adhesions and limited retrolental space, limbal vitrectomy with lensectomy can be performed [36].

For advanced disease, open-sky vitrectomy has also been described with limited success [31, 38]. Although less commonly performed these days, open-sky vitrectomy allows direct visualization of posterior structures after removal of the cornea and lens. This has the advantage of easier access for surgical instruments to the area of pathology, and anterior structures are more readily accessible and more visible; however, this technique risks intraoperative hypotony, choroidal hemorrhage, and globe instability [39].

Lifting the posterior hyaloid membrane is often difficult and complete PVD might not be achieved, and some recommend limiting attempts at PVD induction to avoid iatrogenic breaks [35]. Triamcinolone acetonide can be used intraoperatively to help visualize residual vitreous and assist in removal of persistent tractional membranes. Enzyme-assistant vitrectomy with tissue plasminogen activator [40], autologous plasmin [41], or Ocriplasmin [42] are still being investigated for pediatric vitrectomy but their utility remains to be elucidated. If full vitrectomy or membranectomy is unable to be achieved, silicone oil may be used for endotamponade with fair results [43], however there is the risk of subretinal migration of silicone oil if retinal breaks are present [36].

SB still is advantageous as a primary treatment or adjunct. Several case reports have described the use of SB in IP to minimize tractional forces anterior to the equator [15, 24, 31]. In stage 4A ROP, SB has been shown to prevent further progression of RD and may limit ischemia in the detached retina [44]. It is unclear whether this would apply to IP but extraordinary efforts are often required for disease control. Unlike in adults, the induced myopic shift from SB in pediatrics is large (−11 diopters) and risks refractive amblyopia [45]. Moreover, buckle division or removal is required typically within 6 months for children below the age of 2 years [36]. The role of SB in IP remains uncertain but may be helpful in select cases.

Anatomic success in repair of tractional RDs in IP is uncommon, estimated between 28 and 50% [12, 31], and multiple surgeries are often required. Moreover, many patients are poor surgical candidates at initial presentation due to advanced disease and poor visual potential, highlighting the need for early diagnosis and frequent monitoring.

Rhegmatogenous RD Repair

Rhegmatogenous RDs generally occur in the older subset (31.5 years of age) [15] and may be amenable to standard repairs. Rhegmatogenous RDs have been described in adult ROP and often require multiple surgeries. Patients with IP have been found to have retinal tears at the border of the vascular and avascular retina and therefore require lifelong follow up [15, 26, 46]. Some cases may even spontaneously resolve on their own without intervention [47], although this is an exception to the rule. As with routine rhegmatogenous RD repair, SBs can be used as well [48].

Conclusion

IP is an aggressive disease that leads to progressive retinal ischemia which may be blinding. Management of IP ultimately relies on early screening, frequent monitoring, and low threshold to treat retinal ischemia with laser photocoagulation, anti-VEGF agents or cryotherapy early during the course of the disease. Should these methods fail, and tractional RD develop, surgical management can be undertaken but outcomes are generally poor.

Review Questions

1. A 2-month-old male infant presents with a vesicular rash, suspicious for IP. What is the likely genetic karyotype of this patient?

a. 46, XX or somatic mosaicism
b. 47, XXY or somatic mosaicism
c. Somatic mosaicism
d. None of the above: the patient does not have IP as all male carriers die in utero

2. An infant is referred for ophthalmic evaluation of incontinentia pigmenti. Fundus exam reveals stage 1 IP. What is the recommended management approach?

a. 360° panretinal photocoagulation
b. FA guided laser photocoagulation
c. Cryotherapy
d. Prophylactic scleral buckle

3. What type of retinal detachment is most commonly seen in adult patients with incontinentia pigmenti?

a. Tractional
b. Rhegmatogenous
c. Both
d. Neither are seen

Answers

1. **(B)** Incontinentia pigmenti is an autosomal dominant X-linked disorder. 90–97% of patients with this disorder are female, however, at least 120 reports of males with incontinentia pigmenti have been reported. Male infants with incontinentia pigmenti typically have Klinefelter's syndrome (47, XXY) or somatic mosaicism.

2. **(B)** Stage 1 incontinentia pigmenti, per the grading scheme devised by Montezuma et al. is incomplete peripheral vascularization, abnormal arteriovenous connections, tortuosity and/or engorgement of retinal vessels. These patients benefit from laser photocoagulation. However, FA guided laser therapy is recommended because peripheral areas of retina avascularity and neovascularization can often be difficult to identify.

3. **(B)** 31% of patients with IP develop retinal detachments. The pathophysiology of the retinal detachment appears to follow a bimodal distribution with tractional detachments occurring more commonly in children (median age 1.5 years) and rhegmatogenous detachments occurring more commonly in adults (median age 31.5).

References

1. Garrod A. Peculiar pigmentation of the skin of an infant. 1906;39:216.
2. B B. Eigentumliche bischer nicht beschriebene pigmentaffektion (incontinentia pigmenti). Schweiz Med Wochenschr 1926;7:404–5.
3. Sulzberger M. Uber eine bischer nicht beschriebene congenitale pigmentanomalie (incontinentia pigmenti). Arch Dermatol Syph (Berl). 1928; v. 154.
4. Buinauskiene J, Buinauskaite E, Valiukeviciene S. Incontinentia pigmenti (Bloch-Sulzberger syndrome) in neonates. Medicina. 2005;41(6):496–9.
5. Fusco F, Paciolla M, Conte MI, et al. Incontinentia pigmenti: report on data from 2000 to 2013. Orphanet J Rare Dis. 2014;9:93.
6. Carney RG. Incontinentia pigmenti. A world statistical analysis. Arch Dermatol. 1976;112 (4):535–42.
7. Minić S, Obradović M, Kovacević I, Trpinac D. Ocular anomalies in incontinentia pigmenti: literature review and meta-analysis. Srpski arhiv za celokupno lekarstvo;138(7–8):408–13.
8. Adam MP, Ardinger HH, Pagon RA, et al. GeneReviews. 1993.
9. Cammarata-Scalisi F, Fusco F, Ursini MV. Incontinentia Pigmenti. Actas Dermosifiliogr (Engl Ed). 2019;110(4):273–8.
10. Fusco F, Pescatore A, Bal E, et al. Alterations of the IKBKG locus and diseases: an update and a report of 13 novel mutations. Hum Mutat. 2008;29(5):595–604.

11. Swinney CC, Han DP, Karth PA. Incontinentia Pigmenti: a comprehensive review and update. Ophthalmic Surg Lasers Imaging Retina. 2015;46(6):650–7.

12. Huang NT, Summers CG, McCafferty BK, et al. Management of Retinopathy in Incontinentia Pigmenti: a systematic review and update. Los Angeles, CA: Sage; 2018. v. 2.

13. O'Doherty M, Mc Creery K, Green AJ, et al. Incontinentia pigmenti–ophthalmological observation of a series of cases and review of the literature. Br J Ophthalmol. 2011; 95(1):11–6.

14. Hahn P, Kim JE, Stinnett S, et al. Aflibercept-related sterile inflammation. Ophthalmology. 2013;120(5):1100-1.e1.

15. Chen CJ, Han IC, Tian J, et al. Extended follow-up of treated and untreated retinopathy in Incontinentia Pigmenti: analysis of peripheral vascular changes and incidence of retinal detachment. JAMA Ophthalmol. 2015;133(5):542–8.

16. Catalano RA, Lopatynsky M, Tasman WS. Treatment of proliferative retinopathy associated with incontinentia pigmenti. Am J Ophthalmol. 1990;110(6):701–2.

17. Michel S, Reynaud C, Daruich A, et al. Early management of sight threatening retinopathy in incontinentia pigmenti. Orphanet J Rare Dis. 2020;15(1):223.

18. Nguyen JK, Brady-Mccreery KM. Laser photocoagulation in preproliferative retinopathy of incontinentia pigmenti. J AAPOS. 2001;5(4):258–9.

19. Watzke RC, Stevens TS, Carney RG. Retinal vascular changes of incontinentia pigmenti. Arch Ophthalmol. 1976;94(5):743–6.

20. Jandeck C. Successful treatment of severe retinal vascular abnormalities in incontinentia pigmenti. Retina. 2004;24(4):631.

21. Jalali S, Azad R, Trehan HS, et al. Technical aspects of laser treatment for acute retinopathy of prematurity under topical anesthesia. Indian journal of ophthalmology;58(6):509–15.

22. Rahi J, Hungerford J. Early diagnosis of the retinopathy of incontinentia pigmenti: successful treatment by cryotherapy. Br J Ophthalmol. 1990;74(6):377–9.

23. Yu YS, Cho BJ. Cryotherapy for retinopathy of incontinentia pigmenti. Korean journal of ophthalmology: KJO. 1991;5(1):47–50.

24. Ann C. Incontinentia pigmenti: a florid case with a fulminant clinical course in a newborn. Retina. 2000;20(5):558.

25. Ng EYJ, Connolly BP, McNamara JA, et al. A comparison of laser photocoagulation with cryotherapy for threshold retinopathy of prematurity at 10 years: part 1. Visual function and structural outcome. Ophthalmology 2002;109(5):928–34; discussion 35.

26. Greven CM, Tasman W. Rhegmatogenous retinal detachment following cryotherapy in retinopathy of prematurity. Arch Ophthalmol. 1989;107(7):1017–8.

27. Ho M, Yip WWK, Chan VCK, Young AL. Successful treatment of refractory proliferative retinopathy of incontinentia pigmenti by intravitreal ranibizumab as adjunct therapy in a 4-year-old child. Retinal cases & brief reports;11(4):352–5.

28. Shah PK, Bachu S, Narendran V, et al. Intravitreal bevacizumab for incontinentia pigmenti. Journal of pediatric ophthalmology and strabismus 2013;50 Online:e52-e4.

29. Ni Y, Huang X, Ruan L, et al. Intravitreal injection of ranibizumab in severe retinopathy of incontinentia pigmenti. J AAPOS. 2018;22(4):325-7.e3.

30. Avery RL. What is the evidence for systemic effects of intravitreal anti-VEGF agents, and should we be concerned? Br J Ophthalmol. 2014;98(Suppl 1):i7-10.

31. Wald KJ, Mehta MC, Katsumi O, et al. Retinal detachments in incontinentia pigmenti. Arch Ophthalmol. 1993;111(5):614–7.

32. Fard AK, Goldberg MF. Persistence of fetal vasculature in the eyes of patients with incontinentia pigment. Arch Ophthalmol. 1998;116(5):682–4.

33. Goldberg MF. The blinding mechanisms of incontinentia pigmenti. Ophthalmic Genet. 1994;15(2):69–76.

34. Goldberg MF. Macular vasculopathy and its evolution in incontinentia pigmenti. Trans Am Ophthalmol Soc 1998;96:55–65; discussion-72.

35. Roohipoor R, Karkhaneh R, Riazi-Esfahani M, et al. Surgical management in advanced stages of retinopathy of prematurity; our experience. J Ophthalmic Vis Res. 2009;4(3):185–90.
36. Gan NY, Lam W-C. Special considerations for pediatric vitreoretinal surgery. Taiwan J Ophthalmol;8(4):237–42.
37. Lightfoot D, Irvine AR. Vitrectomy in infants and children with retinal detachments caused by cicatricial retrolental fibroplasia. Am J Ophthalmol. 1982;94(3):305–12.
38. Hirose T, Katsumi O, Mehta MC, Schepens CL. Vision in stage 5 retinopathy of prematurity after retinal reattachment by open-sky vitrectomy. Arch Ophthalmol. 1993;111(3):345–9.
39. Schepens CL. Clinical and research aspects of subtotal open-sky vitrectomy. XXXVII Edward Jackson Memorial Lecture. American journal of ophthalmology 1981;91(2):143–71.
40. Chuang CC, Chen SN. Induction of posterior vitreous detachment in pediatric vitrectomy by preoperative intravitreal injection of tissue plasminogen activator. J Pediatr Ophthalmol Strabismus. 2016;53(2):113–8.
41. Wu WC, Drenser KA, Lai M, et al. Plasmin enzyme-assisted vitrectomy for primary and reoperated eyes with stage 5 retinopathy of prematurity. Retina. 2008;28(3 Suppl):S75-80.
42. Drenser K, Girach A, Capone A. A randomized, placebo-controlled study of intravitreal ocriplasmin in pediatric patients scheduled for vitrectomy. Retina. 2016;36(3):565–75.
43. Scott IU, Flynn HW, Azen SP, et al. Silicone oil in the repair of pediatric complex retinal detachments: a prospective, observational, multicenter study. Ophthalmology 1999;106 (7):1399–407; discussion 407.
44. Hinz BJ, de Juan E, Repka MX. Scleral buckling surgery for active stage 4A retinopathy of prematurity. Ophthalmology. 1998;105(10):1827–30.
45. Chow DR, Ferrone PJ, Trese MT. Refractive changes associated with scleral buckling and division in retinopathy of prematurity. Arch Ophthalmol. 1998;116(11):1446–8.
46. Equi RA, Bains HS, Jampol L, Goldberg MF. Retinal tears occurring at the border of vascular and avascular retina in adult patients with incontinentia pigmenti. Retina. 2003;23(4):574–6.
47. Fekrat S, Humayun MS, Goldberg MF. Spontaneous retinal reattachment in incontinentia pigmenti. Retina. 1998;18(1):75–7.
48. Chen CJ, Han IC, Goldberg MF. Variable expression of retinopathy in a pedigree of patients with incontinentia pigmenti. Retina. 2015;35(12):2627–32.

Norrie Disease

S. Tammy Hsu, Grant Justin, and Lejla Vajzovic

Abstract

Norrie disease disease is a rare X-linked recessive disorder characterized by abnormal retinal development and manifesting as congenital blindness or early childhood blindness in male infants. This chapter discusses the clinical features, genetic testing, differential diagnoses, and management of Norrie disease.

Keywords

Norrie disease · Retinal detachment · NDP

Introduction

Norrie disease is a rare X-linked recessive disorder characterized by abnormal retinal development and manifesting as congenital blindness or early childhood blindness in male infants. The etiology is due to mutations in the Norrie Disease Pseudoglioma (NDP) gene, which codes for the norrin protein that is involved in vascular development and the neural differentiation in the retina and inner ear [1]. Patients with Norrie disease may develop cataracts, vitreous hemorrhage, and

S. T. Hsu · G. Justin
Duke Ophthalmology, Durham, NC, USA
e-mail: s.tammyhsu@duke.edu

G. Justin
e-mail: grant.justin@duke.edu

L. Vajzovic (✉)
Ophthalmology, Adult and Pediatric Vitreoretinal Surgery and Disease, Duke Ophthalmology, Durham, NC, USA
e-mail: lejla.vajzovic@duke.edu

© The Author(s), under exclusive license to Springer Nature Switzerland AG 2023
Ş. Özdek et al. (eds.), *Pediatric Vitreoretinal Surgery*,
https://doi.org/10.1007/978-3-031-14506-3_28

retinal detachments, and eyes often become phthisical in childhood [2–4]. Furthermore, as the norrin protein is also expressed in other parts of the body, the patients may develop other extraocular manifestations including progressive hearing loss and intellectual disability [5].

Diagnosis

Clinical Features

The phenotype for Norrie disease varies, but findings in each person are usually bilateral and symmetric.

Ocular features

- Congenital blindness or early childhood blindness from retinal detachment
- Vitreous hemorrhage
- Posterior synechiae
- Elevated intraocular pressure
- Corneal opacification
- Phthisis bulbi

Extraocular features

- Hearing loss (median age: 12 years old; 85–90% experience hearing loss by mid-20 s) [5]
- Cognitive impairment (28% [5])
- Behavioral disturbances (45% [5])
- Peripheral vascular disease (50% between 16–30 years old, none under 15 years old) [5]

Genetic Testing

Genetic testing can provide definitive diagnosis of Norrie disease. Molecular genetic testing can identify the mutation causing the disease in most affected males. Referral to a genetic counselor or specialist can help identify the proper testing needed.

Prenatal Testing

Norrie disease may be able to be detected on prenatal tests. Genetic testing by amniocentesis may detect mutations suggestive of Norrie disease, thus enabling early intervention with prophylactic laser [6, 7]. Prenatal ultrasound in the third trimester may show bilateral intraocular hyperechogenic vitreous opacities indicative of persistent hyperplastic primary vitreous and retinal detachment [8–10].

Differential Diagnosis

The differential diagnoses for Norrie disease include those that may present with leukocoria in infancy or early childhood. Notably, many of the differential diagnoses are the NDP-related retinopathies, a group of pediatric retinal vascular disorders with etiologies also based in mutations in the NDP gene.

Differential Diagnosis	Differentiating factors from Norrie disease
Persistent fetal vasculature	– Typically unilateral, sporadic – Due to persistence of intraocular fetal vasculature
Familial exudative vitreoretinopathy	– Can be autosomal dominant or X-linked – Progresses more slowly; retinal detachment may not occur until later in life
Retinopathy of prematurity	– Occurs in premature infants (usually <32 weeks with low birthweight <1250 g) treated with supplemental oxygen – Can undergo spontaneous regression
Coats' disease	– Typically unilateral, sporadic – Characterized by abnormal development of blood vessel, yellow exudation leading to retinal detachment
Retinoblastoma	– Exam shows white retinal tumors of various sizes and location and may be associated with vitreous or subretinal seeding or retinal detachment – Imaging shows calcifications
Toxocariasis	– Parasitic disease of the eye after exposure to infected puppies – Retinal lesion leading to retinal detachment
Walker-Warburg syndrome	– Presents with hydrocephalus and agyria
Trisomy 13	– Presents with cleft lip/palate, polydactyly, cardiac defects

Management

Currently, no definitive treatments exist for these patients that would restore vision, and the goal of present attempts at medical and surgical management is to optimize anatomic results.

Medical management

- Laser photocoagulation—some experts recommend early prophylactic laser treatment to avascular retina [6, 7, 10]
- Consult with medical geneticist for genetic counseling
- Multidisciplinary approach to evaluation and management of auditory and cognitive/behavioral symptoms
- Consider possible planned preterm delivery for early intervention if Norrie disease is diagnosed in utero [11]

Surgical management

- Early vitrectomy in cases of Norrie disease with incomplete retinal detachment may mitigate the severity of vision loss by transecting residual hyaloidal vessel remnants and thus releasing retinal traction [12]
- Peeling retrolental fibroplasia in eyes with total retinal detachments may allow the retina to reattach, as well as decrease ciliary body traction and improve rates of hypotony

Prognosis

The natural history of Norrie disease is blindness from bilateral no light perception vision and development of phthisis bulbi. However, with early treatment, the visual and anatomic prognosis may be less dismal as patients may be more likely to retain at least light perception vision and are less likely to develop phthisis [12]. Research is underway involving other possible future treatments; a study involving intravitreal injections of Norrin into mouse models of oxygen-induced retinopathy appeared promising [13]. Hopefully the future development of treatments for Norrie disease may improve prognosis.

Clinical Scenario

Case 1

A 3-week-old male infant born full-term with an uncomplicated pregnancy was referred by his local eye doctor for evaluation of congenital glaucoma. The mother had noticed that his right eye appeared larger and cloudier than his left at birth, and that his eyes did not seem to be focusing.

On exam, the infant did not seem to have any convincing response to light in either eye and did not have an OKN response. Pupils were sluggish bilaterally. Intraocular pressure was 29 in the right and 16 in the left. Portable slit lamp exam

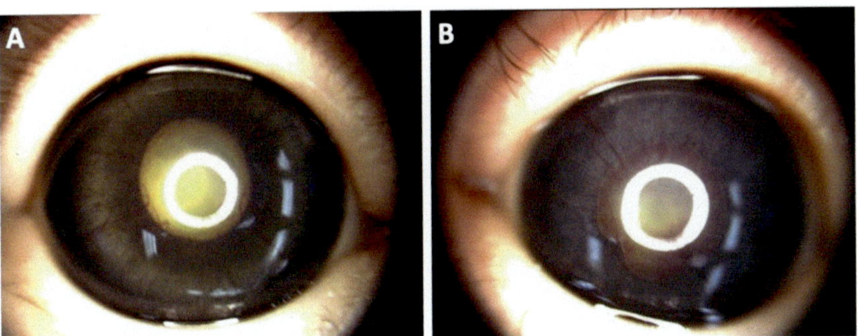

Fig. 28.1 Photographs of the right and left eyes (**A** and **B**, respectively) showing prominent iris vessels growing onto the anterior lens capsules and bilateral retrolental opacities

was notable for buphthalmos in the right eye with trace corneal edema, shallow anterior chambers bilaterally, 360-degree iris bombe in the right eye and iridocorneal apposition in the left eye, bilateral iris transillumination defects and prominent iris vessels growing onto the anterior lens capsules, and bilateral retrolental opacities (Fig. 28.1). Dilated fundus exam was obscured by the retrolental opacities, but the retina appeared to be adherent to the posterior lens capsule (Fig. 28.2). B-scan ultrasonography showed bilateral funnel retinal detachments (Fig. 28.3). B-scan ultrasound biomicroscopy showed the iris bombe with anterior lens dislocation of the right eye (Fig. 28.4A), and iridocorneal apposition with anterior lens dislocation of the left eye (Fig. 28.4B).

To treat the iris bombe, the retinal surgeon performed a 25G lensectomy, peripheral iridotomy, and anterior membrane peel. Post-operatively, the patient's intraocular pressures normalized with IOP-lowering drops. He was then monitored regularly. At the follow-up visits, vision still remained at no light perception.

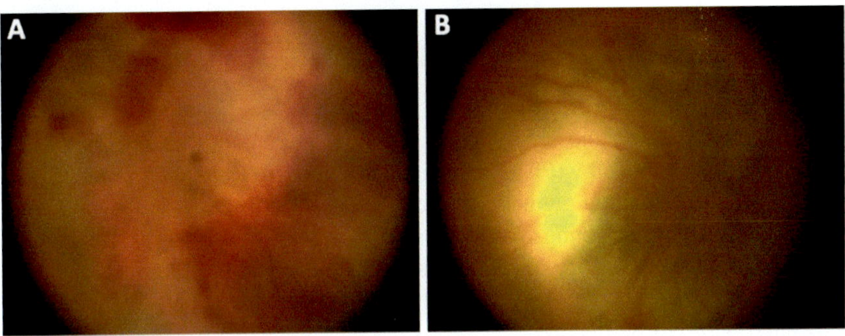

Fig. 28.2 Retcam images of the right and left eyes (**A** and **B**, respectively) showing retina adherent to the posterior lens capsule

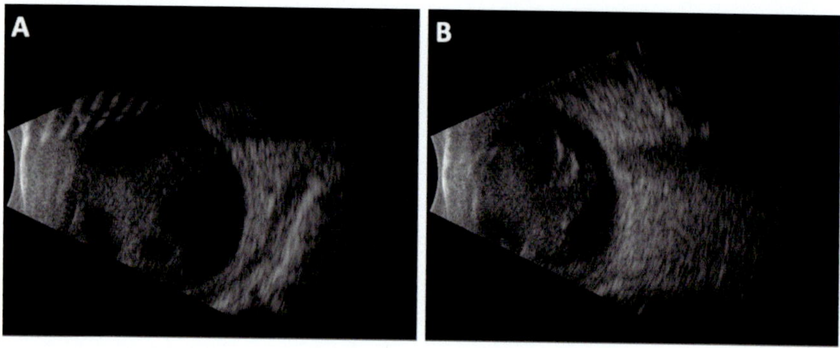

Fig. 28.3 B-scan ultrasonography showing funnel retinal detachments of the right and left eyes (**A** and **B**, respectively). No masses or calcifications were noted

Fig. 28.4 B-scan ultrasound biomicroscopy showed iris bombe with anterior lens dislocation of the right eye (**A**), and iridocorneal apposition with anterior lens dislocation of the left eye (**B**)

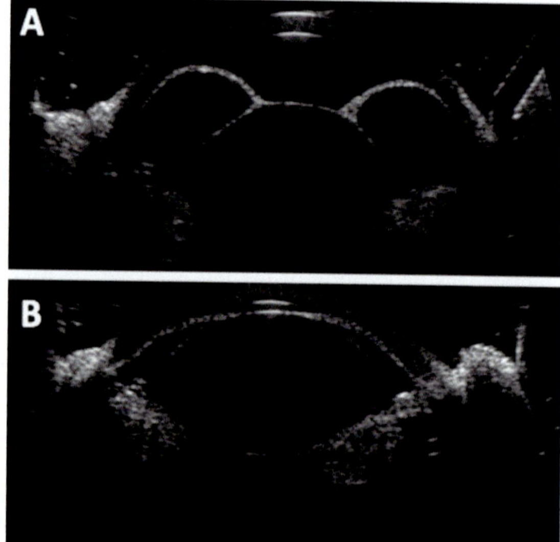

The differential diagnoses for this patient's presentation included familial exudative vitreoretinopathy (FEVR), Norrie disease, persistent hyperplastic primary vitreous and incontinentia pigmenti. Genetic testing showed a pathological variant of the NDP gene, confirming Norrie disease. The patient's family was counseled regarding the poor visual prognosis and hereditary nature of the disease. The patient was also referred for audiology evaluation given the extraocular comorbidities associated with Norrie disease.

Case 2

A 5-month-old male, born full-term with an uncomplicated pregnancy, with bilateral retinal detachments and the presumptive diagnosis of either FEVR or Norrie disease had undergone vitrectomy for repair of retinal detachment in the right eye was referred for further evaluation and care. Family history was notable for maternal great-uncle and maternal male cousin who both also had history of early retinal detachments. Exam showed response to the preferential looking test in the right eye, and unclear response to light in the left eye. Dilated fundus exam of the right eye showed severe disc dragging with retinal fibrosis and scarring mid-periphery, retinal folds emanating and following the vascular arcades, and a grayish retina. B-scan ultrasonography of the left eye revealed a funnel retinal detachment. Genetic testing showed a missense mutation in exon 2, a mutation previously reported in Norrie patients.

The patient had fix and follow vision in the right eye after the operation. He then developed a recurrent tractional retinal detachment at 3 years of age. The surgeon performed a vitrectomy, scleral buckle, membrane peel, endolaser, and silicone oil. Afterward silicone oil removal, his vision remained stable at 20/200 in the right eye for years. At 10 years old, the patient was noted to have VMT/TRD in the right eye (Fig. 28.5A), which was managed with a membrane peel. His vision continued to remain stable. A progressive cataract in the eye was removed and an intraocular lens placed.

At 14-years-old, no extraocular manifestations of Norrie disease had been noted yet, however he had recurrent tractional membranes in his right eye that were

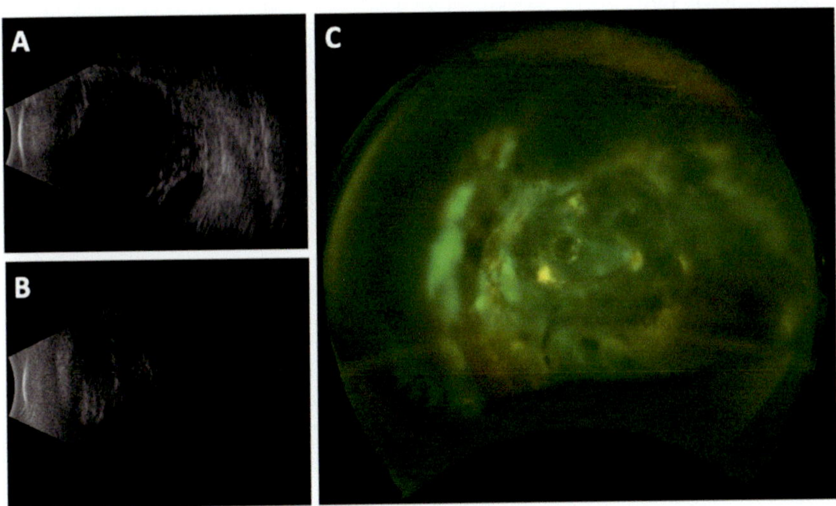

Fig. 28.5 B-scan ultrasonography of the right eye showing a tractional retinal detachment (**A**) and phthisical left eye (**B**). Optos photo taken at the one-month post-op visit (**C**). Photo courtesy of Dr. Cynthia Toth

peeled again. His exam was notable for temporal retinoschisis and a retinal break that was barricaded with laser. The left eye was phthisical and undergoing symptomatic management (Fig. 28.5B). At his one-month post-op visit, visual acuity was 20/400 and the subretinal fluid had greatly improved (Fig. 28.5C).

Conclusion

Norrie disease is a devastating disease that typically leads to blindness (no light perception) in childhood. However, advances in prenatal testing may offer allow for improved prognosis with early intervention.

Revision Questions

1. What is the inheritance pattern of Norrie disease?

a. Autosomal dominant
b. Autosomal recessive
c. X-linked dominant
d. X-linked recessive

2. Which of the following is *not* a common extraocular clinical manifestation of Norrie disease?

a. Aortic aneurysm
b. Behavioral or cognitive challenges
c. Hearing loss
d. Peripheral vascular disease

3. Mutations in what gene are implicated in Norrie disease?

a. IKBKG
b. NDP
c. PAX6
d. RB1

Answers

1. D
2. A
3. B

References

1. Meindl A, Berger W, Meitinger T, et al. Norrie disease is caused by mutations in an extracellular protein resembling C-terminal globular domain of mucins. Nat Genet. 1992;2(2):139–43. https://doi.org/10.1038/ng1092-139.
2. Drenser KA, Fecko A, Dailey W, Trese MT. A Characteristic phenotypic retinal appearance in norrie disease. Retina. 2007;27(2):243–6. https://doi.org/10.1097/01.iae.0000231380.29644.c3.
3. Wu W-C, Drenser K, Trese M, Capone A Jr, Dailey W. Retinal phenotype-genotype correlation of pediatric patients expressing mutations in the Norrie disease gene. Arch Ophthalmol. 2007;125(2):225–30. https://doi.org/10.1001/archopht.125.2.225.
4. Norrie Disease. National organization for rare disorders, rare disease database.
5. Smith SE, Mullen TE, Graham D, Sims KB, Rehm HL. Norrie disease: Extraocular clinical manifestations in 56 patients. Am J Med Genet A. 2012;158A(8):1909–17. https://doi.org/10.1002/ajmg.a.35469.
6. Chow CC, Kiernan DF, Chau FY, et al. Laser photocoagulation at birth prevents blindness in Norrie's disease diagnosed using amniocentesis. Ophthalmology. 2010;117(12):2402–6. https://doi.org/10.1016/j.ophtha.2010.03.057.
7. Kiernan DF, Blair MP, Shapiro MJ. In utero diagnosis of Norrie disease and early laser preserves visual acuity. Arch Ophthalmol. 2010;128(10):1382. https://doi.org/10.1001/archophthalmol.2010.207.
8. Dubucs C, Merveille M, Kessler S, Sevely A, Chassaing N, Calvas P. Prenatal diagnosis of Norrie disease based on ultrasound findings. Ultrasound Obstet Gynecol. 2019;54(1):138–9. https://doi.org/10.1002/uog.20097.
9. Wu LH, Chen L-H, Xie H, Xie Y-J. Prenatal diagnosis of a case of norrie disease with late development of bilateral ocular malformation. Fetal Pediatric Pathol. 2017;36(3):240–245. https://doi.org/10.1080/15513815.2017.1307474.
10. Redmond RM, Vaughan JI, Jay M, Jay B. In-utero diagnosis of Norrie disease by ultrasonography. Ophthalmic Paediatr Genet. 1993;14(1):1–3. https://doi.org/10.3109/13816819309087615.
11. Sisk RA, Hufnagel RB, Bandi S, Polzin WJ, Ahmed ZM. Planned preterm delivery and treatment of retinal neovascularization in Norrie disease. Ophthalmology. 2014;121(6):1312–3. https://doi.org/10.1016/j.ophtha.2014.01.001.
12. Walsh MK, Drenser KA, Capone A Jr, Trese MT. Early vitrectomy effective for Norrie disease. Arch Ophthalmol. 2010;128(4):456–60. https://doi.org/10.1001/archophthalmol.2009.403.
13. Dailey WA, Drenser KA, Wong SC, et al. Norrin treatment improves ganglion cell survival in an oxygen-induced retinopathy model of retinal ischemia. Exp Eye Res. 2017;164:129–38. https://doi.org/10.1016/j.exer.2017.08.012.

Sickle Cell Retinopathy

29

Ishrat Ahmed and Adrienne W. Scott

Abstract

Sickle cell disease is the most common inherited hematological disorder worldwide. Ocular manifestations of SCD include sickle cell retinopathy (SCR) and maculopathy, which are commonly observed in pediatric and adult patients with SCD. Although patients are often asymptomatic, significant vision loss and blindness can occur from complications of sea fan neovascularization, including vitreous hemorrhage and tractional and rhegmatogenous retinal detachment. This chapter reviews the clinical features of SCR and maculopathy and focuses on the medical and surgical management of SCR.

Keywords

Sickle cell disease · Non-proliferative sickle cell retinopathy · Proliferative sickle cell retinopathy · Sea fan neovascularization · Goldberg staging · Scatter laser photocoagulation · Segmentation technique

Supplementary Information The online version contains supplementary material available at https://doi.org/10.1007/978-3-031-14506-3_29.

I. Ahmed (✉)
Retina Service, Massachusetts Eye and Ear, Harvard Medical School, 243 Charles Street, Boston, MA 02114, USA
e-mail: IAHMED4@meei.harvard.edu

A. W. Scott
Retina Division, Wilmer Eye Institute, Johns Hopkins University School of Medicine, 600 North Wolfe Street, Maumenee 719, Baltimore, MD 21287, USA
e-mail: ascott28@jhmi.edu

Introduction

Background

Sickle cell disease (SCD) is a group of hemoglobinopathies characterized by mutations in the β-globin gene. Patients with SCD can present with various systemic complications, including painful vaso-occlusive crises, acute chest syndrome, pulmonary hypertension, stroke, splenic sequestration, aplastic crisis, and premature death [1]. SCD also results in various ocular manifestations, including dilation of small conjunctival vessels [2], segmental iris atrophy [3, 4], hyphema resulting in ocular hypertension [5–7], and ischemic optic neuropathy [8]. This chapter will focus mainly on the retinal manifestations of SCD, the most common cause of vision loss in these patients.

Epidemiology

SCD is the most common inherited hematological disorder worldwide. The birth prevalence of SCD is highest in Africa with 1,125 cases per 100,000 live births [9, 10]. The global prevalence of SCD and sickle cell trait is 3.2 million and 43 million, respectively [10]. Although patients with sickle cell trait are asymptomatic, they may have systemic manifestations under severe conditions such as hypoxia [11]. Newborn screening guidelines have led to improvements in the early diagnosis and management of patients with SCD [12].

Pathophysiology

Adult hemoglobin (Hb A) consists of two α-globin subunits, two β-globin subunits, and a central heme molecule. Point mutations in the sixth position of the β-globin gene result in the production of Hb S (glutamic acid to valine mutation) or Hb C (glutamic acid to lysine mutation) [1, 13, 14]. Furthermore, mutations that impair β-globin production result in β-thalassemia. Combinations of these mutations result in sickle cell anemia (homozygous HbSS disease) and the less common sickle cell variants (heterozygous HbSC disease and HbSβ-thalassemia) [1, 14].

The systemic complications of SCD result from impaired oxygen transport and abnormal Hb S polymerization, which increases cellular rigidity causing sickling and hemolysis [15]. Polymerization occurs under abnormal stimuli, such as hypoxia, dehydration, acidosis, and infection. These intracellular changes, as well as vascular endothelial dysfunction, lead to tissue ischemia and necrosis [15].

Clinical Features

Non-proliferative sickle cell retinopathy (NPSR) includes salmon patch lesions (Fig. 29.1A), angioid streaks (Fig. 29.1B), iridescent spots, and black sunbursts (Fig. 29.1C–E), and typically do not cause vision loss. Salmon patch lesions are localized accumulations of blood between the retina and internal limiting membrane and result from hemorrhage from an occluded or necrotic arteriole [16, 17]. Angioid streaks are more frequently noted in patients with HbSS disease and rarely lead to choroidal neovascularization [18, 19]. Iridescent spots consist of hemosiderin-laden macrophages within a schisis cavity following arteriolar occlusion [16]. Black sunbursts consist of retinal pigment epithelium (RPE) hypertrophy due to intraretinal hemorrhage tracking into the subretinal space [16]. Additional findings include increased vascular tortuosity [18, 20, 21].

The Goldberg classification (Table 29.1) describes additional non-proliferative and proliferative vascular changes in SCD, observed as stepwise vascular remodeling in the retinal periphery. Stage I retinopathy consists of peripheral arteriolar occlusions, which may present as silver-wiring of arterioles (Fig. 29.1D, E) [22]. Stage II retinopathy is defined by the presence of arteriovenous anastomoses. Sea

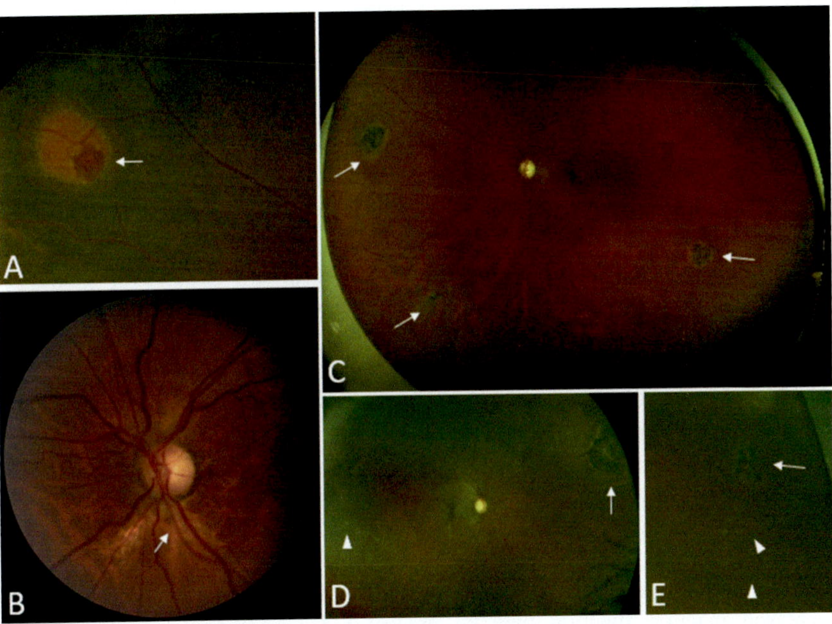

Fig. 29.1 Retinal biomarkers of non-proliferative sickle cell retinopathy are demonstrated. **A** Salmon patch (arrow) in the left eye of a 20-year-old male with HbSC disease. **B** Angioid streak (arrow) in a 45-year-old patient with HbSS disease. **C** Peripheral sunburst lesions (arrows) in a 16-year-old patient with HbSS disease. **D** Right eye and **E** close-up of left eye of a 24-year-old patient with HbSS disease with prominent peripheral black sunbursts (arrows) and ischemic vessels (arrowheads)

Table 29.1 Goldberg classification of sickle cell retinopathy

Stage	Sickle cell retinopathy findings
I	Peripheral arterial occlusions
II	Peripheral arteriovenous anastomoses
III	Neovascular and fibrous proliferations
IV	Vitreous hemorrhage
V	Retinal detachment

fan neovascularization (Fig. 29.2A–D), noted in stage III retinopathy, is the hallmark finding in proliferative sickle cell retinopathy (PSR) [22, 23]. Stage III retinopathy can lead to vitreous hemorrhage (Stage IV) and tractional and/or rhegmatogenous retinal detachments (TRD) most frequently involving the peripheral retina (Stage V) (Fig. 29.2B, F). Vitreous membrane formation from chronic vitreous hemorrhage can cause traction whereas retinal breaks are caused by retinal ischemia and atrophy [22, 23]. Interestingly, compared to proliferative diabetic retinopathy (PDR), PSR does not extend into deep retinal tissues and instead remains localized to the nerve fiber layer and ganglion cell layer on optical coherence tomography (OCT). This results in less vitreoretinal traction compared to PDR, and therefore, decreased risk of tractional detachment in PSR compared to PDR [24].

Overall, the prevalence of PSR is higher in patients with HbSC disease (approximately 43%) compared to HbSS disease (approximately 14%), and usually occurs in younger patients, by 24 to 26 years of age [25]. PSR can also rarely occur in patients with sickle cell trait who also have co-morbidities such as diabetes, syphilis, tuberculosis or sarcoidosis [26]. Loss of visual acuity occurs in 10–12% of eyes with untreated PSR, most frequently from vitreous hemorrhage and retinal detachment [27, 28].

Although peripheral retinal changes are the hallmark features of sickle cell retinopathy, the vascular and anatomical structures of the macula are also affected by episodes of retinal ischemia from repetitive vaso-occlusions in the macular microvasculature. The most common macular findings include enlarged foveal splaying, foveal avascular zone [29], and macular retinal thinning [30], particularly in the temporal macula due to involvement of the watershed zone near the horizontal raphe (Fig. 29.2E) [31–33]. Sickle cell maculopathy, including temporal thinning, can also occur in younger patients (Fig. 29.3). Flow deficits on OCT angiography as shown in Fig. 29.3C occur commonly in pediatric patients with SCD as young as age 5 [31]. Most patients with SCD and macular thinning maintain good distance visual acuity and remain clinically asymptomatic, although decreased macular function may be present [34]. Additional macular findings include paracentral acute middle maculopathy (PAMM) and acute macular neuroretinopathy (AMN) [35]. These macular findings can present as sudden onset of central scotomas, metamorphopsia, and reduced contrast sensitivity [36, 37].

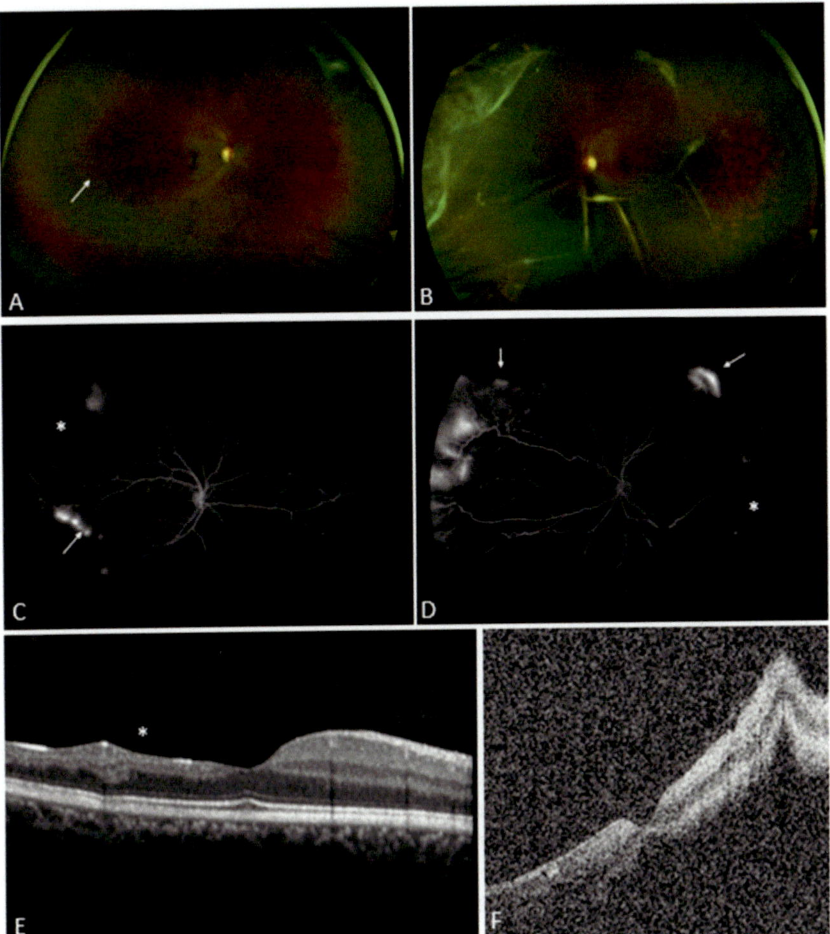

Fig. 29.2 24-year-old patient with HbSC disease with 20/16 vision in the right eye and 20/125 vision in the left eye. Ultra-widefield fundus photos demonstrate **A** stage III retinopathy, or sea fan neovascularization (arrow), in the right eye, and **B** stage V retinopathy, or retinal detachment, in the left eye. **C, D** Fluorescein angiogram highlights areas of leakage from sea fan neovascularization (arrows) and peripheral ischemia (asterisks) in both eyes. Optical coherence tomography in the same patient demonstrates **E** temporal macular thinning (asterisk) in the right eye, and **F** macula-involving retinal detachment in the left eye

Medical Management

Currently, scatter laser photocoagulation remains the gold-standard treatment for stage III PSR to prevent progression to vitreous hemorrhage or retinal detachment. Small peripheral sea fan neovascular complexes can be observed in select cases, as

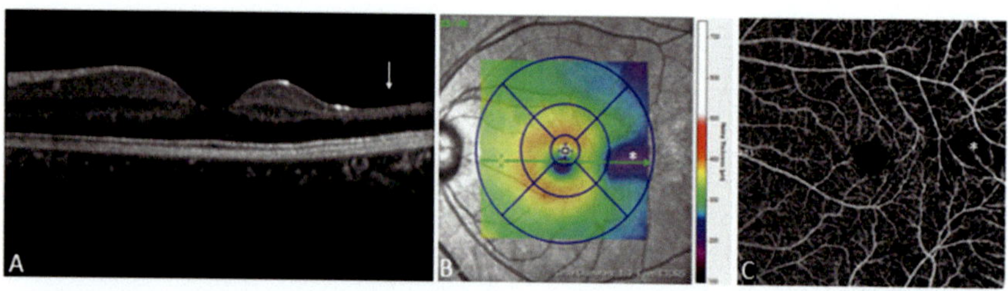

Fig. 29.3 14-year-old male with HbSS disease with **A** temporal macular thinning noted on SD-OCT (arrow) and **B** focal retinal thinning on OCT thickness map (asterisk). **C** *En face* optical coherence tomography angiography demonstrates capillary dropout (asterisk) corresponding to the area of retinal thinning

these neovascular lesions may auto-infarct and regress without visual consequence in upwards of 32% of eyes [25]. Observation with deferral of laser treatment can be considered if the sea fan neovascular complexes are small, and if a patient is likely to adhere to follow up recommendations for serial exams and imaging to monitor the neovascularization for progression. Initiation of laser treatment is recommended if close follow up with serial fundus exams and imaging is not feasible, in monocular patients, if sea fan complexes appear to enlarge or cause progressive retinal traction, or in case of progression to vitreous hemorrhage. Figure 29.4 demonstrates bilateral auto-infarcted sea fan neovascular complexes in an asymptomatic patient 14-year-old patient with HbSC disease.

Scatter laser photocoagulation is the main treatment modality for large and rapidly growing neovascular lesions and could also be considered for the patient in Fig. 29.4. Although laser treatment does not reduce the incidence of neovascularization, it has been shown to improve PSR regression, reduce sea fan recurrence, and decrease the risk of vision loss from vitreous hemorrhage compared to untreated eyes [38]. Laser treatment reduces expression of hypoxia-inducible factor 1α (HIF-1α) and vascular endothelial growth factor (VEGF) from ischemic retina. As such we recommend barricading the neovascular complex and treating the areas of peripheral ischemia as well as the area bordering ischemic retina as demonstrated in Fig. 29.5 [39]. Ultra-widefield fluorescein angiogram (FA) is useful to guide laser treatment.

Off-label use of intravitreal bevacizumab has been used as an adjunct to laser photocoagulation to treat vitreous hemorrhage in several case reports and small series [40–42]. Pre-operative administration of intravitreal bevacizumab has also been shown to facilitate retinal detachment repair in a case report [43]. It is important to note that intravitreal anti-VEGF injections may lead to further fibrosis and rapid contraction of sea fan neovascular complexes thereby increasing retinal traction [44].

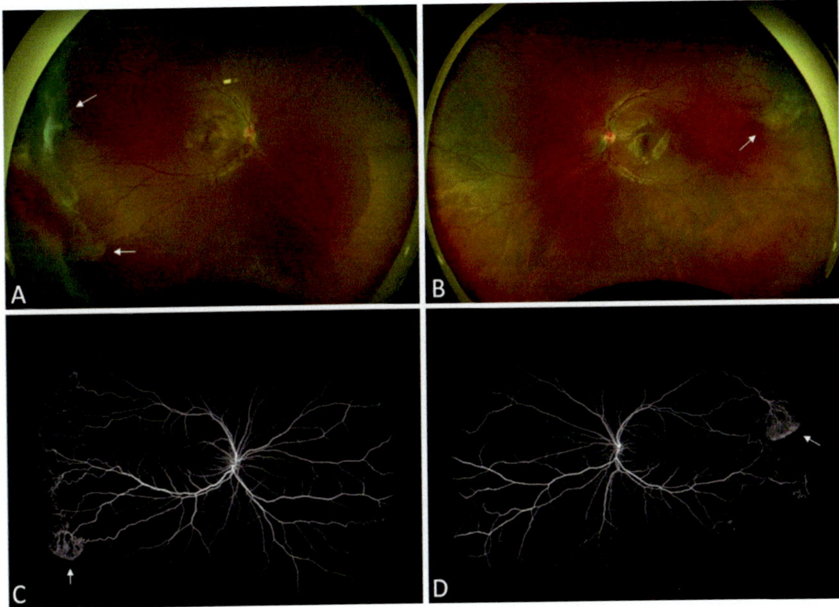

Fig. 29.4 14-year-old patient with HbSC disease who is asymptomatic with 20/20 vision in both eyes. **A, B** Fundus photos show extensive auto-infarcted sea fan neovascularization, with greater involvement in the right eye than left eye. **C, D** Fluorescein angiogram shows extensive peripheral retinal non-perfusion and leakage from sea fan complexes. Close observation with deferral of scatter laser treatment was considered in this case given the sea fan lesions appear to be nearly completely auto-infarcted, and the patient and his family agreed to close follow up and monitoring. *Images courtesy of Nicholas C. Farber, M.D*

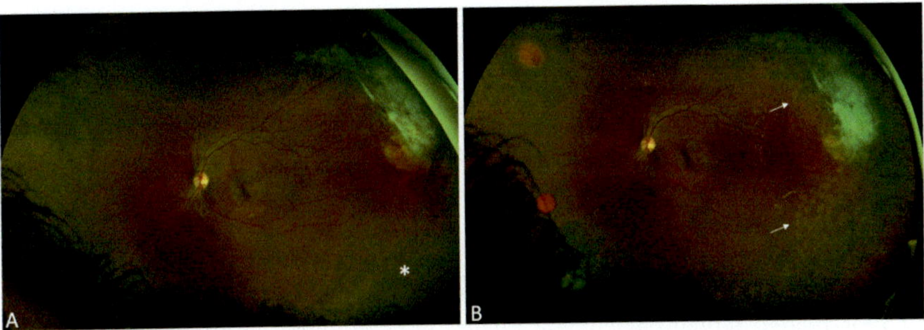

Fig. 29.5 20-year-old male with HbSC disease who presented with **A** a large fibrotic sea fan neovascular lesion in the temporal periphery of the left eye and peripheral retinal ischemia (asterisk). **B** The neovascular lesion was treated with scatter laser photocoagulation. Laser was applied to ischemic retina peripherally and to a border of perfused retina posterior to the neovascular lesion (arrows). A close-up of the salmon patch lesion is shown in Fig. 29.1A

Surgical Management

Indications for surgical management of Stage IV and V PSR include non-clearing vitreous hemorrhage, bilateral vitreous hemorrhage, vitreous hemorrhage in the better-seeing eye of a monocular patient, and retinal detachment. PSR-related retinal complications, such as visually-significant epiretinal membrane (ERM), vitreomacular traction (VMT) (Fig. 29.6) and full-thickness macular holes (FTMH), also warrant repair [28].

Peri-Operative Considerations

Patients with SCD require adequate hydration, supplemental oxygen delivery, and a warm operating room to prevent sickle cell-related adverse events. Pre-operative exchange transfusion may be considered in consultation with a hematologist [45, 46]. Adequate post-operative analgesia is also essential in patients who are prone to systemic vaso-occlusive pain crises under conditions of stress or dehydration.

Careful intraocular pressure monitoring is also required to prevent central retinal artery occlusion. As such, general anesthesia or local anesthesia with a sub-Tenon's block is recommended instead of a retrobulbar block [47]. Carbonic anhydrase inhibitors should be avoided in the post-operative management of ocular hypertension in patients with sickle cell disease as this may promote an acidotic environment in the anterior chamber which may pre-dispose to further sickling of red blood cells [46, 48].

Surgical Considerations

The most common ocular surgical complications in patients with Stage V PSR include iatrogenic retinal breaks and anterior segment ischemia [49, 50]. Scleral buckling was previously associated with anterior segment ischemia. However, scleral buckling has been used safely by avoiding broad and high encircling bands, extraocular muscle injury, compression of posterior ciliary vessels, and excessive cryopexy [46, 48].

Pars plana vitrectomy has also been used frequently for the management of Stage V PSR [48]. The **Surgical Video** demonstrates the 23-gauge vitrectomy setup for PSR-related retinal detachment repair. Triamcinolone is used to highlight the vitreous followed by posterior hyaloid elevation and trimming to the retinal periphery. Diathermy is then applied to sea fan neovascular complexes and any visible breaks. In our experience, small breaks are usually located under the neovascular complexes. The segmentation (rather than delamination) technique is recommended to reduce fibrovascular traction This is achieved by cutting fibrovascular tissue vertically rather than tangentially, thereby eliminating traction on ischemic retina [51]. Using a chandelier and under high magnification, we recommend using bimanual technique with a 25-gauge cutter and either the lighted pick or vertical scissors to segment and remove fibrovascular tissue. Fluid air exchange and draining is then completed through breaks. Endolaser is subsequently applied surrounding breaks and to ischemic peripheral retina guided by pre-operative fluorescein angiography. Gas is generally the preferred tamponade agent, although silicone oil is used if the pathology is located inferiorly or if patient is not able to position post-operatively. We also recommend treating the contralateral eye with scatter laser photocoagulation if indicated while the patient is under general anesthesia.

Surgical Video. *23-gauge pars plana vitrectomy for combined tractional and rhegmatogenous retinal detachment repair of a 24-year-old patient with HbSC disease.* **Video courtesy of Christopher B. Toomey, MD, PhD and Adrienne W. Scott, MD.**

Data on surgical outcomes following PSR-related surgery remain limited. In a recent study of 38 eyes with tractional, rhegmatogenous, and combined retinal detachments in pts with PSR, the anatomic success rate was 79% [52]. Improved visual acuity has been reported in several case series and case reports for retinal detachment, ERM and FTMH repairs [48, 52–55]. Figure 29.7 demonstrates successful primary reattachment at post-operative month one of the patient depicted in Fig. 29.2 under silicone oil tamponade.

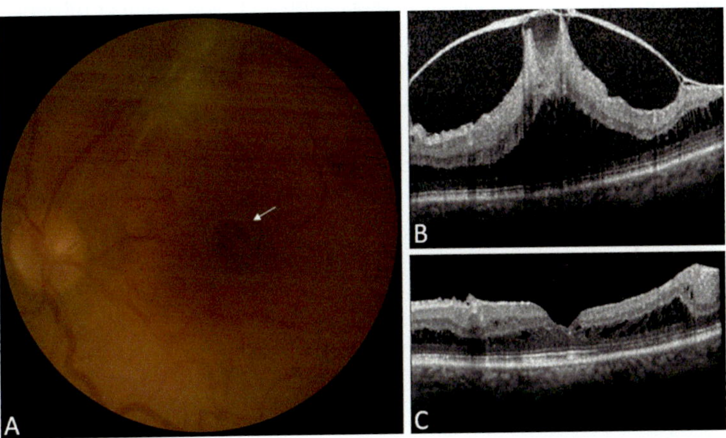

Fig. 29.6 44-year-old patient with HbSC disease who was treated by scatter laser photocoagulation in the left eye for PSR developed **A, B** vitreomacular traction and macular schisis observed on 30-degree fundus photo and OCT. **C** There is significant improvement in foveal contour evidenced by post-operative OCT six months following vitrectomy with membrane peeling

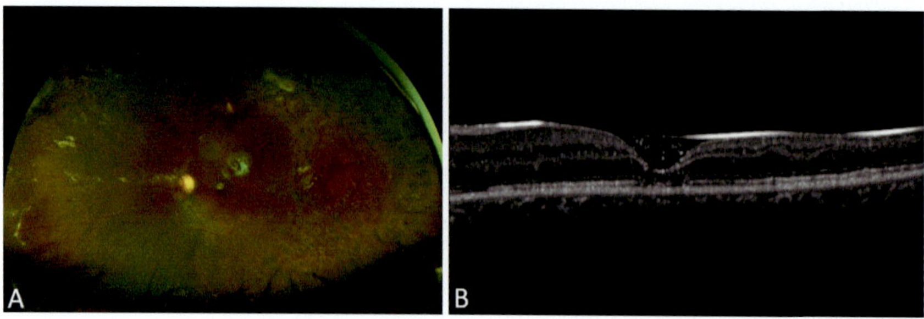

Fig. 29.7 24-year-old patient with HbSC disease following repair of the left eye retinal detachment shown in Fig. 29.2B. **A** The retina remains attached at post-operative month 1 after 23-gauge pars plana vitrectomy and silicone oil tamponade. **B** Optical coherence tomography demonstrates a normalization of foveal contour with focal areas of subfoveal ellipsoid zone disruption

Conclusion

Patients with SCD generally maintain good vision. Macular thinning and loss of vascular density are commonly observed at an early age and are progressive through life in patients with SCD. Vision loss typically occurs from sequelae of PSR advancing to vitreous hemorrhage or retinal detachment. The main treatment modalities for PSR are scatter laser photocoagulation, with adjunct off-label use of intravitreal anti-VEGF agents for persistent vascularization of sea fan complexes, in cases of vitreous hemorrhage, and for pre-operative surgical management of vitreous hemorrhages and retinal detachments. Surgeries in patients with PSR are complex but can be successful with outcomes optimized by careful pre-operative planning with respect to systemic SCD status and peri-operative monitoring of intraocular pressure. Regular retinopathy screening exams with early detection of PSR and treatment when indicated, may help reduce progression of PSR and improve visual outcomes.

Review Questions

1. What is the most likely genotype for a patient presenting with proliferative sickle cell retinopathy?

A. SS
B. SC
C. Sβ-thalassemia
D. AS (sickle cell trait)

2. A 23-year-old asymptomatic patient with HbSS disease presents for a sickle cell retinopathy surveillance exam. Fundus examination reveals a small sea fan neovascular complex in the right eye. What is the recommended first-line management approach?

A. Observation with close monitoring
B. Scatter laser photocoagulation
C. Intravitreal anti-VEGF injection
D. A and B
E. A and C

3. All of the following may be considered for peri-operative management of PSR except?

A. Exchange transfusion
B. Diuresis
C. Hyperoxygenation
D. Pre-operative consultation with hematology
E. Intravenous hydration

Answers

1. B
2. D
3. B

References

1. Elagouz M, Jyothi S, Gupta B, Sivaprasad S. Sickle cell disease and the eye: old and new concepts. Surv Ophthalmol. 2010;55(4):359–77.
2. Condon PI, Serjeant GR. Ocular findings of elderly cases of homozygous sickle-cell disease in Jamaica. Br J Ophthalmol. 1976;60(5):361–4.
3. Chambers J, Puglisi J, Kernitsky R, Wise GN. Iris atrophy in hemoglobin SC disease. Am J Ophthalmol. 1974;77(2):247–9.
4. Galinos S, Rabb MF, Goldberg MF, Frenkel M. Hemoglobin SC disease and iris atrophy. Am J Ophthalmol. 1973;75(3):421–5.
5. Goldberg MF. Sickled erythrocytes, hyphema, and secondary glaucoma: IV. The rate and percentage of sickling of erythrocytes in rabbit aqueous humor, in vitro and in vivo. Ophthalmic Surgery. 1979;10(4):62–69.
6. Goldberg MF. Sickled erythrocytes, hyphema, and secondary glaucoma: I. The diagnosis and treatment of sickled erythrocytes in human hyphemas. Ophthalmic surgery. 1979;10(4): 17–31.
7. Goldberg MF, Dizon R, Raichand M. Sickled erythrocytes, hyphema, and secondary glaucoma: II. Injected sickle cell erythrocytes into human, monkey, and guinea pig anterior chambers: the induction of sickling and secondary glaucoma. Ophthalmic surgery. 1979;10 (4):32–51.
8. Perlman JI, Forman S, Gonzalez ER. Retrobulbar ischemic optic neuropathy associated with sickle cell disease. J Neuro-ophthalmol Official J North Amer Neuro-Ophthalmol Soc. 1994;14(1):45–8.

9. Wastnedge E, Waters D, Patel S, et al. The global burden of sickle cell disease in children under five years of age: a systematic review and meta-analysis. J Glob Health. 2018;8 (2):021103–021103.

10. Global, regional, and national age-sex specific all-cause and cause-specific mortality for 240 causes of death, 1990–2013: a systematic analysis for the Global Burden of Disease Study 2013. The Lancet. 2015;385(9963):117–171.

11. Serjeant GR SB. Sickle cell disease. 3 ed: Oxford University Press; 2001.

12. Benson JM, Therrell BL Jr. History and current status of newborn screening for hemoglobinopathies. Semin Perinatol. 2010;34(2):134–44.

13. Pauling L, Itano HA, Singer SJ, Wells IC. Sickle cell anemia, a molecular disease. Science. 1949;110(2865):543–8.

14. Ashley-Koch A, Yang Q, Olney RS. Sickle Hemoglobin (Hb S) allele and sickle cell disease: a HuGE review. Am J Epidemiol. 2000;151(9):839–45.

15. Sundd P, Gladwin MT, Novelli EM. Pathophysiology of sickle cell disease. Annu Rev Pathol. 2019;14:263–92.

16. Romayanada N, Goldberg MF, Green WR. Histopathology of sickle cell retinopathy. Trans Amer Acad Ophthalmol Otolaryngol Amer Acad Ophthalmol Otolaryngol. 1973;77(5): Op652–676.

17. DA Gagliano JL, Rabb M. Sickle cell disease. In: Tasman WSJE, editor. Duane's clinical ophthalmology, vol. 3. Philadelphia: Lippincott Raven; 1996. p. 1–40.

18. Condon PI, Serjeant GR. Ocular findings in homozygous sickle cell anemia in Jamaica. Am J Ophthalmol. 1972;73(4):533–43.

19. Clarkson JG. The ocular manifestations of sickle-cell disease: a prevalence and natural history study. Trans Am Ophthalmol Soc. 1992;90:481–504.

20. Condon PI, Serjeant GR. Ocular findings in hemoglobin SC disease in Jamaica. Am J Ophthalmol. 1972;74(5):921–31.

21. Welch RB, Goldberg MF. Sickle-cell hemoglobin and its relation to fundus abnormality. Arch Ophthalmol (Chicago, Ill : 1960). 1966;75(3):353–362.

22. Nagpal KC, Goldberg MF, Rabb MF. Ocular manifestations of sickle hemoglobinopathies. Surv Ophthalmol. 1977;21(5):391–411.

23. Goldberg MF. Retinal neovascularization in sickle cell retinopathy. Trans Sect Ophthalmol Amer Acad Ophthalmol Otolaryngol. 1977;83(3 Pt 1):Op409–431.

24. Folgar FA, Reddy S. An in vivo morphologic comparison of retinal neovascularization in sickle cell and diabetic retinopathy. Retinal cases & Brief Reports. 2012;6(1):99–101.

25. Downes SM, Hambleton IR, Chuang EL, Lois N, Serjeant GR, Bird AC. Incidence and natural history of proliferative sickle cell retinopathy: observations from a cohort study. Ophthalmology. 2005;112(11):1869–75.

26. Nagpal KC, Asdourian GK, Patrianakos D, et al. Proliferative retinopathy in sickle cell trait: report of seven cases. Arch Intern Med. 1977;137(3):325–8.

27. Goldberg MF. Retinal vaso-occlusion in sickling hemoglobinopathies. Birth Defects Orig Artic Ser. 1976;12(3):475–515.

28. Moriarty BJ, Acheson RW, Condon PI, Serjeant GR. Patterns of visual loss in untreated sickle cell retinopathy. Eye (Lond). 1988;2(Pt 3):330–5.

29. Sanders RJ, Brown GC, Rosenstein RB, Magargal L. Foveal avascular zone diameter and sickle cell disease. Arch Ophthalmol (Chicago, Ill : 1960). 1991;109(6):812–815.

30. Hoang QV, Chau FY, Shahidi M, Lim JI. Central macular splaying and outer retinal thinning in asymptomatic sickle cell patients by spectral-domain optical coherence tomography. Am J Ophthalmol. 2011;151(6):990-994.e991.

31. Ong SS, Linz MO, Li X, Liu TYA, Han IC, Scott AW. Retinal thickness and microvascular changes in children with sickle cell disease evaluated by optical coherence tomography (OCT) and OCT angiography. Am J Ophthalmol. 2020;209:88–98.

32. Lynch G, Scott AW, Linz MO et al. Foveal avascular zone morphology and parafoveal capillary perfusion in sickle cell retinopathy. Brit J ophthalmol. 2019.

33. Martin GC, Albuisson E, Brousse V, de Montalembert M, Bremond-Gignac D, Robert MP. Paramacular temporal atrophy in sickle cell disease occurs early in childhood. Br J Ophthalmol. 2019;103(7):906–10.

34. Chow CC, Genead MA, Anastasakis A, Chau FY, Fishman GA, Lim JI. Structural and functional correlation in sickle cell retinopathy using spectral-domain optical coherence tomography and scanning laser ophthalmoscope microperimetry. Am J Ophthalmol. 2011;152 (4):704-711.e702.

35. Ong SS, Ahmed I, Scott AW. Association of acute macular neuroretinopathy or paracentral acute middle maculopathy with sickle cell disease. Ophthalmology Retina. 2021;5(11): 1146–55.

36. Martin GC, Denier C, Zambrowski O, et al. Visual Function in asymptomatic patients with homozygous sickle cell disease and temporal macular atrophy. JAMA Ophthalmol. 2017;135 (10):1100–5.

37. Sambhav K, Grover S, Chalam KV. Temporal thinning in sickle cell retinopathy is associated with diminished perfusion on OCTA and dense scotoma on microperimetry. Retinal Cases Brief Reports. 2019;13(4):308–13.

38. Farber MD, Jampol LM, Fox P, et al. A randomized clinical trial of scatter photocoagulation of proliferative sickle cell retinopathy. Arch Ophthalmol. 1991;109(3):363–7.

39. Rodrigues M, Kashiwabuchi F, Deshpande M, et al. Expression pattern of HIF-1α and VEGF supports circumferential application of scatter laser for proliferative sickle retinopathy. Invest Ophthalmol Vis Sci. 2016;57(15):6739–46.

40. Siqueira RC, Costa RA, Scott IU, Cintra LP, Jorge R. Intravitreal bevacizumab (Avastin) injection associated with regression of retinal neovascularization caused by sickle cell retinopathy. Acta Ophthalmol Scand. 2006;84(6):834–5.

41. Shaikh S. Intravitreal bevacizumab (Avastin) for the treatment of proliferative sickle retinopathy. Indian J Ophthalmol. 2008;56(3):259–259.

42. Cai CX, Linz MO, Scott AW. Intravitreal bevacizumab for proliferative sickle retinopathy: a case series. J VitreoRetinal Diseases. 2017;2(1):32–8.

43. Moshiri A, Ha NK, Ko FS, Scott AW. Bevacizumab presurgical treatment for proliferative sickle-cell retinopathy-related retinal detachment. Retinal Cases Brief Reports. 2013;7 (3):204–5.

44. Zhao Y, Singh RP. The role of anti-vascular endothelial growth factor (anti-VEGF) in the management of proliferative diabetic retinopathy. Drugs Context. 2018;7: 212532.

45. Howard J. Sickle cell disease: when and how to transfuse. Hematol Am Soc Hematol Educ Program. 2016;2016(1):625–31.

46. Pulido JS, Flynn HW, Jr, Clarkson JG, Blankenship GW. Pars plana vitrectomy in the management of complications of proliferative sickle retinopathy. Archives of ophthalmology (Chicago, Ill : 1960). 1988;106(11):1553–1557.

47. Roth SE, Magargal LE, Kimmel AS, Augsburger JJ, Morrison DL. Central retinal-artery occlusion in proliferative sickle-cell retinopathy after retrobulbar injection. Ann Ophthalmol. 1988;20(6):221–4.

48. Chen RW, Flynn HW Jr, Lee WH, et al. Vitreoretinal management and surgical outcomes in proliferative sickle retinopathy: a case series. Am J Ophthalmol. 2014;157(4):870-875.e871.

49. Walkden A, Griffin B, Cheng C, Dhawahir-Scala F. Gross anterior segment ischaemia following vitreoretinal surgery for sickle-cell retinopathy. BMJ Case Reports. 2019;12(1): e227541.

50. Jampol LM, Green JL Jr, Goldberg MF, Peyman GA. An update on vitrectomy surgery and retinal detachment repair in sickle cell disease. Arch Ophthalmol. 1982;100(4):591–3.

51. Williamson TH, Rajput R, Laidlaw DA, Mokete B. Vitreoretinal management of the complications of sickle cell retinopathy by observation or pars plana vitrectomy. Eye (Lond). 2009;23(6):1314–20.

52. Ho J, Grabowska A, Ugarte M, Muqit MM. A comparison of 23-gauge and 20-gauge vitrectomy for proliferative sickle cell retinopathy—clinical outcomes and surgical management. Eye (Lond). 2018;32(9):1449–54.
53. Rajagopal R, Apte RS. Full-thickness macular hole in a patient with proliferative sickle cell retinopathy. Retina (Philadelphia, Pa). 2010;30(5):838–9.
54. Mason JO 3rd. Surgical closure of macular hole in association with proliferative sickle cell retinopathy. Retina (Philadelphia, Pa). 2002;22(4):501–2.
55. Brazier DJ, Gregor ZJ, Blach RK, Porter JB, Huehns ER. Retinal detachment in patients with proliferative sickle cell retinopathy. Trans Ophthalmol Soc U K. 1986;105(Pt 1):100–5.

Persistent Fetal Vasculature Syndrome

30

Ece Özdemir Zeydanlı and Şengül Özdek

Abstract

Persistent fetal vasculature (PFV) syndrome represents a broad spectrum of abnormalities that involve varying degrees of fetal hyaloid system remnants and affect almost all parts of the eye. Although the disease has long been recognized in the differential diagnosis of leukocoria, and diagnostic and treatment modalities, as well as our understanding for PFV, have evolved over the years, the full spectrum of findings is still not fully appreciated and the disease continues to present with surprises. This heterogeneity of the disease makes the diagnosis and the management challenging. This chapter presents the current information on important aspects of PFV and provides a comprehensive guide for ophthalmologists, from the recognition of PFV and associated anatomic variations to surgical indications and techniques, and postoperative expectations.

Keywords

Persistent fetal vasculature · Persistent hyperplastic primary vitreous · Microphthalmia · Tractional retinal detachment · Leukocoria · Peripheral retinal elongation · Lens sparing vitrectomy · Lensectomy · Vitrectomy · Amblyopia management · Closed funnel retinal detachment · Tent like tractional retinal detachment · Combined hamartoma of retina and retina pigment epithelium

Supplementary Information The online version contains supplementary material available at https://doi.org/10.1007/978-3-031-14506-3_30.

E. Özdemir Zeydanlı (✉) · Ş. Özdek
Gazi University, Ankara, Turkey
e-mail: ece.ozdmir@gmail.com

Introduction

Persistent fetal vasculature (PFV) syndrome is a congenital developmental abnormality caused by failure of programmed involution of the primary vitreous and hyaloid vasculature. It was first described by Reese in 1955 as a congenital malformation of the anterior portion of the primary vitreous and referred as "persistent hyperplastic primary vitreous" for a long time [1]. However, because "primary vitreous" refers only to retrolental hyaloid vessels, and the condition involves the persistence of both hyaloid vessels and tunica vasculosa lentis (TVL), Goldberg renamed the condition with the more comprehensive term "persistent fetal vasculature" in 1997 [2].

PFV typically presents unilaterally in full-term infants without associated systemic findings, but rarely it may occur in conjunction with systemic syndromes such as Walker- Warburg syndrome [3], Aicardi syndrome [4], trisomy 13, 15, 18 [2, 5] and may be bilateral [6]. Overall, bilateral cases account for less than 10% of the cases. The exact etiology of PFV is still largely unknown. Most of the cases are sporadic. However, rare cases of autosomal dominant and autosomal recessive inheritance have been reported related to the genes NDP and ATOH7 [7, 8].

Normal Embryology

In order to appreciate the disease process of PFV, it is necessary to understand the development and normal regression of the entire fetal intraocular vasculature, the primary function of which is presumed to nourish the developing lens prior to the production of aqueous humor [9] (see also Sect. 1, Chap. 1).

The development of intraocular vascularization is initiated when the hyaloid artery, which is the distal portion of the ophthalmic artery, enters the eye via the fetal fissure at 3 weeks' gestation [10]. The artery traverses to the developing lens over the course of the next week and arborizes to eventually form the posterior tunica vasculosa lentis, a capillary meshwork closely surrounding the posterior pole of the developing lens [9, 11, 12]. The posterior TVL passes along the lens equator as a set of parallel, straight, nonbranching vessels, forming the lateral tunica vasculosa lentis, also known as iridohyaloid vessels (normal regression of which allows space for the development of zonular apparatus). Concurrently, at the anterior edge of the optic cup, vessels form anastomoses to create annular vessel. By 5 weeks' gestation, the hyaloid artery gives off multiple branches 3–4 mm behind the lens which resemble struts of an umbrella and develop into the vasa hyaloida propria [9–11]. At this stage, the primary vitreous is also developing as the hyaloid artery system develops. By 6–7 weeks' gestation, the anterior TVL forms on the anterior surface of the lens by the looping branches of the annular vessel and associated mesoderm [9]. The mesodermal elements are destined to grow into the pupillary area to form pupillary membrane while the vascular loops regress [2].

From 8 to 12 weeks' gestation, this complex vascular system reaches its most extensive state of development, and the lens is completely encircled by the TVL [13].

Subsequently, at the beginning of the second trimester, regressive events initiate posteriorly, first in the hyaloid artery and in the vasa hyaloida propria, then the posterior TVL, and the iridohyaloid vessels [2, 13]. As the hyaloid system starts to involute, the secondary vitreous continues to grow and primary vitreous assumes a cone shape with an apex at the disc and a base at the posterior surface of the lens.

During the fifth month, the anterior TVL disappears, and the pupillary membrane continues to develop. The primary vitreous retracts further centrally creating Cloquet's canal. The hyaloid system continues to involute and is usually totally regressed at 28 to 30 weeks' gestation [2, 14]. However, the remnants of the hyaloid vessels can exist within the Cloquet canal after birth. The pupillary membrane shows variable regression and may also persist normally after birth [2].

Clinical Presentation

PFV syndrome has a spectrum of presentations determined by the degree of involution of the hyaloid and TVL. Although most of the spectrum affects both anterior and posterior segments to some extent, eyes with the persistence of predominantly hyaloid vasculature are classified as posterior PFV, and those with the persistence of predominantly TVL as anterior PFV [2]. Nevertheless, most of the cases exhibit features of both anterior and posterior forms and classified as mixed or combined PFV [6, 9]. The disease can also occur in conjunction with other ocular abnormalities, including Peter's anomaly, microcornea, uveal coloboma, and morning glory disc anomaly [2, 15–18]. Variety of such presentations makes PFV challenging for surgical management.

1. Anterior PFV

The predominantly anterior form characteristically presents with leukocoria shortly after birth (Fig. 30.1a, b). Leukocoria is often due to a retrolental fibrovascular membrane, either alone or in combination with a cataractous lens. The retrolental membrane is caused by the persistence of posterior TVL and may vary in size and shape (Figs. 30.1c–e, 30.4c, 30.10, 30.12, 30.13 and 30.14) [2]. It may incorporate into elongated and centrally dragged ciliary processes and peripheral retina (Figs. 30.10, 30.11, 30.12, 30.13 and 30.14) [5, 15, 16, 18]. The eye is often microphthalmic (Fig. 30.1a, b); however, this may be subtle. Persistent pupillary membrane and strands, prominent and dilated radial iris vessels, and hairpin loops may be observed in some cases (Figs. 30.1c–e and 30.14), related to the persistence of anterior TVL and iridohyaloid vessels. Occasionally, the pupil may be deformed by the arborizing iris vessels, leading to small sphincter notches, corectopia, or congenital ectropion uveae [14]. The anterior chamber may be shallow due to swollen and anteriorly-shifted lens, extensive posterior synechiae (Fig. 30.1c–e),

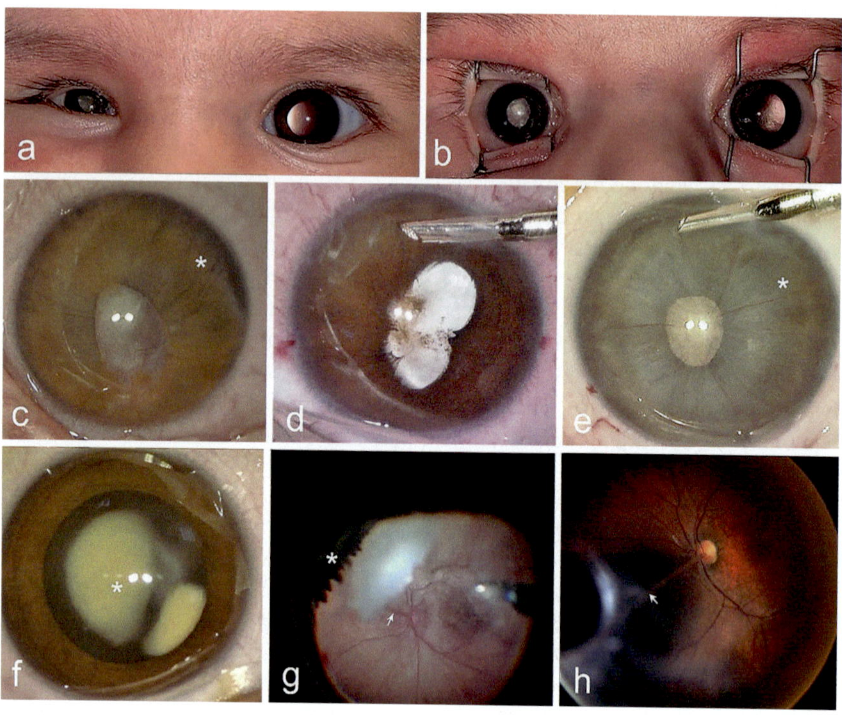

Fig. 30.1 Anterior segment findings of PFV: (**a, b**) Microphthalmia and leukocoria. (**c–e**) Severe anterior PFV cases with radial iris vessels (*), posterior synechia and totally white opaque lens including vascular elements in it. (**f**) Anterior PFV presenting with whitening at the back of the lens that is secondary to an old dehemoglobinized retrolental hemorrhage (*). Note the periphery of the lens is mostly clear. (**g**) Prominent ciliary processes (*) and a thin hyaloid remnant (arrow) in an anterior PFV case (**h**) Mild anterior PFV with a thin and eccentric hyaloid artery connection to the back of the lens (arrow)

and peripheral anterior synechiae, which often progress to secondary angle-closure glaucoma. Unlike the common observation of microphthalmos, patients who develop glaucoma may present with normal-sized or buphthalmic eyes (Fig. 30.9).

Hyphema may be found in some cases, associated with the fine vessels of persistent anterior TVL. Retrolental hemorrhage (between the posterior lens surface and the fibrovascular plaque) may also be seen in some of the cases during the course (Figs. 30.1f and 30.2). Congenital lens subluxation may rarely occur if zonular maldevelopment due to persistent iridohyaloid vessels is severe. Posterior lenticonus may also develop because of hyaloid artery traction on an inherently weak posterior capsule [19]. Although quite infrequent, the hyaloid artery may cause enough traction to cause a full-thickness posterior capsule defect yet it may still resorb during development. This may cause migration of lens particles through a defective posterior capsule, producing a pseudo-hyaloidal stalk appearance (Fig. 30.15, see **Video** 1) [20]. On rare occasions, the lens may contain

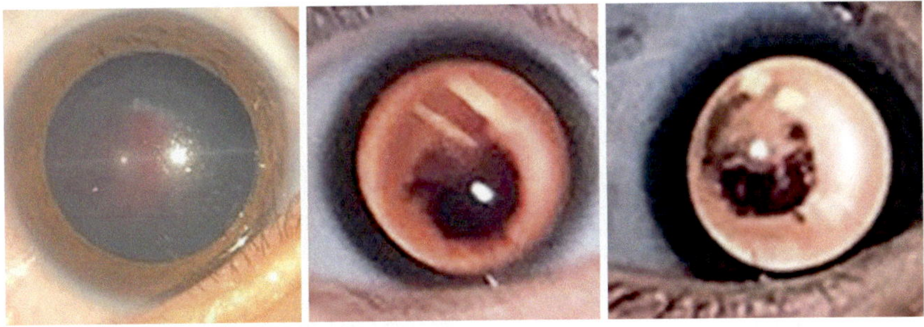

Fig. 30.2 Hemorrhage at the back of the lens which cleared totally leaving a clear lens within time following a lens sparing vitrectomy for the tent-like TRD associated with PFV

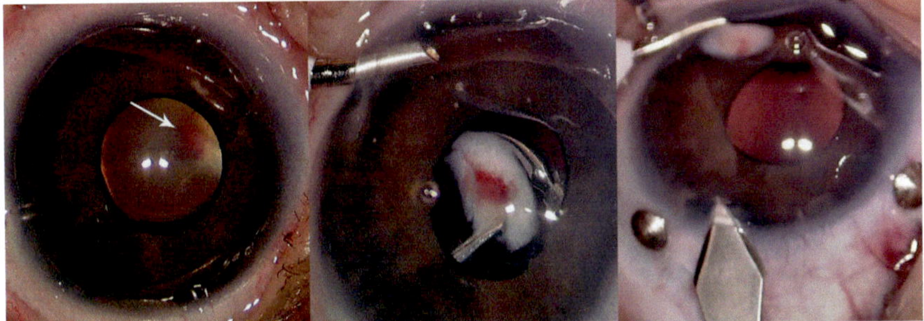

Fig. 30.3 Removal of a choristomatous (cartilage-like) plaque (arrow) through the anterior chamber as a foreign body, which could not be eaten with a vitreous cutter during lensectomy and had to be cut from the sides with curved scissors and to be removed from a limbal corneal incision

choristomatous tissue such as cartilage which cannot be removed with a vitreous cutter and require removal through the anterior chamber as a foreign body (Fig. 30.3). The posterior pole, optic nerve, and macula may be normal in the purely anterior forms without any evidence of a retinal fold. However, a thin hyaloid stalk generally extends from the optic nerve head with the anterior end lying freely in the vitreous gel even in purely anterior forms (Fig. 30.1g, h).

2. **Posterior PFV**

The posterior subtype consists of an elevated epiretinal or vitreous membrane and a stalk from the optic nerve, retinal fold, or tractional retinal detachment (TRD). The stalk itself may be a simple column-like structure extending between the lens and the optic nerve or posterior retina, or it can be an inverted Y shaped with a second or even third arm attaching to the disc and other areas of the retinal surface (Figs. 30.4, 30.5a, 30.6 and 30.16, see **Video** 2). The stalk exerts traction on the retina, resulting in areas of tent-shaped TRD. Some of these cases show overlapping features with the peripapillary combined hamartoma of the retina and retinal

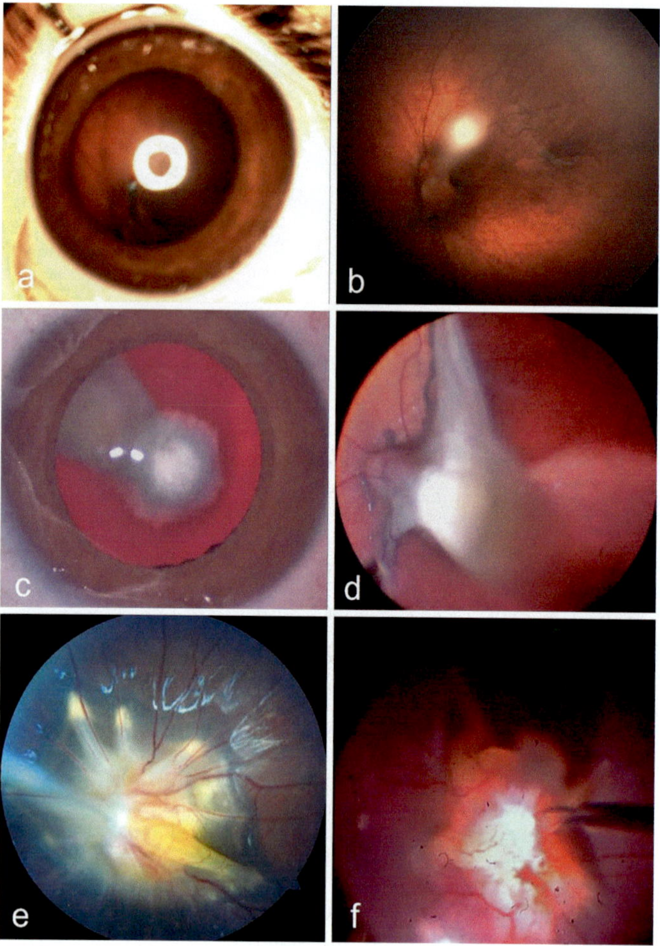

Fig. 30.4 Posterior PFV cases of varying severity: (**a, b**) An isolated mild posterior PFV case with a hyaloid stalk that has a narrow base and apex, causing a peripapillary limited tenting and a tiny retrolental opacity. (**c, d**) A mixed type PFV with centrally located retrolental plaque and multiple attachment points on the retina. (**e, f**) Examples of moderate tent-shaped posterior PFV cases

pigment epithelium (CHRRPE). Both of the diseases have an appearance of elevated mass lesion at the optic nerve that extends in a fanlike projection towards the periphery and associated with greyish pigmented dysplastic retina and tortuous retinal vessels (Fig. 30.5). Differently than CHRRPE, we see a stalk extending anteriorly from the apex of the elevated tissue in PFV cases. This phenotypic similarity between the diseases may suggest a shared origin of disturbance in the development period and may represent different ends of a disease spectrum and needs further investigation.

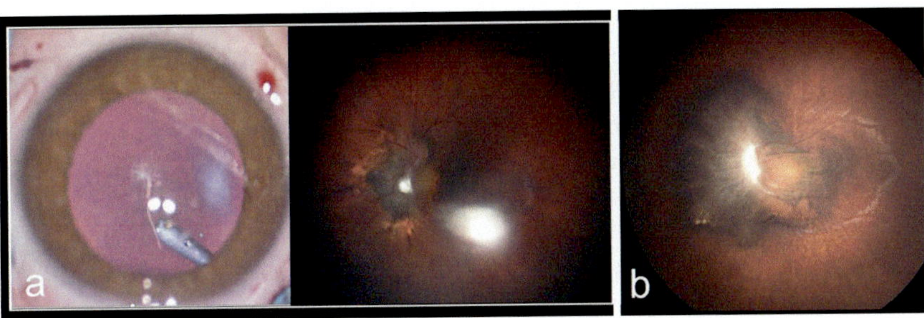

Fig. 30.5 Phenotypic similarity between posterior PFV (**a**) and combined hamartoma of the retina and retinal pigment epithelium (**b**)

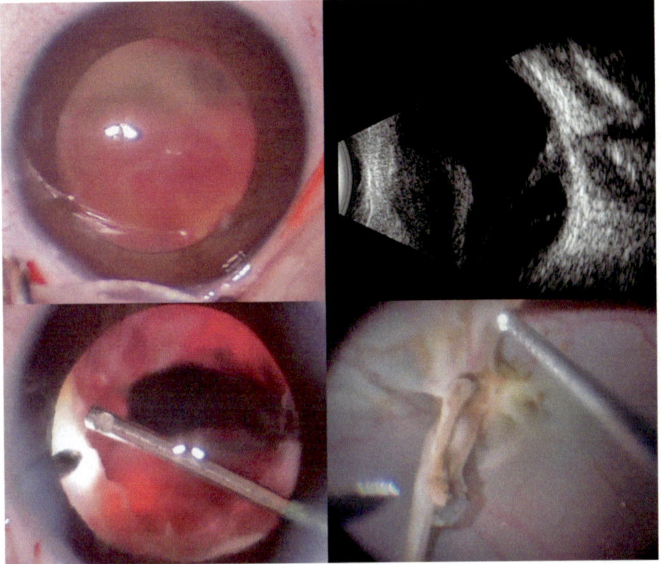

Fig. 30.6 Posterior PFV case presenting with retrolental and vitreous hemorrhage. B-scan ultrasonography revealed multi-rooted stalk and vitreous membranes. A limbal lensectomy vitrectomy surgery was performed. Following layer-by-layer removal of dense hemorrhagic membranes, a hyaloid stalk was observed extending from the optic nerve head and forming retinal folds in all directions

Although the type of retinal detachment in PFV is primarily tractional in origin due to the adhesion of fetal tissue to the developing retina, it may subsequently develop rhegmatogenous characteristics as well. Patients may also develop vitreous hemorrhages (Fig. 30.6). The optic nerve and macula may be primarily hypoplastic or dysplastic. Traction from posterior components of the primary vitreous may further contribute to these structures' dysfunction and abnormal shape, causing changes such as macular ectopia or failure of development of foveal pit.

The eye is usually microphthalmic but may be of normal size. The lens is often clear in the purely posterior subtype; however, it may be associated with a focal lens opacity at the site of attachment of the stalk (Figs. 30.4a, 30.5a and 30.16) or become cataractous over time if the vessels from the membrane expand forward enough to enter the lens via the posterior capsule.

3. Mixed Type PFV

The posterior subtype rarely presents as a pure posterior form with no anterior involvement. Rather, it is often accompanied with persistence of TVL and/or some degree of lens opacity. The eyes that harbor both anterior and posterior segment involvement to a clinically significant extent are classified as *mixed PFV subtype*. As described in the previous paragraphs, the hyaloid stalk exerts traction on the retina causing TRD. The TRD most commonly presents in a *tent-like configuration* (Figs. 30.4, 30.5a, 30.7a and 30.16) and rarely in a *closed-funnel* configuration in the most severe forms of the disease (Figs. 30.7b and 30.17, see **Video** 3).

Tent-shaped morphology is the most typical and common presentation of the posterior disease and shows a better prognosis than the closed funnel form. The release of tractions with surgery often allows the anteriorly pulled-tented retina to return to a more normal anatomical position and function. Literature data show significant reversal of dragging and reattachment of the retina in up to 77% to 91% of these cases and gaining of counting fingers or better vision that range between 42–82% [17, 21–24]. In our series of 30 eyes with tent-shaped posterior PFV, 27 (90%) showed significant reversal of tenting. Except for two cases with persistent macular folds, complete macular reattachment was obtained in all, and 21 eyes (70%) achieved counting fingers or better vision in a follow-up over one year [18].

Closed-funnel shaped posterior PFV, on the other hand, is a rare phenotype associated with very poor prognosis. These cases tend to be bilateral and mostly associated with total cataractous/membranous lens, posterior synechia, shallow anterior chamber, corneal opacification and microphthalmia. Literature research suggests that these cases are often enucleated with the concern of retinoblastoma or

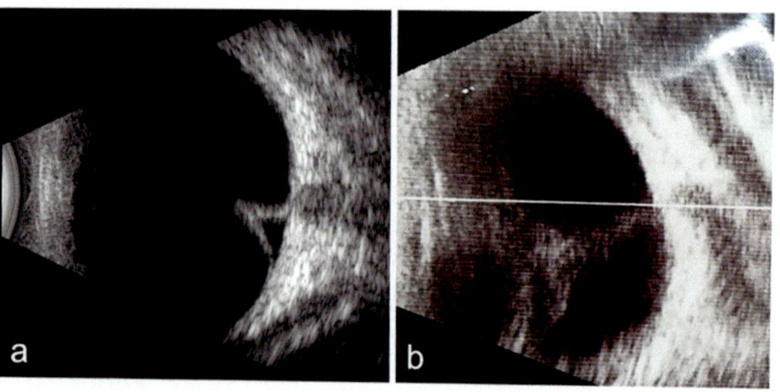

Fig. 30.7 B-scan ultrasonography shows tent-shaped retinal detachment (**a**) and closed funnel-shaped retinal detachment (**b**) in two cases with mixed type PFV

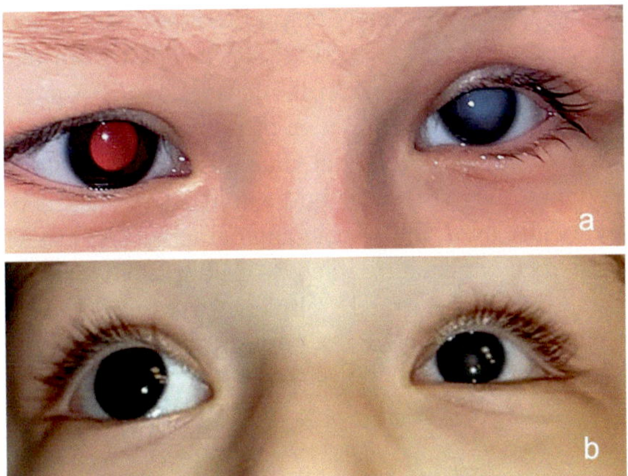

Fig. 30.8 An 18-month-old baby girl with severe form of mixed PFV coming for a second opinion to reverse the increasing corneal opacification in the left eye that causes worsening cosmetic problem every month. B-scan ultrasonography revealed a closed funnel retinal detachment. Note the large central corneal opacification (**a**) secondary to irido-lenticulo-corneal adhesion, which was significantly reversed after lensectomy done for cosmesis. (**b**) Picture taken 6 months after the operation shows a central leukocoria with very mild corneal edema in the left eye. The parents were very satisfied with the cosmetic result

considered inoperable [1, 25–27]. However, the natural course of untreated closed-funnel posterior disease is characterized with progressive deterioration of the globe [1, 16, 25, 28]. These eyes eventually develop corneal opacification, glaucoma, or phthisis bulbi if left untreated. Surgery may prevent these complications and maintain the globe in a more acceptable cosmesis (Figs. 30.8, 30.17). In eyes with shallow anterior chamber, even lensectomy with synechiolysis may prevent further corneal opacification and partially reverse pre-existing opacities. In our series of 22 eyes with closed funnel-shaped PFV, 73% had a formed globe with acceptable cosmesis; apparent leukocoria resolved in 41%; and 45% achieved light perception vision after surgery [18].

Diagnosis

The best diagnostic method is the direct visualization of any component of the persistent vascular remnants. While visualization of the retrolental area may frequently be blocked due to cataracts or synechiae, careful examination of the iris may reveal an iridohyaloid vessel, a small notch or indentation at the pupil margin, or a pupillary membrane. Although not pathognomonic, elongated and prominent ciliary processes are also particularly specific. Presence of such signs should raise the clinician's suspicion, especially when combined with microphthalmia or microcornea.

B-scan ultrasonography is extremely helpful to assist with diagnosis of the eyes with a limited or absent fundus view (Fig. 30.7). Apart from demonstrating the vitreous stalk from the posterior pole to the lens, it can also provide information about the axial length, lens status, presence of retinal detachment and calcification which is very important for differential diagnosis of retinoblastoma. However, B-scan ultrasonography may still miss the hyaloid artery stalk if it is very thin.

Although infrequently used, fluorescein angiography (FA) can also be helpful to delineate abnormal fetal vasculature such as iridohyaloid vessels, hairpin loops around the pupil, radially oriented retrolental vessels (also known as the brittle-star), remnants of vasa hyaloidea propria and hyaloid artery. It may also assist in the differential diagnosis.

Differential Diagnosis

Since the most widely recognized clinical presentation of PFV is leukocoria, the differential diagnosis should include diseases causing a white pupil.

- The most important of these is undoubtedly retinoblastoma, which is the most common intraocular tumor of childhood, and delayed or erroneous diagnosis can lead to grave consequences. In general, PFV eyes are often microphthalmic, while eye size is normal in retinoblastoma. In case of diagnostic difficulty, B-scan ultrasonography and computed tomography (CT) may be helpful. Calcification observed on these imaging studies suggests malignancy; however, magnetic resonance imaging (MRI) may be a better alternative to CT scans because of the potential increased risk of malignancy with ionizing radiation (Table 30.1).
- Other causes of leukocoria; congenital cataracts, familial exudative vitreo-retinopathy (FEVR), Coats' disease, retinopathy of prematurity (ROP), ocular toxocariasis, and rarely, uveitis and incontinentia pigmenti should be considered in the differential diagnosis.
- In particular, it is important to differentiate severe posterior PFV presenting as bilateral closed-funnel retinal detachment from the Norrie disease. Norrie disease is more hemorrhagic and vascular lesions are more prominent. It occurs in boys and has a very poor prognosis. Genetic analysis is the best way for differentiation. Table 30.1 shows the key clinical features for differential diagnosis.

Natural Course of the Disease

The natural course of untreated PFV is often ill-fated due to the changing nature of the process, resulting in sequelae and complications [1, 16, 25]. Exception to this is mildly affected incomplete forms, for example, when only a small patch of fetal

Table 30.1 Key differentiating features of persistent fetal vasculature and simulating disorders

PFV	• Dx within weeks of birth • Unilateral (90%), mostly sporadic • Microphthalmos, microcornea • Prominent iris vessels, posterior synechia, ectropion uvea, shallow AC, elongated ciliary processes, ACG, cataract, retrolental fibrovascular membrane, stalk emanating from the disc (often with TRD) • RD is tractional and often tent-shaped where the peripheral retina is attached (seldom funnel-shaped RD). Fibrotic attachment to the back of the lens more at the nasal side • Retrolental vessels are typically oriented in a radial pattern, and may anastomose with other vasculature in the iris, ciliary body, or circumlental space
Retinoblastoma	• Dx within months/years of birth (average: 1.5 y of age) • Sporadic (90%) or familial (AD inheritance, 10%) • Unilateral (60%) or bilateral (40%) • Normal-sized eye and cornea (may have buphthalmos) • May have white, fluffy seeds on the iris or in the AC (pseudohypopyon), no cataract • NVI is common and the most frequent reason of secondary glaucoma • RD is exudative with subretinal fluid and seeds • Calcification on ultrasonography and CT scan • FA shows dilated and tortuous vessels diving into the RD and feed the hyperfluorescent tumor • MRI: Iso/hyperintense mass in T1, hypointense mass in T2 sections. Pinealoma may may also be present
Norrie disease	• Dx within weeks of birth • Bilateral, X-linked recessive inheritance, male • Mostly associated with progressive hearing loss and mental retardation • Microphthalmos, iris atrophy and synechiae, shallow AC • Severely dysplastic retina (often with severe subretinal hemorrhage and lipid) • RD is often hemorrhagic and vascular lesions more prominent than PFV • Confirmation by molecular genetic testing
ROP (Stage 4 or 5)	• Dx at birth/within weeks of birth • History of prematurity/low birth weight/neonatal oxygen therapy • Bilateral, may be asymmetric • Normal-sized eye (may have microphthalmos) • Elongated ciliary processes, pupillary membrane and TVL may be seen; however, vascular pattern is more irregular than the radially-oriented retrolental vasculature in PFV • Straightening of the vascular arcades with macular and optic disc dragging is typical • RD is generally tractional with a concave configuration, "peripheral trough" (fold between vascular-avascular retina) is characteristic in stage 5 and leads to funnel-shaped RD
FEVR	• Dx within years of birth (average: 6 years) • Mostly AD inheritance (Examination of asymptomatic family members is helpful) • Bilateral and often asymmetric • Normal-sized eye and cornea

(continued)

Table 30.1 (continued)

	• Peripheral avascular retina, straightening of the vascular arcades with macular and optic disc dragging (ROP-like appearance but slower progression), with or without retinal folds (falciform retinal folds extending mostly to the temporal periphery to the back of the lens), as well as pre-, intra-, or subretinal exudation • RD is typically tractional, but may subsequently develop exudative and/or rhegmatogenous components • FA is essential for accurate dx—peripheral nonperfusion, vessel straightening and anastomoses, telangiectasias and neovascularization are typical
Coats' disease	• Dx at 5–10 y of age • Unilateral (90%), male (80%), sporadic • Normal-sized eye and cornea (may have buphthalmos) • Pupillary reflex is more yellow than white (xanthocoria) • Subretinal lipid exudates with telangiectatic retinal blood vessels • RD is typically exudative
Toxocariasis	• Dx at childhood (usually > 3 years) • History of exposure to puppies, eating dirt • Unilateral • Normal-sized eye and cornea • Granuloma with a stalk can be mistaken for a fibrovascular stalk. However, there is often a significant component of posterior uveitis

PFV persistent fetal vasculature; *Dx* diagnosis; *AC* anterior chamber; *ACG* angle-closure glaucoma; *RD* retinal detachment; *TRD* tractional retinal detachment; *AD* autosomal dominant; *NVI neovascularization of iris; CT computed tomography; FA fluorescein angiography; ROP retinopathy of prematurity; FEVR familial exudative vitreoretinopathy*

tissue is found on the posterior lens surface as an isolated finding, it may follow a relatively benign natural course and may never require a surgical intervention [1, 2, 29]. However, the vast majority of PFV eyes appear to undergo secondary changes, which may eventually lead to loss of the eye (Figs. 30.8 and 30.9). Reese expressed this as " I have never seen, a single case of uncomplicated full-blown persistent hyperplastic vitreous in an adult, and neither have any of my colleagues" [1].

Clinical observations and pathology findings in the early literature have expanded our understanding of progressive changes in untreated PFV eyes [1, 16]. We know that the fibrovascular plaque undergoes progressive contracture. This contracture likely causes a break in the posterior capsule, thereby causing

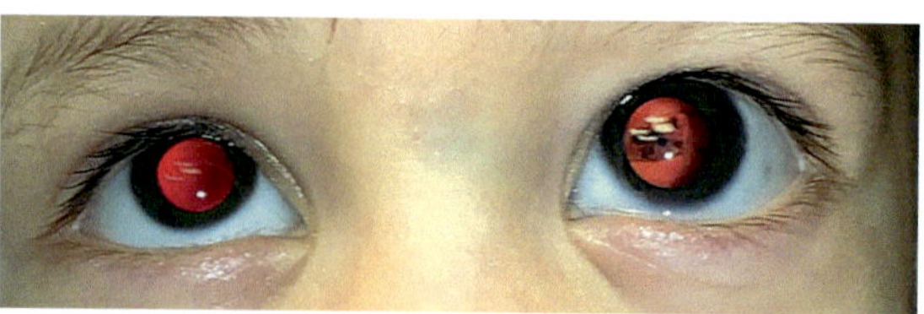

Fig. 30.9 Left eye has mixed PFV with secondary glaucoma causing buphthalmos in an infant

cataractous changes in the lens. This is accompanied by a swelling of the lens, which often comes forward together with the iris and touches the cornea, causing angle-closure glaucoma, corneal edema, scarring and opacification (Fig. 30.8) [1, 2, 6, 16, 25]. Only rarely, instead of swelling, the lens may absorb, partially or totally, and harbor capsular remains. Or it may shrink to a small, white, calcified lesion. These eyes may avoid secondary glaucoma and corneal changes [1]. The progressive contraction of the plaque also exerts constant traction on the ciliary body, which may lead to intraocular hemorrhage, ciliary body detachment, hypotonia, and eventually loss of the eye [1, 2, 6, 16, 25]. Surgery allows us to remove these tractional forces and gives us a chance to change this ill-fated course of the disease.

Treatment

A broad spectrum of presentation translates into a similarly broad range of treatment options and outcomes. At one end of the spectrum, an eye may have only minor sequelae from the fetal vascular structures such as a Bergmeister's papilla (persistent epipapillary fibrovascular tissue), a Mittendorf dot (small retrolental opacity caused by the anterior termination of the hyaloid artery), or persistent pupillary loops and strands. Such eyes, which are minimally affected, with normal visual function or clear visual axis, and without progressive anatomical changes such as shallowing of the anterior chamber or retinal traction, follow an uncomplicated course and remain stable without surgery. Surgery may also be avoided for those at the other end of the spectrum of severity, particularly when PFV is associated with systemic syndromes, such as trisomy 13, or Walker-Warburg syndrome, and the globe is extremely microphthalmic, undifferentiated, and disorganized. Yet for the majority of the PFV cases, surgery is the only treatment option.

- PFV surgery addresses two main problems: One is the media opacities that need to be cleared to prevent amblyopia, and the other is the tractional forces that need to be released to prevent secondary complications such as retinal detachment, glaucoma, ciliary body detachment and phthisis. Because the hyaloidal stalk remains rigid in the growing eye, it exerts anterior, posterior, and circumferential traction on the retina, lens and ciliary body, causing such complications. By releasing the connections of the hyaloid stalk to these structures and clearing the axis, the eye has a chance to grow and achieve acceptable anatomy and function [17, 21, 23, 30, 31].
- In mild to moderate cases, the goal of surgery is to restore vision as much as possible. In severe cases, the primary goal is to salvage the eye and achieve as good cosmesis as possible (Figs. 30.8 and 30.17) and then, if possible, restore some vision. Visual gain is also limited by the degree of retinal dysplasia and optic nerve hypoplasia. To maximize the visual potential, it is essential to coordinate with a pediatric ophthalmologist and combine early surgery with early and aggressive management of amblyopia. The importance of visual

rehabilitation after surgery should be also clearly explained to parents because surgical technique alone will not result in full visual potential without appropriate postoperative rehabilitation.

- One should not forget that these are only spare eyes not normal eyes.

The treatment of PFV was extremely conservative in the early years with the primary aim being the prevention of complications and anatomical preservation of the globe. Although vitrectomy was used in the 1980s, the visual expectations were very limited and severe cases, especially posterior ones have been deemed inoperable for a long time. However, advancements in surgical instruments and technology and greater awareness and understanding of PFV among ophthalmologists over the last decade have changed the disease course. Now, visual gain after surgery is not uncommon for many cases. Reported rates of useful vision (20/400 or better) after surgery ranges from 18 to 79% according to the literature [15, 17, 21–24, 31]. Eyes with anterior PFV, in particular, benefit most from surgery and have been generally associated with more favorable outcomes, when managed properly. In a series of 81 eyes, Sisk et al. [23] reported that 96% of the anterior PFV eyes having undergone surgery achieved counting fingers or better vision at the final follow-up, versus 55% of those with the posterior disease. Similarly, our group reported that 37% of the anterior PFV cases had a final visual acuity of 20/200 or better, and 79% achieved counting fingers or better, whereas respectively 7% and 60% of the cases with posterior involvement achieved the same [15].

Although surgical outcomes in posterior disease still appear somewhat limited, more data has supported the concept of retinal plasticity, even in severe cases. Bosjolie and Ferrone [24] suggested that surgical intervention for posterior PFV eyes up to 1 year of age provided significant reversal of retinal dragging and folds and improvement of visual acuity. The authors emphasized the importance of early intervention before fibrotic retinal changes occur. Walsh et al. investigated the prognosis of bilateral, more severe type mixed PFV eyes. In their study of 22 eyes, 69% maintained at least light perception vision in at least 1 eye, and no more than 11% ended up with phthisis bulbi [30]. The authors advocated surgery in eyes with severe posterior cases who would have likely had poor visual and anatomical outcomes.

Recently, our group have delved into the full spectrum of posterior PFV and investigated outcomes of surgical intervention according to the disease severity, including the ones at the most severe end of the spectrum [18]. In the first group of eyes presenting with typical tent-shaped retinal detachment, the results were comparable to the results of the previous literature, with 90% of the eyes achieving complete or near-complete retinal reattachment and 70% obtaining counting fingers or better vision. Similar to Walsh et al. [30], functional outcomes were limited to light perception vision at best in severe forms of this group who had optic nerve/macula pathologies or severe retinal dysplasia. However, surgery assured a cosmetically acceptable, formed globe in most of them, and only 7% became phthisical. The second group consisted of eyes presenting with leukocoria and closed funnel-shaped RD, which deemed inoperable to date and natural history inevitably leads to secondary complications and loss of the eye [18]. Surgery restored light perception in 45%; this meant that 70% of patients with bilateral pathology had light perception in at least one eye. Even more importantly, anatomical preservation of the globe was possible in most cases; only 14% resulted in phthisis bulbi, and one required enucleation. These results show that even when a postoperative improvement in visual function is not expected in severe cases, removal of tractions via surgery may allow the relieved retina to settle down over time, prevent hypotony and phthisis, decrease the leukocoric appearance and may even enable some light perception (Fig. 30.8).

PFV Surgery: General Considerations

PFV surgery broadly includes vitrectomy with transection of the persistent hyaloid stalk, with or without lensectomy, and the release of tractions on the ciliary body and the retina by excision of the retrolental tissue and removal of epiretinal membranes. Due to the clinical heterogeneity among PFV cases, each case also brings unique challenges that should be addressed. Before moving on to discuss surgical approaches in different clinical scenarios, the following paragraphs focus on key points for a successful PFV surgery:

1. **Make sure the parents have realistic expectations before surgery**
   Parents of children with vitreoretinal diseases such as PFV often find it difficult to accept that their child may experience permanent vision impairment as a result of the disease. They may perceive the surgery as a miraculous solution and might be eager to proceed. Taking time to discuss the goals, risks, and benefits of surgery, the necessity of postoperative rehabilitation, and set realistic expectations is as important as the surgery. The surgeon should explain the natural course of the untreated disease and the expected benefit-risk ratio of the surgery, but should not promise the outcomes.
2. **Examine the ora serrata-pars plicata area for anatomical variations before placing sclerotomies and use limbal entries until safe**
   The surgeon should be aware that peripheral retinal anomalies are quite common in eyes with PFV, particularly in the anterior form of the disease. The peripheral retina may be dragged anteriorly, replace the pars plana in some parts, and elongate as finger-like extensions; or sometimes it may circumferentially extend beyond the ora serrata and become continuous with the retrolental tissue (Figs. 30.10, 30.11 and 30.12, see **Video** 4). We have previously documented that more than 80% of the anterior PFV cases [15], and up to 27% of the posterior cases [18] with tent-shaped retinal detachment had this anomaly. Therefore, once the child is under anesthesia, a thorough examination is crucial before beginning the surgery. If there is an extensive fibrovascular membrane obscuring the view, it would be safer to use limbal entries for the entire

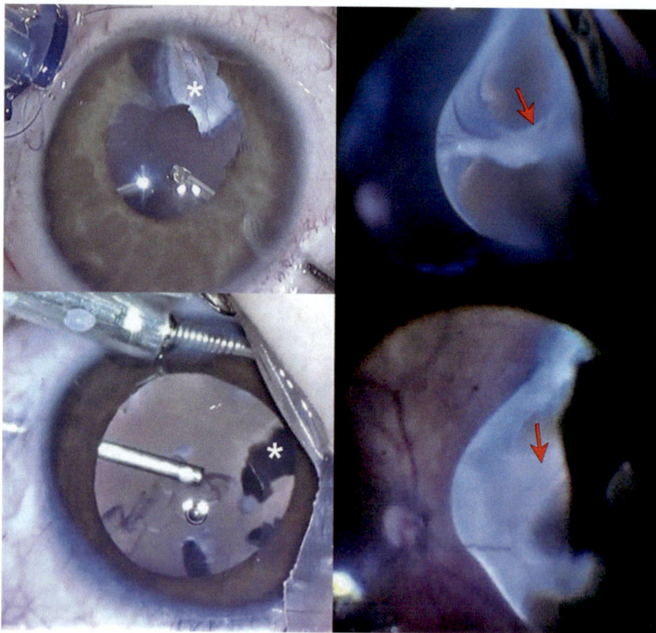

Fig. 30.10 Examples of elongated peripheral retina parts (arrows) that insert into the ciliary processes or more anteriorly, into the retrolental plaques (*)

procedure or until an adequate view of the peripheral retina is achieved. Some clues may also guide the surgeon to detect areas of retinal elongation; nasal and inferiorly localized pigmented or fibrovascular plaques are the places where elongated retina parts are most commonly found (Fig. 30.10).

3. **Always prioritize complete removal of retrolental fibrovascular tissue rather than preservation of the capsule to avoid potential complications**
Rare cases with localized avascular plaque located centrally behind the lens, leaving the peripheral parts of the lens clearer, may allow safe removal of the entire lens opacity while preserving the peripheral capsule for a secondary intraocular lens implantation. However, in cases with extensive and eccentric fibrovascular tissue, complete removal of this tissue should be targeted, as residual fibrovascular tissue contracts over time, leading to pupillary obliteration, angle-closure glaucoma, and chronic peripheral TRD (Fig. 30.11).

4. **Check for the possible continuity of the fibrovascular tissue with the retina before attempting complete removal and be prepared in advance**
As essential as it is to completely remove the fibrovascular tissue, the surgeon should not rush through it. First, the central portion of the fibrovascular tissue should be sufficiently cleared to examine the peripheral retina (Figs. 30.1g and 30.13). If there is an extensive anterior retinal elongation, the possibility of leaving a thin circle of the peripheral fibrovascular tissue remnant which is

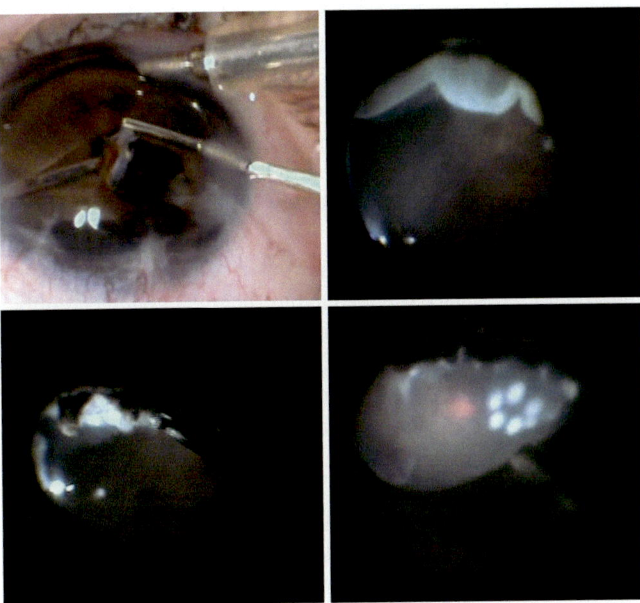

Fig. 30.11 An 8-month-old infant with anterior PFV who had previously undergone lensectomy followed by several operations for pupillary obliteration; There was iris neovascularization and the pupillary aperture was obliterated by a thick and tenacious membrane that was hard to separate. Peripheral retina was detached. The pupillary membrane was continuous with the detached retina in some parts, causing traction. Removal of residual fibrous membranes, 360° retinotomy, photocoagulation and silicone oil tamponade resulted in retinal reattachment

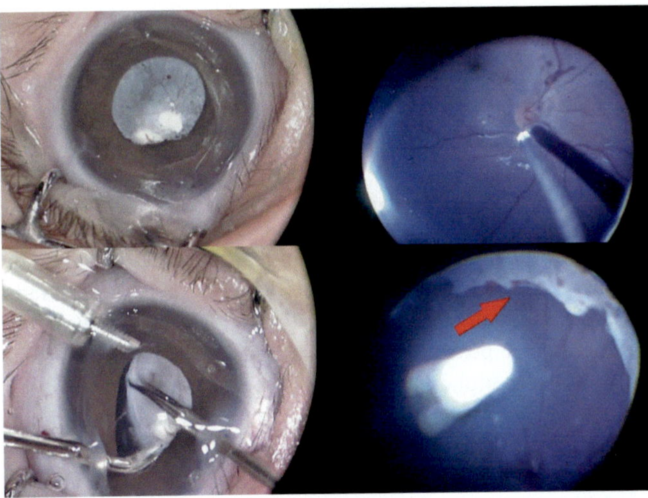

Fig. 30.12 Anterior PFV case in which the peripheral retina was continuous with the anterior fibrovascular tissue. Cutting the fibrovascular tissue resulted in an iatrogenic retinotomy (arrow). In this case, posterior hyaloid was separated, 360° laser photocoagulation and silicone tamponade were applied

segmented with multiple radial incisions should be weight against total removal of that tissue which ends up with retinotomy. When total removal leading to retinotomy is planned, the posterior hyaloid should be separated first to get prepared for retinal breaks before clearing the entire fibrovascular tissue-capsule complex. Otherwise, posterior hyaloid separation may be extremely difficult once an extensive retinotomy has occurred (Figs. 30.12 and 30.14).

5. **Carefully examine the hyaloid stalk for the presence of retinal tissue or vessels**

   The surgeon should be aware that the retinal tissue and vessels may be pulled up and dragged onto the stalk tissue. To avoid rhegmatogenous complications, it is crucial to examine the stalk before transecting it. Aside from direct examination, pushing the stalk from side to side and observing how this alters the retinal circulation can be used as a guide to understand whether or not there are vessels in the stalk. If this occurs, the stalk can be left longer to be on the safe side. There is no need to remove the entire stalk since both ends of the stalk regress postoperatively.

6. **Plan for a staged surgery rather than risking the eye with a retinal break in case of closed funnel RD in eyes with severe mixed PFV**

   In these eyes, surgery starts with limbal entry and lensectomy. Retrolental membranes are dissected starting from the center, layer by layer, to reach the retina as it is done for stage 5 ROP to open the funnel (Fig. 30.17). It is often not possible to completely flatten the retina in such cases of closed funnel posterior PFV. The goal is to dissect the membranes and release tractional forces to allow the retina to gradually go backwards and flatten over time. The surgeon should always remain on the safe side during dissections, as a single retinal break often renders the pediatric eye inoperable. A second surgery may be planned for further membrane dissection 3-6 months later when the retina settles down and go backwards as in stage 5 ROP.

Clinical Scenarios and Surgical Strategies

Case Presentation 1. Mild Anterior PFV

A 2-year-old boy presented for a routine ophthalmological examination. He was born full term by normal vaginal delivery and otherwise healthy. The family history was unremarkable. He was able to fix and follow objects with both eyes. Ocular examination revealed a posterior polar cataract and a retrolental fibrous tissue located nasally at the periphery of the lens capsule in the left eye (Fig. 30.13). A thin hyaloid remnant was observed extending nasally from the optic nerve head and attaching to the retrolental plaque (Fig. 30.13b). There was no microphthalmia. Examination of the right eye was normal. A diagnosis of unilateral mild anterior PFV was made and she underwent lensectomy-vitrectomy surgery. In this case,

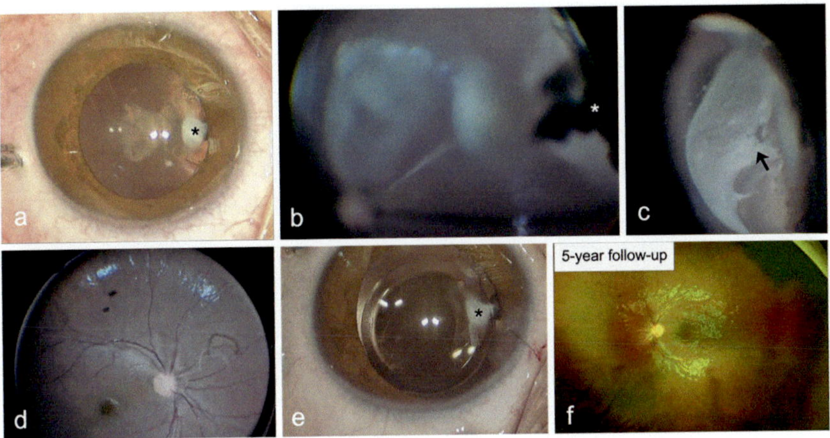

Fig. 30.13 Ocular findings of Case 1 at surgery and at 5-year postoperative follow-up. Note the avascular plaque (*) that had been left in place and mild peripheral retinal elongations (arrow) located in that area

although there was a central opacity of the lens, the retrolental fibrous plaque was small, avascular and attached to the nasal paracentral lens. Although the peripheral retina adjacent to the fibrous plaque had some thin projections anteriorly; none of them was a broad connection (Fig. 30.13c). Because the avascular plaque did not carry a risk for future contraction, it was left in place, the peripheral capsule could be preserved and an IOL was implanted at the time of surgery (Fig. 30.13e). After 5 years of follow-up, visual acuity was 20/50. Visual axis remained clear without secondary proliferation of the residual membrane. Retina was completely attached as seen on the color fundus image (Fig. 30.13f).

Case Presentation 2. Severe Anterior PFV

A 2-month-old boy presented with unilateral leukocoria. He was born full term by normal vaginal delivery and otherwise healthy. The family history was unremarkable. He did not respond to light stimulus in the left eye. Ocular examination showed microphthalmia, retrolental fibrovascular membrane, and a typical radial iris vessel (Fig. 30.14). The pupillary dilation was poor due to posterior synechia. The posterior segment view was obscured and there was a very thin hyaloid artery connection which was barely visualized on ultrasonography (Fig. 30.14b). Examination of the right eye was normal. A diagnosis of unilateral severe anterior PFV was made and he underwent vitreoretinal surgery. Limbal entries were made. Adequate pupillary aperture was achieved with synechiolysis and insertion of the iris retractors. Vascularized, dense, fibrous tissue with elongated and centrally dragged ciliary processes are seen in the image (Fig. 30.14c). The fibrovascular plaque was opened centrally in the first stage and the peripheral part was left in

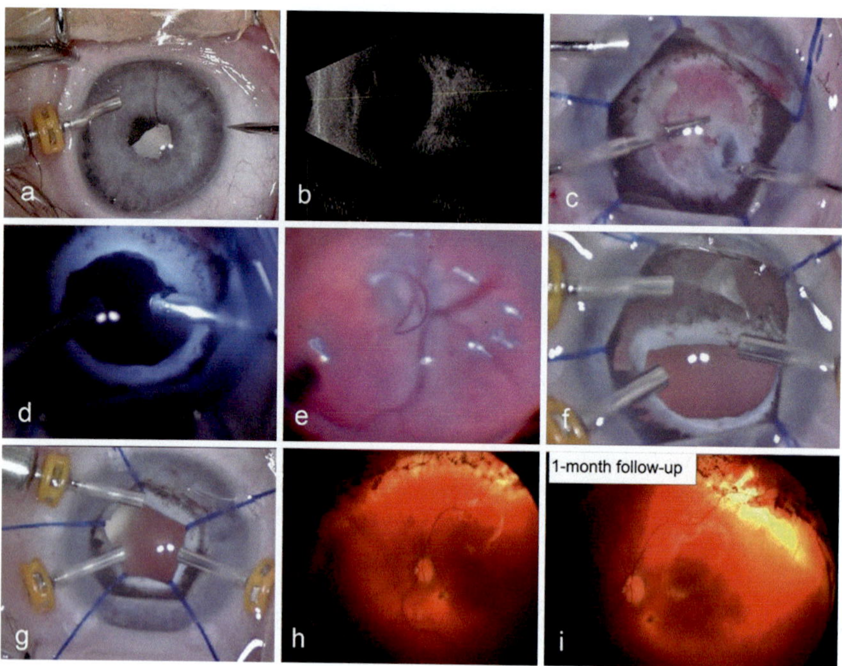

Fig. 30.14 Ocular findings of case 2 during surgery and at early postoperative follow-up

place in case there was a peripheral retinal anomaly (Fig. 30.14d). Retina was attached and there was a thin hyaloid artery connection (Fig. 30.4e). However, since a 360° peripheral retinal extension and direct continuity of the retina with the fibrovascular plaque were detected, preparations were made for a 360° retinotomy by separating the posterior hyaloid first. At this point, the ciliary body and retina, which are the continuation of the ring-shaped fibrovascular tissue remnant, were dramatically detached just before the retinotomy was made (Fig. 30.14f) and the operation could only be continued by holding this tissue with the iris retractors (Fig. 30.14g). Retinal detachment surgery was terminated with 360° retinotomy and silicone tamponade (Fig. 30.14h). At postoperative 1 month, the retina was attached with 360° laser retinotomy margins (Fig. 30.14i). However, this eye was lost to become phthisic because of hypotonia.

Case Presentation 3. Anterior PFV Presenting with a Pseudo-Hyaloidal Stalk [20]

2-month-old boy was referred for bilateral congenital cataracts. He was born full term via normal spontaneous delivery. Systemic evaluation yielded no associated systemic anomalies. The family history was remarkable for an older sibling who had bilateral congenital cataracts, clinical and surgical details of which were not known. Ocular examination revealed near-total white cataract with only a thin rim

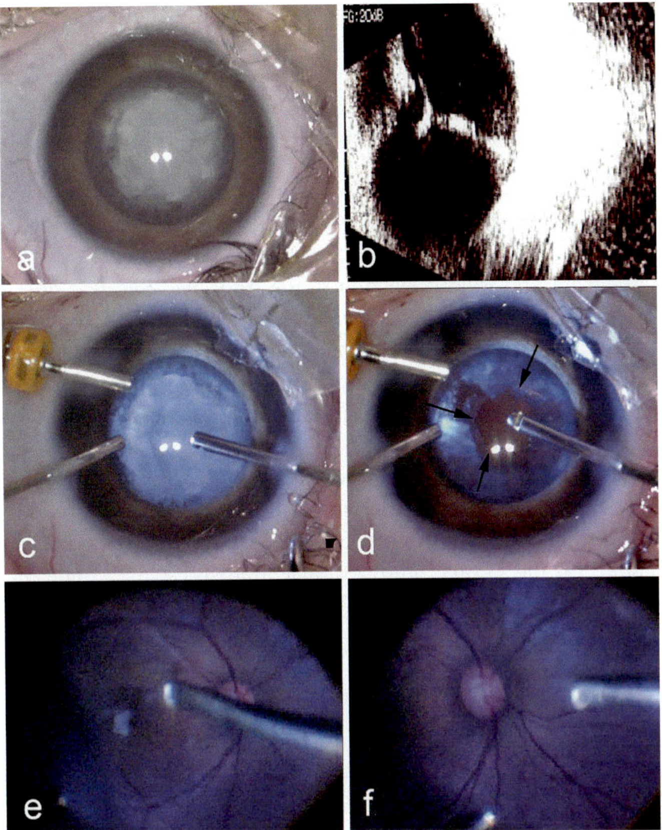

Fig. 30.15 Surgical findings of Case 3 presenting with pseudo-hyaloidal stalk

of clear zone at periphery in both eyes (Fig. 30.15a). There was no fibrovascular structure visible within or behind the lens. The corneas were of equal and normal size, and no associated microphthalmia was present. B-scan ultrasonography showed a hyperechoic band extending from the optic nerve head to the posteriorly-bulged back surface of the lens in each eye, representing a persistent hyaloidal stalk and leading to the diagnosis of bilateral anterior PFV (Fig. 30.15b). Cataractous lens was noticed to be located relatively posteriorly, in the anterior vitreous, at surgery (Fig. 30.15c). During lensectomy, lens particles were noticed to be moving anteriorly from central mid-vitreous towards the aspiration port and the central part of posterior capsule was observed to be developmentally- defective with accompanying white dots (Fig. 30.15d). Lens particles along the Cloquet's canal were removed during central core vitrectomy (Fig. 30.15e). Retina was attached and the optic disc was totally normal even without any stalk (Fig. 30.15f). The peripheral capsule was preserved for future IOL implantation. Both eyes were fitted with contact lenses in the postoperative period and followed up for 2 years. The patient had secondary proliferation of the capsular epithelium blocking the visual axis in the right eye within 4 months and required a second surgery. Visual acuity was central steady maintained in both eyes at final exam.

Case Presentation 4. Posterior PFV with Tent-Shaped TRD

A 14-month-old female infant presented with strabismus in the right eye for several months. She was born full term by normal vaginal delivery and otherwise healthy. The family history was unremarkable. She had esotropia and responded to light stimulus without fix and follow reaction in the right eye. She was able to fix and follow objects with the left eye. Ocular examination revealed microphthalmia and a hyaloid remnant extending between the back of the lens (narrow attachment seen as mittendorf dot, Fig. 30.16a) and the retina (causing peripapillary tent-like retinal detachment, Fig. 30.16b, c). Examination of the left eye was normal. A diagnosis of unilateral posterior PFV was made and she underwent lens-sparing vitrectomy and patching of the left eye for amblyopia treatment. After 8 years of follow-up, visual axis remained clear with a very small opacity at the back of the lens and the acuity was 20/100. Color fundus and optical coherence tomography images show complete flattening of the retina with residual fibrosis at the optic nerve head (Fig. 30.16d).

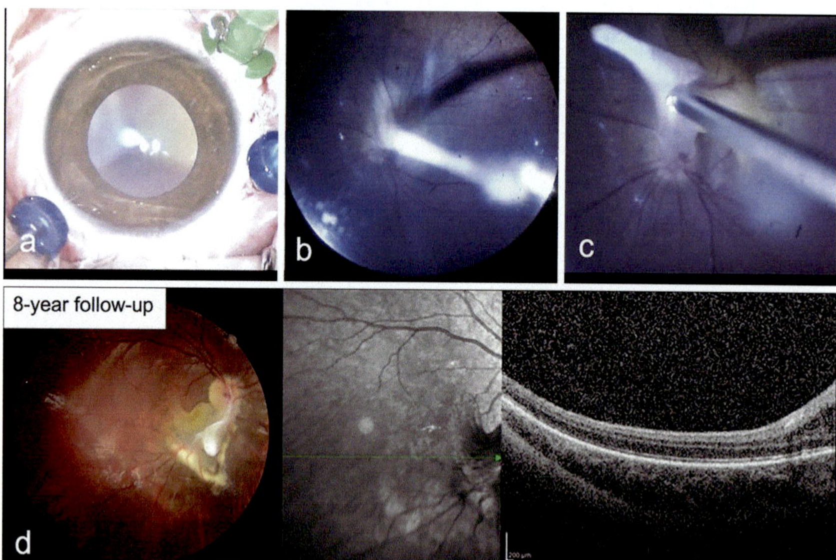

Fig. 30.16 Ocular findings of Case 4 at surgery and at 8-year postoperative follow-up

Case Presentation 5. Severe Mixed PFV with Closed Funnel-Shaped TRD

A 3-month-old boy was referred with the suspicion of bilateral retinoblastoma. The family had noticed white pupils in both eyes a month ago. He was born full term by normal vaginal delivery and otherwise healthy. The family history was unremarkable. He did not respond to light stimulus in either eye. Ocular examination showed microphthalmia, microcornea with corneal diameters of 9 mm, and leukocoria in both eyes (Fig. 30.17a). The posterior segment view was totally obscured. There was no sign of a mass in orbital MRI. Ultrasonography revealed closed funnel-shaped retinal detachment in both eyes. A diagnosis of bilateral severe mixed PFV was made and he underwent limbal lensectomy-vitrectomy. Although retina was severely dysplastic, wide opening of the funnel was possible with meticulous dissection of retrolental and preretinal membranes in both eyes (Fig. 30.17b–e). Retina was partially attached in the posterior pole at 6-month follow-up and light perception vision was achieved in both eyes (Fig. 30.17f).

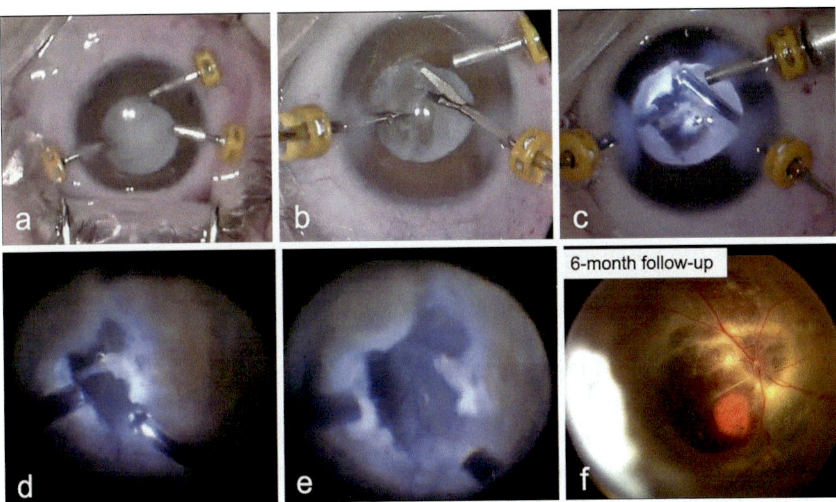

Fig. 30.17 Ocular findings of Case 5 at surgery and at 6-month postoperative follow-up

Conclusions

PFV represents a broad spectrum of anomalies and presentations, which translates into a wide variety of potential outcomes. In general, purely anterior PFV cases have better visual potential than those with posterior malformations; however, many cases with posterior PFV may also achieve useful vision with proper care.

Severe cases may benefit from surgery in terms of anatomic preservation. Peripheral retinal anomalies are much more common than previously thought. Keeping this in mind, extra care should be taken to avoid complications in cases that might otherwise have good visual and anatomical outcomes. All in all, prognosis depends on the severity and type of the disease as well as early diagnosis and intervention, careful planning of the surgical technique, frequent follow-ups, family education and postoperative management of amblyopia.

Review Questions

1. Which of the following statements is true about PFV?

a. Consanguinity is a significant risk factor for the disease development.
b. A meticulous systemic work-up is crucial following the diagnosis of PFV.
c. Ultrasonography and direct visualization are usually enough for PFV diagnosis.
d. Most of the cases remain stable throughout life without surgery.

2. Peripheral retinal anomalies and anterior elongations are most commonly seen in which type of PFV?

a. Predominantly anterior PFV
b. Predominantly posterior PFV
c. Mixed PFV
d. b and c

3. Which of the following statements is true about PFV?

a. Peripheral remnant of retrolental fibrovascular tissue can be left in place and serve as a bed for secondary IOL implantation.
b. Severe mixed type PFV with closed-funnel shaped TRD often presents with bilateral involvement.
c. The growth of the microphthalmic globe to normal dimensions after the operation is an indicator of surgical success.
d. It is necessary to remove the entire hyaloid stalk to prevent its later contraction.

Answers

1. **(C)** Although autosomal dominant or recessive inheritance has been reported in very few cases, PFV is mostly a sporadic non-heritable disease. PFV typically presents without associated systemic findings and routine systemic work-up is not required. Diagnosis of the disease is based on ocular examination and visualization of fetal vascular remnants. Except for the very mild forms, the majority of PFV cases undergo progressive anatomic changes and end up with secondary glaucoma, corneal opacification, and eventual phthisis bulbi.

2. **(A)** Peripheral retinal anomalies are quite common in eyes with PFV, particularly in the anterior form of the disease reaching up to 80% of the cases [15]. It is crucial to check for possible anomalies before placing sclerotomies or to use limbal entries until safe. The nasal and inferior quadrants adjacent to localized pigmented or fibrovascular plaques are the most common sites where retinal elongations are detected.

3. **(B)** Retrolental fibrovascular tissue should be completely removed as residual tissue contracts over time, causing pupillary obliteration, angle-closure glaucoma, and chronic peripheral TRD. Mixed anterior–posterior PFV with closed funnel-shaped TRD is a rare form of PFV and often presents with bilateral involvement (2/3 of this form in our practice). Enlargement of the microphthalmic globe to normal size should alert the physician to the possible development of glaucoma. It is often sufficient to transect the stalk to release antero-posterior traction. The surgeon can shorten the stalk it as long as it is safe. As retinal tissue and vessels are often dragged up to the stalk tissue, attempting a complete removal is very risky and often not possible.

References

1. Reese AB. Persistent hyperplastic primary vitreous. Trans Am Acad Ophthalmol Otolaryngol. 1955.
2. Goldberg MF. Persistent fetal vasculature (PFV): An integrated interpretation of signs and symptoms associated with persistent hyperplastic primary vitreous (PHPV) LIV Edward Jackson Memorial Lecture. Amer J Ophthalmol. 1997.
3. Levine RA, Gray DL, Gould N, Pergament E, Stillerman ML. Warburg syndrome. Ophthalmology. 1983.
4. Marshman WE, Jan JE, Lyons CJ. Neurologic abnormalities associated with persistent hyperplastic primary vitreous. Can J Ophthalmol. 1999.
5. Haddad R, Font RL, Reeser F. Persistent hyperplastic primary vitreous. A clinicopathologic study of 62 cases and review of the literature. Surv Ophthalmol. 1978.
6. Pollard ZF. Persistent hyperplastic primary vitreous: Diagnosis, treatment and results. Trans Amer Ophthalmol Soc. 1997.
7. Galal AH, Kotoury AIS, Azzab AA. Bilateral persistent hyperplastic primary vitreous: an Egyptian family supporting a rare autosomal dominant inheritance. Genet. Couns. 2006.
8. Khaliq S, Hameed A, Ismail M, Anwar K, Leroy B, Payne AM, et al. Locus for autosomal recessive nonsyndromic persistent hyperplastic primary vitreous. Investig Ophthalmol Vis Sci. 2001.
9. Ko MK, Chi JG, Chang BL. Hyaloid vascular pattern in the human fetus. J Pediatr Ophthalmol Strabismus. 1985.
10. Verdijk RM, Herwig-Carl MC. Development of the human eye. In: Fetal and neonatal eye pathology. 2020.
11. Mutlu F, Leopold IH. The structure of fetal hyaloid system and tunica Vasculosa Lentis. Arch Ophthalmol. 1964.
12. Sellheyer K, Spitznas M. Ultrastructure of the human posterior tunica vasculosa lentis during early gestation. Graefe's Arch Clin Exp Ophthalmol. 1987.
13. Barishak YR. Embryology of the eye and its adnexae. Dev. Ophthalmol. 1992.
14. Meisels HI, Goldberg MF. Vascular anastomoses between the iris and persistent hyperplastic primary vitreous. Am J Ophthalmol. 1979.

15. Ozdek S, Ozdemir Zeydanli E, Atalay HT, Aktas Z. Anterior elongation of the retina in persistent fetal vasculature: emphasis on retinal complications. Eye. 2019.
16. Federman JL, Shields JA, Altman B, Koller H. The surgical and nonsurgical management of persistent hyperplastic prima vitreous. Ophthalmology. 1982.
17. Karacorlu M, Hocaoglu M, Sayman Muslubas I, Arf S, Ersoz MG, Uysal O. Functional and anatomical outcomes following surgical management of persistent fetal vasculature: a single-center experience of 44 cases. Graefe's Arch Clin Exp Ophthalmol. 2018.
18. Ozdemir Zeydanli E, Ozdek S. Surgical results of posterior persistent vasculature syndrome. In: Turkish ophthalmological association virtual national congress and live surgery compound meeting; 2020.
19. Kilty LA, Hiles DA. Unilateral posterior lenticonus with persistent hyaloid artery remnant. Am J Ophthalmol. 1993.
20. Ozdemir Zeydanli E, Tefon AB, Atalay HT, Ozdek S. Pseudo-hyaloidal stalk in anterior persistent fetal vasculature: a report of two cases. Turkish J Ophthalmol. 2021;51:407–11.
21. Hunt A, Rowe N, Lam A, Martin F. Outcomes in persistent hyperplastic primary vitreous. Br J Ophthalmol. 2005.
22. Alexandrakis G, Scott IU, Flynn HW, Murray TG, Feuer WJ. Visual acuity outcomes with and without surgery in patients with persistent fetal vasculature. Ophthalmology. 2000.
23. Sisk RA, Berrocal AM, Feuer WJ, Murray TG. Visual and anatomic outcomes with or without surgery in persistent fetal vasculature. Ophthalmology. 2010.
24. Bosjolie A, Ferrone P. Visual outcome in early vitrectomy for posterior persistent fetal vasculature associated with traction retinal detachment. Retina. 2015.
25. Scuderi G, Balestrazzi E, Ranieri G. Destructive and conservative treatment of persistent hyperplastic primary vitreous and retinal dysplasia. Ophthalmologica. 1976.
26. Dawson DG, Gleiser J, Movaghar M, Patel SM, Albert DM. Persistent fetal vasculature. Arch Ophthalmol. 2003; 121(9):1340–1341. Available at: https://doi.org/10.1001/archopht.121.9.1340.
27. Soheilian M, Vistamehr S, Rahmani B, Ahmadieh H, Azarmina M, Mashayekhi A, et al. Outcomes of surgical (pars plicata and limbal lensectomy, vitrectomy) and non-surgical management of persistent fetal vasculature (PFV): An analysis of 54 eyes. Eur J Ophthalmol. 2002.
28. Pollard ZF. Persistent hyperplastic primary vitreous: diagnosis, treatment and results. Trans Am Ophthalmol Soc. 1997.
29. Gulati N, Eagle RC, Tasman W, Tornambe PE, France TD, Stager DR, et al. Unoperated eyes with persistent fetal vasculature. Trans Amer Ophthalmol Soc. 2003.
30. Walsh MK, Drenser KA, Capone A, Trese MT. Early vitrectomy effective for bilateral combined anterior and posterior persistent fetal vasculature syndrome. Retina. 2010.
31. Anteby I, Cohen E, Karshai I, BenEzra D. Unilateral persistent hyperplastic primary vitreous: course and outcome. J AAPOS. 2002.

Retinochoroidal Coloboma

31

Shunji Kusaka

Abstract

Retinochoroidal coloboma is a rare congenital anomaly that is often accompanied by various other ocular anomalies, including iris coloboma, cataract, lens coloboma, optic disc coloboma, microphthalmos, and microcornea. Rhegmatogenous retinal detachment is the most serious vision-threatening complication. Retinal breaks are often located inside colobomas. Pars plana vitrectomy with or without lensectomy and laser ablation around the coloboma and peripheral breaks (if present), followed by silicone oil or long-acting gas tamponade, are commonly performed with relatively good outcomes. However, redetachment is common.

Keywords

Retinochoroidal coloboma · Pediatric rhegmatogenous retinal detachment · Retinal break · Vitrectomy · Silicone oil tamponade · Gas tamponade

Supplementary Information The online version contains supplementary material available at https://doi.org/10.1007/978-3-031-14506-3_31.

S. Kusaka (✉)
Faculty of Medicine, Kindai University, Osakasayama, Osaka, Japan
e-mail: skusaka@gmail.com

Introduction

Background

During the fifth to seventh week of fetal life, malclosure of the embryonic fissure results in coloboma [1, 2]. If it occurs at the anterior end of the embryonic fissure, coloboma of the iris, ciliary body, and choroid in the inferonasal quadrant (Figs. 31.1, 31.2 and 31.3). In contrast, malclosure of the posterior end of the embryonic fissure results in coloboma of the optic disc (Figs. 31.3 and 31.4). A retiochoroidal coloboma occurs when both the neurosensory elements and the retinal pigment epithelium (RPE) precursors fail to fuse. The choroid also fails to differentiate as normal choroidal differentiation requires a normal RPE [1].

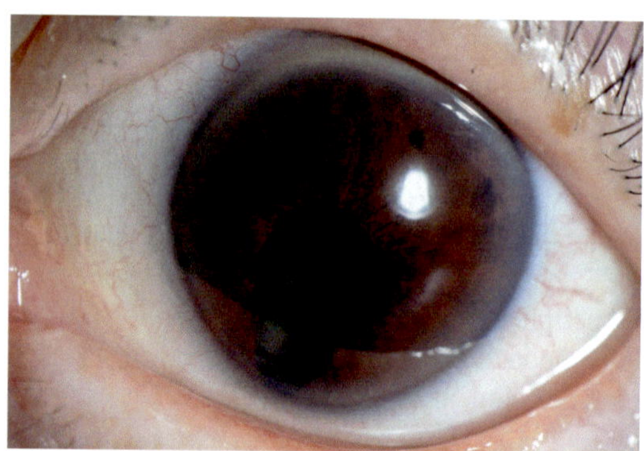

Fig. 31.1 Iris coloboma is seen in the inferonasal quadrant of the left eye

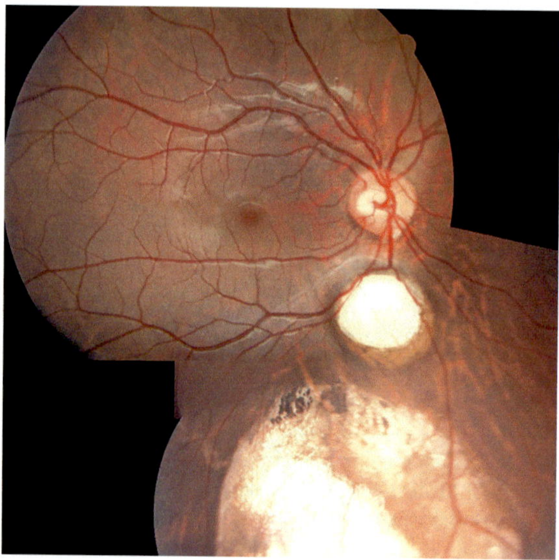

Fig. 31.2 Multiple retinochoroidal colobomas (courtesy of Dr. Kazuki Kuniyoshi)

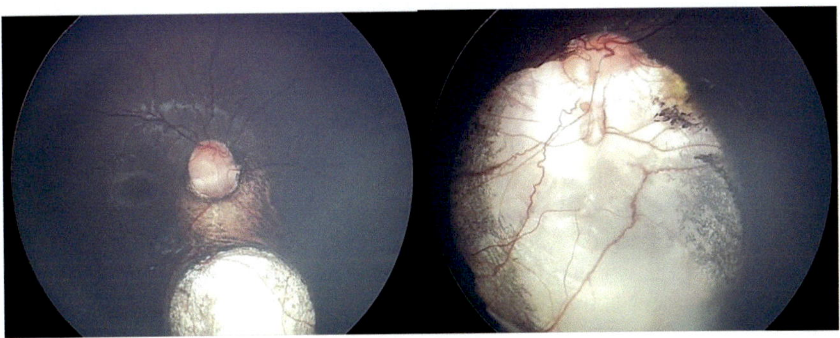

Fig. 31.3 Bilateral retinochoroidal coloboma involving the optic disc. (left panel, OD) (right panel, OS)

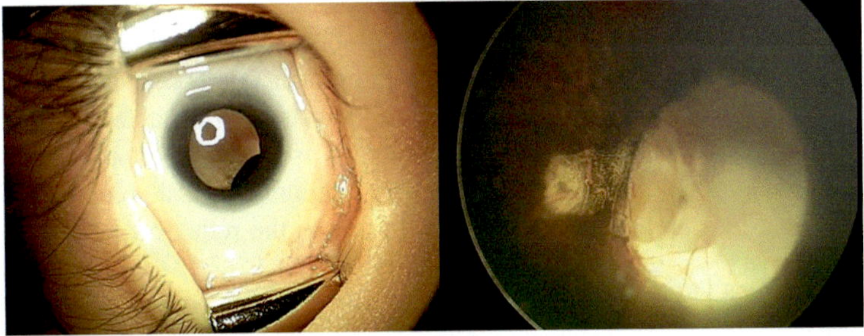

Fig. 31.4 Microcornea and retinochoroidal coloboma involving the optic disc with macular atrophy

Epidemiology

The reported incidence of coloboma ranges from 0.2 to 1.4 per 10,000 births [2–5] with bilateral cases seen in about 50% of cases [4, 6]. Blindness due to coloboma has been reported to occur in 0.7% of 24,605 blind patients of all generations in Canada [7] and 1.3% of all blind children from 26 countries [8].

Typical/Atypical

"Typical" coloboma is the most common. It is caused by malclosure of the embryonic fissure and is located in the inferonasal quadrant. The cause of "atypical" coloboma remains unclear, and its location can be anywhere, except for the inferonasal quadrant [2].

Histopathology of Retinochoroidal Coloboma

The term "retinochoroidal coloboma" is essentially synonymous with "choroidal coloboma". The inner part of the retinochoroidal coloboma is called the intercalary membrane, which is a monolayer of atrophic neurons and glial structures, sometimes with retinal vessels. The underlying RPE is absent, and the choroid is either hypoplastic or absent. At the margin of the coloboma, the retinal layers become reversed, the outer retinal layers are duplicated, and the inner retinal layers are adjacent to the RPE, which is defined as the point of reversal [9]. In the center of the coloboma, the sclera is thin and may protrude posteriorly, forming a staphyloma [10].

Clinical Features

Retinochoroidal coloboma and optic nerve coloboma are more frequently associated with poor visual function than anterior segment coloboma. Retinochoroidal colobomas usually appear as glistening white defects with clear margins, rimmed by pigment clumps. The bottom of the coloboma is often irregular and protrudes posteriorly. An iris coloboma may accompany a retinochoroidal coloboma, but not always. Sometimes parents notice leukocoria due to the reflex of the coloboma in the affected eye.

Microphthalmos and microcornea (Fig. 31.4) are also congenital ocular malformations. They sometimes coexist with retinochoroidal colobomas [11]. A macular and/or optic disc coloboma can be accompanied by a retinochoroidal coloboma. The visual acuity of patients with retinochoroidal coloboma is dependent on the presence and degree of involvement of the optic disc, macula, and other congenital ocular malformations, such as microphthalmos [11, 12].

Vitreoretinal Complications

The most frequent vitreoretinal complication of retinochoroidal coloboma is retinal detachment. Rhegmatogenous retinal detachment is observed in 30–40% of cases with long-term follow-up [10, 13].

Retinal Breaks

Histopathological studies indicated that both a central break in the inner layer and a break in the outer layer at the margin of the coloboma are necessary for the development of retinal detachment [10] (Fig. 31.5). A break in the inner layer may be the result of ischemia or scleral stretching. A break in the outer layer may be

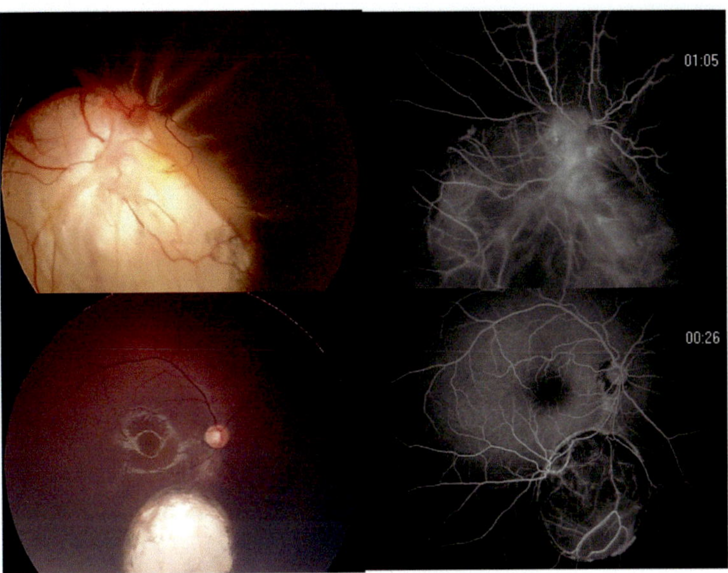

Fig. 31.5 A large retinochoroidal coloboma involving the optic disc with retinal detachment in the temporal and superior quadrants in the left eye. The right eye also has retinochoroidal coloboma. (Upper left panel: color fundus image of the left eye, upper right panel: fluorescein angiography image of the left eye. Lower left panel: color fundus image of the right eye. Lower right panel: fluorescein angiography image of the right eye). No retinal breaks outside of the coloboma are observed. Note the presence of vasculature inside the colobomas

explained by vitreous traction on the margin of the coloboma or extension of the formerly isolated detachment through the outer marginal zone of decreased glial support [10].

Wang et al. [14] reported that of 26 eyes with retinal detachment, retinal breaks were located inside (breaks in the intercalary membrane), outside, both inside and outside of the coloboma, and unidentified, in nine, seven, one, and nine eyes, respectively. Hanneken et al. [15] reported that in five of eight eyes with retinal detachment associated with retinochoroidal coloboma, retinal breaks were identified within the coloboma in four eyes. Corcostegui et al. [16] reported that in seven eyes, all retinal breaks were inside the coloboma, except for one eye with a peripheral retinal break. Gopal et al. [17] reported that out of 47 retinal breaks in 36 eyes (one to four breaks, with a mean of 1.3 breaks per eye), 64% of breaks were located within 2-disc diameters of the margin of coloboma, and the remaining 36% were located in the central portion. Hussain et al. [13] reported that in 15 retinal detachment cases, retinal breaks were identified inside, outside, and both inside and outside of the coloboma in four, five, and four eyes, respectively. No retinal breaks were identified in the remaining two eyes. Thus, the most frequent location of retinal breaks is within or adjacent to the coloboma. Retinal breaks remote from the

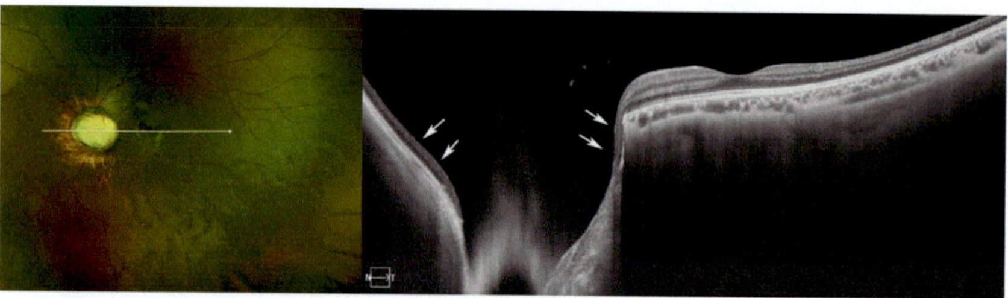

Fig. 31.6 Color fundus photograph of the left eye with optic disc coloboma (left panel). Swept-source OCT image showing a deep excavation of the optic disc and monolayer of the intercalary membrane inside the coloboma (arrows) (right panel)

coloboma are less common. Visualization of the break inside the coloboma is sometimes difficult ophthalmoscopically due to lack of contrast as a result of the RPE being absent in the coloboma (Fig. 31.5). Optical coherence tomography may be useful for identifying breaks inside the coloboma or revealing the detailed structure of the retinochoroidal coloboma [18, 19] (see Fig. 31.6).

Surgery for Retinal Detachment

Scleral buckling may be indicated for eyes with peripheral retinal breaks. In a previous study, even with breaks inside the coloboma, an attempt was made to use two radial scleral buckles on either side of the coloboma, but successful retinal reattachment was achieved in only 6 of 14 eyes [14]. More recently, pars plana vitrectomy has been the preferred technique for the treatment of retinochoroidal coloboma with breaks inside the coloboma. After the posterior vitreous detachment, the subretinal fluid is aspirated from the break inside the coloboma during fluid/air exchange. Then, to create a barrier to prevent the migration of fluid from the space between the detached intercalary membrane and the underlying sclera to the subretinal space, laser ablation is performed around the coloboma. Silicone oil or long-acting gas is used for tamponade.

Even with these surgical techniques, the retinal reattachment rate is not always high, and redetachment seems to be relatively common. Hanneken et al. [15] reported that final reattachment was achieved in seven of eight eyes with an average of three procedures. Gopal et al. [20] reported that final reattachment was achieved in 81.2% of 85 treated eyes. Recurrent retinal detachment was more common in gas-filled eyes than in silicone oil-filled eyes (60% vs. 16.3%). Abouammoh et al. [21] reported a final reattachment rate of 87.4% of 119 eyes. They suggested that encircling does not affect the final anatomical outcome, and that cryopexy is associated with poor surgical results.

Case Presentation (see the Video)

A 16-year-old girl with total retinal detachment and mild proliferative vitreo-retinopathy, retinochoroidal coloboma involving the optic disc, microcornea, and persistent pupillary membrane in the left eye was referred to our clinic for treatment. The patient's right eye was normal. Vitrectomy and lensectomy were performed using a 23-gauge system. There were no visible breaks inside or outside the coloboma. During detachment of the posterior vitreous, which adhered tightly to the retina, perfluoro-*n*-octane was used to stabilize the posterior retina. Iatrogenic retinal breaks were created in the inferior retina during membrane peeling, through which the subretinal strands were removed. During fluid/air exchange, exudation of the fluid from inside the coloboma was found, which suggested the presence of a break. Laser ablation was performed around the coloboma and all retinal breaks, followed by a 14% C_3F_8 gas tamponade. The retina was successfully reattached postoperatively.

Conclusion

Rhegmatogenous retinal detachment sometimes occurs in eyes with retinochoroidal coloboma. Even with recent pars plana vitrectomy techniques, redetachment is relatively common. A better understanding of the pathology to further improve surgical treatment is necessary.

Review Questions

1. Which statement is correct for typical retinochoroidal coloboma?

a. It is most likely to be seen in both eyes.
b. It is likely to be seen in the inferonasal quadrant.
c. Retinal detachment occurs in fewer than 10% of cases.
d. Vasculature is not usually seen inside the coloboma.

2. Which is the most common location of retinal breaks in eyes with retinal detachment and retinochoroidal coloboma?

a. Inside the coloboma
b. Inferonasal quadrant, outside the coloboma
c. Superotemporal quadrant, outside the coloboma
d. Inferotemporal quadrant, outside the coloboma

Answers

1. B
2. A

References

1. Pagon RA. Ocular coloboma. Surv Ophthalmol. 1981;25(4):223–36.
2. Onwochei BC, Simon JW, Bateman JB, Couture KC, Mir E. Ocular colobomata. Surv Ophthalmol. 2000;45(3):175–94.
3. Stoll C, Alembik Y, Dott B, Roth MP. Congenital eye malformations in 212,479 consecutive births. Ann Genet. 1997;40(2):122–8.
4. Shah SP, Taylor AE, Sowden JC, Ragge NK, Russell-Eggitt I, Rahi JS, et al. Anophthalmos, microphthalmos, and typical coloboma in the United Kingdom: a prospective study of incidence and risk. Invest Ophthalmol Vis Sci. 2011;52(1):558–64.
5. Nakamura KM, Diehl NN, Mohney BG. Incidence, ocular findings, and systemic associations of ocular coloboma: a population-based study. Arch Ophthalmol. 2011;129(1):69–74.
6. Morrison D, FitzPatrick D, Hanson I, Williamson K, van Heyningen V, Fleck B, et al. National study of microphthalmia, anophthalmia, and coloboma (MAC) in Scotland: investigation of genetic aetiology. J Med Genet. 2002;39(1):16–22.
7. Ae M. Causes of blindness in Canada: an analysis of 24,605 cases registered with the Canadian national institute for the blind. Can Med Assoc J. 1965;92(6):264–79.
8. Hornby SJ, Gilbert CE, Rahi JK, Sil AK, Xiao Y, Dandona L, et al. Regional variation in blindness in children due to microphthalmos, anophthalmos and coloboma. Ophthalmic Epidemiol. 2000;7(2):127–38.
9. Schubert HD. Schisis-like rhegmatogenous retinal detachment associated with choroidal colobomas. Graefes Arch Clin Exp Ophthalmol. 1995;233(2):74–9.
10. Jesberg DO, Schepens CL. Retinal detachment associated with coloboma of the choroid. Arch Ophthalmol. 1961;65:163–73.
11. Shah SP, Taylor AE, Sowden JC, Ragge N, Russell-Eggitt I, Rahi JS, et al. Anophthalmos, microphthalmos, and Coloboma in the United kingdom: clinical features, results of investigations, and early management. Ophthalmology. 2012;119(2):362–8.
12. Gopal L, Badrinath SS, Kumar KS, Doshi G, Biswas N. Optic disc in fundus coloboma. Ophthalmology. 1996;103(12):2120–7.
13. Hussain RM, Abbey AM, Shah AR, Drenser KA, Trese MT, Capone A Jr. Chorioretinal coloboma complications: retinal detachment and choroidal neovascular membrane. J Ophthalmic Vis Res. 2017;12(1):3–10.
14. Wang KHGF. Retinal detachment associated with coloboma of the choroid. Trans Am Ophthalmol Soc. 1985;83:49–62.
15. Hanneken A, de Juan E, McCuen BW. The management of retinal detachments associated with choroidal colobomas by vitreous surgery. Am J Ophthalmol. 1991;111(3):271–5.
16. Corcostegui B, Guell JL, Garcia-Arumi J. Surgical treatment of retinal detachment in the choroidal colobomas. Retina. 1992;12(3):237–41.
17. Gopal L, Badrinath SS, Sharma T, Parikh SN, Biswas J. Pattern of retinal breaks and retinal detachments in eyes with choroidal coloboma. Ophthalmology. 1995;102(8):1212–7.
18. Jain S, Kumar V, Salunkhe N, Tewari R, Chandra P, Kumar A. Swept-source OCT analysis of the margin of choroidal coloboma: new insights. Ophthalmol Retina. 2020;4(1):92–9.
19. Tanaka S, Yokoi T, Katagiri S, Yoshida-Uemura T, Nishina S, Azuma N. Structure of the retinal margin and presumed mechanism of retinal detachment in choroidal coloboma. Ophthalmol Retina. 2021;5(7):702–10.
20. Gopal L, Badrinath SS, Sharma T, Parikh SN, Shanmugam MS, Bhende PS, et al. Surgical management of retinal detachments related to coloboma of the choroid 11. The authors have no proprietary interest in any of the materials used in this study. Ophthalmology. 1998;105(5):804–9.
21. Abouammoh MA, Alsulaiman SM, Gupta VS, Younis A, Chhablani J, Hussein A, et al. Surgical outcomes and complications of rhegmatogenous retinal detachment in eyes with chorioretinal coloboma: the results of the KKESH international collaborative retina study group. Retina. 2017;37(10):1942–7.

Optic Nerve Head-Related Maculopathy

32

Chen Yen-Ting and Wei-Chi Wu

Abstract

Optic nerve head-related maculopathy (ONHM) is a group of diseases of excavated optic disc anomalies including optic disc pit (ODP), optic disc coloboma (ODC), and morning glory disc anomaly (MGDA) that lead to maculopathy caused by prolonged existing subretinal fluid. If symptoms are less severe in patients with ONHM, observation may be an option and spontaneous resolution can be possible. In ONHM patients with more severe symptoms, vitrectomy is well-accepted as the first treatment option, either alone or in combination with other adjuvant procedures. In patients who are refractory to primary vitrectomy, fovea-sparing internal limiting membrane (ILM) flap, autologous blood, scleral flap, or autologous fibrin can be considered as salvage therapies.

Keywords

Optic pit · Optic pit maculopathy · Morning glory disc anomaly · Optic disc coloboma · Macular detachment · Vitrectomy · Fovea sparing internal limiting membrane flap · Autologous fibrin

Supplementary Information The online version contains supplementary material available at https://doi.org/10.1007/978-3-031-14506-3_32.

C. Yen-Ting (✉) · W.-C. Wu
Department of Ophthalmology, Chang Gung Memorial Hospital, Taoyuan, Taiwan
e-mail: gradychen1107@gmail.com

College of Medicine, Chang Gung University, Taoyuan, Taiwan

Introduction

Congenital excavated optic disc anomalies such as ODP, ODC, and MGDA may lead to maculopathies such as macular detachment, retinoschisis-like separation of retinal layer, ellipsoid zone disruption, outer layer lamellar macular hole, full-thickness macular hole, etc. [1]. The defective closure of the embryonic fissure or an impaired differentiation of the peripapillary sclera from the primary mesenchyme has been suggested to cause these congenital excavated optic disc anomalies [2, 3]. The pathophysiology of the fluid origin is not completely understood. It has been proposed that the fluid may have a double source of origin: vitreal and cerebrospinal [1]. Fluid leaking from the vessels or choroid has also been reported with less evidences [4]. In most cases, the fluid first creates a schisis-like separation of the inner retina and then reaches to the subretinal space creating a macular neuroepithelial detachment. The subsequent ellipsoid zone disruption, outer layer lamellar or full-thickness macular hole formation have been recognized as predictors for poor visual acuity gain [1].

Optic Disc Pits

ODPs are rare congenital disc abnormalities appearing as solitary round or oval gray-white excavations that are typically unilateral (85%) and usually located at the inferotemporal margin of the optic disc [5]. Although they are most frequently observed in early adulthood, ODPs can occur as early as 3 years of age [6]. The exact pathogenesis of ODPs remains unclear, and the source of the accumulating subretinal and intraretinal fluid (IRF) is still debated [4]. Histologically, ODP consist of herniations of dysplastic retina into a collagen-lined pocket extending posteriorly, often into the subarachnoid space, through a defect in the lamina cribrosa [2]. ODPs are usually asymptomatic. However, 25–75% of patients with ODP can experience vision loss at some stage of their lives when serous detachment or retinoschisis affects the central macula, developing into ODP maculopathy (ODPM) [4].

Studies describing the natural history of ODPM in children are scarce; therefore, no consensus exists regarding the optimal indications or timeline for surgical treatment. Although ODPM can spontaneously resolve, observation or conservative treatments such as those involving the administration of systemic carbonic anhydrase inhibitors (CAIs; e.g., acetazolamide, methazolamide, ethoxzolamide, or dichlorophenamide) or topical CAIs (e.g., dorzolamide or brinzolamide) constitute a reasonable first step for patients with a relatively favorable initial visual acuity and less severe symptoms [7–10]. However, for patients with poor initial visual acuity, persistent or progressive subretinal fluid (SRF), or decreased vision during follow-up, surgical intervention may be required because persistent SRF may engender outer retinal atrophy and poor visual outcomes [6]. Studies have suggested the following treatment options: juxtapapillary laser photocoagulation (JLP);

pneumatic tamponade with or without JLP; trans-pars plana vitrectomy (TPPV) with or without ILM peeling; optic disc plugging with an ILM flap, autologous blood, autologous fibrin, fibrin glue, or a scleral flap; and macular buckling [4, 11–18].

Of these options, TPPV with posterior vitreous detachment (PVD) induction, either alone or in combination with other adjuvant procedures (e.g., JLP, pneumatic tamponade, ILM peeling), is currently the mainstay surgical procedure for ODPM treatment. These procedures were reported to have high anatomical success rates (50–90%) and comparable functional outcomes (>50% of cases exhibiting visual improvement) [11]. Nevertheless, the benefits of the adjuvant procedures have yet to be proven. A multi-centered retrospective study showed that JLP and ILM peeling provided no additional anatomical or functional benefit [1]. JLP can cause damage to the maculopapular bundle and subsequent visual field defects. ILM peeling may increase the risk of macular hole formation because of unroofing of the fovea, especially in cases with outer lamellar macular hole [1, 6, 11, 19, 20]. To eliminate the tangential traction caused by the ILM and prevent making a macular hole at the same time, fovea-sparing ILM peeling may be a reasonable technique [21].

Macular buckling was reported to achieve a success rate of 85%, in addition to providing long-term visual improvement and achieving low rates of complications and recurrence [4, 11, 22]. However, this technique is difficult and involves a steep learning curve, thus limiting its application. A case series focusing on ODPM in pediatric patients revealed that TPPV performed along with two partial-thickness inner retinal fenestrations that were created using a 25-gauge MVR blade provided promising results [23]. This case series reported that the mean preoperative best-corrected visual acuity (BCVA) was logMAR 0.71 ± 0.29 (20/100), and the corresponding range was 0.3–1.0 (20/40–20/200); the mean postoperative BCVA was logMAR 0.49 ± 0.30 (20/70) at 2 weeks, 0.35 ± 0.33 (20/50) at 3 months, 0.26 ± 0.32 (20/40) at 6 months, and 0.16 ± 0.29 (20/32) at 1 year. The case series also indicated anatomical success with progressive resolution of IRF and SRF in all six eyes that underwent the procedure, and no complication or recurrence was observed [23]. Nevertheless, additional studies are required to validate this new technique.

Because pediatric vitrectomy is often difficult to perform, weighing the benefits against the risks associated with surgery in children with ODPM is critical. Medical treatment is always the most preferable option. Surgeons should carefully consider visual acuity, SRF fluctuations, disease progression, patient's subjective symptoms, and other systemic and ocular comorbidities when exploring the possibility of surgical treatment. The willingness to undergo surgery and the expectations of surgical outcomes on the part of patients and their families should also be taken into account when determining the appropriacy of surgical intervention. When surgery is chosen, we recommend a complete vitrectomy, PVD induction assisted by tri-amcinolone acetonide for vitreous staining, and tamponade with long-acting gas to ensure surgical outcomes. Optic pit plugging with a fovea-sparing ILM flap or faint JLP along the optic disc margin can be utilized in these cases but not mandatory.

Silicone oil migration to the subretinal space has been reported in studies using silicone oil tamponade [24]. Hence, silicone oil tamponade should be avoided in the treatment of ODPM. For those ODPM patients that were unresponsive to or recurred after vitrectomy, successful treatments had been reported using the autologous blood, scleral flap, or autologous fibrin to seal the ODP (**see the video 1**, video courtesy of Prof. Dr. Şengül Özdek). Despite anatomical successes, the visual improvement in these patients was still limited [1, 14, 17, 18].

Video 1: *Describes a 10 year old boy with an optic pit maculopathy who had been operated once with ILM grafts over the pit area but had a recurrent maculopathy and a secondary macular hole formation. The video shows the second surgery with use of autologous fibrin for optic pit together with macular hole surgery.*

Clinical Case Scenario

An 8.5-year-old girl without any systemic or previous ocular disease presented with acute-onset blurred vision in her left eye after a pillow fight. Her initial BCVA was 0.2, with a moderate degree of myopia (−2.50D). Slit lamp examination results and intraocular pressure were normal. Fundus examination revealed an ODP at the inferotemporal margin with inferior serous retinal detachment (RD; Fig. 32.1A). Optical coherence tomography (OCT) revealed marked SRF with foveal detachment, some IRF, and ellipsoid zone (EZ) disruption (Fig. 32.1B). The right eye was unremarkable. After 6 months of observation, follow-up OCT indicated gradually decreased SRF with some restoration of EZ and an improvement in BCVA to 0.4 (Fig. 32.1C). With treatment with acetazolamide 250 mg four times a day, the SRF decreased further, and the patient's BCVA reached 0.7 at the 1-year follow-up (Fig. 32.1D). The drug was discontinued after 3 months of administration.

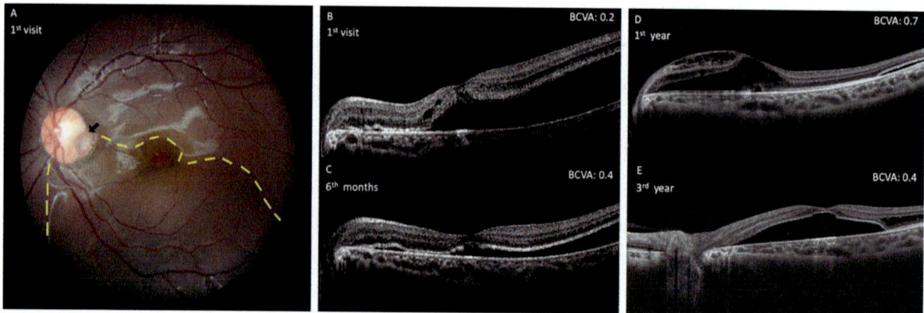

Fig. 32.1 Color fundus and serial optical coherence tomography (OCT) images of an 8.5-year-old girl. **A** An optic disc pit was observed at the inferotemporal margin of the optic disc, appearing as a gray-white oval excavation (arrow). Inferior shallow serous retinal detachment involving the fovea was also observed (yellow bar). **B** Macular OCT revealed marked subretinal fluid (SRF) at initial presentation. **C** The SRF decreased with some ellipsoid zone restoration and visual acuity improvement during follow-up. **D** The SRF further decreased and the best corrected visual acuity (BCVA) improved to 0.7 after 1 year. **E** The SRF and BCVA fluctuated at the 3-year follow-up

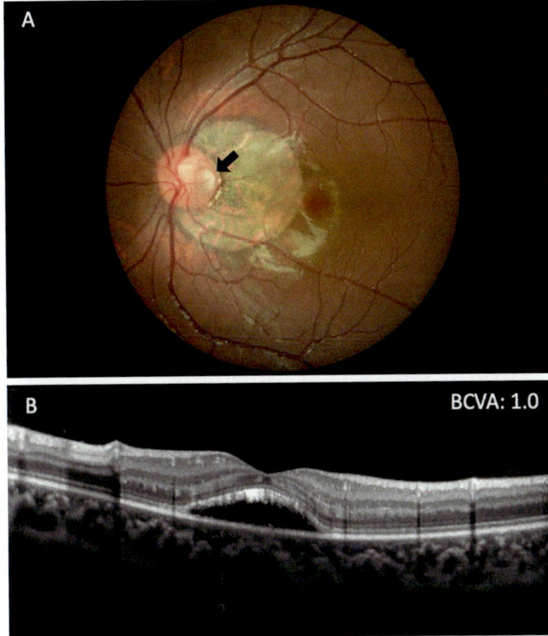

Fig. 32.2 Color fundus and optical coherence tomography (OCT) images of a 6.5-year-old boy with an optic disc pit (ODP). **A** Gray-white ODP at the temporal margin of the optic disc surrounded by a circular zone of depigmentation. **B** OCT image revealed shallow subretinal fluid under the fovea

However, at the 3-year follow-up, the patient's SRF was again remarkable and her BCVA decreased to 0.4 (Fig. 32.1E). Currently, the patient is still under follow-up; close observation and surgical management may be required if her BCVA deteriorates or if the SRF persists.

In another case, a 6.5-year-old boy without any systemic or previous ocular disease was referred to our department for an accidental finding of an ODP in his left eye. Fundus examination showed an ODP at the temporal margin surrounded by a circular zone of depigmentation (Fig. 32.2A). OCT indicated shallow SRF with foveal detachment (Fig. 32.2B). Despite these findings, his left-eye BCVA was 1.0 and no treatment was required during follow up.

Optic Disc Coloboma

Optic disc coloboma (ODC) is a congenital anomaly characterized by a sharply delimited, glistening white, bowl-shaped excavation occupying an enlarged optic disc [2]. The excavation is usually decentered inferiorly, reflecting the position of incomplete closure of the embryonic fissure during the 5th–7th week of intrauterine life [25]. The prevalence of ODC was reported to be 8.9/100.000 in one population-based cross-sectional study [26]. It may be unilateral or bilateral and may occur in association with other ocular colobomas, microphthalmia, or congenital disc anomalies such as ODP and MGDA. The visual function of the affected eye may be significantly impaired if the macula was also colobomatous or presented with maculopathies caused by retinal detachment. ODC most commonly occurs sporadically and may be associated with conditions such as CHARGE syndrome (coloboma, heart defects, nasal choanal atresia, growth/developmental retardation, genitourinary anomalies, and ear defects/hearing loss), Goldenhar syndromes, and chromosomal anomalies such as Edwards and Patau syndrome [27]. ODC was also in association with congenital craniofacial anomalies such as basal encephalocoeles, cleft lip and palate, agenesis of the corpus colosum, defects in the sella turcica, and endocrine dysfunction [25].

Morning Glory Disc Anomaly

MGDA is a rare congenital developmental optic nerve anomaly characterized by a funnel-shaped excavation of the posterior fundus that incorporates the optic disc, with a central tuft of white glial tissue overlying the central portion of the disc, peripapillary pigmentations, and straightened vessels developing from the rim of the optic disc in a radial pattern [25]. MGDA has been observed to be associated with basal encephalocele, Aicardi syndrome, neurofibromatosis type 2, Chiari malformation type 1, and PHACE (Posterior fossa brain malformations, Hemangioma, Arterial lesions, Cardiac abnormalities, and Eye abnormalities) syndrome (a neurocutaneous disorder) [3]. MGDA is nonprogressive and usually does not require treatment unless when it occurs in combination with other ocular comorbidities such as congenital cataracts, persistent hyaloid remnants, lid hemangioma, preretinal gliosis, posterior lenticonus, or RD. RD is present in one-third of patients with MGDA [28, 29]. The precise mechanisms underlying MGDA-associated RD remain unclear, although vessel exudation, vitreous traction, retinal breaks on the optic disc, and cerebrospinal fluid migration from the subarachnoid space have all been suggested as potential mechanisms [30].

The management of MGDA-associated RD poses a unique set of challenges during surgery [31]. First, the lack of contrast between the white scleral background and the anomalous disc as well as the presence of breaks within the overlying fibroglial tissue increases the difficulty of surgery. A careful preoperative or intraoperative OCT can assist in identifying the breaks and enhance safety during fibroglial tissue removal, epiretinal membrane (ERM) peeling, and ILM peeling. Second, inducing PVD in pediatric patients with MGDA-associated RD is difficult because of the tight vitreoretinal adhesion and frequently accompanying vitreoschisis. ERM and ILM peeling can ensure complete removal of the posterior hyaloid membrane. Third, patients with MGDA-associated RD often present late, which may lead to a higher rate of proliferative vitreoretinopathy (PVR) changes. Fourth, abnormal communication between the subretinal space and the subarachnoid space or vitreous cavity can cause serous RD. Plugging the disc with an ILM flap or a scleral flap leads to a resolution of fluid in congenital cavitary optic disc anomalies such as ODPM. However, the large MGDA size renders complete plugging difficult. The use of perfluorocarbon liquids (PFCLs) or silicone oil in MGDA-associated RD should be approached with caution because of the risk of PFCL or oil migration into the subretinal and subarachnoid spaces [30, 31].

Currently, no standard treatment for MGDA-associated RD exists, although TPPV, JLP, and silicone oil tamponade have been frequently attempted [30, 32]. Triamcinolone acetonide is recommended for vitreous staining. The epipapillary fibroglial tissue should be removed or trimmed to remove all the tractional elements. The use of an additional encircling scleral buckle helps in peripheral vitreous base shaving and relieves anterior traction in cases of PVR. Despite an anatomical success rate of 66% (6/9) in a recent case series using TPPV with or without JLP, silicone oil or C3F8 tamponade, visual prognosis in these patients is often guarded due to the inherent pathology of the optic disc, other ocular comorbidities, and amblyopia [32, 33].

Clinical Scenario

A 4-year-old boy was diagnosed as having a left-eye MGDA with a BCVA of 0.04 and shallow SRF at initial presentation (Fig. 32.3A, B). Intermittent exophoria was noted. Left-eye slit lamp examination results, intraocular pressure, and right-eye

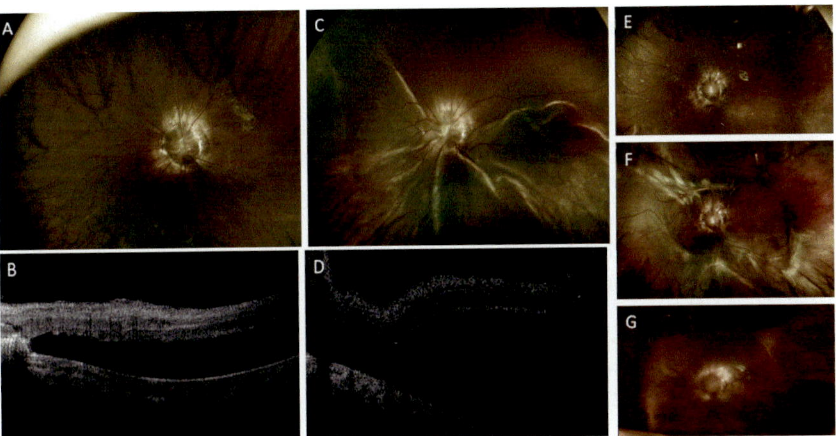

Fig. 32.3 Color fundus and optical coherence tomography (OCT) images of a patient with a morning glory disc anomaly (MGDA). **A** MGDA with classic funnel-shaped excavation of the optic disc, straightening of vessels, central glial tuft, and peripapillary pigmentations was noted. The image was obtained with an Optos ultra-widefield imaging system. **B** Retinal detachment (RD) with shallow subretinal fluid was also observed through OCT. **C** Progression to bullous RD from 2.5 to 10.5 o'clock with foveal involvement and proliferative vitreoretinopathy (PVR) were noted during follow-up. **D** Marked subretinal fluid and retinal undulation were observed through OCT. **E** Reattached retina after the surgery under silicone oil tamponade. **F** Recurrent retinal detachment with proliferative vitreoretinopathy grade CP10 with subretinal bands developed after silicon oil removal. **G** Retinal reattachment was achieved after membrane peeling, 360° retinectomy, subretinal band removal, laser photocoagulation, and silicone oil re-tamponade

examination results were all unremarkable. At 5.5 years old, MGDA-associated RD and PVR changes developed with macular involvement, and his BCVA decreased to 0.01 (Fig. 32.3C, D). He then received 23-gauge TPPV combined with an encircling scleral buckle. During the surgery, PVD was induced through the use of a lighted pick as a second instrument. Membrane peeling was performed with intraocular forceps. PFCLs were used, and a retinotomy was performed to drain the SRF through fluid–air exchange. JLP was applied around the disc margin as well as retinotomy. The eye was tamponaded with 20% C3F8 (**Video** 2).

However, recurrent RD developed 1.5 month after the initial surgery. After the execution of TPPV with membrane peeling and silicone oil tamponade, his retina reattached successfully (Fig. 32.3E). Seven months later, retinal re-detachment was noted again during silicone oil removal. Despite C3F8 tamponade, the retina remained detached, and PVR grade CP10 with subretinal bands developed (Fig. 32.3F). Additional TPPV with lensectomy, membrane peeling, subretinal band removal, 360° retinectomy, laser photocoagulation, and silicone oil tamponade were performed. Subsequently, the retina was attached under silicone oil tamponade (Fig. 32.3G). However, his BCVA was classified as hand motion only.

Take Home Messages

1. Congenital excavated optic disc anomalies may lead to maculopathies causing by the accumulation of fluid that originated from the vitreous or subarachnoid space.
2. Although the surgical standard for the ODPM has not been well established, vitrectomy with long-term gas tamponade can generally lead to good outcomes. The benefit of additional techniques such as JPL or ILM peeling is still under debate.
3. For ODPM cases unresponsive to or recurred after vitrectomy, fovea-sparing ILM flap, autologous blood, scleral flap, or autologous fibrin can be considered.

Review Questions

1. Which of the following is not a typical characteristic of an optic disc pit?

a. Optic disc pits involve gray-white excavation
b. Optic disc pits are typically located at the inferonasal margin of the optic disc
c. Optic disc pits are most commonly unilateral
d. Optic disc pit maculopathy develops in 25–75% of patients

2. A 7-year-old girl was accidentally found to have asymptomatic optic disc pit maculopathy with a best-corrected visual acuity of 20/25 in her right eye. Shallow subretinal fluid was detected with optical coherence tomography. What is the first recommended treatment approach?

a. Trans–pars plana vitrectomy
b. Pneumatic tamponade
c. Barricade laser treatment along the optic disc margin
d. Observation

3. Which congenital abnormality has not been reported to be associated with a morning glory disc anomaly?

a. Aicardi syndrome
b. Basal encephalocele
c. Apert syndrome
d. PHACE syndrome

Answers

1. B
2. D
3. C

References

1. Iros M, Parolini B, Ozdek S, et al. Management of optic disc pit maculopathy: the European VitreoRetinal society optic pit study. Acta Ophthalmol. 2021.
2. Ohno-Matsui K, Hirakata A, Inoue M, Akiba M, Ishibashi T. Evaluation of congenital optic disc pits and optic disc colobomas by swept-source optical coherence tomography. Invest Ophthalmol Vis Sci. 2013;54:7769–78.
3. Ceynowa DJ, Wickstrom R, Olsson M, et al. Morning glory disc anomaly in childhood-a population-based study. Acta Ophthalmol. 2015;93:626–34.
4. Kalogeropoulos D, Ch'ng SW, Lee R, et al. Optic disc pit maculopathy: a review. Asia Pac J Ophthalmol (Phila). 2019;8:247–55.
5. Chatziralli I, Theodossiadis G, Panagiotidis D, Emfietzoglou I, Grigoropoulos V, Theodossiadis P. Long-term changes of macular thickness after pars Plana vitrectomy in optic disc pit maculopathy: a spectral-domain optical coherence tomography study. Semin Ophthalmol. 2017;32:302–8.
6. Steel DHW, Suleman J, Murphy DC, Song A, Dodds S, Rees J. Optic disc pit maculopathy: a two-year nationwide prospective population-based study. Ophthalmology. 2018;125:1757–64.
7. Benatti E, Garoli E, Viola F. Spontaneous resolution of optic disk pit maculopathy in a child after a six-year follow-up. Retin Cases Brief Rep. 2021;15:453–6.
8. Bloch E, Georgiadis O, Lukic M, da Cruz L. Optic disc pit maculopathy: new perspectives on the natural history. Am J Ophthalmol. 2019;207:159–69.
9. Al-Moujahed A, Callaway NF, Vail D, Ludwig CA, Ji MH, Moshfeghi DM. Resolution of optic disc pit-associated macular retinoschisis after topical carbonic anhydrase inhibitor treatment: report of a case. Eur J Ophthalmol 2021;31:NP25–28.

10. Osigian CJ, Gologorsky D, Cavuoto KM, Berrocal A, Villegas V. Oral acetazolamide as a medical adjuvant to retinal surgery in optic disc pit maculopathy in a pediatric patient. Am J Ophthalmol Case Rep. 2020;17: 100599.

11. Pastor-Idoate S, Garcia-Arumi Fuste C, Garcia-Onrubia L, Copete S, Garcia-Arumi J. Surgical options for optic disc pit maculopathy: perspectives and controversies. Clin Ophthalmol. 2020;14:1601–8.

12. Caporossi T, Finocchio L, Barca F, Franco F, Tartaro R, Rizzo S. 27-gauge via pars Plana vitrectomy with autologous ILM transplantation for optic pit disc maculopathy. Ophthalmic Surg Lasers Imaging Retina. 2018;49:712–4.

13. Nawrocki J, Boninska K, Michalewska Z. Managing optic pit. Right Stuff! Retina. 2016;36:2430–2.

14. Travassos AS, Regadas I, Alfaiate M, Silva ED, Proenca R, Travassos A. Optic pit: novel surgical management of complicated cases. Retina. 2013;33:1708–14.

15. D'Souza P, Babu U, Narendran V. Autologous free internal limiting membrane flap for optic nerve head pit with maculopathy. Ophthalmic Surg Lasers Imaging Retina. 2017;48:350–3.

16. Almeida DRP, Chin EK, Arjmand P, Velez G, Evans LP, Mahajan VB. Fibrin glue and internal limiting membrane abrasion for optic disc pit maculopathy. Ophthalmic Surg Lasers Imaging Retina. 2018;49:e271-7.

17. Ozdek S, Ozdemir HB. A new technique with autologous fibrin for the treatment of persistent optic pit maculopathy. Retin Cases Brief Rep. 2017;11:75–8.

18. Rosenthal G, Bartz-Schmidt KU, Walter P, Heimann K. Autologous platelet treatment for optic disc pit associated with persistent macular detachment. Graefes Arch Clin Exp Ophthalmol. 1998;236:151–3.

19. Hirakata A, Inoue M, Hiraoka T, McCuen BW 2nd. Vitrectomy without laser treatment or gas tamponade for macular detachment associated with an optic disc pit. Ophthalmology. 2012;119:810–8.

20. Teke MY, Citirik M. 23 gauge vitrectomy, endolaser, and gas tamponade versus vitrectomy alone for serous macular detachment associated with optic disc pit. Am J Ophthalmol. 2015;160:779–85 e2.

21. Roy R, Saurabh K, Thomas NR, Das K. Surgical management of optic disc pit maculopathy with a fovea sparing internal limiting membrane flap. Indian J Ophthalmol. 2017;65:420–2.

22. Theodossiadis GP, Chatziralli IP, Theodossiadis PG. Macular buckling in optic disc pit maculopathy in association with the origin of macular elevation: 13-year mean postoperative results. Eur J Ophthalmol. 2015;25:241–8.

23. Wong SC, Scripsema NK. Inner retinal fenestration for paediatric optic disc pit maculopathy: a case series. Eye (Lond). 2021.

24. Kuhn F, Kover F, Szabo I, Mester V. Intracranial migration of silicone oil from an eye with optic pit. Graefes Arch Clin Exp Ophthalmol. 2006;244:1360–2.

25. Onwochei BC, Simon JW, Bateman JB, Couture KC, Mir E. Ocular colobomata. Surv Ophthalmol. 2000;45:175–94.

26. Skriapa Manta A, Olsson M, Ek U, Wickstrom R, Tear FK. Optic Disc Coloboma in children-prevalence, clinical characteristics and associated morbidity. Acta Ophthalmol. 2019;97:478–85.

27. Brodsky MC. Congenital anomalies of the optic disc. In: Miller NR, Newman NG, editors. Walsh & Hoyt's clinical neuro-ophthalmology. 5th ed., Ch. 18. Baltimore, MO: Williams & Wilkins; 1998. p. 775–823.

28. Fei P, Zhang Q, Li J, Zhao P. Clinical characteristics and treatment of 22 eyes of morning glory syndrome associated with persistent hyperplastic primary vitreous. Br J Ophthalmol. 2013;97:1262–7.

29. Haik BG, Greenstein SH, Smith ME, Abramson DH, Ellsworth RM. Retinal detachment in the morning glory anomaly. Ophthalmology. 1984;91:1638–47.

30. Sakamoto M, Kuniyoshi K, Hayashi S, Yamashita H, Kusaka S. Total retinal detachment and contractile movement of the disc in eyes with morning glory syndrome. Am J Ophthalmol Case Rep. 2020;20: 100964.

31. Babu N, Kohli P. Surgical challenges in the management of morning glory disc anomaly-associated retinal detachment. Indian J Ophthalmol. 2021;69:2540–1.

32. Sen P, Maitra P, Vaidya H, Bhende P, Das K. Outcomes of vitreoretinal surgery in retinal detachment associated with morning glory disc anomaly. Indian J Ophthalmol. 2021;69:2116–21.

33. Yang XL, Zhang X. Vitrectomy of rhegmatogenous retinal detachment in morning glory syndrome. Int J Ophthalmol. 2010;3:89–91.

Genetic Diseases Causing RRD: Marfan, Stickler and Wagner Syndrome

33

Ana Bety Enriquez and Caroline R. Baumal

Abstract

Pediatric rhegmatogenous retinal detachment (RRD) is an uncommon but serious event, with potential for permanent lifelong visual loss. Pediatric RRD accounts for 0.5–12.6% of all RRD cases. The etiology of pediatric RRD may include congenital and developmental abnormalities. Marfan syndrome, Stickler syndrome and Wagner syndrome constitute the inherited vitreoretinal syndromes most frequently associated with RRD.

Keywords

Marfan syndrome · Pediatric rhegmatogenous retinal detachment · Stickler syndrome · Wagner syndrome

Pediatric rhegmatogenous retinal detachment (RRD) is a serious and fortunately uncommon retinal disorder that accounts for 0.5–12.6% of all RRD cases [1, 2]. It has an annual incidence of 0.38–0.69 per 100,000 individuals and has been associated with poor visual outcomes [1–3]. The anatomy, tissue characteristics, ocular and systemic comorbidities and delayed detection in this age group make pediatric

Supplementary Information The online version contains supplementary material available at https://doi.org/10.1007/978-3-031-14506-3_33.

A. B. Enriquez (✉)
Clínica Oftalmológica Durango, Hospital de Especialidades AMCCI, Durango, México
e-mail: dra.enriquez.amcci@gmail.com

C. R. Baumal
Professor of Ophthalmology, Department of Ophthalmology, New England Eye Center, Tufts University School of Medicine, Boston, MA, USA

"

RRD management extremely challenging. However, careful evaluation and prompt treatment can reduce the morbidity of this major cause of blindness in childhood [1, 2].

Predisposing factors for pediatric RRD include myopia, trauma, previous intraocular surgery and congenital and developmental abnormalities [1]. High myopia has been reported as one of the major etiological factors for pediatric RRD, with an incidence rate in pediatric cases that ranges from 23 to 37.5% [1]. Of note, myopia is also a characteristic of many congenital and developmental abnormalities. If considered alone, simple myopia would not be among the leading reasons for RRD in children and the frequency of congenital and developmental abnormalities related to RRD would increase to percentages as high as 56% [1, 2]. Bilateral retinal detachment (RD) is also more common in children. Up to 30% of children with RRD present with bilateral involvement or develop it over short period of time [2–4].

The detection of congenital and developmental abnormalities is of utmost importance. Along with a thorough history and diligent ocular and systemic examination, genetic testing may help distinguish patients with simple myopia from patients with congenital or developmental diseases [1, 2]. Examination of family members may also be helpful and should be considered when possible, especially given the increased incidence of retinal pathology associated to inherited disorders (sibling RRD risk ratio of 2.1 and parent–offspring RRD risk ratio of 2.9) [2, 4].

Among the congenital and developmental abnormalities, Marfan syndrome, Stickler syndrome and Wagner syndrome constitute the inherited vitreoretinal syndromes most frequently associated with RRD [3].

Marfan Syndrome

Marfan syndrome is the second most common inherited connective tissue disorder, after osteogenesis imperfecta. Cardiovascular, skeletal, pulmonary, cutaneous, dural and ocular abnormalities may be features of Marfan syndrome [5–9].

Epidemiology

The estimated incidence of Marfan syndrome is 1–3 in 10,000 live births. It affects both sexes equally, it is present in all races and its distribution is equal throughout the world [7, 9]. Approximately 50% of patients with Marfan syndrome are initially diagnosed by an ophthalmologist [9].

Pathophysiology/Genetics

Marfan syndrome is caused by autosomal dominant mutations in the fibrillin-1 gene (located on chromosome 15), which encodes for an extracellular matrix protein involved in the deposition of elastin [2, 4, 10]. About 75% of patients with classic Marfan syndrome have a positive family history of the disease. Moreover, this syndrome has high penetrance with variable manifestation of features among family members [7–9, 11] (Table 33.3).

Clinical Features

Systemic features of this syndrome may include the following: tall stature, increased length of extremities, arachnodactyly, hyperextendable joints, high arched palate, prognathism, long and thin face, scoliosis or kyphoscoliosis, pectus deformities, mitral and tricuspid valve prolapse, pulmonary artery dilatation, spontaneous pneumothorax, cutaneous striae, hernias and lumbosacral dural ectasia (Table 33.3 and Fig. 33.5) [2, 6, 7, 9, 11, 12]. Aortic aneurysm/dissection is the most serious complication of Marfan syndrome and it is found in 50% of children and up to 70–80% of adults.

Ocular findings of Marfan syndrome include axial myopia (in 34–44% of cases, 20% with more than 7 diopters), flat cornea, non-traumatic subluxation of the lens (in 50–80% of cases), and posterior segment pathology (in 18–70% of cases) (Table 33.3). When ectopia lentis is associated with Marfan syndrome, it usually presents as bilateral, symmetric, non-progressive and superotemporal displacement. Other features that have been described include strabismus, megalocornea, hypoplastic iris or ciliary muscle, deep anterior chamber, glaucoma, early cataract and capsule opacities [9, 11, 13].

Posterior segment pathology includes early vitreous liquefaction (involving the central and posterior vitreous body), posterior vitreous detachment (PVD), vitreous traction syndromes in the peripheral retina, retinal thinning, choroidal thinning, scleral crescents, posterior staphyloma, white-without-pressure, atrophic holes, lattice degeneration, chorioretinal pigment proliferation, peripheral breaks or RRD [2, 4, 8–14]. The retinal breaks are typically multiple and located anterior to the equator in 69% of cases [8].

RRD constitutes one of the most serious ocular complications of this disease. It has been reported in 5–25.6% of patients, with an increase of incidence up to 38% in patients with ectopia lentis (Fig. 33.1) [8, 9, 11–14]. It predominantly affects men and usually occurs in the mid-twenties [9, 11, 14, 15]. High myopia (reported in 90% of Marfan syndrome patients with RD) combined with other ocular features like ectopia lentis (which exerts traction on the vitreous base), vitreous liquefaction, PVD and prior ocular surgery for the ectopia lentis may predispose to multiple, large and irregular retinal breaks leading to complex RRD. At initial presentation, complete RD has been reported in 75% of cases, RD involving the macula has been observed in 90% of cases and 50% of eyes with RD have been found with more

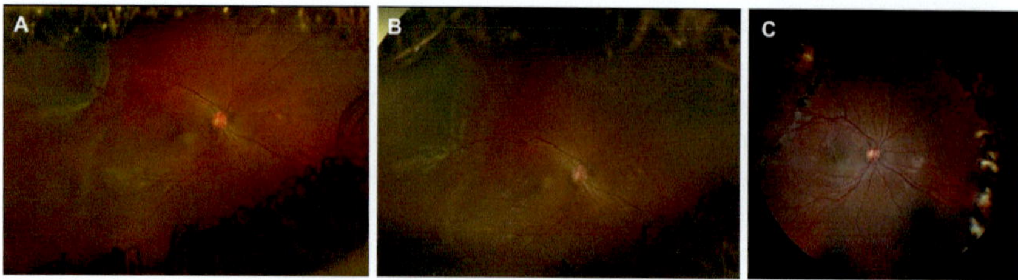

Fig. 33.1 Clinical course of rhegmatogenous retinal detachment in a 27-year-old female with Marfan Syndrome. **A** One year following pars plana lensectomy and sutured IOL for a subluxated lens, she presented with a symptomatic superotemporal RRD. PVD was not observed despite the presence of RRD. **B** The patient initially opted for laser demarcation and deferred pars plana vitrectomy. However, RRD progressed beyond laser. **C** Pars plana vitrectomy was performed to remove preretinal membranes. While scleral bucking was attempted this could not be performed due to anomalous fibrosis of the patient's extraocular muscles. Following pars plana vitrectomy, endolaser and intraocular gas the retina reattached

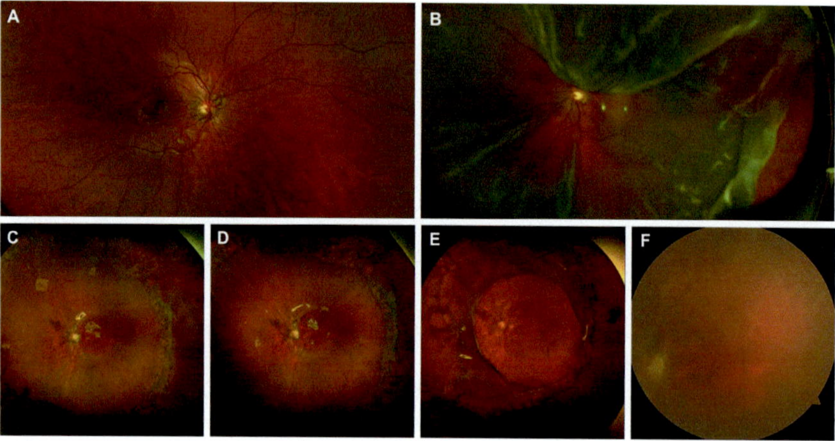

Fig. 33.2 Clinical course of an aphakic 6-year-old male with Marfan Syndrome. **A** Right eye without retinal pathology. **B** Left eye with RRD secondary to a giant retinal tear. **C** Two-weeks following surgical repair with pars plana vitrectomy, brilliant blue, perfluorocarbon liquid, triamcinolone, endolaser and silicone oil retina remains attached (**Video** 1). **D** Six-week post-operative follow-up, the retina remains attached. **E** Three-month post-operative follow-up, before silicone oil removal, retina presents some PVR. **F** Left-eye follow-up after silicone oil removal, retina remains attached. Case courtesy of Prof. Dr. Şengül Özdek

than 2 retinal breaks [14]. Giant retinal tears (Fig. 33.2, **Video** 1) are the cause of RD in 11% of eyes and bilateral RD have been reported in 30–70% of Marfan syndrome cases with RD [2, 9–14].

Clinical diagnosis of Marfan syndrome depends on major and minor criteria, as defined in the updated 2010 Ghent criteria (Table 33.1) [6, 7, 16]; however, some individuals may present only with isolated ocular signs suggestive of Marfan syndrome [13].

Table 33.1 Updated 2010 Ghent criteria for Marfan syndrome diagnosis

In the absence of family history:
1. Aortic Root Dilatation Z score $\geq$ 2 AND Ectopia Lentis = Marfan syndrome
2. Aortic Root Dilatation Z score $\geq$ 2 AND FBN1 mutation = Marfan syndrome
3. Aortic Root Dilatation Z score $\geq$ 2 AND Systemic Score $\geq$ 7pts = Marfan syndrome
4. Ectopia lentis AND a FBN1 mutation associated with Aortic Root Dilatation = Marfan syndrome
Ectopia lentis with or without Systemic Score AND with an FBN1 mutation not known with aortic root dissection or no FBN1 mutation = Ectopia lentis syndrome
Aortic Root Dilatation Z score < 2 AND Systemic Score $\geq$ 5 with at least one skeletal feature without Ectopia lentis = Myopia, mitral valve prolapse, borderline (Z score < 2) aortic root dilatation, striae, skeletal findings phenotype
Mitral valve prolapse AND Aortic Root Dilatation Z score < 2 AND Systemic Score < 5 without Ectopia lentis = Mitral valve prolapse syndrome
In the presence of family history:
5. Ectopia lentis AND Family History of Marfan syndrome = Marfan syndrome
6. A systemic score $\geq$ 7 points AND Family History of Marfan syndrome = Marfan syndrome
7. Aortic Root Dilatation Z score $\geq$ 2 above 20 yrs. old, $\geq$ 3 below 20 yrs. old + Family History of Marfan syndrome = Marfan syndrome

Systemic score
• Wrist AND thumb sign – 3
(Wrist OR thumb sign – 1)
• Pectus carinatum deformity – 2
(Pectus excavatum or chest asymmetry – 1)
• Hindfoot deformity – 2 (plain pes planus – 1)
• Pneumothorax – 2
• Dural ectasia – 2
• Protrusio acetabuli – 2
• Reduced upper segment/lower segment ratio AND increased arm/height AND no severe scoliosis – 1
• Scoliosis or thoracolumbar kyphosis – 1
• Reduced elbow extension – 1
• Facial features (3/5) – 1
(dolichocephaly, enophthalmos, down-slanting palpebral fissures, malar hypoplasia, retrognathia)
• Skin striae – 1
• Myopia > 3 diopters – 1
• Mitral valve prolapse (all types) – 1
Maximum total: 20 points; score $\geq$ 7 indicates systemic involvement

FBN1 = fibrillin-1 gene

Table 33.2 Principles for pediatric retinal detachment repair

Principles for pediatric retinal detachment repair
Pre-operative
Obtain history of current symptoms, past medical history (including perinatal history), allergies, medications, familiar history, review of systems
Ocular examination, if possible, of both eyes • Visual acuity • Refractive error • Amblyopia • Axial length • Strabismus • Nystagmus • Anterior segment • Intraocular pressure • Lens status • Posterior segment with dilation of pupils
Investigate etiology and mechanism of retinal detachment
Examine family members
Evaluate genetics if relevant
Imaging • B-scan ultrasound • Widefield imaging: color and fluorescein angiography (oral) • Optical coherence tomography (OCT) • ERG, EOG • Consider CNS imaging if associated optic nerve abnormalities, i.e.: morning glory anomaly
Intraoperative
Careful examination ± imaging of both eyes
Flexibility for management of findings
Basic surgical principles: • Find all retinal breaks consistent with the appearance of the RRD • Relief of traction on the retinal breaks • Creation of adhesion between neurosensory retina and retinal pigment epithelium • Re-approximation of neurosensory retina to retinal pigment epithelium
Consider scleral buckle alone if all breaks can be supported as the vitreous is adherent and can serve as internal tamponade
If PVR or vitreous traction is present, consider addition of vitrectomy to relieve traction internally
Preplan: Use adjuvants to delineate the vitreous and membranes, silicone oil, lensectomy, additional adjuvants could be used
A staged surgical approach may be discussed Initial scleral buckle → PPV if scleral buckle alone is not successful
Postoperative
Corticosteroids topical. May be intensive or add systemic to minimize fibrin formation
Cataract removal if needed
Visual rehabilitation to avoid amblyopia, team management

(continued)

Table 33.2 (continued)

Principles for pediatric retinal detachment repair
Always
Involve caregivers
Amblyopia management
Monocular safety precautions
Remember
Children are not little adults

Table 33.3 Marfan syndrome, Stickler syndrome and Wagner syndrome genetic characteristics and distinguishing features

Syndrome	Gene	Cytogenetic location	Inheritance	Distinguishing features
Marfan syndrome	FBN1	15q21.1	Autosomal dominant	<u>Systemic</u>: Tall stature, long extremities, arachnodactyly, joint laxity, pectus deformities, scoliosis, aortic aneurism/dissection, mitral valve prolapse, pneumothorax, hernia, lumbosacral dural ectasia <u>Ocular</u>: Ectopia lentis, flat cornea, axial myopia, peripheral breaks, retinal detachment
Stickler syndrome				
Type 1	COL2A1	12q13.11	Autosomal dominant	<u>Systemic</u>: mid-face hypoplasia, cleft palate, sensorineural hearing loss, premature osteoarthritis, scoliosis <u>Ocular</u>: membranous vitreous (Type 1), myopia, early cataract, glaucoma, lattice degeneration, chorioretinal degeneration, retinal detachment
Type 2	COL11A1	1p21.1	Autosomal dominant	<u>Systemic</u>: mid-face hypoplasia, cleft palate, sensorineural hearing loss, premature osteoarthritis, scoliosis <u>Ocular</u>: Beaded vitreous (Type 2), myopia, early cataract, glaucoma, lattice degeneration, chorioretinal degeneration, retinal detachment
Type 4	COL9A1	6q13	Autosomal recessive	<u>Systemic</u>: conductive and/or sensorineural hearing loss, mid-face hypoplasia and cleft palate (either alone or as part of

(continued)

Table 33.3 (continued)

Syndrome	Gene	Cytogenetic location	Inheritance	Distinguishing features
				the Robin sequence), mild spondyloepiphyseal dysplasia, precocious arthritis Ocular: myopia, cataract, vitreoretinopathy, retinal detachment
Type 5	COL9A2	1p34.2	Autosomal recessive	Systemic: conductive and/or sensorineural hearing loss, mid-face hypoplasia and cleft palate (either alone or as part of the Robin sequence), mild spondyloepiphyseal dysplasia, precocious arthritis Ocular: myopia, cataract, vitreoretinopathy, retinal detachment
Type 6	COL9A3	20q13.33	Autosomal recessive	Systemic: sensorineural hearing loss, mid-face hypoplasia, mild epiphyseal changes, tibial and femoral bowing Ocular: myopia
Ocular only	COL2A1	12q13.11	Autosomal dominant	Systemic: None Ocular: membranous vitreous (Type 1), myopia, early cataract, glaucoma, lattice degeneration, chorioretinal degeneration, retinal detachment
Wagner syndrome	VCAN	5q14.2-q14.3	Autosomal dominant	Systemic: None Ocular: optically empty vitreous, avascular vitreous veils, pre-retinal membranes from posterior pole to periphery, progressive chorioretinal atrophy, optic atrophy, retinal detachment

Management

Initial evaluation of Marfan syndrome includes specialist referral involving a pediatrician/internist, cardiologist and medical geneticist. If family history is present, ocular examinations should start at 3–6 months of age [13]. Due to the risk of RRD, patients with Marfan syndrome should have a complete bilateral dilated ophthalmologic examination at least yearly and anytime there are ophthalmic complaints. Widefield image can be helpful for retina examination in younger patients, patients with limited cooperation and/or patients with ocular abnormalities (such as miotic pupils or lens abnormalities) [5, 10, 11, 13–15]. Either in the clinic or, more likely, under anesthesia in the operating room, both eyes of pediatric patients with RRD should be examined in detail with careful attention to location and extent of detachment and retinal breaks [2] (Table 33.2).

The same underlying surgical principles that guide the repair of adult RRD (find, treat and support all retinal breaks) should be followed for pediatric RRD:

- Careful bilateral examination which may require anesthesia in the operating room to find any retinal breaks and ocular pathology.
- Relief of traction on the retinal defect causative of RRD.
- Re-approximation of the neurosensory retina to the retinal pigment epithelium (RPE).
- Creation of adhesion between neurosensory retina and RPE.

However, differences in anatomy and function of pediatric eyes may require change in the techniques employed to achieve those goals [2] (Table 33.2).

The initial consideration for treatment of pediatric RRD especially in eyes with congenital abnormalities should include scleral buckling procedure. The strong internal adhesion of the hyaloid to the retinal surface, the firm consistency of the vitreous and the potential for cataract formation (with reduced accommodation and amblyopia risk) are some of the factors complicating pediatric vitrectomy. Scleral buckling can be successful for 70–80% of simple pediatric RRD cases [2]. However, in complex RRD, vitrectomy may be necessary, often combined with scleral buckling procedure. Vitrectomy may require release of traction for closure of multiple retinal breaks to re-approximate the neurosensory retina to RPE, posterior drainage retinotomy, larger retinectomies, intraoperative perfluorocarbon liquid, lensectomy and silicone oil tamponade [2].

Characteristic of Marfan syndrome patients, the thin and collapsible sclera, ectopia lentis, poorly dilating pupils and the multiple retinal breaks can lead to challenging surgery [2, 10, 12]. The decision of the surgical technique used to repair the RD should depend on the age of the patient, complexity of the detachment, status of the vitreous, severity of lens displacement and fellow eye status [9, 11]. Scleral buckling can be considered with retinal breaks at or anterior to the equator that have undergone pars plana lensectomies, eyes with a clear normal lens or a clear mildly subluxated lens with no interference of visualization [9, 10]. In eyes with giant retina tear (GRT), multiple irregular tears with traction or proliferative vitreoretinopathy (PVR), vitrectomy or combined scleral buckling and vitrectomy should be considered (**Video** 1. Vitrectomy for complex RRD with GRT in Marfan syndrome) [10, 13]. Lensectomy, iris retractors, sphincterotomies, pupillary-stretching techniques, iridectomy, epiretinal and subretinal membrane peeling, retinotomies, use of perfluorocarbon and/or retinal tamponade with long-acting gases or silicone oil may increase surgery success rates by improving visualization of the periphery, facilitating finding retinal breaks, helping to reattach the retina and reducing the risk of recurrence of RD [8, 9, 11, 14]. Difficulties during placement of scleral buckle or wound closure are common in Marfan syndrome patients due to the altered scleral structure [2].

In addition, if retinal breaks or peripheral pathology is present in the fellow eye, then retinopexy with cryotherapy, laser or scleral buckling should be considered to prevent RD. Up to date, no studies have addressed the best methodology for RRD prophylaxis in Marfan patients [2, 8, 10].

Children with Marfan syndrome require routine screening for amblyopia, which may arise due to axial myopia, astigmatism, anisometropia, subluxated lens and/or as a sequelae of RRD (due to longstanding RRD, aphakia, long-term tamponade, induced refractive changes, etc.). Permanent ametropic functional amblyopia, despite good conservative management, has been reported in up to 50% of cases and can increase if lens dislocation approaches the center of the pupil [2, 9].

Prognosis

Prognosis depends on the extent and location of RD, the time between symptoms and surgery and the lens condition (phakic versus aphakic) [10]. Modern surgical techniques and instrumentation have improved outcomes for RRD in Marfan syndrome [9, 10]. For the pediatric population evaluating all causes of RRD, the retinal reattachment rate with a single surgery is 50–80% and the final anatomic reattachment rate is 70–80% [2, 3, 8, 11]. Specifically in Marfan syndrome patients, successful reattachment of the retina has been reported between 56 and 89% and surgical failure reported in 25% of cases has been attributed to poor visualization of retinal periphery and/or PVR [5, 8–11].

Visual outcomes are worse in pediatric RRD than in adult RRD, where 30–40% of cases have a final acuity of 20/200–20/400. The visual potential can be compromised by cataract, aphakia, silicone oil tamponade, strabismus or amblyopia. RRD with macular involvement, giant retinal tears or PVR, have poorer anatomic success rates and visual outcomes [2]. Specifically in Marfan syndrome, visual outcomes have been reported in some series as better than 20/125 in 67% of eyes [8].

Stickler Syndrome

The most common genetic disorder to cause pediatric and adult RRD is Stickler syndrome (SS) [2, 3, 17, 18]. Initially described in 1965, it is an arthro-ophthalmopathy, consisting of connective tissue disorder characterized by craniofacial (84% of cases), musculoskeletal (90% of cases), auditory (70% of cases), and ocular abnormalities (95% of cases) [3, 17, 19].

Epidemiology

Stickler syndrome has an incidence of 1 in 7,500–10,000 live births, with complete penetrance, genetic heterogeneity and marked inter and intrafamilial phenotypic variability [3, 18, 20, 21]. Ocular involvement is the main feature leading to the diagnosis of SS [22].

Pathophysiology

Stickler syndrome is a disorder that can be classified into 5 types (Table 33.3):

- Type I (STL1) accounts for 70–75% of SS cases and is secondary to autosomal dominant frameshift mutations in the COL2A1 gene (located on chromosome 12), which encodes collagen type II. It is most commonly due to haploinsufficiency through nonsense or frameshift mutations and it has the highest incidence of unilateral RRD (as high as 73%) and bilateral RD [2, 4, 17, 21, 23–26].
- Type II (STL2) accounts for 10–20% of SS cases and is secondary to autosomal dominant missense mutations in the COLA11A1 gene, which encodes for collagen type XI [2, 17, 23, 24]. It has an RRD risk between 40–50% [19, 21, 25, 26].
- Type IV (SLT4). It is caused by autosomal recessive mutations in the COL9A1 [23] gene [4, 26].
- Type V (SLT5). It is the result of autosomal recessive mutations in the COL9A2 gene [21, 25, 26].
- Type VI (SLT6). It is secondary to autosomal recessive mutations in the COL9A3 gene [21, 26, 27].

Previously, an autosomal dominant disease caused by COL11A2 mutations was classified as a subtype of SS (Type III or STL3). It was thought to constitute the non-ocular form of the disease; however, it has been reclassified and it is now known as Weissenbacher-Zweymuller syndrome or autosomal dominant oto-spondylomegaepiphyseal dysplasia [2, 17, 23, 25].

In addition, autosomal dominant mutations in exon 2 of the COL2A1 gene (exon splicing, mosaicism and compound heterozygosity) can cause SS with predominant ocular characteristics in absence of detectable systemic features [4, 21, 23, 25, 26] (Table 33.3).

Mutations in the COL2A1 and the COL11A1 genes may also present in other chondrodysplasias that are also accompanied by vitreoretinal degeneration. These include [2, 3, 23]:

- Kniest dysplasia, characterized by shortened limbs, prominent joints with restricted mobility, short trunk dwarfism, kyphoscoliosis orofacial abnormalities and hearing loss, due to autosomal dominant COL2A1 mutations.

- Phalangeal epiphysial dysplasia with brachydactyly, result of autosomal dominant COL2A1 mutations.
- Marshall syndrome, distinguished by early and severe hearing loss, myopia, clear vitreous, congenital cataract and pronounced facial abnormalities including severe mid-face hypoplasia, short nose and anteverted nares, secondary to dominant mutations of the COL11A1 gene.
- Knobloch syndrome, a rare syndrome characterized by congenital occipital defects (from scalp defects to encephalocele and ectopic gray matter in the brain), high myopia and vitreoretinal degeneration that arises from autosomal recessive mutations in the COL18A1 gene, which encodes for type XVIII collagen.

Clinical Features

The phenotype of SS can be highly variable and, in some cases, may not distinguish between the five forms of the disease or even between affected and unaffected family members [17, 23]. SS with ocular involvement usually presents with a combination of mid-face hypoplasia and small chin; bifid uvula, and submucous or frank cleft palate; early cataract; high myopia; congenital abnormalities of the vitreous; lattice degeneration and high rate of RRD [4, 23]. Other features of the disease include micrognathia, Pierre Robin Sequence, sensorineural and conductive hearing loss, mild spondyloepiphyseal dysplasia, spinal abnormalities (such as scoliosis, kyphosis, and platyspondyly), joint hypermobility and precocious osteoarthritis [20–22, 25] (Table 33.3 and Fig. 33.5).

Ocular manifestations of STL1 and STL2 have variable severity, are highly penetrant and, in some patients, an ophthalmological examination is essential not only for making the diagnosis but also for directing genetic testing [23].

The vitreous cavity of SS patients is partially filled with vitreous from birth; therefore, in this disease the central vitreous does not liquify but rather never forms. The remaining vitreous adheres anomalously and unpredictably to the retina [24]. These characteristics, combined with the abnormal vitreous base (which is located more posterior than usual), can lead to the development of retinal tears independently of PVD. In fact, at initial examination less than half of SS patients with RD have PVD [2, 19, 24, 28]. Moreover, vitreous characteristics may enable differentiation between COL2A1 and COL11A1 mutations (Table 33.3 and Fig. 33.5):

- COL2A1 patients have a folded retro-lenticular membrane appearance of the vitreous, which extends to pars plana and peripheral retina vitreous (membranous or type I vitreous) [23].
- COL11A2 patients have a fibrillar and beaded appearance of the vitreous (fibrillar or type II vitreous) [23].

Other ocular features of SS include [2, 3, 19–25] (Table 33.3 and Fig. 33.5):

- High myopia. It is a non-progressive congenital feature of the disease that has been reported in 89% of SLT1 and 88% of SLT2 patients.
- Early cataract. It has a prevalence rate of 11–40% (with a greater proportion of presentation in SLT2 patients than in STL1 patients, 59% versus 36%, respectively), can present congenitally or in childhood and is often described as comma or wedge-shaped.
- Glaucoma. Usually secondary to prior ocular surgery and, more rarely, due to malformations of the iridocorneal angle (in which can cause infantile-onset glaucoma).
- Circumferential lattice degeneration. It is accompanied by vitreous condensations overlying the atrophic retina.
- Radial perivascular chorioretinal degeneration. It presents in adults and lacks overlying vitreous condensations.
- RRD. It commonly occurs in the first two decades of life, even in the infancy. It has a prevalence rate of 41.7–73%, it is usually bilateral (43.3–75% of cases) and it is usually secondary to anterior giant retinal tears or posterior breaks (Fig. 33.3).

Although genetic analysis can confirm the diagnosis, SS is diagnosed clinically. Different sets of diagnostic criteria have been proposed, and the 2005 Rose et al. score is the most widely used; however, there is no consensus for minimal clinical diagnostic criteria for the disease [3, 21, 25]. Molecular genetic testing (that may include chromosomal microarray, gene panels or exome/genome sequencing) is recommended in any patient with suspicion of SS, given that the mutation detection rate for SS is reported to be as high as 96.6% and that a correct diagnosis is fundamental for timely referral to clinicians with expertise [3, 18, 21, 23].

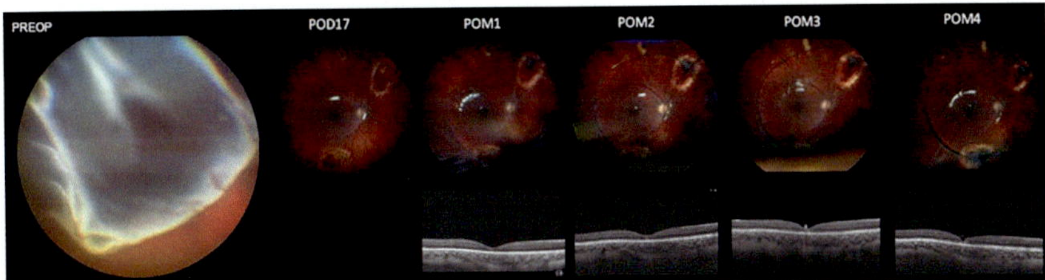

Fig. 33.3 Clinical course following surgical repair of complex RRD in the right eye of a 6-year-old male with Stickler Syndrome. He had a history of Pierre Robin syndrome at birth and positive maternal family history for Stickler Syndrome. His vision was hand motion when he presented with macula off RRD. Surgical repair included combined scleral buckle and pars plana vitrectomy, triamcinolone enhanced staining of the vitreous, endolaser and 5000-centistoke silicone oil tamponade. During follow-up, the inferior retina re-detached then spontaneously improved but a lamellar macular hole developed over time. Final visual acuity was 20/200 with silicone oil tamponade

Management

Fifty percent of patients with SS will experience disease-related ocular and /or systemic complications over their lifetime. For this reason, it is essential to start dilated fundus examinations at 6 months of age, with follow-up every 3–4 months (assisted with ocular ultrasound or exams under anesthesia), as well as perform yearly audiological evaluations and rheumatologic exams on all SS patients [3, 24, 29].

RRD repair for SS is challenging because of the young age when RD may develop, the propensity for giant retinal tears and PVR, and the abnormal vitreous development [19, 30]. Some studies have reported higher anatomic success with pars plana vitrectomy when compared to scleral buckling while others have recommended combined scleral buckling and pars plana vitrectomy with silicone oil tamponade [19, 30]. The choice of surgical intervention is still based on the preference of the vitreoretinal surgeon and individualized to the patients pathology (Figs. 33.3, and 33.4, **Video** 2) [3].

Due to the high rate of PVR (reported in up to 75% of cases), many cases may initially be treated with a combination of scleral buckling and vitrectomy [3, 19, 30]. Posterior RRD could be managed with advanced vitreoretinal techniques including scleral buckle, vitrectomy, release of peripheral traction, completion of PVD, perfluorocarbon-mediated retinal re-attachment, laser retinopexy and tamponade with gas or silicone oil [23]. If multiple breaks are present, or a giant retinal tear caused the RD, silicone oil could be helpful. Also, there could be uncommon cases in which scleral buckle alone would be enough for RRD repair (single tear RD) [19]. Cataract should be managed with phacoemulsification and low fluidics due to the lack of vitreous support [23]. Lensectomy is not usually indicated but could be performed if necessary [19]. In addition, intensive postoperative steroid treatment (topical and by mouth) could help minimize fibrin formation [19] (Table 33.2).

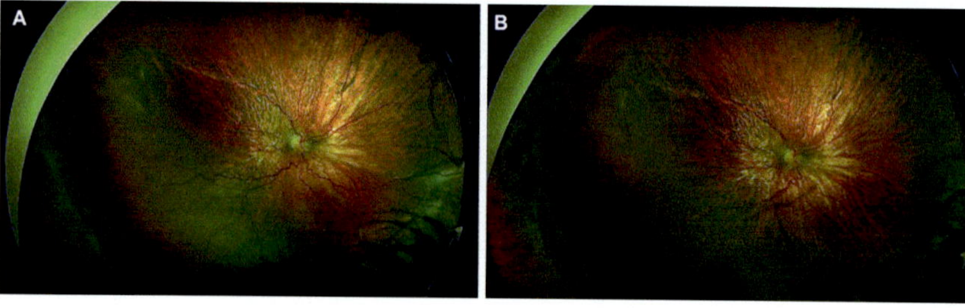

Fig. 33.4 Clinical course of chronic rhegmatogenous retinal detachment in the right eye of a 6-year-old child with Stickler Syndrome. **A** Pre-operatively the RRD is prominent inferotemporally with a retinal hole at 8 o'clock position and with subretinal bands. Surgical repair included scleral buckling procedure with chandelier visualization, external drainage of subretinal fluid and cryotherapy (**Video** 2). **B** Three-month postoperatively, the retina remains attached, and the scleral buckle is visible temporally. Courtesy of Dr. Şengül Özdek

In patients with unilateral RD, the contralateral eye has been reported to have an 89% risk of RRD, at a median of 4 years after the first RD, in the absence of prophylaxis [24]. Therefore, early prophylaxis is a fundamental action in SS ophthalmological management [21] and could be achieved by:

- Peripheral cryopexy. As reported in the Cambridge protocol, it is an effective prophylactic measure against RRD secondary to giant retinal tears in STL1 patients (eight-fold reduction of risk) [2, 18, 19, 23, 30]. It should be applied in a contiguous fashion at the junction of the posterior retina with the pars plana [18, 23]. This technique has a reported failure rate of 9%, at an average of 5.6 years after treatment [18, 24].
- Laser prophylaxis. Some authors favor peripheral laser retinopexy as a preventive action, especially in cases in which tears posterior to the ora serrata must be prevented [24]. It can be applied as follows:
  - Focal retinopexy limited to visible retinal lesions. Successful in skilled hands.
  - Standard fashion, also known as Ora Secunda Cerclage. It consists of grid treatment, from the ora serrata halfway to the vortex vein ampullae. The laser intensity needed is moderate with one to two spot width separation. This creates a "second ora" behind the posterior vitreous base, 3 mm posterior to the ora. This technique has a reported failure rate of 36% [24].
  - Ora Secunda Cerclage modified for SS. It tries to encompass the ora serrata, the anterior vitreous base, as well as posterior retina [24]. Recommended to be applied in two phases:

    Phase 1 (essential): Laser burns are placed in a grid pattern from 2 mm onto the pars plana to the ora serrata, and approximately 4 mm posteriorly, halfway to the vortex vein ampullae. Laser intensity should be moderately high and should have one spot width separation. This may protect against giant retinal tears and anterior breaks.

    Phase 2 (optional): Placed three months after initial treatment. The laser grid is extended posteriorly to and between the vortex vein ampullae. This may protect against giant retinal tears and posterior breaks.

    This technique requires a total of 2000–4000 spots, has been reported to cause an asymptomatic reduction of the visual field (average of 50 degrees in each quadrant) and transient pupillary mydriasis. A 100% of success rate for preventing RD and retinal breaks has been described (average follow-up of 8.7 years) [24].

- Scleral buckling. It is a more invasive method for prophylaxis but is effective in patients with a previous giant retinal tear in the fellow eye [3, 19].
- Vitrectomy. May carry less than 1% risk when performed with specific precautions, modern techniques and special instrumentation, such as wide-field microscopes, small gauge vitrectomy (e.g. 27-gauge), ultra-high-speed probes, low-end suction control and chromovitrectomy [24]. Suitable for very posterior high-risk retinal lesions that may not be covered by laser prophylaxis.

Up to date, there is no consensus or guidelines for prophylaxis for SS RRD [3, 29]. Some authors recommend offering RRD prophylaxis around the age of 2 years, while others indicate that it could be applied at any age [18, 23]. Also, a randomized trial has yet to be published comparing the multiple prophylaxis methods [3, 23].

Prognosis

Studies have reported that success after one RRD repair surgery in patients with SS ranges between 19 and 78%. Most re-detachments have been reported to occur between 2.6 and 9.2 months after the first surgery typically due to PVR. However, with an average of 2.3 surgeries, including silicone oil removal, most patients (93–100%) will achieve retinal reattachment [19].

Final visual acuity reported has been variable [19, 21, 24, 30]. Presenting visual acuity appears to be a prognostic indicator and improvement in visual acuity has been reported post-operatively in 33–64% of cases [3, 30].

Wagner Syndrome

Wagner Syndrome was initially reported in 1938 and represents an uncommon cause of pediatric RRD. However, it will be addressed here as Wagner syndrome (WS) and SS were historically thought as being one entity and previously received the name of Wagner-Stickler syndrome. Over the years, different genotypes and phenotypes have been identified to differentiate these disorders [2, 31].

Epidemiology

WS is a rare inherited vitreoretinopathy with an estimated prevalence less than 1:1,000,000 [32, 33]. It has almost complete penetrance and its expressivity is age-dependent [31–33]. However, due to its phenotypic variation, WS is often overlooked or misdiagnosed [33].

Pathophysiology

WS is an autosomal dominant condition that results from mutations of the gene that encodes for a large extracellular matrix proteoglycan known as chondroitin sulfate proteoglycan type II or Versican (CSPG2) (on chromosome 5). Up to date, at least 9 different mutations in the Versican gene have been reported [33]. CSPG2 interacts with hyaluronan in the vitreous and form large aggregates that support vitreous integrity [2, 4, 23]. It is unknown if the altered protein isoforms that may arise due to abnormal splicing can account for the variability in phenotype expression or in the congenital and acquired features of the disease [23] (Table 33.3).

Clinical Features

WS is not associated with any systemic abnormalities and is characterized by an optically empty central vitreous cavity with avascular fibrillary vitreous veils and pre-retinal membranes extending from the posterior pole towards the periphery [2, 31–34] (Table 33.3 and Fig. 33.5). Most of the patients have normal vision up to the third decade of life; however, over time, progressive chorioretinal atrophy (often starting in the periphery), optic atrophy and RD will develop [2, 23]. The rate of RD varies from 14 to 75%, its mechanism can be rhegmatogenous as well as tractional and can lead to severe loss of vision [4, 23, 31–33]. Bilateral RD is rarely observed in WS [33], and some authors have suggested that the progressive chorioretinal atrophy and subsequent scarring may be a protective factor against RD [31].

Mild myopia, anterior segment dysgenesis, early cataracts, retinal pigment epithelium clumping, uveitis, glaucoma (congenital, neovascular or chronic angle-closure), nyctalopia in early life and pseudo-strabismus (due to congenital temporal displacement of the fovea) may also present in WS [4, 23, 31, 33, 34]. Congenital abnormalities such as microphthalmia, ectopia lentis, iris atrophy and persistent hyperplastic primary vitreous have been described in some families [23, 32].

Jansen Syndrome and Erosive Vitreoretinopathy Syndrome are some of the other chromosome 5 retinopathies that share clinical and allelic features with Wagner syndrome [31, 32, 35]. Retinal detachment is predominant in Jansen Syndrome [32, 35]. Erosive vitreoretinopathy presents with a more marked chorioretinal atrophy, progressive nyctalopia and visual field constriction [4, 23, 31]. The risk for RRD in erosive vitreoretinopathy is between 11 and 15% [34].

Electrophysiologic abnormalities are found in 87% of WS cases [33]. ERG may be normal early in life; however, a reduction in the scotopic B-wave and final dark adaptation thresholds increases over time [2, 23, 34, 36]. A diffuse cone-rod loss ensues as chorioretinal atrophy develops [23]. These characteristics make ERG useful for diagnosis and evaluation of chorioretinal atrophy progression [32]. Fundus autofluorescence highlights the progressive peripheral chorioretinal atrophy and the visual field can show a ring scotoma or advanced loss as the chorioretinal atrophy progresses [23, 36].

Management

Cataract and retinal detachment in WS patients are managed using standard approaches [23] (Table 33.2). The utility of prophylactic treatment for RRD in WS has not been well defined [32].

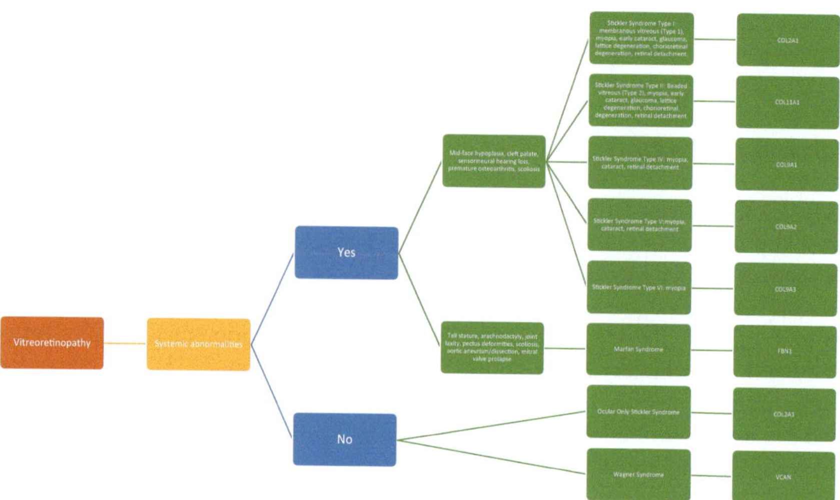

Fig. 33.5 Clinical and genetic characteristics of Marfan syndrome, Stickler Syndrome and Wagner Syndrome

Review Questions

1. A 27-year-old woman comes to your office, with her newborn baby, asking for your professional opinion. She is worried her baby could develop RD because she has a diagnosis of Marfan syndrome, presented RRD on both eyes and, despite treatment, her vision is poor. Which is the recommended age to start ocular examinations on the baby?

(a) At birth
(b) 3–6 months of age
(c) 6–12 months of age
(d) 12–36 months of age

2. Which of the following is not a characteristic of Type II Stickler Syndrome?

(a) Accounts for 10–20% of Stickler Syndrome cases
(b) Autosomal dominant inheritance
(c) It is secondary to mutations in COLA11A1 gene, which encodes for collagen type IX.
(d) It has an RRD risk between 40 and 50%

3. A 33-year-old male presents to your clinic with unilateral RRD. He has two brothers with a history of unilateral RRD and one sister with chorioretinal optic atrophy, but no genetic tests have been done on them yet. You suspect WS. Which of the following is not a characteristic of electrophysiologic abnormalities found in patients with WS?

(a)   Electrophysiologic abnormalities are present in only 25% of the cases.
(b)   A reduction in the scotopic B-wave and final dark adaptation thresholds would increase overtime.
(c)   A cone-rod loss ensues as chorioretinal atrophy develops.
(d)   It is useful for diagnosis and progression evaluation of chorioretinal atrophy.

Answers

1. B
2. C
3. A

References

1. Chen C, Huang S, Sun L, et al. Analysis of etiologic factors in pediatric rhegmatogenous retinal detachment with genetic testing. Am J Ophthalmol. 2020;218:330–6.
2. Wenick AS, Baranano DE. Evaluation and management of pediatric rhegmatogenous retinal detachment. Saudi J Ophthalmol. 2012;26(3):255–63.
3. Coussa RG, Sears J, Traboulsi EI. Stickler syndrome: exploring prophylaxis for retinal detachment. Curr Opin Ophthalmol. 2019;30(5):306–13.
4. Johnston T, Chandra A, Hewitt AW. Current understanding of the genetic architecture of rhegmatogenous retinal detachment. Ophthalmic Genet. 2016;37(2):121–9.
5. Federici TJ, Willson RL, Gitter KA. Pneumatic retinopexy for primary repair of rhegmatogenous retinal detachment in marfan syndrome. Retin Cases Brief Rep. 2007;1 (1):44–5.
6. Konradsen TR, Zetterstrom C. A descriptive study of ocular characteristics in Marfan syndrome. Acta Ophthalmol. 2013;91(8):751–5.
7. von Kodolitsch Y, Robinson PN. Marfan syndrome: an update of genetics, medical and surgical management. Heart. 2007;93(6):755–60.
8. Abboud EB. Retinal detachment surgery in Marfan's syndrome. Retina. 1998;18(5):405–9.
9. Nemet AY, Assia EI, Apple DJ, Barequet IS. Current concepts of ocular manifestations in Marfan syndrome. Surv Ophthalmol. 2006;51(6):561–75.
10. Esfandiari H, Ansari S, Mohammad-Rabei H, Mets MB. Management strategies of ocular abnormalities in patients with Marfan syndrome: current perspective. J Ophthalmic Vis Res. 2019;14(1):71–7.
11. Remulla JF, Tolentino FI. Retinal detachment in Marfan's syndrome. Int Ophthalmol Clin. 2001;41(4):235–40.
12. Loewenstein A, Barequet IS, De Juan E, Jr, Maumenee IH. Retinal detachment in Marfan syndrome. Retina. 2000;20(4):358–63.
13. Nahum Y, Spierer A. Ocular features of Marfan syndrome: diagnosis and management. Isr Med Assoc J. 2008;10(3):179–81.
14. Sharma T, Gopal L, Shanmugam MP, et al. Retinal detachment in Marfan syndrome: clinical characteristics and surgical outcome. Retina. 2002;22(4):423–8.

15. Lee SY, Ang CL. Results of retinal detachment surgery in Marfan syndrome in Asians. Retina. 2003;23(1):24–9.
16. Loeys BL, Dietz HC, Braverman AC, et al. The revised Ghent nosology for the Marfan syndrome. J Med Genet. 2010;47(7):476–85.
17. Richards AJ, Scott JD, Snead MP. Molecular genetics of rhegmatogenous retinal detachment. Eye (Lond). 2002;16(4):388–92.
18. Fincham GS, Pasea L, Carroll C, et al. Prevention of retinal detachment in Stickler syndrome: the Cambridge prophylactic cryotherapy protocol. Ophthalmology. 2014;121(8):1588–97.
19. Lee AC, Greaves GH, Rosenblatt BJ, et al. Long-term follow-up of retinal detachment repair in patients with stickler syndrome. Ophthalmic Surg Lasers Imaging Retina. 2020;51 (11):612–6.
20. Wang DD, Gao FJ, Hu FY, Zhang SH, Xu P, Wu JH. Mutation spectrum of stickler syndrome type i and genotype-phenotype analysis in East Asian population: a systematic review. BMC Med Genet. 2020;21(1):27.
21. Boothe M, Morris R, Robin N. Stickler syndrome: a review of clinical manifestations and the genetics evaluation. J Pers Med. 2020;10(3).
22. Huang L, Chen C, Wang Z, et al. Mutation spectrum and de novo mutation analysis in stickler syndrome patients with high myopia or retinal detachment. Genes (Basel). 2020;11(8).
23. Edwards AO. Clinical features of the congenital vitreoretinopathies. Eye (Lond). 2008;22 (10):1233–42.
24. Morris RE, Parma ES, Robin NH, et al. Stickler syndrome (SS): laser prophylaxis for retinal detachment (Modified Ora Secunda Cerclage, OSC/SS). Clin Ophthalmol. 2021;15:19–29.
25. Boysen KB, La Cour M, Kessel L. Ocular complications and prophylactic strategies in Stickler syndrome: a systematic literature review. Ophthalmic Genet. 2020;41(3):223–34.
26. Snead M, Martin H, Bale P, et al. Therapeutic and diagnostic advances in Stickler syndrome. Ther Adv Rare Dis. 2020;1:2633004020978661.
27. Hanson-Kahn A, Li B, Cohn DH, et al. Autosomal recessive Stickler syndrome resulting from a COL9A3 mutation. Am J Med Genet A. 2018;176(12):2887–91.
28. Alshahrani ST, Ghazi NG, Al-Rashaed S. Rhegmatogenous retinal detachments associated to Stickler syndrome in a tertiary eye care center in Saudi Arabia. Clin Ophthalmol. 2016;10:1–6.
29. Shapiro MJ, Blair MP, Solinski MA, Zhang DL, Jabbehdari S. The importance of early diagnosis of Stickler syndrome: finding opportunities for preventing blindness. Taiwan J Ophthalmol. 2018;8(4):189–95.
30. Reddy DN, Yonekawa Y, Thomas BJ, Nudleman ED, Williams GA. Long-term surgical outcomes of retinal detachment in patients with Stickler syndrome. Clin Ophthalmol. 2016;10:1531–4.
31. Graemiger RA, Niemeyer G, Schneeberger SA, Messmer EP. Wagner vitreoretinal degeneration. Follow-up of the original pedigree. Ophthalmology. 1995;102(12):1830–9.
32. Araujo JR, Tavares-Ferreira J, Estrela-Silva S, et al. WAGNER syndrome: anatomic, functional and genetic characterization of a Portuguese family. Graefes Arch Clin Exp Ophthalmol. 2018;256(1):163–71.
33. Acon D, Hussain RM, Yannuzzi NA, Berrocal AM. Complex combined tractional and rhegmatogenous retinal detachment in a twenty-three-year-old male with Wagner syndrome. Ophthalmic Surg Lasers Imaging Retina. 2020;51(8):467–71.
34. Meredith SP, Richards AJ, Flanagan DW, Scott JD, Poulson AV, Snead MP. Clinical characterisation and molecular analysis of Wagner syndrome. Br J Ophthalmol. 2007;91 (5):655–9.
35. Ronan SM, Tran-Viet KN, Burner EL, Metlapally R, Toth CA, Young TL. Mutational hot spot potential of a novel base pair mutation of the CSPG2 gene in a family with Wagner syndrome. Arch Ophthalmol. 2009;127(11):1511–9.
36. Thomas AS, Branham K, Van Gelder RN, et al. Multimodal imaging in Wagner syndrome. Ophthalmic Surg Lasers Imaging Retina. 2016;47(6):574–9.

Pediatric Traumatic Retinal Detachments

34

Sandra Hoyek, Grace Baldwin, and Nimesh A. Patel

Abstract

Trauma-related retinal detachment (RD) is the leading cause of acquired monocular blindness in the pediatric population globally. It also represents the most common cause of RD in this age group. Diagnosis of traumatic RD is usually delayed in children and predispose to complications, including macular detachment, multiple quadrant involvement, and proliferative vitreoretinopathy development (PVR). Therefore, initial evaluation should be meticulous and holistic, followed by short-interval re-evaluations. Special attention should be paid to nonaccidental trauma and projectile impact, as well as to conditions that can predispose to traumatic detachment including myopia, hereditary vitreo-retinopathies, and prematurity. Appropriate timely management of pediatric traumatic RD is pivotal to optimize anatomic and visual outcomes. In this chapter, we discuss clinical pearls in diagnosis and treatment of trauma-associated RD in children, specifically timing to surgery, treatment choice, intraoperative considerations, and surgical outcomes.

Supplementary Information The online version contains supplementary material available at https://doi.org/10.1007/978-3-031-14506-3_34.

S. Hoyek · N. A. Patel (✉)
Department of Ophthalmology, Massachusetts Eye and Ear, Harvard Medical School, 243 Charles St, Boston, MA 02114, USA
e-mail: nimesh_patel2@meei.harvard.edu

S. Hoyek
e-mail: salhoyek@meei.harvard.edu

G. Baldwin
Harvard Medical School, 25 Shattuck St, Boston, MA 02115, USA
e-mail: grace_baldwin@hms.harvard.edu

Keywords

Trauma · Retinal detachment · Pediatric · Scleral buckle · Pars plana vitrectomy · Proliferative vitreoretinopathy · Self-mutilation

Introduction

Eye trauma is the leading cause of acquired monocular blindness in children worldwide. Further complications include deprivation amblyopia and long-term bilateral visual impairment [1]. In the United States, the incidence of ocular injuries is estimated to be 2.4 million cases annually. One-third of serious ocular injuries occur in the pediatric population at a rate of one injury every three minutes [2].

Of paramount importance is trauma-related retinal detachment (RD), which occurs in approximately 2.5–2.9 per 100,000 children annually and represents the most common cause of RD in this age group [3, 4]. RD is prevalent among pediatric penetrating open globe injuries (OGI), occurring in up to 31% of these cases [5]. RD can also develop from closed globe injury (CGI) secondary to retinal dialysis or breaks that may initially go unnoticed. Predictors of RD include mechanism of trauma (rupture or perforation), large wound size, poor initial visual acuity (VA), hyphema, lens injury, and the development of endophthalmitis.

Children with traumatic RD are more likely to develop complications, including proliferative vitreoretinopathy and a progression to phthisis. Therefore, appropriate timely management is crucial for anatomic and functional success, which can minimize morbidity, psychological impact, and occupational burden.

In this chapter, we discuss clinical pearls in diagnosis and treatment of trauma-associated RD in children and present the surgical outcomes.

Diagnosis

Clinical Profile

As stated above, trauma related RD is the most common cause of RD in children. Pediatric traumatic detachments occur predominantly in boys. Of all forms of detachments, the rhegmatogenous type is the most common [3].

At initial presentation, diagnosis is missed in almost half of all cases [3]. Late diagnosis can occur in up to 85% of OGI, and represents a significant challenge to ophthalmologists [5]. Multiple factors are culpable, including poor fundus visualization due to vitreous hemorrhage, lens opacification, poor mydriasis, corneal scar, or hyphema. Children may not complain initially about decreased vision, especially in unilateral cases. Development of RD might be delayed in children due to firm vitreoretinal adhesion and lack of vitreous liquefaction and posterior vitreous detachment (PVD). The solid vitreous gel can act as a tamponade to retinal breaks leading to slow and shallow progression of RD.

Delayed RD presentation is correlated with a higher incidence of macular detachment, multiple quadrant involvement, and proliferative vitreoretinopathy development (PVR). Therefore, initial evaluation should be meticulous and holistic, followed by short-interval re-evaluations.

Assessment

Assessment clinical pearls:

- History to assess for any underlying predisposition
- Bilateral eye examination
- Careful attention for macular hole
- Fluorescein angiogram consideration if no break or limited history
- B-scan to assess for presence of choroidal detachment
- CT scan if suspicion for open globe or foreign body.

When a pediatric patient presents with traumatic eye injury, the first step is hemodynamic stabilization followed promptly by a complete history with a focus on the mechanism of injury. Specific causes to consider include nonaccidental trauma (abuse, self-injurious behavior, eye rubbing, etc.) and projectile impact. Projectile injury may suggest possible OGI. It is important to assess for myopia, hereditary vitreoretinopathies, and prematurity as these conditions can predispose to traumatic detachment and increase the risk of detachment in the contralateral eye.

With examination, an attempt to record VA is important, as it is one of the clearest predictors of functional outcome. Ocular mobility, pupillary light reflex, and confrontational visual fields should be evaluated. Careful examination of the peripheral retina is imperative to identify location, number, and size of retinal dialysis or breaks. B-scan ultrasonography can be valuable in diagnosing a RD, choroidal detachment, or intraocular foreign body (IOFB), especially if there is media opacity. In pediatric patients the history is often unreliable or a break may not be visible. In these cases, it is prudent to consider fluorescein angiography to evaluate for non-traumatic causes of RD, such as exudative, uveitic, retinopathy of prematurity, and familial exudative vitreoretinopathy.

There are coexisting clinical signs that can alter the surgical plan including vitreous hemorrhage, choroidal detachment, and macular hole. When a slit-lamp evaluation cannot be completed, examination under anesthesia of both eyes should be considered. At the time of general anesthesia, baseline measurements of axial length should be obtained. This can help to assess progression to phthisis in the future and guide the utility of further intervention.

If there is any suspicion for an OGI or IOFB, the authors recommend coronal and axial CT scan of the orbits with thin 0.5–1 mm cuts. This is often required to be specified in the imaging order or discussed with the radiologist. Hounsfield units quantitatively measure radiodensity and can assist in identifying the substance of an IOFB. It is best to avoid MRI in the context of a suspected IOFB as a metallic foreign body may react to the imaging magnet. Gentle ultrasound may be performed if the globe is stable to assist in IOFB localization.

Management

Surgical Tips

- Scleral buckle is often the best primary surgery.
- Anterior approach with lensectomy may be beneficial in cases with funnel retinal detachment or choroidal detachment.
- Posterior vitreous detachment creation can be assisted by triamcinolone staining and flexible loop scraping.
- Due to strong vitreoretinal adhesion in children, segmentation can be an alternative to delamination for pre-retinal fibrous tissue removal.
- Same-day bilateral surgery may be considered in select cases: difficult anesthesia, systemic comorbidities, or amblyopia risk.

Timing to Surgery

In pediatric traumatic RD, timing to surgery is dependent on various factors. If there is a known recent injury and the macula is attached, then an early intervention is indicated. Data suggests that surgery performed four days post-trauma reduces PVR [6]. Immediate surgery is indicated in the context of reactive IOFBs and endophthalmitis. When there is a coexisting hyphema, the intraocular pressure (IOP) should be carefully monitored and surgery prior to corneal blood staining should be considered as this can avoid need for a concurrent corneal transplant.

Reasons to delay intervention include corneal edema, hemodynamic instability, more pressing need for other procedures, and limited access to required resources or surgical team. In the setting of an OGI, often the goal is primary closure with RD repair performed secondarily.

Treatment Choice

The goal of surgery is to reestablish retina-RPE adhesion through scleral buckling procedures (SB) and/or pars plana vitrectomy (PPV). Primary SB is the first line treatment choice. Due to the solid state of the pediatric hyaloid, SB indentation relieves vitreoretinal traction and allows the vitreous gel to tamponade the retinal break. Subsequently, subretinal fluid is progressively resorbed, which can take months in a chronic RD. SB is associated with lower risks of endophthalmitis and cataract formation and has a reasonable rate of anatomic success [7].

While SB constitutes an effective approach in managing uncomplicated CGI-related RD, PPV appears to be required in more severe OGI-related damage [3]. PPV constitutes an unavoidable choice in the following more complex situations: coexistence of cataract or lens subluxation, vitreous hemorrhage or haze, multiple or posterior retinal breaks, giant retinal tear, PVR, retinal or vitreous incarceration, and the need for long term tamponade [8]. In addition, combining PPV with SB may help to decrease retinectomy need, manage incomplete vitreous removal, and preserve crystalline lens [9].

In cases with OGI and RD, SB may be placed at the time of repair since peritomy and rectus muscle isolation has already been performed. Care must be taken to ensure the globe is well closed and not to expulse intraocular contents when tightening the buckle. If planning for a SB as a secondary procedure, it is ideal to return to the operating room within one to two weeks to avoid conjunctival and tenon scarring and minimize the risk of permanent vision loss.

Intraoperative Considerations

Incision

During incision, special attention should be paid to pediatric anatomic characteristics. The pars plana may be partially formed in infants less than seven years old requiring anterior incisions at the iris root or limbus to avoid iatrogenic retinal breaks. In general, incision 4 mm from the limbus should solely be used in children aged four years and older. Adding 1 mm distance from the limbus for each year of age, starting at age one, is a practical approach. Trans-scleral illumination can be considered as it may help perform safe sclerotomy through the pars plana.

Management of the Lens

Management of the lens in pediatric traumatic RD has some considerations. If vitrectomy is required, a lens sparing approach is ideal. This is key in the prevention of amblyopia and glaucoma.

In cases with choroidal detachment, the ciliary body may be anteriorly rotated, which can lead to inadvertent subretinal or suprachoroidal trocar entry. If this occurs, a low threshold for lensectomy is advised. Additionally, a 6 mm trocar may be used to ensure intravitreal placement. Likewise, in cases with a funnel RD, lensectomy may be required.

With trauma, placement of an intraocular lens is usually not advisable at the time of lensectomy. It can serve as a scaffold for proliferative vitreoretinopathy or inflammatory membranes. Due to similar concerns, a capsulectomy is often required. Secondary lenses or contact lenses may be used once the eye is stable for the management of aphakia.

Management of the Posterior Hyaloid

During surgical management of RD, it is advisable to perform a complete vitrectomy with depressed shave after lifting of the posterior hyaloid. This is assisted with the use of triamcinolone and a flexible loop scraper. However, in cases with an adherent hyaloid, focal detachment, or a difficult view, one must consider the benefit of removing all the vitreous traction compared to the risk of iatrogenic retinal breaks. (See supplementary video and caption).

Another option, although controversial and not commonly performed, is preoperative vitreolysis through intravitreal injection of plasmin enzyme for posterior hyaloid separation. This is usually performed after induction of general anesthesia and 30 min prior to surgery [10].

Proliferative Vitreoretinopathy

If proliferative vitreoretinopathy (PVR) is noted during surgery for pediatric traumatic RD, vitrectomy and membrane peeling may be required. Due to firm vitreoretinal adhesion, segmentation can be an alternative to complete delamination for pre-retinal fibrous tissue removal. If the PVR is mild, starting with a scleral buckle without vitrectomy is an option and can lead to reattachment. If using SB for PVR, larger buckle elements (42 band, 287 tires, etc.) tightened to a significant indentation may be required to alleviate the retinal contraction.

Despite best efforts with a SB and membrane peeling, retinectomies are required in up to 38% of cases [11]. In the pediatric population, this results in PVR development at higher rates than adults due to the robust inflammatory response in children.

Tamponade Choice

Tamponade choice during vitrectomy typically constitutes silicone oil for traumatic pediatric RD. Maintenance of postoperative positioning and monitoring IOP are often challenging, thus long-lasting tamponade is frequently needed for complex cases with PVR [8]. Visual rehabilitation is achieved early when silicone oil is used, which reduces the likelihood of amblyopia.

Aphakia is common in traumatic cases, which may result in silicone oil migration to the anterior chamber leading to corneal decompensation, secondary glaucoma, and band keratopathy. In aphakic patients with a gas or oil tamponade, peripheral iridectomy is recommended to avoid pupillary block. Band keratopathy can be managed with ethylene-diamine-tetra-acetic acid (EDTA) chelation with or without oil removal.

Self-inflicted RD

Self-inflicted RD is a rare form of self-mutilation often associated with severe psychiatric and developmental comorbidities. Self-inflicted RD creates unique considerations. Surgical treatment is challenging due to bilateral injury, late diagnosis, limited child cooperation, continuous traumatic behavior, and recurrent RD

[12]. PVR, funnel-shaped RD, and giant retinal breaks are frequent features. Despite complex presentation, SB use as primary treatment can lead to an acceptable outcome. However, when PPV is unavoidable, the authors suggest leaving intraocular silicone oil for a longer duration to ensure retinal healing. Immediate bilateral sequential surgery could be considered when there is significant risk or if there are challenges with repeated general anesthesia [13]. Further, in cases of unilateral RD, repetitive self-injurious behavior may warrant a prophylactic scleral buckle with laser in the fellow eye. In addition, behavioral and occupational therapy, psychiatric medications, and protective devices such as braces, helmets, and mittens help mitigate traumatic reinjury [14].

Outcomes

Pediatric traumatic RD portends a worse postoperative anatomic and functional outcome than adults, due to higher incidence of delayed presentation, macular involvement, and PVR.

Complications

Potential complications in the postoperative course of SB include scleral rupture, buckle extrusion, diplopia, and nerve ischemia. PPV-associated complications include iatrogenic retinal break, retinal and vitreous bleeding, band keratopathy, lens opacification, and silicone oil emulsification. Retinal incarceration, endophthalmitis, and episcleritis can also present following PPV or SB [15].

Predictors of Visual and Anatomic Success

Anatomic and visual outcomes following surgery are tightly bound. The former is defined as final retinal reattachment and is observed in up to 86% of cases [5]. However, redetachment is reported in up to 53% of cases and is more likely to occur in the context of OGI, PPV treatment, and preoperative complications, such as choroidal detachment, PVR, and endophthalmitis [16].

Anatomic success is correlated with improved functional outcomes and cosmetic results, including lower progression to painful blind eye and phthisis. Predictors of suboptimal functional success include young age, delayed presentation, initial low VA (hand motion or less), IOFB, anterior segment scarring, total RD, macular involvement, PVR, choroidal detachment, retained silicone oil, vitrectomy in CGI, amblyopia, and recurrent detachment [17]. According to Soheilian et al., the most important factor that affects both anatomic and visual outcome is advanced PVR [18]. Importantly, a mismatch between functional and anatomic success can be observed, largely due to amblyopia (Table 34.1).

Table 34.1 Pediatric Traumatic Retinal Detachments: Surgery, Success Rate, and Recurrence

PMID	Date	Journal	Period	Characteristics of Series	Number of Trauma-Related RD			Surgery (%)			Success Rate (%)			Recurrence (%)
					Total #	Total | Partial (%)	Mac-On | Mac-Off (%)	SB	PPV	Combined	Total	OGI	CGI	
33358673	2021	Canadian Journal. Ophthalmology	2010–2018	Pediatric traumatic RD	32	20 (63) | 12 (37)	5 (16) | 27 (84)	9 (28)	23 (72)	0	24 (75)	NR	NR	17 (53)
33892134	2021	Ophthalmology Retina	2012–2020	Pediatric traumatic RD	23	NR	7 (32) | 15 (68)	0	13 (93)	0	86%	86%	NR	7 (50%)
30046466	2018	Journal of Ophthalmology	2013–2016	Pediatric traumatic RD	57	NR	35 (63) | 22 (37)	0	57 (100)	0	41 (72)	NR	NR	22 (39)
28858062	2018	Retina	2002–2013	Pediatric RD	60	NR	NR	5 (8)	11 (18)	44 (74)	39 (65)	16 (50)	23 (82)	37 (62)
28195617	2017	Ophthalmic Surgery, Lasers and Imaging Retina	2010–2013	Pediatric traumatic RD	110	34 (31) | 76 (69)	14 (13) | 96 (87)	5 (5)	105 (95)	0	85 (77)	66 (76)	19 (83)	NR
17579292	2007	Ophthalmologica	1983–2003	Pediatric traumatic RD	33	18 (55) | 15 (45)	10 (30) | 23 (70)	4 (12)	10 (30)	19 (58)	12 (36)	12 (36)	NR	NR
16601744	2006	Eye	1991–1999	Pediatric ocular trauma	47	NR	NR	17 (36)	30 (64)	0	55%	PPV 14 (47)	SB 12 (71)	NR
15183788	2004	American Journal of Ophthalmology	1980–2000	Pediatric traumatic RD	60	16 (27) | 44 (73)	25 (42) | 35 (58)	0	0	57 (95)	48%	16 (46)	13 (65)	25 (42)

#: Number, CGI: Closed Globe Injury, Mac-Off: Macula-Off, Mac-On: Macula-On, NR: Not Reported, OGI: Open Globe Injury, PMID: PubMed Identifier, PPV: Pars Plana Vitrectomy, RD: Retinal Detachment, SB: Scleral Buckle

Conclusion

To conclude, despite advances in surgical modalities and visual rehabilitation, functional and anatomic success in pediatric traumatic RD remains a challenge. In order to achieve functional rehabilitation each case requires a thorough and thoughtful pre-operative assessment and an individualized surgical plan.

Video *Caption*

A 10-year-old patient presented with traumatic retinal detachment, cataract, and vitreous hemorrhage in the setting of cerebral palsy and self-injurious behavior. He had a history of congenital cytomegalovirus (CMV) infection. Scleral buckle was placed and lensectomy was performed. Vitreous hemorrhage was removed and an inferior giant retinal tear was found. The posterior hyaloid was helping to maintain the attachment of the macula. The hyaloid was not removed and a focal retinectomy was performed. Silicone oil was placed. An arm brace was placed to prevent recurrent injury. The vision improved and the retina remained attached at one year follow up.

Review Questions

1. What is the best primary surgery for uncomplicated pediatric traumatic retinal detachment?

a. Scleral buckle
b. Pars plana vitrectomy
c. Pars plana vitrectomy and scleral buckle
d. Pars plana vitrectomy and lensectomy

2. What are the indications for an immediate surgery to repair a pediatric traumatic retinal detachment?

a. Intra-ocular foreign body
b. Hyphema
c. Corneal edema
d. Endophthalmitis

3. What are the indications for an anterior approach with lensectomy for the management of pediatric traumatic retinal detachment?

a. Vitreous hemorrhage
b. Funnel retinal detachment
c. Choroidal detachment
d. All cases of open-globe injuries-related retinal detachment

4. What tools are available for posterior vitreous detachment creation in children?

a. Triamcinolone staining
b. Flexible loop scraping
c. Intravitreal injection of plasmin enzyme
d. High aspiration through smaller gauge instrumentation

Answers

1. A
2. A, D
3. B, C
4. A, B, C

References

1. Puodžiuvienė E, Jokūbauskienė G, Vieversytė M, Asselineau K. A five-year retrospective study of the epidemiological characteristics and visual outcomes of pediatric ocular trauma. BMC Ophthalmol. 2018;18(1):10.
2. Matsa E, Shi J, Wheeler KK, McCarthy T, McGregor ML, Leonard JC. Trends in US emergency department visits for pediatric acute ocular injury. JAMA Ophthalmol. 2018;136 (8):895–903.
3. Sarrazin L, Averbukh E, Halpert M, Hemo I, Rumelt S. Traumatic pediatric retinal detachment: a comparison between open and closed globe injuries. Am J Ophthalmol. 2004;137(6):1042–9.
4. Rahimi M, Bagheri M, Nowroozzadeh MH. Characteristics and outcomes of pediatric retinal detachment surgery at a tertiary referral center. J Ophthalmic Vis Res. 2014;9(2):210–4.
5. Portney DS, Jacobson A, Liles N, Bohnsack BL, Besirli CG. Characteristics of retinal detachment after pediatric open-globe injuries. Ophthalmol Retina. 2021;S2468–6530 (21):00128–37.
6. Wang N-K, Chen Y-P, Yeung L, Chen K-J, Chao A-N, Kuo Y-H, et al. Traumatic pediatric retinal detachment following open globe injury. Ophthalmol J Int Ophtalmol Int J Ophthalmol Z Augenheilkd. 2007;221(4):255–63.
7. Nuzzi R, Lavia C, Spinetta R. Paediatric retinal detachment: a review. Int J Ophthalmol. 2017;10(10):1592–603.
8. Sheard RM, Mireskandari K, Ezra E, Sullivan PM. Vitreoretinal surgery after childhood ocular trauma. Eye Lond Engl. 2007;21(6):793–8.
9. Ghoraba HH, Mansour HO, Abdelhafez MA, El Gouhary SM, Zaky AG, Heikal MA, et al. Comparison between pars plana vitrectomy with and without encircling band in the treatment of pediatric traumatic rhegmatogenous retinal detachment. Clin Ophthalmol Auckl NZ. 2020;14:3271–7.
10. Turgut B, Demir T, Çatak O. The recommendations for pediatric vitreoretinal surgery. Adv Ophthalmol Vis Syst. 2019.
11. Gonzales CR, Singh S, Yu F, Kreiger AE, Gupta A, Schwartz SD. Pediatric rhegmatogenous retinal detachment: clinical features and surgical outcomes. Retina Phila Pa. 2008;28(6): 847–52.
12. Liu Q, de Alba Campomanes AG, Stewart JM. Outcomes after Retinal Detachment Resulting from Self-Inflicted Injury. Ophthalmol Retina. 2019;3(8):690–3.

13. Yonekawa Y, Wu W-C, Kusaka S, Robinson J, Tsujioka D, Kang KB, et al. Immediate sequential bilateral pediatric vitreoretinal surgery: an international multicenter study. Ophthalmology. 2016;123(8):1802–8.
14. Rossin EJ, Tsui I, Wong SC, Hou KK, Prakhunhungsit S, Blair MP, et al. Traumatic retinal detachment in patients with self-injurious behavior: an international multicenter study. Ophthalmol Retina. 2021;5(8):805–14.
15. Sul S, Gurelik G, Korkmaz S, Ozdek S, Hasanreisoglu B. Pediatric traumatic retinal detachments: clinical characteristics and outcomes. Ophthalmic Surg Lasers Imaging Retina. 2017;48(2):143–50.
16. Sindal MD, Gondhale HP, Srivastav K. Clinical profile and outcomes of rhegmatogenous retinal detachment related to trauma in pediatric population. Can J Ophthalmol J Can Ophtalmol. 2021;56(4):231–6.
17. Read SP, Aziz HA, Kuriyan A, Kothari N, Davis JL, Smiddy WE, et al. Retinal detachment surgery in a pediatric population: visual and anatomic outcomes. Retina Phila Pa. 2018;38(7):1393–402.
18. Soheilian M, Ramezani A, Malihi M, Yaseri M, Ahmadieh H, Dehghan MH, et al. Clinical features and surgical outcomes of pediatric rhegmatogenous retinal detachment. Retina Phila Pa. 2009;29(4):545–51.

Retinopathy of Prematurity Related Late Rhegmatogenous Retinal Detachment

Dhariana Acón and Audina M. Berrocal

Abstract

Retinopathy of prematurity is a neovascular disease of premature infants and the natural history of this disease has been extensively described. Long term sequelae and complications has been less investigated. Retinal detachment is vision threating in these patients; tractional and exudative retinal detachments are usually presented earlier in age; rhegmatogenous detachments tent to occur more commonly later in life secondary to abnormal vitreoretinal interface changes. Different surgical approaches can be used to treat this complication. Either vitrectomy, scleral buckle or combination of both techniques are recommended depending on the case.

Keywords

Prematurity · Retinopathy · ROP · Retinal detachment · Rhegmatogenous · Laser · Vitrectomy · Buckle

Supplementary Information The online version contains supplementary material available at https://doi.org/10.1007/978-3-031-14506-3_35.

D. Acón (✉)
Retina and Pediatric Retina Specialist: National Children Hospital Costa Rica, Asociados de Macular Vitreo y Retina de Costa Rica, San Jose, Costa Rica

Universidad de Ciencias Médicas, San Jose, Costa Rica

National Children Hospital, San Jose, Costa Rica
e-mail: dhariaconr@gmail.com

A. M. Berrocal
Medical Director of Pediatric Retina and Retinopathy of Prematurity, Vitreoretinal Fellowship Director Retina Department, Bascom Palmer Eye Institute, Miami, FL, USA

Introduction

Advanced cases of ROP can lead to severe visual impairment and even complete blindness. With the improved technology of the pediatric field and the nursing system, the survival rate in premature infants has increased markedly since the late 1960s. This increased survival rate has resulted in the apparent increase of the incidence of ROP [1]. Retinopathy of prematurity is a neovascular disease of premature infants, and while much work has been done in screening and treating ROP in infancy, not much is reported about the late manifestations, findings and complications; specifically for untreated ROP, eyes that don't meet type 1 ROP with persistent avascular retina [2]. The natural history and characteristics of tractional retinal detachment associated with ROP in both neonates and infants have been extensively described; however later sequelae of ROP has been less investigated [3].

Background

In the majority cases of ROP the acute changes resolve without an initial loss of vision. Residual cicatricial vitreoretinal changes are frequently observed in the eyes with more severe stages of ROP [1].

Retinal detachment presents at all ages. The main causes of retinal detachment depend on patients' ages. In patients with regressed ROP either treated with laser or cryotherapy, progressive traction bands with tractional components are the main cause of retinal detachment between 2 and 4 years of age. However, the main cause of late retinal detachment occurred after the age of 6 years are retinal tears [1].

Despite CryoROP and ETROP many of neonatal eyes that have significant ROP disease not meet threshold for any form of treatment. Understanding the anatomical and functional outcomes in a long term basis of these group of eyes is important because many have significant amount of avascular retina, and retinal detachment is the most concerning cause of visual loss in these eyes.

Previous reports by Farris and Tasman stated that late RRD due to ROP occurred between the 5 and 15 years of age; and tractional or exudative retinal detachment occurred earlier. Other authors reported that these complications could be also encountered in adulthood; Machemer reported cases occurring later in life as a sequel to cicatricial ROP. Kaiser et al. showed that RRD occurred in 13.9% of adults who had cicatricial changes of ROP. Smith, et al. reported a detachment rate of 25.6% in their retrospective observational series [8–11]. There are differences in population studied regarding of patients born prior or after Cryo-ROP.

Clinical Features

Previous studies have reported findings and clinical sequelae of regressed ROP such as:

- Retinal tears (34.7%)
- Atrophic holes (54%)
- Tractional retinoschisis (12.1%)
- Macular dragging (12.1%)
- Vitreous condensation ridge like interface (30.9%)
- Displacement of retinal vessels
- Peripheral vascular changes (incompletely vascularized peripheral retina, telangiectatic vessels, vascular arcades with circumferential interconnection, and abnormal branching of retinal vessels)
- Vitreoretinal interface changes (pigmentary changes, peripheral folds, vitreous membranes, lattice like degeneration)
- Retinal detachment in adults and children (38.6%)

Other late findings in patients with regressed ROP are:

- High Myopia
- Strabismus
- Nystagmus
- Diffuse retina atrophy
- Vitreous Hemorraghe
- Peripheral exudates.

Retinal Detachment

Rhegmatogenous retinal detachment can present at all ages but is most commonly manifested later in life. The average age of presentation of retinal detachment is 34.5 years and the average gestational age is 26.6 weeks, with and average birth weight of 875 g. (1) 57.9% of RD occur by the age of 30, and 27.1% by age 18. 13.6% of eyes presents with purely tractional retinal detachment, and 86.4% of RD are rhegmatogenous or combined rhegmatogenous/tractional RDs. Patients with gestational age of 29 wks or less are more likely to have retinal detachments compared to gestational age of 30–34 and eyes with furthest vascularization to posterior zone 2 are more likely to have retinal detachments compared to zone 3 eyes. Unilateral detachments are more frequent, but patients can present with bilateral affection. Six percent of the eyes with RRD have a single break and 52% of cases have multiple breaks; in 12% of the cases the break might not be found but clinical features corroborate the RRD. The most common type of breaks are retina holes that can be present in up to 69% of cases; 28% have retinal tears with traction and 8% of cases have both types. Most commonly breaks are located in the temporal quadrants of the eye (69%) but can be found in any quadrant [6].

Although cryotherapy has been replaced by laser and anti- VEGF treatment it is still used in different countries to treat type 1 ROP. The immediate ocular complications of cryotherapy for ROP are well documented and include conjunctival and subconjunctival hemorrhage, conjunctival laceration and vision threatening retinal, preretinal and vitreous hemorrhage. Longterm complications of transcleral cryotherapy have been less well characterized. Rhegmatogenous retinal detachment can develop as soon as 1–3 years after, a retinal tear adjacent to the cryotherapy area is the most frequent cause associated in these patients [12].

Pathophysiology

Retinopathy of Prematurity is a developmental vasoproliferative retinal disorder that occurs fundamentally in premature infants. The pathophysiology of ROP stems from a hypoxic-anoxic phenomenon in which high intraocular oxygen tension and fluctuations in oxygenation damage newly developed retinal vasculature and delay normal vascular development leading to ischemia, vasoproliferation, and ultimately fibroblastic overgrowth.

Retinal detachment is a possible complication of regressed ROP. It is uncertain whether retinal breaks and RD in regressed ROP are secondary to ongoing changes of ROP, to abnormal vitreoretinal interface changes caused by ROP, or to other unrecognized factors. Tasman speculated that as a result of vitreous traction, retinal vessels sometimes pulled into the vitreous cavity because of shrinking vitreous gel. He implied that temporal vitreous traction on the retina is the rule and proposed that this occurs because the temporal retina, even in full-term infants, is the last area to become vascularized and is thus more sensitive to changes in oxygen concentration [4, 5].

Machemer suggested that the vitreoretinal membrane originated on the surface of retina and this proliferation appeared to be stimulated by chronic exudation similar to other forms of vitreoretinal proliferation such as Coats disease, von Hippel disease, and exudative vitreoretinopathy.

Several known factors can increase the risk of rhegmatogenous or combined retinal detachments such as [2, 8]:

- Persistent peripheral avascular retina (atrophic holes commonly occurred)
- Vitreoretinal traction (vitreous condensation ridge-like interface from areas of old regressed fibrovascular tissue or reactivated neovascularization)

- Vitreous liquefaction,
- high myopia
- Lattice degeneration

Most eyes that develop a retinal tear or detachment have peripheral lattice and avascular retina, without posterior cicatricial ROP; however, patients without severe retinal cicatrization are still at risk of developing retinal detachment.

Management

In the older reported series vitrectomy was not available and only scleral buckle procedure was used to treat retinal detachment associated with regresses ROP. Final success rates reported ranged from 63 to 94%, these good results may be owing to the exclusion of inoperable eyes because of severe vitreoretinal involvement [4].

With the development of vitrectomy, surgeons are operating in more severe ROP retinal detachment cases that could not have been treated by scleral buckling [6].

Literature on this topic is scanty. Sneed et al. reported that retinal detachment with significant traction and or posterior retinal breaks may be treated by closed vitrectomy in conjunction with scleral buckling [7].

Rhegmatogenous RDs associated with regressed ROP and peripheral retinal breaks can often be successfully managed with traditional scleral buckling encircling procedures. However, if posterior retinal breaks, significant vitreoretinal traction, or proliferative vitreoretinopathy with marked tractional membrane are present, a pars plana vitrectomy combined with a scleral buckling procedure may be necessary to successfully reattach these retinas. Silicon oil tamponade may be needed in severe cases [13] (Figs. 35.1, 35.2, 35.3 and 35.4).

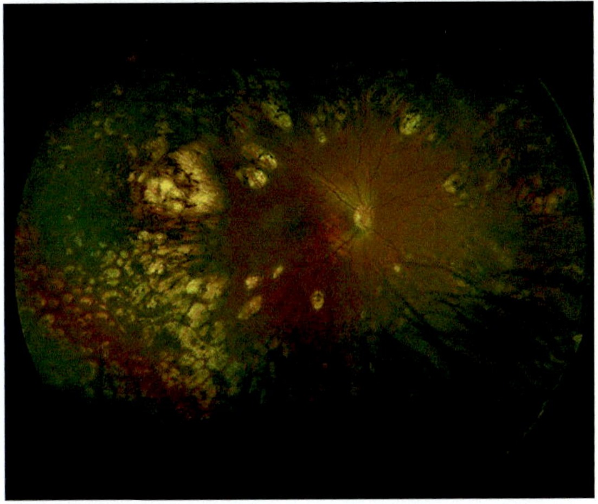

Fig. 35.1 Color photograph of the right eye of a patient born at 23 wks treated with laser and intravitreal anti VEGF

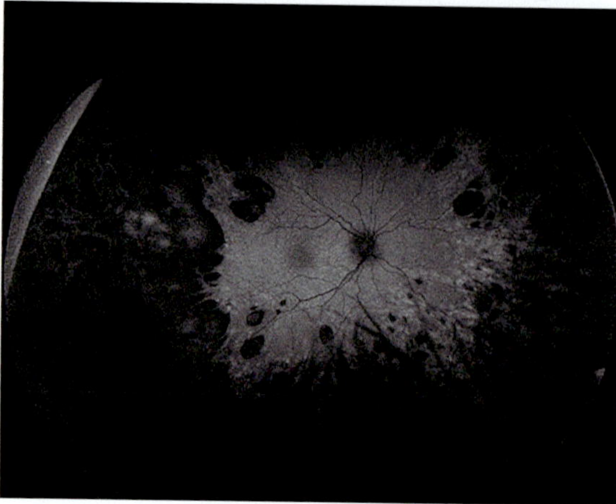

Fig. 35.2 Autofluorescence of the right eye of a patient born at 23 wks treated with laser and intravitreal anti VEGF

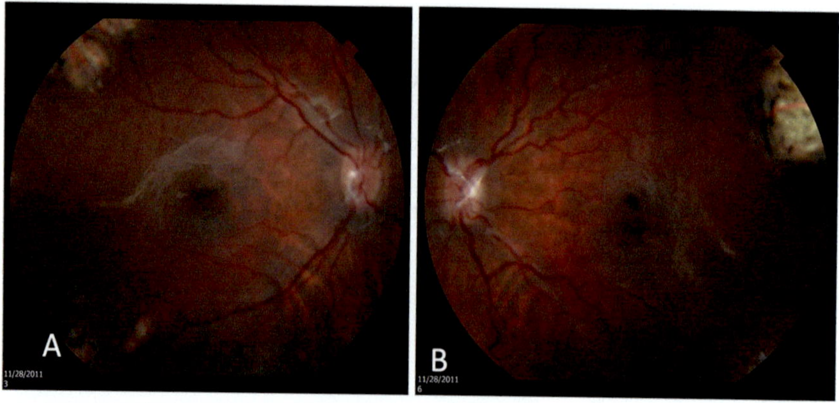

Fig. 35.3 **A–B** Color photographs of a premature patient treated with laser; vascular changes and laser can be seen

Video: *shows the surgery of an 11-year-old prematurely born boy with RRD in the left better seeing eye, who was not screened and did not have any treatment for ROP during neonatal period. Surgery involved encircling band and lens sparing vitrectomy with silicone oil tamponade (Video case courtesy of Dr. Şengül Özdek).*

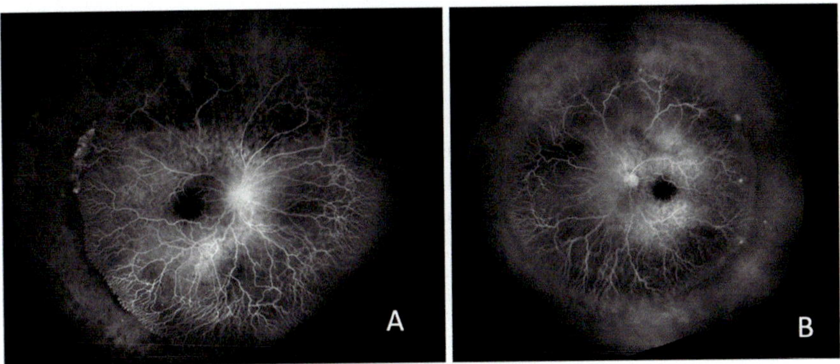

Fig. 35.4 **A–B** Widefield fluorescein angiography of a premature patient treated with intravitreal anti VEGF. These years after follow up photographs shows avascular periphery, telangiectatic vessel and an area of reactivation in the right eye

Conclusion

Patients with premature birth should be monitored regularly for retina complications; ultra widefield fluorescein angiography should be considered as part of the monitoring. Patients should be informed about the possibility and symptoms for retinal detachment. When retinal detachment occurs pars plana vitrectomy, scleral buckle or combination or both can be performed to achieve successful retinal reattachment. Laser barricade can me consider for specific cases. Prospective randomized studies are needed to truly explore the incidence and prognosis of this complication.

Review Questions

1. Known risk factors to that can increase the incidence of RRD or combined RD are:

A. Vitreous Traction
B. Avascular periphery
C. High Myopia
D. All of the above

2. Regarding retinal detachment in ROP:

A. Tractional detachments are commonly presented earlier in life and RRD later in life
B. Tracional detachments are commonly presented later in life and RRD earlier in life

C. Exudative detachment is the most common type of RD in ROP patients
D. None of the above

3. RRD in ROP patients:

A. Can present at all ages but is more common later in life
B. It can affect patients that were not treated because didn't met criteria but had significant amount of avascular periphery.
C. Can be treated with scleral buckle, vitrectomy or both
D. All of the above.

Answers

1. D
2. A
3. D

References

1. Sneed SR, Pulido JS, Blodi CF, et al. Surgical management of late-onset retinal detachments associated with regressed retinopathy of prematurity. Ophthalmology. 1990;97:179–83.
2. Park KH, Hwang J-M, Choi MY, Yu YS, Chung H. Retinal detachment of regressed retinopathy of prematurity in children aged 2 to 15 years. Retina. 2004; Jun 24(3):368–75. https://doi.org/10.1097/00006982-200406000-00006. PMID: 15187658.
3. Hamad AE, Moinuddin O, Blair MP, Schechet SA, Shapiro MJ, Quiram PA, Mammo DA, Berrocal AM, et al. Late-onset retinal findings and complications in untreated retinopathy of prematurity. Ophthalmol Retina. 2020;4(6):602–12. https://doi.org/10.1016/j.oret.2019.12.015 Epub 2019 Dec 24 PMID: 32059986.
4. Tufail A. Late onset vitreoretinal complications of regressed retinopathy of prematurity. Br J Ophthalmol. 2004;88(2):243–6. https://doi.org/10.1136/bjo.2003.022962.
5. Jandeck C. Late retinal detachment in patients born prematurely. Arch Ophthalmol. 2004;122 (1):61–. https://doi.org/10.1001/archopht.122.1.61.
6. Tasman W. Retinal detachment in retrolental fibroplasia (RLF). Mod Probl Ophthalmol. 1969;8:371–6.
7. Hiroko T, Tatsuo H. Late-onset retinal detachment associated with regressed retinopathy of prematurity. 2003;47(5):492–7. https://doi.org/10.1016/s0021-5155(03)00088-1.
8. Retinal detachment of regresses retinopathy of prematurity in children aged 2 to 15 years. Retina. 24(3):368–75. https://doi.org/10.1097/00006982-200406000-00006.
9. Faris BM. Retinopathy of prematurity: part II. Ocular complications. J Med Liban. 1972;25:379–84.
10. Tasman W. Late complications of retrolental fibroplasia. Ophthalmology. 1979;86:1724–40.
11. Kaiser RS, Trese MT, Williams GA, Cox MS Jr. Adult retinopathy of prematurity: Outcomes of rhegmatogenous retinal detachments and retinal tears. Ophthalmology. 2001;108:1647–53.
12. Sneed SR, Pulido JS, Blodi CF, Clarkson JG, Flynn HW, Mieler WF. Surgical management of lateonset retinal detachments associated with regressed retinopathy of prematurity. Ophthalmology. 1990;97(2):179–83. https://doi.org/10.1016/S0161-6420(90)32607-6.
13. Greven CM, Tasman W. Rhegmatogenous retinal detachment following cryotherapy in retinopathy of prematurity. Arch Ophthalmol. 1989;107:1017–8.

Congenital X-Linked Retinoschisis and Retinal Detachment

36

Hüseyin Baran Özdemir and Şengül Özdek

Abstract

Congenital X-linked retinoschisis is a common degenerative retinopathy characterized by bilateral mild to severe visual loss in males with splitting of retinal layers. Onset of the disease is usually during the first decade of life. The most common type is the complex type, and it is also the type in which complications are most common. Visual acuity remains stable in most of the patients however it may deteriorate during the first and second decades of life because of the sight-threatening complications like vitreous hemorrhage, rhegmatogenous retinal detachment, tractional retinal detachment, bullous retinoschisis involving the macula in some of the cases. These complications should be managed appropriately with advanced vitreoretinal surgical techniques. This chapter aimed to cover all aspects of the disease and provide information on the management of complications requiring surgery.

Keywords

Congenital X-linked retinoschisis · CXLR · Pediatric retinal detachment · Foveal cyst · Vitreous hemorrhage · Rhegmatogenous retinal detachment · Tractional retinal detachment · Exudative retinal detachment · Bullous retinoschisis · Inherited retinal diseases · Vitrectomy · Inner layer retinectomy · External drainage · Gene therapy

Supplementary Information The online version contains supplementary material available at https://doi.org/10.1007/978-3-031-14506-3_36.

H. B. Özdemir · Ş. Özdek (✉)
School of Medicine, Ophthalmology Department, Gazi University, Ankara, Turkey
e-mail: sozdek@gazi.edu.tr

Background

Congenital X-linked retinoschisis (CXLR) is a hereditary progressive retinal degenerative disorder characterized by splitting of the layers of the retina, first identified by Haas at 1898 [1, 2]. The disease has been termed differently over time, including neuroretinal disease in males, congenital cystic detachment of the retina, juvenile macular degeneration, and congenital vascular veils [3]. Jager proposed the word "retinoschisis" in 1953 [4]. Since then, the names "juvenile retinoschisis" and "sex-linked retinoschisis" as well as CXLR have been used frequently.

Epidemiology

CXLR prevalence varies between 1:5000 and 1:20,000 [5]. Since it is inherited as X-linked recessive pattern, it primarily affects men. Female carriers rarely show fundus and electrophysiological abnormalities, however heterozygotes with clinical symptoms have been reported [6, 7]. The age of onset is bimodal, with one group of patients emerging in infancy with strabismus and nystagmus and a second group presenting at school age with reduced vision and reading difficulties [8, 9]. Severe forms of the disease with vision-threatening complications usually present before the age of ten [1, 5]. The average visual acuity in young adults is 20/70 ranging from 20/200 to 20/20 [10].

Pathophysiology

CXLR is caused by mutations in the retinoschisin 1 (RS1) gene on chromosome Xp22.13 [11, 12]. RS1 gene encodes retinoschisin, which is involved in cell to cell adhesion and neurotransmission [13–16]. Mutations may affect the adhesive properties of retinoschisin in the different cell types of the neurosensorial retina, including photoreceptors, ganglion cells, amacrine cells, and bipolar cells [17]. The RS1 gene has been shown to have over 200 mutations [18]. The predominant mutations are missense mutations but no significant consistency has been found in visual impairment depending on the mutation type [12, 18].

Although the disease is caused by the same RS1 mutation, the severity of CXLR might vary significantly [19–22]. The underlying pathophysiologic mechanism of schisis cavity formation remains unknown. Joshi et al. proposed that a combination of vitreous tractional forces and intrastructural retinoschisin deficiencies may contribute to cavity formation at the structural level [23]. Molday et al. suggested that interactions between retinoschisin and intracellular Na/K + ATPase pumps modify ionic gradients and tissue balance, resulting in extracellular fluid accumulation in schisis cavities, at the functional level [1].

Clinical Findings

Clinical appearance of the patients may vary among patients, even in siblings with the same mutation. The most characteristic sign of CXLR, foveal schisis, is present in nearly all patients [24]. Foveal schisis has a distinctive clinical appearance. On examination, it is seen as small cysts located in the fovea, and grouped in stellate pattern or radial lines, also called as spoke-wheel pattern (Fig. 36.1). Foveal schisis may not be present in some patients who develop foveal atrophy during the course of the disease [25].

Peripheral retinoschisis (Fig. 36.2A) is present in 33–71% of patients and is most commonly located in the inferotemporal quadrant [26–28]. Other relatively common peripheral fundus changes are vitreous veils (Fig. 36.2B), metallic sheen, white spiculations (Fig. 36.2C, D), and pigmentary changes (Fig. 36.2A) [29, 30].

Bullous retinoschisis is a rare subtype of CXLR (Fig. 36.3) [31–33]. These cases usually present at earlier ages, usually during the first years of life. The most common presentation is strabismus. Nystagmus may also develop during the first year which suggests that the bullous retinoschisis may not have been present at birth [31]. Bullous retinoschisis is mostly bilateral and may involve fovea or overhang on

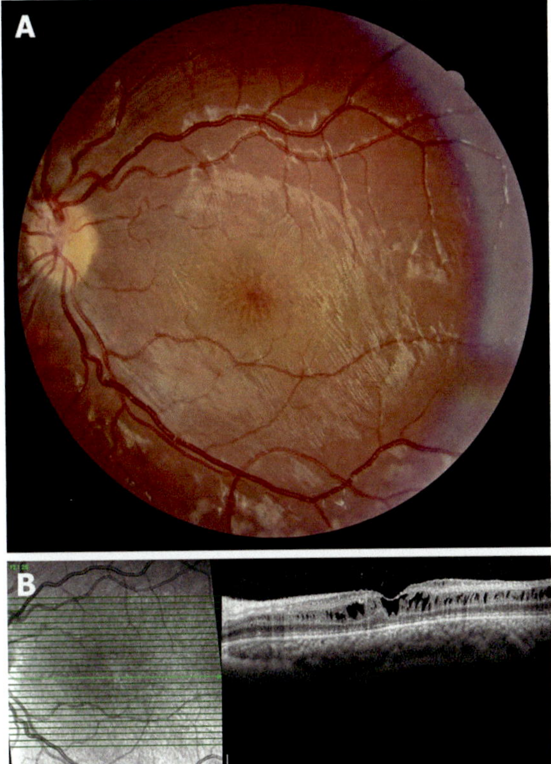

Fig. 36.1 Eight-year-old boy with congenital x-linked retinoschisis. Fundus photography **A** and optical coherence tomography **B** of the left eye (A) showing foveal schisis. Foveal cysts in the fovea form radial lines and appear as spokes-wheel pattern in the fundus photography

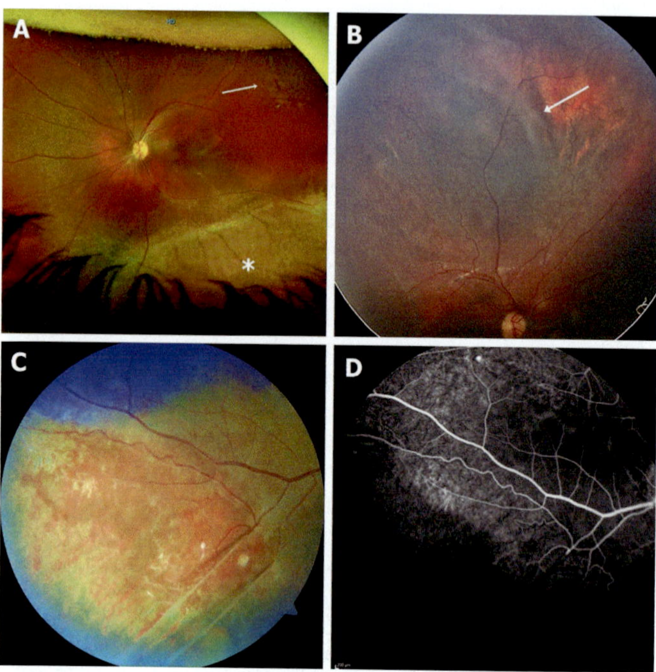

Fig. 36.2 Fundus examination findings of congenital X-linked retinoschisis (CXLR). **A** Ultra-widefield fundus photography of a 10-year old boy with CXLR showing inferotemporal peripheral retinoschisis in the left eye (marked with white asterisk) and pigmentary changes (marked with white arrow) at the upper-temporal quadrant. **B** Wide-field fundus photography of a one-year-old boy with CXLR shows vitreus veils (white arrow) at superior retina. **C** Fundus photography of a 19-year-old male with congenital X-linked retinoschisis showing white spiculations, sclerotic vessels, vascular traction with vitreous veils at the temporal quadrant. **D** Fluorescein angiography of the same patient (**C**) showing retinal non-perfusion areas in the temporal periphery

fovea, and may be highly elevated to become in contact with the back of the lens (see the case presentation). Hemorrhage may present within the schisis cavity or the vitreous. Previous papers reported that bullous schisis cavities may spontaneously resolve, leaving a pigmented demarcation line in most of the cases [31, 32].

Retinal vascular changes such as retinal ischemia (Figs. 36.2C, D and 36.4), optic disc and retinal neovascularization, vitreous hemorrhage and intraschitic hemorrhage (Fig. 36.5) may develop in patients with CXLR [29, 34–42]. The splitted retinal layers can cause stretching and ruptures with retinal vessels, which can lead to circulatory defects in the superficial and deep capillary plexus [40]. Stretched vascular structures may separate over time and cause bleeding into the vitreous or between the retinal layers.

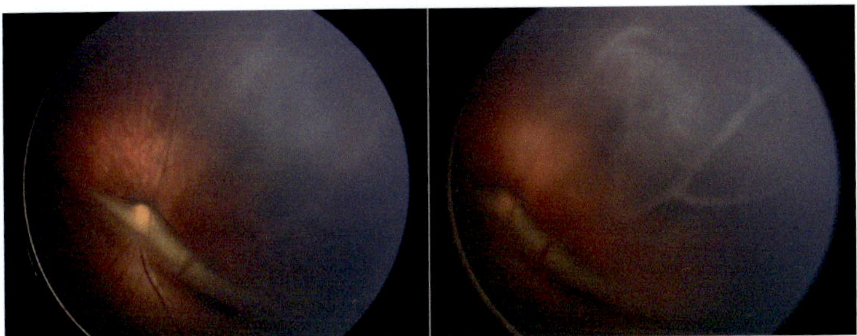

Fig. 36.3 Wide-field fundus photography of a 6-month-old infant showing bullous retinoschisis overhanging macula

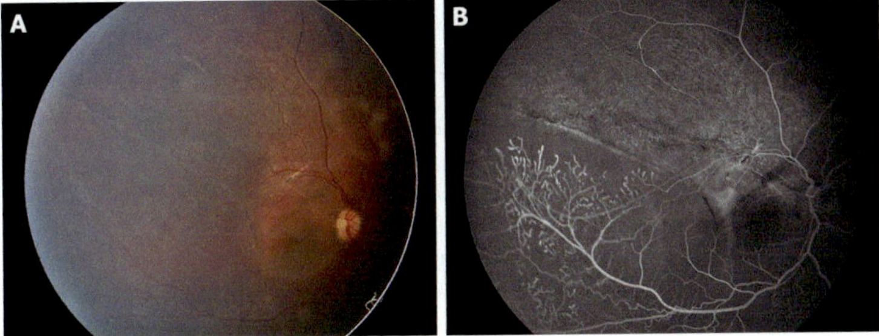

Fig. 36.4 A Widefield fundus photography of a five-year-old boy with congenital X-linked retinoshisis showing retinoschisis in the temporal and inferior-temporal quadrants in the right eye. **B** Fluorescein angiography of the same eye showing ischemic retina at the schitic areas and vascular changes. Note the leakage at the borders of retinoschisis area

Subretinal exudation or exudative retinal detachment may accompany with retinoschisis (Fig. 36.5) [43–46]. Clinical manifestation of exudation may be misdiagnosed with pediatric vascular diseases such as Coats disease or familial exudative vitreoretinopathy [43, 44]. The pathopshyiology of exudation is unclear. Retinal ischemia and neovascularization are not uncommon in CXLR, and exudation is likely to develop after these vascular pathologies secondary to retinoschisis.

Sight-threatening complications such as rhegmatogenous retinal detachment (RRD), tractional retinal detachment (TRD), vitreous hemorrhage, intraschitic hemorrhage within large schisis cavity, bullous retinoschisis and retinoschisis involving the macula may develop in patients with CXLR and these findings may be present at the initial examination [1, 3, 22, 26, 47–50].

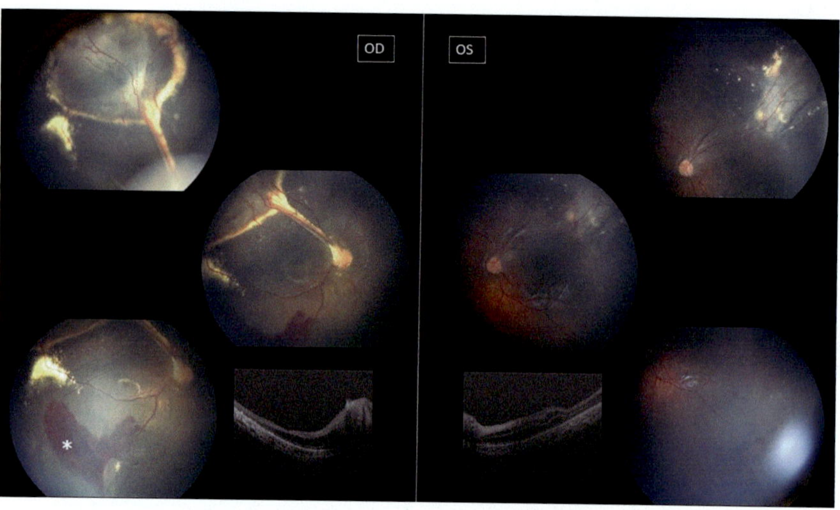

Fig. 36.5 A 2-year old boy presented with bilateral combined exudative and tractional retinal detachment with temporal retinal fold. FEVR and Coats' disease were considered in the differential diagnosis due to macular dragging and retinal exudation in both eyes. OCT revealed foveal schisis. The hemorrhage (white asterisk) below the inferior arcuate vessel, which was thought to be subretinal, was found to be intraschitic. His younger brother was also examined during diagnosis process and bullous retinoschisis was found. The patient was diagnosed as congenital X-linked retinoschisis. (**see the video** 1)

Classification

The classification of CXLR (Table 36.1) is suggested by Prenner et al. by using OCT and clinical examination (Figs. 36.6, 36.7, 36.8 and 36.9) [51]. Foveal schisis is the main finding in all types. Macular lamellar schisis represents schisis within the macula, which appears normal on clinical examination but is indicated by OCT. Type 3 (Complex) CXLR is the most common type and found to be a risk factor for the development of a combined retinoschisis-RD during follow-up [3, 52]. The type of classification may change during follow up in 17% of patients of cases [52].

Table 36.1 Congenital X-linked retinoschisis classification [52]

CXLR type	Foveal cystic Schisis	Macular lamellar Schisis	Peripheral schisis
Type 1: Foveal	Yes	No	No
Type 2: Foveo-lamellar	Yes	Yes	No
Type 3: Complex	Yes	Yes	Yes
Type 4: Foveo-peripheral	Yes	No	Yes

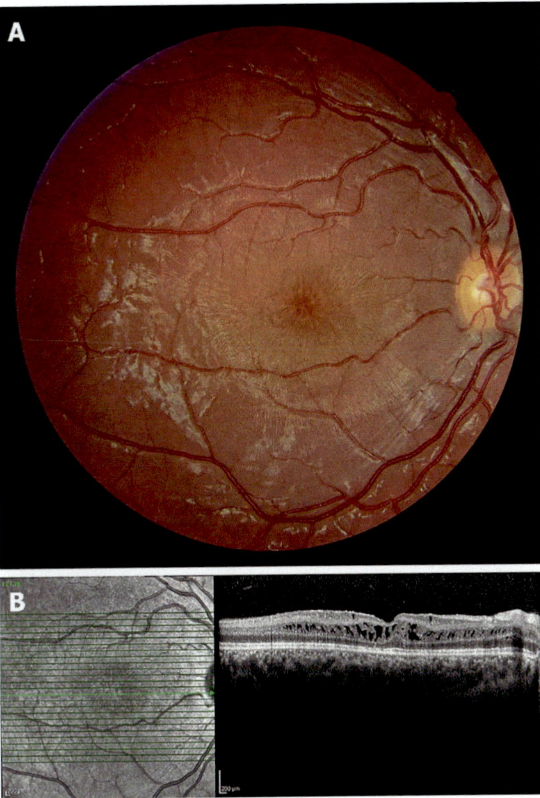

Fig. 36.6 Right eye of an eight-year-old boy who has type 1 (foveal) CXLR

Imaging and Electrophysiology

In addition to clinical examination findings, imaging, electrophysiological tests and, if necessary, genetic tests can be used for the diagnosis of CXLR. In fact, the diagnosis can be made with examination in male patients with a typical clinical appearance, but additional tests and imaging may be needed for the diagnosis in atypical presentations.

OCT is a valuable imaging method to evaluate pathological changes in the macula. Classification of CXLR also requires OCT findings. Schitic changes can be seen on OCT, even if the fovea appears normal on examination. Schisis can be seen in all retinal layers with OCT [3, 53, 54]. Schitic spaces are observed to be predominantly within the inner nuclear layer [53, 55]. No correlation was found between foveal thickness and presence of cysts in OCT and visual acuity [56, 57]. OCT-based studies showed that a decrease in foveal photoreceptor outer segment length, and a compromised integrity of external limiting membrane, ellipsoid portion of inner segment, and the cone outer segment tips are correlated with poor vision in patients with CXLR [44, 56, 58]. Foveal schisis may progress to foveal

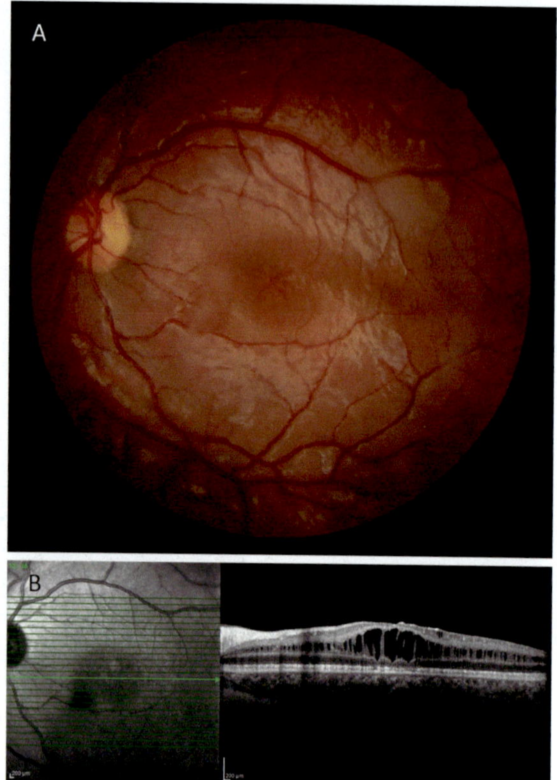

Fig. 36.7 Left eye of a 12-year-old boy who has type 2 (foveo-lamellar) congenital X-linked retinoschisis. Retinoschisis beyond the area of foveal schisis visible in the fundus photograph (**A**) and observed on the optical coherence tomography (**B**) is called macular lamellar schisis

atrophy within years in elderly patients [59]. Visual loss in these patients is correlated with the outer segment atrophy [60].

Although fluorescein angiography (FA) is not a "must" as a diagnostic tool, vascular changes can be observed during the course of the disease where FA may be helpful [61]. There is typically no leakage in FA of foveal cysts. Vascular leakage, retinal non-perfusion areas and neovascularization may be observed in a minority of the cases [62]. Peripheral vascular leakage may indicate increased vascular permeability as a potential source of intraretinal fluid [37, 63, 64]. Splitting retinal layers can lead to rupture of the vascular structures between the retinal layers and ischemic findings. These ischemic changes may result in neovascularization [35, 65].

Electroretinography (ERG) is another important diagnostic tool for CXLR [66]. There is a reduction in the dark-adapted b-wave amplitude in almost all patients [1]. Reduced b-wave amplitude with relatively preserved a-wave amplitude and altered b/a ratio (electronegative waveform) are the most significant findings for CXLR (Fig. 36.10) [67–71]. Increasing age causes a significant delay in XLRS b-wave onset, suggesting that the dysfunction of photoreceptor synapses or bipolar cells increases with age of XLRS subjects [69]. ERG findings are correlated with severity

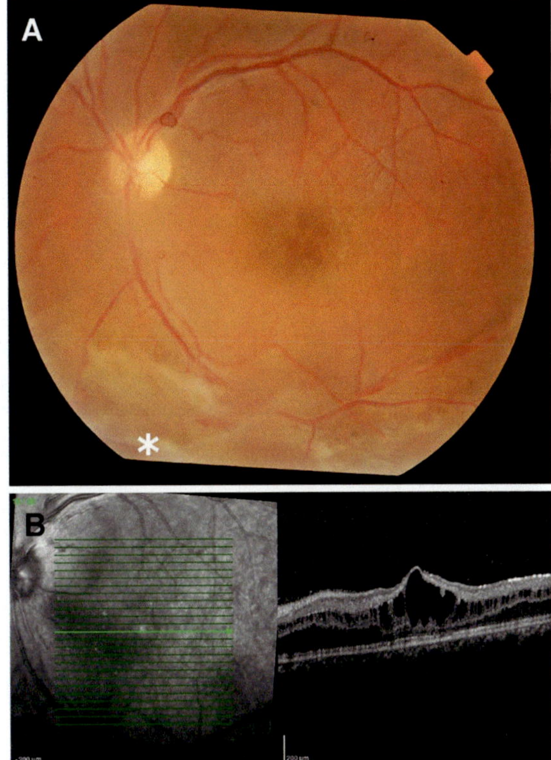

Fig. 36.8 A 16-year-old boy with type 3 (complex) congenital X-linked retinoschisis. **A** Fundus photography showing foveal schisis and peripheral schisis (white asteriks) vith vitreus veils. **B** Optical coherence tomography showing both foveal and macular lamellar schisis

of the disease. A study on phenotype-genotype correlation in CXLR reported that; nonsense, splice-site, or frame-shifting mutations in RS1 consistently caused electronegative bright-flash ERG, delayed flicker response, and abnormal pattern ERG; missense mutations result in a broader range of ERG abnormalities [72].

Genetics

Hemizygous pathogenic variant in RS1 gene identified by molecular genetic testing in a male patient with suggestive findings confirms the diagnosis of CXLR (Table 36.2). Depending on the phenotype, molecular genetic testing may include a combination of gene-targeted testing (single-gene testing and multigene panels) and complete genomic testing (exome sequencing, genome sequencing) [73]. Gene-targeted testing can be used if a clinical manifestation of CXLR typical, but comprehensive genomic testing should be performed if atypical findings are accompanied and if there is a doubt in the differential diagnosis. Single-gene testing

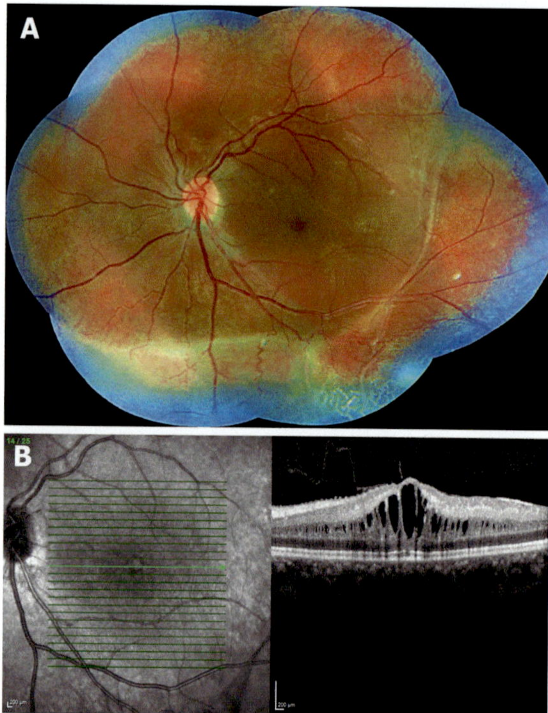

Fig. 36.9 A 19-year-old male with type 4 (foveo-peripheral) congenital X-linked retinoschisis. **A** Composed fundus photography showing peripheral retinoschisis at the inferior and temporal retina. Note the sclerotic vessels and white spiculations at the inferior-temporal quadrant. **B** Optical coherence tomography showing foveal schisis without lamellar component

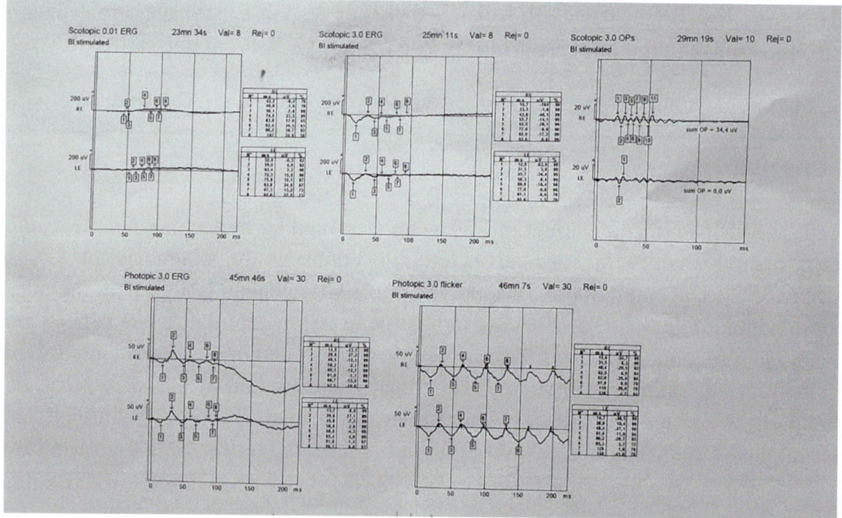

Fig. 36.10 An electroretinogram (ERG) of a 17-year-old boy with congenital X-linked retinoschisis. The patient's dark-adapted (scotopic 3.0) ERG has reduced b-wave amplitude with relatively preserved a-wave amplitude and altered b/a ratio, indicating an electronegative ERG

Table 36.2 Important RS1 mutations [74]

DNA Nucleotide change	Predicted Protein change	Single Nucleotide Polymorphism
c.286 T > C	p.TRP96ARG	rs61752063
c.304C > T	p.ARG102TRP	rs61752067
c.214G > A	p.GLU72LYS	rs104894928
c.216G > T	p.GLU72ASP	rs104894932
c.221G > T	p.GLY74VAL	rs104894933
c.325G > A	p.GLY109ARG	rs104894934
c.38 T > C	p.LEU13PRO	rs104894935
c.667 T > C	p.CYS223ARG	rs104894929
c.160_163dup	p.Thr55fs (4-BP INS)	rs281865342
c.608C > T	p.PRO203LEU	rs104894930
c.305G > A	p. ARG102GLN	rs61752068

includes sequence analysis of RS1 which aims detect small intragenic deletions/insertions and missense, nonsense, and splice site variants. If no variant is detected by the sequence analysis, gene-targeted deletion/duplication analysis should be performed to detect exon and whole-gene deletions or duplications.

Differential Diagnosis

Clinical diagnosis of CXLR may be challenging due to high variability of phenotype. The disease may present with exudative or non-exudative changes. Exudation and vascular changes may mimic Coats disease, FEVR, uveitis-related exudative retinal detachment, or retinoblastoma.

Goldmann–Favre Vitreoretinal Degeneration also known as the severe form of Enhanced S-Cone Syndrome is caused by autosomal recessive (AR) NR2E3 mutations. Intraretinal cystoid changes may occur with peripheral retinoschisis besides severe visual loss, peripheral pigmentary changes and night blindness. ERG shows significantly reduced a- and b-waves. Cystoid macular edema may also occur in patients with retinitis pigmentosa (RP), however, typical clinical findings of RP like optic nerve pallor, narrowing of retinal vessels, and "bone spicule" pigmentary clumping with a severely affected full-field ERG help in differential diagnosis. Diseases with electronegative ERG such as congenital stationary night-blindness is another entity to be considered in the differential.

CXLR and VCAN vitreoretinopathies can be confused due to vitreous abnormalities. Chronic retinal detachment may present with peripheral retinoschisis and cystoid macular edema and should be considered.

Management

The majority of patients have slowly progressive disease with stable visual acuity [52]. Wood et al. reported that most of the patients who do not present with complications requiring treatment remains stable without conversion between type or development of a complication requiring surgical intervention [52].

No treatment is recommended for foveal schisis. There is no correlation between the height of foveal schisis and visual acuity [75]. Foveal thickness and the volume of cysts may reduce with topical or oral carbonic anhydrase inhibitors [76–80]. Increase in visual acuity may be observed in some patients but there is no high-level evidence or prospective study on carbonic anhydrase inhibitors [75]. Cases in which cysts were observed to increase paradoxically after carbonic anhydrase inhibitor were also reported in the literature [81]. Abalem et al. reported that the central foveal thickness varies during daytime hours in patients with CXLR [82]. They indicated that this variation may explain the inconsistent and heterogeneous responses to treatment with carbonic anhydrase inhibitors and suggests standardization of measurement times in treatment trials for CXLR as well as in the routine ophthalmic evaluation of these patients. Our clinical observation is parallel to Abalem et al. that these foveal cysts may spontaneously become higher and lower during follow up.

Resolution of foveal schisis and decrease in foveal cysts after PPV have been reported before [83–86]. Induction of PVD seems to be useful to resolution of foveal cysts but the role ILM peeling is controversial [86]. ILM peeling was suggested beneficial for flattening of foveal schisis, but the risk of macular hole formation secondary to unroofing of the cyst should be kept in mind. Some authors reported recurrence of foveal schisis after silicone oil removal [87].

Surgical interventions such as argon laser photocoagulation (ALPC), pars plana vitrectomy (PPV) or scleral buckle (SB) may be used for the complications of CXLR. The incidence of sight-threatening complications is reported to be between 18–50% [47, 52]. The most common cause of surgery in patients with CXLR is RRD which has been reported in up to 20% of patients (Fig. 36.11). Occurrence of vitreous hemorrhage was reported in 40% of patients [5]. Other sight-threatening complications that needed surgery are retinoschisis involving macula, tractional RD, macular dragging, intraretinal hemorrhage spilled over the vitreous, and bullous retinoschisis. Surgery is often required before the age of 10 due to bullous retinoschisis and vitreous hemorrhage, and RDs secondary to inner and outer layer tears are seen at the second-third decades of life.

Prophylactic ALPC to the borders of peripheral retinoschisis should be considered in case of progressive retinoschisis but this treatment is controversial [36]. ALPC may induce RRD secondary to iatrogenic breaks or RRD/TRD due to vitreoretinal proliferation, especially in early post-operative period [88, 89]. Patients should be followed closely after ALPC to detect such complications. ALPC is not recommended for non-progressive retinoschisis.

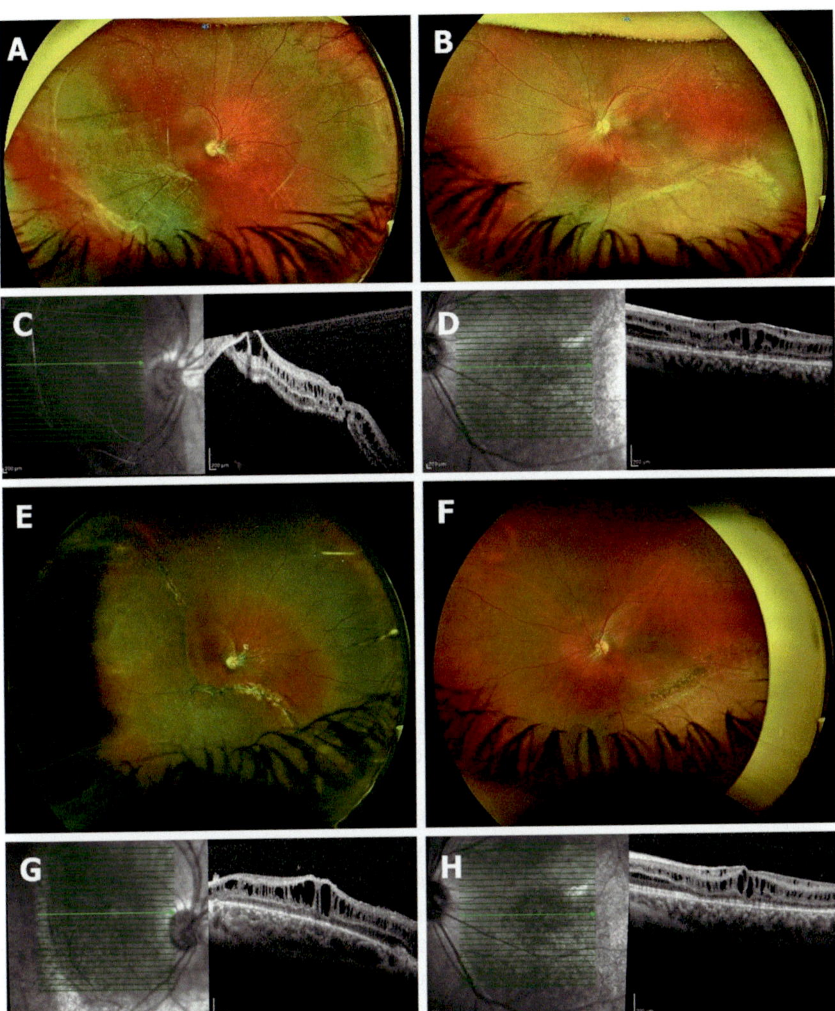

Fig. 36.11 A 10-year-old boy is referred to our center with retinal detachment in the right eye (RE). Visual acuity was 20/400 in RE and 20/100 in the left (LE). Macula off retinal detachment was seen in the inferotemporal quadrant in the RE (**A**). Peripheral retinoschisis is present in the lower temporal quadrant of LE (**B**). Optical coherence tomography images showed retinal detachment with retinoschisis in RE (**C**), and foveal schisis in LE (**D**). Pars plana vitrectomy, inner-layer retinectomy and endolaser surgery was performed with silicone oil exchange to RE. Prophylactic argon laser photocoagulation was applied to the borders of retinoschisis borders in LE. After the silicone removal, the retina was attached and the visual acuity increased to 20/100 in RE (**E, G**). LE remained stable during follow-up (**F, H**). **(see the video 1)**

Another option for progressive peripheral retinoschisis is vitreoretinal surgery. Removal of the posterior hyaloid membrane relieves tractional forces on retinoschisis and may help in preventing the progression of retinoschisis. The most important maneuver of the surgery is the posterior hyaloid detachment and removal of the inner leaflet. Incomplete removal of hyaloid may cause posterior hyaloidal contraction and retinal detachment. In cases where the highly elevated inner wall is left, it may contract and cause tractional RD. Inner layer retinectomy is crucial in preventing and treating this PVR (Fig. 36.12, see **video** 2).

The most common sight-threatening complication in patients with CXLR is RRD [5]. Tears or holes only in the inner layer of the retina do not cause RRD. Anteroposterior or tangential traction forces over the schitic retina may lead to development of outer retinal holes. Presence of both inner and outer retinal layer tears are necessary for the development of RRD in CXLR.

Localization of outer retinal break is very important to determine the type of vitreoretinal surgery in CXLR patients with RRD. Scleral buckling (SB) may be a good option in young, phakic patients if outer retinal break that cause RRD can be found and if there is no associated significant traction [38]. The success of the vitreoretinal surgery is relatively low, reported to range between 72 to 88% [34, 86, 90–93]. SB can be performed alone or combined with vitrectomy. The most common causes of surgical failure after SB are missed outer retinal breaks and PVR [94]. Vitreoretinal proliferation may cause hyaloidal traction and tractional retinal detachment, vitreous hemorrhage besides surgical failure [92, 94]. PPV should be added to SB in the presence of PVR, significant vitreous traction, vitreous hemorrhage, or if outer retinal break cannot be seen [93]. Removal of posterior hyaloid is very essential to decrease the rate of surgical failure and PVR. In cases with bullous peripheral retinoschisis and RRD, inner wall retinectomy must be done to prevent future contraction and traction on outer retinal layers and prevent PVR. Inner wall retinectomy does not have a negative effect on peripheral vision since these patients already have an absolute scotoma in peripheral retinoschisis areas. Adjuvant use of autologous plasmin is another technique to facilitate the induction of PVD [95]. After removal of the posterior hyaloid, localization of the outer retinal break(s) and internal drainage of the subretinal fluid, endolaser should be performed around the breaks, retinotomy holes, and to the border of schisis cavities or inner wall retinectomy. Silicone oil is the most preferred endotamponade for RRD in CXLR patients. Perfluoropropane and sulfur hexafluoride can also be used as endotamponade in selected cases.

Extramacular bullous retinoschisis cases may be followed up conservatively. Spontaneous regression of bullous schisis cavities were reported up to 85–100% of cases [31, 32]. Recent study conducted by Hinds et al. reported fewer spontaneous regression rates [33]. Other indication is bullous schisis involving the fovea which causes permanent visual deterioration [33]. The main question is to save or not to save the inner layer. Since the connection between the retinal layers has already been lost, there is no meaning of conserving the inner layer which may contract and cause complications like intraschitic hemorrhage, tractional and RRD. However, if one still wants to preserve it, intraschitic fluid drainage can be performed externally

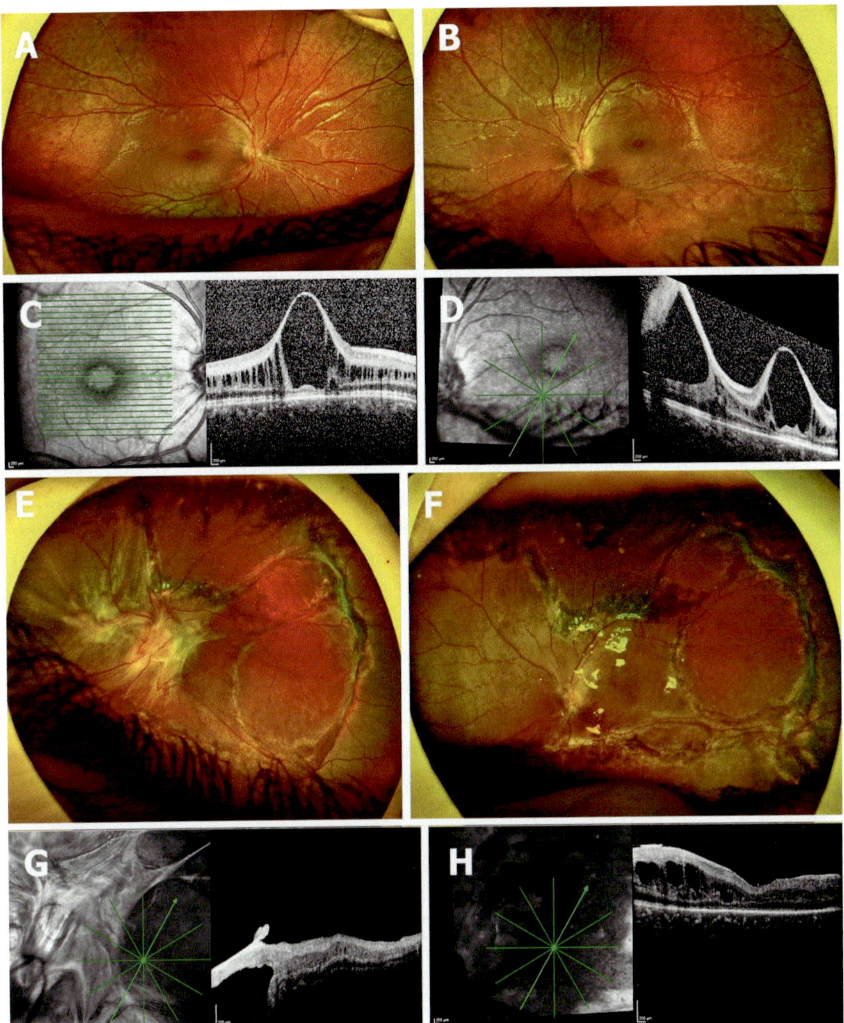

Fig. 36.12 An 8-year-old male patient with congenital X-linked retinoschisis (CXLR) type 3 (complex) in both eyes was followed in our clinic. Visual acuity was 20/70 in the right eye (RE) and 20/400 in the left eye (LE). The retinoschisis in the inferior half of RE stayed stable during follow up (**A**). However, retinoschisis in the inferior retina progressed to involve the macula in the left eye (**B**). Optical coherence tomography showed foveolamellar schisis in RE (**C**) and foveal schisis with inferonasal macular traction caused by the inner retinal leaflet of the peripheral retinoschisis in LE (**D**). Pars plana vitrectomy with perfluoropropane gas tamponade was performed to LE without any complication. However, proliferative vitreoretinopathy (PVR) was seen to develop following resorption of the gas (**E, G**). A second surgery with membrane peeling, inner-wall retinectomy and silicone oil tamponade was performed for PVR which resulted in attachment of the retina very nicely (**F, H**)

through a sclero-choroido-outer retinotomy without vitrectomy or through a small inner layer retinotomy with a 41-gauge cannula during vitrectomy. When an external drainage is preferred, cryotherapy to the drainage retinotomy and local external buckle should be added to the procedure. This procedure may be preferred especially for those severe cases where bullous inner retinal height reaches to the back of the lens (see the case presentation). By performing an external drainage, inner retina goes backwards which may allow a lens sparing vitreoretinal surgery if needed (**see the video** 2). However, the reattached inner retina may contract later to form PVR and traction during follow up which necessitates vitrectomy. Vitrectomy with an inner layer retinectomy may be effective during the first surgery both to prevent and treat such complication. In our experience, retinal detachment, vitreous hemorrhage or progression of retinoschisis may occur with vitreous contraction. We recommend lens sparing vitrectomy with inner layer retinectomy in selected cases (**see the case presentation and video 2**).

Vitreous hemorrhage is usually caused by rupture of strained retinal vessels in the schitic retina or rarely secondary to neovascularization in CXLR patients [3, 41, 96]. In some cases, strained retinal vessels lead to intraretinal (intraschisis) hemorrhage and this hemorrhage may spill over vitreous through an inner retinal break. After excluding RRD, vitreous hemorrhage can be observed for a month due to high rate of spontaneous resolution. Dense and non-resolving hemorrhages should be treated with vitrectomy. During vitrectomy, the cause of vitreous hemorrhage should be evaluated; if the cause is rupture of strained intraschitic vessels, induction of posterior hyaloid detachment and inner wall retinectomy will prevent recurrent vitreous hemorrhage. Endolaser should be performed to the presumed non-perfusion areas if sclerotic vessels and neovascularization are present (Fig. 36.13).

Case Presentation: (See Video 2)

A 5-month-old full term baby boy was referred to our clinic with the diagnosis of retinal detachment. Family history was negative for any ocular diseases. On initial examination, anterior segment examination revealed bilateral retinal vessels behind the lens (Fig. 36.14A). Bilateral bullous retinoschisis was noticed in fundus examination and he was diagnosed as CXLR (Fig. 36.14).

Vitreoretinal surgery was planned because of bullous retinoschisis and macular involvement in both eyes. Since the inner leaflet of the retina was behind the lens, an external drainage of the intraschitic fluid through a sclero-choroido-outer retinotomy, cryotherapy to the drainage site and local scleral buckle was performed to avoid lensectomy in both eyes (**see the video**). Retina was totally attached at the postoperative first month (Fig. 36.15).

At the postoperative first month of the left eye, retina was attached in both eyes although some signs of posterior hyaloidal contraction was seen in the LE (Fig. 36.15B). Follow-up without intervention was planned.

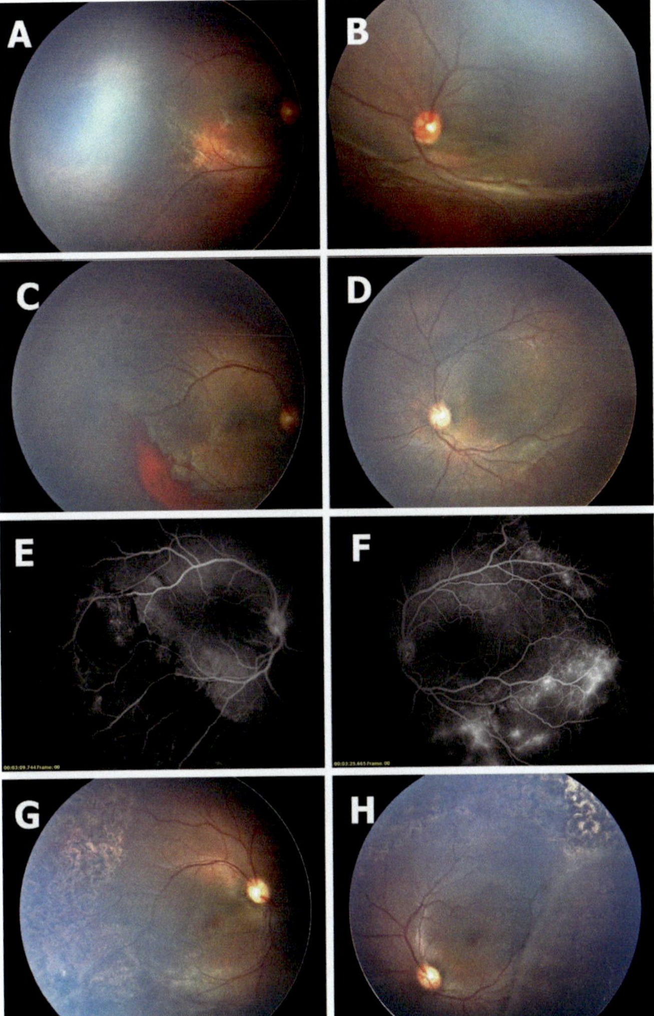

Fig. 36.13 A 6-month-old male patient was referred to our center with the diagnosis of retinal detachment after routine examination. On initial examination, the patient was found to have retinoschisis at the inferotemporal quadrants of the right eye (RE) (**A**) and the left eye (LE) (**B**). A clinical diagnosis of congenital X-linked retinoschisis was made and genetic testing was requested. In the examination under general anesthesia performed 2 months later, intraschitic hemorrhage infiltrating the vitreous was observed in the RE (**C**). Retinoschisis in the LE was found to regress partially (**D**). Fluorescein angiography showed temporal retinal ischemia with hyperfluorescent dots in RE (**E**), and diffuse leakage with peripheral retinal ischemia in LE (**F**). A bilateral argon laser photocoagulation treatment to the ischemic retina was performed in both eyes. Note that, RE is stable but there is progression of the retinoschisis inferotemporally in the LE during follow up (**G**, **H**)

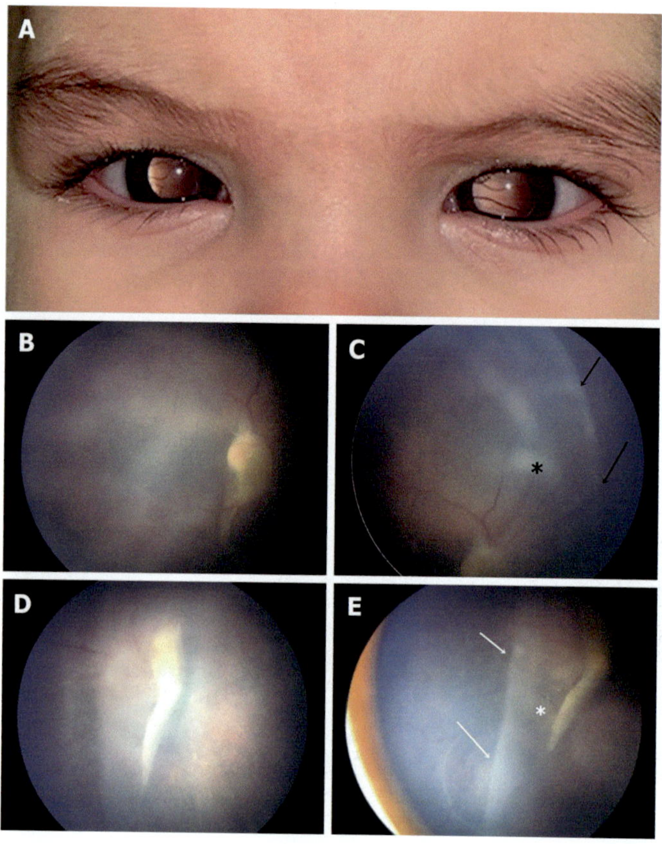

Fig. 36.14 Wide-field fundus images of a 5-month-old baby boy with bullous retinoschisis. **A** In the right eye, fundus examination revealed that, bullous retinoschisis involved the macula pushing it over the optic nerve to form a fold. **B** Borders (black arrow) of bullous retinoshisis (black asterisk) can be noticed with fundus examination in the right eye. **C, D** Similar appearance of bullous retinoshisis (white asteriks) was seen in the LE. White arrows indicate the borders of schisis

Five months later, retina stayed attached in the right eye but vitreous hemorrhage with inner layer contraction developed in the left eye (Fig. 36.16). Vitrectomy with inner-wall retinectomy, endolaser to the borders of retinoschisis with air tamponade was performed which resulted in the reattachment of the retina (**Video** 2, Fig. 36.17).

Similar inner retinal layer contraction was detected in the RE within a month and vitrectomy with inner-wall retinectomy was performed to the right eye similarly with success (**see the video** 2 and Fig. 36.17). Retina stayed attached with a small foveal fold in both eyes during follow-up with a good ambulatory vision (Fig. 36.18).

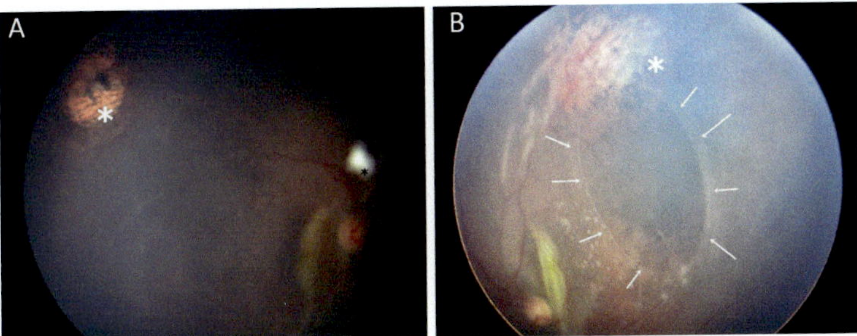

Fig. 36.15 Postoperative first month fundus pictures of both right (**A**) and left (**B**) eyes. A) Retina was attached leaving only a foveal fold in the right (**A**) and left eyes (**B**). Note the cryotherapy scarring (white asterisk in both eyes) at the drainage site and lens opacity (black asterisk) in the right eye. Some signs of posterior hyaloidal contraction in the left eye has started as indicated with white arrowheads

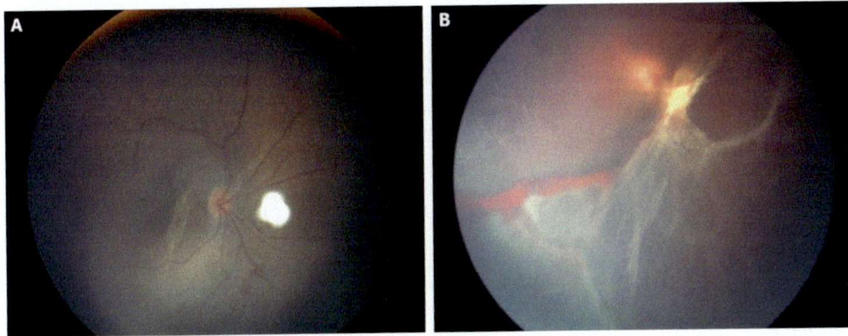

Fig. 36.16 Right postoperative 7th month, left postoperative 6th month wide-field fundus photography. **A** Retina is attached in the right eye. **B** Inner retinal layer contraction with vitreous hemorrhage was seen also in the left eye

Gene Therapy

Along with gene therapy for Leber congenital amaurosis (voretigene neparvovec-rzyl), whose phase III study was completed and approved by FDA, gene therapy studies for many inherited retinal diseases speeded up. CXLR is a monogenic disease and has become a suitable target for gene therapy.

Subretinal injection of an adeno-associated viral (AAV) serotype 5 vector containing the human RS1 gene under the control of the mouse opsin promoter (AAV5-mOPs-RS1) resulted in significant morpho-functional improvement in the retinoschisin knockout (Rs1-KO) mouse [97, 98]. Intravitreal administration of a self-complementary AAV delivering a human retinoschisin (RS1) gene under control of the RS1 promoter and an interphotoreceptor binding protein enhancer (AAV8-scRS/IRBPhRS) vector also showed morpho-functional improvement in the retinoschisin knockout (Rs1-KO) mouse [99]. After preclinical studies [99,

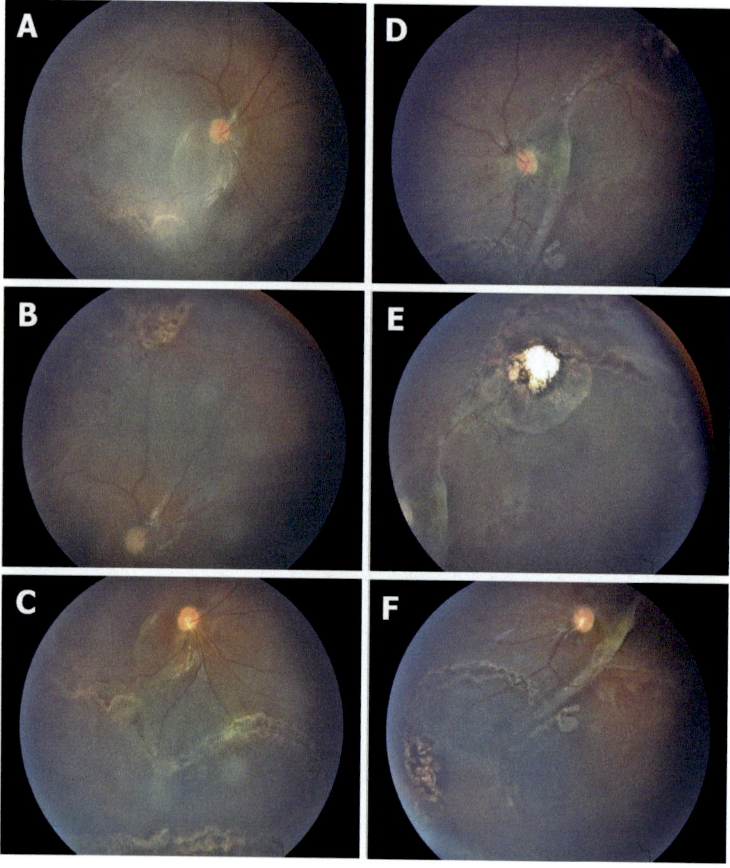

Fig. 36.17 Wide-field fundus images of the patient undertaken at final examination. **A–C** Retina was attached in the right eye with laser scars at the borders of inner-wall retinectomy. **D–F** Retina was attached in the left eye with laser scars at the borders of inner-wall retinectomy

100], FDA approved phase I/IIa dose-escalation trial of AAV8-*RS1* retinal gene transfer by intravitreal injection. In the phase I/IIa single-center, prospective, open-label, three-dose-escalation clinical trial, AAV8-RS1 vector was administered to nine participants with pathogenic *RS1* mutations and it was generally well tolerated in all but one individual [101]. A dose-dependent increase in ocular inflammation occurred in one participant which resolved with topical and systemic steroids. Cavity closure in one participant provided the first signal of possible efficacy. A second trial (NCT02416622) evaluating the safety and efficacy of intravitreally injected recombinant AAV vector, expressing retinoschisin (rAAV2tYF-CB-hRS1) in patients with X-linked retinoschisis continues [102].

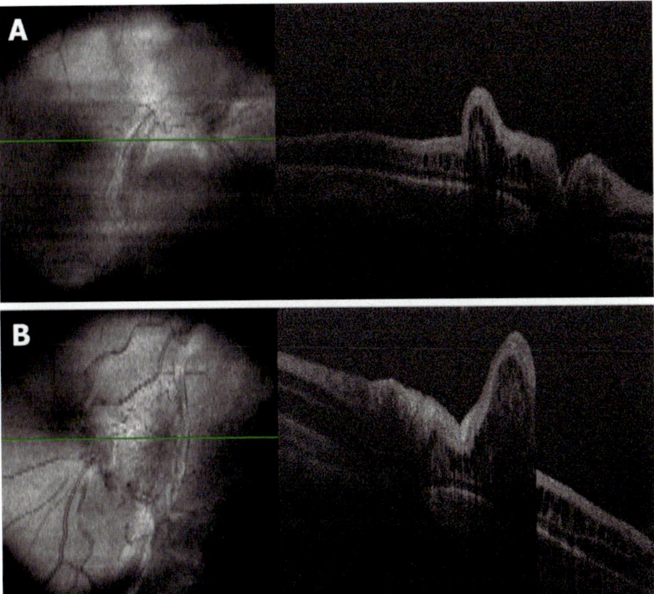

Fig. 36.18 Hand-held optical coherence tomography (OCT) images of the patient undertaken at final examination. Retina was atttached with foveal fold and foveolamellar retinvoschisis in both right (**A**) and left eye (**B**)

Conclusions

- CXLR is generally stable in long term, however, complications mostly occurring in the first two decades, may compromise vision.
- Clinical course of CXLR is highly variable with a wide range of RS1 gene variants, and there is no clear genotype–phenotype correlation.
- Vision-threatening complications are most common in Type 3 (Complex) CXLR.
- RRD is the most important complication causing loss of vision.
- In cases complicated by RRD, vitreous hemorrhage, TRD or bullous retinoschisis, vitreoretinal surgery is required to provide anatomical and functional restoration.
- Scleral buckle may be suitable for selected RRD cases, but most cases require a combined vitrectomy with posterior hyaloid removal, inner wall retinectomy and frequently silicone oil as endotamponade.
- Inner wall retinectomy, especially in cases with RRD and bullous retinoschisis is essential to prevent contraction of schitic inner retinal layer and PVR.
- Developing gene therapies are encouraging especially for uncomplicated CXLR patients.

Review Questions

1. Which of the following is not a complication of congenital X-linked retinoschisis?

a. Rhegmatogenous retinal detachment
b. Cystoid macular edema
c. Vitreous hemorrhage
d. Tractional retinal detachment
e. Retinal neovascularization

2. Which of the following is true regarding congenital X-linked retinoschisis?

a. The most common sight-threatening complication is vitreous hemorrhage.
b. Internal limiting membrane peeling is a recommended treatment for foveal retinoschisis.
c. Inner retinal breaks are the main cause for rhegmatogenous retinal detachment.
d. Performing an inner wall retinectomy may prevent retinal contraction and proliferative vitreoretinopathy even if posterior hyaloid is peeled off.
e. Vitreoretinal surgery should always be performed in bullous retinoschisis.

3. Which of the following is false regarding congenital X-linked retinoschisis?

a. Type 3 (Complex) is the most common type and found to be a risk factor for the development of rhegmatogenous retinal detachment.
b. Reduced b-wave amplitude with relatively preserved a-wave amplitude and altered b/a ratio (electronegative waveform) are the most significant findings.
c. Both optical coherence tomography and fluorescein angiography are required for classification of congenital X-linked retinoschisis.
d. Vitreous hemorrhage is usually caused by rupture of strained retinal vessels in the schitic retina or rarely secondary to neovascularization.
e. There is no clear genotype–phenotype correlation demonstrated in the literature.

Answers

1. B
2. D
3. C

References

1. Molday RS, Kellner U, Weber BH. X-linked juvenile retinoschisis: clinical diagnosis, genetic analysis, and molecular mechanisms. Prog Retin Eye Res. 2012;31(3):195–212.
2. Haas J. Ueber das zusammenvorkommen von Veranderungen der retina und choroidea. Arch Augenheilkd. 1898;37:343–8.
3. Rao P, Dedania VS, Drenser KA. Congenital X-linked retinoschisis: an updated clinical review. Asia-Pacific J Ophthalmol. 2018;7(3):169–75.

4. Jager G. A hereditary retinal disease. Trans Ophthalmol Soc UK. 1953;73:617–9.
5. George N, Yates J, Moore A. X linked retinoschisis. Br J Ophthalmol. 1995;79(7):697.
6. Kim LS, Seiple W, Fishman GA, Szlyk JP. Multifocal ERG findings in carriers of X-linked retinoschisis. Documenta Ophthalmologica Adv Ophthalmol. 2007;114(1):21–6.
7. Booth AP, Trump D, George ND. A manifesting female heterozygote in x-linked retinoschisis: clinical and genetic study. Invest Ophthalmol Vis Sci. 2003;44(13):1484.
8. Deutman AF, Pinckers AJ, Aan de Kerk AL. Dominantly inherited cystoid macular edema. Amer J Ophthalmol. 1976;82(4):540–8.
9. Sikkink SK, Biswas S, Parry NR, Stanga PE, Trump D. X-linked retinoschisis: an update. J Med Genet. 2007;44(4):225–32.
10. Meier P, Wiedemann P. Surgery for pediatric vitreoretinal disorders. In: Schachat AP, editor. Ryan's retina. Sixth edition. ed. Edinburgh ; New York: Elsevier; 2018. p. 2170–93.
11. Sauer CG, Gehrig A, Warneke-Wittstock R, Marquardt A, Ewing CC, Gibson A, et al. Positional cloning of the gene associated with X-linked juvenile retinoschisis. Nat Genet. 1997;17(2):164–70.
12. Functional implications of the spectrum of mutations found in 234 cases with X-linked juvenile retinoschisis. The Retinoschisis Consortium. Human molecular genetics. 1998;7 (7):1185–92.
13. Wang T, Zhou A, Waters CT, O'Connor E, Read RJ, Trump D. Molecular pathology of X linked retinoschisis: mutations interfere with retinoschisin secretion and oligomerisation. Br J Ophthalmol. 2006;90(1):81–6.
14. Wu WW, Wong JP, Kast J, Molday RS. RS1, a discoidin domain-containing retinal cell adhesion protein associated with X-linked retinoschisis, exists as a novel disulfide-linked octamer. J Biol Chem. 2005;280(11):10721–30.
15. Wu WW, Molday RS. Defective discoidin domain structure, subunit assembly, and endoplasmic reticulum processing of retinoschisin are primary mechanisms responsible for X-linked retinoschisis. J Biol Chem. 2003;278(30):28139–46.
16. Grayson C, Reid SN, Ellis JA, Rutherford A, Sowden JC, Yates JR, et al. Retinoschisin, the X-linked retinoschisis protein, is a secreted photoreceptor protein, and is expressed and released by Weri-Rb1 cells. Hum Mol Genet. 2000;9(12):1873–9.
17. Rahman N, Georgiou M, Khan KN, Michaelides M. Macular dystrophies: clinical and imaging features, molecular genetics and therapeutic options. Br J Ophthalmol. 2020;104 (4):451–60.
18. Chen J, Xu K, Zhang X, Pan Z, Dong B, Li Y. Novel mutations of the RS1 gene in a cohort of Chinese families with X-linked retinoschisis. Mol Vis. 2014;20:132–9.
19. Eksandh LC, Ponjavic V, Ayyagari R, Bingham EL, Hiriyanna KT, Andréasson S, et al. Phenotypic expression of juvenile X-linked retinoschisis in Swedish families with different mutations in the XLRS1 gene. Archives of ophthalmology (Chicago, Ill : 1960). 2000;118 (8):1098–104.
20. Shinoda K, Ishida S, Oguchi Y, Mashima Y. Clinical characteristics of 14 japanese patients with X-linked juvenile retinoschisis associated with XLRS1 mutation. Ophthalmic Genet. 2000;21(3):171–80.
21. Simonelli F, Cennamo G, Ziviello C, Testa F, de Crecchio G, Nesti A, et al. Clinical features of X linked juvenile retinoschisis associated with new mutations in the XLRS1 gene in Italian families. Br J Ophthalmol. 2003;87(9):1130–4.
22. Pimenides D, George ND, Yates JR, Bradshaw K, Roberts SA, Moore AT, et al. X-linked retinoschisis: clinical phenotype and RS1 genotype in 86 UK patients. J Med Genet. 2005;42 (6): e35.
23. Joshi MM, Drenser K, Hartzer M, Dailey W, Antonio Capone J, Trese MT. Intraschisis cavity fluid composition in congenital X-linked retinoschisis. Retina. 2006;26(7):S57–S60.
24. Tantri A, Vrabec TR, Cu-Unjieng A, Frost A, Annesley WH Jr, Donoso LA. X-linked retinoschisis: a clinical and molecular genetic review. Surv Ophthalmol. 2004;49(2):214–30.

25. Doğuizi S, Şekeroğlu MA, Çolak S, Anayol MA, Yılmazbaş P. Assessment of spectral-domain optical coherence tomography findings in three cases of X-linked Juvenile Retinoschisis in the same family. Turkish J Ophthalmol. 2017;47(5):302–5.

26. George NDL, Yates JRW, Moore AT. Clinical features in Affected males With X-linked Retinoschisis. Arch Ophthalmol. 1996;114(3):274–80.

27. Kousal B, Hlavata L, Vlaskova H, Dvorakova L, Brichova M, Dubska Z, et al. Clinical and genetic study of X-linked Juvenile Retinoschisis in the Czech population. Genes. 2021;12 (11).

28. Eksandh LC, Ponjavic V, Ayyagari R, Bingham EL, Hiriyanna KT, Andréasson S, et al. Phenotypic expression of juvenile x-linked Retinoschisis in Swedish families with different mutations in the XLRS1 gene. Arch Ophthalmol. 2000;118(8):1098–104.

29. Fahim AT, Ali N, Blachley T, Michaelides M. Peripheral fundus findings in X-linked retinoschisis. Br J Ophthalmol. 2017;101(11):1555–9.

30. Juvenile X-Linked Retinoschisis. In: Levin AV, Zanolli M, Capasso JE, editors. Wills Eye Handbook of Ocular Genetics. New York: Thieme Medical Publishers; 2018. p. 241–7.

31. George ND, Yates JR, Bradshaw K, Moore AT. Infantile presentation of X linked retinoschisis. Br J Ophthalmol. 1995;79(7):653–7.

32. Mosin IM, Moshetova LK, Mishustin VV, Letneva IA. Bullous form of X-linked congenital retinoschisis in infants. Vestn oftalmol. 2001;117(1):40–3.

33. Hinds A-M, Fahim A, Moore AT, Wong SC, Michaelides M. Bullous X linked retinoschisis: clinical features and prognosis. Br J Ophthalmol. 2018;102(5):622–4.

34. Savoie BT, Ferrone PJ. Complicated congenital retinoschisis. Retinal Cases Brief Reports. 2017;11(Suppl 1):S202–10.

35. Ando A, Takahashi K, Sho K, Matsushima M, Okamura A, Uyama M. Histopathological findings of X-linked retinoschisis with neovascular glaucoma. Graefe's archive for clinical and experimental ophthalmology = Albrecht von Graefes Archiv fur klinische und experimentelle Ophthalmologie. 2000;238(1):1–7.

36. Brockhurst RJ. Photocoagulation in congenital retinoschisis. Arch Ophthalmol. 1970;84 (2):158–65.

37. Ewing C. Juvenile hereditary retinoschisis. Trans Ophthalmol Soc UK. 1970;89:29–39.

38. Kellner U, Brümmer S, Foerster MH, Wessing A. X-linked congenital retinoschisis. Graefes Arch Clin Exp Ophthalmol. 1990;228(5):432–7.

39. Kim SY, Ko HS, Yu YS, Hwang JM, Lee JJ, Kim SY, et al. Molecular genetic characteristics of X-linked retinoschisis in Koreans. Mol Vis. 2009;15:833–43.

40. Murro V, Caputo R, Bacci GM, Sodi A, Mucciolo DP, Bargiacchi S, et al. Case report of an atypical early onset X-linked retinoschisis in monozygotic twins. BMC Ophthalmol. 2017;17(1):19.

41. Ibad S, Wilkins CS, Pinhas A, Sun V, Wieder MS, Deobhakta A. Acute vitreous and intraretinal hemorrhage with multifocal subretinal fluid in Juvenile X-Linked Retinoschisis. Case Reports Ophthalmol Med. 2020;2020:6638553.

42. Conway BP, Welch RB. X-chromosone-linked juvenile retinoschisis with hemorrhagic retinal cyst. Am J Ophthalmol. 1977;83(6):853–5.

43. Fan KC, McAllister MA, Yannuzzi NA, Patel NA, Prakhunhungsit S, Negron CI, et al. X-linked Retinoschisis and a coats-like response in the setting of retinopathy of prematurity. J Vitreoretinal Diseases. 2020;4(6):525–9.

44. Hahn LC, van Schooneveld MJ, Wesseling NL, Florijn RJ, ten Brink JB, Lissenberg-Witte BI, et al. X-linked Retinoschisis: novel clinical observations and genetic spectrum in 340 patients. Ophthalmology. 2022;129(2):191–202.

45. Keunen JE, Hoppenbrouwers RW. A case of sex-linked juvenile retinoschisis with peripheral vascular anomalies. Ophthalmologica Journal international d'ophtalmologie International journal of ophthalmology Zeitschrift fur Augenheilkunde. 1985;191(3):146–9.

46. Shukla D, Rajendran A, Gibbs D, Suganthalakshmi B, Zhang K, Sundaresan P. Unusual manifestations of x-linked retinoschisis: clinical profile and diagnostic evaluation. Am J Ophthalmol. 2007;144(3):419–23.

47. Georgiou M, Finocchio L, Fujinami K, Fujinami-Yokokawa Y, Virgili G, Mahroo OA, et al. X-linked Retinoschisis: deep Phenotyping and genetic characterization. Ophthalmology. 2021.

48. Xu F, Sui R, Dong F. Thirty-two years follow-up of X-linked juvenile retinoschisis in a Chinese patient with RS1 mutation. Ophthalmic Genet. 2012;33(2):77–82.

49. Ip M, Garza-Karren C, Duker JS, Reichel E, Swartz JC, Amirikia A, et al. Differentiation of degenerative retinoschisis from retinal detachment using optical coherence tomography. Ophthalmology. 1999;106(3):600–5.

50. Gao FJ, Dong JH, Wang DD, Chen F, Hu FY, Chang Q, et al. Comprehensive analysis of genetic and clinical characteristics of 30 patients with X-linked juvenile retinoschisis in China. Acta Ophthalmol. 2021;99(4):e470–9.

51. Prenner JL, Capone A Jr, Ciaccia S, Takada Y, Sieving PA, Trese MT. Congenital X-linked retinoschisis classification system. Retina. 2006;26(7 Suppl):S61–4.

52. Wood EH, Lertjirachai I, Ghiam BK, Koulisis N, Moysidis SN, Dirani A, et al. The natural history of congenital X-Linked Retinoschisis and conversion between phenotypes over time. Ophthalmology Retina. 2019;3(1):77–82.

53. Ling KP, Mangalesh S, Tran-Viet D, Gunther R, Toth CA, Vajzovic L. Handheld spectral domain optical coherence tomography findings of x-linked retinoschisis in early childhood. Retina. 2020;40(10):1996–2003.

54. Yu J, Ni Y, Keane PA, Jiang C, Wang W, Xu G. Foveomacular schisis in juvenile X-linked retinoschisis: an optical coherence tomography study. Am J Ophthalmol. 2010;149(6):973-8.e2.

55. Han IC, Whitmore SS, Critser DB, Lee SY, DeLuca AP, Daggett HT, et al. Wide-field swept-source OCT and Angiography in X-linked Retinoschisis. Ophthalmology Retina. 2019;3(2):178–85.

56. Yang HS, Lee JB, Yoon YH, Lee JY. Correlation between spectral-domain OCT findings and visual acuity in X-linked retinoschisis. Invest Ophthalmol Vis Sci. 2014;55(5):3029–36.

57. Hu QR, Huang LZ, Chen XL, Xia HK, Li TQ, Li XX. X-Linked Retinoschisis in Juveniles: follow-up by optical coherence tomography. Biomed Res Int. 2017;2017:1704623.

58. Padrón-Pérez N, Català-Mora J, Díaz J, Arias L, Prat J, Caminal JM. Swept-source and optical coherence tomography angiography in patients with X-linked retinoschisis. Eye (Lond). 2018;32(4):707–15.

59. Andreoli MT, Lim JI. Optical coherence tomography retinal thickness and volume measurements in X-linked retinoschisis. Am J Ophthalmol. 2014;158(3):567-73.e2.

60. Tsang SH, Vaclavik V, Bird AC, Robson AG, Holder GE. Novel phenotypic and genotypic findings in X-linked retinoschisis. Archives of ophthalmology (Chicago, Ill: 1960). 2007;125(2):259–67.

61. Souied EH, Goritsa A, Querques G, Coscas G, Soubrane G. Indocyanine green angiography of juvenile X-linked retinoschisis. Am J Ophthalmol. 2005;140(3):558–61.

62. Rao P, Robinson J, Yonekawa Y, Thomas BJ, Drenser KA, Trese MT, et al. Wide-field imaging of nonexudative and exudative congenital x-linked retinoschisis. Retina. 2016;36(6):1093–100.

63. Green JL, Jampol LM. Vascular opacification and leakage in X-linked (juvenile) retinoschisis. Br J Ophthalmol. 1979;63(5):368–73.

64. Fong DS, Frederick AR, Blumenkranz MS, Walton DS. Exudative retinal detachment in X-linked retinoschisis. SLACK Incorporated Thorofare, NJ; 1998. p. 332–5.

65. Strupaitė R, Ambrozaitytė L, Cimbalistienė L, Ašoklis R, Utkus A. X-linked juvenile retinoschisis: phenotypic and genetic characterization. Int J Ophthalmol. 2018;11(11):1875–8.

66. Neriyanuri S, Dhandayuthapani S, Arunachalam JP, Raman R. Phenotypic characterization of X-linked retinoschisis: Clinical, electroretinography, and optical coherence tomography variables. Indian J Ophthalmol. 2016;64(7):513–7.

67. Ambrosio L, Hansen RM, Kimia R, Fulton AB. Retinal Function in X-Linked Juvenile Retinoschisis. Invest Ophthalmol Vis Sci. 2019;60(14):4872–81.

68. Khan NW, Jamison JA, Kemp JA, Sieving PA. Analysis of photoreceptor function and inner retinal activity in juvenile X-linked retinoschisis. Vision Res. 2001;41(28):3931–42.

69. Bowles K, Cukras C, Turriff A, Sergeev Y, Vitale S, Bush RA, et al. X-Linked Retinoschisis: RS1 mutation severity and age affect the ERG Phenotype in a Cohort of 68 affected male subjects. Invest Ophthalmol Vis Sci. 2011;52(12):9250–6.

70. Peachey NS, Fishman GA, Derlacki DJ, Brigell MG. Psychophysical and electroretinographic findings in X-linked juvenile retinoschisis. Archives of ophthalmology (Chicago, Ill: 1960). 1987;105(4):513–6.

71. McAnany JJ, Park JC, Fishman GA, Collison FT. Full-field electroretinography, Pupillometry, and luminance thresholds in X-linked Retinoschisis. Invest Ophthalmol Vis Sci. 2020;61(6):53.

72. Vincent A, Robson AG, Neveu MM, Wright GA, Moore AT, Webster AR, et al. A phenotype-genotype correlation study of X-linked retinoschisis. Ophthalmology. 2013;120(7):1454–64.

73. PA S, IM M, SH. Congenital Retinoschisis. In: MP A, HH A, RA P, editors. GeneReviews® [Internet]. Seattle (WA): University of Washington, Seattle2003.

74. Stickler GB, Belau PG, Farrell FJ, Jones JD, Pugh DG, Steinberg AG, et al. Hereditary progressive arthro-ophthalmopathy Mayo Clinic Proc. 1965;40:433–55.

75. Pennesi ME, Birch DG, Jayasundera KT, Parker M, Tan O, Gurses-Ozden R, et al. Prospective evaluation of Patients With X-linked Retinoschisis during 18 months. Invest Ophthalmol Vis Sci. 2018;59(15):5941–56.

76. Genead MA, Fishman GA, Walia S. Efficacy of sustained topical dorzolamide therapy for cystic macular lesions in patients with X-linked Retinoschisis. Arch Ophthalmol. 2010;128(2):190–7.

77. Coussa RG, Kapusta MA. Treatment of cystic cavities in X-linked juvenile retinoschisis: The first sequential cross-over treatment regimen with dorzolamide. Amer J Ophthalmol Case Reports. 2017;8:1–3.

78. Thangavel R, Surve A, Azad S, Kumar V. Dramatic response to topical dorzolamide in X-linked retinoschisis. Indian J Ophthalmol. 2020;68(7):1466–7.

79. Andreuzzi P, Fishman GA, Anderson RJ. Use of a carbonic anhydrase inhibitor in x-linked retinoschisis: effect on cystic-appearing macular lesions and visual acuity. Retina. 2017;37(8):1555–61.

80. Apushkin MA, Fishman GA. Use of dorzolamide for patients with X-linked retinoschisis. Retina. 2006;26(7):741–5.

81. Menke B, Walters A, Payne JF. Paradoxical anatomic response to topical carbonic anhydrase inhibitor in X-linked Retinoschisis. Ophthalmic Surg Lasers Imaging Retina. 2018;49(2):142–4.

82. Abalem MF, Musch DC, Birch DG, Pennesi ME, Heckenlively JR, Jayasundera T. Diurnal variations of foveoschisis by optical coherence tomography in patients with RS1 X-linked juvenile retinoschisis. Ophthalmic Genet. 2018;39(4):437–42.

83. Gupta MP, Parlitsis G, Tsang S, Chan RV. Resolution of foveal schisis in X-linked retinoschisis in the setting of retinal detachment. J AAPOS: Official Publication Amer Assoc Pediatric Ophthalmol Strabismus. 2015;19(2):172–4.

84. Iordanous Y, Sheidow TG. Vitrectomy for X-linked retinoschisis: a case report and literature review. Can J Ophthalmol. 2013;48(4):e71–4.

85. Ikeda F, Iida T, Kishi S. Resolution of retinoschisis after vitreous surgery in X-linked retinoschisis. Ophthalmology. 2008;115(4):718–22. e1.

86. Yu H, Li T, Luo Y, Yu S, Li S, Lei L, et al. Long-term outcomes of vitrectomy for progressive X-linked retinoschisis. Amer J Ophthalmol. 2012;154(2):394–402. e2.

87. Goel N, Ghosh B. Temporary resolution of foveal schisis following vitrectomy with silicon oil tamponade in X-linked retinoschisis with retinal detachment. Indian J Ophthalmol. 2015;63(11):867–8.

88. Turut P, François P, Castier P, Milazzo S. Analysis of results in the treatment of peripheral retinoschisis in sex-linked congenital retinoschisis. Graefes Arch Clin Exp Ophthalmol. 1989;227(4):328–31.

89. Sobrin L, Berrocal AM, Murray TG. Retinal detachment 7 years after prophylactic schisis cavity excision in juvenile X-linked retinoschisis. Slack Incorporated Thorofare, NJ; 2003. p. 401–2.

90. Rosenfeld PJ, Flynn HW Jr, McDonald HR, Rubsamen PE, Smiddy WE, Sipperley JO, et al. Outcomes of vitreoretinal surgery in patients with X-linked retinoschisis. Ophthalmic Surg Lasers. 1998;29(3):190–7.

91. Ferrone PJ, Trese MT, Lewis H. Vitreoretinal surgery for complications of congenital retinoschisis. Am J Ophthalmol. 1997;123(6):742–7.

92. Sen P, Agarwal A, Bhende P, Gopal L, Bhende M, Rishi P, et al. Outcome of vitreoretinal surgery for rhegmatogenous retinal detachment in X-linked juvenile retinoschisis. Indian J Ophthalmol. 2018;66(12):1825–31.

93. Schulman J, Peyman GA, Jednock N, Larson B. Indications for vitrectomy in congenital retinoschisis. Br J Ophthalmol. 1985;69(7):482–6.

94. Regillo CD, Tasman WS, Brown GC. Surgical management of complications associated with X-linked retinoschisis. Archives of ophthalmology (Chicago, Ill : 1960). 1993;111 (8):1080–6.

95. Wu WC, Drenser KA, Capone A, Williams GA, Trese MT. Plasmin enzyme-assisted vitreoretinal surgery in congenital X-linked retinoschisis: surgical techniques based on a new classification system. Retina. 2007;27(8):1079–85.

96. Lee JJ, Kim JH, Kim SY, Park SS, Yu YS. Infantile vitreous hemorrhage as the initial presentation of X-linked juvenile retinoschisis. Korean J Ophthalmol KJO. 2009;23(2): 118–20.

97. Janssen A, Min SH, Molday LL, Tanimoto N, Seeliger MW, Hauswirth WW, et al. Effect of late-stage therapy on disease progression in AAV-mediated rescue of photoreceptor cells in the retinoschisin-deficient mouse. Molec Therapy J Amer Soc Gene Therapy. 2008;16 (6):1010–7.

98. Min SH, Molday LL, Seeliger MW, Dinculescu A, Timmers AM, Janssen A, et al. Prolonged recovery of retinal structure/function after gene therapy in an Rs1h-deficient mouse model of x-linked juvenile retinoschisis. Molec Therapy J Amer Soc Gene Therapy. 2005;12(4):644–51.

99. Bush RA, Zeng Y, Colosi P, Kjellstrom S, Hiriyanna S, Vijayasarathy C, et al. Preclinical dose-escalation study of intravitreal AAV-RS1 gene therapy in a mouse model of x-linked retinoschisis: dose-dependent expression and improved retinal structure and function. Hum Gene Ther. 2016;27(5):376–89.

100. Marangoni D, Bush RA, Zeng Y, Wei LL, Ziccardi L, Vijayasarathy C, et al. Ocular and systemic safety of a recombinant AAV8 vector for X-linked retinoschisis gene therapy: GLP studies in rabbits and Rs1-KO mice. Molec Therapy Methods Clin Dev. 2016;5:16011.

101. Cukras C, Wiley HE, Jeffrey BG, Sen HN, Turriff A, Zeng Y, et al. Retinal AAV8-RS1 Gene Therapy for X-Linked Retinoschisis: initial findings from a phase I/IIa trial by intravitreal delivery. Molec Therapy J Amer Soc Gene Therapy. 2018;26(9):2282–94.

102. Safety and Efficacy of rAAV-hRS1 in Patients With X-linked Retinoschisis (XLRS). ClinicalTrials.gov Identifier: NCT02416622. Available from: https://clinicaltrials.gov/ct2/show/NCT02416622. Accessed 23 Jan 2022.

Congenital Glaucoma Related Retinal Detachment

37

Supalert Prakhunhungsit and Audina M. Berrocal

Abstract

Congenital glaucoma is a rare inherited condition in which the increased intraocular pressure is detected shortly after birth. The retinal detachment related to this condition is rare but it can lead to a poor visual outcome if left untreated. The awareness of this condition by the treating physicians leads to the early detection and treatment. Therefore, the patients can maintain their useful visions afterwards. This chapter will discuss in details of congenital glaucoma related retinal detachment and the applications for ophthalmologists.

Keywords

Congenital glaucoma · Primary congenital glaucoma · Secondary glaucoma · Retinal detachment · Trabeculectomy · Surgical technique · Vitrectomy · Silicone oil

Supplementary Information The online version contains supplementary material available at https://doi.org/10.1007/978-3-031-14506-3_37.

S. Prakhunhungsit (✉)
Faculty of Medicine Siriraj Hospital, Department of Ophthalmology, Mahidol University, Bangkok, Thailand
e-mail: supalert.pra@gmail.com

A. M. Berrocal
Medical Director of Pediatric Retina and Retinopathy of Prematurity, Vitreoretinal Fellowship Director Retina Department, Bascom Palmer Eye Institute, Miami, FL, USA

Ş. Özdek et al. (eds.), *Pediatric Vitreoretinal Surgery*,
https://doi.org/10.1007/978-3-031-14506-3_37

Introduction

Congenital glaucoma is defined as the presence of glaucoma at birth; however, the term developmental glaucoma is also sometimes interchangeably used to describe this condition. Previous study alternatively defined congenital glaucoma as glaucoma that presents within 3 years after birth [1]. Primary congenital glaucoma is defined as idiopathic glaucoma with no intraocular abnormalities except for trabecular meshwork malformation. Secondary congenital glaucoma is glaucoma that is associated with other ocular disorders, such as aniridia, Sturge-Weber syndrome, and Axenfeld-Rieger syndrome [1]. Congenital glaucoma is a major cause of blindness in pediatric population with an incidence 1:10,000 births. Sixty-five percent of those with congenital glaucoma are male, and 75% have bilateral disease [2].

Retinal detachment in congenital glaucoma was first reported by Axenfeld [3]. Retinal detachment is a rare complication in patients with congenital glaucoma with a reported incidence ranging from 3 to 12% among all retinal detachment cases [2, 4–6]. During the first 2 decades of life, retinal detachment in congenital glaucoma was found in approximately 0.15% of all retinal detachments [7]. The prevalence of retinal detachment in primary congenital glaucoma patients was reported to range from 4.0% to 6.3% [1, 7]. In some reviews of pediatric rhegmatogenous retinal detachment, the disorder associated with congenital glaucoma or buphthalmos included only a small number of children in each study [4, 8, 9]. Therefore, data specific to congenital glaucoma related retinal detachment remains relatively scarce.

Pathophysiology

Congenital glaucoma is usually associated with myopia [7]. In a case series of primary congenital glaucoma, all eyes in the study were highly myopic with an average of refractive errors of approximately −8.00 diopters [5, 10]. In general pediatric population, myopia, untreated peripheral retinal degeneration, and ocular trauma have been recognized as the factors that predispose a patient to retinal detachment [1]. Although myopia is usually related to longer axial length that can lead to myopic change of the fundus, including retinal thinning and degeneration, the cause of myopia in congenital glaucoma is mainly due to corneal curvature change and posterior location of the lens [7]. A more recent study investigated the effect of axial length on the development of retinal detachment in primary congenital glaucoma, and they found patients with an axial length longer than 26 mm to be at 24.4 times higher risk of having pathologic peripheral retinal degeneration when compared to those with an axial length less than 26 mm [1]. These patients generally tend to have an axial length longer than that found in normal population. This is supported by the findings of a case series that reported axial lengths ranging from 25–33 mm in congenital glaucoma patients [10]. Fifteen percent of primary congenital glaucoma patients had peripheral retinal degeneration, which is defined as lattice degeneration with or without holes, and isolated holes or tears [1]. The increased axial length of these buphthalmic eyes with high myopia and peripheral retinal degeneration may be one of the causes of retinal detachment [1, 10].

Posterior vitreous detachment caused by vitreous syneresis following myopic progression and prior intraocular surgeries are important causes of retinal tear, which can lead to the development of retinal detachment in buphthalmic eyes [5, 11]. Therefore, eyes with a history of previous intraocular surgeries, such as cataract surgery or glaucoma-related surgeries, are thought to be at risk for the development of retinal detachment [11]. The risk of prior glaucoma surgeries was evaluated in a series of 350 patients with complicated glaucoma who underwent Molteno shunt implantations. Those authors found 5% risk of rhegmatogenous retinal detachment post-surgery, and in 70% of the cases, the condition was detected within the first 4 months after surgery. Another study found some retinal detachment cases after glaucoma drainage device implantation, but no retinal detachment cases in the trabeculectomy group among a cohort of 212 glaucoma surgeries with a 5-year follow-up [12]. However, that study included only non-buphthalmic eyes, which means that the risk of prior glaucoma surgeries leading to retinal detachment could be higher in vulnerable subjects, such as those with buphthalmic eyes [11].

Clinical Characteristics

Although retinal detachment in this setting is associated with a congenital disorder, a large number of congenital glaucoma related retinal detachment patients are not in their childhood. The median age of patients with retinal detachment was reported to range from 38 to 43 years [5, 10]. The diagnosis of retinal detachment was made from 6 to 16.7 years after glaucoma diagnosis (mean: 8.1 years) [13], and affected patients were mostly males (72–84%) [2, 7]. Almost 50% of cases had a prior history of retinal detachment [13].

Due to the natural course of congenital glaucoma, most patients do not have good preexisting vision and/or visual field. The deterioration of vision or visual field caused by retinal detachment is frequently detected late [5, 13]. Furthermore, poor posterior segment visualization and lack of comprehensive examination data in these patients due to congenital glaucoma sequelae, such as photophobia, nystagmus, corneal opacity, and/or cataract, often results in delayed diagnosis of retinal detachment. Persistent ocular hypotony with or without choroidal detachment and/or a sudden decrease in vision heightens suspicion of retinal detachment in congenital glaucoma patients [11, 13]. Al-Harthi, et al. reported that 92% of cases presented with ocular hypotony [13]. Another case series reported that all 5 patients with sudden loss of vision [10]. Therefore, a complete ocular examination or further investigations are indicated when these symptoms and signs present. Other signs that can be associated with retinal detachment in congenital glaucoma include vitreous hemorrhage, secondary lens subluxation, and abnormal red reflex noted during distant direct ophthalmoscopy, especially when patients had a history of multiple previous intraocular surgeries [1, 5, 7].

Although retinal detachment following filtering surgery or previous intraocular surgery is uncommon in general population [8, 12], nearly all congenital glaucoma related retinal detachment patients had a history of previous intraocular surgeries [1, 5, 7], especially in cases with perioperative complications, such as vitreous loss, vitreous hemorrhage, or choroidal detachment [13]. However, miotic drugs for use in the filtering procedure were not found to be significantly associated with the development of retinal detachment [7]. The surgeries most commonly reported to precede retinal detachment are listed in Table 37.1.

The proportion of retinal tear detection in these cases was reported to range from 50% to 73.7% [2, 7]. The corneal opacity resulting from long-standing congenital glaucoma prevents complete peripheral retina examination, which means that retinal breaks often cannot be detected. Multiple retinal breaks, giant retinal tears, and flap tears were most commonly found in these cases [2, 5, 7, 10] (Fig. 37.1). In contrast, retinal dialysis was found to be correlated with post-Molteno shunt implantation [11]. A retinal dialysis may occur during tube insertion through the sclera or during a pars plana sclerotomy at the time of shunt implantation [11]. Satofuka et al. reported that the most common area of retinal break was around the equator [5].

Proliferative vitreoretinopathy (PVR) was found in 40–80% of cases [10, 11, 13]. Some PVR was found in the area of the trabeculectomy site, which was believed to be related to the filtering procedure [10]. A higher rate of PVR incidence correlated with a larger number of previous glaucoma surgeries, which suggests a link with postoperative inflammation induced by the multiple previous operations [11].

In secondary congenital glaucoma, such as aniridia, Cooling, et al. reported that peripheral retinal abnormalities, such as multiple small circumferential white spots in the post-ora serrata, retinal strands entering the anterior vitreous, and abnormal vitreoretinal adhesion, may be related to retinal detachment in these cases [7]. However, retinal detachment in secondary congenital glaucoma may not always be

Table 37.1 Intraocular surgeries that were reported to be most commonly performed prior to the development of congenital glaucoma related retinal detachment [2, 5, 10]

Glaucoma surgery
• Trabeculectomy /trabeculotomy (n = 49)
• Goniotomy (n = 4)
• Iridencleisis (n = 4)
• Cyclocryotherapy (n = 3)
• Glaucoma drainage device (n = 1)
• Laser trabeculoplasty (n = 1)
Lens surgery
• Intracapsular cataract extraction (ICCE) (n = 3)
• Extracapsular cataract extraction (ECCE) (n = 2)
• Phacoemulsification (n = 1)

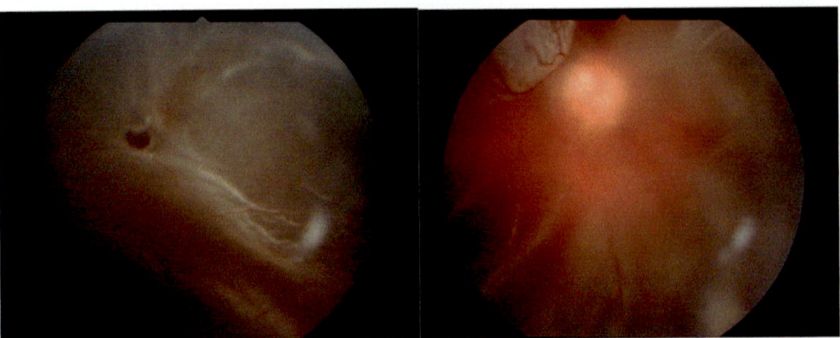

Fig. 37.1 Bilateral retinal detachment after an ocular injury in a 15-year-old boy with history of congenital glaucoma, congenital nystagmus, and high myopia is demonstrated. The retinal breaks found in this case comprised a small flap tear and lattice degeneration in the right eye, and temporal lattice degeneration with retinal holes in the left eye

rhegmatogenous in origin. A case with congenital glaucoma and Sturge-Weber syndrome presenting with bilateral exudative retinal detachment has also been reported [7]. However, in most cases, rhegmatogenous retinal detachment should be first ruled out so that patients can be surgically treated without delay.

Investigations

Ocular ultrasonography is beneficial in cases with corneal opacities, cataract, and dense vitreous opacity that prevents posterior segment examination. High-amplitude membrane attached to the optic nerve head with reduced mobility on eye movement indicates retinal detachment. Ocular ultrasonography is also recommended in chronic retinal detachment cases because choroidal detachment is often discovered in these cases. This information will provide the surgeon with a complete preoperative view that will facilitate surgical planning, as well as patient and family counselling. During the postoperative period, ocular ultrasonography is helpful for detecting re-detachment of the retina under the silicone oil in silicone filled eyes. However, the silicone oil slows the speed of sound, so derived images of the globe will be longer than normal.

Ultrawide-field fundus photography is very helpful in cases with nystagmus and small pupils. This fundus imaging method can be used for urgent examination in some pediatric cases before advancing them for examination under general anesthesia. Moreover, this camera can capture retinal pathology even in cases with small pupils caused by multiple previous surgeries. The wider photographic field of up to 200° delivered by this camera yields clear details of the peripheral retina without the need for scleral indentation or general anesthesia. Therefore, the rate of retinal break detection can be improved. The fine clinical details that can be extracted from these wide-field photographs are essential for both treatment planning and patient/family counselling. However, physicians should interpret distorted peripheral images with caution. The relationship between the lesion and the surrounding anatomy could be altered by the gaze direction and the location on the retina.

Examination Under General Anesthesia and Treatment Planning

Once retinal detachment is suspected, the patient should be advanced for comprehensive ocular investigations. Examination under general anesthesia will yield essential retinal pathology-related details that the physician will need for treatment planning. Repeat ocular ultrasonography and/or fundus photography should also be performed to document and collect as much up-to-date case-related detail as possible.

Surgical Indications and Surgical Challenge

Poor visualization due to the sequelae of congenital glaucoma often results in delayed diagnosis of retinal detachment. Some patients present with persistent hypotony and choroidal detachment, which greatly complicates surgery. In the past, patients with significant corneal or lens opacity and limited potential for useful vision were often prohibited from receiving retinal surgery [7]. However, improvements in surgical instruments and vitrectomy platforms have made surgery more feasible in complicated cases. The greatest surgical challenge in these cases is poor visualization. Obscuration caused by anterior segment pathologies, such as corneal epithelial edema, corneal haab striae, central corneal opacity, small pupil, and pupil distortion or decentration, can lead to problematic surgery [5, 7, 10, 13]. Therefore, complete preoperative evaluation and meticulous presurgical planning for the entire operation is highly recommended.

Due to the poor visualization, scleral indentation to identify causative holes or retinal breaks and complete peeling of proliferative vitreoretinopathy might prove very challenging. Therefore, the encircling procedure might be helpful in these cases [10]. However, scleral band would be infeasible in cases with a preexisting glaucoma drainage device or trabeculectomy bleb and scleral thinning or ectasia due to buphthalmic condition [2].

Due to the elongation of these buphthalmic eyes, sclerotomy placement and surgical instrument length must be considered in advance. More posterior placement of sclerotomies will allow the surgeon closer access to more posterior pathology. However, the risk of causing an iatrogenic retinal break at the ora serrata must also be considered. The removal of cannulas to allow closer access of instruments to the retina is beneficial in cases with a very long axial length. A contact viewing system could be used instead of a non-contact viewing platform to avoid contact between surgical instruments and the non-contact lens.

If visualization is obscured by iris tissue, the surgeon may need to remove the iris tissue or enlarge the pupil. Sterile topical glycerine during the surgery might be required if corneal stromal haze occurs. Advance preparation of this medication may improve intraoperative visualization.

Surgery combined with lensectomy might be beneficial in cases with a subluxated lens or cataract. Pars plana lensectomy can be performed without intraocular lens implantation. Triamcinolone can then be used to retrieve the posterior vitreous detachment while performing the core vitrectomy. Perfluorocarbon liquid can be used to stabilize the retina while shaving the peripheral vitreous base. In cases with massive subretinal fibrosis or severe proliferative vitreoretinopathy, perfluorocarbon liquid can also help to flatten the retina, and retinectomy might be performed to remove all traction. Air-fluid exchange and endolaser retinopexy are then performed around the retinal breaks and retinotomy. A full 360 degrees of laser retinopexy can be considered.

The most commonly used vitreous substitute for complex cases is silicone oil. In cases that require a long-term tamponade, 5,000-centistoke silicone oil should be used, and an inferior surgical peripheral iridectomy must be performed in every aphakic patient. Gas tamponade is sometimes alternatively used by some surgeons. An overview of the commonly reported retinal surgeries and vitreous substitutes used to treat these patients is shown in Table 37.2. Moreover, the surgeon needs to maintain appropriate intraocular pressure during the operation in eyes with compromised optic nerve perfusion and low scleral rigidity [10]. Intraoperative pulsation of optic nerve head vessels or optic nerve head pallor should be of concern.

Often times, repeated retinal surgeries might be needed to reflatten the retina and to maintain retinal stabilization. In these cases, a relaxing retinotomy and/or retinectomy of the immobilized and shorten retina should be performed.

Special Instruments in Congenital Glaucoma Related Retinal Detachment Surgery

Temporary keratoprosthesis is a device that is used to achieve a better surgical view in cases with severe corneal pathologies. The procedure requires the replacement of the cloudy cornea with a clear prosthesis at the beginning of surgery. Then, all standard surgical steps of conventional pars plana vitrectomy can be

Table 37.2 Commonly reported retinal surgeries and vitreous substitutes used to treat congenital glaucoma related retinal detachment [2, 5, 7, 10]

Retinal surgeries
• Pars plana vitrectomy (PPV) (n = 50)
• Encircling (n = 20)
Vitreous substitutes
• Silicone oil (n = 27)
• Sulfurhexafluoride (SF_6) (n = 2)
• Perfluoropropane (C_3F_8) (n = 1)

performed, including vitrectomy, fluid-air exchange, endo-laser retinopexy, and silicone oil injection. Globe stability during the vitrectomy can be achieved with tight corneal sutures. The peripheral retina can also be thoroughly examined and treated. Prakhunhungsit, et al. described a novel vitrectomy technique using Eckardt keratoprosthesis without the need for sclerotomies. Alternatively, the surgical instruments are introduced through the preexisting holes of the prothesis. The benefit of this prosthesis was well demonstrated in a post-trauma case with a large corneal wound [14]. However, once a temporary keratoprosthesis is used, a penetrating keratoplasty with a donor cornea must be performed at the end of surgery.

Endoscopic vitrectomy is another valuable treatment option in cases with severe corneal pathology, and endoscopic vitrectomy was proven effective in a selected case of adult vitreoretinal surgery. The endoscope can bypass the preexisting corneal lesions and directly enter the vitreous cavity. The surgery could then be performed via visualization from the monitor. Endoscopic vitrectomy is currently available only in 20G and 23G platforms. Of note, the side-on perspective produced by the endoscope would be challenging for surgeons who are unfamiliar with its use [15].

Postoperative Follow-Up

The issue of main concern during the postoperative period in these patients is inability by the physician to clearly visualize the posterior segment due to the preexisting corneal problems. Moreover, visual acuity in these patients cannot be precisely and accurately assessed since there are other factors that influence the functional outcome—not only the reattachment of the retina. Therefore, the use of special investigations, such as ultrawide-field fundus photography or ocular ultrasonography can be used to assess the surgical outcome.

Silicone oil filling of the anterior chamber might be encountered in aphakic eyes, eyes without an iris, and in eyes with hypotony resulting from ciliary body insufficiency. Long-standing filling of silicone oil in the anterior chamber could lead to further corneal problems, such as band keratopathy [2]. Silicone oil filling in trabeculectomy resulting in an increase of intraocular pressure has also been reported [10]. To avoid these complications, iris diaphragm implantation was reported to be advantageous [16].

Surgical Outcomes

In the past, the surgical outcomes in these cases were often guarded. The use of new surgical instruments, such as small-gauge vitrectomy platform, and improved understanding of the pathogenesis in these cases have improved postoperative outcomes [2]. However, visual function measurement might be challenging since there are many factors that influence postoperative vision, such as preoperative vision, amblyopia, severity of preexisting glaucoma, and corneal abnormalities [1, 10]. The visual outcome varied widely among studies. Ambulatory vision was achieved postoperatively in 42–50% of cases [2, 5]. Long-term silicone oil tamponade can facilitate at least ambulatory vision in these patients. However, vision deterioration or no light perception was reported in 25–50% of cases [2, 5, 10, 13]. Prior poor retinal perfusion, dense amblyopia, band keratopathy, advanced glaucomatous optic neuropathy, retinal re-detachment, proliferative vitreoretinopathy, and postoperative intraocular pressure fluctuation are poor prognostic factors for visual improvement [2, 7, 10].

Concerning anatomical outcome in a series of 26 patients, re-detachment of the retina was found in 9 cases (34%) after a mean follow-up duration of 3 years [13]. Compared to the rate of final reattachment of rhegmatogenous retinal detachment in general pediatric population, the reattachment rate in congenital glaucoma related retinal detachment was reported to be very low [6, 17, 18]. The major factors contributing to poor anatomical reattachment were poor visualization of the peripheral retina to identify and adequately treat the retinal breaks during the surgery, severe intraocular hemorrhage, and severe proliferative vitreoretinopathy. Twenty-one percent of cases transitioned to phthisis bulbi at various times during follow-up [2].

Even though the functional and anatomical outcomes are generally low in these patients, retinal surgery can preserve the globes, which helps to circumvent the social and psychological impact of phthisis bulbi in the non-surgical eye. The rate of globe preservation in congenital glaucoma related retinal detachment was 79% compared to 86% in general pediatric rhegmatogenous retinal detachment patients [2].

Long-Term Follow-Up

Since congenital glaucoma was found bilaterally in the majority of cases, periodic screening with dilated fundus examination or ocular ultrasonography in cases with inadequate visualization of the posterior segment should be performed in both eyes for preexisting retinal pathology, especially in cases with high axial length [1]. Prophylactic treatment, such as laser photocoagulation or cryotherapy, for lesions that predispose a patient to retinal detachment should be considered. Patients and family members should both be informed that significant visual deterioration is an important sign of possible retinal detachment, so urgent medical attention recommended to rule out this condition.

Surgical Case Example

Case 1: a 10-year-old boy with a history of congenital glaucoma and cataract in both eyes presented with sudden visual deterioration from 20/80 to 20/200 and ocular hypotony after a blunt ocular injury to the left eye. He also had a history of multiple ocular surgeries, including multiple diode laser transscleral cyclophotocoagulations, lensectomy with anterior vitrectomy in both eyes, and glaucoma drainage device implantation in the left eye (Fig. 37.2). The ocular ultrasonography of the left eye showed a total retinal detachment without choroidal detachment (Fig. 37.3). Then, a 25G pars plana vitrectomy, retinotomy, air-fluid exchange, 360 degrees of endolaser photocoagulation, and heavy silicone oil injection were performed. The retinal break could not be identified intraoperatively due to the poor visualization; however, the retinal reattachment was achieved after the surgery. The silicone oil was left inside the eye for 6 months. After the silicone oil was removed, the retina was still attached and the patient's vision remained stable at 20/200 (Fig. 37.4). The ultrawide-field fluorescein angiography was performed to clearly depict peripheral retinal pathologies in this patient (Fig. 37.5). However, the patient's intraocular pressures were high, so multiple glaucoma surgeries had to be performed.

Case 2: a surgical video of a 10-month old male infant who had vitreous hemorrhage and rhegmatogenous retinal detachment following a trabeculotomy for congenital glaucoma was presented. Lensectomy and vitrectomy were performed. Intraoperatively, a retinal incarceration to the trabeculotomy wound was found with surrounding scar formation. The rhegmatogenous retinal detachment was repaired with the use of perfluorocarbon liquid to completely peel the vitreous cortex and a retinectomy was performed. Perfluoropropane (C_3F_8) was then used as a tamponade. (**Video 1,** Courtesy of Prof. Dr. Şengül Özdek).

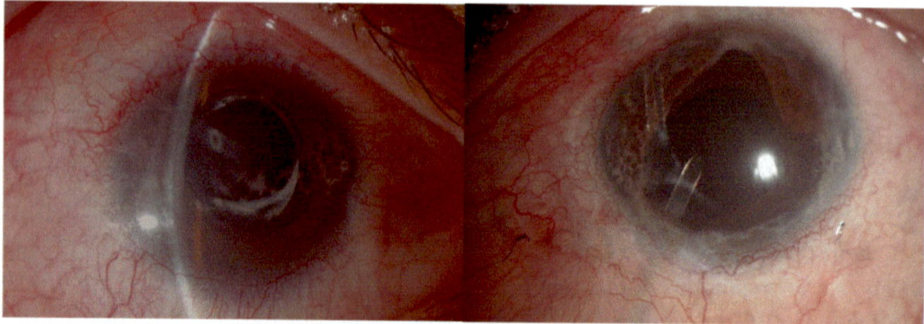

Fig. 37.2 Anterior segment photographs of a 10-year-old boy with history of congenital glaucoma. (Left) The right eye shows band keratopathy, a glaucoma drainage device tube behind the iris, and small pupil size from multiple previous surgeries. (Right) The left eye shows generalized conjunctival scar, early band keratopathy, peripheral anterior synechiae, and multiple glaucoma drainage device tubes in the anterior chamber. Poor visualization resulting from the corneal pathologies, and miosis resulting from multiple previous surgeries must be of concern and the surgical steps should be planned in advance in such a case

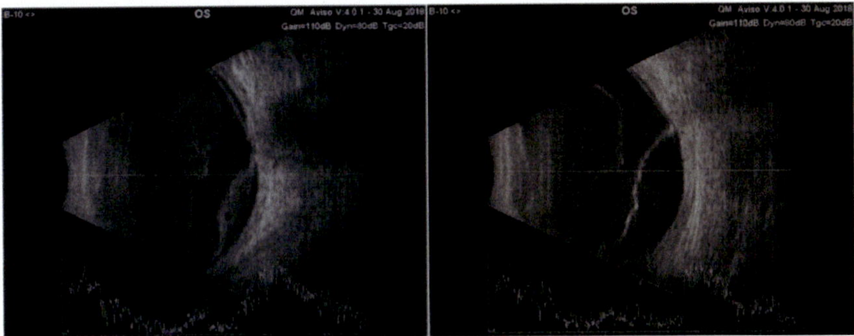

Fig. 37.3 Ocular ultrasonography of the left eye shows a high spike membrane-like lesion attached to the optic nerve head with negative after movement. Total retinal detachment with complete posterior vitreous detachment of the left eye was suspected. There was no choroidal detachment detected on ocular ultrasonography. The patient and parents were counselled with a recommendation for surgical intervention

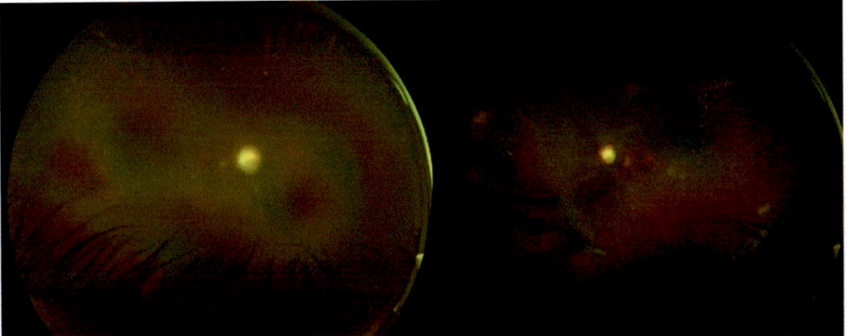

Fig. 37.4 The retina of the left eye was reattached after a pars plana vitrectomy with long-term silicone oil tamponade for six months (Right). Note the poor visualization of the retina of the right eye resulting from anterior segment pathologies (Left). An inability to appropriately and adequately visualize the retina in such a case prevents early detection of retinal detachment

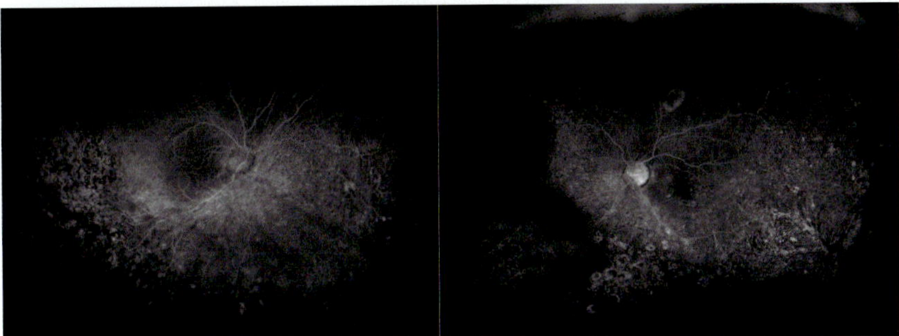

Fig. 37.5 After reattachment of a retina, ultrawide-field fluorescein angiography could be performed because this imaging technique can be used to more clearly depict peripheral retinal pathologies in patients with congenital glaucoma. Retinal lesions that predispose a patient to retinal detachment should be treated, and regular follow-up is recommended

Conclusion

Congenital glaucoma related retinal detachment is a rare disorder with a poor visual outcome. Early detection of the disease by the patient, family members, or physician can lead to early intervention resulting in better surgical outcomes. Sudden visual deterioration and ocular hypotony should alert the treating physicians to investigate and rule out this condition. If congenital glaucoma related retinal detachment is diagnosed and the surgical procedure is planned, visualization for the surgery must be a high priority concern. Detailed retinal examination and treatment of predisposing lesions of the fellow eye are recommended to prevent the development of retinal detachment.

Review Questions

1. What are the most common symptoms and signs indicating retinal detachment in congenital glaucoma patients?

1. Flashes of light
2. Sudden decreased vision
3. Ocular hypotony
4. Visual field defect

a. 1,2
b. 1,3
c. 2,3
d. 1,2,4

2. What should be concerned in regard to surgical intervention in the congenital glaucoma related retinal detachment?

a. Poor visualization
b. The long axial length of the globe
c. Proliferative vitreoretinopathy
d. All of above

Answers

1. (**C**) The most common symptoms and signs suspicious for retinal detachment in congenital glaucoma patients are sudden decreased vision and ocular hypotony.

2. (**D**) The main concerns during the surgical intervention include the following:

- The poor visualization resulted from corneal problems, miosis and cataract could make the surgery difficult.
- Surgeon might require special techniques and instruments during the surgery in the very long eyes.
- Longstanding retinal detachment often leads to severe proliferative vitreo-retinopathy which could make the surgery complicated.

References

1. Gupta S, Gogia V, Jose C, Chanana B, Bypareddy R, Kapoor KS, Gupta V. Peripheral retinal degenerations and rhegmatogenous detachment in primary congenital glaucoma. Retina. 2016;36(1):188–91.
2. Ghoraba HH, El Gouhary SM, Ghali AA, Abdelhafez MA, Zaky AG, Leila M, Heikal MA, Mansour HO. Pars plana vitrectomy with/without encircling scleral band for treatment of retinal detachment associated with buphthalmos. Int J Retina Vitreous. 2021;7(1):1–5.
3. Axenfeld T. Uber das Vorkommen von Netzhautablosung und uber die Bedeutung allgemeiner vasomotorischer Storungen beim Hydrophthalmus. Klin Monbl Augenheilkd. 1903;41:1–6.
4. Akabane N, Yamamoto S, Tsukahara I, Ishida M, Mitamura Y, Yamamoto T, Takeuchi S. Surgical outcomes in juvenile retinal detachment. Jpn J Ophthalmol. 2001;45(4):409–11.
5. Satofuka S, Imamura Y, Ishida S, Ozawa Y, Tsubota K, Inoue M. Rhegmatogenous retinal detachment associated with primary congenital glaucoma. Int Ophthalmol. 2008;28(5): 369–71.
6. Gonzales CR, Singh S, Yu F, Kreiger AE, Gupta A, Schwartz SD. Pediatric rhegmatogenous retinal detachment: clinical features and surgical outcomes. Retina. 2008;28(6):847–52.
7. Soheilian M, Ramezani A, Malihi M, Yaseri M, Ahmadieh H, Dehghan MH, Azarmina M, Moradian S, Peyman GA. Clinical features and surgical outcomes of pediatric rhegmatogenous retinal detachment. Retina. 2009;29(4):545–51.
8. Cooling RJ, Rice NS, Mcleod D. Retinal detachment in congenital glaucoma. Br J Ophthalmol. 1980;64(6):417–21.
9. Wang NK, Tsai CH, Chen YP, Yeung L, Wu WC, Chen TL, Lin KK, Lai CC. Pediatric rhegmatogenous retinal detachment in East Asians. Ophthalmology. 2005;112(11):1890–5.
10. Weinberg DV, Lyon AT, Greenwald MJ, Mets MB. Rhegmatogenous retinal detachments in children: risk factors and surgical outcomes. Ophthalmology. 2003;110(9):1708–13.
11. Wiedemann PE, Heimann KL. Retinal detachment in eyes with congenital glaucoma. Retina (Philadelphia, Pa.). 1992;12(3 Suppl):S51–4.
12. Waterhouse WJ, Lloyd MA, Dugel PU, Heuer DK, Baerveldt G, Minckler DS, Liggett PE. Rhegmatogenous retinal detachment after Molteno glaucoma implant surgery. Ophthalmology. 1994;101(4):665–71.
13. Gedde SJ, Schiffman JC, Feuer WJ, Herndon LW, Brandt JD, Budenz DL, Tube versus Trabeculectomy study group. Treatment outcomes in the Tube Versus Trabeculectomy (TVT) study after five years of follow-up. Amer J Ophthalmol. 2012;153(5):789–803.
14. Al-Harthi E, Al-Shahwan S, Al-Turkmani S, Khan AO. Retinal detachment and congenital glaucoma. Ophthalmology. 2007;114(8):1590–1.
15. Prakhunhungsit S, Yannuzzi NA, Berrocal AM. Vitrectomy using the Eckardt temporary keratoprosthesis. Am J Ophthalmol Case Rep. 2020;19:100709. Published 2020 May 1.
16. Prakhunhungsit S, Berrocal AM. Diagnostic and management strategies in patients with persistent fetal vasculature: current insights. Clin Ophthalmol. 2020;14:4325–4335. Published 2020 Dec 10.

17. Thumann G, Kirchhof B, Bartz-Schmidt KU, Jonescu-Cuypers CP, Esser P, Konen W, Heimann K. The artificial iris diaphragm for vitreoretinal silicone oil surgery. Retina (Philadelphia, Pa.). 1997;17(4):330–7.
18. Read SP, Aziz HA, Kuriyan A, Kothari N, Davis JL, Smiddy WE, Flynn Jr HW, Murray TG, Berrocal A. Retinal detachment surgery in a pediatric population: visual and anatomic outcomes. Retina (Philadelphia, Pa.). 2018 Jul;38(7):1393.

Non-syndromic Pathologic Myopia Associated Rhegmatogenous Retinal Detachment in Pediatric Eyes

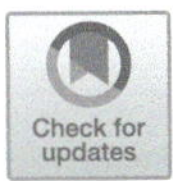

Abdussalam M. Abdullatif, Tamer A. Macky, and Hassan A. Mortada

Abstract

Pediatric rhegmatogenous retinal detachment (RRD) is associated with a relatively poorer prognosis compared to adults. This is mainly due to the relatively higher incidence of more advanced PVR at the time of the child presentation with subsequent higher rates of severe PVR and recurrent retina detachments postoperatively. Thus the initial standard intervention in non-syndromic myopic pediatric RRD should be buckle surgery, yet in certain cases vitrectomy is needed as eye with posterior breaks, ultra-thin sclera, media opacity, and high grades of PVR. We have described a surgical technique called 'extended ILM peeling' in which we peel the ILM to at least 2 disc diameters outside the retinal vascular arcades. We found this surgical technique helpful to reduce postoperative fibrous proliferation on retinal surface in the peeled area. We believe that the extended ILM peeling surgical technique might help to reduce the rate of recurrences and vitrectomy failures in pediatric RRD.

Keywords

Internal limiting membrane · Non-Syndromic Pathologic Myopia · Pediatric rhegmatogenous retinal detachment · Pars plana vitrectomy

---

Supplementary Information The online version contains supplementary material available at https://doi.org/10.1007/978-3-031-14506-3_38.

A. M. Abdullatif · T. A. Macky · H. A. Mortada (✉)
Department of Ophthalmology, Kasr El Aini Hospital, Cairo University, Cairo, Egypt
e-mail: has.mortada@gmail.com

Ş. Özdek et al. (eds.), *Pediatric Vitreoretinal Surgery*,
https://doi.org/10.1007/978-3-031-14506-3_38

Introduction

Myopia is currently considered as a significant public health issue causing significant visual loss as well as a risk factor for a range of other serious ocular conditions. The prevalence of this condition is increasing on a global basis, for reasons that still are not understood. Although the definition of myopia varies in different reports [1, 2], a refraction greater than—6.00D is defined as high myopia.

High myopia is associated with progressive and excessive elongation of the eyeball, which results in various posterior segment changes [3, 4]. These changes include areas of atrophy of the retinal pigment epithelium and choroid, lacquer cracks in Bruch's membrane, subretinal hemorrhage, and macular neovascularization. In addition, a large peripapillary crescent is considered a hallmark of highly myopic eyes [5]. Studies have found that the prevalence of these myopic fundus changes increases gradually with age. Curtin and Karlin [5] demonstrated that the incidence of chorioretinal atrophy in highly myopic eyes increases in patients 40 years and older, suggesting that these myopic fundus changes might be rare in children.

Pathological myopia, on the other hand, is defined as excessive axial elongation associated with high myopia that leads to further structural changes in the posterior segment of the eye. These changes are posterior scleral staphyloma, myopic maculopathy, and myopic traction maculopathy; which are macular retinoschisis; lamellar or full thickness macula hole; and/or foveal retinal detachment, and high myopia-associated optic neuropathy. All these changes contribute to the reduced best corrected visual acuity potential in these eyes. Prevalence of these pathological myopia fundus changes are less commonly seen in children with high myopia compared to adults with high myopia. This may be explained by the fact that axial length elongation is relatively limited in highly myopic children eyes compared to the highly myopic adult eyes. In addition, even among those patients with an axial length longer than 25.5 mm, the prevalence of posterior staphyloma or severe chorioretinal atrophy is relatively low. This is due to the fact that a long time period is necessary for the excessive eyeball stretching to cause the described fundus changes [6]. Data collected during the long-term development of myopia in experimental animals suggest that although the sclera thins rapidly and alters its material properties during the early stages, shifts in the collagen fibril diameter are not apparent until later in myopia development [7]. So, it is not only simple mechanical stretching but also long-term, continual mechanical stretching or aging that might be necessary for the development of myopic fundus changes.

Non Syndromic Pathologic Myopia: Although pathologic myopia could occur as part of a congenital-developmental hereditary anomalies as Stickler or Marfan syndrome in 53% of eyes [8] or as part of acquired disorder as cicatricial retinopathy of prematurity, yet it could be as the only ocular pathology. We will refer to this type of pathologic myopia without any associated disease entity as "Non Syndromic". This type of non syndromic pathologic myopia has been found to be a risk factor in the development of pediatric pediatric rhegmatogenous retinal detachment (RRD) in 9.5–41.4% of cases [2, 8, 10]. In addition, as myopia is more prevalent in Eastern Asian countries, it was reported to be more commonly involved as a risk factor for the development of RRD (23–38%) in studies from Taiwan [1, 9] and Japan [10, 11]. In contrast, in the United States, Weinberg et al. [12] reported the absence of myopia as the sole risk factor for pediatric RRD in their series, while other studies reported myopia to be involved in 17–34% of their pediatric RRD series [2, 9].

In recent years, it has become increasingly clear that there may be strong genetic components influencing the development of non syndromic forms of pathologic myopia and RRD. Non syndromic pathologic myopia may be inherited in autosomal dominant, autosomal recessive, or X-linked recessive modes [13]. To date, autosomal recessive mutations in 3 genes Cathepsin H (CTSH, Online Mendelian Inheritance in Man [OMIM] 116,820), low-density lipo-protein receptor related protein-associated protein 1 (LRPAP1, OMIM 104,225), and LEPREL1 (Prolyl 3 Hy- droxylase 2, OMIM 610,341) have been associated with largely non syndromic pathologic myopia [14–18].

Non Syndromic Pathologic Myopia as Risk factor for pediatric RRD: Risk factors for the development of RRD in eyes with pathologic myopia include peripheral retinal abnormalities such as lattice degeneration, retinal holes, and tears [19]. Although peripheral retinal features in highly myopic adults have generally been well characterized [20–23], there are very few studies that specifically describe the peripheral retinal findings in highly myopic children. It was reported that in children with pathologic myopia and RRD, peripheral retinal abnormalities were found in approximately one third of the eyes and lattice degeneration in 20%, white without pressure (11%), and retinal holes with subretinal fluid (4%) [24], while one study showed a prevalence of lattice degeneration to be 0.15% [25].

Clinical Features

Symptoms

Compared with adults, children with RRDs are less likely to report symptoms, present later with more chronic detachments, and are more difficult to examine in an office setting with a thorough examination of the peripheral retina may not be possible without general anesthesia in many cases [1, 9, 12, 26, 27]. Thus children with pathologic myopic pose an exceptional clinical dilemma, and consequently their RRDs may be more chronic and have more severe proliferative vitreoretinopathy (PVR) resulting in poorer surgical and visual outcomes [1, 9, 12, 26, 27]. Given these differences in the pediatric population, especially in children ≤ 10 years of age, examination under anesthesia (EUA) with prophylactic treatment of lesions predisposing to retinal detachment may be warranted in some cases.

Examination

Diligent attempts should be made to assess the child visual acuity in each eye. Inability to determine pre-operative acuity has been reported as a poor prognostic factor [12]. Ocular alignment should be noted as strabismus may indicate chronicity. Also the presence of cataract, hypotony, choroidals, and uveitis all are suggestive of a long- standing detachment and are poor prognostic indicators. Nystagmus may also indicate long-term and congenital vision loss, and also may help point to a specific underlying disease or syndrome. The refractive error in the unaffected eye can also be useful in the determination of etiologic factors, which has implications for determining the risk of detachment in the fellow eye. Thus a thorough examination of the peripheral retina of the fellow eye is vital given the high incidence of bilateral detachments. This can sometimes be accomplished in the clinic in older pediatric patients, but warrants an EUA in most younger pediatric patients which is usually done in conjunction with surgery of the fellow eye if surgery is planned [28].

On ophthalmoscopy, myopic temporal crescent is found to be associated with mean spherical equivalent and axial eye length. Increased peripapillary atrophy (PPA)-to-disk area ratio was associated with increased axial length, increased myopia severity, and increasing age. Cup-to-disk ratios is smaller in subjects with myopia compared with those with emmetropia, but this did not correlate with severity of myopia. In subjects with severe myopia, the upper pole of the disk was rotated away from the fovea but to lesser extent than in those with emmetropia or milder myopia [25]. Progression of myopia and the growth of axial length, β-PPA and optic disc ovality index also changed [29].

Ultrasonography is essential with insufficient view of the retina due to cataract, ectopia lentis, or poorly dilating pupil. It is also helpful to delineate areas of schisis and detachment in combined schisis/RRD. Ultrasonography is also critical in pediatric RRDs with suboptimal view to search for a mass or calcification, as the diagnosis of retinoblastoma must be excluded in a timely fashion. Optical coherence tomography can often be performed even on small children and help to differentiate juvenile X-linked retinoschisis based on the characteristic macular cystoid schisis [28].

Management

Prophylactic treatment

In prophylactic treatment for peripheral retinal pathology in adults, there are sufficient data to support the treatment only of symptomatic flap tears [30]. However, no recommendations or evidence are found regarding the long-term benefit of prophylactic treatment of the different retinal lesions that could predispose to RRDs in children. In addition, as the posterior hyaloid is tightly adherent to the retina in children, prophylactic retinopexy may lead to the development of new retinal breaks at the edge of the retinopexy scar when posterior vitreous detachment occurs later on. This limits the recommendation for any unproven application of prophylactic retinopexy in children. So, we advocate no treatment for lattice degeneration (with or without round holes). Retinopexy is recommended only for tears with vitreoretinal traction, and prophylactic encircling band may be considered for such tears in the fellow eyes of non-syndromatic RRDs.

Surgery

Buckle surgery should be considered the first line treatment in children with RRDs due to the high risk of PVR development and other considerations that will be discussed later. Those considerations favor the scleral buckle as the treatment of choice for pediatric RRD. Vitrectomy is reserved only for cases with posterior breaks, ultra-thin sclera, media opacity, high grades of PVR. Even in some cases of PVR, scleral buckle still has a role such as in cases with inferior PVR.

The role of adding scleral buckling to vitrectomy is still controversial. On one side, some surgeons consider it a beneficial procedure to aid in the attachment of the retina by counteracting the early and late vitreoretinal tractions, supporting the vitreous base with any unrecognized retinal breaks that may develop after surgery, and reducing any late tractions on peripheral retina from residual vitreous gel contractures. On the other hand, other surgeons believe that proper complete vitreous base shaving with the relieve of all traction forces is sufficient to guard against recurrence, and to avoid scleral buckle drawbacks as globe distortion, secondary axial lengthening, redundant retinal folds, and fish mouthing. However, a recent meta-analysis of randomized clinical trials showed low-certainty evidence of benefit in placement of a scleral buckle during vitrectomy for management of RRDs, however no similar studies is present in the pediatric age group [31]. Addition of a encircling scleral buckle may support the vitreous base better especially in phakic eyes since vitreous base cleaning could not be performed as good as in pseudophakic or aphakic eyes.

Buckle surgery is discussed in Sect. 5 Chap. 8, and here we will discuss our recently described pars plana vitrectomy with extended internal limiting membrane (ILM) peeling for pediatric RRDs [32].

Considerations for Vitreoretinal Surgery on Pediatric RRDs

When managing pediatric retina patients, certain anatomical differences compared to adult eyes as well as other issues should be considered:

1. **The Crystalline Lens**: in very young children, the eye is grossly smaller than the adult eye and the ratio of the size of the lens to the eye is larger. Thus pediatric vitreoretinal surgeons should be very mindful of the lens during intravitreal injections, trocar insertion, and instrument manipulation in order to minimize the risk of traumatic lens injury.
2. **The Sclera**: It has a different elasticity compared to adults, and sclerotomy sites may not always be amenable to being sutureless after vitrectomy.

3. **The Cortical Vitreous**: The attachment of the pediatric cortical vitreous to the internal limiting lamina of the retina is known to be much stronger in younger patients [33]. This contributes to challenges in removing the vitreous, and increased difficulty with inducing a posterior vitreous detachment (PVD). In a recent randomized clinical trial, intravitreal ocriplasmin administered 30–60 min prior to vitrectomy did not exhibit clear efficacy with inducing PVD before vitrectomy or during application of suction [34].

4. **PVR**: Postoperatively, younger patients can have a more robust inflammatory response, potentially resulting in higher rates of PVR and associated complications [35, 36].

5. **Post-Operative Positioning**: The possibility that children will not comply with appropriate postoperative head positioning may favor the use of silicone oil over intraocular gases as intraocular tamponades [37].

Surgical Technique

ILM peeling had been shown to minimize epiretinal membrane (ERM) formation during primary vitrectomy for RRD improving the anatomical outcome [13, 32]. In this technique, we perform an extended of ILM peeling up to 2-disc diameter beyond the vascular arcades in the management of complex pediatric RRDs [32].

(A)   Settings:

1. All these type of surgeries are performed under general anesthesia.
2. Vitrectomy System: 23 gauge valved cannula system.
3. The vitrectomy machine settings are: fixed high cutting rate (7500 cuts/min) and vacuum adjusted at 650 mmHg with linear control using foot-switch. The infusion pressure is kept between 25–30 mmHg.
4. Viewing System: is a non-contact HD wide angle viewing system.
5. Illumination System: a 25 gauge Chandelier light is always fixed to the lower nasal quadrant in these eyes.

(B)   **Management of the crystalline lens**: Lensectomy is performed in presence of lens opacity. All capsular remnants should be removed, with vitrectomy probe and using deep scleral indentation. Care should be taken to avoid injury to the iris and ciliary processes. Lens sparing vitrectomy may be performed in presence of clear lens

(C)   **The Vitreous Gel**: Excision of the vitreous gel proceeds from anterior to posterior with removing the equatorial gel. Almost all cases have tightly adherent posterior hyaloid, and thus extreme care should be taken to avoid retinal injury during excision of the gel as the retina may be aspirated with the gel towards the aspiration port. In the presence of dangerously mobile and high detached retina, it is recommended to stop the cutting and move the probe posteriorly towards the optic disc and start first by detaching the posterior hyaloid.

(D)   **Posterior hyaloid (PH) detachment, peeling, and excision** (Fig. 38.1): The probe is positioned just above the optic disc with the aspiration port directed

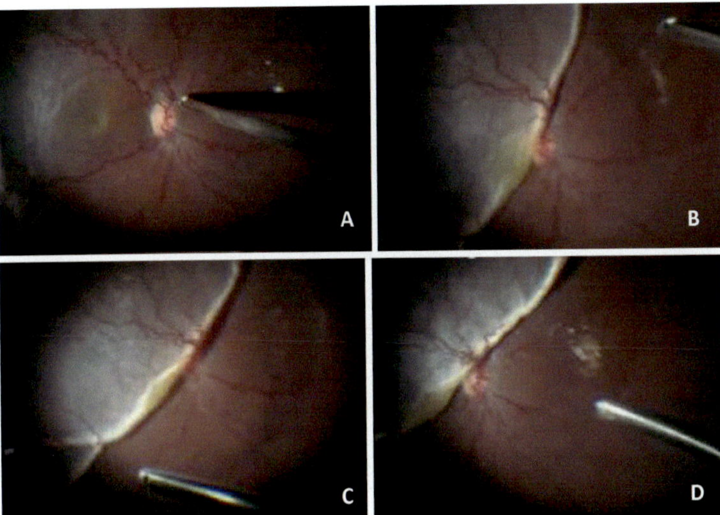

Fig. 38.1 Posterior Hyaloid Detachment: **A** The probe is positioned just above the optic disc with the aspiration port directed nasally. **B** Slowly move the probe anteriorly away from the optic disc. **C, D** Engage the vitreous gel with the probe in different quadrants and repeat the pull with careful observation of the retina to avoid retinal breaks development

nasally. Gradually activate the linear vacuum to aspirate and catch the posterior cortical vitreous. Slowly move the probe anteriorly away from the optic disc, carefully observing the behavior of the nearby retina. You may have to repeat this maneuver several times before you can observe separation of the PH from the edge of the optic disc and nearby surrounding retina. Move the aspiration port with the caught gel further away from the disc and detach the PH over a larger area of posterior retina. This is observed as spreading circular wave centered over the optic disc. Activate cutting to release the gel. Activate vacuum only to re-aspirate the detached gel, move the probe anteriorly towards the retinal periphery to further induce PH detachment. This maneuver is repeated in all quadrants. Careful observation of the vitreoretinal interface during PH peeling is critical to avoid creating retinal tears at areas of strong or abnormal vitreoretinal attachment.

(E) **Tightly adherent PH**: In eyes with strongly adherent PH, the above technique may fail to induce PH detachment. In this case, injection of Triamcinolone Acetonide aqueous suspension will help to highlight the PH. Then the now more visible PH can again be aspirated, detached, and peeled with the probe, as described above. Other helpful options are a diamond dusted Tano scrapper to swipe it off the retinal surface or a serrated forceps to grasp, detach, and peel.

(F) **Extended ILM peeling** (Figs. 38.2, 38.3): In most cases, the PH can be peeled beyond the temporal vascular arcades and may be up to or beyond the equator. Once this is achieved, an extended ILM peeling is the next step. The

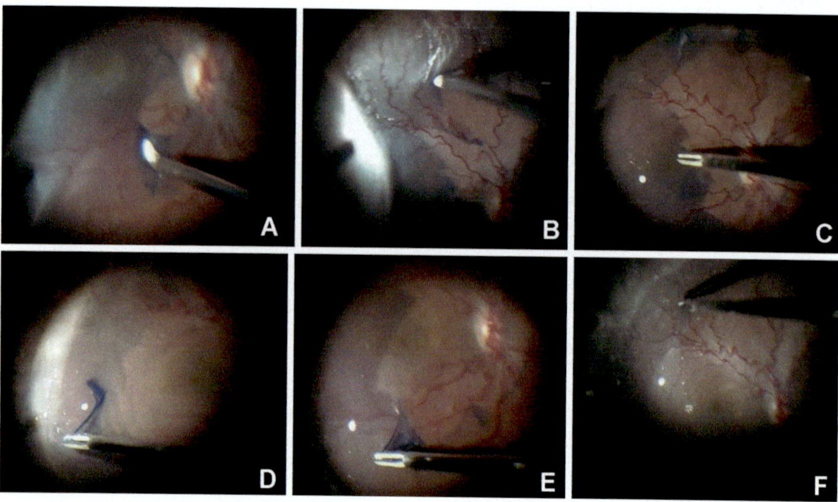

Fig. 38.2 Intraoperative fundus pictures showing steps of ILM peeling. **A** Initiation of an Internal Limiting Membrane (ILM) flap by Dimond dusted tano scraper. **B** Extending the ILM flap above and below the arcades by the scrapper. Using ILM forceps, ILM is peeled over the macular (**C**), beyond the macula (**D**), 2-disc diameter beyond the arcades (**E**), (**F**)

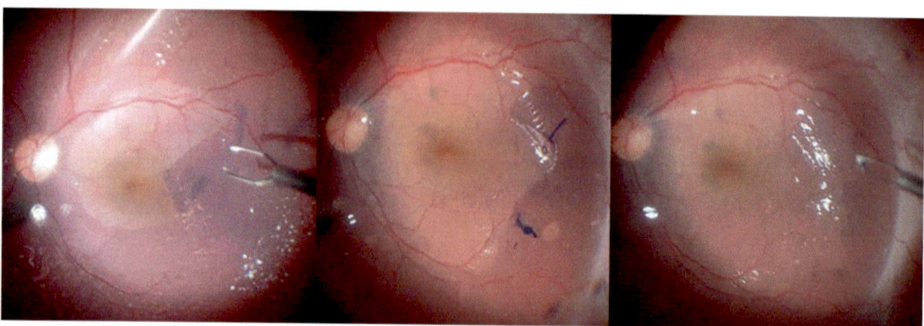

Fig. 38.3 Show the same steps described in Fig. 38.2 in a different patient

infusion is stopped; cooled Brilliant Blue (BB) is injected over the posterior pole and left for 30 s. The infusion is restored, excess BB is aspirated. It is preferred to start ILM peeling on the temporal side of the optic disc (OD) or just inside the lower temporal arcade. Using an ILM forceps, the ILM is pinched, slightly elevated, and moved side way till a break is made in the stained ILM and a free edge is created, the ILM is now released. The forceps re-grasp the free edge of the ILM, and peel it working parallel to the retinal surface, using the OD as an anchor. If the detached retina is mobile, Perfluorocarbon Liquid (PFCL) is injected to stabilize the posterior retina and facilitate peeling. ILM peeling is extended over the largest area possible, reaching up to 2 disc diameters beyond the temporal vascular arcades. BB may have to be injected more than once to augment staining and improve visibility.

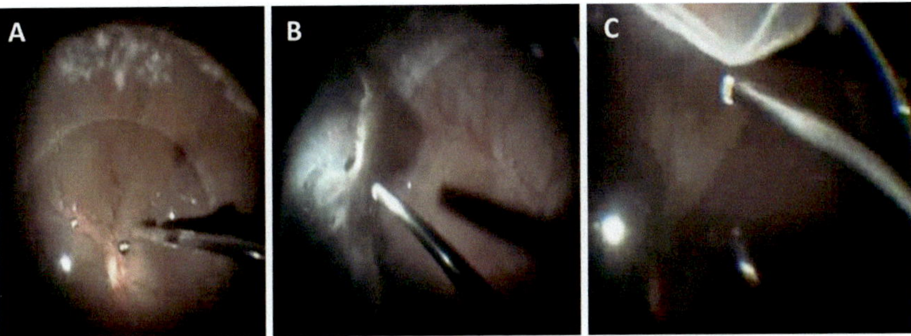

Fig. 38.4 A More perflourocarbon liquid injection to support the posterior retina up to the posterior border of peripheral break in **B, C** Shaving the vitreous base 360°

(G) **Peripheral Retina and Vitreous Base** (Fig. 38.4): Once the posterior ILM peeling is completed and the posterior retina stabilized with PFCL, more peripheral peeling of the PH is performed. In eyes with strongly adherent PH, bimanual surgery using 2 serrated forceps or a forceps and vitrectomy probe can be used to achieve more peripheral PH peeling. Attempts at PH peeling are carried out till the posterior border of the vitreous base is reached. Great care should be taken not to create iatrogenic tearing of the retina. More PFCL is injected as the PH peeling proceeds peripherally, till the posterior border of the most posterior retinal break is reached. Under illumination provided with Chandelier light, 360 degrees shaving of basal vitreous gel is next performed using deep scleral indentation.

(H) **Peripheral Circumferential Retinotomy**: may be performed to help complete retinal attachment in the following situations: (1) Subretinal proliferation interfering with retinal attachment (2) Severe anterior PVR that cannot be removed without irregular tearing of the retinal (3) Antero-posterior retinal shortening not relieved with PH and membrane peeling. Retinectomy of the anterior flap should be accomplished.

(I) **Peripheral Laser Photocoagulation**: More PFCL is injected to achieve complete retinal attachment. Then endolaser photocoagulation is applied to all retinal breaks, retinotomies, and to the retinal periphery for 360 degrees sparing the 3 and 9 o'clock meridians.

(J) **Silicone Oil Injections**: In aphakic eyes, the pupil is constricted and an inferior (6 o'clock) peripheral iridectomy is performed. Direct PFCL/Silicone oil (2000 Cs.) is slowly performed.

(K) **Sclerotomies**: The sclerotomies are always closed with 8/0 Vicryl.

Unlike posterior hyaloid peeling, which is difficult and challenging in children, ILM peeling is feasible in children with the same surgical difficulty as in adults. The ILM in children is more elastic and not friable which aid in peeling with less retinal trauma. Using this technique, we do not find clinically epiretinal

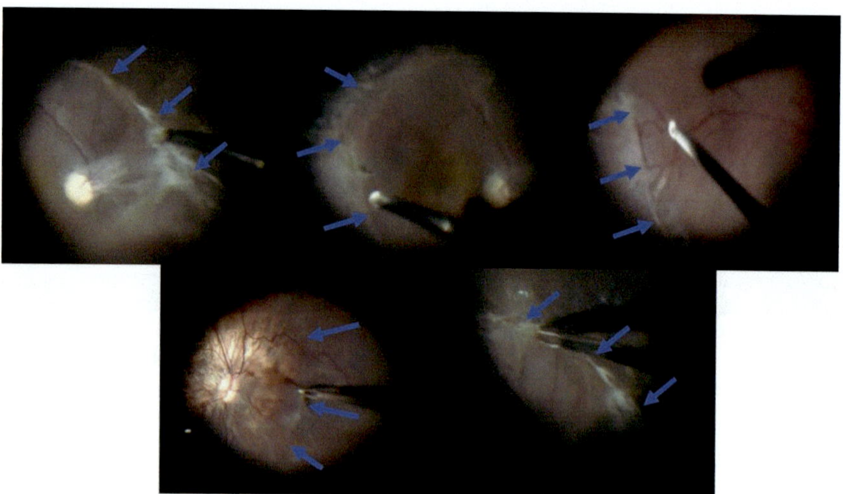

Fig. 38.5 Fundus pictures at the time of silicone oil removal showing recurrent proliferation which stops at the edge of the peeled ILM (Blue Arrows)

proliferation over the macula and over the area of peeled ILM in the post-operative period. Even in eyes that develop PVR, proliferation stopped at the edge of the peeled area due to inhibition of the process of visible fibrosis over those areas. Furthermore, when reoperation is needed the macular area is free of any proliferation improving the anatomical and functional outcome as seen in Fig. 38.5.

These findings could be explained by the fact that peeling of ILM ensures complete removal of the posterior cortical vitreous, cellular component, and extracellular matrix. Accordingly, retinal pigment epithelial cells and other proliferating cells are deprived of any scaffold for proliferation preventing the formation of ERM. Also, the absence of ILM at the macula limits the retinal tension that can develops from the peripheral contraction to the posterior pole thus increasing the macular compliance. The combination of these effects may explain the lower re-detachment rate in our published case series.

Needless to say that visual recovery in pediatric RRD is also affected by other factors such as amblyopia, and other congenital anomalies in addition to postoperative complications. In addition, the long term safety of ILM peeling is still controversial. It may result in mechanical trauma to the retina, which could lead to macular thinning, dissociated optic nerve fiber layer, concentric macular dark spots, dimple sign, pitting and forceps-related retinal thinning [22]. Although, the effect of these anatomical damages on visual function is debatable, the long-term effect of ILM peeling in the pediatric age group still needs to be investigated more thoroughly.

Video 1: Pediatric recurrent RD, post SB. *This video demonstrates 23G vitrectomy for management of recurrent total RRD, following scleral buckling procedure, in 10 year old boy. Following core vitrectomy, attempts were made to detach the adherent posterior hyaloid without the use of TA. The vitrectomy probe is positioned just above the optic disc, with the aspiration port directed nasally. Only vacuum is activated to aspirate and catch the the posterior cortical vitreous into the aspiration port. The probe is moved anteriorly, detaching and peeling the posterior hyaloid from the surface of the retina. This can be seen as a spreading and expanding circular wave moving anteriorly across the retinal surface. In this particular case, the posterior hyaloid was not strongly attached to the underlying retina. TA was next injected to highlight and reveal any attached cortical vitreous, which was removed using Tano's scrapper. After staining with Brilliant Blue, extended peeling of ILM was performed. The latter was first performed without PFCL. ILM peeling is usually started on the nasal side of the OD, using the latter as an anchor. ILM peeling is extended to the arcades and on the temporal side. Removing the ILM, the scaffold, protects the macular area from future formation of epi-macular proliferation, a common complication in this age group. Next, meticulous shaving of the basal vitreous gel is done. An area of vireo-retinal incarceration, probably complicated external SRF drainage during the SB procedure, was discovered. This probably was a reason for retinal shortening and traction. This was corrected by performing extensive circumferential retinotomy. Heavy diathermy is done. The retinotomy is done just anterior to the diathermy line and extended to the ora serrata on either side. Retinotomy should be posterior to any retinal break and extended from mobile retina to mobile retina. The goal is to relieve both A/ P and circumferential traction. Retinectomy of the anterior flap is next performed to avoid future anterior proliferation, development of anterior PVR, epi-ciliary proliferation and hypotony. Small radial cuts may be needed to completely relive circumferential shortening. Hydraulic complete retinal re-attachment using PFCL was done. Four raws of endolaser were performed along the retinotomy and extended for 360 degrees along the retinal periphery, sparing the horizontal meridians. Finally, direct PFCL/silicone oil exchange was performed. The patient was instructed to adopt a face down position for 5 days.*

Video 2: Giant Retinal Tear complicating Stickler's syndrome. *This video demonstrates management of 180 degrees GRT in 12 year old boy with Stickler's syndrome and strong family history of RD. During core vitrectomy one can realize the strong vitreoretinal adhesion, which is the case in most cases of Stickler. TA should be injected to highlight the posterior hyaloid. A serrated forceps was used to grasp and peel the thick posterior hyaloid in the area around the optic disc. PH peeling should be done cautiously and slowly, stopping every now and then so as not to exceed the elasticity and tensile strength of the retina. A key point to success in these cases is to avoid creating iatrogenic retinal breaks. Working unimanually, it was possible to detach the PH over the posterior pole. Brilliant blue assisted peeling of ILM was next performed, first without and then under PFCL. With the posterior retina stabilized by PFCL, further dissection of the PH was performed bimanually* *under Chandelier light. Different tools can be used for bimanual dissection of this strongly adherent PH, among them: 2 serrated forceps's, serrated forceps and small gauge probe, spatula and forceps. The PH is held with one serrated forceps while the other forceps or probe is used as a spatula to undermine and push the retina. The key point is to peel the PH over the largest area possible without inflicting iatrogenic retinal breaks. The more this goal could be achieved, the less the risk for future recurrence of proliferation and recurrence of RD. More PFCL may be injected to further stabilize the posterior retina, allowing more anterior dissection of the posterior hyaloid. This was continued till reaching the posterior border of the vitreous base, where one cannot peel more. Complete hydraulic retinal re-attachment is done with PFCL. Four raws of endolaser applications were applied to the edge of the GRT and to retinal periphery for 360 degrees. Finally, direct PFCL/silicone oil exchange was performed and the patient is instructed to adopt a face down position for 5 days. Silicone oil is planned to be removed after 3 months.*

Take Home Message: Pediatric RRD is associated with a relatively poorer prognosis compared to adults. This is mainly due to the relatively higher incidence of more advanced PVR at the time of the child presentation with subsequent higher rates of severe PVR and recurrent retina detachments postoperatively. Thus the initial standard intervention in non-syndromic myopic pediatric RRD should be buckle surgery, yet in certain cases vitrectomy is needed as eye with posterior breaks, ultra-thin sclera, media opacity, and high grades of PVR. We have described a surgical technique called 'extended ILM peeling' in which we peel the ILM to at least 2 disc diameters outside the retinal vascular arcades. We found this surgical technique helpful to reduce postoperative fibrous proliferation on retinal surface in the peeled area. We believe that the extended ILM peeling surgical technique might help to reduce the rate of recurrences and vitrectomy failures in pediatric RRD.

Review Questions

1. Which of the following could be considered the hallmark of high myopia:

A. Retinal pigment epithelium atrophy.
B. Macular neovascularization.
C. Sub-retinal hemorrhage.
D. Peripapillary crescent of chorioretinal atrophy.

2. Pathological myopia fundus changes are less common in children due to:

A. Early recognition in children.
B. Thinner sclera in children.
C. Limited axial elongation.
D. Glaucomatous optic neuropathy.

3. Myopia is more prevalent in:

A. Eastern Europe.
B. North America.
C. Africa.
D. Eastern Asia.

4. Pediatric RRDs have poorer prognosis compared to adults due to:

A. Presenting later with more chronic RRD and worse PVR.
B. Have higher incidence of posterior staphyloma.
C. Have higher incidence of cataracts.
D. Have higher incidence of myopic tractional maculopathy.

5. Pediatric eyes compared to adults have relatively:

A. Smaller crystalline lens
B. More adherent posterior hyaloid.
C. Less post-operative inflammatory response.
D. Longer axial length.

6. Extended ILM peeling in pediatric RRD helps to reduce post-operative:

A. Epiretinal membrane formation.
B. Cataract development.
C. Inflammation.
D. Intraocular pressure.

7. The PH could be detached and peeled using any of the following except:

A. Vitrectomy probe.
B. Retinal forceps.
C. Tano scrapper.
D. Retinal scissors.

8. The ILM peeling could need any of the following except:

A. Retinal forceps
B. Tano scrapper
C. Brilliant blue stain
D. Vitrectomy probe

Answers

1. D
2. C
3. D
4. A

5. B
6. A
7. D
8. D

References

1. Chen SN, Jiunn-Feng H, Te-Cheng Y. Pediatric rhegmatogenous retinal detachment in Taiwan. Retina. 2006;26:410–4.
2. Fivgas GD, Capone A Jr. Pediatric rhegmatogenous retinal detachment. Retina. 2001;21:101–6.
3. Curtin BJ. Ocular findings and complications. In: Curtin BJ, editor. The myopias. Philadelphia: Harper & Row; 1985. p. 277–347.
4. Steidl SM, Pruett RC. Macular complications associated with pos- terior staphyloma. Am J Ophthalmol. 1997;123:181–7.
5. Curtin BJ, Karlin DB. Axial length measurement and fundus changes of the myopic eye. Am J Ophthalmol. 1971;71:42–53.
6. Kobayashi K, Ohno-Matsui K, Kojima A, et al. Fundus characteristics of high myopia in children. Jpn J Ophthalmol. 2005;49(4):306–11.
7. McBrien NA, Gentle A. Role of the sclera in the development and pathological complications of myopia. Prog Retin Eye Res. 2003;22:307–38.
8. Soheilian M, Ramezani A, Malihi M, et al. Clinical features and surgical outcomes of pediatric rhegmatogenous retinal detachment. Retina. 2009;29:545–51.
9. Chang PY, Yang CM, Yang CH, et al. Clinical characteristics and surgical outcomes of pediatric rhegmatogenous retinal detachment in Taiwan. Am J Ophthalmol. 2005;139:1067–72.
10. Nagpal M, Nagpal K, Rishi P, et al. Juvenile rhegmatogenous retinal detachment. Indian J Ophthalmol. 2004;52:297–302.
11. Okainami S, Ogino N, Nishimura T, et al. Juvenile retinal detachment. Ophthalmologica. 1987;194:95–102.
12. Weinberg DV, Lyon AT, Greenwald MJ, et al. Rhegmatogenous retinal detachments in children: risk factors and surgical outcomes. Ophthalmology. 2003;110:1708–13.
13. Li J, Zhang Q. Insight into the molecular genetics of myopia. Mol Vis. 2017;23:1048e1080.
14. Jiang D, Li J, Xiao X, et al. Detection of mutations in LRPAP1, CTSH, LEPREL1, ZNF644, SLC39A5, and SCO2 in 298 families with early-onset high myopia by exome sequencing. Invest Ophthalmol Vis Sci. 2014;56:339e345.
15. Mordechai S, Gradstein L, Pasanen A, et al. High myopia caused by a mutation in LEPREL1, encoding prolyl 3- hydroxylase 2. Am J Hum Genet. 2011;89:438e445.
16. Khan AO, Aldahmesh MA, Alkuraya FS. Clinical character- ization of LRPAP1-related pediatric high myopia. Ophthalmology. 2016;123:434e435.
17. Muratoglu SC, Belgrave S, Hampton B, et al. LRP1 protects the vasculature by regulating levels of connective tissue growth factor and HtrA1. Arterioscler Thromb Vasc Biol. 2013;33:2137e2146.
18. Aldahmesh MA, Khan AO, Alkuraya H, et al. Mutations in LRPAP1 are associated with severe myopia in humans. Am J Hum Genet. 2013;93:313e320.
19. Straatsma BR, Allen RA. Lattice degeneration of the retina. Trans Am Acad Ophthalmol Otolaryngol. 1962;66:600.
20. Karlin DB, Curtin BJ. Peripheral chorioretinal lesions and axial length of the myopic eye. Am J Ophthalmol. 1976;81:625–35.

21. Lai TY, Fan DS, Lai WW, Lam DS. Peripheral and posterior pole retinal lesions in association with high myopia: a cross-sectional community based study in Hong Kong. Eye. 2008;22:209–13.

22. Celorio JM, Pruett RC. Prevalence of lattice degeneration and its relation to axial length in severe myopia. Am J Ophthalmol. 1991;111:20–3.

23. Pierro L, Camesaca FI, Mischi M, Brancato R. Peripheral retinal changes and axial myopia. Retina. 1992;1:12–7.

24. Bansal AS, Hubbard GB. Peripheral retinal findings in highly myopic children ≤ 10 years of age. Retina. 2010;30(4 SUPPL. 4):9–12.

25. Tong L, Saw SM, Chua WH, et al. Optic disk and retinal characteristics in myopic children. Am J Ophthalmol. 2004;138(1):160–2.

26. Wang NK, Tsai CH, Chen YP, et al. Pediatric rhegmatogenous retinal detachment in East Asians. Ophthalmology. 2005;112:1891–6.

27. Gonzales CR, Singh S, Yu F, et al. Pediatric rhegmatogenous retinal detachment: clinical features and surgical outcomes. Retina. 2008;28:847–52.

28. Wenick AS, Barañano DE. Evaluation and management of pediatric rhegmatogenous retinal detachment. Saudi J Ophthalmol [Internet]. 2012;26(3):255–63.

29. Zhang JS, Li J, Wang J Da, et al. The association of myopia progression with the morphological changes of optic disc and β-peripapillary atrophy in primary school students. Graefe's Arch Clin Exp Ophthalmol. 2021;(0123456789).

30. Wilkinson CP. Evidence-based analysis of prophylactic treatment of asymptomatic retinal breaks. Ophthalmology. 2000;107:12–5.

31. Rosenberg DM, Ghayur HS, Deonarain DM, et al. Supplemental scleral buckle for the management of rhegmatogenous retinal detachment by pars plana vitrectomy: A meta-analysis of randomized controlled trials. Ophthalmologica 2021.

32. Abdullatif AM, Macky TA, Mortada HA. Extended internal limiting membrane peel in pediatric Rhegmatogenous retinal detachment with severe proliferative vitreoretinopathy. Ophthalmologica. 2021;244(3):223–8.

33. Sebag J. Age-related differences in the human vitreoretinal interface. Arch Ophthalmol. 1991;109(7):966–71.

34. Drenser K, Girach A, Capone A Jr. A randomized, placebo-controlled study of intravitreal ocriplasmin in pediatric patients scheduled for vitrectomy. Retina. 2016;36(3):565–75.

35. Akabane N, Yamamoto S, Tsukahara I, et al. Surgical outcomes in juvenile retinal detachment. Jpn J Ophthalmol. 2001;45(4):409–11.

36. Yokoyama T, Kato T, Minamoto A, et al. Characteristics and surgical outcomes of paediatric retinal detachment. Eye (Lond). 2004;18(9):889–92.

37. Scott IU, Flynn HW Jr, Azen SP, et al. Silicone oil in the repair of pediatric complex retinal detachments: a prospective, observational, multicenter study. Ophthalmology. 1999;106 (7):1399–407.

Giant Retinal Tear Related Retinal Detachment

Anne L. Kunkler, J. Daniel Diaz, and Audina M. Berrocal

Abstract

A giant retinal tear (GRT) is defined as a full-thickness retinal break that extends circumferentially for three clock hours. GRT-related retinal detachments constitute a high proportion of pediatric retinal detachments. Repair of a GRT-related detachment poses technical challenges, especially in in children, due to an increased risk of complications such as proliferative vitreoretinopathy. Advances in surgical techniques over the years has resulted in improved surgical success. This chapter reports on pediatric giant retinal tears-related retinal detachments, as well as a case presentation with an example surgical video.

Keywords

Pediatric retina · Retinal detachment · Giant retinal tear · Stickler syndrome · Myopia · Scleral buckling · Vitrectomy · Proliferative vitreoretinopathy

Supplementary Information The online version contains supplementary material available at https://doi.org/10.1007/978-3-031-14506-3_39.

A. L. Kunkler (✉) · J. D. Diaz
Bascom Palmer Eye Institute, Department of Ophthalmology, University of Miami, Miami, FL, USA
e-mail: alk145@miami.edu

A. M. Berrocal
Medical Director of Pediatric Retina and Retinopathy of Prematurity, Vitreoretinal Fellowship Director Retina Department, Bascom Palmer Eye Institute, Miami, FL, USA
e-mail: aberrocal@med.miami.edu

Introduction

A giant retinal tear (GRT) is defined as a full-thickness retinal break that extends circumferentially for three clock hours (>90°) [1]. Repair of a GRT-related retinal detachment (RD) is challenging due to technical complexity and post-operative complications such as proliferative vitreoretinopathy (PVR). A GRT-related detachment in children poses additional challenges due later presentation of detachment, lack of a posterior vitreous detachment (PVD) with stronger vitreo-retinal interface adhesions, difficulties with post-operative positioning, associated systemic or ocular conditions, and amblyopia therapy. Advances in vitreoretinal surgery techniques with small gauge vitrectomy and perfluorocarbon liquid (PFCL) have improved the success rate of GRT surgery, but pediatric GRT-related RDs continue to pose a unique and challenging scenario.

Epidemiology

Pediatric rhegmatogenous retinal detachment (RRD) is relatively rare, representing approximately 2–6% of all cases of RRD and with an incidence range of 0.38–0.69 per 100,000 children [2, 3]. GRT-related detachments comprise a small portion of pediatric RDs. In a report by Hasan et al., 5.6% of all pediatric retinal detachments were related to GRTs, but this number has been higher in other series ranging from 15 to 20% [4–7]. In comparison, the percentage of GRT-related detachments in adults is even lower around 1.9% [8]. The overall average age of incidence is 42 years [9]. In children, GRTs have a male preponderance, which is similar to adults [4, 9, 10].

Pathophysiology

The etiology and risk factors for GRTs include idiopathic, trauma, myopia, lattice degeneration, hereditary conditions, and iatrogenic. In children, the most common cause of GRT is myopia (32%) and trauma (29%) [4]. In adults, most cases of GRTs are idiopathic (50–66%) [10]. GRTs can also be iatrogenic and develop as a complication to certain surgical procedures, such as pars plana vitrectomy (PPV), and is associated with a variety of other surgical and refractive procedures [9].

GRTs occur due to liquefaction of the central vitreous with associated peripheral vitreous condensation and subsequent vitreotraction in the area of the vitreous base [11]. The retina tears circumferentially along the attached vitreous base, leaving the posterior flap of retina to move freely and fold upon itself while the anterior flap stays flat [8, 11]. This is different from a retinal dialysis, in which the retina is separated from the pars plana at the ora serrata and vitreous is adherent to the posterior aspect of the retinal tear [12, 13]. In a retinal dialysis, the retina is not very mobile, making repair easier than a GRT.

In children there is a strongly adherent vitreoretinal interface, and vitreous syneresis and liquefaction is typically not present. In cases of trauma, it is theorized that the formation of a GRT is related to abnormal vitreous traction on an area of weak peripheral retina [14]. However, in hereditary vitreoretinopathies and pathological myopia, there is vitreous liquefaction and fibrillar collagen condensation that may explain the occurrence of GRTs in younger age [15]. The most commonly associated hereditary vitreoretinopathies include Stickler syndrome, Marfan syndrome, Wagner syndrome, and familial exudative vitreoretinopathy (FEVR) [4]. Additionally, developmental anomalies associated with GRTs include aniridia, buphthalmos, and micros) pherophakia [16–18]. These genetic disorders lead to vitreous and retinal abnormalities that increase the risk of GRT formation. The BGEEs study reported 14.5% of GRTs in all age groups to be related to hereditary vitreoretinopathies and which is similar to the 12.6% of all pediatric GRTs reported by Hasan et al. [4, 9].

Surgical Treatment

Surgical management of GRTs in the pediatric age group is especially challenging due to many potential factors, including but not limited to: a more adherent vitreous gel, absence of a posterior vitreous detachment, high rate of association of systemic diseases (high myopia or hereditary vitreoretinopathies such as stickler's syndrome), and a more limited ability to position postoperatively. Furthermore, trauma is a major risk factor for GRTs in this age group, and associated comorbidities including cataract, subluxated lens, or glaucoma can contribute to the surgical complexity.

Pediatric eyes present unique issues for the vitreoretinal surgeon. In infants, the volume of the vitreous cavity is significantly less than the adult eye, limiting safe maneuvers during surgery and increasing the risk of iatrogenic lenticular trauma and retinal breaks. PVD induction also often requires the use of adjuvant surgical instruments such as intraocular picks or loop scrapers. In cases of hereditary vitreoretinopathies, the abnormal vitreoretinal adhesions can also severely limit how complete the hyaloid can be lifted without risking iatrogenic retinal breaks.

The use of scleral buckling continues to be a matter of debate, even in the adult population. Given the potential for development of PVR in GRT-associated detachments, surgeons may argue that scleral buckling, by creating peripheral scleral indentation, can theoretically decrease the rate of recurrent detachments from secondary contraction of the vitreous base [19]. Others favor more thorough vitreous base dissection without adjuvant scleral buckling in order to avoid potential complications such as slippage or choroidal hemorrhage.

Overall, it appears that the recent trend is to manage GRT-related retinal detachments with PPV alone. The British Giant Retinal Tear Epidemiology Eye Study (BGEES), which primarily looked at adult eyes, for example reported that 93.5% of cases were managed with primary PPV [9].

Visualization is extremely important in these cases. Intraoperative use of triamcinolone can aid in highlighting the vitreous and to facilitate trimming the vitreous skirt. Perfluorocarbon liquid (PCFL) can help stabilize the posterior retina as the peripheral vitreous is further mechanically stripped.

If a scleral buckle was placed, one should be mindful of the height of the buckle, as this could encourage posterior slippage. Retinal slippage remains one of the more difficult intraoperative complications to manage. Peripheral slippage leading to a retinal fold is not a huge concern, however in posterior GRT-related detachments, slippage resulting in macular folds can lead to poor final visual acuity outcomes if not treated appropriately. Ensuring that as much fluid as possible has been aspirated prior to removing PFCL during fluid-air exchange is crucial in limiting the chances of slippage occurring. Also, if adjuvant scleral buckling is used, it is important to ensure that the buckle is not too high, as a steep posterior slope may more easily allow for retinal slippage to occur.

Direct PFCL-silicone oil exchange is an important tool to have at the ready when retinal slippage is a concern, such as in cases of GRT-associated retinal detachments. It is possible to under- or over-fill the eye with silicone oil during this maneuver, therefore it is extremely important to ensure that the intraocular pressure remains within normal limits following the exchange. If operating unassisted, it may be advised to use a chandelier endo-illuminator and the oil-infusion kit in one hand with the extrusion in the other through the superior trocars. If assisted, one can replace the infusion line with the oil-infusion cannula and using the light pipe and extrusion line under passive aspiration in the other hand to remove the PFCL as the oil infuses. Surgeons must ensure that all residual PFCL following direct PFCL-silicone oil exchange is removed, as subretinal migration can result in permanent retinal damage.

Like adult GRTs, removal of all vitreous traction around the edges or horns of the giant retinal tear is crucial to achieving anatomical success. The presence of a crystalline lens may make it difficult to achieve a thorough peripheral vitreous base removal, especially if there is no concomitant scleral buckle placement. In adult eyes, several studies have advocated for lens removal at the time of PPV, either via phacoemulsification or pars plana lensectomy, but this would not generally be recommended for children unless there is an associated traumatic cataract [20, 21].

The adult literature reports that silicone oil remains the most used tamponade agent during repair of GRT-related retinal detachments. Children, being more prone to PVR formation, are also likely to benefit from silicone oil insertion. One can consider insertion of higher viscosity silicone oil (5000 centistoke) as the pediatric age group is known to be inconsistent with postoperative positioning and it is also less likely to emulsify. Overall, the high rate of postoperative PVR and risk of intraoperative retinal slippage are likely the major forces driving the use of silicone oil [22]. However, one must balance this with the risk of developing silicone oil related complications. Unexplained vision loss and maculopathy, both resulting in poor vision, have been reported with long-term silicone oil use [23, 24]. Gas tamponade, with its higher surface tension compared to oil, has also been used successfully. A recent study from Bascom Palmer found no difference in anatomical success or final visual acuity between C3F8 or silicone oil tamponade after PPV for GRT in adult patients [25].

Outcomes and Potential Complications

The surgical success and functional outcomes in pediatric GRT-related detachments are lower compared to those of adult GRTs. Ambulatory vision ($\geq$ counting fingers) can be achieved in 41–54.8% of children, which may be accounted for by both poor vision at presentation and delayed time of presentation [4, 26]. Primary reattachment rates in the pediatric population have been reported around 63.4–68% [4, 26]. For comparison, in adults the primary reattachment rates after PPV alone vary from 87 to 100% with small gauge vitrectomy [27, 28]. Though Hasan et al. achieved final anatomic success of 63.4%, the single operation success was 40.2%. Hasan et al. found retinal reattachment chances were increased with early diagnosis, surgery within 10 days of symptom onset, lack of PVR, and presence of a PVD. Recurrent retinal detachment occurred in nearly 60%. In general, children are also more prone to PVR than adults. In an eye with GRT, the risk of PVR increases as a large area of bare RPE cells is exposed to fluid currents and these cells can migrate, proliferate and form membrane on the surface of the retina as well as in the subretinal space [8]. Recurrent PVR-related retinal detachments are more common in the pediatric patient population, as well as in patients with chronic GRT-related detachments, traumatic GRTs, or in those with already present PVR. Adjuvant scleral buckling in these cases can be considered in order to better support the vitreous base in the event of postoperative contraction [9, 21, 25].

Additionally, emulsified silicone oil can lead to postoperative intraocular pressure elevation. As such, silicone oil removal 3–6 months following reattachment is usually advocated. In adults, unexplained vision loss and maculopathy related to silicone oil tamponade has also been reported.

Patients with GRT-related detachments are at risk for detachment and breaks in the fellow eye. The rate of retinal detachment in fellow eyes in children has been reported as high as 33%, which is more than the 16% rate reported in the adult population [9, 29]. In adults, the presence of a break in the fellow eye has also been reported as high as 36% [30]. There is a lack of consensus regarding prophylactic treatment with laser retinopexy or cryopexy in the fellow eye. Prior studies have shown no benefit to prophylactic laser retinopexy while others have shown laser to lower the rate of retinal detachment in the fellow eye [9, 31]. In cases of hereditary vitreoretinopathy like Stickler syndrome, prophylactic cryopexy has been shown to prevent retinal detachment [32, 33].

Case Presentation

A 13-year-old male with a history of myopia presented with blurred vision in the right eye for 1 week. The patient and family denied a history of trauma. Presenting visual acuity was 20/800 in the right eye and 20/40 in the left eye. Intraocular pressures were normal in both eyes. Anterior segment exam was unremarkable in both eyes. Fundus examination of the right eye revealed a 270-degree GRT-RRD with the retina folded inferiorly and overhanging optic nerve (Fig. 39.1A). Fundus examination of the left eye revealed a nasal GRT-RRD extending 4 clock hours (Fig. 39.1B).

The patient was taken for bilateral surgery. The right eye was repaired with 25-gauge pars plana vitrectomy (**supplemental video**). After core vitrectomy, PFCL was used to unfurl the folded retina and a thorough peripheral shave was performed (Fig. 39.2A, B). A direct PFCL to silicone oil exchange was performed to avoid retinal slippage with aid of a 27-gauge chandelier (Fig. 39.2C, D). Endolaser was applied 360°. The left eye was then repaired with primary scleral buckle and external drainage of the subretinal fluid. Diode indirect laser was also applied 360 to the peripheral retina.

Given the history of myopia with GRT-RRDs in both eyes, genetic testing was performed on the patient. Testing revealed a heterozygous pathogenic variant in COL2A1 gene, and the patient was diagnosed with Stickler syndrome and referred to genetic counseling. There was no family history of retinal detachment. At follow up 10 months after initial presentation, the retina remained attached in both eyes as seen on fundus photos and OCT (Fig. 39.3A, B). Best corrected visual acuity at last follow up was 20/300 in the right eye and 20/50 in the left eye.

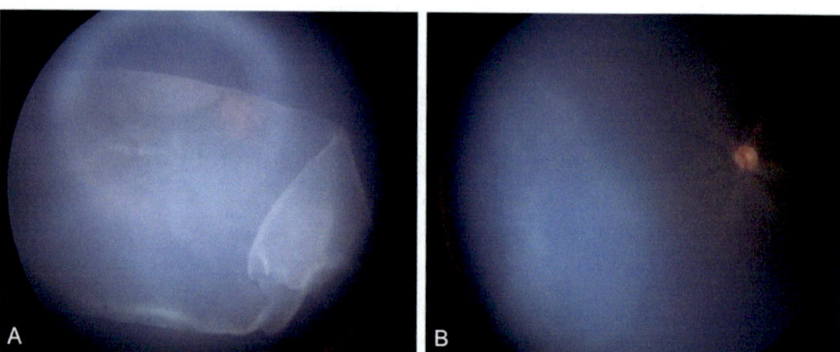

Fig. 39.1 Intraoperative fundus photograph of the right eye demonstrating a superior giant retinal tear with the retina folded over obscuring the optic nerve (**A**). Intraoperative fundus photograph of the left eye showing a nasal giant retinal tear with surrounding retinal detachment (**B**)

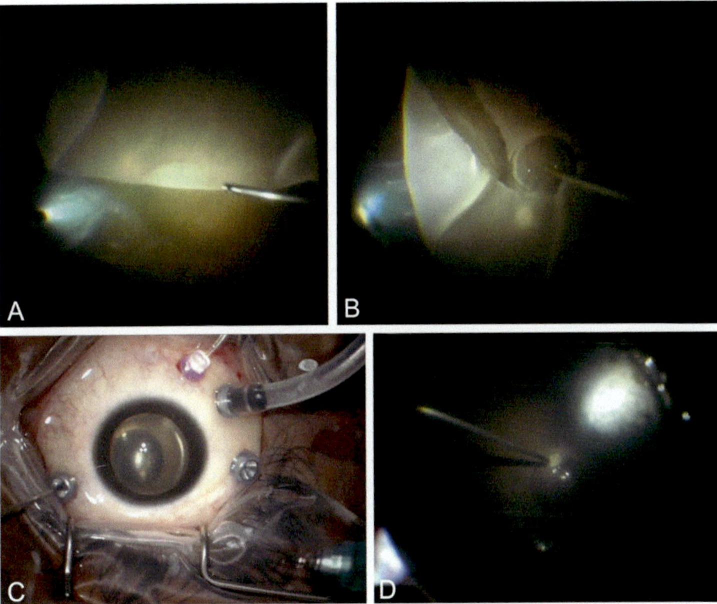

Fig. 39.2 Surgical repair of giant retinal tear-related retinal detachment. A core vitrectomy was performed with 25-guage pars plana vitrectomy (**A**). The retina was flattened using perfluorocarbon liquid and endolaser was applied to the periphery 360° (**B**). A 27-guage chandelier was inserted to aid in endoillumination (**C**). Finally, a direct perfluorocarbon liquid to silicone oil exchange was performed to avoid retinal slippage (**D**)

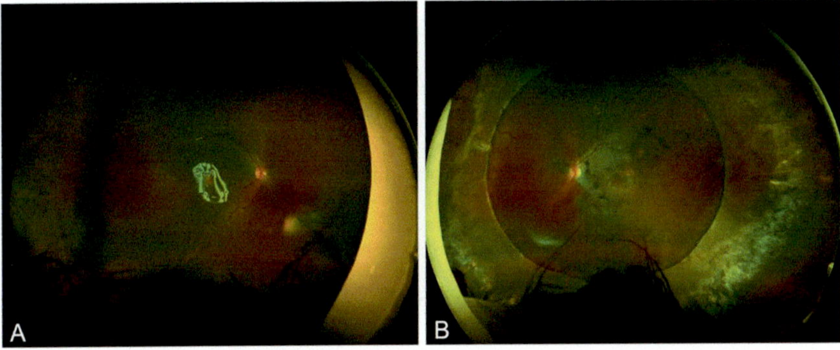

Fig. 39.3 Postoperative wide-field fundus photograph of the right eye demonstrating an attached retina (**A**). Postoperative wide-field fundus photograph of the left eye demonstrating an attached retina with scleral buckle and endolaser (**B**)

Conclusions

GRT-related detachments in children are most commonly due to myopia, trauma, and hereditary vitreoretinopathies. Surgical repair is challenging due to high rates of intra-operative and post-operative complications, such as high rates of PVR formation. The surgical success and visual outcomes in children are less than adults. There is a lack of consensus on prophylactic management of fellow eyes. It is important to build the family-physician relationship and to set expectations for prognosis, clinical outcomes, and need for visual-rehabilitation and amblyopia therapy.

Review Questions

1. By definition, a giant retinal tear extends circumferentially for at least how many clock hours?

a. 1
b. 3
c. 6
d. 9

2. What is the most common cause of a GRT-related detachment in children?

a. Myopia
b. Hereditary vitreoretinopathy
c. Trauma
d. Idiopathic

3. Why are visual outcomes generally worse in pediatric GRT-related detachments compared to adults?

a. High rates of proliferative vitreoretinopathy
b. Poor postoperative positioning
c. Delayed presentation
d. All of the above

Answer

1. B
2. A
3. D

References

1. Schepens CL, Dobble JG, Mc MJ. Retinal detachments with giant breaks: preliminary report. Trans Am Acad Ophthalmol Otolaryngol Am Acad Ophthalmol Otolaryngol. 1962;66:471–9.
2. Winslow RL, Tasman W. Juvenile rhegmatogenous retinal detachment. Ophthalmology. 1978;85(6):607–18.
3. Fivgas GD, Capone Jr A. Pediatric rhegmatogenous retinaldetachment. Retina. 2001;21 (2):101e106.
4. Hasan N, Azad SV, Kaginalkar A, et al. Demography, clinical profile and surgical outcomes of paediatric giant retinal tear related retinal detachments. Eye (Lond). 2021;35(11):3041–8. https://doi.org/10.1038/s41433-021-01621-y.
5. Weinberg DV, Lyon AT, Greenwald MJ, Mets MB. Rhegmatogenous retinal detachments in children: risk factors and surgical outcomes. Ophthalmology. 2003;110:1708–13.
6. Gonzalez MA, Flynn HW Jr, Smiddy WE, Albini TA, Tenzel P. Surgery for retinal detachment in patients with giant retinal tear: etiologies, management strategies, and outcomes. Ophthalmic Surg Lasers Imaging Retina. 2013;44(3):232–7. https://doi.org/10. 3928/23258160-20130503-04.
7. Read SP, Aziz HA, Kuriyan A, et al. Retinal detachment surgery in a pediatric population: visual and anatomic outcomes. Retina. 2018;38(7):1393–402. https://doi.org/10.1097/IAE. 0000000000001725.
8. Shunmugam M, Ang GS, Lois N. Giant retinal tears. Surv Ophthalmol. 2014;59:192–216.
9. Ang GS, Townend J, Lois N. Epidemiology of giant retinal tears in the United Kingdom: the British Giant Retinal Tear Epidemiology Eye Study (BGEES). Invest Ophthalmol Vis Sci. 2010;51:4781–7.
10. Ghasemi Falavarjani K, Alemzadeh SA, Modarres M, Alemzadeh SA, Parvarash MM, Naseripour M, et al. Outcome of surgery in patients with giant retinal tear: 10 years experience. Eye Lond Engl. 2017;31:1284–9.
11. Berrocal MH, Chenworth ML, Acaba LA. Management of giant retinal tear detachments. J Ophthalmic Vis Res. 2017;12(1):93–7. https://doi.org/10.4103/2008-322X.200158.
12. Scott JD. Retinal dialysis. Trans Ophthalmol Soc U K. 1977;97:33–5.
13. Smiddy WE, Green WR. Retinal dialysis: pathology and patho- genesis. Retina. 1982;2:94–116.
14. Savastano A, Barca F, Tartaro R, Caporossi T, Rizzo S. Post- traumatic giant retinal tear without posterior vitreous detachment: a case series. Ophthalmic Surg Lasers Imaging Retin. 2018;49:686–90.
15. Bishop PN, Holmes DF, Kadler KE, McLeod D, Bos KJ. Age- related changes on the surface of vitreous collagen fibrils. Invest Ophthalmol Vis Sci. 2004;45:1041–6.
16. Pal N, Sharma YR, Azad R, Chandra P. Isolated bilateral microspherophakia with giant retinal tear and rhegmatogenous retinal detachment. J Pediatr Ophthalmol Strabismus. 2005;42 (4):238–40.
17. Cooling RJ, Rice NS, Mcleod D. Retinal detachment in congenital glaucoma. Br J Ophthalmol. 1980;64(6):417–21.
18. Dowler JG, Lyons CJ, Cooling RJ. Retinal detachment and giant retinal tears in aniridia. Eye (Lond). 1995;9(Pt 3):268–70.
19. Gutierrez M, Rodriguez JL, Zamora-de La Cruz D, Flores Pimentel MA, Jimenez-Corona A, Novak LC, et al. Pars plana vitrectomy combined with scleral buckle versus pars plana vitrectomy for giant retinal tear. Cochrane database Syst Rev. 2019;12:CD012646.
20. Kreiger AE, Lewis H. Management of giant retinal tears without scleral buckling. Use of radical dissection of the vitreous base and perfluoro-octane and intraocular tamponade. Ophthalmology. 1992;99(4):491–7.
21. Moharram HM, Abdelhalim AS, Hamid MA, Abdelkader MF. Comparison between silicone oil and gas in tamponading giant retinal breaks. Clin Ophthalmol. 2020;14:127–32.

22. Banerjee PJ, Chandra A, Petrou P, Charteris DG. Silicone oil versus gas tamponade for giant retinal tear-associated fovea-sparing retinal detachment: a comparison of outcome. Eye (Lond). 2017;31(9):1302–7.
23. Batman C, Cekic O. Vitrectomy with silicone oil or long-acting gas in eyes with giant retinal tears: long-term follow-up of a randomized clinical trial. Retina. 1999;19(3):188–92.
24. Michel G, Meyer L, Naoun O. Sudden visual loss following silicone oil removal: three patients treated for giant retinal tear. J Fr Ophtalmol. 2009;32(2):104–11.
25. Rodriguez M, Lin J, Townsend JH, Smiddy WE, Albini TA, Berrocal AM, et al. Giant retinal tears: clinical features and outcomes of vitreoretinal surgery at a university teaching hospital (2011–2017). Clin Ophthalmol. 2018;12:2053–8.
26. Scott IU, Flynn HW Jr, Azen SP, Lai MY, Schwartz S, Trese MT. Silicone oil in the repair of pediatric complex retinal detachments: a prospective, observational, multicenter study. Ophthalmology. 1999;106(7):1399–408.
27. Kunikata H, Abe T, Nishida K. Successful outcomes of 25- and 23-gauge vitrectomies for giant retinal tear detachments. Ophthalmic Surgery Lasers Imaging Retina. 2011;42(6): 487–92.
28. Randolph JC, Diaz RI, Sigler EJ, Calzada JI, Charles S. 25-gauge pars plana vitrectomy with medium-term postoperative perfluoro-n-octane for the repair of giant retinal tears. Graefes Arch Clin Exp Ophthalmol. 2016;254(2):253–7.
29. Lee SY, Ong SG, Wong DWK, Ang CL. Giant retinal tear management: an Asian experience. Eye Lond Engl. 2009;23:601–5.
30. Freeman HM. Fellow eyes of giant retinal breaks. Trans Am Ophthalmol Soc. 1978;76: 343–82.
31. Verhoekx JSN, van Etten PG, Wubbels RJ, van Meurs JC, van Overdam KA. Prophylactic laser treatment to decrease the inci- dence of retinal detachment in fellow eyes of idiopathic giant retinal tears. Retin Philos Pa. 2020;40:1094–7.
32. Fincham GS, Pasea L, Carroll C, et al. Prevention of retinal detachment in Stickler syndrome: the Cambridge prophylactic cryotherapy protocol. Ophthalmology. 2014;121(8):1588–97. https://doi.org/10.1016/j.ophtha.2014.02.022.
33. Ang A, Poulson AV, Goodburn SF, Richards AJ, Scott JD, Snead MP. Retinal detachment and prophylaxis in type 1 Stickler syn- drome. Ophthalmology. 2008;115:164–8.

Scleral Buckling Surgery for Pediatric RRD

40

Ulrich Spandau

Abstract

A rhegmatogenous retinal detachment in children can be operated with episcleral buckling and vitrectomy. This chapter shows step-by-step the surgical technique of episcleral buckling.

Keywords

Episcleral buckling · Pediatric retinal detachment · RRD · Scleral buckling

Introduction

Vitrectomy for primary repair of retinal detachment has become the preferred choice for vitreoretinal surgeons. Several studies, however, reveal the importance of avoiding a primary vitrectomy in the majority of pediatric RRD cases [1–3]. A recent study demonstrates the unfavourable outcome and increased PVR rate of vitrectomy for pediatric RRD surgery [4].

The most retinal detachments in children are caused by trauma or myopia. The vast majority of these detachments can be operated with an episcleral buckling. The vitreous in children is intact and attached. The silicone sponge reattaches the retinal tear and the pediatric vitreous serves as a good tamponade. Removing the vitreous in a vitrectomy means the loss of this tamponade plus an increased risk for PVR because the vitreous has to be removed and a complete PVD is warranted. In contrast, the complication spectrum and PVR risk for episcleral buckling is low.

U. Spandau (✉)
St Eriks Eye Hospital, University of Stockholm, Stockholm, Sweden
e-mail: ulrich_spandau@yahoo.de

© The Author(s), under exclusive license to Springer Nature Switzerland AG 2023   581
Ş. Özdek et al. (eds.), *Pediatric Vitreoretinal Surgery*,
https://doi.org/10.1007/978-3-031-14506-3_40

The Surgical Technique

The surgery of traumatic RD in children using vitrectomy technique is very difficult, the risk of PVR redetachment is high, the likelihood of several surgeries is also high and the outcome is poor [1–4]. In contrast, the surgery of traumatic RD using episcleral buckling is easier and the outcome in almost all cases excellent. Why? A common retinal finding after trauma is an ora dialysis. Ora dialysis has a 100% attachment rate with scleral buckling. Other common pediatric detachments are giant tears with more or less focal detachments. The vitreous may be detached at the area of a giant tear and removing this attached vitreous with vitrectomy creates only problems and complications. The vitreous in children is dense and attached. It serves as a scaffold for growth of scaring tissue and its occurrence is common. In buckling surgery, the vitreous is not removed. Place a buckle on the sclera and seal the retinal break, that's all.

The surgery

For children we use the conventional surgical technique with panophthalmoscope because the view to retina in children is excellent. The cornea, the lens and the vitreous are clear. For the suturing of the silicone sponge, we use the microscope. We use only segmental buckles and not encircling bands for episcleral buckling of children. In case of a combined vitrectomy-buckle procedure we always use an encircling band.

The surgery step-by-step:

1. Limbal peritomy
2. 3 holding sutures
3. Cryopexy of the retinal break
4. Marking of the break
5. Choice of silicone sponge regarding on a retinal break size
6. Suturing of the silicone sponge
7. Inspection of retina
8. In case of detached retinal edges inject 0,5 ml air.

Material: Silicone sponge:

(1) 5 × 3.77 mm partial thickness sponge (Labtician, Canada). Our most common used silicone sponge. Indication: Ora dialysis, all normal size breaks. This sponge requires a 7 mm marking.
(2) 7.0 × 5.28 mm partial thickness sponge (Labtician, Canada). Less commonly used silicone sponge. Indication: Large breaks. This sponge requires a 9.0 mm marking.

The surgery step-by-step:

1. **Limbal peritomy**
2. **3 holding sutures**

This part is done under the microscope: Start with limbal peritomy and dissect the thick Tenon's capsule from the sclera. Then place three holding sutures on the recti muscles closest to the break.

3. **Cryopexy of the retinal break**
4. **Marking of the break**
5. **Choice of silicone sponge regarding on a retinal break size**

This part is done with the panophthalmoscope: Place a cryopexy on the retinal break until you see a white bleaching of the retina. Leave the cryopexy tip on the sclera, insert an orbita spatula behind the cryopexy tip and rotate the globe towards you. Dry the sclera around the cryo tip, remove it and mark the sclera. In children the sclera is often bluish after cryopexy. Continue with cryopexy and marking of the complete retinal break. At the end the retinal break is marked on the sclera and you can choose a silicone sponge. If you are insecure then measure how wide the break is with help of a caliper. If the break is 3 mm wide than a 5 mm wide sponge is sufficient. If the break is 5 mm wide, then a 7 mm wide sponge is required.

Tipps and tricks

A cryopexy is also diagnostic for finding of a retinal break: When the retina becomes white from cryopexy, then you see the dark break inside the white retina.

6. **Suturing of a silicone sponge**

This part is done under the microscope: Suture the sponge onto the sclera so that the sponge covers the complete break. Mark first the location of the sutures with the caliper. Tipp: Mark the tips of the caliper with the pen so that the sclera is marked by the caliper.

Then place two sutures. Before placing the sponge, we need a hypotensive globe. Take a syringe with 30G cannula and remove aqueous from the anterior chamber. If you use a paracentesis knife then you must suture the paracentesis because this is a child's eye.

Then place the sponge and tie the knot with 2-1-1 throws in case of Supramid suture and 3-1-1 in case of Mersilene.

7. **Inspection of retina**
8. **In case of detached retinal edges inject 0,5 ml air**.

This part is done with the panophthalmoscope: Observe if the sponge covers the break and observe if the retinal edges are very elevated. If the latter is the case, then inject 0,5 ml air into the eye. Remark: Air is inside the eye for 3–5 days and this is sufficient to tamponade the break. SF_6 is not necessary because it stays too long time in the eye, causes ocular irritation and PVR and may result in a tractive detachment. An external drainage is not performed.

Case Presentations

Case 1: (Figs. 40.1 and 40.2)

An 18 y/o male patient was hit in his left eye by a hockey stick. Due to the visual acuity decrease he visited an optician the following week. The optician stated a visual acuity decrease to 0.2 uncorrected and submitted him to the local eye clinic. Three weeks later he was examined at the local eye clinic and a PVR detachment with a large ora dialysis was detected. The macula was shallowly detached and the

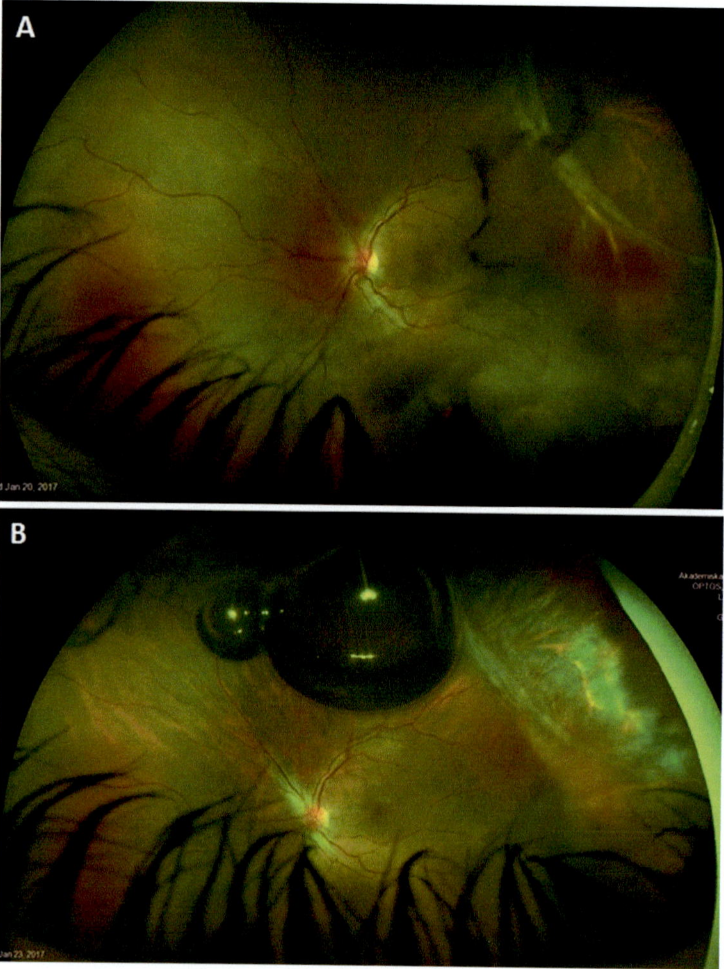

Fig. 40.1 **A** 18 y/o male patient with a 4 weeks old traumatic retinal detachment secondary to an Ora dialysis with rolled edges. **B** 4 days postoperative view to fundus. Operated with scleral buckle and air injection

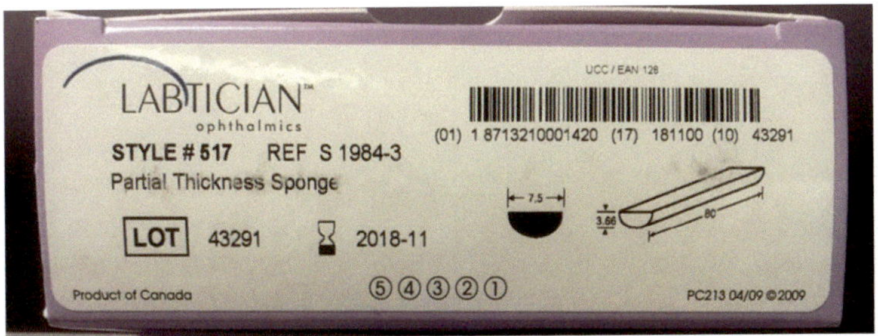

Fig. 40.2 A 7,5 mm wide silicone sponge was used for this case

retinal edges of the ora dialysis were rolled in. The visual acuity was +3.0sph = 0.1 and the IOP was 0 mmHg. referred to us for surgery (Fig. 40.1A).

The operation was performed with binocular indirect ophthalmoscope, cryopexy and the 9 × 5,77 sponge from Labtician, Canada (Fig. 40.2) was used. The intraoperative retinal inspection showed small tear at 11:45, large ora dialysis from 12 to 3 o'clock and subretinal PVR from 3 to 6 o'clock. The segmental buckle was placed under the superior and lateral recti muscles sutured at 11:30, 1:30 and 3:30. The suture at 1:30 was necessary to achieve sufficient scleral depression. A 0.4 cc anterior chamber tap was done. 0.5 ml air was injected to attach the enrolled retinal edges. In addition, triamcinolone was injected subconjunctivally to reduce the risk of PVR and to increase the IOP.

The 3-days follow-up showed completely attached retina, VA was 0.2 without correction, 20% of the vitreous cavity was filled with air and IOP was 18 mmHg. The enrolled edges persisted, and the choroid was visible (Fig. 40.1B).

The 1-month follow-up showed completely attached retina, VA was 0.2 with −3.0D an IOP was 16 mmHg. The retina was completely attached. The enrolled edges persisted.

Case 2: (Figs. 40.3 and 40.4)

A 5 y/o boy was injured with a stick. At examination an inferior detachment with a large tear from 7:30 to 9:15 was detected. A cryopexy of the retinal edges was performed and a silicone sponge was placed from 7:30 to 9:30. The upper edge of the silicone sponge was 1–2 mm below the muscle insertion. The retina was reattached within 2 days. If one chooses a vitrectomy the surgery becomes difficult. Why? (1) The risk of natural lens opacification. If you remove it then the eye will become severe amblyopic. (2) The removal of the dense pediatric vitreous which serves as a scaffold may result in inferior PVR detachment. Additionally, silicone oil would be needed which would necessitate the need another surgery for removal.

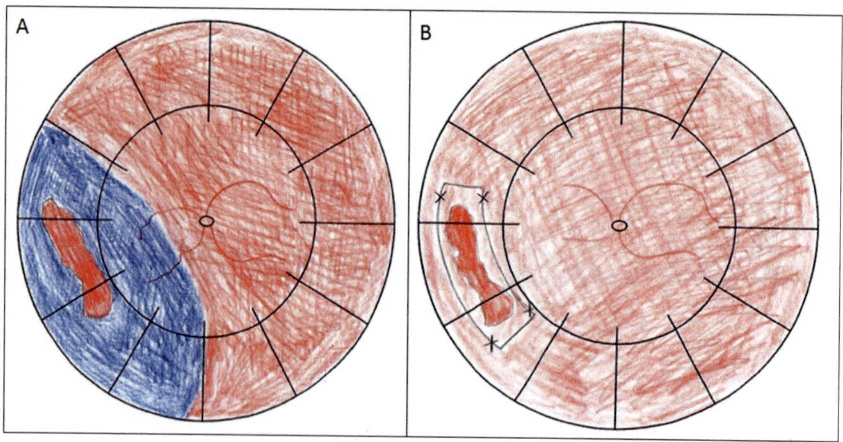

Fig. 40.3 **A** and **B** A 4 y/o boy with traumatic retinal detachment (**A**). A giant tear from 7:30 to 9:15. A vitrectomy in this case is very difficult and has a large complication spectrum. Try first a scleral buckle and in the most cases you will succeed with one surgery. The retina was attached after 2 days (**B**)

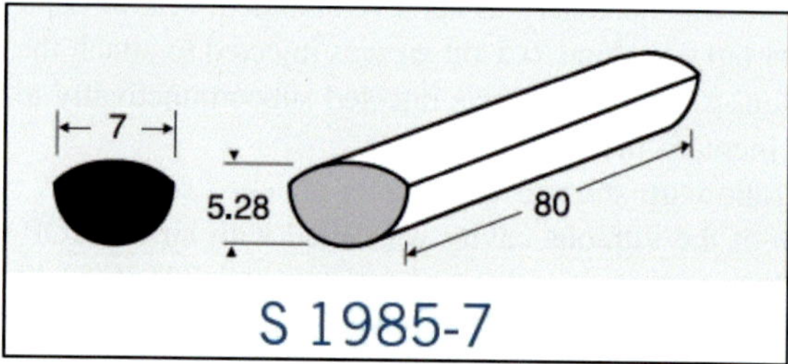

Fig. 40.4 This silicone sponge was used (Labtician, Canada)

Case 3: (**Figs.** 40.5, 40.6 **and** 40.7)

A 11 y/o boy was hit in left eye by a soccer ball. Ophthalmological examination revealed an ora dialysis. A silicone sponge (Fig. 40.5) was placed under the inferior rectus muscle. The upper edge of the sponge was in height with the muscle insertion. No drainage was necessary.

Fig. 40.5 A 8 y/o boy with ora dialysis secondary to a football

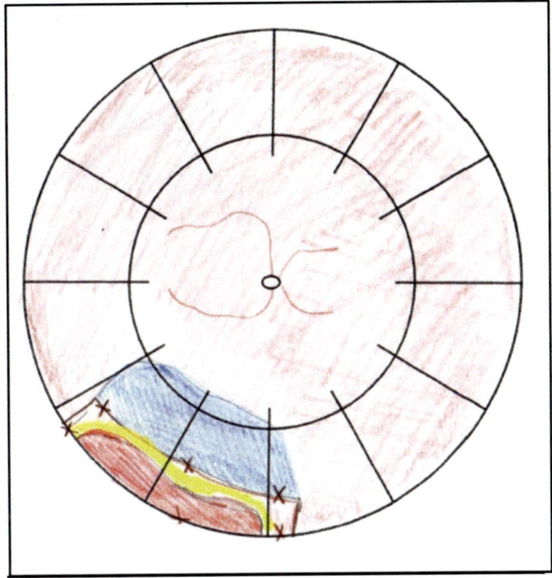

Fig. 40.6 The retina is attached after 2 days

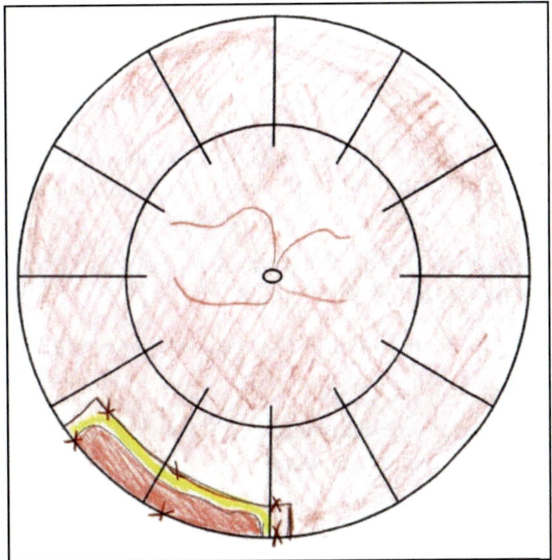

Fig. 40.7 The silicone sponge was placed under the inferior rectus muscle. The muscle indents the sponge

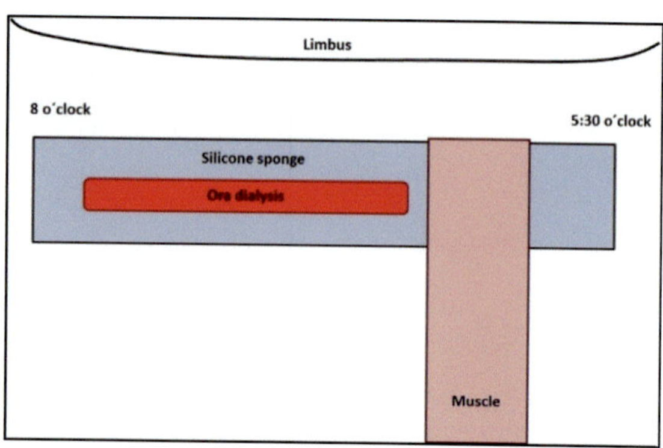

Conclusion

Episcleral buckling is an effective surgical technique and the method of choice for a pediatric detachment. The PVR risk and complication spectrum are low.

Review Questions

1. What is the most common cause for a pediatric retinal detachment?

(a) An idiopathic rhegmatogenous retinal detachment
(b) A traumatic rhegmatogenous retinal detachment
(c) An exudative retinal detachment

2. Right or Wrong: Vitrectomy has a higher PVR risk than episcleral buckling for pediatric RRD?

3. What technique has the most unfavourable outcome in pediatric RRD?

(a) Vitrectomy alone
(b) Vitrectomy with buckle
(c) Episcleral buckle alone

Answers

1. B
2. Right
3. A

References

1. Drenser K. Pearls for managing pediatric retinal detachments. Ophthalmology. 2019;126(9):1271–2. https://doi.org/10.1016/j.ophtha.2019.03.022. PMID: 31443787.
2. Carranza-Casas M, Quiroz-González E, Hernández-Reyes A, Matsui-Serrano R, Ariza-Camacho E, Graue-Wiechers F. Pediatric rhegmatogenous retinal detachment: predictors of anatomic and functional success. Int Ophthalmol. 2021;41(8):2777–88. https://doi.org/10.1007/s10792-021-01834-w Epub 2021 Apr 11 PMID: 33840049.
3. Smith JM, Ward LT, Townsend JH, Yan J, Hendrick AM, Cribbs BE, Yeh S, Jain N, Hubbard GB 3rd. Rhegmatogenous retinal detachment in children: clinical factors predictive of successful surgical repair. Ophthalmology. 2019;126(9):1263–70. https://doi.org/10.1016/j.ophtha.2018.11.001. Epub 2018 Nov 10. PMID: 30419297; PMCID: PMC6510644.
4. Rejdak R, Nowakowska D, Wrona K, Maciejewski R, Junemann AG, Nowomiejska K. Outcomes of vitrectomy in pediatric retinal detachment with proliferative vitreoretinopathy. J Ophthalmol. 2017;2017:8109390.

Combined Buckling-Vitrectomy Surgery for Pediatric Rhegmatogenous Retinal Detachment

41

Safa Rahmani

Abstract

Pediatric rhegmatogenous retinal detachments (RRD) is often chronic and advanced at presentation due to the unique etiologies and population. This chapter explores the various surgical consideration for repair of RRD in pediatric population including pre-op, intraop decision making and post op follow up. Special emphasis is placed on discussion and literature that supports used of combined scleral buckle vitrectomy surgery for these difficult to repair retinal detachments.

Keywords

Combined surgery · Pediatric rhegmatogenous retinal detachments · Buckling-vitrectomy surgery

Supplementary Information The online version contains supplementary material available at https://doi.org/10.1007/978-3-031-14506-3_41.

S. Rahmani (✉)
Vitreoretinal Surgery, Northwestern University, Chicago, IL, USA
e-mail: safa.rahmani@northwestern.edu

Pediatric Vitreoretinal Surgery, Ann and Robert H. Lurie Children's Hospital of Chicago, 225 East Chicago street, Box 70, Chicago, IL 60611, USA

Introduction

Pediatric rhegmatogenous retinal detachments (RRD) are relatively rare occurrences that are complex and frequently require challenging surgical management. Children often do not report visual symptoms or decreased vision, thus at presentation the pediatric retinal pathology is usually more chronic and advanced, with more significant proliferative vitreoretinopathy, and poor visual acuity. This chapter will focus on surgical considerations for repair of RRD in the pediatric population with combined scleral buckle and vitrectomy. Many of the etiologies and surgical details presented here are covered in depth elsewhere in the book (see Table 41.1).

General Considerations for Surgery

Pre-operative Evaluation

Pediatric patients have different anatomical considerations compared to adults including size of the eye, density of vitreous gel, increased vitreoretinal adhesion and increased risk of membrane formation. An important aspect of successful surgery is clear surgical planning. A thorough clinical exam is needed for decision of surgical technique. Kids that are too young often need exam under anesthesia in order to accurately assess the clinical presentation and perform any specialized testing that may aid in management. Widefield fundus photography, optical coherence tomography and B-scan ultrasound are often critical for detailed assessment of the detachment. In many cases a thorough history and exam of not only child but also other family members may aid in eliciting the etiology of the detachment. For example, in FEVR, a widefield fluorescein angiogram of parents may aid in diagnosis and proper care of the pediatric patient.

Table 41.1 Adapted and modified from Chen et al. [1]

Common etiologies of nontraumatic rhegmatogenous retinal detachment

(a) *Congenital/developmental anomalies*
     Stickler syndrome
     Familial exudative vitreoretinopathy
     Marfan syndrome
     Ehlers-Danlos Syndrome
     Morning glory syndrome
     X-linked retinoschisis
     Retinopathy of prematurity
     Choroidal coloboma

(b) *Simple myopia (not related to congenital abnormalities)*
(c) *Previous intraocular surgery (i.e., congenital cataracts)*

Counseling patient family and setting expectations of possible outcomes is also an important step in management. Although good anatomical outcomes can be achieved, it may often take multiple surgeries [2]. Even after successful anatomical outcome, visual recovery may be impaired due to permanent damage seen in these RRDs.

Scleral buckle

Scleral buckle is generally preferred as the first line approach for many pediatric retinal detachments as it avoids having to induce posterior vitreous detachment and manipulate the very adherent vitreoretinal interface. It also minimizes risk of iatrogenic retinal breaks, and avoids complications related to tamponade agents. Yet, scleral buckle is not adequate if there is vitreous hemorrhage, significant traction or advanced PVR. A combined approach will allow for support of all elements of vitreoretinal interface to achieve improved outcomes. For example, in PVR cases all the epiretinal proliferation may not be safely removed with vitrectomy and placement of a buckle can be very helpful in relieving tractional forces secondary to PVR [3].

Another common indication of SB is to maximize preservation of native lens whenever possible in these pediatric patients. The placement of scleral buckle supports the vitreous base of these eyes and allows safer vitrectomy if/when a full posterior separation is not able to be completed [4].

Scleral buckle can be placed sequential or concurrent with vitrectomy depending on the pathology addressed.

When combined with vitrectomy, scleral buckle placement is usually circumferential to provide full broad and low support anterior to the equator. In younger children, smaller bands are used. Additional elements can be used to provide further support of the retinal breaks.

Vitrectomy

Once decision is made to proceed with vitrectomy, initial port placement is of critical importance in pediatric patients. Based on the pathology, the decision to place ports at limbus or pars plana need to be considered carefully. In some cases, avoiding cannulas completely may be the best option. Even in anatomically normal eyes, the pars plana/plicata complex of younger children is not as wide as adult and explicit care must be taken to ensure safe entry sites are available prior to surgery [5]. For example, in significant portion of persistent fetal vasculature cases the pars plicata may be absent, and anterior projections of retina beyond the pars can lead to devastating outcomes if a retinal break is created at the entry site [6].

Addressing the lens is often one of the early decisions when planning for detachment repair. Leaving a child phakic, pseuodophakic or aphakic can have significant impact on the surgery and visual outcomes. Considering the status of the other eye and amblyopia can also effect decision making. In addition, choice of tamponade for the cases and ultimately assessing if the lens remains stable in the long term (such as in trauma or self-injurious behavior) may impact lens status. Those considerations in addition to retinal pathology need to be carefully reviewed prior to surgery. Specific details of vitrectomy are covered in other chapters of this book.

Intraoperative Considerations for Vitrectomy

Posterior Hyaloid Separation and Membranes

Elevation of the hyaloid is a critical step in vitrectomy surgery. Although essential, it is often very challenging to accomplish in pediatric eyes due to presence of pathology (such as stickler) or naturally adherent and dense vitreous at younger age. The usual induction of PVD with suction and cutter may not be effective in children. Staining the vitreous with triamcinolone can be valuable with viewing the planes, and use of flex loop and forceps can be used to initiate hyaloid separation with goal of extending it past the equator [7]. In many of these eyes, safe separation without causing iatrogenic breaks is extremely difficult. Thus sometimes partial vitreous removal without risk of breaks is preferred.

In the same context, removal of epiretinal tractional membranes have to be done carefully as to not cause retinal breaks (and possibly worsening PVR). Flex loop, bimanual technique, and using lighted picks can be useful in safely separating membranes. Due to the firm vitreoretinal adhesions, it is often preferable to perform segmentation instead of delamination. Perfluorocarbon liquid (PFCL) can assist in flattening the retina and avoiding retinotomies. Again, in children it is best to avoid any breaks (or use the existing breaks from the original retinal pathology). In complete detachments, partial PFCL can also provide stability to the posterior retina and counter traction as anterior membranes are removed and retinal flattened [8].

Tamponade Considerations

The decision to use gas versus oil in children depends on the etiology of the detachment, length of desired tamponade, and age of the child. Gas provides better short term tamponade without the need for second surgery. In pediatric patients that are difficult to position, silicone oil may be a much better alternative [9]. Oil also provides long term tamponade that may be needed in successful repair. Cataracts are less likely to form with oil and because kids can see through the oil it may be less amblyogenic, especially in younger kids. Depending on the etiology of the detachment both gas and oil can be effective tools for tamponade. Oil (and PFCL) should be avoided in coloboma associated detachments due to risk of oil/PFCL migration into subretinal space or intracranial cavity [10, 11].

Post-Operative Considerations

In children, post-operative care often lasts much longer than the immediate operative window. Even with good surgical outcome, risk of amblyopia is significant and involving the pediatric ophthalmologist for aggressive amblyopia management and visual rehab is crucial. If visual prognosis is poor, connecting families with community resources of visually impaired can be helpful to the patient and family and improve the child's chance of integration in the society. In monocular patients or patients at high risk of detachments (Sticker) using protective glassware and sports goggles is highly recommended and counseling patients on long term need for follow up can help mitigate late complications.

Surgical Outcomes

RRD in children is a distinct and challenging condition to treat. Compared with adult RRD, pediatric detachments tend to present late due to lack of visual complaints, and subsequent management often is complicated by more advanced proliferative vitreoretinopathy (PVR). Compared to adults, there is lower rates of primary reattachment after a single operation. The tendency for late diagnosis is an important characteristic that leads to macular involvement in 60–85% of the cases and PVR grade C or worse in 25–60% [1–3, 12–22].

Additional challenges more unique to the pediatric population are posed by poor cooperation for examinations and difficulty with postoperative positioning. Addressing the systemic comorbidities (prematurity, connective tissue disorders) can also pose a significant intraoperative challenge. Despite the higher risk, successful reattachment of the retina is possible in most patients.

Single surgery anatomical success rates vary largely in literature depending on patient groups and surgical instrumentations available; it generally ranges from 40 to 90% [16, 18, 23]. Due to heterogeneity of etiology and rarity of RRD in pediatric population, what has been less clear in literature is the type of operation most likely to result in retinal reattachment. There are no randomized clinical trials that compare surgical procedures in this population. However, systematic analysis of retrospective surgical outcomes studies provides important support in identifying factors predictive of successful surgical outcomes.

In pediatric RRDs without significant PVR scleral buckle continues to be the most prevalent surgical procedure with reattachment outcomes >80% for single surgery success [8]. Even in cases with chronic inferior retinal detachments with subretinal bands, scleral buckle alone can yield excellent surgical outcomes [24]. Some factors associated with failure of scleral buckles include multiple breaks, three or more quadrants of detachment; horseshoe tears; and Stickler syndrome [25].

For complex cases that include total retinal detachment, extensive PVR, trauma, and giant retinal tear, primary scleral buckle (SB) is not sufficient. Pars plana vitrectomy (PPV) is a critical component of successful outcomes.

In multiple studies, there were higher success rates of RRD repair with combined scleral buckle and Vitrectomy compared to vitrectomy alone or primary buckle alone, although most were not statistically significant [1–3, 12–14, 17–20, 26]. Consistent risk factors across most studies that resulted in poor outcomes was total retinal detachment and advanced PVR [1–3, 13–20, 23, 26, 27]. The tendency toward performing combined SB/PPV was increased in these studies if there was extensive detachment (total vs partial), more advanced PVR, trauma, vitreous hemorrhage and history of previous intraocular surgery [3, 14–17, 26]. Smith et al. reported the final surgical success rate in a large cohort of pediatric RRD patients was highest in combined SB/PPV, followed by primary SB, and lowest for primary vitrectomy [14].

In a retrospective study of traumatic RRD from self-injurious behavior (SIB) authors found low rates of single surgery success (37%) but final outcomes (average of 2 surgeries) were about 80% anatomical success (including partial attachments). They found significant association between final attachment rates and the use of a SB at any surgery. Although the eyes that underwent primary SB showed less PVR, more eyes in the SB plus PPV group (71.9%) demonstrated grade C PVR than did eyes in the vitrectomy only group (47.3%). The more severe the preoperative presentation of detachment the more likely choice of SB/PPV for attempted repair [28, 29].

Most recently, Carranza-Casas et al. completed multivariate analysis on their large cohort of RRD that included factors such as age, initial procedure, lens status, macula status, subtotal/total RD, and PVR. Study found presenting macular status and choosing SB or SB/PPV as the initial procedure when compared with PPV alone were significantly associated with better outcomes. In addition, patients who were candidates for scleral buckling as a first surgery tend to have better long-term results, and there is an advantage of SB/PPV over PPV alone as an initial procedure to predict surgical success [26]. Table 41.2 summarizes indications for consideration of combined scleral buckle with vitrectomy.

Table 41.2 Indications for consideration of combined Scleral buckle with Vitrectomy	
	Advanced proliferative Vitreoretinopathy (PVR)
	Vitreous hemorrhage
	Posterior retinal breaks
	Significant vitreoretinal traction
	Previous failed vitrectomy
	Giant retinal tear

Conclusions

Pediatric rhegmatogenous retinal detachments are rare occurrences that require complex surgical management. They are often associated with trauma and hereditary conditions such as Stickler and Marfan Syndrome and can present as bilateral cases. Scleral buckle with vitrectomy is a superior option for many RRD cases that have total retinal detachment and more advanced PVR. Multiple surgeries may be necessary for anatomical success. Counseling of children and their parents is important in successful management of these patients as they often require long term multifaceted care in addition to our surgical repairs (see Figs. 41.1, 41.2 and 41.3).

Surgical Video Courtesy of Prof. Dr. Şengül Özdek

The video describes a 7-year-old boy with an infantile high myopia associated RRD who had been previously treated with a combined surgery with an encircling band, lens sparing vitrectomy and silicone oil tamponade and ended up with PVR related recurrence in inferior half of the retina. The video shows the second surgery with addition of a local 5 mm scleral sponge with a groove to be placed under the preexisting encircling band together with PVR surgery.

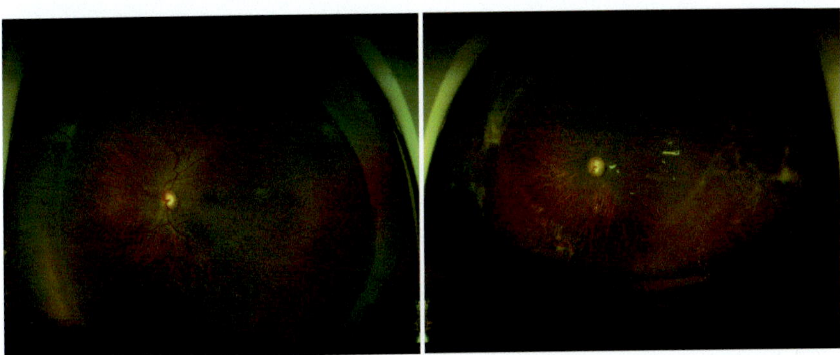

Fig. 41.1 15-year-old with stickler syndrome. Initial presentation of bilateral retinal detachment. **Picture on the left**: Right eye had small localized supertemporal detachment with a hole that reattached well with primary scleral buckle. This eye has remained stable during the 3-year follow-up. **Picture on the right**: Left eye presented with vitreous hemorrhage and 200 degree temporal giant retinal tear with total retinal detachment. The left eye first underwent lensectomy/scleral buckle/ Vitrectomy with silicone oil. Retina re-detached temporally 2 months after the first operation. A repeat vitrectomy with further membrane removal was successful. Retina has remained attached for the two-year follow-up with silicone oil

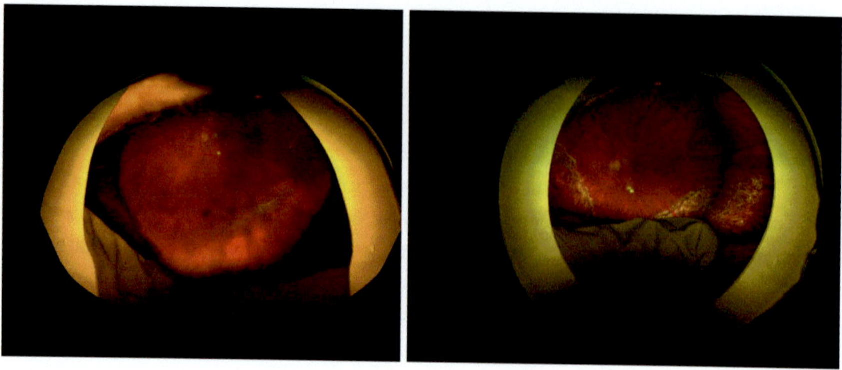

Fig. 41.2 16-year-old Ehlers-Danlos Syndrome. Initial presentation of near total retinal detachment with large posterior break through lattice inferotemporal (picture on the left). Patient underwent scleral buckle with vitrectomy. He developed nasal contraction away from original detachment. He subsequently underwent repeat vitrectomy and nasal relaxing retinectomy with cataract extraction and IOL placement. He remained attached at 1 year follow-up with stable inferior scar that attaches to stable nasal retinectomy (picture on the right)

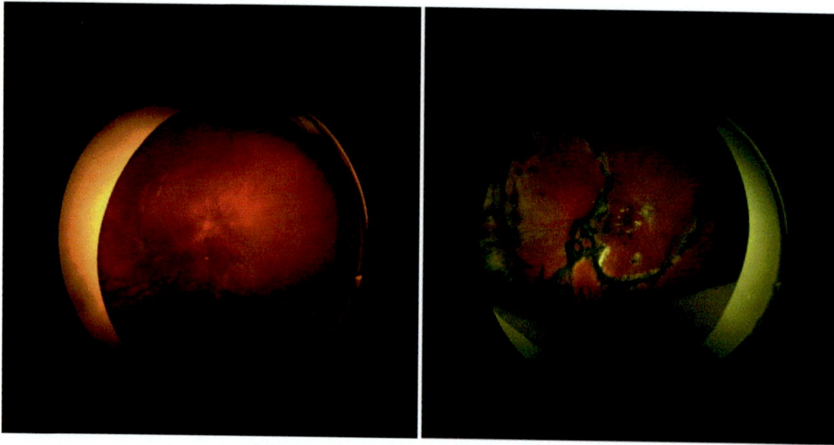

Fig. 41.3 17-year-old non-verbal autistic self-injurious patient. He presented with total right eye retinal detachment and pre-phthisical left eye from chronic retinal detachment with neovascularization. **Picture on the left**: Initial presentation of the right eye. During exam under anesthesia patient was found to have >10 tears. He underwent primary scleral buckle that failed after 1 month due to worsening PVR. He then underwent vitrectomy with lens extraction and IOL with silicone oil. He learned to wear helmet for protection. He remained attached for 1 year. After oil removal he had psychotic episode and severely injured himself again, causing a traumatic very posterior giant retinal tear. Repeat vitrectomy with large relaxing retinectomy was needed to repair retina. **Picture on the right**: Final attached retina at 2 years under oil. He underwent weekly Electroconvulsive Therapy to decrease his violent psychotic episodes. He has done remarkably well and is independent with daily activities in group home

Review Questions

1. Which of the below is one of the most common causes of pediatric rhegmatogenous retinal detachment?

a. Congenital cataracts
b. Retinitis pigmentosa
c. Ocular trauma
d. Congenital glaucoma

2. What intraocular pathology will push surgeon to consider vitrectomy with scleral buckle for pediatric retinal detachment

a. Proliferative vitreoretinopathy
b. Retinal dialysis
c. Macular hole
d. Pseudophakia

Answers

1. (**C**) Ocular trauma is one of the most common causes of pediatric retinal detachment.
2. (**A**) Proliferative Vitreoretinopathy is a strong indication for performing combined SB/PPV.

References

1. Chen C, Huang S, Sun L, Li S, Huang L, Wang Z, Ding X. Analysis of etiologic factors in pediatric rhegmatogenous retinal detachment with genetic testing. Am J Ophthalmol2020. https://doi.org/10.1016/j.ajo.2020.02.015.
2. Yokoyama T, Kato T, Minamoto A, et al. Characteristics and surgical outcomes of paediatric retinal detachment. Eye (Lond). 2004;18:889–92.
3. Read SP, Aziz HA, Kuriyan A, Kothari N, Davis JL, Smiddy WE, Berrocal A. Retinal detachment surgery in a pediatric population. Retina. 2018;38(7):1393–402.
4. Haring G, Wiechens B. Long-term results after scleral buckling surgery in uncomplicated juvenile retinal detachment without proliferative vitreoretinopathy. Retina. 1998;18(6):501–5.
5. Wright LM, Harper CA 3rd, Chang EY. Management of infantile and childhood retinopathies: optimized pediatric pars plana vitrectomy sclerotomy nomogram. Ophthalmol Retina. 2018;2(12):1227–34.
6. Ozdek S, Ozdemir Zeydanli E, Atalay HT, Aktas Z. Anterior elongation of the retina in persistent fetal vasculature: emphasis on retinal complications. Eye (Lond). 2019;33(6): 938–47.
7. Cernichiaro-Espinosa LA, Berrocal AM. Novel surgical technique for inducing posterior vitreous detachment during pars plana vitrectomy for pediatric patients using a flexible loop. Retin Cases Brief Rep. 2020;14:137–40.
8. Ung C, Laíns I, Papakostas TD, Rahmani S, Miller JB. Perfluorocarbon liquid-assisted intraocular foreign body removal. Clin Ophthalmol. 2018;12:1099–104. Published 2018 Jun 18. https://doi.org/10.2147/OPTH.S159509.

9. Moisseiev J, Vidne O, Treister G. Vitrectomy and silicone oil injection in pediatric patients. Retina. 1998;18:221–7.

10. Kuhn F, Kover F, Szabo I, et al. Intracranial migration of silicone oil from an eye with optic pit. Graefe's Arch Clin Exp Ophthalmo. 2006;244:1360–2.

11. Johnson TM, Johnson MW. Pathogenic implications of subretinal gas migration through pits and atypical colobomas of the optic nerve. Arch Ophthalmol. 2004;122(12):1793–800.

12. Weinberg DV, Lyon AT, Greenwald MJ, Mets MB. Rhegmatogenous retinal detachments in children: risk factors and surgical outcomes. Ophthalmology. 2003;110:1708–13.

13. Lee RW, Mayer EJ, Markham RH. The aetiology of pediatric rhegmatogenous retinal detachment: 15 years experience. Eye (Lond). 2008;22(5):636–40.

14. Smith JM, Ward LT, Townsend JH, Yan J, Hendrick AM, Cribbs BE, Hubbard GB. Rhegmatogenous retinal detachment in children: clinical factors predictive of successful surgical repair. Ophthalmology. 2019;126(9):1263–70.

15. Gurler B, Coskun E, Öner V, et al. Clinical characteristics and surgical outcomes of pediatric rhegmatogenous retinal detachment. Int Ophthalmol 2016;36:521–5.

16. Soheilian M, Ramezani A, Malihi M, et al. Clinical features and surgical outcomes of pediatric rhegmatogenous retinal detachment. Retina 2009;29:545–51.

17. Wang NK, Tsai CH, Chen YP, et al. Pediatric rhegmatogenous retinal detachment in East Asians. Ophthalmology 2005;112:1890–5.

18. Al-Zaaidi S, Al-Rashaed S, Al-Harthi E, Al-Kahtani E, Abu El-Asrar AM. Rhegmatogenous retinal detachment in children 16 years of age or younger. Clin Ophthalmol. 2013;7:1001–14.

19. Gonzales CR, Singh S, Yu F, et al. Pediatric rhegmatogenous retinal detachment: clinical features and surgical outcomes. Retina. 2008;28:847–52.

20. Butler TKH, Kiel AW, Orr GM. Anatomical and visual outcome of retinal detachment surgery in children. Br J Ophthalmol. 2001;85:1437–9.

21. Huang Y-C, Chu Y-C, Wang N-K, Lai C-C, Chen K-J, Hwang Y-S, Wu W-C (2017) Impact of etiology on the outcome of pediatric rhegmatogenous retinal detachment. Retina.

22. McElnea E, Stephenson K, Gilmore S, O'Keefe M, Keegan D. Paediatric retinal detachment: aetiology, characteristics and outcomes. Int J Ophthalmol. 2018;11(2):262–6.

23. Oono Y, Uehara K, Haruta M, Yamakawa R. Characteristics and surgical outcomes of pediatric rhegmatogenous retinal detachment. Clin Ophthalmol. 2012;6:939–43.

24. Ozdek S, Kiliç A, Gurelik G, Hasanreisoglu B. Scleral buckling technique for longstanding inferior rhegmatogenous retinal detachments with subretinal bands. Ann Ophthalmol (Skokie). 2008 Spring;40(1):35–8.

25. Errera MH, Liyanage SE, Moya R, Wong SC, Ezra E. Primary scleral buckling for pediatric rhegmatogenous retinal detachment. Retina. 2015;35(7):1441–9.

26. Carranza-Casas M, Quiroz-González E, Hernández-Reyes A, et al. Pediatric rhegmatogenous retinal detachment: predictors of anatomic and functional success. Int Ophthalmol. 2021;41:2777–88.

27. Rossin EJ, Tsui I, Wong SC, Hou KK, Prakhunhungsit S, Blair MP, Shapiro MJ, Leishman L, Nagiel A, Lifton JA, Quiram P, Ringeisen AL, Henderson RH, Arruti N, Buzzacco DM, Kusaka S, Ferrone PJ, Belin PJ, Chang E, Hubschman JP, Murray TG, Leung EH, Wu WC, Olsen KR, Harper CA 3rd, Rahmani S, Goldstein J, Lee T, Nudleman E, Cernichiaro-Espinosa LA, Chhablani J, Berrocal AM, Yonekawa Y. Traumatic retinal detachment in patients with self-injurious behavior: an international multicenter study. Ophthalmol Retina. 2021;5(8):805–14.

28. Chang PY, Yang CM, Yang CH, et al. Clinical characteristics and surgical outcomes of pediatric rhegmatogenous retinal detachment in Taiwan. Am J Ophthalmol. 2005;139:1067–72.

29. Al Taisan AA, Alshamrani AA, AlZahrani AT, Al-Abdullah AA. Pars plana vitrectomy vs combined pars plana vitrectomy-scleral buckle for primary repair of pediatrics retinal detachment. Clin Ophthalmol. 2021;15:1949–55.

Pneumatic Retinopexy: Is There a Role in Pediatric Rhegmatogenous Retinal Detachment (RRD)?

42

Wei Wei Lee and Rajeev H. Muni

Abstract

Pneumatic retinopexy is an elegant office-based procedure that can be very useful in the management of select pediatric rhegmatogenous retinal detachments. Specifically, children meeting morphological clinical trial criteria (PIVOT) can have superior functional outcomes and faster recovery while minimizing potential morbidity with more invasive procedures. Success with pneumatic retinopexy is dependent on thorough baseline clinical evaluation, proper technique, and careful follow-up with timely transition to an operating room procedure when required. All pediatric vitreoretinal surgeons should gain training and experience so that they are comfortable and competent at performing pneumatic retinopexy in appropriate pediatric cases.

Keyword

Pneumatic retinopexy · pediatric retinal detachment

Case presentations

Case 1: PIVOT criteria

A 15-year-old boy presented with reduced vision in the left eye for one day. Examination revealed a left fovea split rhegmatogenous retinal detachment (RRD) from 9 to 2 o'clock with a retinal break at the 10 o'clock position (Fig. 42.1).

Supplementary Information The online version contains supplementary material available at https://doi.org/10.1007/978-3-031-14506-3_42.

W. W. Lee · R. H. Muni (✉)
Department of Ophthalmology and Vision Sciences, University of Toronto, Toronto, Canada
e-mail: rajeev.muni@gmail.com

601

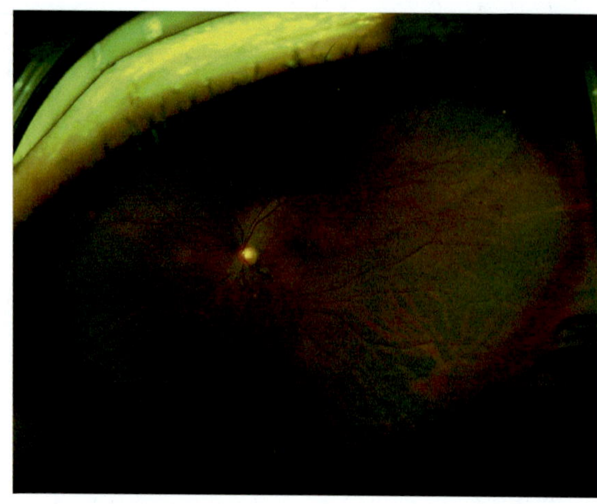

Fig. 42.1 PIVOT criteria retinal detachment. Ultra-widefield color fundus photo of left eye demonstrating fovea split rhegmatogenous retinal detachment from 9 to 2 o'clock

Case 2: Extended criteria

A 16-year-old boy presented with reduced vision in the left eye for two days. Examination revealed a left fovea off RRD from 8 to 2 o'clock with 4 clock hours retinal dialysis superiorly (Fig. 42.2).

Case 3: Complex case with PIVOT criteria

A 12-year-old boy with Marfan syndrome and subluxated lens, underwent a right lensectomy and sutured Gortex intraocular lens by anterior segment surgeon with no vitrectomy. He presented with a right fovea on RRD from 2 to 9 o'clock with a retinal tear at the 3 o'clock position (Fig. 42.3).

Case 4: Complex case with Extended criteria

A 12-year-old girl with Stickler syndrome presented with sudden onset reduced vision in the left eye that morning. Examination revealed a left total retinal detachment and giant retinal tear from 10 to 5 o'clock (Fig. 42.4).

Introduction

Pediatric rhegmatogenous retinal detachment (RRD) is a sight-threatening condition which may require urgent surgical intervention. There are several methods of repairing a pediatric retinal detachment including scleral buckle, pars plana vitrectomy, pneumatic retinopexy and combined vitrectomy and scleral buckle. Traditionally, scleral buckle has been the most common method that has been utilized for repairing a pediatric RRD. This is because vitreous removal in children can be fraught with technical difficulty which can lead to surgical failure and sight-threatening complications. This particularly applies to patients who have an

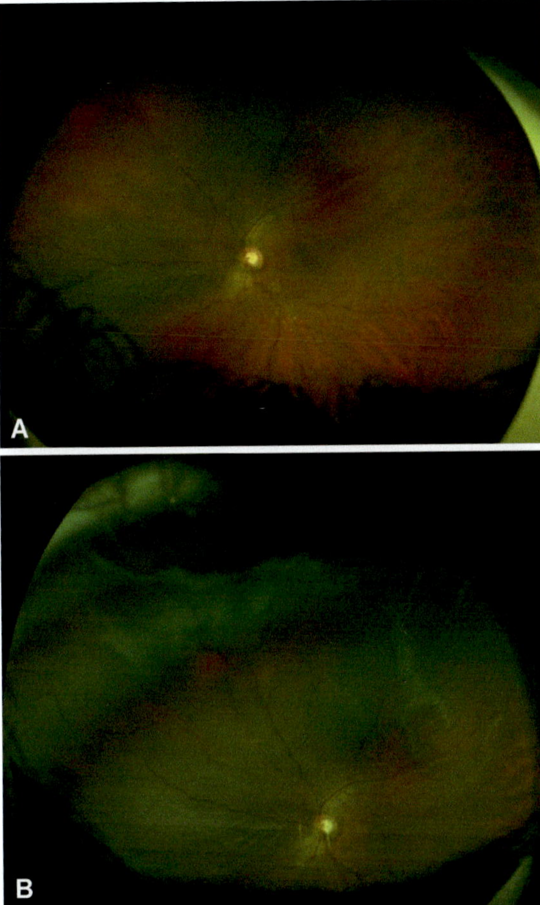

Fig. 42.2 Extended criteria retinal detachment with 4 clock hours retinal dialysis. Ultra-widefield color images demonstrating left fovea off retinal detachment from 8 to 2 o'clock **A** with a 4-clock hour retinal dialysis extending from 10 to 1 o'clock **B**

attached posterior hyaloid, where addressing the peripheral break with a scleral buckle can be a relatively simple and elegant solution. However, there are some limitations of scleral buckle, and like all surgical procedures there are some risks. These risks include the possibility of scleral perforation with possible supra-choroidal or subretinal hemorrhage. Patients who undergo an external drainage procedure can also have hemorrhagic complications or retinal incarceration. These complications can lead to recurrent retinal detachment and proliferative vitreo-retinopathy, which leads to a very guarded prognosis, particularly in children. Other post-operative complications can include choroidal effusions, diplopia, and ptosis. Despite, all of these potential risks and complications with scleral buckle, this is still the most popular treatment, especially compared to vitrectomy which would be considered to have greater risks as a result of difficulty associated with vitreous removal and greater risk of failure. We will not discuss all the potential risks of vitrectomy in this chapter.

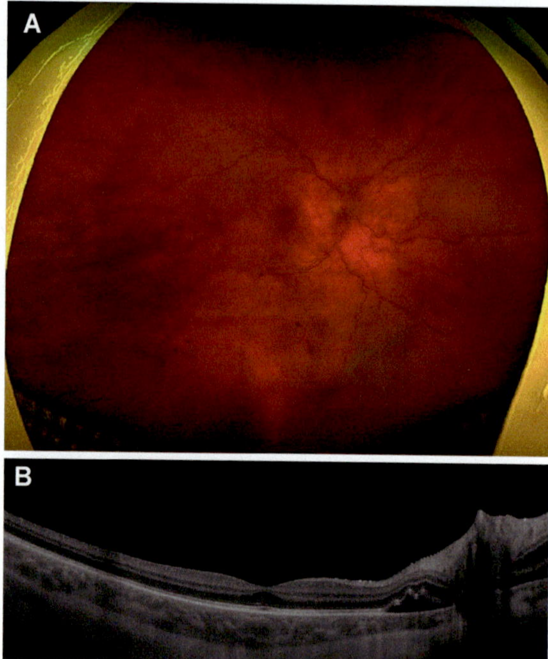

Fig. 42.3 Right fovea on retinal detachment in Marfan syndrome. Ultra-widefield color fundus image of the right eye upon presentation demonstrating retinal detachment from 2 to 9 o'clock **A**. Retinal break at 3 o'clock is very close to the ora, not visible on this image. Swept-source optical coherent tomography of the right eye at presentation demonstrating subretinal fluid nasally and temporal to the disc **B**

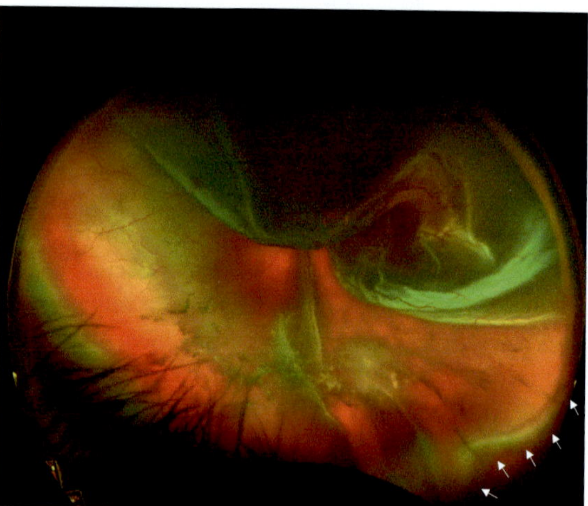

Fig. 42.4 Left total retinal detachment with giant retinal tear in Stickler syndrome. Ultra-widefield color fundus imaging of the left eye upon presentation demonstrating bullous total retinal detachment with giant retinal tear from 10 to 5 o'clock (white arrows) and vitreous veils

Role of Pneumatic Retinopexy

Pneumatic retinopexy is an elegant and minimally invasive office-based technique that can be used to repair certain pediatric RRDs. There are several reasons why pneumatic retinopexy should be considered in selected cases.

- It can be performed immediately in the office.
- Immediate access to the procedure with appropriate positioning can allow the fovea to be protected in macula-on cases and can allow rapid foveal reattachment in approximately 2 hours in patients who carry out face down positioning. This allows reattachment of the photoreceptors and reestablishment of normal photoreceptor-RPE exchange.
- Pneumatic retinopexy is a less invasive procedure, it avoids many of the potential complications that come with operating room procedures such as scleral buckle or vitrectomy.

The youngest patient that the authors have treated in the clinic with subconjunctival anesthesia was 9 years old. One of the drawbacks of pneumatic retinopexy is the potentially lower single-procedure reattachment rate. In the pneumatic retinopexy trial that compared scleral buckle vs pneumatic retinopexy, although scleral buckle had a higher single-procedure reattachment rate, the difference was not statistically significant [1]. At the same time, patients in the pneumatic group had better visual acuity outcomes, particularly in macula-off patients. It is also important to note that patients who failed a pneumatic retinopexy and went on to have a subsequent scleral buckle, did just as well as patients in the primary scleral buckle group. In other words, a pneumatic attempt did not jeopardize future success. Another recent trial involving pneumatic retinopexy was the PIVOT trial that compared pneumatic retinopexy to pars plana vitrectomy [2]. This trial demonstrated that patients in the pneumatic group achieved superior ETDRS visual acuity at every time point including the one-year primary endpoint. Furthermore, patients in the PPV group had more vertical metamorphopsia and worse vision-related quality of life in the first 6 months. There was a 12% lower risk of a single-procedure reattachment in the pneumatic group. However, like the pneumatic retinopexy trial, patients who did not achieve reattachment with pneumatic retinopexy, went on to have reattachment with subsequent vitrectomy. Again, the failure of pneumatic retinopexy did not compromise future success and future functional outcomes.

There have also been a whole host of studies that have assessed the "integrity" of retinal reattachment that have demonstrated that pneumatic retinopexy is associated with better anatomic outcomes, such as less retinal displacement, less discontinuity of the outer retinal bands and less outer retinal folds compared to vitrectomy [3–6]. This is likely related to the minimally invasive procedure with a smaller gas fill, where the retinal reattachment is achieved by a slow and natural reabsorption of subretinal fluid by the retinal pigment epithelial pump, rather than forced internal drainage during vitrectomy. It is likely that scleral buckle also shares many of these "integrity" advantages with pneumatic retinopexy when compared to vitrectomy.

With an understanding of the current evidence surrounding pneumatic retinopexy in comparison to scleral buckle and vitrectomy, it seems logical that pneumatic retinopexy should be considered in specific pediatric patients that meet clinical trial criteria. The fear of an initial pneumatic failure should not dissuade pediatric retina specialists from attempting the procedure in suitable candidates. The potential for successful reattachment, with a minimally invasive procedure is enticing and should not be left off the table. In a recent retrospective study that assessed the outcomes following pneumatic retinopexy in children that met PIVOT trial criteria, we found a single-procedure reattachment rate of 85% at 3 months and 75% at final follow-up with excellent visual acuity outcomes [7]. These results compared favorable to published data following retinal detachment repair with other techniques such as scleral buckle and vitrectomy in children.

It is also important to consider some of the anatomic and physiologic aspects that make pneumatic retinopexy a potentially suitable procedure in children. Firstly, in children the vitreous is formed. It may seem somewhat counterintuitive, but this can be a substantial advantage. The formed vitreous can potentially help tamponade the retinal break internally once the gas bubble is injected, much like how it may help to occlude the break with scleral buckle surgery where the break may be rotated into the peripheral vitreous. Secondly, children have very strong RPE pump activity and simply occluding the break with the gas bubble can quickly result in retinal reattachment in a few hours. Thirdly, children are very healthy and flexible, making posturing easily achievable. Children also have the benefit of parental supervision to ensure positioning compliance.

Selection Criteria

We recommend that all pediatric patients who meet PIVOT trial criteria [2] and can be properly examined in the clinic be considered for pneumatic retinopexy. These patients are likely to do very well with the procedure. Of note, lens status, posterior vitreous detachment status, extent, and location of the RRD do not factor into the decision. Break location is a critical factor.

PIVOT Trial criteria:

- A single retinal break or group of breaks, no larger than one clock hour (30^0), in detached retina
- All breaks in the detached retina to lie above the 8 and 4 o'clock meridian
- Breaks or lattice degeneration in attached retina at any location (even inferior) were permitted

Furthermore, in some cases, with appropriate patients, extended criteria can be utilized. Extended criteria:

- Multiple retinal tears larger than one clock hour in detached retina above the 8 and 4 o'clock meridian
- Retinal dialysis
- Giant retinal tears

In selected cases, pneumatic retinopexy can also be used in complex cases.

- Myopic retinal detachment
- Traumatic retinal detachment
- Retinal detachment after cataract surgery (pseudophakic, sutured intraocular lenses, aphakic)
- Systemic conditions (Marfan syndrome, Stickler syndrome)

Regardless of the indication, these are few important points:

- Laser retinopexy or cryotherapy should be performed on all retinal tears, holes, or lattice degeneration in the attached retina before gas injection.
- Thorough scleral depressed fundus examination to identify all breaks prior to gas injection is the key to a successful treatment
- To follow patients carefully with thorough fundus examination at every visit following pneumatic retinopexy
  - It is important to determine if there is adequate tamponade of the break
- Residual subretinal fluid can take time to go away.
  - As long as the break is closed and treated, it is important to be patient to allow the fluid to resorb.
- It is important to recognize when the procedure is failing.
  - If the break remains open after a few days
  - When the retinal detachment is worsening
  - In some instances, this can be the result of misunderstanding regarding positioning instructions and sometimes revisiting compliance can be helpful.
- However, if it is clearly failing and not salvageable, then it is important to swiftly proceed to another procedure.
  - This would usually be a scleral buckle. Scleral buckle is carried out with the usual technique. It is important to keep the patient face down prior to surgery to protect the macula and the lens. Also, although we generally prefer non-drainage procedures, if external drainage is required, it is important to be cautious to keep the bubble away from the drainage site as this could force the retina into the sclerotomy. This can be avoided by not rotating the eye with the traction sutures too much during this step.

Pneumatic Retinopexy Technique (see **Video** 1, 2)

The pneumatic retinopexy technique in children has some variations, although the technique is largely the same as that described in the supplementary appendix of the PIVOT trial [2]. Although laser retinopexy following gas injection is generally preferred; in children, always try to use pre-gas injection cryopexy. This relates to the fact that we never know for certain if a child will cooperate with laser retinopexy after the initial pneumatic retinopexy procedure. Often supplement laser retinopexy can be performed at a later date if possible, however the cryopexy treatment can be sufficient in most cases. If laser retinopexy is used instead of cryotherapy, it is usually performed 24–48 h after gas injection. Pneumatic retinopexy is almost always performed under local anesthesia (subconjunctival anesthesia) with no sedation. This can be usually done by talking the child through the procedure and getting buy-in from the parents who can encourage the child. It is important to try to minimize any discomfort for the child, as pain can lead to them no longer cooperating. This is achieved by initially putting topical anesthesia and then subconjunctival anesthesia, which can usually be done with no discomfort. The cryopexy is then performed which can have some minimal discomfort, but this can be minimized by accurate probe placement for efficient treatment without wasted cryotherapy applications. Once the cryotherapy is performed, an anterior chamber paracentesis is performed which is usually painless. Here, special care is taken to avoid touching the lens with the needle. We recommend entering at the inferior limbus parallel to the iris plane and always keeping the 30G needle (attached to a 1°cc syringe with the plunger removed) over the iris to avoid lens contact. The plunger is used for counterpressure to stabilize the eye for entry and to dome up the cornea over the needle tip. Firm counterpressure at the limbus also encourages liquified vitreous to come anteriorly. It is helpful to tap as much fluid as possible, allowing for a larger gas fill. The amount of gas injected is the anterior chamber tap volume plus 0.3cc. So, for example, if 0.4cc is removed from the anterior chamber then 0.7cc is injected. Regardless of how much is removed from the anterior chamber, the minimum volume of 100% sulfur hexafluoride (SF6) gas injected is 0.6cc. During gas injection, the 30G needle (1/2 inches long, on a 3-cc syringe) is advanced to 50% length and then pulled back so the tip is barely in the eye. The gas is then injected in a brisk constant pace from one of the superior quadrants. This technique is to ensure that the gas is injected into the enlarging gas bubble to prevent fish eggs. After gas injection, the central retinal artery is examined. If the artery is occluded or remains pulsatile after 5 min, a repeat anterior chamber tap is performed to reduce the intraocular pressure. On rare occasions, additional anterior chamber paracenteses are required as the anterior chamber reforms. Once the central retinal artery is patent (i.e., it only pulsates with digital pressure), then the patient is given a prescription of antibiotic and steroid eyedrops 4X/day for 5 days and given positioning instructions. Positioning instructions are given in detail to both the child and the family to insure buy-in and compliance. The child is examined daily for the first few days and as the retina reattaches additional laser retinopexy can be applied.

SF6 gas is preferred as it only lasts for 12 days, versus 38 days for perfluoropropane (C3F8) gas. 12 days duration is ideal for pneumatic retinopexy where you want the gas to be used and dissipate quickly once it is no longer required. Leaving the gas in for 38 days in a vitreous filled eye as would be the case with C3F8 is not ideal. In some complex cases, a larger gas bubble is required, in which case sequential gas bubbles of SF6 can be injected (the second bubble usually injected on day 2–3). The second bubble is injected with the exact same technique as the first bubble. In some situations C3F8 may be used, and in those cases 0.3cc of pure gas is injected first, and an anterior chamber paracentesis only performed if required.

Positioning can be with the steamroller maneuver (described in the supplementary appendix of the PIVOT trial [2]) to expedite macular reattachment by expressing some of the subretinal fluid through the retinal break; or support the break positioning where the bubble is immediately placed such that is covers the break and subretinal fluid is pumped out by the retinal pigment epithelium pump. For positioning, we currently recommend the steamroller maneuver where patient is required to be face down for the first 4 h in macula-on cases and 6 h in macula-off cases. We then ask patients to raise their head slowly over a few hours until they reach the head elevated position. This encourages subretinal fluid to be displaced by the buoyant force of the gas bubble through the retinal break. The patient is then advised to position with the bubble on the break for 23 out of 24 h per day for one week. It is important to advise the patient and the family that strict positioning compliance is essential day and night.

Potential Complications

Like all procedures, pneumatic retinopexy can be associated with certain complications. This includes fish eggs or subretinal gas. Fish eggs on their own do not generally compromise success, although it is important to avoid fish eggs from entering the subretinal space. This can be managed by keeping the patient face down for the first 24 h. Usually, most of the fish eggs coalesce as the gas expands. Fish eggs can be avoided with proper technique, where only the needle tip is in the eye, so that the gas is injected at the highest point into an ever-expanding gas bubble. A small amount of subretinal gas does not generally impact successful reattachment, if it is away from the retinal break. Subretinal gas can often be expressed from the subretinal space with scleral depression and specific head movements. If subretinal gas cannot be removed and prevents closure of the retinal break, then the pneumatic retinopexy has failed and another surgical procedure should be carried out. Fortunately, this is a rare occurrence. In another rare circumstance, the gas can be injected into the canal of petit. Anterior hyaloidal gas can be managed by keeping the patient face down. Often the gas will break through the anterior hyaloid face as the bubble expands. In rare cases, the gas needs to be removed with a needle in the office or in the operating room with additional surgical procedures to achieve retinal reattachment.

Other complications including lens touch during the procedure, vitreous hemorrhage/hyphema or suprachoroidal gas injection, all of which can initially be observed, and which may not compromise success. As with all RRD repair procedures, it is possible that the retina fails to reattach or re-detaches in the future. Data from clinical trials suggests that pneumatic retinopexy is a durable treatment, with a low proportion of patients having a redetachment after 3 months with pneumatic retinopexy compared to vitrectomy or scleral buckle. It is particularly important to follow patients with pneumatic retinopexy very carefully in the first few months to insure successful reattachment. Inadequate follow-up and redetachment can lead to poor outcomes with proliferative vitreoretinopathy.

Pneumatic Retinopexy Follow-up

Regardless of the indication, it is important to follow patients carefully. We suggest follow-up daily for the first 2 days or more until the laser is successfully completed around all the retinal breaks, then at 1 week, 3 weeks and 2 months post-pneumatic.

At every visit, it is important to determine if there is adequate tamponade of the breaks and if all breaks have been identified. This requires careful examination at every visit. In some cases, patients have residual subretinal fluid that can take time to fully resorb. As long as the break is closed and treated, it is important to be patient to allow the fluid to resorb naturally by the RPE pump. At the same time, if the break remains open after a few days and the detachment is worsening, it is important to recognize that the pneumatic retinopexy is failing. In some instances, this can be the result of misunderstanding regarding positioning instructions and sometimes revisiting compliance can be helpful. However, if the pneumatic is clearly failing and not salvageable, then it is important to swiftly proceed to another procedure. This would usually be a scleral buckle in children for the reasons mentioned above. Scleral buckle is usually carried out with the usual technique. It is important to keep the patient face down prior to surgery to protect the macula and the lens. Also, although we generally prefer non-drainage procedures, if external drainage is required, it is important to be cautious to keep the bubble away from the drainage site as this could force the retina into the sclerotomy. This can be avoided by not excessively rotating the eye with the traction sutures during the drainage step.

Summary

In conclusion, pneumatic retinopexy is an elegant and useful technique for RRD repair in certain children. Pneumatic retinopexy should be considered for certain pediatric RRDs, as it is an excellent minimally invasive procedure with superior functional outcomes for patients who have the most to gain in terms of years of quality vision. Success is dependent on thorough clinical examination, proper technique, and careful follow-up. We suggest that all pediatric vitreoretinal surgeons gain experience with the procedure so that they can include it in their armamentarium for pediatric RRD.

Return to Case Presentation

Case 1: PIVOT Criteria

This 15-year-old boy with left fovea-split RRD from 9 to 2 o'clock with a retinal break at 10 o'clock position underwent a pneumatic retinopexy (PnR) on the same day. 0.3cc anterior chamber tap was performed and 0.6cc of 100% SF6 was injected. He was positioned with the steamroller maneuver and once upright, he was then positioned with the head tilted to the left at 45 degrees daytime and lying on his left side with 2 pillows at night. Day 1 after PnR, retina was fully attached (Fig. 42.5) and remained attached during long-term follow-up.

Case 2: Extended Criteria

This 16-year-old boy with fovea-off RRD with a 4-clock hour retinal dialysis underwent cryopexy and pneumatic retinopexy on the day of presentation. 100% SF6 was used as the tamponade and the patient positioned upright after the steamroller maneuver. Day 1 after PnR, there was a residual pocket of subretinal fluid temporally, but the retinal dialysis was attached (Fig. 42.6). The retina was fully attached 2 days after PnR and remained attached long-term (Fig. 42.7).

Case 3: Complex case with PIVOT criteria

This 12-year-old boy with macula on retinal detachment with a retinal break at the 3 o'clock position, underwent cryopexy and pneumatic retinopexy on the same day under local anaesthesia with no sedation (**Video** 1). 0.4cc anterior chamber tap was performed and 0.7cc of 100% SF6 was injected. He was positioned face down for

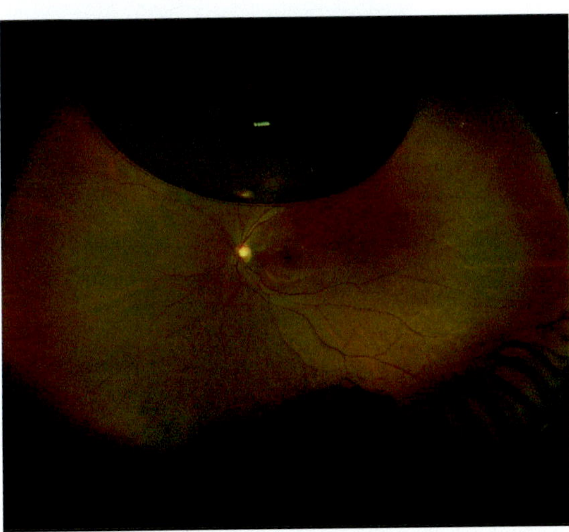

Fig. 42.5 Day 1 after Pneumatic Retinopexy. Ultra-widefield color fundus photo demonstrated that the retina was reattached with a single gas bubble in the eye

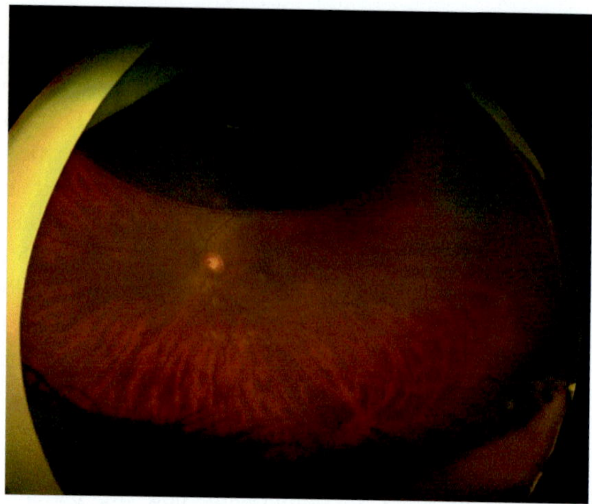

Fig. 42.6 Day 1 post pneumatic retinopexy. Color fundus image demonstrating retinal reattachment at 1 day following pneumatic retinopexy

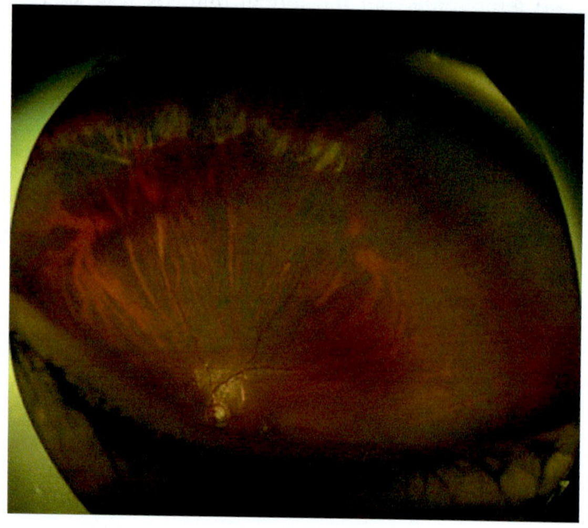

Fig. 42.7 Week 2 post pneumatic retinopexy. Ultra-widefield color image demonstrating an attached retina with cryopexy scars superiorly over area of retinal dialysis

the first 4 h and then lying on his right side. 2 days following PnR, his retina was attached and laser retinopexy was added in the location of the retinal break (Fig. 42.8). He remained attached at 6 months.

Case 4: Complex case with Extended criteria

This 12-year-old girl with a one-day history of vision loss and a left total retinal detachment and giant retinal tear from 10 to 5 o'clock underwent a left pneumatic retinopexy under local anaesthesia with no sedation (**Video** 2). She was positioned face down for the first 6 h then the right side down with the head overhanging the edge of the bed. A day after PnR, the macula was attached, and the retina was attached temporal and inferiorly (Fig. 42.9). Laser retinopexy was performed from

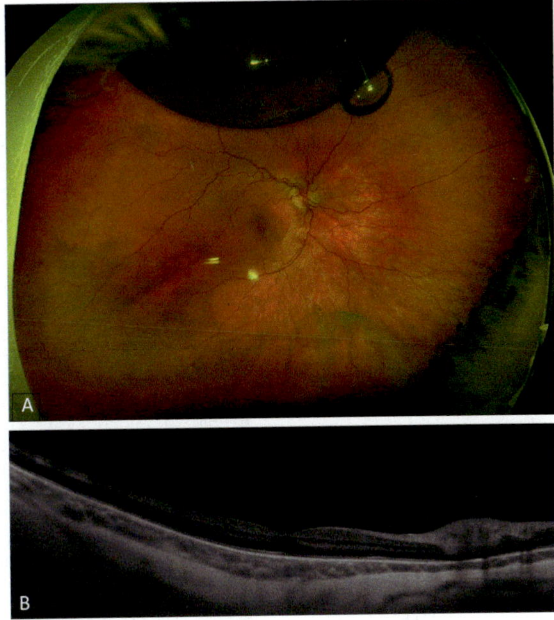

Fig. 42.8 Day 2 after pneumatic retinopexy. Ultra-widefield color fundus imaging of the right eye demonstrated attached retina with gas bubble in eye **A.** Swept-source optical coherence tomography of the fovea demonstrated that the fovea was attached **B**

2 to 5 o'clock posterior to the edge of the GRT in attached retina. 2 days after PnR, laser was completed temporal and inferiorly (Fig. 42.10) and the child was required to alter her position to upright in order to tamponade the GRT superiorly. Laser retinopexy was added superiorly and completed surrounding the GRT from 10 to 5 o'clock on day 4. 6 days after PnR, the retina was fully attached, and laser completed 360 degrees (Fig. 42.11). She remained attached at 4 months (Fig. 42.12) when this chapter was concluded.

Review Questions

1. Pediatric pneumatic retinopexy can be successful in children because

(a) Cooperative children can position very well
(b) Parents generally supervise the positioning
(c) There is a very competent retinal pigment epithelial pump in children
(d) Many children over the age of 9 can tolerate the procedure well
(e) All of the above

2. Pediatric pneumatic retinopexy can be considered in children with

(a) A one traumatic clock-hour superior dialysis
(b) High myopia with superior atrophic holes within one clock hour and inferior lattice in attached retina

Fig. 42.9 Day 1 after pneumatic retinopexy. Ultra-widefield color imaging demonstrates attached retina temporal **A** and inferiorly **B** with laser marks seen at the posterior edge of the giant retinal tear from 2 to 5 o'clock. Swept-source optical coherence tomography of the macula demonstrated an attached fovea with intact ellipsoid zone **C**

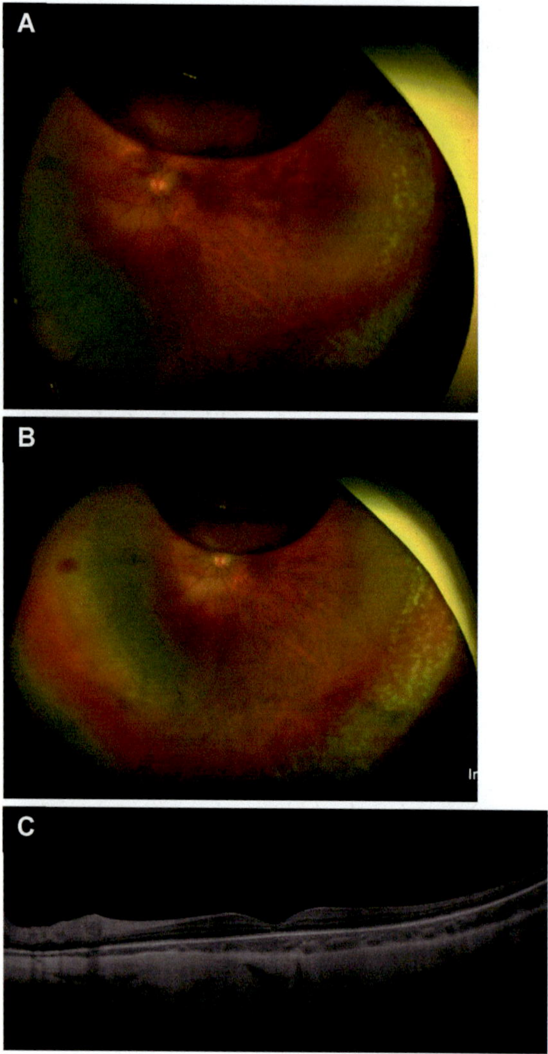

(c) Marfan syndrome with a superior horseshoe tear

(d) Stickler syndrome with multiple breaks within one clock at 9 o'clock

(e) All of the above

Answers

1. E
2. E

Fig. 42.10 Day 2 after pneumatic retinopexy. Ultra-widefield color imaging demonstrates attached retina temporal and inferiorly with laser marks seen over the posterior edge of the giant retinal tear from 1 to 5 o'clock

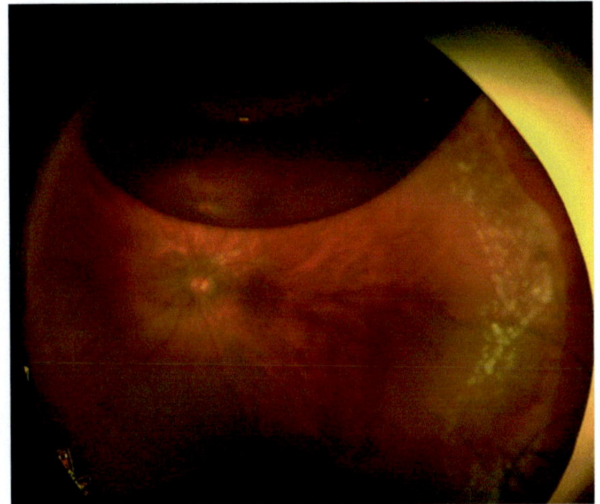

Fig. 42.11 Day 6 after Pneumatic Retinopexy. Ultra-widefield color imaging demonstrates attached retina with laser marks seen over the posterior edge of the giant retinal tear from temporal **A** and superiorly **B**

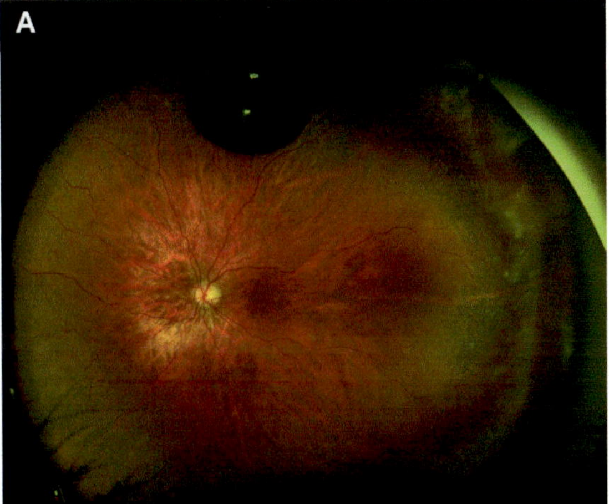

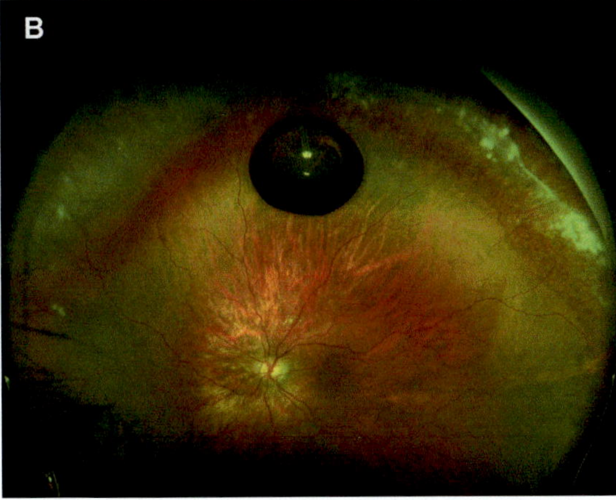

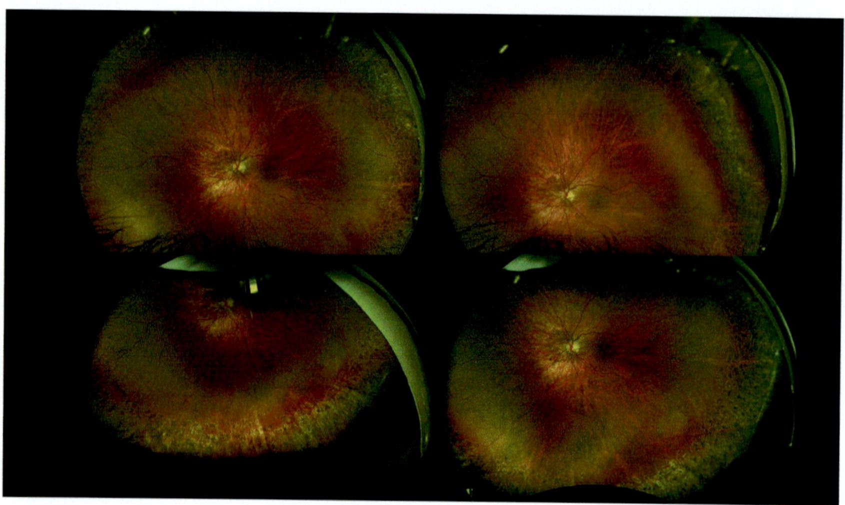

Fig. 42.12 Month 4 after Pneumatic Retinopexy. Ultra-widefield color imaging demonstrates attached retina with 360 degrees laser

References

1. Tornambe PE, Hilton GF. Pneumatic retinopexy. A multicenter randomized controlled clinical trial comparing pneumatic retinopexy with scleral buckling. The Retinal Detachment Study Group. Ophthalmology 1989;96(6):772–83; discussion 784. https://doi.org/10.1016/S0161-6420(89)32820-X
2. Hillier RJ, Felfeli T, Berger AR, Wong DT, Altomare F, Dai D, Giavedoni LR, Kertes PJ, Kohly RP, Muni RH. The pneumatic retinopexy versus vitrectomy for the management of primary rhegmatogenous retinal detachment outcomes randomized trial (PIVOT). Ophthalmology. 2019;126(4):531–9. https://doi.org/10.1016/j.ophtha.2018.11.014.
3. Francisconi CLM, Marafon SB, Figueiredo NA, Juncal VR, Shaikh S, Bhambra N, Ta Kim DT, Brosh K, Qian J, Chaudhary V, Berger AR, Giavedoni LR, Wong DT, Altomare F, Chow DR, Di Simplicio S, Kadhim MR, Deonarain D, Hillier RJ, Muni RH. Displacement following pneumatic vs vitrectomy for retinal detachment (ALIGN). Ophthalmology 2021; S0161–6420(21)00943-X. https://doi.org/10.1016/j.ophtha.2021.12.007.
4. Brosh K, Francisconi CLM, Qian J, Sabatino F, Juncal VR, Hillier RJ, Chaudhary V, Berger AR, Giavedoni LR, Wong DT, Altomare F, Kadhim MR, Newsom RB, Marafon SB, Muni RH. Retinal displacement following pneumatic retinopexy vs pars plana vitrectomy for rhegmatogenous retinal detachment. JAMA Ophthalmol. 2020;138(6):652–9.
5. Muni RH, Felfeli T, Sadda SR, Juncal VR, Francisconi CLM, Nittala MG, Lindenberg S, Gunnemann F, Berger AR, Wong DT, Altomare F, Giavedoni LR, Kohly RP, Kertes PJ, Sarraf D, Hillier RJ. Postoperative photoreceptor integrity following pneumatic retinopexy vs pars plana vitrectomy for retinal detachment repair: a post hoc optical coherence tomography analysis from the pneumatic retinopexy versus vitrectomy for the management of primary rhegmatogenous retinal detachment outcomes randomized trial. JAMA Ophthalmol. 2021;139 (6):620–7. https://doi.org/10.1001/jamaophthalmol.2021.0803.

6. Lee WW, Bansal A, Sadda SR, Sarraf D, Berger AR, Wong DT, Kertes PJ, Kohly RP, Hillier RJ, Muni RH. Outer retinal folds after pars plana vitrectomy vs. pneumatic retinopexy for retinal detachment repair: post hoc analysis from PIVOT. Ophthalmol Retina 2021;S2468-6530(21)00284-0. https://doi.org/10.1016/j.oret.2021.09.001.
7. Figueiredo N, Warder DC, Muni RH, Lee WW, Yong SO, Kertes PJ. Pneumatic retinopexy as a treatment for rhegmatogenous retinal detachment in pediatric patients meeting PIVOT criteria. Can J Ophthalmol. 2021;S0008-4182(21):00214-23. https://doi.org/10.1016/j.jcjo.2021.06.007.

Closed Globe Injuries

43

Umut Karaca, Murat Kucukevcilioglu, and Ali Hakan Durukan

Abstract

Closed globe injuries are an important cause of acquired visual impairment and monocular blindness in childhood age that can lead to a variety of social and economic results. Accidental occurrence, single eye involvement, and preventable trauma are the common characteristics of closed globe injuries. As a result of direct and indirect contusion forces, the cornea and sclera remain largely intact, while other eye structures of anterior and posterior segment can be significantly damaged. Diagnosis, treatment, and management are challenging when compared with the adult age group.

Keywords

Blunt ocular trauma · Closed globe injuries · Pediatric age · Posterior segment · Vitreous hemorrhage · Retinal tear · Retinal detachment

Supplementary Information The online version contains supplementary material available at https://doi.org/10.1007/978-3-031-14506-3_43.

U. Karaca
Department of Ophthalmology, School of Medicine, Suleyman Demirel University, Isparta, Turkey

M. Kucukevcilioglu · A. H. Durukan (✉)
Department of Ophthalmology, Gulhane School of Medicine, University of Health Sciences, Ankara, Turkey
e-mail: drahdurukan@yahoo.com

Introduction

Background

Ocular trauma remains the leading cause of monocular vision loss and blindness, particularly in pediatric patients. Data from the American Academy of Pediatrics (AAP) show that two-thirds of ocular injuries occur in the pediatric age group (under 16 years) (most often in the 9–11 age range). Closed-globe injuries are generally caused by blunt objects, in which the cornea and sclera remain intact, while other eye structures can be damaged to various degrees. The terminology and classification necessary for the assessment of trauma and consensus on therapeutic interventions are well defined by the Birmingham Eye Trauma Terminology (BETT) and Ocular Trauma Score System [1–3].

Epidemiology

Closed-globe injuries constitute approximately half of all ocular traumas in the pediatric age group. Statistically, the male sex is affected three to five times more in injuries. In a cohort analysis of 12,687 patients by Shah et al., 41.9% of the cases were closed globe injuries, with a mean age of 10.2 and an m/f ratio of 2.3/1 [4]. Madan et al. determined the rate of closed globe injury to be 24.9% in a series of 350 cases and showed that most of them were sports injuries [5]. Although there was no statistically significant difference in the total number of accidental eye injuries during the Covid-19 lockdown, the rate of closed globe injuries accounted for almost two-thirds of all injuries [6]. Closed-globe injuries can occur in daily life, often at home or at school, during sports or play, most commonly as a result of a thrown object or struck in the eye (finger, fist, or ball) [7]. Child abuse or shaken baby syndrome is another important cause of asymmetric bilateral closed-globe trauma in children [8]. Despite the primary standard treatment, glaucoma or vitreous hemorrhage, which may develop due to the late effects of trauma, may threaten vision. Although there is no full-thickness perforation after direct impact of mostly blunt objects on the eye, the involvement of posterior segment structures such as the retina and optic nerve may result in severe vision loss [9].

Pathophysiology

The pathophysiological mechanism underlying the damage after blunt object crush is a sudden increase in pressure worldwide, transmission of pressure within the globe, and contraction—reexpansion of the equatorial region. Damage may occur at the contact point (coup) or opposite the contact point (contrecoup).

Clinical Features

Anterior and posterior segment pathologies that may develop due to closed-eye trauma can be classified as shown in Table 43.1. In this section, the current approach for posterior segment pathologies due to closed-globe injuries is examined.

1. Vitreous

1.1 Vitreous Hemorrhage

Traumatic vitreous hemorrhage is the most common posterior segment pathology in closed-globe injuries and is accompanied by retinal pathology in approximately half of the cases. In contrast, the most common cause of vitreous hemorrhage in the pediatric age group is closed-globe trauma. In contrast to adults, diagnosis is challenging due to poor patient cooperation, difficulty in anamnesis, and examination. On the other hand, the presence of comorbidities, necessity of general anesthesia, and refractive rehabilitation present a challenge to comprehensively manage this condition.

Following the post-traumatic hemorrhage, coagulation (1–2 days) was followed by fibrinolysis and phagocytosis (5–10 days). Spontaneous resolution of the coagulum from the vitreous cavity may occur within a period–1–6 months, depending on the amount of hemorrhage. Prolonged retention of vitreous hemorrhage is associated with other complications such as proliferative vitreoretinopathy and ghost cell glaucoma [10].

It is difficult to establish a consensus on the approach and treatment plan for children with vitreous hemorrhage. Initially, the possibility of globe rupture and other pathologies accompanying the hemorrhage (such as retinal detachment) should be excluded. Within this period, the patient should be examined at regular

Table 43.1 Closed globe injuries

Anterior segment	Posterior segment	
1. Hyphema	**Vitreous**	1. Vitreous Hemorrhage
2. Cataract		2. Vitreous base avulsion
3. Zonular dialysis/Iridodialysis		3. Posterior vitreous detachment
4. Angle recession/Trabecular Hemorrhage	**Retina**	1. Commotio Retina
5. Corneal/Scleral Lamellar Laceration		2. Retinal tears/Dialysis
6. Hyphema		3. Retinal detachment
		4. Pre/intra/subretinal Hemorrhage
		5. Epiretinal membrane/Macular hole
	Choroid	1. Choroidal rupture
		2. Choroidal Hemorrhage

intervals, followed by B-scan ultrasonography, and bed rest should be recommended by increasing head height. B-scan ultrasonography performed at regular intervals is important in terms of showing both the condition of the vitreous and additional posterior segment pathologies, such as retinal tear or detachment. Regular fundoscopic examination is important for the presence of retinal tears or detachment.

Treatment options can be classified into three subgroups: observation/medical therapy, nonsurgical therapy (laser/cryotherapy), and surgery. A review of the existing literature revealed that almost half of the cases were treated with observation or medical therapy. However, surgery is often preferred in cases of prolonged hemorrhage, bilateral involvement, retinal dialysis/detachment, ghost cell glaucoma, and subretinal/suprachoroidal hemorrhage. Early surgery may be considered in patients under the age of seven because of the risk of amblyopia. The most appropriate treatment option should be determined by performing a detailed assessment, including the patient's age, severity of the trauma, and risks of general anesthesia.

1.2 Vitreous Base Avulsion

Vitreous base avulsion is the breakup of the anterior portion of the vitreous from the retina or pars plana. It is also defined as the 'bucket-handle symptom' due to opacities circulating in the peripheral retina. In general, there is no need for surgical intervention. However, owing to the risk of retinal tears or retinal dialysis, peripheral retinal monitoring is recommended.

2 Retina

2.1 Commotio Retina

The commotio retina (Berlin edema in macular involvement) is characterized by gray-white opacification of the retina following blunt ocular trauma. Histopathologically, it is associated with the disruption of the photoreceptor outer segment and retinal pigment epithelium. Recent optical coherence tomography angiography studies have revealed foveal avascular zone enlargement and microvascular injuries. There is no proven effective treatment for commotio retinas. The prognosis may vary depending on the severity of trauma. Permanent vision loss may develop in the presence of concomitant subretinal/choroidal hemorrhage.

2.2 Retinal Tears/Dialysis

Retinal tears are tractional retinal injuries that occur after vitreous mobilization due to coup and counter-coup effects after closed-globe trauma. Tears that exceed three clock hours (90°or more) are called giant retinal tears. Dialysis is often seen in the lower temporal quadrant as a result of detachment of the vitreous base and rupture of the ora serrata. In contrast to adults, posttraumatic tear and detachment development are more common in children and young adults. Retinal dialysis, which is

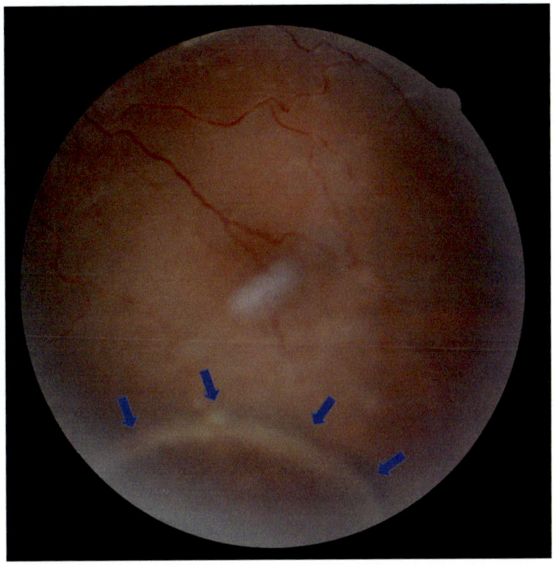

Fig. 43.1 Color fundus photograph of the right eye showing a retinal dialysis in the temporal periphery with adjacent retinal detachment. Blue arrows indicate the border of the dialysis

one of the rarest causes of retinal detachment, is also considered one of the leading causes of traumatic retinal detachment in children and young adults (Fig. 43.1).

Early diagnosis of retinal tears/dialysis is key to avoiding intensive treatment and permanent vision loss. In the pediatric age group, both the detection of retinal tears and management of retinal detachment that may develop due to tears are challenging. In some cases, indirect ophthalmoscopy can be performed under general anesthesia in young patients. Re-examination may be required at intervals, as vitreous or preretinal hemorrhage may obscure the view.

Healthy and formed vitreous gel, absence of PVD, strong vitreoretinal interface association, surgical difficulties, associated ocular or systemic disease (high myopia or Stickler syndrome), accompanying traumatic/subluxed cataract or glaucoma, postoperative positioning, and visual rehabilitation should be considered in the management. Detachment prophylaxis can be performed using transscleral cryoretinopexy or laser retinopexy. Scleral buckling surgery is a highly successful surgical option, especially in young patients, because it provides anatomical integrity and increases postoperative visual acuity. Fortunately, advances in instrumentation, visualization, illumination, and manipulation of detached retinas have contributed significantly to improved surgical success (Fig. 43.2).

2.3 Pre/Intra/Subretinal Hemorrhage

After closed-globe injury, retinal vascular damage or retinal tears may result in anterior, intraretinal, and/or posterior retinal hemorrhages. Extensive fundoscopy and optical coherence tomography (OCT) can be used in this location.

It is important to determine the location in terms of treatment planning.

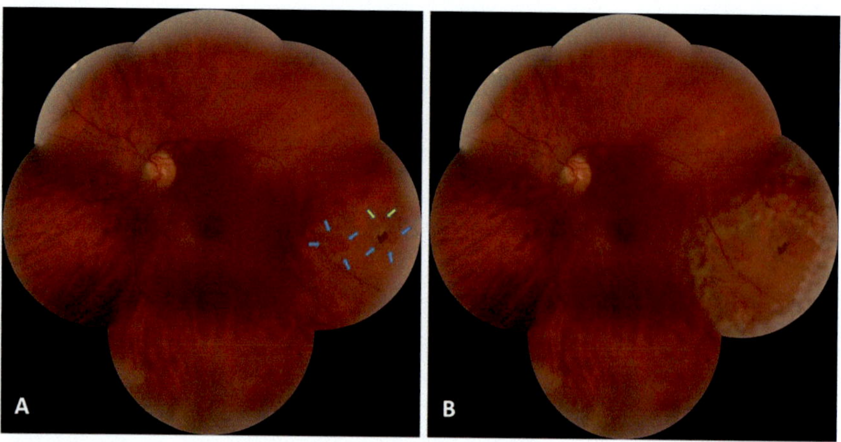

Fig. 43.2 **A**. Two horseshoe retinal tears (blue arrows) and a retinal hole (yellow arrow) in the temporal periphery of the left eye due to closed globe injury. **B**. Laser photocoagulation around the tears and hole

- Preretinal (sub-hyaloid/sub-ILM) hemorrhage can lead to retinal toxicity and epiretinal membrane development. Extensive sub-hyaloid hemorrhages (greater than 2-disc diameter hemorrhages within 3 weeks after trauma) should be treated with YAG laser hyaloidotomy. The injection of tissue plasminogen activator (tPA) and/or gas into the vitreous is another treatment option.
- Intraretinal hemorrhages should be followed up to spontaneous resolution.
- Subretinal hemorrhage should be evaluated for accompanying choroidal pathologies. Submacular hemorrhage should be treated immediately to prevent photoreceptors.

2.4 Traumatic Macular Hole

Pediatric MHs are generally much less common than in adults. However, trauma is a more common predisposing factor for MHs in children than in adults. The incidence of macular hole after closed-globe injury in adults is 1%; this rate is 5% in the pediatric age group [11]. Although the mechanism of macular hole development after blunt trauma has not been fully elucidated, the tensile force due to equatorial expansion following the axial compression of the globe is thought to be responsible [12].

During treatment, follow-up is usually sufficient. In the literature, it has been reported that approximately two-thirds of cases are closed within 3 months and almost all within 6 months without any treatment [13, 14]. The visual prognosis is better in younger patients. Spontaneous closure is more common in younger patients, those with small macular hole diameters, and in the absence of posterior vitreous detachment [15].

Since many publications have reported spontaneous closure in the first three months after trauma, there is no consensus on when to operate on traumatic MHs that do not close [16]. Although it seems appropriate to wait three months before deciding on surgery, there is no clear information about how long to wait. It has been reported that traumatic holes that underwent delayed vitrectomy one year later were less likely to be closed than those that underwent earlier surgery [17]. We should try to compensate for waiting long enough for spontaneous closure, but not so long as it significantly reduces the likelihood of an anatomically successful outcome. TGF-beta 2, platelet concentrate, serum, and amniotic membranes can be used during surgery. Plasmin-assisted vitreolysis can be performed for tight posterior hyaloids and ILM in children [18, 19] (Fig. 43.3).

2.5 Retinal Detachment

Retinal detachment (RD) is a serious complication of ocular trauma. Although the incidence in the general population is approximately 1 in 10,000 per year, only 1% of these cases are secondary to trauma. The incidence is much lower in children. Retinal detachment can be seen in approximately 0.028% of children aged 17–19 years, and two-thirds of these cases are due to trauma [20]. In children, male sex and open globe injuries are more prone to retinal detachment, and almost half of them are diagnosed at the time of first presentation.

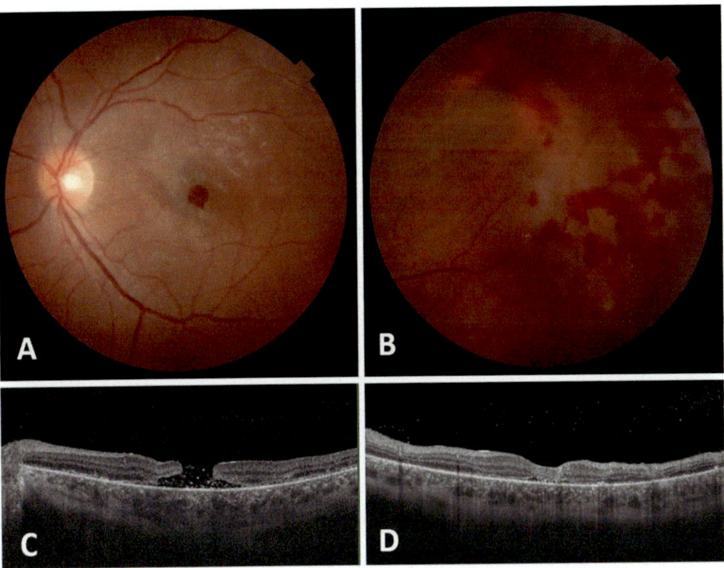

Fig. 43.3 A. (fundus photograph) and **C.** (optical coherence tomography), taken two days after closed globe injury showing a full-thickness macular hole. **B.** (fundus photograph), showing commotio retina in the temporal periphery of the same eye. **D.** (optical coherence tomography), taken 9 days after trauma, showing spontaneous closure of the macular hole with residual subretinal fluid

Detachments that develop as a result of closed globe injuries are often rhegmatogenous, and approximately half of them have a single tear. Retinal tears are generally observed immediately following trauma. However, in young patients, RD usually does not develop immediately due to the tamponading effect of the formed vitreous. The average interval between trauma and diagnosis of detachment is 17.3 months in cases of closed-globe injury [21]. Although retinal dialysis with vitreous base avulsion is typical for detachment in closed-globe injuries, it is rarely encountered in pediatric patients.

To prevent or minimize vision loss, retinal detachment should be repaired using surgical intervention as soon as possible. Although there is no consensus on the choice of surgical method in the pediatric and young populations, the decision can be made depending on the characteristics of the retinal tear, the condition of the lens, the adaptation to the post-surgical position, and the experience and preference of the surgeon [22].

Scleral buckling surgery is the primary treatment modality for 70% of childhood primary rhegmatogenous retinal detachment. Technical difficulty in completing vitrectomy in children, high incidence of post-vitrectomy cataract development, and scleral buckling as the first choice. However, potentially partially damaged thin sclera and muscles, increased intraocular pressure, and risk of back-and-forth shift of the iris lens diaphragm complicate scleral buckling surgery. Pneumatic retinopexy is preferred only in adolescent patients who can adapt to postoperative stabilization.

Pars plana vitrectomy or combined PPV—scleral buckle surgery may be considered for traumatic cases with giant retinal tears, very large or posteriorly located tears, severe PVR, and redetachment following scleral buckling [23]. Induction of posterior vitreous detachment is the most important step that must be completed successfully with successful retinal reattachment. Preoperative enzyme-assisted vitreolysis or intraoperative use of triamcinolone acetonide helps clear the posterior hyaloid. Iatrogenic retinal breaks, which may trigger the development of PVR, should be avoided during pediatric vitrectomy. Silicone oil is preferred over intraocular gas as a tamponading agent in children. Despite improvements in surgical techniques and instruments, the outcomes of pediatric traumatic retinal detachment repair have been poor. Although anatomical success can be achieved in more than half of the cases, it is not possible to reach the expected level of recovery according to the ocular trauma score. PVR is the main cause of late surgical failure in children.

2.6 Proliferative Vitreoretinopathy

Proliferative vitreoretinopathy (PVR) is the formation of abnormal cellular deposits in the vitreous and subretinal spaces produced by the retinal pigment epithelium and Müller cells. The risk of PVR increases with vitreous and subretinal hemorrhage, choroidal detachment, prolonged retinal detachment, and excessive laser/cryo-retinopexy after trauma. When we look at the literature, trauma was the etiologic factor in more than half of pediatric rhegmatogenous retinal detachments that developed PVR [24].

PVR is the most common cause of surgical failure following traumatic retinal detachment surgery. Strong vitreoretinal adhesions complicate surgery in children Surgical timing and planning vary according to the degree of PVR (Table 43.2) and surgeon's experience [25]. The difficulty in relieving traction during surgery has led to increased research on the chemical inhibition of cell proliferation and membrane contraction [26].

3 Choroid

3.1 Choroid Rupture

It is a rupture of the choroid, Bruch's membrane, and retinal pigment epithelium, often after closed globe injury in approximately 5% of patients [27]. Rupture can be seen either directly at the impact site close to the limbus or indirectly adjacent to the optic disc, away from the impact area, as a contrecoup injury. Direct choroidal rupture is rarely observed.

Diagnosis can be made using an indirect ophthalmoscope. The diagnosis may be delayed in the presence of concomitant vitreous hemorrhage, commotio retinae, or suprachoroidal hemorrhage. Visual acuity is usually worse in multiple ruptures complicated by intraocular hemorrhage and located in the maculopapular region [28].

Choroid rupture does not require treatment alone; however, strict follow-up should be performed in patients with large ruptures located close to the fovea because of the high risk of choroidal neovascularization [29].

3.2 Chorioretinitis Sclopetaria

Full-thickness rupture of the choroidal and retinal tissues due to trauma named as "sclopetaria." It occurs as a result of high-energy bullet trauma that does not penetrate the eye [30]. It can also be associated with diffuse intraocular hemorrhage (subretinal, intraretinal, and vitreous hemorrhage). Histopathologically, irreversible Bruch's membrane, choroid, and photoreceptor damage occur in patients. Fibrotic tissue replaces the damaged retina and the choroid [31]. The final visual acuity is low because of extensive fibrovascular proliferation and scar formation [32].

Table 43.2 Proliferative vitreoretinopathy classification [25]

Grade	Features
A	Vitreous haze; vitreous pigment clumps; pigment clusters on inferior retina
B	Wrinkling of inner retinal surface; retinal stiffness; vessel tortuosity; rolled and irregular edge of retinal break; decreased mobility of vitreous
C P 1–12*	Posterior to equator: focal, diffuse, or circumferential full-thickness folds; subretinal strands
C A 1–12*	Anterior to equator: focal, diffuse, or circumferential full-thickness folds; subretinal strands; anterior displacement; condensed vitreous with strands

* Expressed as the number of clock hours involved

Special Cases for Pediatric Closed Globe Injury

1. Nonaccidental Trauma (Child Abuse)

Child abuse or abusive head trauma, and related retinal hemorrhage should be considered under this section. Shaken-baby syndrome causes more than 1,200 infant deaths per year in the United States [33]. It should be considered in male infants younger than 3 years of age, in the presence of bilateral retinal hemorrhage involving the posterior pole. Retinal hemorrhage has a sensitivity and specificity of 75 and 93%, respectively, for the diagnosis of child abuse [34]. Fortunately, they usually heal spontaneously and do not cause permanent vision loss (Fig. 43.4).

2. Sports Injuries

Sports-related eye injuries account for 8.3–17% of eye injuries in adults, whereas this rate is almost 30% in the pediatric age group [35, 36]. Among these cases, open globe injuries constituted only 0.01% of the eye injuries presenting to the emergency department; all others were closed globe injuries. Protective eyewear is critical to prevent sports-related eye trauma in baseball, paintball, soccer, and ice hockey.

3. Self-Inflicted/Home Injuries

At the pediatric age, approximately two-thirds of closed-globe injuries occur at home and during games. Traumas caused by oneself, or a sibling/friend are especially common in children under 7 years old and especially in male gender. Elastic bands should be kept out of the reach of children at home, and children should be closely followed [37].

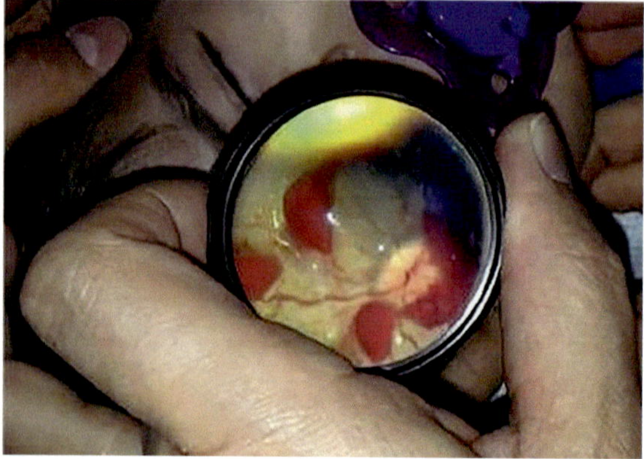

Fig. 43.4 Retinal hemorrhages on indirect ophthalmoscopy in a 4-month-old boy with abusive head trauma

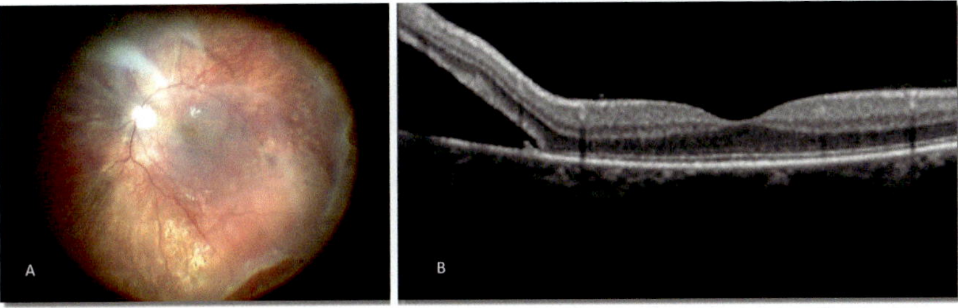

Fig. 43.5 Preoperative **A.** (fundus photograph), and **B.** (optical coherence tomography) of the patient. Temporal macula-on retinal detachment due to multiple traumatic temporal tears can be seen

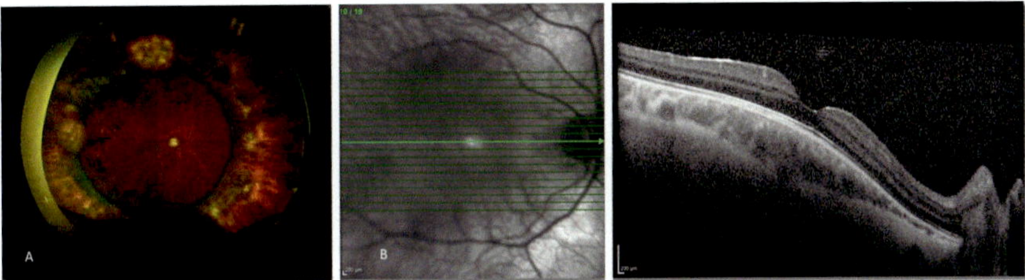

Fig. 43.6 Postoperative **A.** (fundus photograph), and **B.** (optical coherence tomography) of the patient. The retina is observed to be attached, and peripheral chorioretinal scars due to cryotherapy and compression of the scleral buckle can be seen

Case Report: *A 13-year-old man stated that his complaints started after he was punched in the right eye about a month prior to his argument at school. Best-corrected visual acuity was 0.6 (Snellen) in his right eye with high myopic correction (−6.00 Dpt). Ophthalmic examination of the right eye revealed a macula-on temporal retinal detachment with multiple tears (Fig. 43.5). The patient underwent a chandelier-assisted scleral buckle surgery.* **Supplemental digital video clips of the surgery are available.** *The best-corrected visual acuity was 0.8 (Snellen) in his right eye with high myopic correction (−7.00 Dpt) and the retina was attached at the postoperative 3rd-month examination (Fig. 43.6).*

Review Questions

1. A 13-year-old boy sustained blunt trauma to his right eye while playing football. Six months later, he presented with blurred vision in his right eye. His right visual acuity was 20/200, and there was a macular-off retinal detachment with inferior dialysis. What is the most appropriate surgical repair method?

a. Pars plana vitrectomy and 12% C3F8
b. Pars plana vitrectomy and silicone oil
c. PP Lensectomy with vitrectomy and silicone oil tamponade
d. Scleral buckling with cryotherapy with/without subretinal fluid drainage

2. All of the below can be listed in the differential diagnosis of Shaken Baby Syndrome except:

a. Valsalva retinopathy
b. Retinal macroaneurysm
c. Purtscher's retinopathy
d. Central retinal vein occlusion

3. Which of the following retinal injuries is the most frequent following closed globe injury?

a. Tears around lattice
b. Giant retinal tears
c. Inferotemporal dialysis
d. Retinal Holes

Answers

1. (**D**) Scleral buckle surgery is the most appropriate surgery for traumatic retinal detachment due to retinal dialysis at pediatric age.
2. (**B**) Fundoscopic examination of shaken baby syndrome reveals retinal hemorrhages and cotton wool spots. Similar findings are also seen in conditions such as central retinal vein occlusion, Purtsher retinopathy and Valsalva retinopathy.
3. (**C**) Inferotemporal retinal dialysis is the most frequent retinal injury.

References

1. Kuhn F, Morris R, Witherspoon CD. Birmingham eye trauma terminology (BETT): terminology and classification of mechanical eye injuries, Vol. 15. Ophthalmology Clinics of North America; 2002. p. 139–43.
2. Kuhn F, Maisiak R, Mann LR, Mester V, Morris R, Witherspoon CD. The ocular trauma score (OTS) [Internet]. Vol. 15, Ophthalmology Clinics of North America; 2002. p. 163–5. https://pubmed.ncbi.nlm.nih.gov/12229231/.
3. Kuhn F, Morris R, Witherspoon CD, Mester V. Birmingham eye trauma terminology system (BETT). J Fr Ophtalmol. 2004;27(2):206–10. https://pubmed.ncbi.nlm.nih.gov/15029055/.
4. Shah S, Shah M, Singh R, Rathod C, Khanna R. A prospective cohort study on the epidemiology of ocular trauma associated with closed-globe injuries in pediatric age group. Indian J Ophthalmol. 2020;68(3):500–3. https://pubmed.ncbi.nlm.nih.gov/32057012/.
5. Madan AH, Joshi RS, Wadekar PD. Ocular trauma in pediatric age group at a tertiary eye care center in central Maharashtra, India. Clin Ophthalmol. 2020;14:1003–9. https://pubmed.ncbi.nlm.nih.gov/32280195/
6. Franchina M, Blaszkowska M, Lewis J, Johnson A, Clark A, Lam G, et al. Paediatric eye injuries during a COVID-19 pandemic lockdown. Clin Exp Optom. 2021. https://www.tandfonline.com/doi/abs/10.1080/08164622.2021.1964921.

7. Kadappu S, Silveira S, Martin F. Aetiology and outcome of open and closed globe eye injuries in children. Clin Exp Ophthalmol. 2013;41(5):427–34. https://pubmed.ncbi.nlm.nih.gov/23145496/.

8. Breazzano MP, Unkrich KH, Barker-Griffith AE. Clinicopathological findings in abusive head trauma: analysis of 110 infant autopsy eyes. Am J Ophthalmol. 2014;158(6):1146-54.e2.

9. Erdurman FC, Sobaci G, Acikel CH, Ceylan MO, Durukan AH, Hurmeric V. Anatomical and functional outcomes in contusion injuries of posterior segment. Eye 2011;25(8):1050–6.

10. Yeung L, Chen TL, Kuo YH, Chao AN, Wu WC, Chen KJ, et al. Severe vitreous hemorrhage associated with closed-globe injury. Graefe's Arch Clin Exp Ophthalmol. 2006;244(1):52–7. https://pubmed.ncbi.nlm.nih.gov/16044322/.

11. Liu J, Peng J, Zhang Q, Ma M, Zhang H, Zhao P. Etiologies, characteristics, and management of pediatric macular hole. Am J Ophthalmol. 2020;210:174–83. https://pubmed.ncbi.nlm.nih.gov/31560879/.

12. Finn AP, Chen X, Viehland C, Izatt JA, Toth CA, Vajzovic L. Combined internal limiting membrane flap and autologous plasma concentrate to close a large traumatic macular hole in a pediatric patient. Retin Cases Brief Rep. 2021;15(2):107–9. https://pubmed.ncbi.nlm.nih.gov/29979253/.

13. Yamashita T, Uemara A, Uchino E, Doi N, Ohba N. Spontaneous closure of traumatic macular hole. Am J Ophthalmol. 2002;133(2):230–5.

14. Sanjay S, Yeo TK, Au Eong KG. Spontaneous closure of traumatic macular hole. Saudi J Ophthalmol. 2012;26(3):343–5. http://www.ncbi.nlm.nih.gov/pubmed/23961017.

15. Mitamura Y, Saito W, Ishida M, Yamamoto S, Takeuchi S. Spontaneous closure of traumatic macular hole. Retina. 2001;21(4):385–9. https://pubmed.ncbi.nlm.nih.gov/11508892/.

16. Budoff G, Bhagat N, Zarbin MA, Azzolini C. Traumatic macular hole: diagnosis, natural history, and management. J Ophthalmol. 2019; 2019. https://pubmed.ncbi.nlm.nih.gov/31016038/.

17. Miller JB, Yonekawa Y, Eliott D, Kim IK, Kim LA, Loewenstein JI, et al. Long-term Follow-up and Outcomes in Traumatic Macular Holes. Am J Ophthalmol. 2015;160(6):1255–8.e1. https://pubmed.ncbi.nlm.nih.gov/26393438/.

18. Wu WC, Drenser KA, Trese MT, Williams GA, Capone A. Pediatric traumatic macular hole: results of autologous plasmin enzyme-assisted vitrectomy. Am J Ophthalmol. 2007;144(5). https://pubmed.ncbi.nlm.nih.gov/17870044/.

19. Glaser BM, Michels RG, Kuppermann BD, Sjaarda RN, Pena RA. Transforming growth factor-β2 for the treatment of full-thickness macular holes: a prospective randomized study. Ophthalmology. 1992;99(7):1162–73.

20. Sarrazin L, Averbukh E, Halpert M, Hemo I, Rumelt S. Traumatic pediatric retinal detachment: A comparison between open and closed globe injuries. Am J Ophthalmol. 2004;137(6):1042–9. https://pubmed.ncbi.nlm.nih.gov/15183788/.

21. Youssri AI, Young LHY. Closed-globe contusion injuries of the posterior segment. Int Ophthalmol Clin. 2002;42:79–86. https://pubmed.ncbi.nlm.nih.gov/12131585/.

22. Sul S, Gurelik G, Korkmaz S, Ozdek S, Hasanreisoglu B. Pediatric traumatic retinal detachments: Clinical characteristics and outcomes. Ophthalmic Surg Lasers Imaging Retina 2017;48(2):143–50. https://pubmed.ncbi.nlm.nih.gov/28195617/.

23. Al Taisan AA, Alshamrani AA, Alzahrani AT, Al-Abdullah AA. Pars plana vitrectomy vs combined pars plana vitrectomy-scleral buckle for primary repair of pediatrics retinal detachment. Clin Ophthalmol. 2021;15:1949–55. https://pubmed.ncbi.nlm.nih.gov/34007147/.

24. Rejdak R, Nowakowska D, Wrona K, Maciejewski R, Junemann AG, Nowomiejska K. Outcomes of vitrectomy in pediatric retinal detachment with proliferative vitreoretinopathy. J Ophthalmol. 2017;2017. https://pubmed.ncbi.nlm.nih.gov/28840039/.

25. Machemer R, Aaberg TM, Freeman HM, Irvine AR, Lean JS, Michels RM. An updated classification of retinal detachment with proliferative vitreoretinopathy. Am J Ophthalmol. 1991;112(2):159–65. https://pubmed.ncbi.nlm.nih.gov/1867299/.

26. Schaub F, Hoerster R, Schiller P, Felsch M, Kraus D, Zarrouk M, et al. Prophylactic intravitreal 5-fluorouracil and heparin to prevent proliferative vitreoretinopathy in high-risk patients with retinal detachment: Study protocol for a randomized controlled trial. Trials 2018;19(1). https://pubmed.ncbi.nlm.nih.gov/30012187/.

27. Lupidi M, Muzi A, Castellucci G, Kalra G, Piccolino FC, Chhablani J, et al. The choroidal rupture: current concepts and insights [Internet]. Surv Ophthalmol. 2021;66:761–70. https://pubmed.ncbi.nlm.nih.gov/33545177/.

28. Patel MM, Chee YE, Eliott D. Choroidal rupture: a review. International Ophthalmology Clinics. 2013;53: 69–78.

29. Lorusso M, Micelli Ferrari L, Nikolopoulou E, Micelli FT. Optical coherence tomography angiography evolution of choroidal neovascular membrane in choroidal rupture managed by intravitreal bevacizumab. Case Rep Ophthalmol Med. 2019;6(2019):1–4.

30. Ludwig CA, Shields RA, Do DV, Moshfeghi DM, Mahajan VB. Traumatic chorioretinitis sclopetaria: risk factors, management, and prognosis. Am J Ophthalmol Case Rep.. 2019; 39–46. https://doi.org/10.1016/j.ajoc.2019.02.004.

31. Evans LP, Newell EA, Mahajan MA, Tsang SH, Ferguson PJ, Mahoney J, et al. Acute vitreoretinal trauma and inflammation after traumatic brain injury in mice. Ann Clin Transl Neurol. 2018;5(3):240–51. https://onlinelibrary.wiley.com/doi/full/10.1002/acn3.523.

32. Rayess N, Rahimy E, Ho AC. Spectral-domain optical coherence tomography features of bilateral chorioretinitis sclopetaria. Ophthalmic Surg Lasers Imaging Retina 2015;46(2):253–5. https://pubmed.ncbi.nlm.nih.gov/25707053/.

33. Narang SK, Sachdev KK, Bertocci K, Pierre-Wright MJ, Kaczor K, Bertocci G, et al. Overturned abusive head trauma and shaken baby syndrome convictions in the United States: Prevalence, legal basis, and medical evidence. Child Abuse Negl. 2021;122:105380. https://pubmed.ncbi.nlm.nih.gov/34743053/

34. Abed Alnabi W, Tang GJ, Eagle RC, Gulino S, Thau A, Levin AV. Pathology of perimacular folds due to vitreoretinal traction in abusive head trauma. Retina. 2019;39(11):2141–8.

35. Zhang J, Zhu X, Sun Z, Wang J, Sun Z, Li J, et al. Epidemiology of sports-related eye injuries among athletes in Tianjin, China. Front Med. 2021;8. https://pubmed.ncbi.nlm.nih.gov/34604250/.

36. Patel PS, Uppuluri A, Zarbin MA, Bhagat N. Epidemiologic trends in pediatric ocular injury in the USA from 2010 to 2019. Graefe's Arch Clin Exp Ophthalmol. 2021. https://pubmed.ncbi.nlm.nih.gov/34536117/.

37. Sharifzadeh M, Rahmanikhah E, Nakhaee N. Pattern of pediatric eye injuries in Tehran, Iran. Int Ophthalmol. 2013;33(3):255–9. https://pubmed.ncbi.nlm.nih.gov/23192721/.

Open Globe Injuries

44

Ferenc Kuhn and Adrienne Csutak

Abstract

Mechanical injuries are an important etiology in vision loss; these young patients are facing several decades of life with visual impairment. This makes the treatment of such patients all the more crucial. The evaluation of the child with an eye injury requires skills beyond ophthalmology. The process should be restricted to the minimal necessary so that the decision whether surgery is necessary and how soon can be made. As a general rule, surgery is best performed on an urgent basis, to prevent infection (especially because the history as provided by the child is often unreliable) and scarring. Surgery is best performed by an ophthalmologist who is well versed in all types of (intra)ocular reconstruction, from corneal suturing to subretinal blood evacuation. Because postoperative scar formation is commonly seen in children and is typically more robust than in adults, the child must be followed closely.

Keywords

History · Corneal suturing · Scarring · Proliferative vitreoretinopathy · Phthisis

F. Kuhn (✉)
Helen Keller Foundation for Research and Education, Birmingham, AL, USA
e-mail: fkuhn@mindspring.com

F. Kuhn · A. Csutak
Department of Ophthalmology, Medical School, University of Pécs, Pécs, Hungary

Introduction

Injury[1] is always unexpected. Ocular trauma is unique because of people's fear of blindness; eye injury in a child[2] is additionally unique due to several factors.

- Adults perceive children as vulnerable and innocent; consequently, an ophthalmologist treating an injured child must be prepared properly to deal with seemingly irrational emotional reactions.
- Because of the long life expectancy of a child, the financial burden on family and society is disproportionate.
- Obtaining a truthful history can be difficult or impossible: the child may be too young or wants to hide/alter what happened for fear of reprisal, or because a perpetrator wants to conceal his involvement in the child's injury to avoid criminal prosecution.
- The young child's visual system is still developing and vulnerable to amblyopia due to reduced input (media opacity) or a refractive error (loss of the lens).
- The child may not co-operate during the examination.
- The eye, reaching 85% of its final axial length by 2 years of age, continues to grow at 1% annually; interventions such as an encircling band can interfere with this growth.
- Intraocular scarring is typically much more rapid and aggressive in a child than in an adult. Another consequence of this enhanced wound healing is that corneal sutures become loose sooner.
- Conversely, the child's eye has increased tolerance (see the *Case report* below).
- The orbital floor is immature before puberty and overlies a small maxillary sinus; the bones bend easily and fracture rather than shatter so that muscle entrapment commonly results.

Terminology

The BETT system (Fig. 44.1) is used to classify the injuries to the eye; the tissue of reference is always the entire globe (e.g., in "corneal penetrating injury" "corneal" refers to the location of the wound, not the depth of the wound within the tissue). An open globe injury can be a rupture (caused by a blunt object) or one caused by a sharp object (penetrating, intraocular foreign body [IOFB], or perforating) [1].

---

[1] Injury in this chapter is understood as one that is serious enough to cause or threaten with severe consequences for the eye's function and/or anatomical integrity.
[2] We define children as those aged 0–18 years ("under 19").

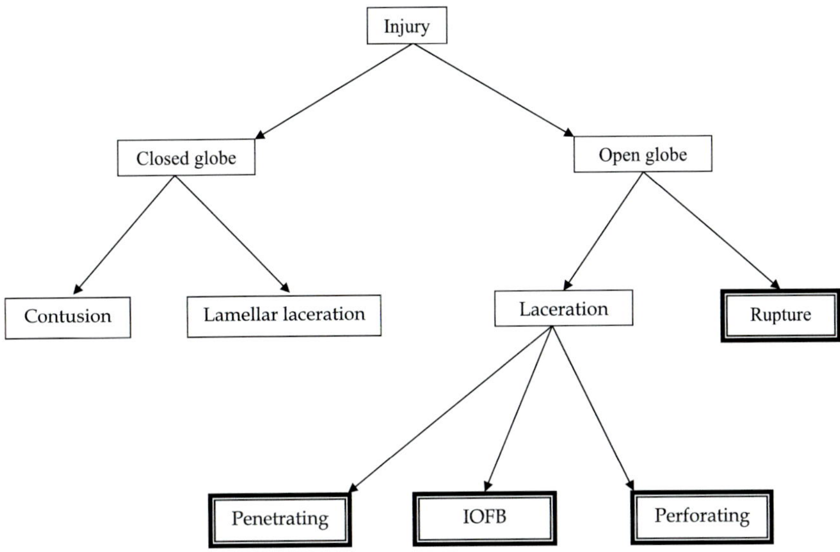

Fig. 44.1 The Birmingham Eye Trauma Terminology (BETT) system. A serious mechanical trauma to the eye causes either a closed globe injury (no full-thickness wound of the eyewall) or an open globe one; in the latter case, two options are possible. Either the causative agent is a blunt object—which causes a *rupture*—or a sharp one (laceration), in which case there are three possibilities. If a single wound is present, the injury is either a *penetrating* one, or an *intraocular foreign body* is also present; if the object exited the eye through a second wound, the injury is a *perforating* one

Epidemiology

Injury is the leading cause of monocular blindness in children, [2] and the risk of injury is greatest in children from poor socioeconomic populations; bystanders represent a significant percentage of the victims.

The home is the most common place for ocular trauma in children, and typically sports are the most common activity resulting in eye injury; sharp objects are the most likely culprit.

Evaluation

Special Recommendations

Not wearing a white coat is very helpful; children commonly associate it with something unpleasant or even pain (see *Counseling* below).

The injuries are bilateral in less than 3% in children. The unaffected eye should serve as control for the injured eye to compare with. If there is a conflict between history and findings, the ophthalmologist should trust the latter.

History

History-taking is an especially complex proposition when a child is injured. Very young children commonly cannot recall the events at all or do so inaccurately; they may be overwhelmed by fright or pain, be in denial, or fear punishment for disclosing the truth. Fabrication (Münchausen syndrome) is rather common even in older children; it is therefore desirable to seek an objective, uninvolved adult eyewitness. Table 44.1 lists the most important issues to cover.

Table 44.1 The most important issues to cover during history-taking for a pediatric eye injury

Question	Comment
What happened?	General circumstances
What object caused the injury?	Rephrase the question if history and findings are in obvious conflict
Can the causative object be located?	A wealth of important information could be uncovered
Any person who played a key role in the injury?	Whether another child or an adult
Any eyewitness?	Is the person reliable?
When did the injury occur?	Two-thirds of children present after the critical first 24 h
Where did the injury take place?	Soil-contamination is of crucial importance
What symptoms occurred instantly and how have they changed since?	Visual deterioration is the most important, followed by pain[3]
Has any treatment been administered?	Local (washout, foreign body removal, bandage) or general (pills etc.)
The time of the last meal and drink?	Anesthesiologists are rarely willing to put the child to sleep if the last meal was within 6 h
Was the eye normal before the injury?	Previous surgery, injury, myopia, and amblyopia
Did the child wear (prescription) glasses or contact lenses when the injury occurred?	Nonsafety glasses may be protective in some cases but can also cause injury by shattering
Any systemic diseases?	If yes, any medications taken for it and when were they taken last?
Any allergies?	If yes, to what?
Tetanus immunization status?	When and what type of tetanus shot was last administered

---

[3] There is an inverse relationship between pain and condition severity: a corneal abrasion causes severe pain while a rupture with extensive tissue prolapse may cause no pain.

General Implications

A systemic examination, with the help of a pediatric specialist or an anesthesiologist if necessary, must never be foregone, and this should include searching for signs of polytrauma. Unique relationships between ocular and systemic symptoms exist, e.g., bradycardia and somnolence being common with hyphema, or the oculocardiac reflex (nausea, bradycardia, and hypotension) with orbital fractures and muscle entrapment.

External Inspection

Examining a very young or uncooperative child may require proper physical restraining, for which at least one assistant (preferably a parent) is necessary. Even if the child is older and does cooperate, the ophthalmologist must always explain what's coming so that the child is prepared. See Table 44.2 for details.

If possible, the visual acuity should be determined in both eyes. If the child is willing to cooperate but cannot read, illiterate charts (Allen cards, or the "E" sign) can be used.

Table 44.2 External inspection of the child with a suspected open globe injury

Examine	Comment
Lids, periocular skin, and bones for injury-related tissue damage, foreign material, and wounds	Under natural light if possible. Small lid wounds may hide thin, long, and potentially life-threatening intraorbital foreign bodies that can protrude intracranially or point to an ocular wound underneath. Dog bites are often restricted to the skin and lacrimal system, yet can cause severe infection
Position of the eyes (exophthalmos, enophthalmos, deviation in primary position) and any asymmetry in the appearance of the eyes or orbits	A recent preinjury picture is useful to allow comparison between "was" and "is"
Globe motility	Restriction presents early in a trap-door type blowout fracture
The globe itself, first with a penlight. Look for large foreign bodies, significant prolapse of intraocular tissues, and large subcutaneous and subconjunctival hemorrhages	Reassure the child that none of what's coming will be painful. Do not try to forcefully try to open lids that are swollen, whether due to edema or hemorrhage
Pupils and their reaction to light	Do not forget to test for an afferent pupillary defect
Bone dislocation, subcutaneous foreign bodies, and crepitus via careful palpation	Not always recommended as it may cause pain and thus be counterproductive

Slit Lamp and Ophthalmoscopy

If the child is cooperative, these can yield crucial information about the nature and extent of the injury; see Table 44.3. for details. As a general rule, if a full-thickness wound has been confirmed, there is no need for such detailed examination; urgent surgery is in order, and all additional details are determined intraoperatively. Forceful opening of the lids, whether because of tightness due to a hemorrhage of to overcome a resisting child, is not only counterproductive but can lead to an expulsive choroidal hemorrhage.

Table 44.3 Slit lamp and ophthalmoscopy of the severely injured eye

Tissue	Comment
Conjunctiva	Large and thick hemorrhages may hide scleral wounds (occult rupture). If it is impossible to determine whether a scleral wound is present, exploratory surgery is indicated
Cornea	Epithelial abrasions and ulcerations, stromal opacities, and wounds are sought; Rose bengal or fluorescein stain may be used. If a corneal laceration is found, it must be verified whether it is of full thickness; the Seidel sign is positive if it is (sometimes slight pressure on the eye is necessary to detect the leakage). It is crucial to determine whether suturing is required[4]
Anterior chamber	Foreign bodies, flare, inflammatory cells, fibrin, pus, blood, lens material, and vitreous may be present. A shallow chamber may signal aqueous loss (open globe injury), although an anteriorly displaced lens or a hemorrhagic/serous choroidal detachment can also be the culprit
Iris	Look under both direct- and retroillumination for full-thickness or stromal defects and sphincter tears, iridodialysis or iridodonesis (eye movement is obviously necessary to detect the latter)
Pupil	Evaluate its shape, size, and location. The two pupils should be of equal size and have identical reaction to direct and consensual light. The presence or absence of an afferent pupillary defect (APD) should also be determined as it's presence signals a poor prognosis
Lens	Determine whether it is present in the eye and if yes, whether it has been sub/luxated (phacodonesis; partial or complete zonular rupture); the capsules have been violated (the posterior[5] is more important); the clarity has been maintained; an intralenticular foreign body (FB) is present. Any of these pathologies can occur in severe trauma, whether the injury is open or closed globe (except the FB type, which naturally signals an open globe in jury)
Vitreous	Foreign bodies, cells, fibrin, membranes, and hemorrhage may be present
Retina	Easily identifiable pathologies (hemorrhage, edema, posterior break such as a macular hole), and detachment should be sought; examination of the periphery is usually deferred until the presence of an open globe injury can be excluded or the wound has been sutured
Intraocular pressure (IOP)	It is rarely measured but assessed digitally. Crucially, neither a low nor an elevated IOP is pathognomic for the presence of an open wound[6]

---

[4] Not all full-thickness wounds need to be sutured; conversely, certain partial-thickness wounds (those with a displaced or very loose flap), do.

[5] Of eyes undergoing surgery for traumatic cataract, up to one half were found to have posterior capsular ruptures [5].

[6] The IOP may be high in an open globe injury because of a severe intraocular hemorrhage; conversely, the IOP may be low in a closed globe injury because a ciliary body shutdown.

Most of the pathologies described in this chapter can occur both in open or closed globe injuries; Table 44.4 helps with the differential diagnosis.

Table 44.4 Differential diagnosis in eyes with severe trauma*

Pathology	Contusion	Rupture	Penetrating injury	IOFB injury	Perforating injury
Subconjunctival hemorrhage	+	++/+++	+/++	±	±
Corneal wound	−	−/+	+	±	+ −/
Limbal wound	−	+	±	±	±
Posterior wound	−	±	−	−	+
Tissue prolapse in wound	−	+/++	±	−/+	±
Hyphema	+	+/++	±	±	±
Vitreous prolapse into anterior chamber	+	+	−	−/+	−
Lens extruded	−	±	−	−	−
Lens sub/luxated	±	±	−	−	−
Cataract	+	+	+	+	+
Vitreous hemorrhage	+	+/+++	+	+	+
Commotio retinae	+	−	−	−	−
Peripheral retinal tear	±	−/+	−/+	−/+	−/+
Direct retinal injury	−	−/+	−/+	±	±
Macular hole	±	−	−	−	−
Retinal detachment	+	+/++	+	+/++	+/++
Choroidal rupture	±	−/+	−	−	−

* −: No or very rare; −/+: rare; ±: relatively common; +: common. An individual's specific injury may be different from the statistical probabilities this Table represents, and some of the pathologies (e.g., retinal detachment) may not present until later in the postinjury period

Imaging Studies

Caveat: No imaging method is 100% accurate, making it all the more important to take history and local findings into account, and maintain a high level of suspicion.

While ultrasonography is helpful to detect foreign bodies, lens sub/luxation and capsular ruptures, posterior full-thickness wounds, vitreous hemorrhage, and retinal detachment, as well as for follow-up, it typically should not be used in eyes with open globe trauma to avoid (further) tissue extrusion.[7]

Computed tomography is the most valuable test as it avoids physical contact with the eye and can detect very small IOFBs as well as very fine intraocular and intraorbital pathologies. Magnetic resonance imaging provides visualization of even finer details of soft tissue lesions but is contraindicated if a ferrous IOFB is suspected.

---

[7] An exception can be made for an eye with a small wound with minimal risk of tissue extrusion in a child who is cooperative, the examiner is experienced, and is aware of the risk.

Counseling

The child must be treated as a person, not as a pathology. The treatment of tissue lesions is insufficient if mental and spiritual support are absent; even the most efficient drug and the most appropriate surgical repair cannot make up for the lack of empathy; offering comfort, hope, understanding, compassion, and affection is as much needed as proper information. "Informed consent" is not a document to sign but a process in which the child and the family are treated as partners, not as objects of an intervention.

In adults, the "target" of counseling is primarily the patient. If the injured person is a child, the task is much more complex because the primary decision-maker is not the child but the parent. How much detail is shared with the child is a choice taken on a case-by-case basis. Often the parent decides whether and how much should be disclosed to the child. Ideally, all decisions regarding therapy are made jointly: family, ophthalmologist, and, if feasible, child. The Ocular Trauma Score is very helpful to guide the prognostic information provided by the surgeon; [3] it is better to be slightly pessimistic than overly optimistic.

Management and Decision-Making

Once the diagnosis of an open globe injury has been confirmed,[8] the surgeon must prepare for the next step. If the three *"E"* questions (*E*xpertise, *E*xperience, and *E*quipment) are answered in the affirmative,[9] the next two issues to deal with are the timing and type/extent of the primary surgery. The overall goal of the intervention is to restore as much of the globe's anatomy as possible - the basis for functional improvement. As a minimum, every effort should be made to preserve a comfortable eye; primary enucleation is acceptable only if there is not enough left of the eye (wall to suture).

Timing

While, as a general rule, surgery should be performed on an urgent basis, in children it is even more so: the risk of postinjury tissue extrusion by eye-rubbing is greater in children than in a co-operative adult. As a minimum, the wound should be sutured as soon as general anesthesia is available, and the child may have to be restrained during the waiting period.

---

[8] Or it cannot conclusively be excluded, in which case exploratory surgery is indicated.
[9] Otherwise urgent referral is in order (see Table 44.5).

Table 44.5 In case of referral of the child with an open globe injury

Do/consider this	Comment
Cover the eye with a firm, resistant shield	A styrofoam cup is just as effective as a proper shield
Restrain a non-co-operative child	Fix the elbow in a stretched position or tie the hands at the wrist; an adult should stay with the child to prevent liberation from the restraining
Start antibiotic therapy	Appropriate if the injury is high risk for endophthalmitis; the medication should be given intravenously
Start tetanus prophylaxis	Unless the last shot is recent
Send along all documentation and a list of medications administered	Include copies of the imaging studies performed (not only their readings)
Leave in situ any protruding IOFB	The child must not be able to self-remove it during transit

The Extent of the Primary Surgery

The surgeon must choose between the minimal or the comprehensive. In the first option, the intervention is restricted to wound closure and occasionally cleaning the anterior chamber and/or removing the lens; a second surgery is then to follow (typically a week or two after the initial one).[10]

In the second option, a "pole-to-pole"[11] surgery is performed: all pathologies are addressed from the cornea to the subretinal space, to restore the anatomy. Obviously, this is where the three "*E*"s come into play; if they are all answered "yes" and a comprehensive primary reconstructive surgery done, the prognosis is improved, and the risk and severity of postoperative complications reduced.

Surgical Reconstruction[12]

Conjunctiva

- Small wounds do not have to be sutured unless surgical intervention is needed anyway.
- 8/0 vicryl is the best suture material.

---

[10] This staged approach has its own problems even in adults; in children the complications due to the delayed secondary surgery are much more severe.

[11] A term coined by the late Cesare Forlini.

[12] Obviously, only a short description of certain variables can be presented in this brief chapter. The list provided here is restricted to the globe itself. What is described here as tissue-specific recommendations apply to any surgery, whether performed primarily or secondarily.

Cornea

- In case of a deep foreign body, a careful decision must be made whether to remove it. If removal is advisable (those of inert material may be left in place if they do not interfere with vision), extreme care is needed to avoid pushing the object intraocularly.
- Prior to suturing, all materials (foreign body, fibrin, uvea, vitreous etc.) must be removed from the wound. To retrieve iris from the wound, a paracentesis should be created at least 90 degrees away from the wound and a spatula used to pull the iris back; this prevents damage to the iris (which would occur by trying to push it back through the wound) and avoids loss of aqueous. For a vitreous prolapse, the vitrectomy probe is preferred to the cellulose sponge/scissors alternative.
- Unlike in an adult, even small and firmly self-sealing wounds should be sutured since a child is more prone to rub the eye and thus reopen the wound.
- The goals of suturing are: to create a watertight wound without causing astigmatism; a regular surface; minimal scarring; and maintaining the normal depth of the anterior chamber. For this, every step of the suturing process must be carefully planned.

Table 44.6 provides important details about suturing. Figure 44.2A and B show examples of how not to suture a corneal wound.

Table 44.6 The rules of suturing corneal wounds

Rule	Comment
The best suture material is 10–0 nylon	
Occasionally a small part of the corneal edge is rolled inward; this must be preserved, not excised, with a suture that incorporates it. If there is true tissue loss, a glue (cyanoacrylate) may be used	A bandage contact lens may have to applied; penetrating keratoplasty is rarely necessary
Unless the wound is limbus-parallel, long, and in the periphery, interrupted—rather than running—sutures are recommended	Using running sutures across the cornea results in a flattened anterior chamber
The sutures should be of full thickness (100% deep)	This achieves proper alignment of all corneal layers; it eliminates posterior gaping and dries the cornea intraoperatively[13]
All sutures should be at a 90-degree angle to the wound edge	This avoid tissue shift, a distortion that is not corrected by suture removal
The first suture should be placed at a landmark	The limbus or the tip of the wound's angle

(continued)

---

[13] More than half of eyes with a corneal wound require vitreoretinal surgery; the 100% deep suture allows the vitrectomy to be performed when it is ideal rather than when it is possible, unhindered by an opaque cornea.

Table 44.6 (continued)

Rule	Comment
If the wound is corneoscleral, the order of suture placement should be: limbus, cornea, sclera	The corneal and scleral aspects of the wound are then treated as a standalone wound would be
If the wound is long and cross-corneal, the suturing should start from the two wound edges and progress symmetrically toward the center	The peripheral bites should be long and become progressively shorter toward the center; avoid suturing in the visual axis
The suture should never be made too tight	It causes a distortion that is not corrected by suture removal
The knot should be firm and small	To avoid loosening and allow burying
All suture knots must be buried	This minimizes irritation and vascularization
Remove the sutures between 3 and 6 months, depending on wound length and the actual situation	Sterilize the surface as if an intraocular injection were to be given. The removal may have to be done under the microscope in sedation

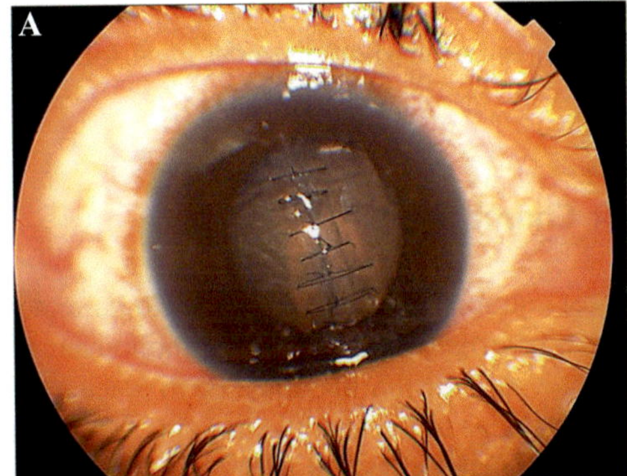
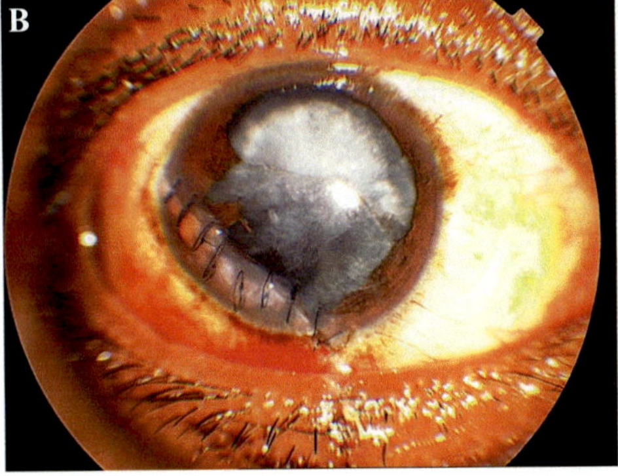

Fig. 44.2 Improper wound closure in the cornea. **A**. The sutures are of equal length and the epicenter is not spared. **B**. Running sutures should have been used here

Sclera

- Vicryl 6–8/0 as a suture material allows sufficient closure without the need for removal.
- If the wound is *anterior*, the conjunctiva should be opened so as to allow visualization of the wound in its entirety. The "50%" rule is ideal regarding the order of suture placement.
- If the wound is *posterior*, it is contraindicated to expose the wound in its entirety; this avoids (additional) tissue loss. The conjunctiva is opened in a small area anteriorly, the underlying scleral wound closed, and this is repeated advancing posteriorly. If it becomes difficult to access the posterior aspect of the wound, the suturing must be stopped, the conjunctiva closed, and the underlying pathologies addressed from the inside during vitreoretinal (VR) surgery.
- If the wound is underneath an extraocular muscle, suturing of the visible parts on either side of the wound should precede disinserting the muscle. If the wound is parallel to the limbus, a suture may be placed through the muscle without taking it off.
- Prophylactic cryopexy over the scleral wound is an option that must be forgotten.
- A prophylactic scleral buckle may be placed, even though it is not known during the primary surgery where its most ideal location would be.[14]

Anterior Chamber

- The most common material that needs to be removed is blood. Hyphema that is liquid can be irrigated out either by a monomanual or a bimanual technique; for a clotted one, an infusion line must be in place and the vitrectomy probe be used, avoiding damage to the endothelium, iris, and the lens. If the intraocular pressure (IOP) is elevated and a total hyphema present, the removal is urgent to prevent corneal blood imbibition.
- If an IOFB is present, viscoelastic use should be considered; creating a removal incision away from the location is preferred to a direct cut-down.

---

[14] Placing the buckle during a secondary surgery is much more difficult due to scarring having developed by then.

Iris and Pupil

- The old rule that any iris that has been prolapsed for over 24 h should be excised no longer applies; it is extremely rare that the iris caught in the wound cannot be retained. Prior to repositioning, the iris surface must be thoroughly cleansed.
- One of the reasons why a pupil remains wide after the trauma is a fibrinous membrane on its back surface; the membrane constricts and pulls the iris toward its root. This is another reason why early surgery is so important: if the iris is pulled carefully centripetally with forceps[15] before the membrane organizes, the pupil's size can still be normalized without suturing (Fig. 44.3A and B).

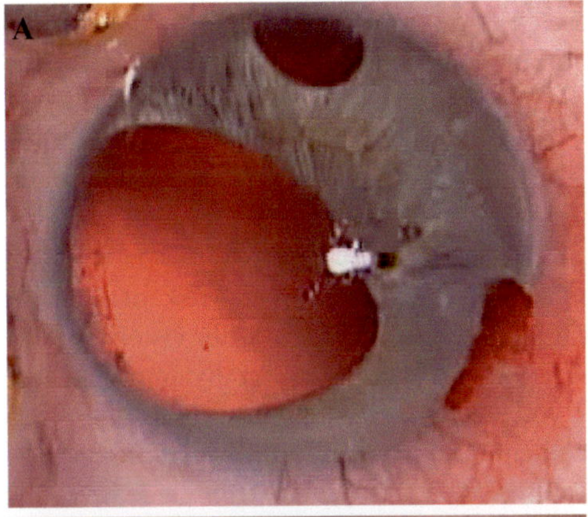

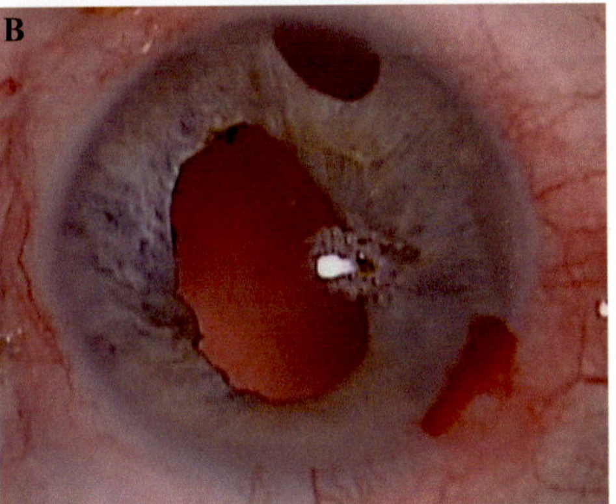

Fig. 44.3 Early intervention for an injury-related pupillary dilation. **A** The pupil remained wide following the trauma. At the completion of the primary, comprehensive surgery, silicone oil has been installed and the iris gently pulled toward the center, 360 degrees, with forceps, aided by a spatula. **B.** Without the need of suturing, the pupil's normal size and central position have been restored

---

[15] A spatula can be used in the surgeon's other hand to swipe the back surface of the iris, helping to break the membrane's grip.

- Lacerations are sutured using the McCannel technique; [4] a similar suture is used to deal with an iridodialysis. The iris does not have a wound and thus does not heal; it is solely the suture that holds it together. The suture must not be too tight, otherwise cheesewiring occurs.
- Transpupillary membranes should be removed as they interfere with the child's vision and can cause pupillary block (even angle closure if they grow) and secondary glaucoma. Fresh synechiae are broken with a blunt tool; chronic ones with a sharp one as they may tear the tissue they are adhering too. Bleeding is common when breaking chronic synechiae.
- If the pupil is permanently dilated, a purse-string suture can be used to constrict it. Restoring pupil size is usually delayed until all other surgeries will have been completed.
- In case of aniridia, an iris diaphragm should be transplanted; it can be combined with an intraocular lens (IOL).

Lens

- Traumatic cataract increases the risk of amblyopia in children under the age of ~6 years, and interferes with vision for the child and visibility for the ophthalmologist. This is especially important because more than half of these eyes will require VR surgery: both the vitreous hemorrhage and retinal detachment rates are significantly higher than in similar injuries without cataract.
- In children with a capsular rupture, lens swelling causing severe secondary glaucoma can develop in a few hours.
- Due to the strong connections between the posterior lens capsule, the anterior hyaloid, and the peripheral retina, intracapsular lens removal must never be attempted in children. For the same reason, in eyes with posterior lens capsule violation, vitrectomy instrumentation must be used (lensectomy). Otherwise, because the lens is soft, simple aspiration is adequate.
- The younger the child, the more pressing the need to remove both lens capsules (see the *Case report* at the end of this chapter) [5]; this reduces the risk of the development of anterior proliferative vitreoretinopathy (PVR) and eliminates the risk of capsular shrinkage, which would lead to phthisis[16] even if the rest of the eye's anatomy has been fully restored. The removal of the capsules is different from how it is performed in adults: the surgeon must cut, not simply pull on, the zonules.
- If the surgeon decides against capsule removal, a posterior capsulectomy and anterior vitrectomy should always be performed, preferably through a pars plana approach, to prevent postoperative opacification.

---

[16] The zonules are very strong; instead of breaking as the capsule shrinks, they transmit the traction force onto the ciliary processes, which start to atrophy within months.

- It should be the exception, rather than the rule, to simultaneously implant an IOL. The risk of inflammation and synechia formation are high and the power of the IOL is not easy to determine. In the amblyopic-age-child, antiamblyopia therapy is necessary until the eye's refractive power is properly restored.
- If the lens is subluxed but no other serious pathologies are present and the vision is good, there is no need for lens removal.
- If the lens is luxated (dislocated) into the vitreous cavity, a complete vitrectomy must be performed along with the lensectomy. In the extremely rare case of an anteriorly dislocated lens, the removal is urgent to prevent endothelial damage and IOP elevation.

Ciliary Body

- In addition to the posterior retina, the ciliary body is the other intraocular structure that determines the long-term outcome of an injury. Many surgeons, unfortunately, neglect this tissue at the time of the initial surgery, and it may be too late to save the ciliary body later in the postinjury period.
- The surface of the ciliary body must be thoroughly cleaned, leaving no fibrin, blood, vitreous on its surface; if the lens is removed in its entirety, the zonules should also be removed. Both sharp tools (e.g., scissors) and blunt ones (vitrectomy probe, spatula) may have to employed. It is crucial not to cut into the ciliary processes as this cause profuse, occasionally uncotnrollable bleeding. Bimanual surgery is a must, and it is preferable to do self-indentation—another argument in favor of removing the lens in its entirety.
- If a cyclodialysis is present and exceeds ~ 2 clock hours, it must be sutured; the McCannel technique is applicable.

Vitreous and Retina

- The most common pathology is hemorrhage. In addition to issues related to vision, there is an increased risk of PVR—a major reason why primary vitrectomy (see above) is recommended.
- Detachment of the posterior cortical vitreous—a crucially important maneuver in traumatology—is very difficult or even impossible in children. Enzymatic vitreolysis may offer a solution in the future [6]. If the posterior cortical vitreous remains undetached, it must be carefully shaved and all obvious traction released; the child must be closely followed. One of the most harmful myths in ocular traumatology is to delay the VR surgery in the (completely false) hope that the delay will achieve spontaneous posterior vitreous detachment (Fig. 44.4).

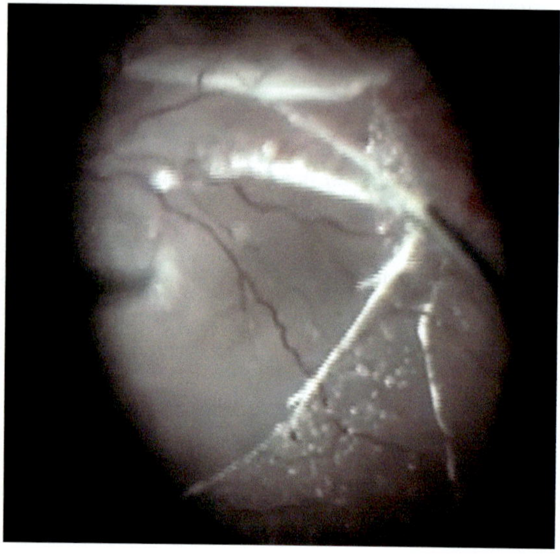

Fig. 44.4 Surgical detachment of the posterior cortical vitreous. Even 4 weeks postinjury,[17] there is a vitreoschisis but not a posterior hyaloid separation. Triamcinolone is used to mark the vitreous to be detached and then removed

- The vitreous base must also be shaved as closely to the retina as possible.
- Fresh IOFBs should be removed; a high level of suspicion (and careful history-taking) must be maintained so that no IOFB gets missed (Fig. 44.5). For a ferrous IOFB, a strong permanent intraocular magnet is the best tool; for the rest, a proper forceps or a lasso may be the best option. Using a heavy liquid to "float" the IOFB is a two-edged sword: the liquid may overflow the IOFB instead or initially keeps pushing it across the retinal surface; the IOFB will also be directed toward the eyewall while the liquid is only partially filling up the vitreous cavity.
- Macular holes[18] should be operated on as soon as possible, even though spontaneous closures have been reported.[19] Removal of the internal limiting membrane measurably increases the success rate but may be difficult in the child. Postoperative positioning is obviously not something that can reasonably be expected.
- Giant tears are rather common in children; the most effective treatment is vitrectomy without a scleral buckle to avoid slippage.
- In eyes with a posterior scleral wound (rupture, penetrating trauma, exit wound of a perforating injury) or an IOFB impact that involves the choroid, prophylactic chorioretinectomy should be performed to reduce the risk of PVR development [7].
- Because of the high risk of causing/increasing myopia, use of an encircling buckle is not a good substitute for a complete vitrectomy.

---

[17] The patient was not referred earlier.

[18] Much less common in open- than in closed globe trauma.

[19] The authors don't prefer waiting for spontaneous hole closure, but it is up to the parents to make the decision, based on counseling.

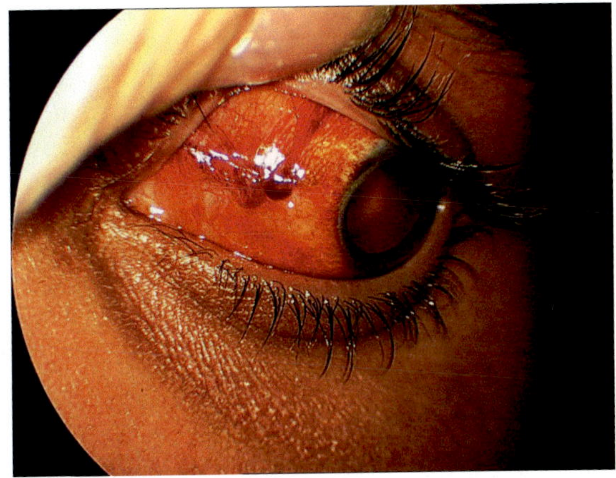

Fig. 44.5 No visible scleral wound in an eye that harbors a fresh intraocular foreign body. The wound is very small and covered up by a small conjunctival hemorrhage

- The risk of PVR is higher in children than in adults; PVR is also more aggressive and appears sooner[20]; again, this argues for primary comprehensive reconstruction, rather than the traditional staged approach with the second surgery delayed for weeks. Subretinal PVR is also more common in children than in adults.

Endophthalmitis

- In addition to using intravitreal antibiotics, vitrectomy should be performed on an emergency basis, and it should be as complete as possible. Pus should not be left on the posterior retina. If a VR surgeon is unwilling to perform vitrectomy early, the child should be referred immediately.

Case Report

History: A 9-year-old child presented with light perception vision[21] following a rupture injury sustained almost a year earlier. No data were available regarding the previous surgeries and although the father went from ophthalmologist to ophthalmologist, no surgery was offered after the early postinjury period.

Evaluation: The eye was phthisical (21 mm axial length) and there was no pupil (virtually nothing but iris was seen behind the cornea (Fig. 44.6A), and the anterior chamber was very shallow); a small corneal scar in the periphery indicated where (part of the) wound had occurred. No further testing was performed.[22]

---

[20] The authors have seen a closed-funnel retinal detachment as soon as 4 days postinjury.

[21] The fact that the media opacity in this case was the iris explains why vision greater than light perception could not be expected.

[22] While ultrasonography and radiological tests could have been done, they would neither have altered the conversation during counseling nor the plan/design for, or technique of, surgery.

Fig. 44.6 Illustrations for the case report; intraoperative images.[23] **A.** The iris is stretched, blocking view of the eye's interior. **B.** Endodiathermia is used to coagulate the iris behind the corneal wound. **C.** The iris is cut with scissors. **D.** The retroiridal membrane is removed, after the retina has been sharply separated from it. The edge of the detached retina is visible inferiorly. **E.** Multiple subretinal scars are removed. **F.** Scirrors, among other tools, is used to remove all tissues covering the ciliary body; a single surviving ciliary process is visible in this area. **G.** The detached ciliary body is being resutured. **H.** The iris is sutured. **I.** The apperance of the front of the eye one day postoperatively. **J.** The silicone-oil-filled eye one day postoperativelyc

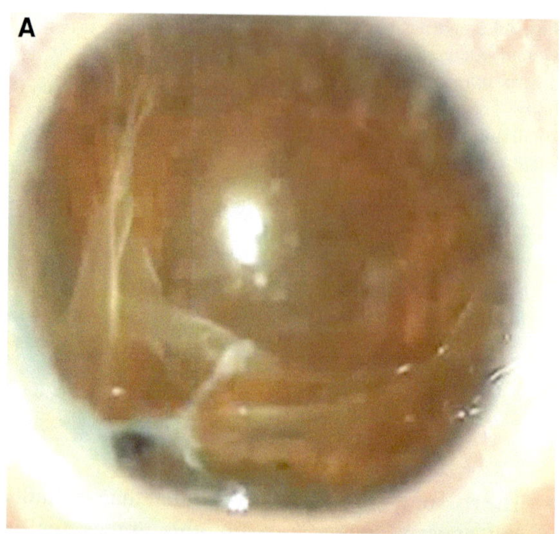

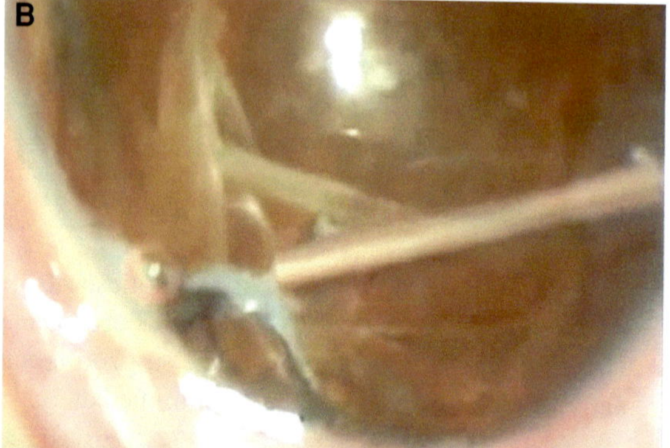

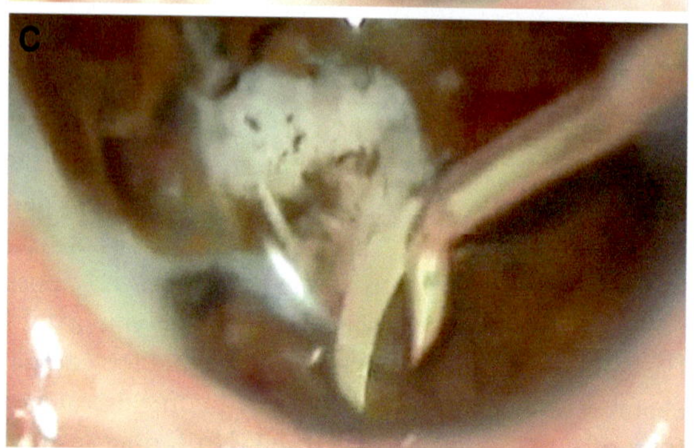

[23] See the text for more details.

Fig. 44.6 (continued)

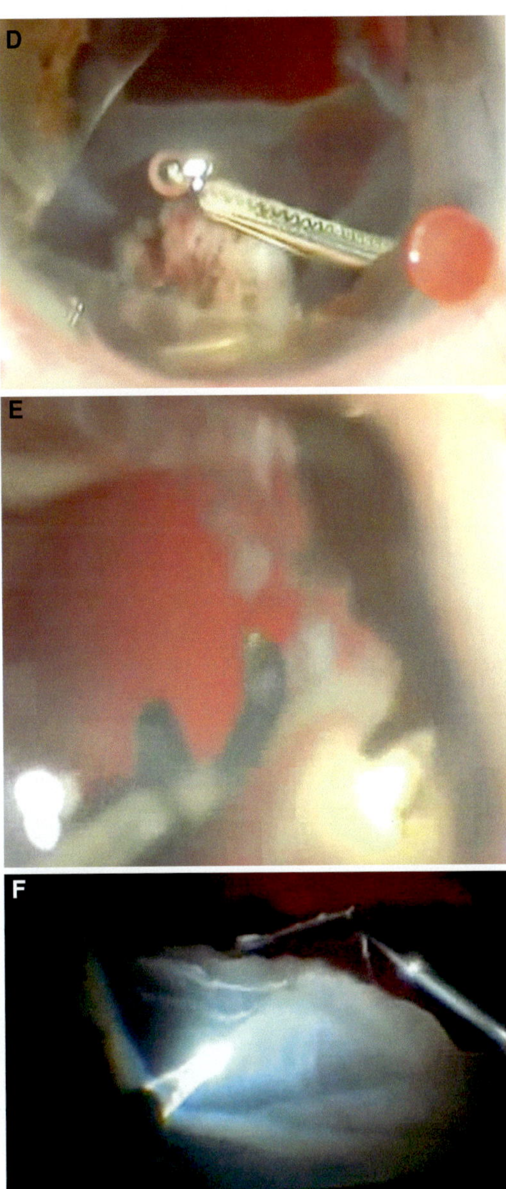

Fig. 44.6 (continued)

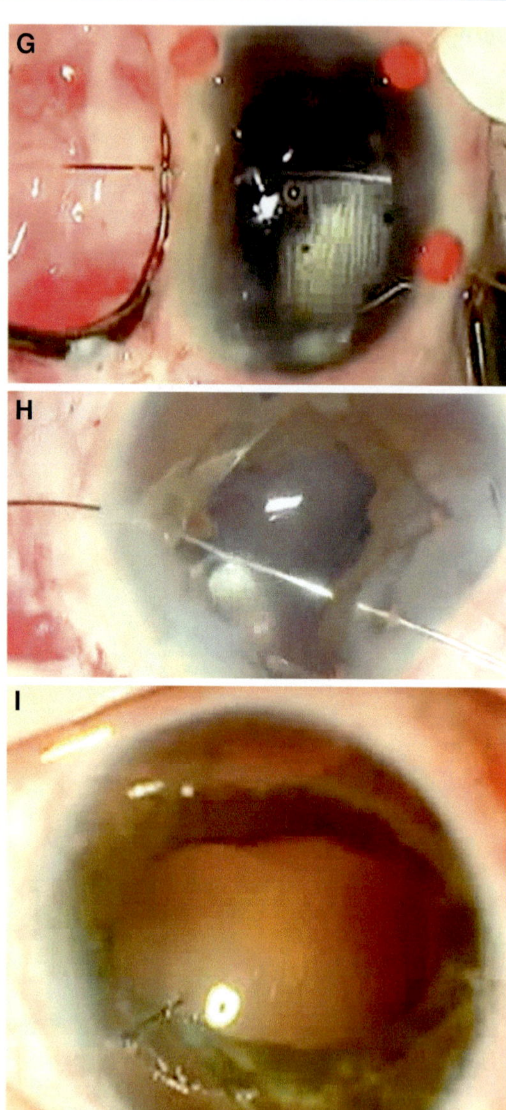

Fig. 44.6 (continued)

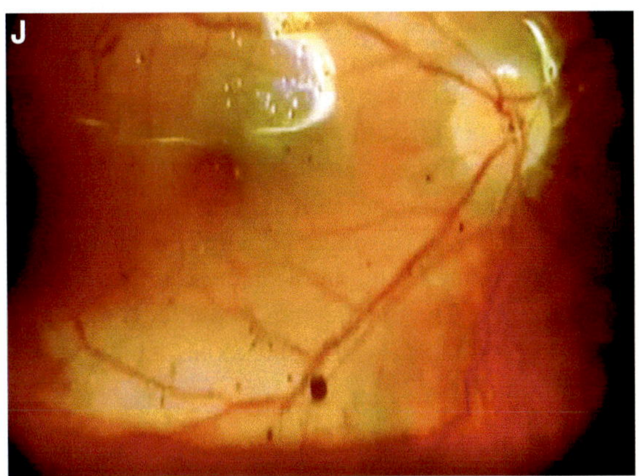

Counseling: The (very mature and intelligent) child and his father really wanted to have another surgery. After we explained that while there was no real risk of further damage to this eye (and a very low risk for sympathetic ophthalmia) but neither was functional improvement likely, and even preserving the eye's current anatomy would be doubtful, the father and child still opted for surgery.

Surgical planning: We decided in favor of a careful anterio-posterior advance. We expected total scarring over the ciliary body (CB) and an at least partially attached retina.[24]

Surgery: In general anesthesia, an anterior chamber maintainer was placed and the anterior synechiae behind the corneal scar endodiathermized (Fig. 44.6B), then cut with scissors (Fig. 44.6C). Iris hooks were then used to create a large and central pupillary opening.

A huge white scar was found behind the iris; as suspected at this point, the retina was adherent to it. After cutting the retina with scissors, the scar was also endodiathermized and then removed through a pars plana incision (Fig. 44.6D). There was no lens in the eye, only a posterior capsule—presumably left behind by the previous surgeon so that an IOL can be subsequently implanted in the bag.

The ciliary body was then inspected; surprisingly, no white scar was found on its surface, only the disappearance of about half of the ciliary processes. The remaning zonules were stretched, exerting tremendous traction on the remaining ciliary processes, which were also were covered by a fine membrane. This tissue complex was removed, 360 degrees, using self-indentation, along with the shrinking capsule; the zonules were cut with scissors and the vitrectomy probe (Fig. 44.6E). It took over 15 min to complete this procedure, with self-indentation.

---

[24] Ultrasonography was not performed as it would not have changed the planning for, or execution of, the surgery. The fact that the eye had light perception vision showed that viable retina was present; in such eyes we always procede assuming that it is detached and may be very anteriorly located.

The retina was indeed partially detached; fortunately, the posterior pole remained attached. There were no signs of PVR on the anterior retinal surface but an extensive network of subretinal strands were found. We removed these by flipping the peripheral retina over (Fig. 44.6F).

We then resutured the ciliary body (Fig. 44.6G), which was detached in almost one quadrant, and recreated the pupil (Fig. 44.6H). The retina was reattached using decaline, and then substituted it with silicone oil. The next day the pupil was round (medically dilated, Fig. 44.6I) and the retina attached (Fig. 44.6J)

Follow-up: The oil was removed after 6 months. At 1 year postoperatively, the eye had normal pressure, the axial length remained 21 mm, and the vision improved to 0,8.

Implications of this case:

- Never give it up; even hopeless cases may have some promise. Proper counseling, however, is mandatory: giving false hope has terrible consequences for the patient (and even for the surgeon if a lawsuit is pursued).
- Preoperative testing that have no impact on the steps to follow are meaningless and thus unnecessary.
- Designing a surgical plan is crucial; the plan, however, must be changed as the findings and the tissues' reaction differ from the expected.
- In a child's eye, the tissues have a wide range of reaction to the action they are exposed to: an obvious example is the iris that was able to stretch all the way across the anterior chamber.
- In an adult's eye, having lost half of the ciliary processes would have sentenced the eye to death by 1 year postinjury.[25] This case illustrates the need to think about "eyeball", rather than "posterior capsule". The child was lucky that the ciliary body was not covered by a white scar—which is what happens in most cases—and that at the time of reconstruction half of the ciliary processes were still viable.
- The child was also lucky that the posterior retina never detached; that the PVR was restricted to the subretinal space; and that these spared the macular area.

Review Questions

1. Does the evaluation of the pediatric patient differ from that of an adult?

A: No; the eye is an eye, regardless of age.
B: Yes: it is more difficult to o a slit-lamp examination.
C: Yes: almost all parts of the process must be adopted to the child, based on his/her age and reaction to the situation.

---

[25] The child was lost to follow-up after 3 years; we do not know how the eye will survive as the child ages.

2. How deep should the corneal sutures be if the wound is full thickness?

A: Whatever works.
B: 100% so that the aqueous access to the stroma is instantly stopped.
C: 90% or just above the Descemet.
D: 2/3.

3. What is the most optimal timing for the intraocular reconstruction?

A: During the primary repair: in the same surgical sitting as the wound closure.
B: During a secondary surgery at least a week later.
C: During a secondary surgery at least two weeks later.

Answers

1. C
2. B
3. A

References

1. Kuhn F, Morris R, Witherspoon CD, Heimann K, Jeffers J, Treister G. A standardized classification of ocular trauma terminology. Ophthalmology. 1996;103:240–3.
2. Jandeck C, Kellner U, Bornfeld N, Foerster M. Open globe injuries in children. Graefe's Arch Ophthalmol. 2000;238:420–6.
3. Kuhn F, Maisiak R, Mann L, Mester V, Morris R, Witherspoon C. The Ocular Trauma Score (OTS). Ophthalmol Clin North Am. 2002;15:163–6.
4. McCannel M. A retrievable suture idea for anterior uveal problems. Ophthalmic Surg Las. 1976;7:8–103.
5. Mester V, Kuhn F. Lens. In: Kuhn F, Pieramici D, editors. Ocular Trauma: principles and practice. New York: Thieme; 2002. p. 180–96.
6. Margherio A, Margherio R, Hartzer M, Trese M, Williams G, Ferrone P. Plasmin enzyme-assisted vitrectomy in traumatic pediatric macular holes. Ophthalmology. 1998;105:1617–20.
7. Ferreira N, Monteiro S, Meireles A, Kuhn F. Outcome of vitrectomy and chorioretinectomy in perforating eye injuries. Ophthalmic Res. 2015;53:200–6.
8. Sul S, Gurelik G, Korkmaz S, Ozdek S, Hasanreisoglu B. Pediatric open-globe injuries: clinical characteristics and factors associated with poor visual and anatomical success. Graefes Arch Clin Exp Ophthalmol. 2016;254(7):1405–10. https://doi.org/10.1007/s00417-015-3087-y Epub 2015 Jul 5 PMID: 26143290.

Posttraumatic Endophthalmitis Management at Pediatric Age

45

Giampaolo Gini

Abstract

Post-traumatic endophthalmitis (PTE) in children is a relatively rare event which must be dealt with rapidly. The approach is almost invariably surgical with the adjunct of systemic medical treatment.

Keywords

Pediatric Post Traumatic Endophthalmitis · Complete early vitrectomy

Introduction

Endophthalmitis is a severe, purulent infection of the intraocular structures. The tissue-destructive effects of the toxins and enzymes released by the infecting organism are exacerbated by the body's immune reaction. Endophthalmitis is generally a complication of either intra-ocular surgery or penetrating injuries. Very rarely it can complicate extra-ocular surgery and in very few cases it can be the result of an endogenous infection. This chapter will focus on post-traumatic endophthalmitis (PTE).

PTE in children is a very serious condition. Its consequences can be devastating, and treatment must be appropriate, aggressive and timely.

Supplementary Information The online version contains supplementary material available at https://doi.org/10.1007/978-3-031-14506-3_45.

G. Gini (✉)
University Hospitals Sussex, Worthing, UK
e-mail: giampaolo.gini@gmail.com

Epidemiology and General Considerations on Pediatric Post-traumatic Endophthalmitis

The incidence of PTE in children affected by ocular trauma is extremely variable and strongly related to the geographic area considered. Environmental and cultural factors account for significant differences in incidence. Pediatric cases account for about 20% of all PTE in western countries whereas this number climbs to over 50% in other areas of the world. As expected, boys are much more at risk than girls representing about 75% of cases.

The modalities with which the trauma occurs are also quite diverse, with scissors and wooden sticks leading the way. The fact that so many injuries in childhood, unlike those of adults, are associated with organic or contaminated material accounts for the relatively high incidence of PTE in pediatric trauma.

Another cause for concern is the fact that scleral wounds with possible intraocular foreign body (IOFB) retention in children may be self-sealing and thus go unnoticed even by ophthalmologists. Finally, children are sometimes slow to realize and to report changes in their visual acuity which can create significant delays in diagnosis and treatment. A detailed slit lamp examination is usually not possible in small children because of cooperation issues which may lead to overlooking the early signs of PTE. All of these elements lead to late diagnosis of PTE in children which definitely worsens the prognosis.

Case Presentation 1 (Fig. 45.1, See the video 1):

A four year old girl accidentally injured her right eye while playing with a sharp pencil. Her mother took her to the local hospital where she was inspected by the on-call ophthalmologist. A small infero-temporal conjunctival hemorrhage was observed and topical Chloramphenicol ointment was prescribed. Three days later the mother noticed that the child was unusually quiet and often rubbed her right eye which appeared bloodshot.

She took her again to hospital where a diagnosis of endophthalmitis was made and the patient was referred to our attention.

Upon examination of the child we found a marked RAPD defect with no red reflex present.

Visual acuity was reduced to light perception. A significant limbal injection was present, no significant corneal oedema and a small hypopion (approx. 3 mm).

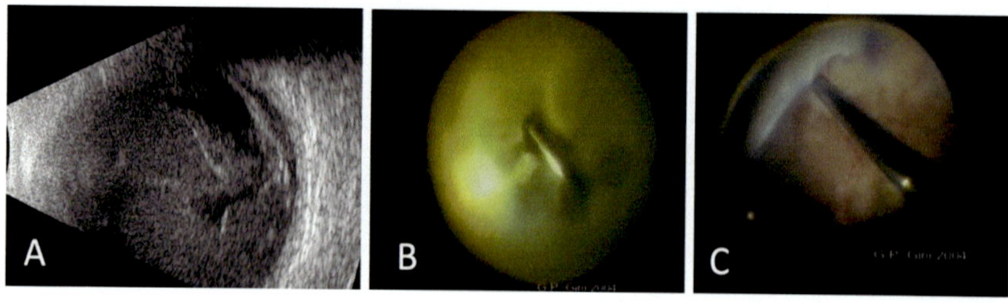

Fig. 45.1 **A** Pre-op U/S **B** Early stages of vitrectomy **C** Late stages of vitrectomy

Slit lamp examination was somewhat difficult as the child had become restless and added little to what was already seen macroscopically.

An Ultrasound scan showed a diffusely hyperechogenic vitreous cavity but failed to identify any foreign body (Fig. 45.1A).

We made a diagnosis of endophthalmitis related to a penetrating injury with possible foreign body retention and proceeded with pars plana vitrectomy with the technique described further on in the text.

After having obtained a vitreous sample for the lab, antibiotics were placed in the infusion bottle and used throughout the procedure. A fragment of what appeared to be the tip of the pencil was seen in the thickened vitreous and removed with the vitreous cutter (the case pre-dates the small gauge era and was done with a 20ga. probe).

Streptococcus Pneumoniae was identified by the lab.

Anatomical success was obtained with a poor visual outcome of counting fingers (CF) vision.

The case we have illustrated highlights the importance of two elements when making a diagnosis:

- Description of the event which determined the trauma both by the child as well as by other witnesses. Traumas with small children involved are generally emotionally challenging and the surgeon must try to reassure both patient and parents so as to obtain the necessary co-operation.
- Imaging to identify possible foreign bodies in what would appear to be a closed-globe injury but where the description of the event suggests otherwise. A plain x-ray and/or ultrasound scan is generally sufficient to provide the necessary information. Occasionally, MRI and to a lesser extent CT scans may be necessary to identify certain IOFBs (i.e. soft organic matter). It should be kept in mind that an MRI scan **should never be performed** before the presence of a metallic foreign body has been ruled out.

Diagnosing PTE

Diagnosing PTE can be much more challenging than doing so in post-interventional cases. This is because the amount of injury suffered by the tissues may be extensive and mask an underlying infection.

Thus:

- Severe open globe injuries with corneal lacerations, uveal prolapse and vitreous hemorrhage should be treated as potentially infected especially if an organic material is involved.
- Open globe injuries with minimal tissue disruption can be treated more conservatively once the presence of an IOFB has been ruled out.

- PTE in these cases will present with the usual symptoms and signs as in post-interventional endophthalmitis.
- A synopsis of the signs and symptoms more readily detectable in children are summarized in the table below.

Post-traumatic Endophthalmitis		
Signs	• Conjunctival/episcleral hyperemia, Conjunctiva edema, hypopyon • Reduction or complete loss of red reflex	Red reflex lost due to corneal edema, AC fibrin, vitreous opacities Easy to perform as it does not require patient co-operation at the slit lamp. Easy to interpret and to follow in time allowing monitoring of progression
Symptoms	Reduced VA, pain	

- The onset of PTE can be acute, often within 24 h from the initial trauma or delayed, even weeks after primary repair has taken place as is the case with slow-growing bacteria and fungi.

Management of PTE

Timing

It must be kept in mind that endophthalmitis is a dynamic rather than a static process.

What we see at presentation might be dramatically different after a few hours due to the exponential growth of pathogens. Unlike post-interventional endophthalmitis, PTE may be associated with more than one pathogen, and these are generally of a more virulent variety.

Therefore, the concept of "mild" as opposed to "severe" endophthalmitis should really be replaced by the terms "early" or "late" to emphasize the importance of immediate action.

PTE is an ophthalmic emergency and must be dealt with as such.

Treatment

Two treatment options are available depending on the stage of PTE at presentation, the type of trauma the eye has suffered and specific circumstances.

1. *Tap and inject procedure:*

- This is generally considered a temporary step if vitrectomy is not readily available. Taken as a stand-alone procedure it should be the exception rather than the rule. (For indications on how to perform tap/inject see Appendix 1)

- The procedure is applicable in specific circumstances where PTE is detected in its very early stages, the extent of the lesions created by the trauma is limited, there has been no lens damage and there has been no need for vitrectomy for globe repair.

- The main reason for foregoing vitrectomy as a first line approach in these cases is essentially to preserve the natural lens.

- The procedure may be associated with the addition of antibiotics in the anterior chamber where a significant AC component is present (i.e. a corneal injury).

- Sufficient material must be obtained from both from the anterior chamber and the vitreous for microbiological assessment.

- Careful close monitoring must be in place so as to detect any worsening of the condition. The patient must be available for examination several times per day and as such should generally be hospitalized. Staff, possibly the same physician for continuity of care, must also be available for repeated patient assessment. Finally, an anesthetist must be present on short notice for sedating the patient for surgery if the condition deteriorates.

- Finding the resources for all this is not a small task in many hospitals and it should be an additional consideration when deciding the most appropriate treatment option.

2. *Vitrectomy*

- We have said before that PTE is to be considered an emergency. We can add here that it should be considered a surgical emergency not a medical one.
- *Complete and Early Vitrectomy* for *Endophthalmitis* (CEVE) is, in our experience, the most effective way of dealing with PTE in general and pediatric PTE in particular.
- Modern vitrectomy is a safe procedure especially if performed in the early stages of PTE when the view is still relatively good.
- It is generally considered safe to place trocars at 4 mm from the limbus in children aged 4 years or older. In younger patients adjustments must be made according to age.
- The advantages of vitrectomy are numerous:
  - Mechanically reduces the pathogenic load
  - Removes toxic elements which cause cellular necrosis

- Allows adequate sample collection **(Please refer to the Dry Tap technique used by the Author and described in Appendix** 1**).**
  - Clears media for retina inspection
  - Allows introduction of drugs (antibiotics and steroids) directly in the anterior chamber and the vitreous cavity. The Author uses antibiotics in the infusion line. During the first part of the surgery, aimed at the anterior segment (see further on) the infusion line is placed in the anterior chamber while the vitreous cutter is used to aspirate all visible pus and fibrin. Once this has been achieved, the infusion line is repositioned through the pars plana.
- Having a clear view during surgery at all steps is crucial for the surgery. No surgical procedure can be successful without having a clear view at all times. This must be kept in mind throughout the procedure and steps must be taken to eliminate those obstacles hindering adequate view of operating field details. Therefore:
  - Remove corneal epithelium if corneal edema is present
  - Use temporary keratoprosthesis (TKP) if excessive corneal scarring is present
  - Remove pus and fibrin from ac
  - Use mechanical devices for dilating the pupil if necessary (iris hooks, Malyugin ring)
  - Remove natural lens if a cataract is present
- Move in an orderly fashion from the anterior to the posterior pole. Once inside the vitreous the following steps must be taken:
  - Make sure you can identify the infusion port
  - Work your way perpendicularly towards the posterior pole remaining on the nasal side of the optic disc
  - Once you have identified the retinal plane you can move out to the periphery more safely and work your way upwards toward the ciliary body.
  - Removing the natural lens will allow efficient ciliary body debulking. A compromise must be reached in phakic eyes.
  - Just how far into the periphery you will want to go depends on your level of expertise and on the case in question. It is important that you remain within your comfort zone.
  - Do not attempt posterior hyaloid detachment which can lead to iatrogenic tears. In cases where a significant macular hypopion is present and greater diffusion of the antibiotic within the retinal tissue is desired, the posterior hyaloid can be "opened" rather than detached with a technique the Author has called "macular fenestration" (Please see **Video** 2).
- Use of antibiotics during vitrectomy: Antibiotics may be either injected into the infusion line at the beginning of the surgery or into the eye at the end of the procedure. The Author prefers to use antibiotics in the infusion line throughout the procedure. This allows rapid diffusion of antibiotics within the eye to all areas reached by the vitreous cutter. The antibiotics are added to the

infusion bottle, in the appropriate concentration, **after** having obtained the necessary samples for microbiology. We regularly use Vancomycin and Ceftazidime.

- There are no definitive studies on the antibiotic dosages to be used within the eye.

  It is generally accepted that 1mg of Vancomycin and 2.25 mg of Ceftazidime are effective and non-toxic. If we consider the volume of the vitreous cavity to be 5 ml on average, the concentration of these antibiotics will be around 0.2 and 0.5 mg/ml for Vancomycin and Ceftazidime respectively.

When using antibiotics placed directly into the infusion, 250 mg of Vancomycin and 250 mg of Ceftazidime are used. The result is a concentration of 0.5mg/ml in the infusion line and ultimately into the eye. These concentrations are somewhat higher for Vancomycin than those normally recommended but the Author has found no toxic effects. In particularly severe infections, the Author has employed 500 mg of Vancomycin in the infusion with no side effects.

If antibiotics are used at the end of the procedure, a recommended dosage of 0.1 ml (1 mg) of Vancomycin and 0.1 ml (2.25 mg) of Ceftazidime is used. Once again, it is our belief that somewhat higher concentrations may be used for severe infections. The Author has used Vancomycin 0.2 ml with no adverse consequences.

The use of intravitreal steroids is optional but strongly recommended except where a fungal endophthalmitis is suspected. (For indications on how to prepare appropriate antibiotic concentrations see Appendix 2).

3. *Additional Medical Therapy*

Both the inflammatory process as well as vitrectomy itself allows greater permeability of the blood brain barrier. The use of systemic antibiotics and steroids is therefore recommended especially when faced with severe open globe injuries and/or when orbital tissue is involved. We generally leave systemic therapy to be decided upon by a pediatrician. In our experience, Ciprofloxacin either I.V. at the dose of 10 mg/kg every 12 h or orally at the dose of 15 mg/kg every 12 h has generally been the antibiotic of choice in severe endophthalmitis. Concerns have been raised over the use of Fluorochinolones in children for the potential musculoskeletal adverse effects. However, recent data has shown that these side effects are reversible following the withdrawal of the drug.

Most third generation cephalosporins (ceftriaxone, cefotaxime, ceftazidime, cefixime and cefepime) as well as carbapenems (imipenem) have been proven to penetrate the B-B barrier to some extent and can be used as alternatives to Fluorochinolones.

Systemic Dexamethasone may be used to reduce the inflammatory response with a regimen of 0.15–0.30 mg/kg per day. The duration of treatment depends on the response to these drugs.

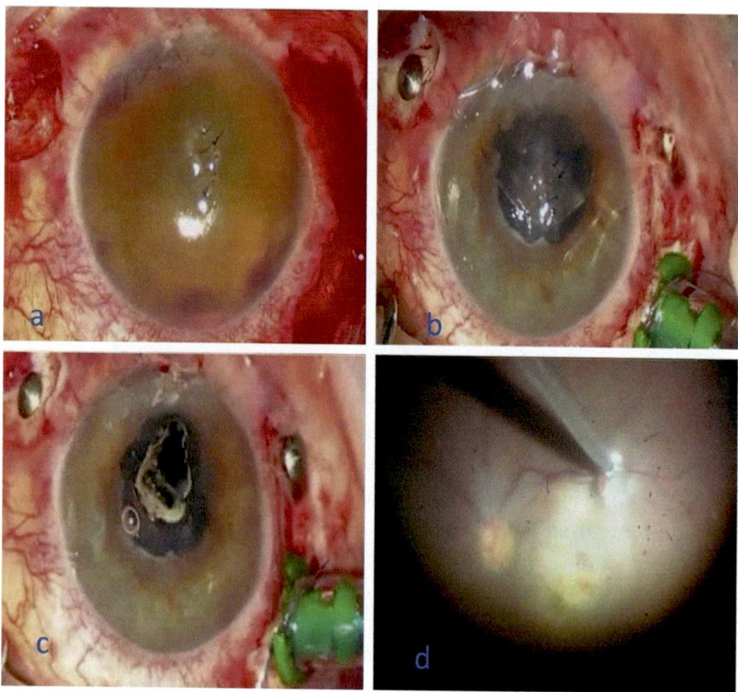

Fig. 45.2 See the case presentation 2 in the text

Case Presentation 2 (Fig. 45.2, See the video 3)

This was a 12-year-old child, who presented elsewhere for a corneal penetrating injury with a small metallic foreign body also penetrating the lens and stopping at the back of the eye. Primary corneal wound repair had been done together with primary cataract surgery with implantation of IOL within 24 h. He presented with a full-blown endophthalmitis 3 days after and was referred to us at this stage for vitrectomy combined with penetrating keratoplasty. Vision was light perception, and the cornea was very cloudy with a central laceration area, there was hypopyon and inflammatory membranes covering and blocking the pupillary area (Fig. 45.1 A). An urgent vitrectomy was performed. After debridement of the corneal epithelium, an aqueous sample was taken for microbiologic examination. Following removal of inflammatory membranes from the anterior chamber the IOL could be identified as an ACIOL. Following pars plana entry, a vitreous sample was obtained and membranes covering the back of the lens in the pupillary area were also removed which made the view clearer (Fig. 45.1B) so that we could proceed with vitrectomy without a penetrating keratoplasty. After removal of the central vitreous opacities, we could reach a small metallic foreign body within the opacities. We extracted the ACIOL to make the view clearer and to take the IOFB out through the same limbal incision (Fig. 45.1C.). The retina could be visualized nicely after these maneuvers and 360-degree peripheral laser was applied. There were edema and scars in the macular area, but the retina was attached (Fig. 45.1D). The eye was left with silicone oil and 1/3 dose of intravitreal vancomycin and ceftazidime at the very end of the procedure. Culture was negative for the case, but infection could be controlled very well after the surgery with the given intravitreal antibiotics and topical moxifloxacin + dexamethasone every hour for the first 5 days which was tapered later. Silicone oil was removed 3 months after and the best-corrected visual acuity remained 20/400 at the last follow up because of the macular scar. The patient was left aphakic. (Case courtesy of Prof. Dr. Şengül Özdek).

Case Presentation 3 (Fig. 45.3)

An 11-year-old boy presented to another clinic with a 2-day history of pencil-tip injury of the left eye. He mentioned about the injury 2 days after the trauma to his parents. When they arrived at the hospital, intravitreal cefazolin and gentamicin were administered following a diagnosis of endophthalmitis. After 3 days of follow-up, hypopyon was still apparent and the patient was referred to us. By then 5 days had passed from the original injury. Visual acuity was hand motion. There was a lead mark in the corneal entry site, corneal edema, and hypopyon (Fig. 45.3A). B-scan ultrasound showed some vitreous opacities (Fig. 45.3B). Urgent vitreous tap and intravitreal injection (vancomycin, ceftazidime, and dexamethasone) were performed. Samples were obtained from the vitreous as well as from the anterior chamber. Postoperative infection was controlled, but visual acuity remained hand motion because of the lens and vitreous opacities (Fig. 45.3C). One week after admission, a pars plana vitrectomy and lensectomy were performed.

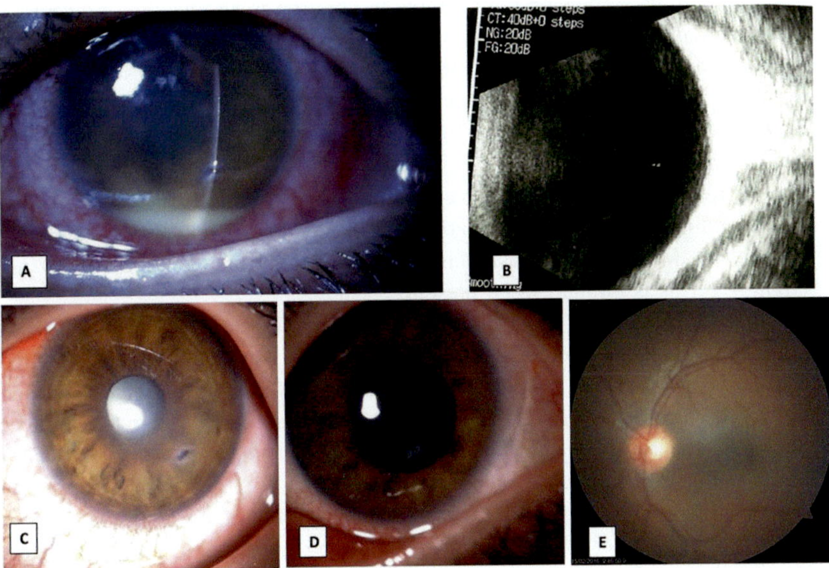

Fig. 45.3 See the text for case presentation 3

During lensectomy posterior lens capsule was defective, and inflammatory material was observed inside the lens capsule. Pars plana lensectomy was performed together with a complete vitrectomy. Posterior hyaloid was not removed because of its strong adhesions to the posterior pole. There was no retinitis. The case ended up with a fluid–air exchange. Two weeks postoperatively, there were no signs of infection (Fig. 45.3D, E). Visual acuity was 0.2 with a refraction of +13 D. (Case courtesy of Prof. Dr. Şengül Özdek).

Prognosis

There is a scarcity of papers in the literature on PTE. This makes statistical conclusions difficult. The prognosis is thought to be poor often resulting in severe visual loss which can sometimes extend to become anatomical damage ending up with a deformed phthisic eye as well.

However, it must be said that some of these papers follow the EVS criteria with mainly intra-vitreal injections and no vitrectomy. Others, where vitrectomy was performed, report a ***median*** time between trauma and intervention ranging from three to twelve days. The Author suggest that early prompt vitrectomy may improve the prognosis.

Conclusions

- Endophthalmitis associated with trauma in children is an uncommon event.
- Environmental and cultural factors account for significant differences in incidence. Ratio of pediatric cases is much less in the western countries as compared to other areas of the world. Boys represent about 75% of the cases. The dynamics involved in the accident and the type of injury also vary with geography.
- The microbiological profile is also extremely variable and related to the nature of the offending agent (organic *versus* non-organic), as well as environmental setting (rural *versus* urban). A fairly equal distribution between Gram- and Gram + germs is thought to be present.
- It is a well-known fact that children are not 'small adults' reacting differently both emotionally as well as clinically to trauma. One of the additional risk factors in children as opposed to adults is the difficulty of obtaining a clear history of the event with the real danger of overlooking minimally invasive penetrating injuries. This is why an ultrasound scan should always be carried out in all pediatric trauma cases which do not present with a manifest open globe injury. In suspicious "fresh" cases a follow-up should be arranged with an ophthalmologist after 24 h and parents should be instructed to roughly evaluate the child's visual acuity, comparing one eye to the other.

- Treatment is prompt and surgical. We advocate **complete and early vitrectomy** with or without lensectomy depending on the stage of the infection and the state of the lens. Saving the eye obviously takes priority over saving the lens.
- Since any procedure on a child must be done under general anesthesia, it is difficult to see the use of intravitreal antibiotics even as a temporary step before vitrectomy. However, exceptional circumstances may exist which justify this approach. Finally, the use of intravitreal antibiotics as a stand-alone procedure aimed at sparing the lens and further surgical trauma, is to be considered only in very limited circumstances.

Review Questions

1. Which of these techniques should be used as a first line approach for the diagnosis of intra-ocular foreign bodies when no fundus view is possible?

A. MRI
B. CT scan
C. Ultrasound scan

2. Which micro-organisms are more likely involved in PTE?

A. Gram negative
B. Gram positive
C. Equal weight between Gram + and Gram −

3. A pars plana vitrectomy for endophthalmitis should be performed

A. When visual deterioration reaches counting fingers at 50 cm
B. When a positive vitreous tap returns from the lab
C. As soon as endophthalmitis is suspected

Answers

1. C
2. C
3. C

Appendix 1: Tap and Inject Technique

- Before the tap is performed you must liaise with the Microbiology laboratory (within working hours) or the on-call biologist (out of hours).
- The specimen must go to microbiology immediately after it has been taken as delay will reduce the chance of microbial isolation.

- If a 24/7 microbiology service is not available, an alternative plan must be in place. The appropriate culture media provided by the microbiology department must be available and in date so that the specimen can be seeded immediately.
- A small-gauge (23/25/27ga.) vitrectomy probe is used. The aspiration tubing is connected to a 1 ml syringe which is operated manually.
- A second trocar is inserted with the infusion line. The infusion line will carry ONLY AIR not water. The use of air to replace the vitreous which is removed allows the harvesting of relatively large, undiluted amounts of vitreous without the risk of hypotony.
- Once the sample has been collected, the antibiotics can be injected in the recommended dosage (see Appendix 2 and Fig. 45.4).

Appendix 2: How to Prepare Intravitreal Antibiotics

To prepare Ceftazidime intravitreal injection 2.5 mg in 0.1 ml:

- Reconstitute a vial of Ceftazidime 500 mg with 4 ml Water for Injections*
- Shake vial thoroughly to dissolve
- Withdraw the entire contents and make up to 5 ml with Water for Injections = 100 mg/ml
- Shake syringe thoroughly to mix

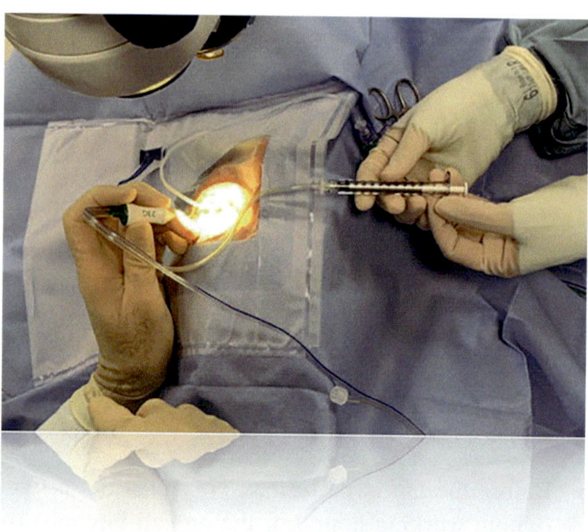

Fig. 45.4 Tap and inject procedure

- Inject 1 ml back into the vial and add 3 ml of sodium chloride 0.9% injection = 25 mg/ml
- Withdraw approximately 0.2 ml (excess to facilitate priming) into a 1 ml syringe
- When ready to inject discard all but 0.1 ml of the solution
- Administer 2.5 mg in 0.1 ml.
- * Indications are based on product packaging available to the Author.

To prepare Vancomycin intravitreal injection 2 mg in 0.1 ml:

- Reconstitute a vial of Vancomycin 500 mg with 5 ml Water for Injections* = 100 mg/ml
- Shake vial thoroughly to dissolve
- Inject 1 ml back into the vial and add 4 ml of sodium chloride 0.9% injection = 20 mg/ml
- Shake vial thoroughly to mix
- Withdraw approximately 0.2 ml (excess to facilitate priming) into a 1 ml syringe.
- When ready to inject discard all but 0.1 ml of the solution
- Administer 2 mg in 0.1 ml.
- * Indications are based on product packaging available to the Author.

To prepare Dexamethasone intravitreal injection 400 µg in 0.1 ml:

- Draw up 0.1 ml of Dexamethasone with a 1 ml syringe from a 4 mg/ml vial.
- Add 0.9 ml of water for injections (bring up to 1 ml).
- When ready to inject discard all but 0.1 ml of the solution.
- Administer 400 µg in 0.1 ml.

Some of these drugs are available in pre-diluted preparations depending on Countries.

Vancomycin is safe to use in patients with penicillin allergy.

Ceftazidime should be used with caution in patients with penicillin allergy and avoided in those with a history of anaphylaxis to penicillin. In these patients Amikacin 400 µg in 0.1 ml is a safe alternative.

References

1. Rishi E, Rishi P, Koundanya VV, Sahu C, Roy R, Bhende PS. Post-traumatic endophthalmitis in 143 eyes of children and adolescents from India. 2016. https://doi.org/10.1038/eye.2016.9.
2. Venkatesh R, Dave AP, Gurav P, Agrawal M. Post-traumatic endophthalmitis in children. Nepal J Ophthalmol. 2019;11(21):55–63. https://doi.org/10.3126/nepjoph.v11i1.25419.
3. Mansouri M, Faghihi H, Hajizadeh F, Rasoulinejad SA, Rajabi MT, Tabatabaey A, et al. Epidemiology of open-globe injuries in Iran: analysis of 2,340 cases in 5 years (report no. 1). Retina 2009;29:1141–9.

4. Junejo SA, Ahmed M, Alam M. Endophthalmitis in pediatric penetrating ocular injuries in Hyderabad. J Pak Med Assoc. 2010;60(7):532–5.
5. Rishi E, Rishi P, Nandi K, Shroff D, Therese KL. Endophthalmitis caused by *Enterococcus faecalis*—a case series. Retina 2009;29:214217.
6. Alfaro DV, Roth DB, Laughlin RM, Goyal M, Liggett PE. Pediatric post-traumatic endophthalmitis. Br J Ophthalmol. 1995;79:888–91.
7. Weinstein GS, Mondino BJ, Weinberg RJ, Biglan AW. Endophthalmitis in a pediatric population. Ann Ophthalmol. 1979;11:935–43.
8. Han DP, Wisniewski SR, Wilson LA, Barza M, Vine AK, Doft BH, et al. Spectrum and susceptibility of microbiologic isolates in the endophthalmitis vitrectomy study. Am J Ophthalmol. 1996; 122(1):1–17.
9. Chhabra S, Kunimoto DY, Kazi L, Regillo CD, Ho AC, Belmont J, et al. Endophthalmitis after open globe injury. Microbiologic spectrum and susceptibilities of isolates. Am J Ophthalmol. 2006;142: 852–4.
10. Kuhn F, Morris R, Witherspoon CD, Mester V. The Birmingham eye trauma terminology system (BETT). J Fr Ophtalmol. 2004;27(2):206–10. https://doi.org/10.1016/s0181-5512(04)96122-0.
11. Kuhn F, Gini G. Vitrectomy for endophthalmitis. Ophthalmology. 2006;113:714.
12. Adefurin A, Sammons H, Jacqz-Aigrain JE, Choonara I. Ciprofloxacin safety in paediatrics: a systematic review. Arch Dis Childhood 2011; 96(9)

Pediatric Intraocular Foreign Body Management

46

Abdulla Shaheen, Julia Hudson, Sarah Read, and Nicolas Yannuzzi

Abstract

Pediatric intraocular foreign body (IOFB) injuries account for approximately one-third of open globe injuries and present distinctive management and ocular morbidity challenges not seen in adults, including a severe inflammatory response and the potential of amblyopia. As a result, a comprehensive clinical examination with ultrasound and CT scan coupled with examination under general anesthesia is required. The perioperative management of IOFB should follow a standardized protocol and be tailored to each patient individually addressing whether and when to operate or not operate, how many surgical stages to undergo, and dealing with any complications. This chapter discusses the management of pediatric posterior segment IOFB injuries management based on current best clinical practices and the author's experience, including pearls for each surgical step and management of unexpected or complex cases.

Keywords

Intraocular foreign body · Posterior segment trauma · Vitrectomy

Supplementary Information The online version contains supplementary material available at https://doi.org/10.1007/978-3-031-14506-3_46.

A. Shaheen · J. Hudson · N. Yannuzzi (✉)
Department of Ophthalmology, Bascom Palmer Eye Institute, Miller School of Medicine, University of Miami, Miami, FL, USA
e-mail: nay7@med.miami.edu

S. Read
Department of Ophthalmology, Miller School of Medicine, Bascom Palmer Eye Institute, Miller School of Medicine, University of Miami, Miami, FA, USA

Retinal Consultants of Hawaii, Honolulu, HI, USA

Introduction

Intraocular foreign body (IOFB) injury accounts for 18% to 41% of all open globe injuries in children [1]. The location and damage caused by an IOFB are determined by the object's physical properties such as size, shape, and composition, and object's momentum at the time of impact. This chapter discusses the clinical assessment and management of IOFB-associated posterior segment traumatic eye injuries.

Assessment

A thorough history of the injury, including the onset, mechanism, and IOFB material and the use of eye protection, prior ocular history or surgeries, tetanus vaccine status, and last oral intake should be obtained. If there is concern for abuse or neglect, a proper investigation should be performed by child protective services.

A thorough ophthalmic examination should then be performed including slit lamp examination and fundoscopy. In many cases, a pediatric patient may be difficult to examine following trauma, and much of the exam may need to be deferred until the patient is under anesthesia. Aggressive manipulation or force during physical examination in the case of an uncooperative child may risk further injury or extrusion of ocular contents.

Adjunctive B-scan ultrasonography may be helpful for the localization of the foreign body or may be deferred until anesthesia induction. A noncontract CT of the orbits with fine cuts through the orbit should be performed preoperatively. The Hounsfield units, attenuation, and imaging artifacts associated with the foreign body may aid in identification of the material (Table 46.1) [2].

Portable metal detectors are becoming obsolete but is still available in some emergency departments. They can be used to detect and localize magnetic metallic foreign bodies, and hence determine the necessity for intraoperative magnets [3].

Management

To operate or not: The decision to take the patient to surgery is the first step in management. Patients with complications from the IOFB should generally undergo surgery. This includes all patients with endophthalmitis, whether suspected or confirmed, those with open globe injury, retinal detachment (RD), retinal tear, or significant lens damage (risk of phacoanaphylaxis). Foreign bodies associated with an inflammatory response should be surgically removed. The amount of inflammation is influenced by the composition of the IOFB and its location within eye. An IOFB embedded in the lens, for example, may cause a minor inflammatory reaction, whereas retinal or choroidal particles can cause an exaggerated response [4]. Some metallic foreign bodies can incite destructive chemical reactions, as will be discussed later in this chapter.

Table 46.1 Imaging features of most commonly encountered intraocular foreign body materials

Foreign body material	Plain film X-ray appearance	Ultrasound ring-down artifact***	CT appearance	Hounsfield Unit (HU)
Metallic				
Aluminum	Moderately Radiopaque	Flashlight	High attenuation without artifact	713.5
Brass*	Radiopaque	Overlapping	High attenuation with shadow artifact and edge streak artifact	3070
Copper	Radiopaque	Overlapping	High attenuation with shadow artifact and edge streak artifact	3062
Silver	Radiopaque	Overlapping	High attenuation with shadow and streak artifact	3052
Steel**	Radiopaque	Overlapping	High attenuation with shadow artifact and edge streak artifact	3060
Lead	Radiopaque	Headlight	High attenuation with shadow and streak artifact	3069
Nonmetallic				
Plastic (polyvinyl chloride [PVC])	Minimally Radiopaque	Overlapping	High attenuation without artifact	484
Plastic (CF6 spectacle plastic)	Radiolucent	Overlapping	Moderate attenuation (similar to retina)	123
Glass (bottle glass)	Radiopaque	Overlapping	High attenuation without artifact	2096
Glass (windshield glass)	Radiopaque	Headlight	High attenuation without artifact	2700
Poplar Wood (dry)	Radiolucent	Overlapping	Low attenuation without artifact	371
Poplar Wood (wet)	Radiolucent	Overlapping	Low attenuation without artifact	102.5
Stone (slate)	Radiopaque	Overlapping	High attenuation without artifact	2615

*Brass is an alloy of zinc and copper; ** Steel is the most common form of iron; *** Ring-down artifact is a solid line or a series of parallel bands emanating behind the IOFB
CT = computed tomography; Headlight shape = broad and dense; Flashlight shape = focused and narrow

Not every patient with an intraocular foreign body requires surgery. Assessment for the possibility of long- or short-term complications can help determine whether to operate or not. For example, a chronic inert IOFB such as glasses can be left without operation in an asymptomatic individual. Uncomplicated inert metallic IOFB in anterior chamber resulting from a self-sterilizing event such as explosive thermal energy with no evidence of inflammation or infection can also be left without surgical intervention. Table 46.2 depicts some of the most common inert

Table 46.2 Intraocular foreign body classified according to their chemical interaction with ocular tissue

	Inert	Toxic
Metallic	Silver Gold Platinum	Iron (magnetic) Nickel (magnetic) Copper Aluminum Mercury Zinc
Nonmetallic	Glass Stone Plastic Porcelain	Vegetable

and toxic IOFBs. In acute traumatic cases, a full comprehensive examination under general anesthesia is required to fully evaluate the extent of ocular injuries.

- **Preoperative protocol**: Patients with suspected IOFBs should be treated with a standardized protocol that include eyeshield protection of the affected eye, update of tetanus prophylaxis, systemic and topical antibiotics, and anesthesia preparation with no oral intake. Infectious endophthalmitis may complicate up to 24% of metallic IOFB injuries [5]. There is no clear consensus on the use of oral antibiotics for open globe injuries, however we recommend a broad spectrum such as amoxicillin/clavulanate to cover the most frequently associated Gram positive and negative organisms involved in posttraumatic endophthalmitis. In particularly high-risk cases where OR access is limited or delayed, the use of intravitreal antibiotics before surgery could be considered but administration should be performed cautiously given the risk of extrusion of ocular contents from an open wound and is rarely performed in a pediatric patient unless highly cooperative. Analgesic and anti-emetic medication should be administered as needed. A retrobulbar block after anesthesia should be considered to assist with post-operative pain management, adjusting the volume of the block to minimize the potential of central nervous system side effects in younger children.
- **Timing to surgery**: Surgical timing for a pediatric intraocular foreign body is determined by several factors and early intervention is the best choice in most circumstances. Toxic IOFBs or endophthalmitis require immediate surgery. Total hyphema with uncontrolled intraocular pressure or high likelihood for corneal staining require surgery. Development of corneal blood staining is an absolute indication for intervention for patients in the amblyopic age range, and a relative indication for older patients to avoid the need for corneal transplantation.
- **Surgical steps**: Following slit-lamp examination, ultrasound, CT scan, and initiation of the preoperative open globe protocol, the patient should be examined under general anesthesia. This should include portable slit lamp exam of the anterior segment, a fundus examination, and B scan ultrasound of the posterior segment or high-resolution ultrasound of the anterior segment if the view is compromised or location of the IOFB cannot be adequately determined. At the

completion of the exam, the surgical plan should be finalized and may include: exploration alone, closure of any globe defects, lensectomy, vitrectomy, IOFB removal, or retinal detachment repair.

- Step 1: Globe exploration
  - 360° conjunctival peritomy and isolation of the muscles with careful inspection of the sclera behind the muscle insertions. If there is concern for posterior rupture, this should be performed gently with limited globe manipulation to limit the risk for posterior extrusion.
- Step 2: Globe closure
  - Corneal lacerations can be closed with 10–0 nylon, limbal lacerations with 9–0 nylon, and scleral lacerations with a mix of 8–0 nylon and 7–0 vicryl suture.
  - If the laceration is under a muscle, the muscle may need to be isolated, secured, and taken down for proper scleral closure and then reattached.
- Step 3: Assess the position of the IOFB
  - 3a: IOFB is outside the globe. The condition is known as intraorbital foreign body injury, and while it is beyond the scope of this chapter, organic FBs are usually removed while inorganic FBs may be left in place depending on patient symptoms and the composition of the FB. Foreign bodies in the anterior orbit are more likely to be removed and those in the posterior orbit or near the optic nerve are more likely to be left in place due to the risk associated with their removal.
  - 3b: IOFB is in the anterior chamber without lens violation or involvement. In these cases, create a paracentesis, reform or stabilize the anterior chamber with an adaptive viscoelastic (Healon5), and remove the foreign body with retinal forceps. Intracameral antibiotics with half dose vancomycin and ceftazidime may be considered after anterior chamber washout is performed.
  - 3c: IOFB is embedded in the lens without suspicion for posterior capsular rupture. In these cases, consider phacoemulsification. The capsule may be left behind for subsequent sulcus lens placement after the eye has healed.
  - 3d: IOFB damaged the lens with anterior and posterior capsular defects suspected. We recommend lensectomy with the cutter or phaco-assisted lens removal in cases where the lens involvement is through and through. If an RD is present, the capsule should be removed. If there is no RD, the capsule can be left in place for future IOL implantation.
  - 3e: IOFB is in the angle. Gonioscopy often provides the best view of the IOFB. It is best to avoid utilizing the entry wound of the IOFB. Instead, a paracentesis 180° from the IOFB should be created and the anterior chamber stabilized with viscoelastic. Using a gonio lens to view the IOFB, often it can then be grasped with intraocular forceps.
  - 3f: IOFB is in the posterior chamber behind the iris. This can be a difficult case and endoscopy often provides the best view of the retroirideal space. A paracentesis should be created, and the anterior chamber stabilized with viscoelastic. Once a view of the IOFB is obtained, often it can be grasped with intraocular forceps, brought into the anterior chamber, and then removed

through the paracentesis. Notably, if the IOFB is contained within the zonules, a pars plana lensectomy will be necessary to get access to it.

- 3g: IOFB is in the mid vitreous cavity. A standard three-port set-up is used and at first a core vitrectomy is performed to allow for manipulation of the IOFB without causing vitreous traction to avoid inducing retinal breaks. Induction of a posterior vitreous detachment should be attempted and vitreous adjacent to the IOFB must be removed before attempting to grasp or remove the IOFB. Pediatric posterior vitreous detachment (PVD) induction can be challenging and the use of dilute triamcinolone to stain the posterior hyaloid for better visualization is often helpful. A flex loop can be used to tease up and create space under the Weiss ring prior to full induction with the cutter.
- 3h: IOFB is resting on the retina. This requires a core vitrectomy and induction of a PVD prior to removal of IOFB. The peripheral retina should be carefully examined for breaks and lasered appropriately.
- 3i: IOFB is subretinal or associated with retinal detachment. This requires a core vitrectomy and PVD induction before attempting manipulation or removal of the IOFB. If the IOFB has caused a large retinal break, extract the IOFB through it; if the break is small, perform localized retinectomy. During removal, perfluoro-N-octane (PFO) may stabilize the retina and avoid posterior hemorrhage migration during IOFB removal. In addition, aggressive diathermy surrounding the IOFB incarceration site within the retina/choroid can help reduce the risk of bleeding.
- After removal of the IOFB, retinal detachment repair can proceed in the usual fashion followed by placement of a gas or oil tamponade.
- Step 4: Removing an IOFB from the vitreous cavity
  - 4a: Determine the site of exit. If lens is being removed, then clear cornea is often the easiest site for removal. If lens is being spared, then the IOFB is typically removed via a pars plana wound and care should be taken to avoid accidental intraoperative lens trauma.

    Preservation of the lens in pediatric cases should be prioritized whenever possible. A small capsular tear may self-seal and the cataract formed can be non-visually significant avoiding lens removal. Unfortunately, severe damage to the lens in the case of large IOFBs or necessity of an anterior approach to address posterior pathology such as funnel detachments or choroidals often necessitate sacrifice of the lens. IOL implantation is rarely indicated at the time of initial repair given the risk of endophthalmitis, however the integrity of the lens capsule and zonules should be assessed to aide in future planning for secondary lens placement.
  - 4b: Lift the IOFB off the posterior segment and secure with forceps. Depending on the location of the IOFB, consider placement of liquid perfluorocarbon (PFO) to protect the macula during removal [6]. One may also consider utilizing a chandelier illuminating system to free the second hand for large IOFBs that may require a two-handed technique. Directly lifting the IOFB with a Maxgrip or Rappazzo intraocular forceps can be attempted although this can be quite challenging. If the IOFB is magnetic and

forceps-assisted removal is unsuccessful, consider lifting the IOFB from the retinal surface with a rare earth magnet and then transferring to a forceps in a two-handed approach. If the IOFB is not magnetic, then one can use suction from the soft tip extrusion cannula to lift from the retinal surface and then likewise pass it to an intraocular forceps with a two-handed approach. If the IOFB is embedded in the choroid or sclera, applying laser around the IOFB can reduce the risk of hemorrhage upon removal.

- 4c: Remove the IOFB via the sclerotomy. Create a sclerotomy with MVR blade or microkeratome that is larger than the combined cross-sectional area of the IOFB and forceps and located roughly 180° from the FB to avoid scraping the retina or the choroid. If bleeding from the retina or choroid is encountered, disengage, use diathermy to control the bleeding, and clear the vitreous hemorrhage before making a second attempt at extracting the FB.
- 4d: Wound closure and retinal inspection. Stabilize the globe but closing the corneal or scleral exit wound. A thorough depressed exam should be performed to inspect the impact site for any whitening, signs of infection, retinal breaks, bleeding and managed according. Given the risk of endophthalmitis we advocate for placement of prophylactic intravitreal antibiotics, typically vancomycin and ceftazidime.

Extra tips and pearls

- If the infusion cannot be visualized, start with the infusion in the AC, remove the lens, then move the infusion back to the pars.
- If the IOFB produced posterior rupture sites that could not be closed, PPV would be challenging because irrigating fluid can flow into the orbit and cause posterior pressure. In these cases, close the wound immediately and postpone vitrectomy for a week to allow for adequate wound closure. Canthotomy and cantholysis are alternatives for dealing with increased posterior pressure.
- Perform a pars plana vitrectomy first, then remove the IOFB. This avoids incarceration of the vitreous into the forceps during extraction, loosens attachments to the IOFB and limits vitreous traction to prevent induction of retinal breaks. Perform a peripheral shave at the site of IOFB removal to prevent vitreous dragging during extraction.
- In children aged 4 years and older, sclerotomies are frequently placed 4 mm from the limbus. The exact location of the sclerotomy may vary according to age, and different techniques may advocate for different cutoff points. Gan et al. recommended an easy-to-remember strategy of following a 1 mm limbus-to-sclerotomy distance for children up to one year of age and adding 1 mm to the limbus for each year thereafter [7].
- Create a sclerotomy that is roughly equal to the cross section of the foreign body (estimated) plus the size of the forceps (known) to avoid traumatic wound distortion when removing the IOFB. The best chance of removing the IOFB is on the first try. It is better to make a larger wound than to go too small and end up with your IOFB stuck in the pars plana.

- For cases of IOFB involving the posterior segment with a very high risk of PVR and retinal detachment, consider placement of a scleral buckle. This is to avoid future difficulty in dissecting and placing a scleral buckle arising from the conjunctival/tenon's capsule scarring after RD repair.
- For anterior lacerations, if there is leakage after closure with the PPV (elevated IOP can stress even a good wound closure), try placing a bandage contact lens (BCL) on the eye during the PPV. It will still seep around the BCL, but you should be able to maintain a reasonable view.
- If the IOFB is metallic, utilize an intraocular magnet to assist transfer to the forceps for extraction. Engage the IOFB with the magnet, bring it to the anterior vitreous, transfer the IOFB to the forceps jaws, and use the forceps to extract the IOFB from the globe. The magnet is intended to be utilized in combination with pars plana vitrectomy during typical 19- or 20-gauge pars plana sclerotomies. While removing tiny foreign bodies using the micromagnet does not need enlarging the sclerotomies, removing large foreign bodies often requires transferring the foreign body from the magnet to a foreign body forceps, which requires enlarging one of the sclerotomies [8].
- Dealing with fluidic stability in the setting of IOFB-induced posterior pole laceration needs careful handling. Switching the mode between vacuum and flow control is required to maintain steady fluidics during vitrectomy. When doing a core vitrectomy, pursue vacuum control mode to remove the vitreous more effectively. Switch to flow control as you get closer to the mobile retina at the retinal break site to avoid surges and turbulence that can occur when using vacuum mode, as the flow control mode does not build up pressure when the tip is occluded, avoiding the formation of a retinal hole that would have occurred with vacuum control [9].

Complications

Complications of IOFB arise from the mechanical damage, infection, toxic, and inflammatory reactions. These include cataract, hyphema, optic neuropathy, and sympathetic ophthalmia, and metallosis bulbi a direct electrolytic toxicity to ocular structures from certain metals. Posterior segment sequelae involve endophthalmitis, proliferative vitreoretinopathy, retinal tear, and retinal detachment. Retinal detachment risk increases with wound size greater than 3 mm and with IOFB located in the posterior segment.

Endophthalmitis risk factors include wound closure more than 24 h after initial injury, wound in zone II, injury in a rural location with soil contamination, ruptured lens capsule, and retained IOFB. The type of the foreign body influences the risk of endophthalmitis, with metallic foreign bodies found to be protective against endophthalmitis due to the self-sterilizing effect of the generated heat. Polymicrobial infection is more common than after an injection or surgery. Bacillus species may complicate soil contaminated IOFB, whereas fungal organisms can be found in organic matter contamination. Visual outcome is better with good VA at presentation and early surgery and worse with delayed removal and/or posterior segment IOFB [10, 11].

Certain metallic IOFBs may be toxic to the retina and optic nerve if not detected during examination. Metallosis bulbi is ocular tissue damage resulting from oxidation and chemical reactions between retained metallic IOFB and ocular tissue and fluids [12, 13]. Except in the case of pure copper IOFBs (>85%), metallosis is an insidious condition that manifests months or years after the initial injury. Therefore, metallosis prevention is not a major concern in the primary surgical care of ocular injuries. Siderosis (iron) and chalcosis (copper) are the two most frequent types of metallosis. Electroretinogram (ERG) reveals changes before clinical presentation. In the early stage of siderosis, both the a- and b-waves may be transiently increased. As the condition progresses, the amplitude of the b-wave diminishes, resulting in a reduction in the b-wave/a-wave ratio [14]. ERG changes in chalcosis are less well documented and compared to siderosis, no supernormal b-waves are seen, and the magnitude of ERG amplitude reduction is less than 50%. Following removal of the IOFB, most cases of siderosis have reversal of the ERG changes [14]. B-wave amplitude reductions of up to 50% are associated with reversible ERG changes; B-wave amplitude reductions of more than 50% are usually permanent [4]. There are no studies documenting reversibility of ERG changes in chalcosis; however, because of milder changes, we would expect most cases to be reversible.

Patients with siderosis initially present with progressive vision loss and nyctalopia with/without dyschromatopsia or scotomas [15]. Anterior segment examination may reveal rust-colored or yellowish pigmentary deposits in the cornea at the level of stroma or endothelium [16], greenish-brown discoloration of the iris [17], reversible fixed dilated pupil [18] and cataract formation [14]. Posterior segment can show pigmentary degeneration of the retina and edema of the optic disc.

Copper-containing IOFB manifests acutely (≤ 3 weeks) as an inflammatory reaction and chronically (≥ 1 year) as ocular tissue degeneration. Presentation includes suppurative endophthalmitis, chronic non-granulomatous inflammation, and disseminated ocular copper deposits (chalcosis). Suppurative endophthalmitis occurs acutely when copper content is more than 85%. Chalcosis occurs with unencapsulated copper IOFBs [19]. Manifestations include Kayser-Fleischer ring, iris discoloration, sunflower cataract, vitreous degeneration, refractile deposits in the macular region sparing the periphery, and retinal degeneration [19, 20].

Visual Outcome

Given that IOFB injuries in the pediatric population are rare, there are no large-scale studies of visual outcomes. In a case series of 11 children with posterior segment IOFB followed for an average of 20 months, 40% achieved 20/40 or better and 70% achieved $\geq 20/200$ or better at the last follow-up [21]. Extrapolating from a study on posterior segment IOFB in adults, 29% of patients can reach a final VA of 20/40 or better, while the rest can achieve less than 20/400. This does not account for the amblyopia period, which may result in a poor prognosis [22]. Furthermore, several factors can influence the visual outcome, with larger entry

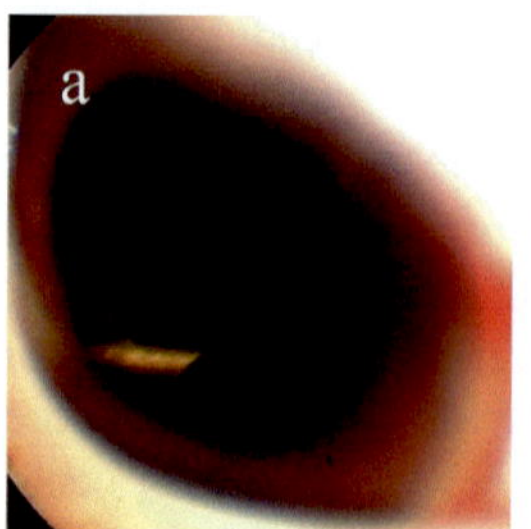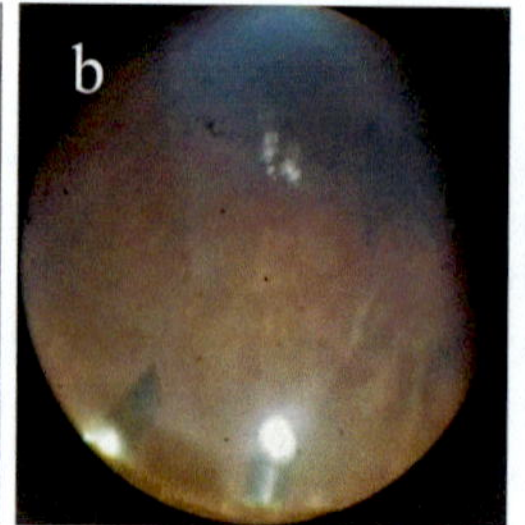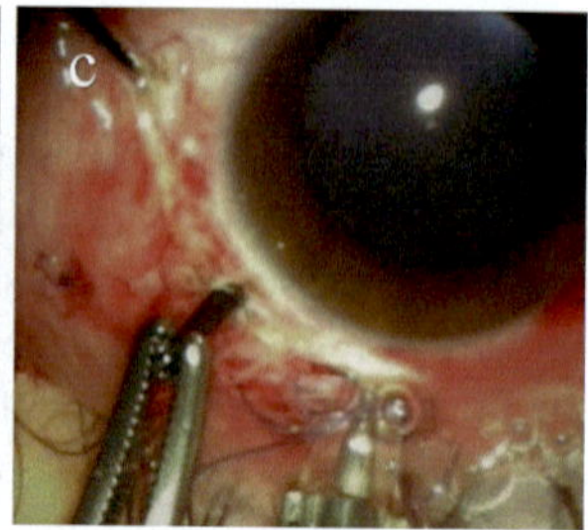

Fig. 46.1 Shows a lens-sparing vitrectomy removal of a pencil tip intraocular foreign body from an eye of a 10-year-old boy. First, the infusion cannula was placed next to the pencil tip (**a**). Next, the inner tip of the IOFB in the vitreous was grasped with forceps to push out through the entry site backward (**b**), and the outgoing part of the pencil tip was grasped outside to remove from the eyewall (**c**)

wounds, entry wound lengths higher than the diameter of the IOFB, IOFB in the posterior segment, and endophthalmitis contributing to a poor prognosis [23].

Case Presentation #1

A 10-year-old boy presented a pencil tip IOFB injury at school. His VA was 20/20, and the pencil tip was stuck into the eye from inferotemporal pars plana (fortunately) without causing damage either to the retina or to the lens (Fig. 46.1, **see video 1**). A lens-sparing vitrectomy was planned. The infusion cannula was placed next to the pencil tip (Fig. 46.1a). The suture of the primary repair at the entry site was cut. The inner tip of the IOFB in the vitreous was grasped with forceps to push out through the entry site backward (Fig. 46.1b). The outgoing part of the pencil tip was grasped outside to remove from the eyewall (Fig. 46.1c). Vision remained full without any complication throughout the four years of follow-up [24]. A video of the operation is included in the chapter. The case and the video courtesy are of Prof. Dr. Şengül Özdek.

Case Presentation #2

A 9-year-old boy presented to the ED with a traumatic cataract and IOFB after a pellet gun injury (Fig. 46.2). Pars plana lensectomy was performed using iris retractors (Fig. 46.2a). Vitreous opacities and posterior hyaloid were removed (Fig. 46.2b). The IOFB was entirely freed by removing any adherent vitreous strands. Then it was transferred to the AC with a passive aspiration of the flute cannula (Fig. 46.2c, d) and extracted via a limbal route with the help of viscoelastic (Fig. 46.2e). Later, vitreous removal was completed at the base, and the peripheral retina was checked to detect any tears (Fig. 46.2f). Retinal tears at the impact site at the superonasal retina were lasered (Fig. 46.2g). Gas tamponade was used at the end of the surgery. A secondary IOL implantation to the sulcus was performed six months later after removing the primary repair sutures [24]. The case is a courtesy of Prof. Dr. Şengül Özdek.

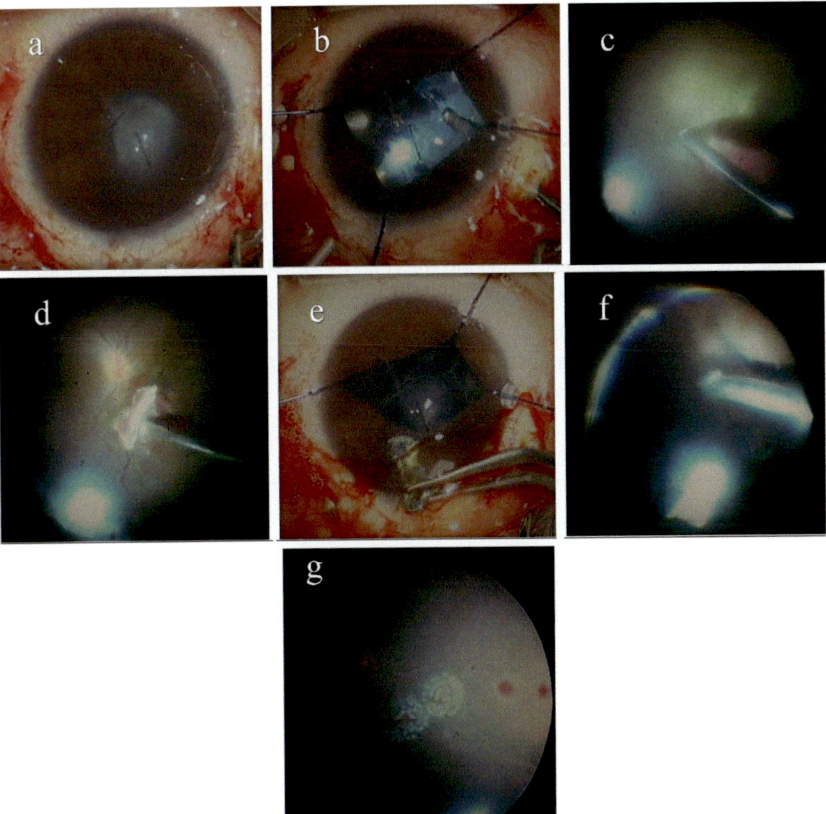

Fig. 46.2 Shows the pars plana vitrectomy removal of an intraocular foreign body (IOFB) from the eye of a 9-year-old boy. Pars plana lensectomy was performed using iris retractors (**a**). Vitreous opacities and posterior hyaloid were removed (**b**). The IOFB was entirely freed by removing any adherent vitreous strands. Then it was transferred to the anterior chamber (AC) with a passive aspiration of the flute cannula (**c, d**) and extracted via a limbal route with the help of viscoelastic (**e**). Next, vitreous removal was completed at the base, and the peripheral retina was checked to detect any tears (**f**). Retinal tears at the impact site at the superonasal retina were lasered (**g**). Gas tamponade was used at the end of the surgery

Video 1: Pencil Tip Intraocular Foreign Body Injury: We demonstrate the management of a pencil tip intraocular foreign body (IOFB) injury. Our approach involved placing an infusion cannula adjacent to the pencil tip and cutting the suture of the primary repair at the entry site. Forceps were utilized to grasp the inner tip of the IOFB, followed by the performance of a sclerotomy. The pencil tip was then carefully grasped and removed through the sclerotomy. Afterward, the sclerotomy was sutured, and the posterior segment appeared normal. The patient's postoperative visual acuity remained unaffected, with no complications observed.

Video 2: IOFB-RD: Combined encircling buckle with PPV, metallic IOFB extraction with silicone oil tamponade. We present a case of an eight-year-old male patient who experienced retinal detachment, metallic intraocular foreign body (IOFB), and siderosis six months after a motor vehicle accident. Our surgical approach involved a 360-degree encircling scleral buckle, core vitrectomy, careful peripheral vitreous removal, and hyaloid lifting. We used dilute Kenalog to stain and remove residual vitreous, ensuring the reduction of proliferative vitreoretinopathy and recurrent detachment risks. To stabilize the posterior retina, perfluorocarbon was injected, followed by diathermy around the IOFB-embedded area. A sclerotomy was performed using an MVR blade, and the IOFB was removed with forceps. After an additional shave and fluid-air exchange, endolaser photocoagulation was applied to surround the retinal break in 360 degrees over the scleral buckle. Finally, silicone oil was injected, and the sclerotomy and conjunctiva were closed.

Conclusion

Pediatric IOFB injuries vary in severity and visual outcome and pose unique diagnostic and surgical challenges. Adjunct pre-operative CT and ultrasound imaging to identify IOFB composition, location, and surrounding ocular injuries, and an examination under general anesthesia are almost always necessary to plan for the management. Management of IOFB-ocular injuries and associated complications should be handled on a case-by-case basis, with consultation with an experienced retinal surgeon for optimal patient care and outcomes.

Review Questions

1. Which of the following intraocular foreign body injury scenarios need not be taken to the operating room?

1. A seven-year-old boy with an iron-containing foreign body embedded in the retina.
2. A nine-year-old girl with an iron-containing foreign body suspended in the vitreous.
3. A nine-year-old boy with a large wound laceration posterior to the limbus.
4. None of the above

2. All the following are true except:

1. An intraocular foreign body injury associated with the inflammatory response should be surgically removed.
2. In general, foreign bodies embedded in the lens elicit a more severe reaction than those embedded in the retina or choroid.

3. Not all patients with foreign bodies require surgical removal.
4. Covering with systemic antibiotics is a good practice for most patients with suspected IOFB.

3. A 3-year-old boy is taken to the operating room for a posterior segment intraocular foreign body. Where to place the sclerotomy?

a. 4 mm posterior to the limbus
b. 1 mm posterior to the limbus
c. 3 mm posterior to the limbus
d. 7 mm posterior to the limbus

Answers

1. (**D**) Patients with retained metallic foreign bodies can experience a delayed reaction known as metallosis. A consequence of metallosis is ocular tissue degeneration. If left untreated, it can result in irreversible ocular tissue damage (Answers A & B). Sutures are required for patients with extensive wound lacerations regardless of the foreign body material (Answer C). Pediatric patients who have experienced a foreign body wound injury should be taken to the operating room, assessed under general anesthesia, and the wound closed. The foreign body is removed at the same surgery (one-stage) or subsequent surgery (two or more staged surgeries).

2. (**B**) Foreign bodies embedded in the retina or choroid causes a more robust reaction due to the increased blood supply.

3. (**C**) In children younger than four years, an easy-to-remember limbus-to-sclerotomy distance is as follows: 1 mm for infants up to one year; 2 mm for two-year-old; and 3 mm for three-year-old.

References

1. Zhang Y, Zhang M, Jiang C, Qiu HY. Intraocular foreign bodies in China: clinical characteristics, prognostic factors, and visual outcomes in 1421 eyes. Amer J Ophthalmol. 2011;152(1):66–73.e1. https://doi.org/10.1016/j.ajo.2011.01.014.
2. Bolliger SA, Oesterhelweg L, Spendlove D, Ross S, Thali MJ. Is differentiation of frequently encountered foreign bodies in corpses possible by hounsfield density measurement? J Forensic Sci. 2009;54(5):1119–22. https://doi.org/10.1111/j.1556-4029.2009.01100.x.
3. Leonardi F. The Berman metal locator for generic and qualitative diagnosis of intra-bulbar foreign bodies in clinical practice. Ann Ottalmol Clin Ocul. 1954;80(10):429–50. Il Berman metal locator per la diagnosi generica e qualitativa dei corpi estranei endobulbari, nella pratica clinica.
4. Lit ES, Young LHY. Anterior and posterior segment intraocular foreign bodies. Int Ophthalmol Clin. 2002;42(3):107–20.
5. Yang Y, Yang C, Zhao R, et al. Intraocular foreign body injury in children: clinical characteristics and factors associated with endophthalmitis. Br J Ophthalmol. 2020;104 (6):780–4. https://doi.org/10.1136/bjophthalmol-2019-314913.

6. Ung C, Laíns I, Papakostas TD, Rahmani S, Miller JB. Perfluorocarbon liquid-assisted intraocular foreign body removal. Clin Ophthalmol. 2018;12:1099–104. https://doi.org/10.2147/OPTH.S159509.

7. Gan NY, Lam W-C. Special considerations for pediatric vitreoretinal surgery. Taiwan J Ophthalmol. 2018;8(4):237–42. https://doi.org/10.4103/tjo.tjo_83_18.

8. McCuen BW II, Hickingbotham D. A new retractable Micromagnet for intraocular foreign body removal. Arch Ophthalmol. 1989;107(12):1819–20. https://doi.org/10.1001/archopht.1989.01070020901036.

9. de Oliveira PRC, Berger AR, Chow DR. Vitreoretinal instruments: vitrectomy cutters, endoillumination and wide-angle viewing systems. Int J Retina Vitreous. 2016;2:28–28. https://doi.org/10.1186/s40942-016-0052-9.

10. Ahmed Y, Schimel AM, Pathengay A, Colyer MH, Flynn HW. Endophthalmitis following open-globe injuries. Eye. 2012;26(2):212–217. https://doi.org/10.1038/eye.2011.313.

11. Chaudhry IA, Shamsi FA, Al-Harthi E, Al-Theeb A, Elzaridi E, Riley FC. Incidence and visual outcome of endophthalmitis associated with intraocular foreign bodies. Graefe's archive for clinical and experimental ophthalmology = Albrecht von Graefes Archiv fur klinische und experimentelle Ophthalmologie. 2008;246(2):181–186. https://doi.org/10.1007/s00417-007-0586-5.

12. Barry DR. Effects of retained intraocular foreign bodies. Int Ophthalmol Clin Spring. 1968;8(1):153–70.

13. Duke-Elder SS, Macfaul PA. Non-mechanical injuries. 1972.

14. Kannan NB, Adenuga OO, Rajan RP, Ramasamy K. Management of ocular Siderosis: visual outcome and Electroretinographic changes. J Ophthalmol. 2016;7272465. https://doi.org/10.1155/2016/7272465.

15. Ballantyne JF. Siderosis bulbi. Br J Ophthalmol. 1954;38(12):727–33. https://doi.org/10.1136/bjo.38.12.727.

16. Talamo JH, Topping TM, Maumenee AE, Green WR. Ultrastructural studies of cornea, iris and lens in a case of siderosis bulbi. Ophthalmology. 1985;92(12):1675–80. https://doi.org/10.1016/s0161-6420(85)34090-3.

17. Barr CC, Vine AK, Martonyi CL. Unexplained heterochromia. Intraocular foreign body demonstrated by computed tomography. Surv Ophthalmol. 1984;28(5):409–11. https://doi.org/10.1016/0039-6257(84)90246-7.

18. Welch RB. Two remarkable events in the field of intraocular foreign body: (1) The reversal of siderosis bulbi. (2) The spontaneous extrusion of an intraocular copper foreign body. Trans Am Ophthalmol Soc. 1975;73:187–203.

19. Rao NA, Tso MOM, Rosenthal AR. Chalcosis in the human eye: a Clinicopathologic study. Arch Ophthalmol. 1976;94(8):1379–84. https://doi.org/10.1001/archopht.1976.03910040247018.

20. Ravani R, Kumar V, Kumar A, Kumar P, Chawla S, Ghosh S. Fleck-like deposits and swept source optical coherence tomography characteristics in a case of confirmed ocular chalcosis. Indian J Ophthalmol. 2018;66(11):1640–2. https://doi.org/10.4103/ijo.IJO_437_18.

21. Zhang T, Zhuang H, Wang K, Xu G. Clinical features and surgical outcomes of posterior segment intraocular foreign bodies in children in East China. J Ophthalmol. 2018;2018:5861043–5861043. https://doi.org/10.1155/2018/5861043.

22. Mukkamala LK, Soni N, Zarbin MA, Langer PD, Bhagat N. Posterior segment intraocular foreign bodies: A 10-Year review. Ophthalmol Retina. 2017;1(4):272–277. https://doi.org/10.1016/j.oret.2017.01.007.

23. Zhang Y, Zhang M, Jiang C, Qiu HY. Intraocular foreign bodies in china: clinical characteristics, prognostic factors, and visual outcomes in 1,421 eyes. Am J Ophthalmol. 2011;152(1):66-73.e1. https://doi.org/10.1016/j.ajo.2011.01.014.

24. Sengul Ozdek. EO. Ocular emergency. Ocular Trauma. In: H Y, ed. Open-Globe Injuries. Springer, Singapore; 2018:175–213.

Management of Proliferative Vitreoretinopathy in Pediatric Trauma Related Vitreoretinal Surgery

47

Gökhan Gürelik

Abstract

Children aged under 10 years account for 6.5% of all eye injuries and ocular trauma is a major cause of non-congenital visual impairment in children. The main indications for vitreoretinal surgery in the pediatric age includes rhegmatogenous retinal detachments (RRD) caused by trauma and in pediatric traumatic retinal detachments, proliferative vitreoretinopathy (PVR) was found to be a significant factor influencing the visual and anatomic outcome. Pediatric vitreoretinal surgery has important differences compared to that in adults and we must keep in mind that 'pediatric eyes are not simply small adult eyes'. First, posterior hyaloid is strongly attached to ILM and second, retinal breaks in children can stimulate strong inflammatory responses and increase the risk of PVR. Treatment of PVR-RD in pediatric ocular trauma is challenging and requires complex vitreoretinal surgery. Choosing the most suitable technique is crucial for a successful, less complicated surgery and better anatomical and functional results.

Keywords

Pediatric ocular trauma · Retinal detachment · Proliferative vitreoretinopathy

Supplementary Information The online version contains supplementary material available at https://doi.org/10.1007/978-3-031-14506-3_47.

G. Gürelik (✉)
Faculty of Medicine, Gazi University, Ankara, Turkey
e-mail: gurelik@gazi.edu.tr

687

Introduction

Ocular trauma is a major cause of non-congenital visual impairment in children. Children aged under 10 years account for 6.5% of all eye injuries [1], but 21–35% of hospital admissions for ocular trauma are from the paediatric age group [2–4] and trauma remains a leading cause of monocular blindness in children [5] because of PVR.

The main indication for vitreoretinal surgery in the pediatric age includes rhegmatogenous retinal detachments (RRD) caused by trauma. In a series of 182 eyes with open globe injury, RD rate was 51.6% and PVR was present in 28.6% [6].

In pediatric traumatic RRD, PVR was found to be a significant factor influencing the visual and anatomical outcome. PVR was the cause of surgical failure in most cases and 'PVR is the only potentially modifiable risk factor for poor outcome' in their study [7]. The PVR process is characterized by formation of periretinal fibrocellular membranes, intraretinal fibrosis, and subretinal bands [8]. PVR often leads to recurrent retinal detachments that are complicated in nature with a tractional component, require additional surgery, and have a guarded visual prognosis.

Pediatric vitreoretinal surgery (PVRS) has important differences compared to that in adults. We have to keep in mind that "pediatric eyes are not simply small adult eyes" [9].

What is Different in Pediatric Eyes Compared to Adults?

Pediatric eyes are smaller than the adult eyes and combined anterior and posterior segment involvement rates are higher in pediatric ocular traumas.

RRD in the adult usually is associated with the posterior vitreous detachment (PVD), but RRD in pediatric age is often caused by trauma or congenital abnormalities and there is no complete PVD in most cases. The vitreous is densely formed and the cortical vitreous is strongly attached to the internal limiting membrane (ILM). Surgical induction of PVD and completely removing the vitreous is usually very difficult. Mechanical traction while creating surgical PVD may result in vitreoschisis or retinal breaks.

As pediatric RRD usually present in late stages and pediatric ocular anatomy is featured, PVRS is more difficult and complex and has greater complication rates. The most common and devastating complication of PVRS is PVR. PVR rate is higher before the surgery and after the surgical intervention as well.

The ocular response to surgical trauma in the pediatric age differs from those of the adults. Retinal breaks in children can stimulate strong inflammatory responses and increase the risk of PVR. In particular, iatrogenic retinal breaks, creating a posterior draining retinotomy or relaxing retinotomy-retinectomy procedures can cause PVR in children because of the strong inflammatory and proliferative response [10–14].

Management of PVR

Treatment of PVR-RD in pediatric ocular trauma is challenging and requires complex vitreoretinal surgery. Choosing the most suitable technique is crucial for a successful, less complicated surgery and better anatomical and functional results.

1. Scleral Buckle Surgery

To avoid surgically induced PVR formation, if possible, do not enter into the vitreous cavity. As the vitreous is densely formed and posterior hyaloid is firmly adherent in children, an attempt to create surgical PVD is nearly impossible in infants and very challenging in younger children. Vitrectomy surgery to repair RRD in children can start PVR because of the residual vitreous and to avoid this complication, scleral buckling surgery (SBS) is a favorable option in selected eyes [15–18].

RD eyes with single retinal breaks, retinal dialysis, no PVR, with clear optical media are good candidates for a scleral buckle surgery with a 70.6% single surgery success rate [7]. If primary vitrectomy surgery was applied to these eyes instead of SBS, surgically induced PVR would occur in a considerable amount of these eyes and require recurrent surgeries.

Even if there is limited PVR (PVR C1), and chronic RD eyes with subretinal bands, a primary buckle is often enough to reattach the retina [9].

Draining or not is up to the surgeon, but we should keep in mind that most RDs in children are chronic [15]. It is not necessary to drain all the subretinal fluid. The residual fluid will be absorbed by RPE in months if the break is completely sealed (Fig. 47.1).

Another advantage of scleral buckling surgery is sparing the lens and preserving accommodation, on the other hand, myopic shift is a negative consequence of this surgery. Vitrectomy becomes necessary if scleral buckling fails.

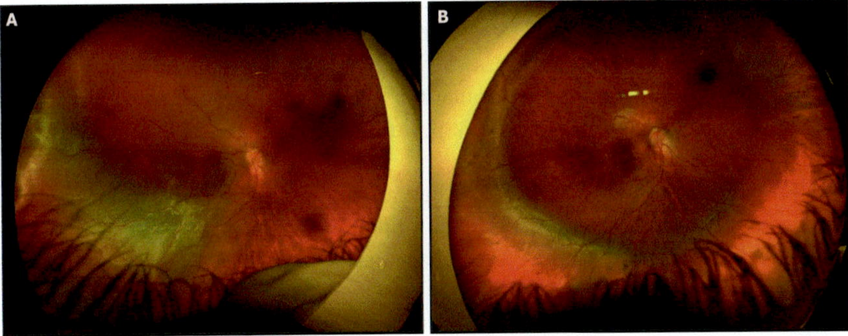

Fig. 47.1 A pediatric traumatic RD with minimal vitreous hemorrhage (**A**), managed with a 360 scleral buckling surgery (**B**)

2. Vitrectomy

Vitreoretinal surgery is the main treatment for complicated RDs with PVR, prior failed SBS, failed vitreoretinal surgery, cataract or lens subluxation, vitreous hemorrhage or haze, multiple retinal breaks, posterior retinal breaks, giant retinal tear and retinal or vitreous incarcerations.

Timing of surgery following trauma depends on the case.

- In early intervention (within the first 4 days after trauma), the risk of a subsequent development of endophthalmitis is eliminated; all tissue pathologies that do not represent irreversible damage may be treated (e.g., lens swelling, vitreous hemorrhage, RD); inflammatory cells are removed and thus the risks of PVR and secondary ciliary body destruction are reduced.
- Deferring the reconstruction for at least one week (days 8–14) is the most common approach. It presents a more comfortable surgery because of the decreased tissue (especially corneal) edema and vascular engorgement, like elective cases. Delaying the surgery leads to the formation of mature membranes, which are generally easier to remove than fragile, immature membranes that are difficult to remove in sheets. However, RD may already have occurred and PVR has started, and the risk of postoperative complications also increase [19]. When the surgery is later, it becomes more comfortable but with the expense of increased PVR.
- In severe penetrating trauma cases, early intervention is recommended.

The severely injured eyes achieve favorable anatomical restoration, with favorable visual outcomes in nearly 70% of the patients. Early vitrectomy means less PVR with a better visual acuity [20].

In patients with advanced PVR-RD, lens removal necessitates a total capsulectomy since the residual capsule serves as a scaffold for membrane proliferation and secondary circumferential vitreoretinal contraction which may end up with ciliary body detachment and hypotony [21].

One of the keys to success, like adult surgery, is to induce a complete PVD. Otherwise, residual vitreous will ease PVR formation. Triamcinolone staining and re-staining may be helpful to ensure that the hyaloid is separated. In circumstances such as vitreoschisis and membranous posterior hyaloid surface, bimanual dissection may be helpful (Fig. 47.2).

Subretinal PVR membranes—if isolated, extrafoveal and not exerting tractional forces—may not need to be removed for retinal reattachment. SBS in combination with vitrectomy may also relieve tractional forces caused by subretinal membranes in selected cases.

Epiretinal membranes frequently causes retinal contraction. To re-attach the retina, meticulous peeling is necessary to relieve all the tractional forces. In the presence of firm vitreoretinal attachments, it is preferable to perform segmentation instead of delamination to avoid iatrogenic retinal tears. Relaxing retinotomy-retinectomies are the last options to relieve the tractions. We must keep

Fig. 47.2 Bimanual thick posterior hyaloidal membrane removal following triamcinolone application which makes it visible

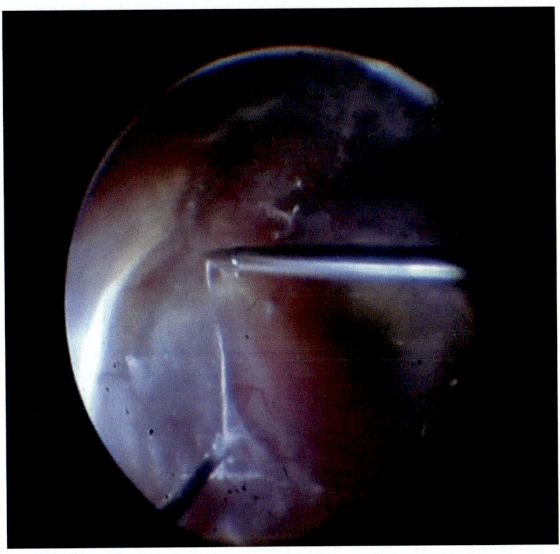

in mind that extensive PVR often develops along retinectomy edges in children. Avoiding from unnecessary retinectomies is one of the important points in traumatic PVR surgery especially in children. After meticulous membrane peeling, if the retina is still stiff and impossible to flatten, then a relaxing retinectomy may be necessary to relieve traction. In severe anterior PVR cases, relaxing retinotomy is generally required. It is recommended to perform the retinectomy as far anterior as possible, to preserve functional retina (**see case presentation and surgical video**). In very severe cases, up to 360° retinectomy may be necessary to achieve retinal flattening but retinal defects will most probably lead to explosive PVR in pediatric cases. To avoid relaxing retinectomies or at least decrease the need for retinectomies, an addition of SBS may be helpful to relieve tractions.

In perforating ocular injuries, when there is a posterior retinal incarceration, inevitably we have to perform retinectomy around the exit site. To avoid PVR formation, retino-choroidectomy around the wound needs to be performed [22] (Figs. 47.3A–C).

In reattaching the retina, decaline may be preferred as the PFCL. Posterior drainage retinotomies are best avoided as extensive fibrous proliferation can occur postoperatively. If a draining retinotomy is unavoidable, it is usually recommended to create one as close to the ora serrata as possible. Finally, as an internal tamponade, C3F8 or 5000 cs silicone oil is preferable.

Although following all the rules for the management of pediatric traumatic RDs, anatomic and functional success rates are lower than adults. In a series of 110 traumatic pediatric retinal detachments, anatomical success rates were 75.9% in open globe injury (OGI) and 82.6% in closed globe injuries (CGI). Advanced PVR was associated with poor anatomical and visual outcome in both OGIs and CGIs [23].

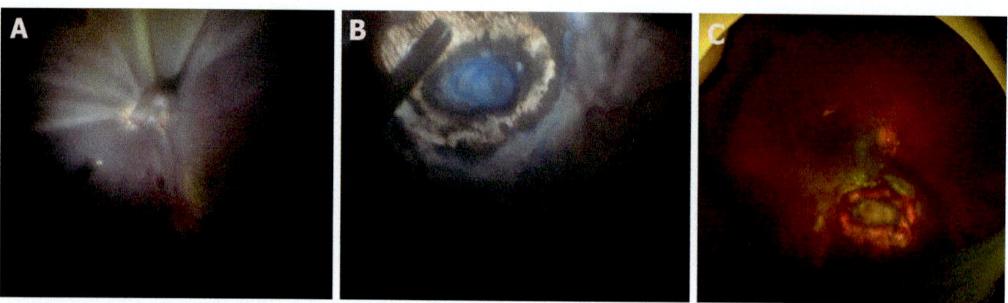

Fig. 47.3 **A** Fundus picture during surgery shows the retinal incarceration and fibrosis at the inferior temporal vascular arcades, total retinal detachment in a pediatric open globe injury. **B** Retino-choroidectomy application during surgery and dense fibrous tissue isolated in the center. **C** Postoperative fundus picture shows attached retina and silicone oil in the eye

Another series of 57 pediatric traumatic RD, 37% of eyes had PVR before the surgeries which ended up with an anatomical success rate of 72% and functional success rate of 37%. The authors comment that baseline visual acuity, the presence of macula-off RD, and PVR at the time of presentation and recurrent retinal detachment during follow-up are all important predictors of final visual acuity [24].

3. Pharmacological Adjuvants and Future Directions

The greatest challenge is to identify a pharmacological approach and adjuvant surgery that could be truly prophylactic for the development of PVR.

Various pharmacological agents have demonstrated potential in reducing post-operative PVR risks, including intravitreal low molecular weight heparin, 5-FU, daunomycin, anti-VEGF drugs, systemic and intravitreal corticosteroids. However, many clinical trials have shown none of these agents are successful in preventing PVR after surgery [25].

Recently we have published the use of intraoperative intravitreal temporary use of Mitomycin-C (MMC) which is shown to effectively treat and prevent PVR formation in a case series of severe traumatic RDs [26]. MMC is applied with a so called 'MMC sandwich technique' which provides protection of posterior and anterior vital structures of the eye from MMC contact. In this technique MMC is temporarily applied during the operation.

A brief explanation of the technique (**see also surgical video and case presentation**):

- After performing complicated vitreoretinal surgical procedures and attaching the retina with perfluorocarbon liquid (PFCL), a partial fluid-air exchange is applied.
- PFCL is partially aspirated below the posterior borders of retinochoroidal wounds, breaks or retinectomy sites (Fig. 47.7A). The remaining PFCL will be enough to cover and prevent MMC contact with optic disc, macula and underlying RPE and major vascular arcades.

- Ciliary epithelium and other anterior segment structures are protected from MMC contact with the air filling the rest of the eye.
- A concentration of 10–20 µg/mL MMC solution is injected carefully above the PFCL bubble until it covers the future possible PVR areas; retinal breaks, retinotomy-retinectomy sites (Fig. 47.7B). Adding 0,05 ml of dual blue or briliant blue dye to the MMC solution before application makes the MMC solution more visible during the operation. MMC solution is totally aspirated after 60 s (Fig. 47.7C).
- Finally, the remaining PFCL is removed, and silicone oil is used as an internal tamponade.

PVR was successfully treated and recurrent PVR formation was prevented with this method in all of the 15 eyes with no ocular toxicity in our pilot study [26].

Another promising agent is the antimetabolite methotrexate. Weekly intravitreal methotrexate injections of 400 mcg/0.05 mL beginning intraoperatively have been successfully employed to reduce PVR- associated recurrent detachment in high-risk patients [27]. Currently, a prospective, randomized clinical trial is under way that aims to assess the efficacy of postoperative intravitreal methotrexate in prevention of PVR-associated re-detachment [28].

Case Presentation

An 8-year-old Caucasian boy had a history of an ocular trauma with a piece of tile hit to his left eye 2 weeks ago. He had a suturation of upper eyelid injury in elsewhere but there was no information about globe perforation or rupture in the referral notes. The patient admitted to our clinic with decreased vision in his left eye. Initial ocular examination at application revealed that uncorrected visual acuity in the right eye (RE) was 20/20 and best corrected visual acuity was 20/200 in the left eye (LE). Intraocular pressure was 15 mmHg in RE and 13 mmHg in LE. Anterior segment examination was unremarkable in RE (Fig. 47.4A). Conjunctiva was slightly hyperemic and temporal subconjunctival hemorrhage was visible in LE, there were no cells or flare in the anterior chamber, the patient was phakic with clear crystalline lens (Fig. 47.4B).

Retinal examination of the RE was normal (Fig. 47.5A). In the LE, nasal retina and posterior pole was detached with nasal dragging of the retina which was incarcerated into the possible globe rupture area (Fig. 47.5B, C). Optical coherence tomography (OCT) revealed normal findings in RE (Fig. 47.6A) but macula was detached with an attached vitreous in the LE (Fig. 47.6B).

Pars plana vitrectomy with relaxing retinotomy & retinectomy was performed to the patient (**see the surgical video**). Adjuvant intraoperative MMC was used to prevent PVR especially at the borders of retinotomy as described in the text above. Roughly PFCL was injected to cover posterior pole and anterior level of PFCL was adjusted below the retinotomy level. Then a fluid-air was performed while keeping

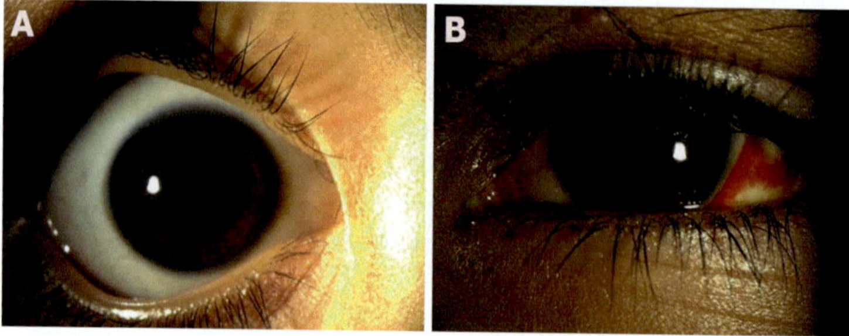

Fig. 47.4 **A** Anterior segment examination was unremarkable in RE, **B** conjunctiva was slightly hyperemic and temporal subconjunctival hemorrhage was visible in LE, there was no cells or flare in the anterior chamber, the patient was phakic with clear crystalline lens

Fig. 47.5 **A** Retinal examination of RE looks normal, **B**, **C** nasal and posterior retinal detachment with dragging-incarceration of the retina to the globe rupture area

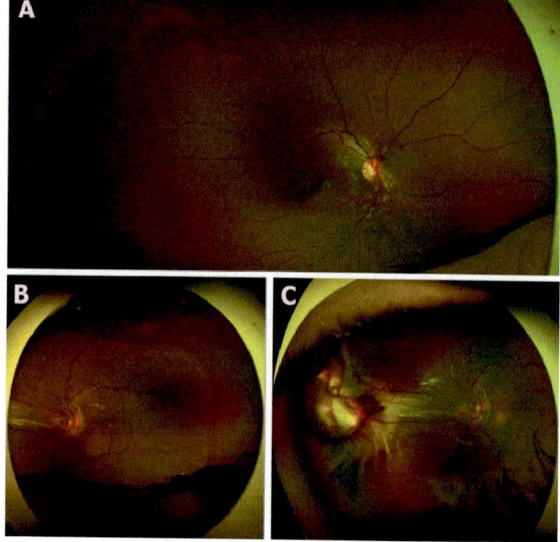

PFCL covering the posterior pole (Fig. 47.7A). MMC was injected over the PFCL until it covers the retinotomy edges (Fig. 47.7B). MMC solution was aspirated back after 60 s (Fig. 47.7C). 5000 cs silicone oil was used as a tamponade. The retina was attached with no PVR at postoperative first (Fig. 47.8A) and third months (Fig. 47.8B). Visual acuity was 20/100 following silicone oil removal.

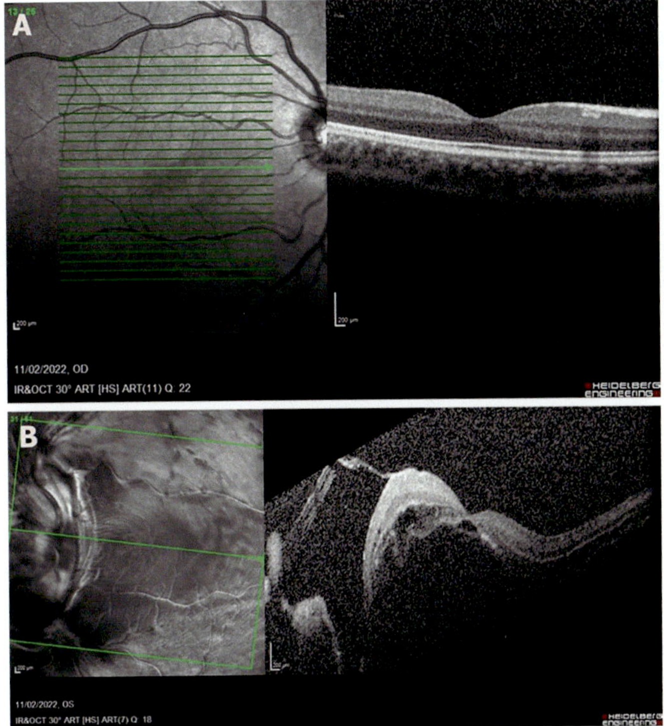

Fig. 47.6 OCT of the **A** RE with normal findings, **B** LE with macular detachment

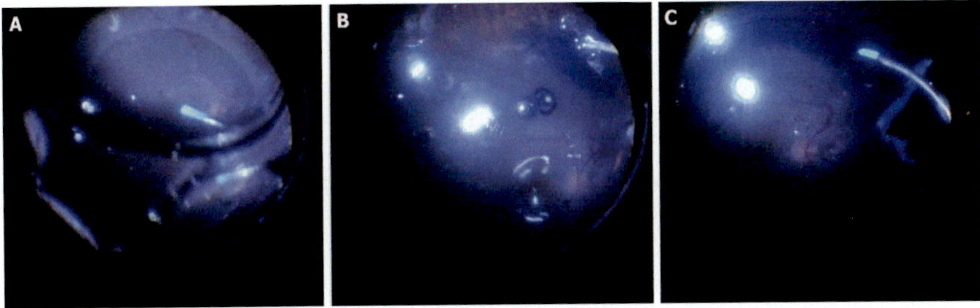

Fig. 47.7 **A**, **B**, **C**: MMC application steps (see the text)

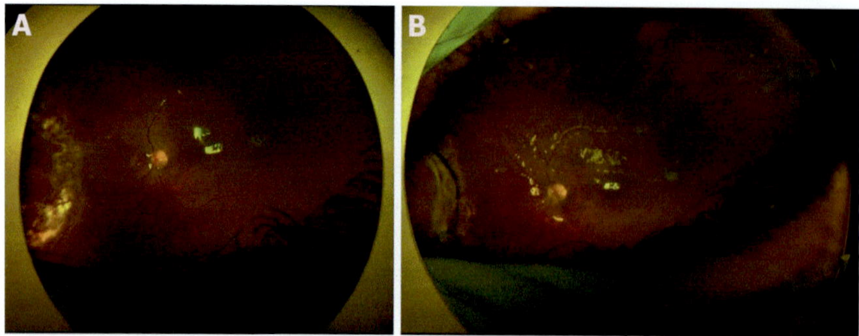

Fig. 47.8 Postoperative fundus pictures of the case. Retina was attached at the postoperative first (**A**) and third months (**B**)

Review Questions

1. What is the most prominent cause of non-congenital visual impairment in children?

a. Herpetic Keratitis
b. Ocular trauma
c. Primary open angle glaucoma
d. Uveitis

2. What is the most important cause of surgical failure in traumatic retinal detachments in the pediatric age?

a. Proliferative Vitreoretinopathy
b. Choroidal effusion
c. Recurent iridocyclitis
d. Chronic hypotony

3. Which one of the following surgical maneuvers is harder in pediatric cases than in adults?

a. Creating posterior draining retinotomy
b. Creating relaxing retinotomy
c. 360 scleral buckling
d. Creating posterior vitreous detachment

Answers

1. B
2. A
3. D

References

1. Katz J, Tielsch JM. Lifetime prevalence of ocular injuries from the Baltimore Eye Survey. Arch Ophthalmol. 1993;111:1564–8.
2. Klopfer J, Tielsch JM, Vitale S, See LC, Canner JK. Ocular trauma in the United States. Eye injuries resulting in hospitalisation, 1984 through 1987. Arch Ophthalmol 1992;110: 838–842.
3. Niiranen M, Raivio I. Eye injuries in children. Br J Ophthalmol. 1981;65:436–8.
4. Zagelbaum BM, Tostanoski JR, Dawnielle JK, Hersh PS. Urban eye trauma. a one year prospective study Ophthalmology. 1993;100:851–6.
5. Strahlman E, Elman M, Daub E, Baker S. Causes of pediatric eye injuries. a population-based study Arch Ophthalmol. 1990;108:603–6.
6. Sul S, Gurelik G, Korkmaz S, Ozdek S, Hasanreisoglu B. Pediatric open-globe injuries: clinical characteristics and factors associated with poor visual and anatomical success. Graefes Arch Clin Exp Ophthalmol.
7. Sheard RM, Mireskandari K, Ezra E, Sullivan PM. Vitreoretinal surgery after childhood ocular trauma. Eye. 2007;21:793–8.
8. Wiedemann P, Yandiev Y, Hui Y-N, Wang Y.Chapter 97—pathogenesis of proliferative vitreoretinopathy. Retina Fifth Edition. 2013;3:1640–1646.
9. Yonekawa Y. Practical pearls in pediatric vitreoretinal surgery.Practical Retina August 2018;49(8):561–565.
10. Al-Zaaidi S, Al-Rashaed S, Al-Harthi E, et al. Rhegmatogenous retinal detachment in children 16 years of age or younger. Clin Ophthalmol. 2013;7:1001–14.
11. Wadhwa N, Venkatesh P, Sampangi R, et al. Rhegmatogenous retinal detachments in children in India: clinical characteristics, risk factors, and surgical outcomes. J AAPOS. 2008;12 (6):551–4.
12. Wenick AS, Barañano DE. Evaluation and management of pediatric rhegmatogenous retinal detachment. Saudi J Ophthalmol. 2012;26(3):255–63.
13. Read SP, Aziz HA, Kuriyan A, et al. Retinal detachment surgery in a pediatric population: visual and anatomic outcomes. Retina. 2018;38(7):1393–402.
14. Gan NY, Lam WC. Retinal detachments in the pediatric population. Taiwan J Ophthalmol. 2018;8(4):222–36.
15. Fivgas GD, Capone A Jr. Pediatric rhegmatogenous retinal detachment. Retina. 2001;21 (2):101–6.
16. Wang NK, Tsai CH, Chen YP, et al. Pediatric rhegmatogenous retinal detachment in East Asians. Ophthalmology. 2005;112(11):1890–5.
17. Errera MH, Liyanage SE, Moya R, Wong SC, Ezra E. Primary scleral buckling for pediatric rhegmatogenous retinal detachment. Retina. 2015;35(7):1441–9.
18. Huang YC, Chu YC, Wang NK, et al. Impact of etiology on the outcome of pediatric rhegmatogenous retinal detachment. Retina. 2017. https://doi.org/10.1097/IAE. 0000000000001908. [Epub ahead of print].
19. Kuhn F. The timing of reconstruction in severe mechanical Trauma. Ophthalmic Res. 2014;51:67–72.
20. Liu X, Wang L, Yang F, et al. Surgical management and outcomes of pediatric open globe injuries requiring vitrectomy. Eur J Ophthalmol. 2022;32(1):546–52.
21. Ranchod TM, Capone A Jr. Tips and tricks in pediatric vitreoretinal surgery. Int Ophthalmol Clin. 2011;51:173–83.
22. Kuhn F, Schrader W. Prophylactic chorioretinectomy for eye injuries with high proliferative-vitreoretinopathy risk. Clin Anat. 2018;31(1):28–38. https://doi.org/10.1002/ca. 22906 Epub 2017 Jun 21.
23. Sul S, Gurelik G, Korkmaz S, Ozdek S, Hasanreisoglu B. Pediatric traumatic retinal detachments: clinical characteristics and outcomes. Ophthalmic Surg Lasers Imaging Retina. 2017;48(2):143–50.

24. Yasa D, Erdem ZG, Urdem U, Demir G, Demircan A, Alkın Z. Pediatric traumatic retinal detachment: clinical features, prognostic factors, and surgical outcomes. J Ophthalmol. 2018;25(2018):9186237. https://doi.org/10.1155/2018/9186237.eCollection2018.
25. Morescalchi F, Duse S, Gambicorti E, et al. Proliferative vitreoretinopathy after eye injuries: an overexpression of growth factors and cytokines leading to a retinal keloid. Mediators Inflamm. 2013;2013: 269787. https://doi.org/10.1155/2013/269787 Epub 2013 Sep 30.
26. Gurelik G, Sul S, Ucgul AY. Intraocular mitomycin C use in the treatment and prophylaxis of proliferative vitreoretinopathy in severe traumatic retinal detachments. Eur J Ophthalmol. 2021;31(6):3284–93. https://doi.org/10.1177/1120672120976038.Epub.
27. Eliott D. Methotrexate for the prevention of PVR: A Phase 1 study. Presented at Vail Vitrectomy, Vail, Colorado, Feb 20, 2016.
28. The GUARD Trial—Part 1: A Phase 3 clinical trial for prevention of proliferative vitreretinopathy. Available at: https://clinicaltrials.gov/ct2/show/NCT04136366. Accessed 6 June 2021.

Pediatric Macular Holes

48

Alay S. Banker, Sejal H. Shah, Deepa Banker, and Şengül Özdek

Abstract

A full-thickness defect in the fovea involving all retinal layers is defined as a macular hole. Idiopathic macular holes are most commonly seen in adult life and is age-related but when seen in pediatric population, it is mostly following trauma though other rare causes like infantile myopia, choroidal coloboma, optic pit maculopathy, X linked retinoschisis, retinitis pigmentosa, Coats disease, Best disease, idiopathic cavitary maculopathy, retinopathy of prematurity, uveitis, laser pointer injury and juvenile idiopathic epiretinal membrane also may be associated with macular holes. Unlike adult macular holes, pediatric macular holes may be associated with other posterior and anterior segment abnormalities secondary to trauma which might be of prognostic importance. Usually, conservative management in the form of observation for a few weeks may result into spontaneous closure of the hole in pediatric cases. However, in very young children and if the hole does not close spontaneously, surgical management in the form of minimal invasive vitrectomy surgery with ILM peeling and internal tamponade is suggested. In most cases, visual prognosis remains good unless there are comorbidities due to the trauma affecting other parts of the eye.

A. S. Banker (✉) · S. H. Shah
Banker's Retina Clinic and Laser Centre, Ahmedabad, India
e-mail: alay.banker@gmail.com

D. Banker
NHL Municipal Medical College, Ahmedabad, India

Ş. Özdek
School of Medicine, Ophthalmology Department, Gazi University, Ankara, Turkey

© The Author(s), under exclusive license to Springer Nature Switzerland AG 2023
Ş. Özdek et al. (eds.), *Pediatric Vitreoretinal Surgery*,
https://doi.org/10.1007/978-3-031-14506-3_48

Keywords

Pediatric macular hole · Blunt trauma · Vitrectomy · ILM peeling · Adjuvants · Infantile myopia · Pars planitis associated macular hole

Introduction

Unlike idiopathic age-related macular holes which are common, pediatric macular holes are rare and mostly associated with blunt trauma. While the incidence of idiopathic macular holes in adults is about 3.3 per 1000, macular holes occur in 0.15% of open-globe injuries and 1.4% of closed-globe injuries [1]. Idiopathic macular hole in pediatric population is extremely rare with only about 19 cases being reported in the literature so far [2]. With the advent of OCT, diagnosis of macular holes even in the pediatric population has become easier and can be done at a very early stage of the disease. Though spontaneous closure of macular holes can occur in pediatric cases following trauma, surgical intervention does give good anatomic and visual results. This chapter will provide an overview of various causes and management of pediatric traumatic macular holes with the help of some representative cases.

Etiology and Pathophysiology

While antero-posterior vitreous traction along with tangential tractional forces are thought to be the main pathogenesis of idiopathic macular holes in adults, the predominant mechanism in pediatric macular holes is mostly following trauma [3]. The impact from the blunt trauma is thought to cause a sudden anterior–posterior reduction and decompression and equatorial expansion of the globe resulting in horizontal forces to the posterior pole that cause a splitting of the inner retinal layers in fovea. Unlike the adult macular holes where vitreous traction and posterior vitreous detachment is thought to play an important role in causing the holes, in most pediatric macular holes, the posterior hyaloid remains attached and hence primary vitreous traction is not thought to be the main implicating factor [4]. Idiopathic macular holes in pediatric population is very rare and may be associated with a congenital abnormality in the development of the fovea. Rarely macular holes in pediatric population may be associated with other retinal diseases like infantile myopia, choroidal coloboma, optic pit maculopathy, X linked retinoschisis, retinitis pigmentosa, Coats disease, Best disease, idiopathic cavitary maculopathy, retinopathy of prematurity, *Bartonella* neuroretinitis, pars planitis and juvenile idiopathic epiretinal membrane [5]. More recently there have been reports of macular holes following laser injury in children [6].

Clinical Features and Diagnosis

Historically, clinical examination with indirect ophthalmoscopy and slit-lamp biomicroscopy reveals a round or ellipsoid full-thickness defect of the neurosensory retina in the fovea with or without a rim of subretinal fluid. In adults, in older times, a Watzke-Allen test, where the patient would appreciate a break/narrowing of the slit beam through the fovea was a characteristic sign. However, it might be difficult to do that in children. Also, with the advent of optical coherence tomography (OCT), it is very easy to demonstrate the full-thickness retinal defect, as well as other features including the shape and size of the hole, status of the hyaloid, and associated macular changes and most importantly all the retinal layers which is a useful guide to the prognosis (Fig. 48.1A) [7]. OCT is also very helpful in serial follow-up examinations to observe the changes that takes place with time (Fig. 48.1B) [8].

Detailed fundus examination with a good indirect ophthalmoscopy is essential. Peripheral examination with good indentation is recommended to find out associated changes as regards to vitreous base avulsion, peripheral retinal tears or dialysis, retinal detachment, choroidal rupture, commotio retinae, subretinal, retinal and vitreous hemorrhage, retinal tears and retinal dialysis may be noted. A good anterior segment examination including gonioscopy in certain cases should be performed to rule out changes related to trauma like pupillary sphincter tears, iridodialysis, traumatic cataract and secondary glaucoma. Microperimetry might be a very useful prognostic tool [9]. Recently, ultra-widefield retinal imaging including autofluorescence demonstrating hyperautofluorescence in the hole has been found to be very useful in pediatric population more so when they are uncooperative to do a physical examination [10]. Wide-field imaging is also helpful in detecting associated retinal changes in the periphery.

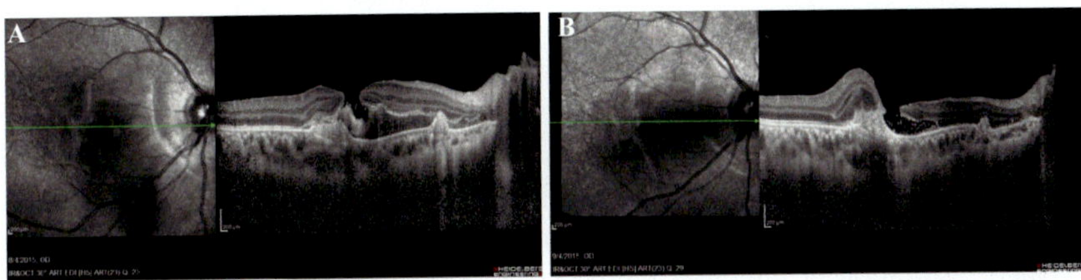

Fig. 48.1 **A** OCT of post-traumatic macular hole demonstrating a full thickness macular hole with a choroidal rupture in the peri-papillary region and at temporal edge of hole and subfoveal hemorrhage under the edges of the hole **B** OCT of the same case one month later showing resolution of the subretinal blood and apposition of the retinal layers making the hole smaller

Management

Vitrectomy surgery is required for the management of idiopathic macular holes in the adults. However, in the pediatric population, the macular hole may close spontaneously within days or months after the trauma. Thus, conservative management in the form of observation is generally recommended, especially in older children who are at a lesser risk of developing amblyopia and in those with good visual acuity, small holes, without any other retinal pathologies, and/or attached posterior vitreous. Spontaneous closure in traumatic macular holes have been reported ranging from 10 to 50%, with higher rates in pediatric cases [11–15]. A systematic review and single-arm meta-analysis of traumatic macular holes found that patients of ≤ 24 years of age with MH sizes of ≤ 0.2 DD were more likely to achieve spontaneous hole closure [15]. Other factors that may increase the likelihood of spontaneous closure include absence of intraretinal cysts on OCT and absence of PVD [8]. Use of topical nonsteroidal anti-inflammatory drugs, resulting in closure of traumatic holes associated with cystoid macular edema have also been described in the literature [1]. Although there are at present no evidence-based guidelines prescribing the optimal duration of observation, since spontaneous closure typically occurs within 3 months and is rare after 6 months, most surgeons prefer to wait for 3 months before surgical intervention unless there are other indications or early surgery [5].

Case Scenario 1: Traumatic Macular Hole

We would like to showcase a representative case of spontaneous closure of traumatic macular hole. A 12-year-old boy presented with dimness of vision, twelve days after a cricket ball injury. Fundus examination revealed a full thickness macular hole with a thin layer of subretinal haemorrhage near the nasal edge of the hole and evidence of choroidal rupture at the temporal edge of the optic disc (Fig. 48.2A). Corresponding OCT also confirmed the clinical findings (Fig. 48.2B). The patient was advised on conservative management. The macular hole closed spontaneously over a period of 3 months, with OCT showing closure of the hole with subfoveal loss of IS-OS layer and mild loss of outer retinal layers (Fig. 48.2C). Six months later there is complete closure of the hole (Fig. 48.2D) and the OCT revealed restoration of the outer retinal layers also (Fig. 48.2E).

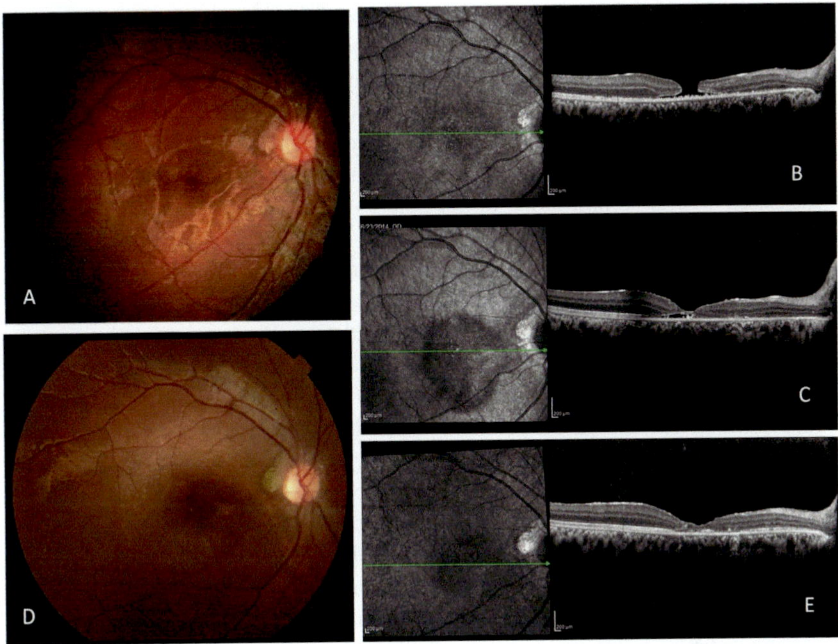

Fig. 48.2 **A** Colour fundus photo showing a full thickness macular hole with a thin layer of subretinal haemorrhage near nasal edge of the hole and choroidal rupture at temporal edge of the optic disc **B** Corresponding OCT confirming full thickness macular hole **C** 3 months follow up OCT showing closure of the hole with loss of IS-OS layer subfoveally and a few deposits overlying the RPE layer and mild loss of outer retinal layers. **D** 6 months fundus colour photo showing complete closure of the hole **E** corresponding OCT showing complete closure of the hole with restoration of outer retinal layers

The basic principles of surgery for macular hole remain the same since it was first described by Kelly and Wendell in the form of doing complete vitrectomy with induction of posterior hyaloid separation, removal of epiretinal membranes and use of internal tamponade (air, gas, or oil) [16]. Since then, various modifications and additions in the surgical techniques have evolved, particularly for traumatic macular holes. Pars plana vitrectomy with smaller gauge micro-incision vitrectomy systems using 23, 25 or 27 g instrumentation has revolutionized the surgical techniques and outcomes [17, 18]. Separation of the posterior hyaloid is one of the most important steps in a macular hole surgery and due to the well-formed vitreous and strong attachment of the posterior hyaloid to the underlying retina in pediatric cases is very challenging. Repeated staining of the vitreous for better visualization with the help of intravitreal triamcinolone suspension has become a very useful tool. It also helps to stain the posterior layer of cortical schisis and also the peripheral vitreous. In some cases where suction alone is not able to induce a posterior hyaloidal separation, a bent microvitreoretinal (MVR) blade, retinal pick and/or forceps may be employed to engage or obtain an opening in the hyaloid from which the PVD can be induced. One must be aware of causing iatrogenic retinal breaks during induction of a PVD, particularly in the pediatric population. Plasmin-assisted vitrectomy by injecting plasmin intravitreally before vitrectomy to weaken the hyaloid-ILM adhesion to make the surgical induction of PVD easier, has also been decribed [19]. Data regarding the use of ocriplasmin, which is a commercially available recombinant truncated form of plasmin in the pediatric population is limited [20]. Various adjuvants have since then been used to facilitate the closure of macular holes in the form of intraoperative transforming growth factor β (TGF-β), platelet concentrates (e.g., autologous platelet-rich plasma) and autologous serum [21–23].

As with idiopathic macular holes, internal limiting membrane (ILM) peeling is also routinely employed for pediatric macular holes and was first described in traumatic macular holes by Kuhn et al. [24]. Recently, various stains like indocyanine green, triamcinolone acetonide, trypan blue and brilliant blue are being used to facilitate the visualization and removal of the ILM [25–27]. Modifications and innovations in using different techniques to remove ILM like inverted ILM, sunflower ILM, flower petal, ILM, free-flap ILM, use of amniotic membrane or lens capsule to bridge the gap of the macular hole have been described with good surgical and visual outcomes [28–35]. In very big holes (>500 microns), use of the Tano's diamond dusted forceps or a Finesse loop (Alcon, Ft. Worth, TX) to gently massage around the hole in order to provide better apposition of the edges of the holes have been described [36]. Injection of fluid under the edges of the holes and also creating relaxing incisions adjacent to the holes to loosed the tissues allowing for larger holes to be closed have also been described [35]. Recently, in a largest series of surgical outcomes in pediatric macular holes, Kothari et al., reported a high single (81%) and final (94%) success rate [17]. Most recently, Cai et al., have shown that intraoperative portable handheld and microscope-integrated OCT enhance the pediatric vitreoretinal surgeon's diagnostic abilities and improve visualization of vitreoretinal anatomic relationships thereby improving surgical safety and efficiency [37]. It has demonstrated value in confirming completion or lack thereof of epiretinal and internal limiting membrane peeling. This could be very useful particularly in pediatric cases where removal of the posterior hyaloid, posterior cortical layer of the vitreous and of the ILM can at times be very difficult. Performing removal of internal limiting membrane (ILM) peeling without vitrectomy has also been described in treatment of laser-induced macular holes in children [38].

Table 48.1 Review of Pediatric Macular Holes: management and outcomes

References	No of cases	Management	Anatomic Hole closure rate	Visual success
Zhou et al. [14]	275 (combined all reviews)	Observation	random-model pooled rate was 0.37	n/a
Kothari et al. [17]	31	Vitrectomy $\pm$ ILM peeling $\pm$ gas/silicone oil	81% first surgery 94% second surgery	65%
Wu et al. [19]	13	Vitrectomy + Plasmin	92%	92%
Wachtlin et al. [21]	4	Vitrectomy + Platelet concentrate	100%	100%
Rubin et al. [22]	12	Vitrectomy + TGF-β2	67%	67%
Kuhn et al. [24]	17	Vitrectomy + ILM peeling	100%	94%
Abou Shousha [28]	12	Vitrectomy + inverted ILM flap	100%	n/a
Chen et al. [38]	2	ILM peeling without vitrectomy	100%	100%

In patients with large holes, recurrent holes, or holes that failed to close with an initial surgery especially in those associated with infantile myopia or significant PVR retinal detachment human amniotic membrane graft may be used as a seal to increase the closure rates (**see the video** in Chap. 49) (case scenario 3, Fig. 48.4).

Internal tamponade using intraocular gas (air, SF6, or C3F8) in conjunction with prone (face-down) positioning for one to two weeks is recommended though the duration of positioning remains controversial [39]. In young children incapable of positioning or in patients with large holes, recurrent holes, or holes that failed to close with an initial surgery, silicone oil tamponade may also be considered, but requires additional surgery to remove the oil. A brief review of literature on pediatric macular holes management and outcomes are shown in Table 48.1.

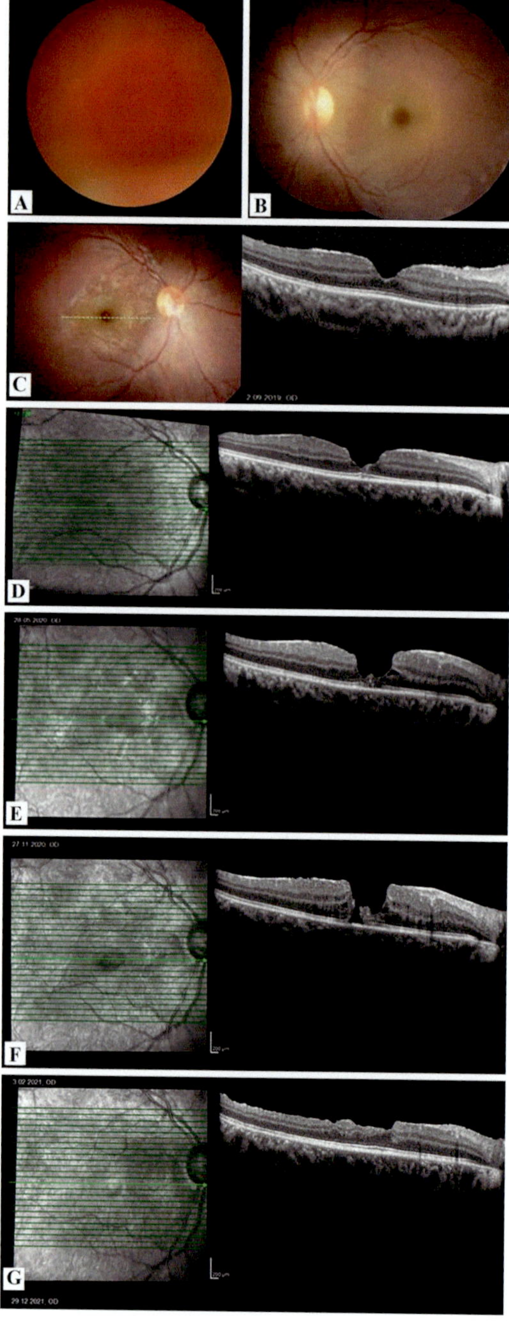

◀ **Fig. 48.3** An 8-year-old girl presenting with sudden visual loss in the right eye (RE) was found to have hand motions vision caused by vitreous hemorrhage in the RE (**A**), and 20/25 vision with +2 *vitreous cells* and perivascular sheathing in the left eye (LE) was diagnosed as bilateral pars planitis (**B**). Following start of immunosupressive treatment including oral prednisolone and azathiopurine, vitreoretinal surgery was performed for unresolved hemorrhage in the right eye. After cleaning the vitreous opacities some inflammatory membranes covering the macula and the optic disc area and snowbanking in the inferior pars plana were observed. Following peeling of the epiretinal membranes, vision increased to 20/25 with a normal foveal contour seen in the early postoperative color fundus photograph and OCT image (**C**). During follow-up, vision started to drop to 20/50 within 1.5 year period and OCT studies showed thinning and disruption of inner retinal layers leading to a lamellar macular hole (**D**, **E**), and eventually evolving into a full-thickness macular defect (**F**). Macular hole could be closed with repeat vitreoretinal surgery with inverted ILM flap and gas (SF6) injection ending up with 20/30 vision which was stable during the 12 month follow up (**G**). (Case courtesy of Prof. Dr. Şengül Özdek)

Case Scenario 2: Macular Hole Secondary to Pars Planitis (Fig. 48.3)

Case Scenario 3

Bilateral retinal detachment associated with macular hole in a 2-year-old boy with infantile myopia which was treated with vitrectomy and amniotic membrane plug (Fig. 48.4).

Visual acuity following spontaneous or vitrectomy-induced closure in cases with traumatic macular holes is usually good. Other factors like the size of the hole, timing of surgery from trauma, restoration of the ellipsoid layer and respective photoreceptors, and presence of other sequela of trauma, including glaucoma, cataract, contusive damage to the retina and subjacent retinal pigment epithelium and amblyopia, may affect the patient's ultimate visual outcome.

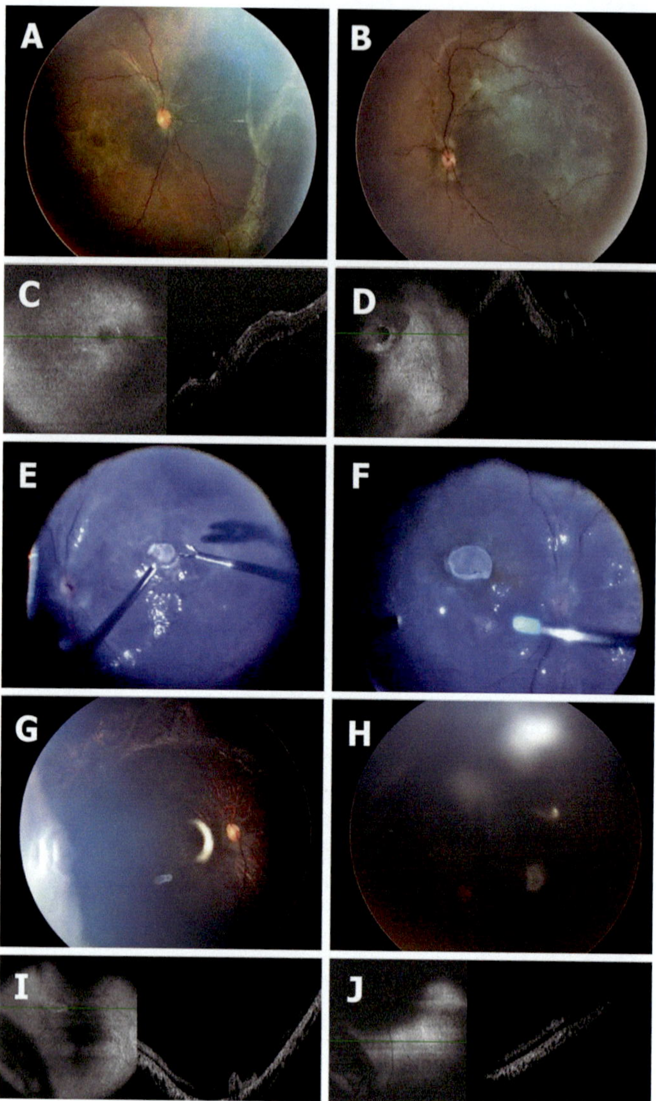

◀ **Fig. 48.4** A 2-year-old baby boy was referred to our clinic for bilateral retinal detachment. He had been using bilateral–10.00 D glasses for a year. On fundus examination, fundus was lightly colored and there was bilateral shallow retinal detachment with subretinal bands and membranes (**A, B**). A macular hole was evident on fundus examination of the left eye (**B**). Hand-held optical coherence tomography (OCT) image of the RE revealed a vague vitreomacular traction associated with a tiny macular hole as a cause of retinal detachment (**C**). Hand-held OCT image of the LE revealed a larger macular hole with vitreomacular traction causing retinal detachment (**D**). Pars plana vitrectomy was performed bilaterally. The remaining posterior hyaloid was very tightly attached to retina and could only be separated with bimanual maneuvers with the help of PFCL after staining with triamcinolone. A piece of human amniotic membrane graft was used to seal the macular hole in both eyes and silicone oil was used as a tamponade (**E, F**). Silicone oil removal was performed two months after the surgery. Examination under general anesthesia was performed one month after silicone oil removal. The refraction in RE was −13.00, but refraction could not be obtained from the left eye due to newly developed cataract. The holes were closed with the amniotic membrane plugs and the retina was attached in both eyes (**G, H**). Hand-held OCT image of RE shows the amniotic membrane covering the hole area with an attached retina (**I**). The OCT of the LE was of low quality because of the newly formed cataract but still the retina seemed to be attached (**J**). (Case courtesy of Prof. Dr. Şengül Özdek)

Conclusion

Unlike macular holes in adults, traumatic macular holes usually result from blunt trauma and is seen more commonly in younger patients. Spontaneous closure can occur within a few weeks to months after the trauma. If the macular hole persists, vitrectomy, induction of PVD, ILM peeling and internal tamponade is associated with very good anatomic and visual outcomes. Newer imaging tools and use of various adjuvants, instruments and intraoperative OCT will result in better final results.

Review Questions

1. A 10 year old boy presented with sudden dimness of vision in his left eye following a blunt injury by tennis ball before 2 days. Examination revealed a full-thickness macular hole with retinal hemorrhages in the periphery and pupillary sphincter tear. How will you manage this case ?

a. Vitrectomy surgery as soon as possible.
b. Conservative management for 8–12 weeks and then possible surgery.
c. Intravitreal gas injection and face down positioning.

2. A 5 year old boy presents with a known diagnosis of post-traumatic macular hole with retinal dialysis and localised retinal detachment of one weeks duration. What is the best way to manage this case.

a. Vitrectomy surgery with ILM peeling with silicone oil/gas temponade
b. Scleral buckle surgery
c. Conservative management.

3. A 12 year old girl presented with a post-traumatic macular hole with surrounding macular pigmentary changes and scar and a healed chorio-retinal rupture through the hole of six months duration. What will you do ?

a. No active intervention will be of any visual potential.
b. Vitrectomy surgery
c. Systemic steroids

Answers

1. (**B**) Spontaneous closure of post-traumatic macular hole is known and also has good visual outcomes. In the absence of major associated comorbidities, early vitrectomy is not indicated.

2. (**A**) In presence of retinal detachment, surgery is indicated to treat post-traumatic macular hole. Doing scleral buckle alone will not lead to closure of traumatic macular hole and hence vitrectomy with ILM peeling with internal temponade is indicated. In very young children, silicone oil might be preferred as they might not be able to maintain face down positioning post-surgery.

3. (**A**) Since the hole is six months old and is associated with macular scar and pigmentary changes along with a chorio-retinal scar through the fovea, the visual potential is not good. Hence no active intervention would be indicated.

References

1. Budoff G, Bhagat N, Zarbin MA. Traumatic macular hole: diagnosis, natural history, and management. J Ophthalmol. 2019;19(2019):1–7.
2. Shaikh N, Kumar V, Salunkhe N, Nayak S, Azad S. Pediatric idiopathic macular hole—a case report and review of literature. Indian J Ophthalmol. 2020;68:241–4.
3. Gass JD. Idiopathic senile macular hole. Its early stages and pathogenesis. Arch Ophthalmol. 1988;106(5):629–39.
4. Johnson RN, Gass JD. Idiopathic macular holes. Observations, stages of formation, and implications for surgical intervention. Ophthalmology. 1988;95(7):917–24.
5. Johnson RN, McDonald HR, Lewis H, Grand MG, Murray TG, Mieler WF, et al. Traumatic macular hole: observations, pathogenesis, and results of vitrectomy surgery. Ophthalmology. 2001;108(5):853–7.
6. Gupta MP, Ferrone PJ. Pediatric Macular Hole. In: Wu WC, Lam WC, editors. A Quick Guide to Pediatric Retina. Springer: Singapore; 2021. p. 978–81.
7. Birtel J, Harmening WM, Krohne TU, et al. Retinal injury following laser pointer exposure. Dtsch Arztebl Int. 2017;114(49):831–7.
8. Huang J, Liu X, Wu Z, Sadda S. Comparison of full-thickness traumatic macular holes and idiopathic macular holes by optical coherence tomography. Graefes Arch Clin Exp Ophthalmol. 2010;248(8):1071–5.

9. Chen H, Chen W, Zheng K, Peng K, Xia H, Zhu L. Prediction of spontaneous closure of traumatic macular hole with spectral domain optical coherence tomography. Sci Rep. 2015;5:12343.

10. Dalan D, Jaishankar D, Madhu A, Mani K, Ratra D. Macular function assessment by multifocal electroretinogram and microperimetry in macular hole and correlation with visual acuity. Nepal J Ophthalmol. 2020;12(23):7–16.

11. Kumar V, Surve A, Kumawat D, et al. Ultra-wide field retinal imaging: a wider clinical perspective. Indian J Ophthalmol. 2021;69(4):824–35.

12. Pediatric Yamashita T, Uemara A, Uchino E, Doi N, Ohba N. Spontaneous closure of traumatic macular hole. Am J Ophthalmol. 2002;133(2):230–5.

13. Miller JB, Yonekawa Y, Eliott D, et al. Long-term follow-up and outcomes in traumatic macular holes. Am J Ophthalmol. 2015;160(6):1255–8.

14. Mitamura Y, Saito W, Ishida M, Yamamoto S, Takeuchi S. Spontaneous closure of traumatic macular hole. Retina. 2001;21(4):385–9.

15. Zhou Q, Feng H, Lv H, Fu Z, Xue Y, Ye H. Vitrectomy vs. spontaneous closure for traumatic macular hole: a systematic review and meta-analysis. Front Med (Lausanne). 2021;8:735968.

16. Gao M, Liu K, Lin Q, Liu H. Management modalities for traumatic macular hole: a systematic review and single-arm meta-analysis. Curr Eye Res. 2017;42(2):287–96.

17. Kelly NE, Wendel RT. Vitreous surgery for idiopathic macular holes. Results of a pilot study. Arch Ophthalmol. 1991;109(5):654–9.

18. Kothari N, Read SP, Baumal CR, et al. A multicenter study of pediatric macular holes: surgical outcomes with microincisional vitrectomy surgery. J VitreoRetinal Diseases. 2020;4(1):22–7.

19. Liu W, Grzybowski A. Current management of traumatic macular holes. J Ophthalmol. 2017;2017:1748135.

20. Wu WC, Drenser KA, Trese MT, at al. Pediatric traumatic macular hole: results of autologous plasmin enzyme-assisted vitrectomy. Am J Ophthalmol. 2007;144(5):668–72.

21. Drenser K, Girach A, Capone A Jr. A randomized, placebo-controlled study of intravitreal ocriplasmin in pediatric patients scheduled for vitrectomy. Retina. 2016;36(3):565–75.

22. Wachtlin J, Jandeck C, Potthofer S, et al. Long-term results following pars plana vitrectomy with platelet concentrate in pediatric patients with traumatic macular hole. Am J Ophthalmol. 2003;136(1):197–9.

23. Rubin JS, Glaser BM, Thompson JT, et al. Vitrectomy, fluid-gas exchange and transforming growth factor–beta-2 for the treatment of traumatic macular holes. Ophthalmology. 1995;102(12):1840–5.

24. Banker AS, Freeman WR, Azen SP, Lai M, and the Vitrectomy for Macular Hole Study Group. A multicentered clinical study of serum as adjuvant therapy for surgical treatment of macular holes. Arch Ophthalmol.1999;117(11):1499–1502.

25. Kuhn F, Morris R, Mester V, Witherspoon CD. Internal limiting membrane removal for traumatic macular holes. Ophthalmic Surg Lasers. 2001;32(4):308–15.

26. Kimura H, Kuroda S, Nagata M. Triamcinolone acetonide-assisted peeling of the internal limiting membrane. Am J Ophthalmol. 2004;137(1):172–3.

27. Enaida H, Hisatomi T, Hata Y, et al. Brilliant blue G selectively stains the internal limiting membrane/brilliant blue G-assisted membrane peeling. Retina. 2006;26(6):631–6

28. Kadonosono K, Itoh N, Uchio E, Nakamura S, Ohno S. Staining of internal limiting membrane in macular hole surgery. Arch Ophthalmol. 2000;118(8):1116–8.

29. Abou Shousha MA. Inverted internal limiting membrane flap for large traumatic macular holes. Medicine. 2016;95(3).

30. Velez-Montoya R, Ramirez-Estudillo JA, Sjoholm-Gomez de Liano C, et al. Inverted ILM flap, free ILM flap and conventional ILM peeling for large macular holes. Int J Retina Vitreous 2018;4:8.

31. Aurora A, Seth A, Sanduja N. Cabbage leaf inverted flap ILM peeling for macular hole: a novel technique. Ophthalmic Surg Lasers Imaging Retina. 2017;48(10):830–2.

32. Morizane Y, Shiraga F, Kimura S, et al. Autologous transplantation of the internal limiting membrane for refractory macular holes. Am J Ophthalmol. 2014;157(4):861–9.
33. Chen SN, Hsieh YT, Yang CM. Multiple free internal limiting membrane flap insertion in the treatment of macular hole-associated retinal detachment in high myopia. Ophthalmologica. 2018;240(3):143–9.
34. Rizzo S, Caporossi T, Tartaro R, et al. A human amniotic membrane plug to promote retinal breaks repair and recurrent macular hole closure. Retina. 2019;39(Suppl 1):S95–103.
35. Grewal DS, Charles S, Parolini B, Kadonosono K, Mahmoud TH. Autologous retinal transplant for refractory macular holes: multicenter international collaborative study group. Ophthalmology. 2019;126(10):1399–408.
36. Charles S, Randolph JC, Neekhra A, Salisbury CD, Littlejohn N, Calzada JI. Arcuate retinotomy for the repair of large macular holes. Ophthalmic Surg Lasers Imaging Retina. 2013;44(1):69–72.
37. Kubota M, Watanabe T, Hayashi T et al. Novel use of finesse flex loop for macular hole retinal detachment. Amer J Ophthalmol Case Reports. 2020;18.
38. Cai S, Therattil A, Vajzovic L. Pediatric vitreoretinal surgery and integrated intraoperative optical coherence tomography. Dev Ophthalmol. 2021;61I15–25.
39. Chen N, Zheng K. Internal limiting membrane peeling without vitrectomy for laser-induced macular holes in two children. Eur J Ophthalmol. 2021;28:1120672121990633.
40. Essex RW, Kingston ZS, Moreno-Betancur M, et al. The effect of postoperative face-down positioning and of long-versus short-acting gas in macular hole surgery: results of a registry-based study. Ophthalmology. 2016;123(5):1129–36.

Shaken Baby Syndrome

49

Kimberly D. Tran and Audina M. Berrocal

Abstract

Shaken baby syndrome (SBS) is a leading cause of childhood trauma and results in significant morbidity and mortality. Systemic evaluation should be performed in any child suspected of SBS including physical exam, fundus photography, skeletal survey, neuroimaging, and serologies. One of the hallmark findings of SBS is innumerable retinal hemorrhages extending anterior to the equator. Treatment of ocular findings centers around amblyopia management and visual development and may require anterior scatter laser in cases of ischemia, or vitrectomy for non-clearing vitreous hemorrhage obstructing the visual axis, macular hole, and retinal detachment. Many infants with SBS may suffer from significant cortical vision loss and bilateral optic atrophy regardless of their ocular findings and treatment. The long-term visual prognosis of SBS is guarded.

Keywords

Shaken baby syndrome · Non-accidental trauma · Abusive head trauma · Retinal hemorrhage

Supplementary Information The online version contains supplementary material available at https://doi.org/10.1007/978-3-031-14506-3_49.

K. D. Tran (✉)
Sanford University of South Dakota Medical Center, Sioux Falls, SD, USA
e-mail: Kimberly.Tran@sanfordhealth.org

1621 S Minnesota Ave., Sioux Falls, SD 57105, USA

A. M. Berrocal
Medical Director of Pediatric Retina and Retinopathy of Prematurity, Vitreoretinal Fellowship Director Retina Department, Bascom Palmer Eye Institute, Miami, FL, USA

Ş. Özdek et al. (eds.), *Pediatric Vitreoretinal Surgery*,
https://doi.org/10.1007/978-3-031-14506-3_49

Introduction

Shaken baby syndrome (SBS), also called abusive head trauma and non-accidental trauma (NAT), results from forcefully shaking an infant or toddler. Sadly, SBS is often one of multiple episodes of child abuse. A child may initially appear normal but over time may develop health or behavioral problems including vision loss, developmental delay, learning and behavioral difficulties, seizure, and cerebral palsy.

Epidemiology

Shaken baby syndrome (SBS) is the leading cause of fatal head injuries in children younger than 2 years old, and is responsible for 53% of serious or fatal traumatic brain injury cases [1]. The United States National Center on Shaken Baby Syndrome estimates that there are approximately 1300 cases in the U.S. per year. The majority of victims are under the age of 1 year old. Approximately 80% of these babies suffer long-term disabilities, and approximately 25% die. Caregivers under stress, domestic violence, and substance abuse may be at higher risk [2].

Pathophysiology

The injuries of SBS are predominantly driven by the coup-contrecoup forces as the brain impacts the inside of the skull. Additionally, the sudden acceleration and deceleration motion in opposing directions can cause shearing and destruction of axons and vascular structures within the central nervous system resulting in hemorrhage and hypoxia. Within the eye, the forces produced during a shaking event cause vitreoretinal traction resulting in bleeding in all three layers of the retina, retinoschisis, traumatic macular hole, or retinal detachment. Peripheral capillary destruction may lead to persistent peripheral nonperfusion resulting in late neovascular complications.

Clinical Features

A child with SBS may initially appear normal without obvious sign of injury or violence. Symptoms are caused by traumatic cerebral edema and can present hours later after injury. Symptoms include fussiness or irritability, difficulty breathing with blue or pale skin, poor eating and vomiting, somnolence, seizure, paralysis, and coma.

On exam, a child may exhibit signs of prior abuse. On skeletal imaging, an infant may be found to have skull fractures and broken long bones such as arms, legs, ribs, or collarbone. On neuroimaging, there may be associated cerebral edema or intracranial hemorrhage. External ocular manifestations of periorbital trauma may be present including ecchymosis, lid edema, orbital fractures. On fundus exam, one of the hallmark findings of SBS are retinal hemorrhages. These retinal hemorrhages involve all three layers, preretinal, intraretinal, and subretinal, and are often too many to count extending anterior to the equator due to vitreoretinal traction along the vitreous base. Additional findings may include peripheral nonperfusion, macular hole, retinoschisis, retinal detachment and evidence of anterior segment trauma.

Differential Diagnoses

There are several differential diagnoses that may mimic SBS.

- Normal birth trauma may result in retinal hemorrhages in newborns born via spontaneous vaginal deliveries. A higher incidence of retinal hemorrhages is found in newborns with history of instrumental deliveries (vacuum extraction or forceps). Retinal hemorrhages are commonly bilateral, intraretinal, posterior, and rarely persist beyond 6 weeks [3]. Similarly, accidental head injury, blunt ocular trauma, a child with seizures or post cardiopulmonary resuscitation may also present with retinal hemorrhages.
- Purtscher retinopathy can often be associated with long bone or thoracic fractures. A skeletal survey should be performed to rule out new or old fractures.
- Terson syndrome with bilateral vitreous hemorrhage can be found in infants with intracranial hemorrhage.
- Anemia and coagulopathies may also be associated with retinal hemorrhages.

Medical Management

A prompt and thorough systemic evaluation should be performed in any child suspected of SBS including physical exam, fundus photography, skeletal survey, neuroimaging, and serologies.

Workup

(1) History / Physical Exam: Is the history provided by caregiver consistent with the child's physical exam findings?
(2) Dilated fundus examination: Any retinal hemorrhage, retinoschisis, retinal detachment, or signs of ischemia should be carefully documented with fundus camera. If fluorescein angiography (FA) is available, this may be used to identify peripheral retinal nonperfusion. Optical coherence tomography

(OCT) may note a small macular hole not otherwise seen on exam, and provides information about the density, thickness, and location of hemorrhage for management decisions.

(3) Skeletal Survey: A series of x-rays of all the bones of the body are used to detect fractures and may be used to differentiate new or old fractures indicative of prior trauma.

(4) Neuroimaging: A skull CT (Computed tomography) scan or head MRI (magnetic resonance imaging) can investigate the extent of intracranial injury.

(5) Laboratory investigation: Bleeding diatheses may be identified by abnormal serologies including Complete blood count (CBC), Prothrombin time (PT), International Normalized Ratio (INR), Activated partial thromboplastin time (APTT), Fibrinogen, coagulation factors, and von Willebrand factor.

Treatment

Health care professionals are legally required to report all suspected cases of child abuse to state authorities, and a multidisciplinary team should follow the patient for systemic co-morbidities. The medical management of ocular findings in SBS centers around visual development and amblyopia management. In cases of persistent peripheral ischemia with neovascular complications, anterior scatter laser may be applied.

Clinical Case

This two-year-old female was admitted to the intensive care unit with loss of consciousness after SBS. One month after trauma, color photographs showed diffuse preretinal, intraretinal and subretinal hemorrhages within the macula and in all four quadrants (A, B). FA showed bilateral leakage from the optic nerve heads and peripheral nonperfusion 360 degrees extending two disc diameters posterior to the ora serrata (C, D). On follow up exam two months later, fundus exam showed fibrosis surrounding the optic nerves, subretinal fluid within the macula, interval improvement in peripheral retinal hemorrhages, but persistent areas of severe retinal ischemia with pinpoint areas of leakage and neovascularization in both eyes (E–H). Both eyes were treated with laser photocoagulation to the peripheral ischemic retina with subsequent regression of neovascularization in both eyes. Over time, both eyes have remained stable with fibrosis and atrophy involving the optic nerve and macula. The patient was followed by pediatric ophthalmology for visual development and remains visually impaired and stable without further need for surgical intervention. (Images courtesy of Audina M. Berrocal, MD. Reproduced from Tran K, Ko A, Read S, et al. The Use of Fluorescein Angiography to Evaluate Pediatric Abusive Head Trauma: An Observational Case Series. *Journal of Vitreoretinal Diseases.* 2017;1(5):321–327.) [4] (Fig. 1).

Surgical Management

The decision for surgery is often directed by concerns for amblyopia. While retinal hemorrhages are expected to clear 4–6 weeks after onset, vitreous or subhyaloid hemorrhage may last several months, putting the child at risk for deprivation amblyopia. In these cases, vitrectomy may be considered to remove blood from the visual axis. A macular hole that does not close with conservative observation may similarly require vitrectomy. Finally, traumatic rhegmatogenous retinal detachment or tractional retinal detachment secondary to neovascularization of the retina may also warrant surgical intervention. The decision for surgery must be weighed against the vision potential of the eye and that status of fellow eye. Many infants with SBS may suffer from significant cortical vision loss and bilateral optic atrophy regardless of their ocular findings.

When pursuing pediatric pars plana vitrectomy, special attention is paid to placement of the trocars to avoid iatrogenic damage to crystalline lens and peripheral retina [5]. Small gauge and short trochars may additionally assist with surgical maneuvers in a small eye. Internal limiting membrane can be peeled to reduce epiretinal proliferation, reduce tractional tangential forces, and release sub-internal limiting membrane hemorrhage. In cases where repeated inductions of general anesthesia are undesirable due to a tenuous clinical status, immediate sequential bilateral vitreoretinal surgery can be considered [6].

Prognosis

The long-term visual prognosis of SBS is guarded. While retinal hemorrhages are expected to clear in the vast majority of patients [7], approximately one fifth of survivors will go on to have lifelong poor vision [8]. Severe neurologic impairment correlates highly with loss of vision largely due to cortical vision impairment and optic atrophy. Retinal fibrosis and amblyopia may further limit visual function.

Surgical Video: *A Shocking Case of Shaken Baby: Giant Macular Tear Treated with Amniotic Membrane.*

This 35-week-old premature female was brought to the emergency room for failure to thrive. She was found to have a subdural hematoma, bruises all over her body, and widespread intraretinal and subretinal hemorrhage in the right eye. In the left eye, she was found to have a retinal detachment associated with temporal retinal dialysis, giant retinal tear, and giant macular hole. She initially underwent lens-sparing vitrectomy with silicone oil tamponade. Postoperatively, she was found to have a persistent shallow retinal detachment due to the giant macular hole. She underwent repeat vitrectomy with human amniotic membrane to plug the giant macular hole resulting in successful reattachment of the retina under silicone oil. Six months later, she underwent lensectomy and silicone oil removal. The retina has remained stable and attached without further need for surgery. (Video courtesy of Şengül Özdek, MD.)

Conclusion

Shaken baby syndrome is a leading cause of childhood trauma and results in significant morbidity and mortality. Systemic evaluation should be performed in any child suspected of SBS including physical exam, fundus photography, skeletal survey, neuroimaging, and serologies. Treatment of ocular findings of SBS centers around amblyopia management and visual development and may require anterior scatter laser in cases of ischemia, or vitrectomy for non-clearing vitreous hemorrhage obstructing the visual axis, macular hole, and retinal detachment.

Review Questions

1. What are components of the workup for a child suspected of shaken baby syndrome?

a. Dilated fundus exam
b. Serologies to rule out mimickers
c. Skeletal survey
d. Neuroimaging
e. All of the above

2. How long do retinal hemorrhages associated with shaken baby syndrome typically last?

a. Less than 24 h
b. 1–7 days
c. 4–6 weeks
d. 2–3 months

3. What is the most important component of management of shaken baby syndrome?

a. Fundus exam
b. Health care professionals are legally required to report all suspected cases of child abuse to state authorities. A multidisciplinary team should follow the patient for multiple co-morbidities.
c. Vitrectomy for non-clearing vitreous hemorrhage
d. Patching for amblyopia management

Answers

1. E
2. C
3. B

References

1. Keenan HT, Runyan DK, Marshall SW, et al. A population-based study of inflicted traumatic brain injury in young children. JAMA. 2003;290(5):621–6.
2. National Center on Shaken Baby Syndrome. Nov 2, 2021. https://www.dontshake.org/.
3. Watts P, Maguire S, Kwok T, et al. Newborn retinal hemorrhages: a systematic review. J AAPOS. 2013;17(3):341.
4. Tran K, Ko A, Read S, et al. The use of fluorescein angiography to evaluate pediatric abusive head trauma: an observational case series. J Vitreoretin Dis. 2017;1(5):321–7.
5. Wright L, Harper C III, Chang E. Management of Infantile and Childhood Retinopathies: Optimized Pediatric Pars Plana Vitrectomy Sclerotomy Nomogram. Ophthalmol Retin. 2018;2:1227–34.
6. Yonekawa Y, Wu WC, Kusaka S, et al. Immediate sequential bilateral pediatric vitreoretinal surgery: an international multicenter study. Ophthalmology. 2016;123(8):1802–8.
7. McCabe CF, Donahue SP. Prognostic indicators for vision and mortality in shaken baby syndrome. Arch Ophthalmol. 2000;118(3):373–7.
8. Kivlin JD, Simons KB, Lazoritz S, Ruttum MS. Shaken baby syndrome. Ophthalmology. 2000;107(7):1246–54.

Management of Vitreous Hemorrhage at Pediatric Age

50

Jessica G. Lee and Philip J. Ferrone

Abstract

Vitreous hemorrhage occurs more rarely in children than in adults. The etiologies of vitreous hemorrhage in pediatric patients can differ from adults, including diagnoses related to retinopathy of prematurity, trauma, congenital malformations, genetic conditions, among others. In pediatric patients, the risk of amblyopia is an important consideration that can affect the management of vitreous hemorrhage. Additionally, the smaller size of the eye as well as the more formed vitreous in young eyes affects the surgical approach.

Keywords

Vitreous hemorrhage · Pediatric retinal surgery · Non-accidental trauma · Trauma · Retinopathy of prematurity · Coats disease · Familial exudative vitreoretinopathy · Pars planitis

Introduction

Vitreous hemorrhage occurs rarely in the pediatric population. The etiologies of vitreous hemorrhage in children tend to be different than in adults and are varied including birth trauma, non-accidental trauma, blunt and/or penetrating trauma,

Supplementary Information The online version contains supplementary material available at https://doi.org/10.1007/978-3-031-14506-3_50.

J. G. Lee · P. J. Ferrone (✉)
Vitreoretinal Consultants of New York, Great Neck, NY, USA
e-mail: pjferrone@gmail.com

retinopathy of prematurity, inflammation, Coats disease, coagulation disorders as well as other less common genetic conditions and congenital malformations of the eye [1, 2]. The presentation and management of vitreous hemorrhages in the pediatric population compared to the adult population can differ for various reasons.

The vitreous in infants and children is more formed and gelatinous than the vitreous in adults, thus when a young eye develops a vitreous hemorrhage it tends to be more consolidated and denser with a lower tendency to disperse than in adults. The spontaneous absorption of vitreous hemorrhage in infants can take much longer than an adult and usually takes from 2 to 13 months [3]. Vitreous hemorrhage in the pediatric age group is most concerning for the potentially irreversible effects of prolonged occlusion of the affected eye leading to deprivational amblyopia. Infants and young children who are unable to express their visual complaints, may present with the sequalae of the vitreous hemorrhage obscuring the central visual axis with symptoms of strabismus, nystagmus, abnormal pupillary reflex or behavioral changes noted by the parents. Older children (>9 years old) tend to present with decreased vision, and floaters [2]. The visual prognosis of vitreous hemorrhage in children and infants is variable and depends on the etiology of the hemorrhage.

The clinical exam of pediatric patients who present with vitreous hemorrhage should importantly assess whether the visual axis is obscured and grade how dense the hemorrhage is. If the vitreous hemorrhage is very dense, there is a higher risk of deprivational amblyopia and this can lead to a poorer visual prognosis. It is important to determine the underlying pathology that led to the development of vitreous hemorrhage. Trauma (both penetrating and nonpenetrating), nonaccidental trauma, and birth trauma have been found to be the most common cause of vitreous hemorrhage in the pediatric population. Of note, in patients who present with bilateral vitreous hemorrhage, non-accidental trauma should be considered especially in very young patients. Other common causes include retinopathy of prematurity, familial exudative vitreoretinopathy, and pars planitis. The more rare causes may include X-linked juvenile retinoschisis, persistent fetal vasculature, Coats disease, Terson syndrome, and coagulation disorders such as disseminated intravascular coagulation disorder, Protein C or Protein S deficiency (Table 50.1) [1, 2, 4].

A thorough exam of the eye is essential, especially in the setting of trauma. However, often in pediatric patients the exam in the office may be limited due to poor cooperation—in such cases, one should have a low threshold to perform an exam under anesthesia, at which time fundus photos and, if necessary, a fluorescein angiography can be performed. If non-accidental trauma is suspected, fundus photos should be taken to document the findings. Fluorescein angiography can be especially helpful in identifying vascular disorders and help guide management in conditions such as Coats disease, Incontinentia Pigmentii, retinopathy of prematurity, and familial exudative vitreoretinopathy amongst other conditions that can affect retinal vasculature. If fluorescein angiography demonstrates areas of capillary non-perfusion or any neovascularization, then laser photocoagulation is usually performed to help prevent recurrence of the vitreous hemorrhage. If the vitreous

Table 50.1 Causes of vitreous hemorrhages in children

Causes of Vitreous Hemorrhage
1. Trauma–
•Nonpenetrating
• Penetrating
• Non-accidental trauma
• Birth trauma
2. Vascular conditions–
• Retinopathy of prematurity
• Coats disease
• Familial Exudative Vitreoretinopathy
• Incontinentia Pigmentii
3. Developmental
• Persistent Fetal Vasculature
4. Inflammatory
• Pars Planitis
• Retinal Vasculitis (Sarcoidosis, Behçet's disease, Lupus-related)
5. Coagulation disorders—
• Disseminated Intravascular Coagulation Disorder
• Protein C/S deficiency
6. Others
• Terson's Syndrome
• Valsalva Retinopathy
• Retinal detachment
• Congenital X-linked retinoschisis

hemorrhage limits the view of the posterior pole, B-scan ultrasonography can be done in the office to help evaluate if retinal pathology is present.

Visual prognosis is highly dependent on the underlying etiology of the vitreous hemorrhage. Additionally, children 6 years old or younger can develop irreversible deprivational amblyopia caused by long standing dense vitreous hemorrhage leading to occlusion of the visual axis. Thus, when evaluating pediatric patients who present with vitreous hemorrhage, especially infants, it is important to assess if the baby and or child would benefit from prompt surgery. With infants it is important to assess for how long after term (the due date) the hemorrhage has been present, and whether the infant is stable enough for surgery. For infantile vitreous hemorrhage, to avoid irreversible vision loss from deprivational amblyopia we extrapolate from congenital monocular and binocular cataract data to guide the timeline for surgery. If there is dense vitreous hemorrhage obscuring the central visual axis, surgery before 6–8 weeks of age may minimize the effects of unilateral deprivation amblyopia [5]. In bilateral dense visual axis obscuring vitreous hemorrhage (assuming there is no underlying pathology that needs sooner treatment) it is acceptable to wait up to 12 weeks to intervene to clear the vitreous hemorrhage (similar to the bilateral congenital cataract data).

In addition to deprivational amblyopia, there can be several other complications of vitreous hemorrhage in the pediatric age group, which can occur as early as 6 weeks after the onset of the vitreous hemorrhage. Occlusion by vitreous hemorrhage can also induce the development of a high degree of ansiometropic myopia which can persist even after the hemorrhage clears. Along with the vitreous hemorrhage some patients may additionally have subhyaloidal and/or subretinal hemorrhage which can lead to epiretinal membrane formation or pigmentary retinopathy and consequently a worse visual outcome [6]. Vitreous hemorrhage can also be associated with vitreous traction and traction retinal detachments [1].

In cases where the vitreous hemorrhage is principally out of the visual axis when the infant or child is upright, observation should be considered. For infants, in their waking hours the infant can be placed upright in a car seat or to help displace the vitreous hemorrhage out of the visual axis by gravity. However, if the vitreous hemorrhage is dense and vision threatening, a lens-sparing pars-plana vitrectomy to clear the vitreous hemorrhage should be considered to avoid amblyopia and potentially other mentioned complications of vitreous hemorrhage. The timing of the surgery needs to be carefully planned to prevent amblyopia while also considering any other comorbidities that need consultation with the child's pediatrician and the anesthesia team.

Surgical management of pediatric vitreous hemorrhage requires special consideration of eye size and axial eye growth in pediatric patients [7]. Scleral thickness is age-dependent and thickens with age. Infants have significantly thinner sclera than older children with an average scleral thickness of approximately 0.4 mm. By 2 years old, the sclera doubles in thickness to approximately 0.8 mm [8]. The pars plana is not fully developed in a full-term infant at birth. In infants, to avoid inadvertent lens and retinal trauma, a safe distance to enter into these eyes is usually at 1 mm posterior to the limbus. The average pars plana/pars plicata size at term in a non-microphthalmic eye is 1.87 mm [9]. As children get older, the safe zone of entry for pars-plana-vitrectomy broadens, but it is still much narrower than in adults. At 6 months of age, the pars plana/pars plicata size on average is approximately 3 mm in a non-microphthalmic eye, so entering this eye at 1.5–2.0 mm posterior to the limbus should be safe [9]. It is important to examine the eye and determine the safe zone of entry into the vitreous cavity in children up to 13 years of age at which time the eye is approximately adult size [7]. In microphthalmic eyes, the safest point of entry may be at half the distances listed above, depending on how dramatically microphthalmia affects the eye.

The goal of the vitrectomy for vitreous hemorrhage is to clear the visual axis, and to perform a limited axial vitrectomy to clear the hemorrhage. The posterior hyaloid is tightly adherent in these young eyes unlike in adult eyes, and in most cases of pediatric vitreous hemorrhage the posterior cortical vitreous does not necessarily need to be detached and removed.

If there is any retrolenticular hemorrhage, the risk of causing inadvertent lens trauma is high. It is often safer to try and clear the retrolenticular hemorrhage indirectly by trimming the peripheral vitreous base. Also, in these young eyes be cognizant of the intraocular pressure (IOP) during surgery. The blood pressure in these young patients runs much lower than in adults, and to allow for adequate perfusion of the retina and optic nerve the IOP setting on the vitrectomy machine may need to be set lower than one might usually set it in adult cases.

We share two cases as clinical examples of pediatric patients who present with vitreous hemorrhage, and detail their clinical history and management course.

Case 1

A 10-week-old female infant, born full term via normal spontaneous vaginal delivery without complications, was referred for evaluation of vitreous hemorrhage in the left eye. The patient's visual acuity was light perception in both eyes, and there was a small-angle esotropia in right eye. There was no afferent pupillary defect, and the anterior exam was normal in both eyes. Fundus exam of the right eye was normal. In the left eye, there was old vitreous hemorrhage with no view of the nerve or macula. B-scan ultrasonography of the left eye was performed to confirm that the retina was attached (Fig. 50.1). The vitreous hemorrhage was consistent with birth trauma. A lens-sparing pars-plana-vitrectomy was performed for non-clearing vitreous hemorrhage. An exam under anesthesia was performed prior to surgery. There was no view to the macula or the optic nerve due to the vitreous hemorrhage and the retina was fully vascularized with scleral depression 360°. Lens-sparing pars-plana-vitrectomy using 25-gauge trocars was performed with placement of the trocars 1 mm posterior to the limbus. Once the vitreous hemorrhage was cleared using the high-speed mechanical vitrector, there was noted to be macular thickening and distortion consistent with old subretinal hemorrhage and likely combined hamartoma of the retina and RPE with retinal distortion and thickening. An epiretinal membrane was peeled. There was no well-defined fovea visible. There were no complications from the surgery. At 1-month postoperatively, vision was still light perception with a clear vitreous cavity, and the patient was recommended to follow-up with a pediatric ophthalmologist for amblyopia and esotropia management. Wide-field fundus photos post-operatively showed clearance of the vitreous hemorrhage (Fig. 50.2).

Fig. 50.1 Pre-operative B-scan ultrasonography showing vitreous hemorrhage

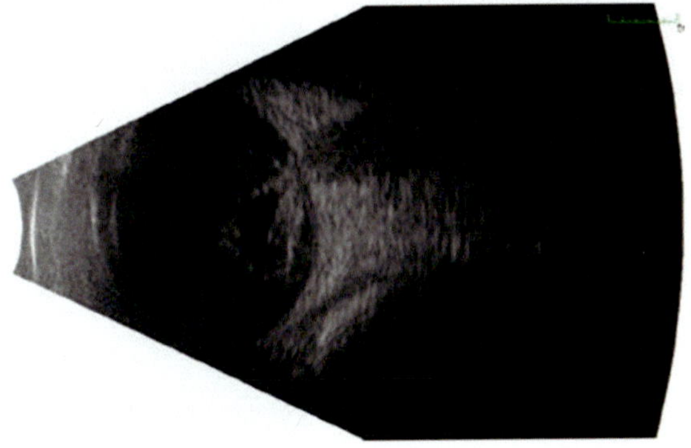

Fig. 50.2 Fundus photo post-vitrectomy showing clearance of vitreous hemorrhage. Nasal macula showing grey pigmentation of combined hamartoma of retina and RPE

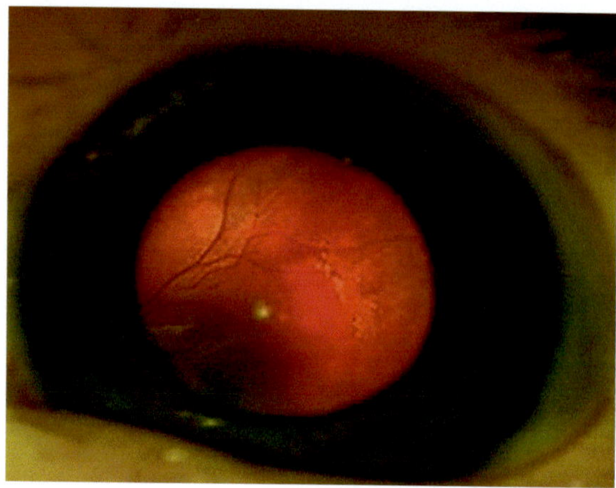

Case 2

Previously healthy 6-year-old boy born full-term without complication suffered non-accidental trauma while with a babysitter, 2 years prior to presentation in our clinic. He had suffered traumatic brain injury and underwent several brain surgeries. He presented with severe upper limb contractures, was nonverbal and wheelchair bound. He reacted to light OU and had exotropia OU. Anterior exam was normal. Fundus exam of the right eye revealed vitreous hemorrhage that did not appear dense and was inferior to the central visual axis (Fig. 50.3). Fundus exam of the left eye was normal. Given the characteristics of the vitreous hemorrhage not being in the visual axis and not being a dense hemorrhage, as well as the child's other comorbidities and anesthesia risk, observation was recommended.

Fig. 50.3 Persistent not visually significant vitreous hemorrhage (not obscuring the visual axis) in a child following non-accidental trauma

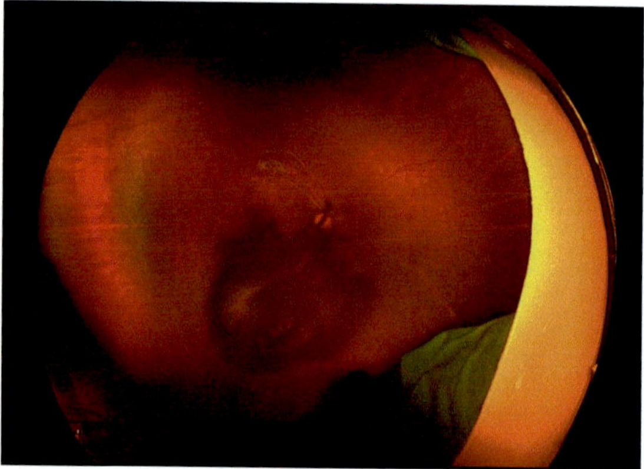

Surgical video: The video shows a vitreoretinal surgery in a 10 months old baby boy with bilateral buphthalmos, total iridocorneal apposition, leukocoria and vitreous hemorrhage associated with possible FEVR (video courtesy of Prof. Dr. Şengül Özdek).

Conclusions

The etiologies, presentation and management of vitreous hemorrhage in pediatric patients can differ from adult patients. The management of pediatric vitreous hemorrhage must consider the risk of amblyopia in these young eyes. The denser vitreous in pediatric patients as well as the smaller size of pediatric eyes affects the surgical approach when performing pars plana vitrectomy for clearance of the vitreous hemorrhage.

Review Questions

1. If there is pediatric patient with dense vitreous hemorrhage obscuring the central visual axis in one eye, to reduce risk of deprivational amblyopia, surgery should be performed:

a. Within 1 week
b. Within 1 month
c. Before 6–8 weeks of age
d. Before child turns 1 year old

2. If a pediatric patient presents with bilateral vitreous hemorrhage, one should suspect:

a. Non-accidental trauma
b. Retinopathy of prematurity
c. Coagulation disorder
d. All of the above

Answers

1. C
2. D

References

1. Ferrone PJ, de Juan E. Vitreous hemorrhage in infants. Arch Ophthalmol Chic Ill 1960. 1994;112(9):1185–9. https://doi.org/10.1001/archopht.1994.01090210069018.
2. Spirn MJ, Lynn MJ, Hubbard GB. Vitreous hemorrhage in children. Ophthalmology. 2006;113 (5):848–52. https://doi.org/10.1016/j.ophtha.2005.12.027.
3. Braendstrup P. Vitreous haemorrhage in the newborn. A rare type of neonatal intraocular haemorrhage. Acta Ophthalmol (Copenh). 1969;47(3):502–13.
4. Rishi P, Rishi E, Gupta A, Swaminathan M, Chhablani J. Vitreous hemorrhage in children and adolescents in India. J Am Assoc Pediatr Ophthalmol Strabismus. 2013;17(1):64–9. https://doi. org/10.1016/j.jaapos.2012.10.013.
5. Birch EE, Stager DR. The critical period for surgical treatment of dense congenital unilateral cataract. Invest Ophthalmol Vis Sci. 1996;37(8):1532–8.
6. Spirn M, Hubbard G. Pediatric vitreous hemorrhages. Invest Ophthalmol Vis Sci. 2004;45 (13):5281.
7. Maldonado RS, O'Connell RV, Sarin N, et al. Dynamics of human foveal development after premature birth. Ophthalmology. 2011;118(12):2315–25. https://doi.org/10.1016/j.ophtha. 2011.05.028.
8. Ryan SJ, Hinton DR, Sadda SR, Schachat AP. Retina. Section 4. In: Chapter 145 Surgical Aspects of Vitreoretinal Disease in Children. Elsevier Health Sciences; 2012. p. 2478.
9. Hairston RJ, Maguire AM, Vitale S, Green WR. Morphometric analysis of pars plana development in humans. Retina. 1997;17(2):135–8.

Part VIII

Inflammatory Disorders in Children

Ocular Toxoplasmosis

Merve İnanç Tekin and Pınar Çakar Özdal

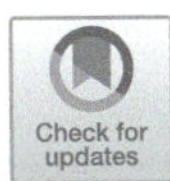

Abstract

Ocular toxoplasmosis is a recurrent retinochoroiditis caused by *Toxoplasma gondii* and is the most common cause of infectious posterior uveitis in children. The most typical clinical manifestation of an active toxoplasmic lesion is whitish and edematous necrotizing retinochoroiditis close to an old pigmented scar. Ocular toxoplasmosis might be associated with vitreoretinal complications including rhegmatogenous and/or tractional retinal detachment (RD), vitreous hemorrhage, epiretinal membrane, choroidal neovascular membranes, and vitreous opacities. All can potentially cause severe visual loss and require vitreoretinal surgery that can be used for both diagnostic and therapeutic purposes.

Keywords

Ocular toxoplasmosis · Pediatric uveitis · Toxoplasma gondi · Vitreoretinal surgery

Supplementary Information The online version contains supplementary material available at https://doi.org/10.1007/978-3-031-14506-3_51.

M. İ. Tekin
Ulucanlar Eye Training and Research Hospital, Ankara, Turkey

P. Ç. Özdal (✉)
Department of Ophthalmology, University of Health Sciences, Ulucanlar Eye Training and Research Hospital, Ankara, Turkey
e-mail: pinarozdal@hotmail.com

Key points

- The most common cause of infectious uveitis in the pediatric age group.
- Causative agent: *Toxoplasma gondii*
- Typical lesion: Focal necrotizing retinochoroiditis (variable in size and location)
- Satellite lesion adjacent to old scar is a common presentation but may also occur primarily
- Vitritis concentrated on the lesion is typical, it may be severe ('headlight in the fog')
- Associated features: Retinal vasculitis, optic disc edema, anterior uveitis.
- Treatment–combination therapy with antiparasitic drugs and corticosteroids.
- During the healing process of the lesion, the center atrophies and a pigmented scar forms on the edges.

Introduction

Toxoplasmosis is an infection caused by the intracellular parasite named *Toxoplasma gondii (T. gondii)* [1]. Infection of *T. gondii* in the eye, also named ocular toxoplasmosis has a worldwide distribution [2, 3]. *T. gondii* infects up to a third of the world's population and is the most frequent etiology of infectious intraocular uveitis in both pediatric and adult age groups [4].

Epidemiology

The incidence of symptomatic ocular toxoplasmosis was estimated to be 0.4 cases per 100,000 population per year in British-born patients and the lifetime risk of disease to be 18 cases per 100,000 population [5]. Seroprevalence in Europe varies. It is high (up to 54%) in Southern European countries, and decreases with increasing latitude to 5–10% in northern Sweden and Norway [6, 7]. *T. gondii* is a common infection in South America, and a study from Brazil found that seroprevalence was high in people from poor socio-economic conditions probably due to waterborne transmission [8]. Epidemiological studies in pediatric uveitis patients report that ocular toxoplasmosis is, as in adults, the most frequent cause of posterior uveitis, and accounts for 3.3 to 21% of the total number of cases in this age group [9–12].

Life Cycle and Mode of Transmission

T. gondii exists in 3 infectious forms including oocysts, tachyzoites and bradyzoites. Oocysts are produced only in cat intestines and require sexual reproduction. Oocysts than spread out with defecation and become infectious in 1–5 days by sporulation. Tachyzoites are the fastest replicating form and responsible for systemic dissemination and active tissue infection in intermediate hosts. Tachyzoites can enter almost any type of host cell and multiply until the host cell is filled with parasites. Lysis of the host cell results in tachyzoite release followed by re-entry into a new host cell. As a result of this cycle, multifocal tissue necrosis may occur. The host usually limits this phase of infection, and the parasite then transforms into dormant form, named bradyzoites. This form of parasite is characteristic for chronic infection, and isolated in tissue cysts which contain hundreds of bradyzoites. These cysts usually do not cause host reaction and may remain asleep throughout the host's life. Cats are the definitive host, whereas humans become intermediate hosts by ingesting the cyst or bradyzoite form. Once ingested, the cyst form can migrate to cardiac, muscular, and neural/retinal tissues. Rupture of the cyst then leads to release of the tachyzoite form, resulting in active disease.

Clinical Presentation and Phenotypes

The infection may be acquired or congenital by vertical transmission to the fetus. Ocular toxoplasmosis has long been regarded as a disease that was mainly caused by congenital infection, while symptomatic ocular infection acquired after birth was considered rare. This paradigm was challenged by data from Brazil showing that ocular toxoplasmosis acquired after birth was much more common compared to congenital infection [13]. This concept was confirmed by other groups and probably applies to many other areas of the world as well [14].

Congenital Ocular Toxoplasmosis

Vertical transmission of toxoplasmosis occurs during primary infection in pregnant women, and generally the maternal disease goes unnoticed. In the first trimester of pregnancy, rates of transplacental infection are around 10–25% and progressively increase to reach 60–80% in the third trimester. Conversely, the potential severity of fetal sequelae typically decreases during pregnancy. Congenital toxoplasmosis is associated with a variety of systemic manifestations ranging from intrauterine death or serious malformations to the neonatal infectious syndrome, including anemia, thrombocytopenia, skin rash, hepatitis, pneumonia, myocarditis, and encephalitis. Sabine tetrad, which is characterized by hydrocephaly or microcephaly, intracranial calcifications, mental retardation, and retinochoroiditis is seen in less than 10% of

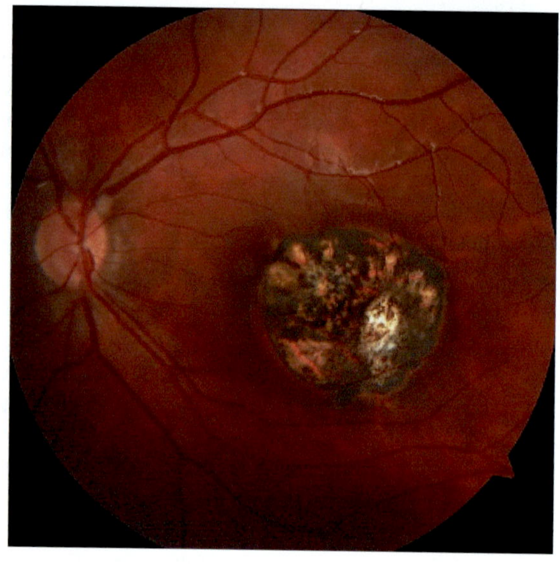

Fig. 51.1 An atrophic hyperpigmented macular scar that is described as 'wagon-wheel' lesion

newborns with congenital toxoplasmosis [15]. Retinochoroiditis is the main finding seen in up to 80% of newborns at birth [16, 17].

Typical presentation of congenital ocular toxoplasmosis is an atrophic hyperpigmented scarred macular lesion that is described as 'wagon-wheel' lesion (Fig. 51.1). It shows a central area composed of glial and pigmented material connected by pigmented strands to a peripheral ring of pigment at the edge of the lesion. A study designed to detect ocular involvement in infants with congenital toxoplasma infection reported that ocular involvement occurred in 70.4% of the cases, with mean age of active lesion at 1.4 months. Bilateral macular scarring has been reported in approximately 15.7% of congenital ocular toxoplasmosis cases and is more common than acquired form [18]. These children may develop recurrent retinochoroiditis lesions later in life, usually before puberty (Fig. 51.2A, B). Retinochoroidal scars, cataract, microphthalmia, optic atrophy, strabismus, nystagmus and even phthisis bulbi are other sequelae ocular findings of congenital disease. Inactive cases are generally noticed during routine eye examinations or when they apply for a reason such as microphthalmia or strabismus.

Acquired Toxoplasma Infection

Acquired infection occurs by consumption of raw meat containing cysts or ingestion of water or food contaminated by oocytes [19, 20]. Once the active parasite has invaded the body, it will spread via the blood stream, and due to a high affinity for cerebrovascular and retinovascular endothelial cells, can become established within the retina. Following invasion of the parasite into the eye, the tachyzoite remains latent in the cyst under the control of the immune response of host. In event

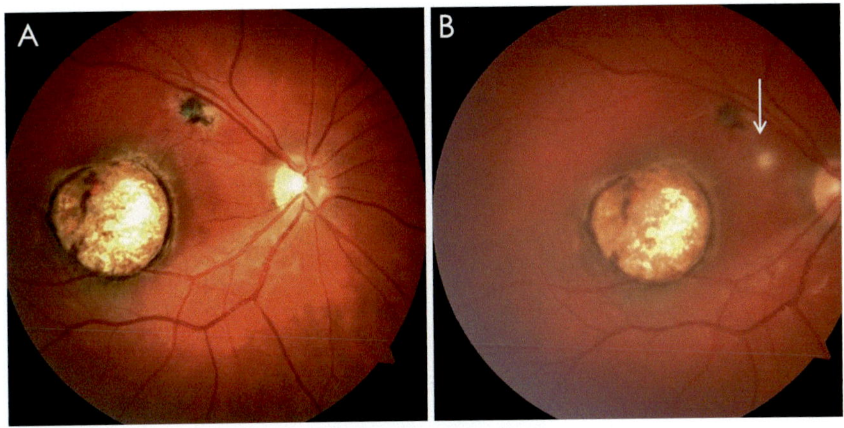

Fig. 51.2 14 y/o male patient with ocular toxoplasmosis **A** Inactive scar lesion **B** Activation adjacent to the scar lesion. Vitreous haze, and active satellite lesion (white arrow) can be seen

triggering the cyst rupture, the tachyzoite is converted to bradyzoite, and the inflammatory response is activated [21, 22].

The typical ocular toxoplasmosis lesion is focal necrotizing retinochoroiditis. It is variable in size and location, and may be located in the posterior pole or the periphery. It may develop primarily or as a satellite lesion adjacent to the old scar. Active lesions appear as an area of focal retinochoroiditis with an overlying vitritis that is either mild or severe ("headlight in the fog") (Fig. 51.3). In more severe cases, anterior chamber might be secondarily involved and manifests mostly with granulomatous anterior uveitis and high intraocular pressure. Retinal vasculitis may also occur to varying degrees. Periphlebitis adjacent or distant to focal

Fig. 51.3 13 y/o male patient having active lesion with an overlying vitritis ("headlight in the fog")

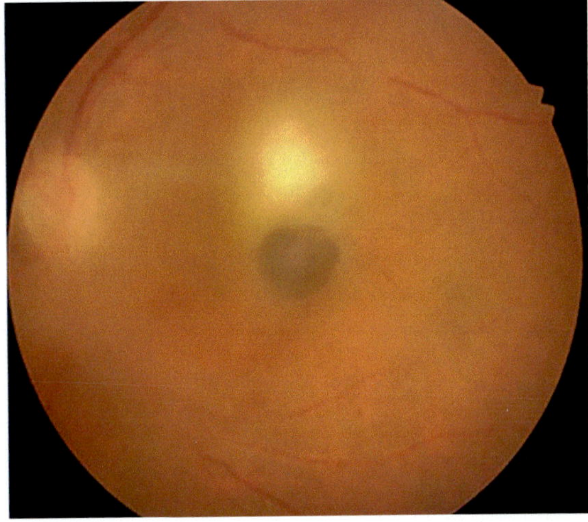

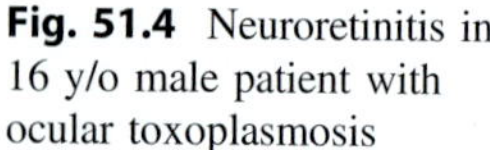

Fig. 51.4 Neuroretinitis in 16 y/o male patient with ocular toxoplasmosis

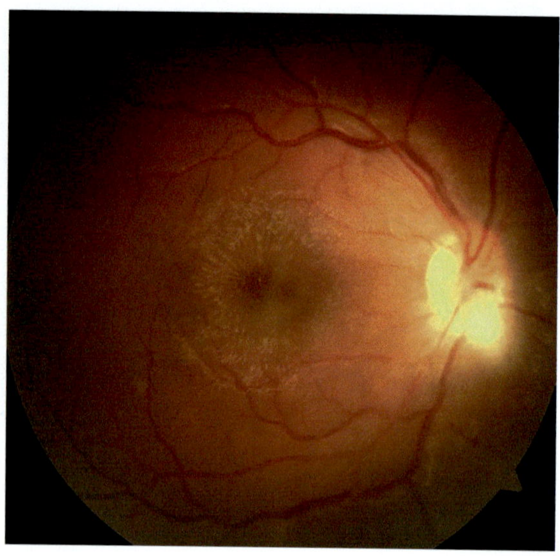

retinochoroiditis is a common manifestation. Periarterial plaques named as "Kyrieleis arteriolitis" is located adjacent to active lesion can also be seen. Ocular toxoplasmosis may also present with atypical presentations. Large, multifocal or even bilateral active lesions can be confused with viral retinitis [23]. Other unusual forms include neuroretinitis (Fig. 51.4), punctate outer retinal toxoplasmosis and various optic nerve pathologies [24–27]. Toxoplasmic intraocular inflammation without necrotizing retinochoroiditis is relatively rare and may present as isolated anterior uveitis, retinal vasculitis, and optic neuritis [28, 29].

Characteristics of Pediatric Cases that Differ from Adults

- Bilaterality is more common (Fig. 51.5)
- Posterior pole involvement is more common
- Cat-dog contact history is more frequent
- Most of them are inactive cases with low vision and strabismus for a long time.
- Visual prognosis is poor because active cases are mostly located in the posterior pole and diagnosed late.

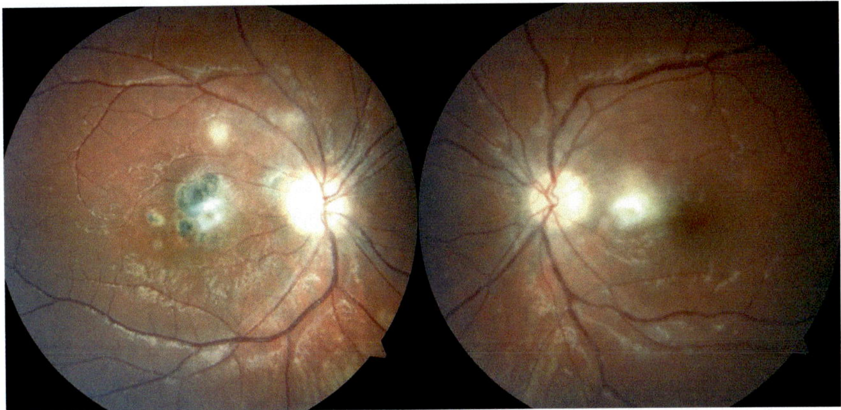

Fig. 51.5 Bilateral involvement in a 15 y/o male patient with ocular toxoplasmosis

Diagnosis

The diagnosis is essentially based on clinical presentation and supported by serological tests. Absence of specific IgG and IgM virtually excludes the possibility of toxoplasmosis, whereas their presence indicates recently acquired disease especially in significant titers. A rise in titer of specific IgG antibodies over a 3-week period and low avidity of specific anti–*T. gondii* IgG antibodies are used for supporting a recent infection. On the other hand, the presence of specific IgG antibodies confirms previous exposure to the parasite but given the worldwide high seroprevalence, it is not enough to make the diagnosis if the clinical manifestations are absent. However, Ig G negativity excludes the diagnosis of toxoplasma infection [30]. Enzyme-linked immunosorbent assay (ELISA), Sabin-Feldman dye study, indirect fluorescent antibody test, complement fixation test, and indirect hemagglutination test are various assays available for detection of serum anti-toxoplasma antibody titers. Polymerase chain reaction (PCR) of aqueous and vitreous specimens or Goldmann-Witmer testing, which compares intraocular antibody production to that of serum, may be helpful to establish a definitive diagnosis [31]. In infants, detection of IgM or IgA is suggestive for prenatal infection.

Management

The aim of medical treatment is to reduce the severity and duration of acute inflammation, and to reduce the size of the scar that may occur. And also, ocular toxoplasmosis may be associated with vitreoretinal complications such as rhegmatogenous and/or tractional retinal detachment (RD), vitreous hemorrhage, epiretinal membrane, choroidal neovascular membranes, and vitreous opacities that can potentially cause severe vision loss and may require vitreoretinal surgery [32, 33]. **(see the video).**

A. *Medical treatment*

Treatment in children is a combination of antiparasitic drugs and systemic corticosteroids as in adults. Topical corticosteroids, mydriatic, and hypotensive agents are also used as needed. Pyrimethamine, sulfonamides, clindamycin, trimethoprim + sulfamethoxazole and spiramycin are the most commonly used agents. The most widely used regimen (called classic therapy) is the combination of sulfadiazine and pyrimethamine [34]. All patients on pyrimethamine should be monitored routinely with complete blood counts and receive supplementation with folinic acid to prevent leukopenia and thrombocytopenia [35]. In the setting of allergy or intolerance to sulfonamides, clindamycin or azithromycin may be employed. Patients with congenital infection require therapy for longer duration (from 2 to 12 month) and typically are treated with pyrimethamine and sulfadiazine. Clindamycin may also be added to this regimen. Oral corticosteroids are used with caution after 24–48 hours of antibiotic treatment, in patients with excessive vitreous haze and lesions adjacent to optic disc, macula, and great vessels [36].

Indications for Medical Treatment

- Lesions involving the macula/papillomacular bundle
- Lesions involving/adjacent to the optic disc
- Intense vitritis, those with vitreous haze
- Progressive peripheral lesions
- Young children in whom ophthalmologic examination is difficult

B. *Surgical treatment*

Vitreoretinal surgery may be used for both diagnostic and therapeutic purposes [33]. Vitrectomy can be beneficial for the management of complications such as persistent vitreous opacification, RD, secondary epiretinal membrane, vitreous hemorrhage and choroidal neovascular membrane.

a. *Therapeutic vitrectomy*

• *Vitreous opacification*

In some cases, vitreous opacification can persist despite intensive antibiotic and steroid treatment. After 2 or 3 months of appropriate treatment, the following conditions should be reviewed; 1. vitreous opacification from inflammatory cells or vitreous degeneration, 2. is it still possible to reduce it with steroids?

If opacification is due to large vitreous cords and secondary vitreous degeneration, steroid therapy is no longer indicated and vitrectomy may be considered to clear the posterior cavity, to improve visual acuity, and to avoid excessive steroid therapy [37].

- ***Retinal detachment***

Retinal detachment in ocular toxoplasmosis is generally thought to be rare (Fig. 51.6). It can be either rhegmatogenous and/or tractional. Though the mechanism of RD in ocular toxoplasmosis is not fully understood, it is thought that vitritis leads to vitreous liquefaction and traction, which results in rhegmatogenous retinal detachment (RRD) and/or tractional retinal detachment (TRD). In the study of Garza-Leon et al. examining pediatric ocular toxoplasmosis cases, RD frequency was found to be 1.8% [38]. In a review of 154 patients with ocular toxoplasmosis by Bosch-Driessen et al., prevalence for RD following ocular toxoplasmosis was reported as 6%, 2 out of 9 patients with RD (22.2%), and 1 out of 7 with retinal breaks (14.2%) were children [19]. In the study of Faridi et al. higher rate of RD (11.4%) was observed [39]. Consistent with the case series of Bosch-Driessen et al. in which patients with ocular toxoplasmosis-related RD had severe intraocular inflammation at baseline, Faridi et al. reported that vitreous inflammation was associated with a higher frequency of RD [19, 39, 40]. Therefore, patients with ocular toxoplasmosis, especially those with vitritis, should be followed carefully. The location of retinitis, that is, extramacular versus macular, was not associated with an increased risk of RD, although extramacular lesions have been associated with greater vitreous inflammation [41]. Because RD in ocular toxoplasmosis can be severe and complicated by recurrent detachments, it can result in severe visual loss [19, 39]. Recurrent RD occurs frequently due to new breaks and/or proliferative vitreoretinopathy [19, 39, 42]. In the review of Bosch-Driessen et al.,

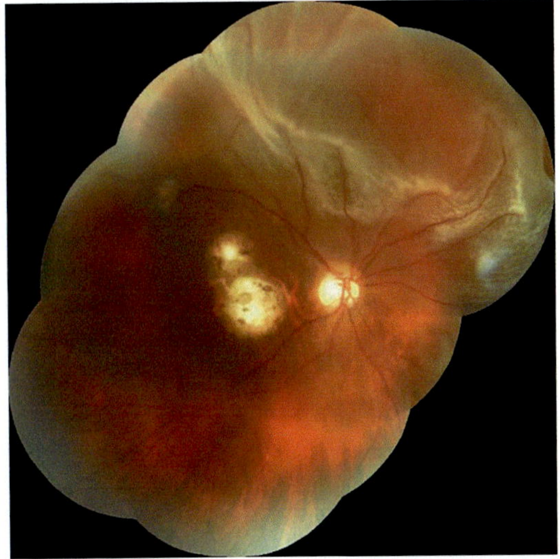

Fig. 51.6 Rhegmatogenous RD developed in the adulthood in a patient thought to have macular scar due to congenital toxoplasma infection

functional prognosis of patients with ocular toxoplasmosis-related RD was poor, with 5 of 9 patients with RD developing legal blindness [19].

Various techniques for retinal repositioning, including retinopexy with scleral buckle (SB) and pars plana vitrectomy (PPV) using gas or silicone oil (SO) injection, have been suggested over time [43]. The postoperative results may vary depending on the condition of the macula, the detachment time, and the presence of proliferative vitreoretinopathy. Previous studies have also examined various surgical techniques using small sample sizes. Adan et al. evaluated 8 patients with RRD treated using SB and PPV, 5 of which were administered long-acting gas tamponade and 3 of which were administered SO tamponade [44]. Papadopoulou et al. examined 2 RRD patients treated with PPV and gas injection and a third patient who underwent PPV and gas injection combined with SB [45]. Bosch-Driessen et al. evaluated 6 patients with RRD, of which 4 patients were treated by SB, one was treated by combined PPV and SO injection, and one was treated using cryocoagulation [40]. All of these studies reported improvements in the functional results, although no statistically significant differences between techniques were observed.

- ***Epiretinal membrane***

Epiretinal membrane (ERM) formation is uncommon in ocular toxoplasmosis, however it is one of the most important causes of reduced vision in patients with healed toxoplasmosis infection [46]. Miranda et al. examined 14 patients who underwent PPV for ERM secondary to ocular toxoplasmosis and reported that PPV is a safe and effective procedure in patients with ERM secondary to ocular toxoplasmosis, improving both visual acuity and anatomical result on macular optical coherence tomography (OCT) [47]. However, this surgery must be done only when the eye is quiet and free of inflammation for a minimum period of 3 months. Raval et al. evaluated 4 patients with ERM secondary to ocular toxoplasmosis and reported that surgery for ERM secondary to healed toxoplasmosis infection has good anatomical outcome and reasonable visual improvement, when the surgery is performed in a quiet eye [48].

- ***Vitreous hemorrhage and choroidal neovascular membrane***

Retinal vasculitis is common in patients with ocular toxoplasmosis and typically occurs in the same quadrant with retinochoroiditis but also can occur remote from the site of infection [49]. In rare cases, the vasculitis may be occlusive, resulting in retinal infarction and retinal ischemia with secondary neovascularization [50, 51].

Choroidal neovascular membrane (CNV) secondary to ocular toxoplasmosis occurs as a late complication of retinochoroiditis [52] (Fig. 51.7). CNV development is more common in children. 75% of ocular toxoplasmosis cases treated with photodynamic therapy are under the age of 15 [53]. Disruption of Bruch's membrane caused by necrotizing chorioretinitis promotes the development of CNV, which may develop adjacent to the retinal scar or at a distant location with feeder vessels originating from the scar. Submacular surgery may represent an option in

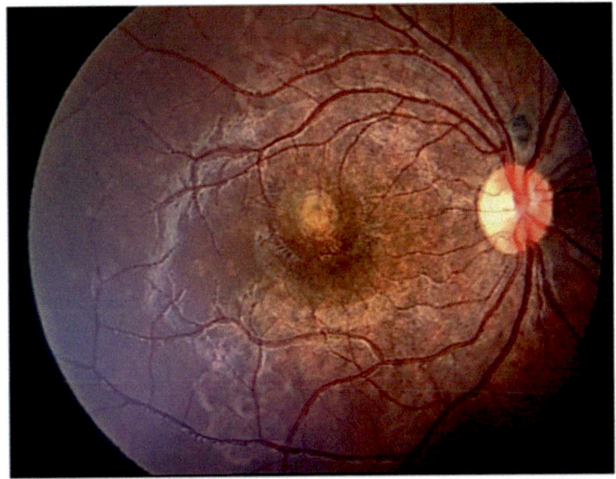

Fig. 51.7 14 y/o male patient with CNV secondary to ocular toxoplasmosis

treatment [54]. Uemura et al. reported one case of surgically treated subfoveal choroidal neovascularization associated with toxoplasmic retinochoroiditis in a pediatric patient. Preoperatively, the best-corrected visual acuity in the affected eye was 20/100. Postoperatively, visual acuity returned to 20/20 and has remained stable during 27 months' follow-up without recurrent CNV [55].

b. *Diagnostic vitrectomy*

Ocular toxoplasmosis most commonly presents with unilateral retinitis adjacent to a chorioretinal scar; however, systemically immunosuppressed individuals may present with atypical presentations, such as bilateral, extensive, or multifocal disease consisting of large areas of retinal necrosis without adjacent retinal scarring [56, 57]. Patients who have received local or systemic corticosteroid without concomitant anti-parasitic therapy have also been reported to develop severe retinal necrosis from toxoplasmosis [36] (Fig. 51.8). Differential diagnosis of such lesions includes acute retinal necrosis syndrome, other necrotizing herpetic retinopathies, cytomegalovirus retinitis, severe panuveitis, fungal infection, and intraocular lymphoma. Early use of invasive diagnostic procedures in patients with undiagnosed sight-threatening chorioretinitis or patients who do not respond to a selected empirical therapy may provide better visual and anatomical outcomes for this devastating ocular infection.

The standard technique for diagnostic vitrectomy is the collection of an undiluted vitreous sample with the cutter attached directly to a syringe. The main difficulty in the technique is the need to obtain an undiluted vitreous sample under sterile conditions. A centrifugation process is required for diluted samples that can be obtained by vitrectomy by opening the infusion, and cells may be damaged during this process. In addition, the risk of microbial contamination increases when collecting the diluted sample. Therefore, undiluted samples should be preferred whenever possible. During sampling, the peripheral retina should be carefully monitored, and the intraocular pressure should be constantly controlled [58, 59].

Fig. 51.8 15 y/o female patient with ocular toxoplasmosis treated with intravitreal triamcinolone acetonide injection and systemic corticosteroid without using antibiotic treatment

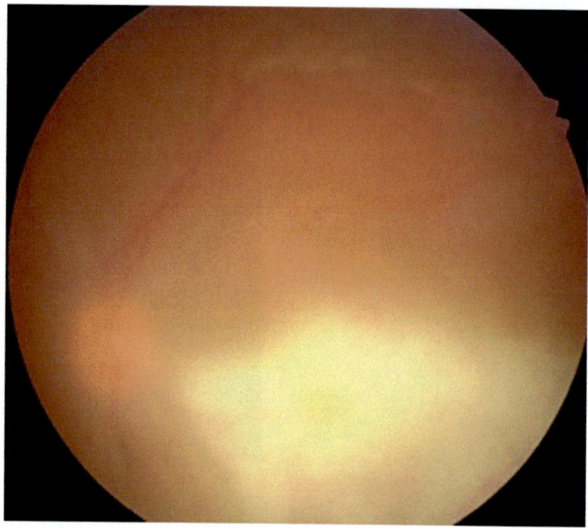

With this material, it is possible to examine the lymphocytes and perform PCR. Viruses can also be detected by PCR. Intraocular antibody production can be detected with the Goldmann-Witmer coefficient determined by comparing the vitreous antibody level with that of the serum.

Conclusion

Toxoplasmosis is one of the most common causes of posterior uveitis in children. The most classic clinical manifestation of an active toxoplasmic lesion is whitish and edematous necrotizing retinochoroiditis close to an old pigmented scar. Ocular toxoplasmosis might be associated with vitreoretinal complications including RRD, TRD, vitreous hemorrhage, epiretinal membrane, choroidal neovascular membranes, and vitreous opacities. All can potentially cause severe visual loss and require vitreoretinal surgery that can be used for both diagnostic and therapeutic purposes.

Clinical Case (With Courtesy of Prof. Dr. Şengül Özdek [43])

A prematurely born baby boy (GA 32 weeks & BW 1590 g) was referred to ophthalmology/uveitis clinic from the neonatology unit for the confirmation of congenital ocular toxoplasmosis. Prenatally, hydrocephaly had been detected. Toxoplasma IgG and IgM antibodies were also detected in his mother during pregnancy. Postnatally, infectious markers in blood samples confirmed the diagnosis of congenital toxoplasmosis. Ophthalmological examination revealed bilateral cataracts and seclusio pupilla. Buphthalmos with Haab's striae was detected in his right eye (corneal diameters: 12 × 12 mm, axial length: 25 mm) and microphthalmos (corneal diameters: 7×8 mm, axial length: 13 mm) in the left eye. Fundus examination was unable to provide clues regarding RD due to cataract and posterior synechia in both eyes. Ultrasonographic examination revealed pre-retinal membranes and freely mobile RD resembling RRD in the right eye and total TRD with dense vitreous membranes causing closed funnel RD appearance in the left eye. Surgery was not suggested for the microphthalmic left eye but lensectomy and vitrectomy were performed on his right eye (**see the video**). During surgery, complete bullous RD was detected, as well as a thick, tight fibrotic membrane extending from the nasal to temporal retina passing superior to optic nerve head (ONH) and over the macular pigmented chorioretinitis scar, ending in a very thick and strong fibrotic adhesion in the temporal equator. The nasal retina was pulled towards the temporal scar tissue over the ONH. There was a large, triangular retinal break at the nasal end of the membrane superior to the ONH, and the peripheral retina was avascular in zone 1 with a stage 2 ROP (Fig. 51.9A). The posterior

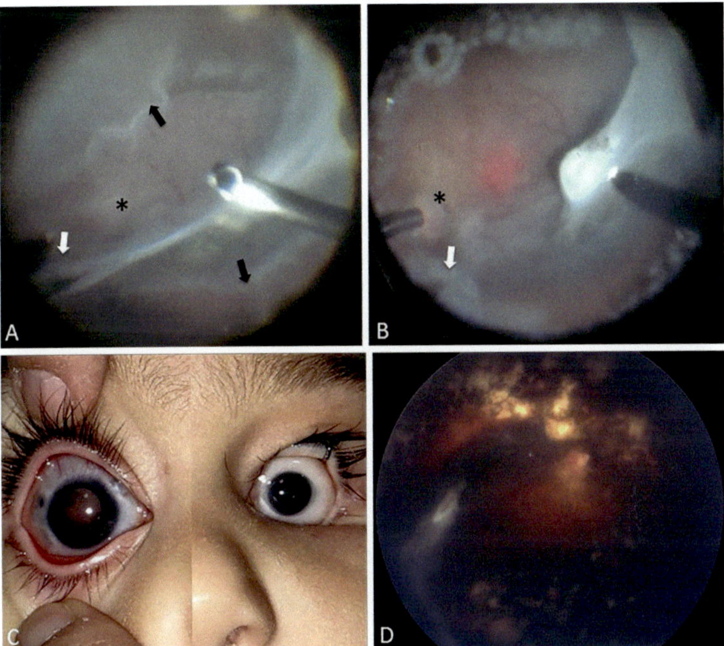

Fig. 51.9 and video **A** Combined rhegmatogenous and tractional RD in the right eye. Note the fibrotic membrane extending from nasal to temporal periphery leading to a large triangular retinal break (white arrow) superior to the optic nerve head (black star), which is barely visible due to the nasal retina pulled over it, and avascular retina in zone 1 with stage 2 retinopathy of prematurity (black arrow); **B** Peroperative fundus image after peeling the fibrotic membranes around the large, triangular retinal break (white arrow) and application of endolaser photocoagulation to avascular retina and around the breaks; **C** Postoperative image showing the buphthalmic appearance of the right eye and microphthalmic appearance of the left eye; **D** Postoperative fundus image of the right eye with attached retina and fibrotic membrane remnants in the temporal area and laser scars visible throughout the periphery. (Courtesy of Prof. Dr. Şengül Özdek)

hyaloid could not be detached because of the highly mobile retina which resulted in a small iatrogenic retinal hole formation in the inferior ridge region. A fluid air exchange was performed to drain the subretinal fluid and to stabilize the retina to prepare for membrane peeling. Perfluorocarbon liquid was injected to assist the removal of posterior hyaloid and fibrotic membranes meticulously around the break to eliminate all the tractions. Endolaser photocoagulation was applied to the retinal tears and avascular retina (Fig. 51.9B), and 16% C3F8 gas was given as tamponade. At 1-year follow-up, mild buphthalmic appearance with minimal corneal edema persisted, with the addition of minimal scleral staphylomas at the previous sclerotomy sites (Fig. 51.9C). Glaucoma could not be controlled with medical treatment and an Ahmed Glaucoma Valve was implanted to prevent further glaucomatous damage. The retina remained attached throughout follow-up (Fig. 51.9D). Vision could not be assessed well because of the mental-motor retardation, but the patient was able to follow light and large objects.

Review Questions

1. Which of the following statements about ocular toxoplasmosis is false?

(A)   The causative agent is *Toxoplasma gondi*.
(B)   Typical lesion is focal necrotizing retinochoroiditis.
(C)   Steroids cannot be used alone for treatment.
(D)   The potential severity of fetal sequelae increases during pregnancy.
(E)   Tachyzoites are the fastest replicating form and responsible for active tissue infection in intermediate hosts.

2. Which is not a treatment indication for ocular toxoplasmosis?

(A)   Lesions involving the macula/papillomacular bundle
(B)   Lesions involving/adjacent to the optic disc
(C)   Intense vitritis, those with vitreous haze
(D)   Progressive peripheral lesions
(E)   Peripheral lesions in advanced age children that can be easily examined.

3. Which of the following statements is incorrect for the diagnosis of ocular toxoplasmosis?

(A)   Anti-Toxo IgG positivity does not indicate the disease.
(B)   Anti-Toxo IgG negativity does not exclude the disease.
(C)   Antibody titers do not correlate with ocular disease.
(D)   The diagnosis is essentially based on clinical presentation.
(E)   In infants, detection of IgM or IgA is suggestive for prenatal infection.

4. Which of the differences between pediatric and adult ocular toxoplasmosis cases is incorrect?

(A) Bilaterality is more common in adult cases.
(B) Posterior pole involvement is more common in pediatric cases.
(C) Cat contact history is more common in pediatric cases.
(D) The macular scar, called 'wagon wheel', is more suggestive of congenital cases.
(E) The visual prognosis is poor since the lesion is mostly located in the posterior pole in pediatric cases.

Answers

1. (**D**) In the first trimester of pregnancy, rates of transplacental infection are around 10–25% and progressively increase to reach 60–80% in the third trimester. Conversely, the potential severity of fetal sequelae typically decreases during pregnancy.

2. (**E**) Peripheral lesions that can be easily examined in older children can be followed without treatment.

3. (**B**) The diagnosis of ocular toxoplasmosis is essentially based on clinical presentation and supported by serological tests. The presence of specific IgG antibodies confirms previous exposure to the parasite but it is not enough to make the diagnosis if the clinical manifestations are absent. However, Ig G negativity excludes the diagnosis of toxoplasma infection.

4. (**A**) Bilateral involvement is observed more frequently in the pediatric age group.

References

1. Pappas G, Roussos N, Falagas ME. Toxoplasmosis snapshots: global status of Toxoplasma gondii seroprevalence and implications for pregnancy and congenital toxoplasmosis. Int J Parasitol. 2009;39:1385–94.
2. McCannel CA, Holland GN, Helm CJ, Cornell PJ, Winston JV, Rimmer TG. Causes of uveitis in the general practice of ophthalmology. UCLA Community-Based Uveitis Study Group. Am J Ophthalmol. 1996;121:35–46.
3. Tran VT, Auer C, Guex-Crosier Y, Pittet N, Herbort CP. Epidemiological characteristics of uveitis in Switzerland. Int Ophthalmol. 1994;18:293–8.
4. Hettinga YM, de Groot-Mijnes JD, Rothova A, de Boer JH. Infectious involvement in a tertiary center pediatric uveitis cohort. Br J Ophthalmol. 2015;99:103–7.
5. Gilbert RE, Dunn DT, Lightman S, Murray PI, Pavesio CE, Gormley PD, Masters J, Parker SP, Stanford MR. Incidence of symptomatic toxoplasma eye disease: aetiology and public health implications. Epidemiol Infect. 1999;123:283–9.
6. Evengård B, Petersson K, Engman ML, Wiklund S, Ivarsson SA, Teär-Fahnehjelm K, Forsgren M, Gilbert R, Malm G. Low incidence of toxoplasma infection during pregnancy and in newborns in Sweden. Epidemiol Infect. 2001;127:121–7.

7. Jenum PA, Stray-Pedersen B. Development of specific immunoglobulins G, M, and A following primary Toxoplasma gondii infection in pregnant women. J Clin Microbiol. 1998;36:2907–13.

8. Bahia-Oliveira LM, Jones JL, Azevedo-Silva J, Alves CC, Oréfice F, Addiss DG. Highly endemic, waterborne toxoplasmosis in north Rio de Janeiro state Brazil. Emerging Infect Dis. 2003;9:55–62.

9. Tugal-Tutkun I, Havrlikova K, Power WJ, Foster CS. Changing patterns in uveitis of childhood. Ophthalmology. 1996;103:375–83.

10. Soylu M, Ozdemir G, Anli A. Pediatric uveitis in southern Turkey. Ocul Immunol Inflamm. 1997;5:197–202.

11. Kump LI, Cervantes-Castañeda RA, Androudi SN, Foster CS. Analysis of pediatric uveitis cases at a tertiary referral center. Ophthalmology. 2005;112:1287–92.

12. Kadayifçilar S, Eldem B, Tumer B. Uveitis in childhood. J Pediatr Ophthalmol Strabismus. 2003;40:335–40.

13. Glasner PD, Silveira C, Kruszon-Moran D, Martins MC, Burnier Júnior M, Silveira S, Camargo ME, Nussenblatt RB, Kaslow RA, Belfort JR. An unusually high prevalence of ocular toxoplasmosis in southern Brazil. Am J Ophthalmol. 1992;114:136–44.

14. Gilbert RE, Stanford MR. Is ocular toxoplasmosis caused by prenatal or postnatal infection? Br J Ophthalmol. 2000;84:224–6.

15. Sabin AB, Eichenwald H, Feldman HA, Jacobs L. Present status of clinical manifestations of toxoplasmosis in man: indications and provisions for routine serologic diagnosis. J Am Med Assoc. 1952;150:1063–9.

16. Koppe JG, Loewer-Sieger DH, de Roever-Bonnet H. Results of 20-year follow-up of congenital toxoplasmosis. Lancet. 1986;1:254–6.

17. Wilson CB, Remington JS, Stagno S, Reynolds DW. Development of adverse sequelae in children born with subclinical congenital Toxoplasma infection. Pediatrics. 1980;66:767–74.

18. Melamed J, Eckert GU, Spadoni VS, Lago EG, Uberti F. Ocular manifestations of congenital toxoplasmosis. Eye. 2010;24:528–34.

19. Bosch-Driessen LE, Berendschot TT, Ongkosuwito JV, Rothova A. Ocular toxoplasmosis: clinical features and prognosis of 154 patients. Ophthalmology. 2002;109:869–78.

20. Jones JL, Kruszon-Moran D, Wilson M, McQuillan G, Navin T, McAuley JB. Toxoplasma gondii infection in the United States: seroprevalence and risk factors. Am J Epidemiol. 2001;154:357–65.

21. Chen KC, Jung JJ, Engelbert M. Single acquisition of the vitreous, retina and choroid with swept-source optical coherence tomography in acute toxoplasmosis. Retin Cases Brief Rep. 2016;10:217–20.

22. Rothova A. Ocular involvement in toxoplasmosis. Br J Ophthalmol. 1993;77:371–7.

23. Johnson MW, Greven CM, Jaffe GJ, et al. Atypical, severe toxoplasmic retinochoroiditis in elderly patients. Ophthalmology. 1997;104:48–57.

24. Moreno RJ, Weisman J, Waller S. Neuroretinitis: an unusual presentation of ocular toxoplasmosis. Ann Ophthalmol. 1992;24:68–70.

25. Fish RH, Hoskins JC, Kline LB. Toxoplasmosis neuroretinitis. Ophthalmology. 1993;100:1177–82.

26. Matthews JD, Weiter JJ. Outer retinal toxoplasmosis. Ophthalmology. 1988;95:941–6.

27. Moraes HV. Punctate outer retinal toxoplasmosis in an HIV-positive child. Ocul Immunol Inflamm. 1999;7:93–5.

28. Rehder JR, Burnier MB Jr, Pavesio CE, et al. Acute unilateral toxoplasmic iridocyclitis in an AIDS patient. Am J Ophthalmol. 1988;106:740–1.

29. Holland GN, Muccioli C, Silveira C, et al. Intraocular inflammatory reactions without focal necrotizing retinochoroiditis in patients with acquired systemic toxoplasmosis. Am J Ophthalmol. 1999;128:413–20.

30. Ronday MJ, Luyendijk L, Baarsma GS, Bollemeijer JG, Van der Lelij A, Rothova A. Arch Ophthalmol. 1995;113:1524–9.

31. Goldmann H, Witmer R. Antibodies in the aqueous humor. Ophthalmologica. 1954;127: 323–30.

32. Rothova A. Ocular manifestations of toxoplasmosis. Curr Opin Ophthalmol. 2003;14:384–8.

33. Smith JR, Cunningham ET. Atypical presentations of ocular toxoplasmosis. Curr Opin Ophthalmol. 2002;13:387–92.

34. Holland GN, Lewis KG. An update on current practices in the management of ocular toxoplasmosis. Am J Ophthalmol. 2002;134:102–14.

35. Dutton GN, McMenamin PG, Hay J, Cameron S. The ultrastructural pathology of congenital murine toxoplasmic retinochoroiditis: part II—the morphology of the inflammatory changes. Exp Eye Res. 1986;43:545–60.

36. Bosch-Driessen EH, Rothova A. Sense and nonsense of corticosteroid administration in the treatment of ocular toxoplasmosis. Br J Ophthalmol. 1998;82:858–60.

37. Bovey EH. Usefulness of vitrectomy in the treatment of ocular toxoplasmosis. Int J Med Sci. 2009;6:139.

38. Garza-Leon M, Garcia LA. Ocular toxoplasmosis: clinical characteristics in pediatric patients. Ocul Immunol Inflamm. 2012;20:130–8.

39. Faridi A, Yeh S, Suhler EB, Smith JR, Flaxel CJ. Retinal detachment associated with ocular toxoplasmosis. Retina. 2015;35:358–63.

40. Bosch-Driessen LH, Karimi S, Stilma JS, Rothova A. Retinal detachment in ocular toxoplasmosis. Ophthalmology. 2000;107:36–40.

41. Dodds EM, Holland GN, Stanford MR, Yu F, Siu WO, Shah KH, Ten Dam-van Loon N, Muccioli C, Hovakimyan A, Barisani-Asenbauer T. International Ocular Toxoplasmosis Research Group. Intraocular inflammation associated with ocular toxoplasmosis: relationships at initial examination. Am J Ophthalmol. 2008;146:856–65.

42. Dodds EM. Toxoplasmosis. Curr Opin Ophthalmol. 2006;17:557–61.

43. Hasanreisoğlu M, Özdek Ş, Gülpınar İkiz GD, Aktaş Z, Atalay T. Effects of congenital ocular toxoplasmosis on peripheral retinal vascular development in premature infants at low risk for retinopathy of prematurity. Turk J Ophthalmol. 2019;49:230–34.

44. Adan A, Giralt J, Alvarez G, Alforja S, Bures-Jesltrup A, Casaroli-Marano RP, Corcostegui B. Pars plana vitrectomy for vitreoretinal complications of ocular toxoplasmosis Eur J Ophthalmol. 2009;19:1039–43.

45. Papadopoulou DN, Petropoulos IK, Mangioris G, Pharmakakis NM, Pournaras CJ. Pars plana vitrectomy in the treatment of severe complicated toxoplasmic retinochoroiditis. Eur J Ophthalmol. 2011;2:83–8.

46. Binder S, Freyler H. Vitrectomy in inflammatory diseases of posterior segment of the eye. Klin Monatsbl Augenheilkd. 1983;183:86–9.

47. Miranda AF, Costa de Andrade G, Novais EA, Maia A, Nascimento H, Muccioli C, Belfort Jr R. Outcomes after pars plana vitrectomy for epiretinal membranes associated with toxoplasmosis. Retina. 2016;36:1713–17.

48. Raval V, Rao S, Das T. Anatomical and functional outcomes of pars plana vitrectomy for inflammatory epiretinal membrane surgery in healed toxoplasmosis infection. Indian J Ophthalmol. 2018;66:1485–9.

49. Theodossiadis P, Kokolakis S, Ladas I, Kollia AC, Chatzoulis D, Theodossiadis G. Retinal vascular involvement in acute toxoplasmic retinochoroiditis. Int Ophthalmol. 1995;19:19–24.

50. Gentile RC, Berinstein DM, Oppenheim R, Walsh JB. Retinal vascular occlusions complicating acute toxoplasmic retinochoroiditis. Can J Ophthalmol. 1997;32:354–8.

51. Gaynon MW, Boldrey EE, Strahlman ER, Fine SL. Retinal neovascularization and ocular toxoplasmosis. Am J Ophthalmol. 1984;98:585–9.

52. Fine SL, Owens SL, Haller JA, Knox DL, Patz A. Choroidal neovascularization as a late complication of ocular toxoplasmosis. Am J Ophthalmol. 1981;91:318–22.

53. Mauget-Faysse M, Mimoun G, Ruiz-Moreno JM, Quaranta-El Maftouhi M, De Laey JJ, Postelmans L, Soubrane G, Defauchy M, Leys A. Verteporfin photodynamic therapy for

choroidal neovascularization associated with toxoplasmic retinochoroiditis. Retina. 2006;26:396–403.

54. Adan A, Mateo C, Woolley-Dod C. Surgery for subfoveal choroidal neovascularization in toxoplasmic retinochoroiditis. Am J Ophthalmol. 2003;135:386–7.

55. Uemura A, Thomas MA. Visual outcome after surgical removal of choroidal neovascularization in pediatric patients. Arch Ophthalmol. 2000;118:1373–8.

56. Gagliuso DJ, Teich SA, Friedman AH, Orellana J. Ocular toxoplasmosis in AIDS patients. Trans Am Ophthalmol Soc. 1990;88:63–88.

57. Fardeque C, Romand S, Narsing RA, Cassoux N, Bettembourg O, Thulliez P, Lehoang P. Diagnosis of toxoplasmic retinochoroiditis with atypical clinical features. Am J Ophthalmol. 2002;134:196–203.

58. Davis JL, Miller DM, Ruiz P. Diagnostic testing of vitrectomy specimens. Am J Ophthalmol. 2005;140:822–9.

59. Margolis R, Brasil OF, Lowder CY, et al. Vitrectomy for the diagnosis and management of uveitis of unknown cause. Ophthalmology. 2007;114:1893–7.

Ocular Toxocariasis

52

Murat Hasanreisoglu, Zahed Chehab, and Şengül Özdek

Abstract

Ocular toxocariasis is an uncommon worldwide parasitic infection that affects mostly children. Parasitic infections of the eye are a major cause of blindness especially in areas with low social economic status and humid environments. The diagnosis of ocular toxocariasis is based on clinical findings, and associated laboratory data such as serum enzyme-linked immunosorbent assay (ELISA) titers and ELISA Toxocara titers; other diagnostic and imaging methods are utilized such as optical coherence tomography, fluorescein angiography, computed tomography, and ocular ultrasound. Treatment may be necessary for ocular complications arising from intraocular inflammation and vitreous membrane traction. Surgical intervention may be of value both diagnostically and therapeutically for selected cases.

Keywords

Pediatric ophthalmology · Retina · Ocular toxocariasis · Vitrectomy · Tractional retinal detachment · Leukocoria · Vitritis · Granuloma · Endophthalmitis

Supplementary Information The online version contains supplementary material available at https://doi.org/10.1007/978-3-031-14506-3_52.

M. Hasanreisoglu (✉) · Z. Chehab
School of Medicine, Ophthalmology Department, Koç University, Istanbul, Turkey
e-mail: rmurat95@yahoo.com

Ş. Özdek
School of Medicine, Ophthalmology Department, Gazi University, Ankara, Turkey

Background

Ocular toxocariasis (OT) is an uncommon worldwide ocular infection that affects mostly children. It is caused by the round worm Toxocara canis or Toxocara cati. It is found in both rural and urban areas. A common way of infection is by ingestion of soil contaminated with Toxocara embryonated eggs and then the toxocora larvae finds its way to ocular circulation. In most cases, the course of the disease is mild, but the spectrum of clinical manifestations and severity is broad, and the potential for uniocular blindness due to this entity is well recognized.

The diagnosis of toxocariasis is essentially clinical, based on the lesion morphology and supportive laboratory data and imaging studies. Differentiation of OT from retinoblastoma is critical to avoid unnecessary enucleation of eyes with OT. It is important to establish an adequate correlation between the clinical findings and diagnostic methods including serum ELISA titers, radiologic evaluation by ultrasound and computed tomography scan, and optical coherence tomography (OCT).

Treatment is directed at complications that are the result of intraocular inflammation and vitreous membrane traction. Vitrectomy may be of value both diagnostically and therapeutically and especially if it is done early in the course of the disease [1].

Epidemiology

It has been estimated that ocular toxocariasis results in 5–20% of blindness secondary to uveitis [1]. The overall estimated prevalence of OT around the world was calculated to be 5% with remarkable variations at regional and national scales possibly due to differences in socio-economic conditions, population sanitation status, and environmental hygiene, as well as the climate [2]. Based on a systematic review and meta-analysis on the seroprevalence estimates for human toxocariasis worldwide, the highest and lowest rates were reported from African (37.7%) and Eastern Mediterranean areas (8.2%), having significant association with lower income level countries [3]. With respect to geographical parameters, the highest prevalence rate of OT was in countries with high geographical longitude and low geographical latitude at 8% [3]. There are several reasons for this finding. First of all, the temperature required for embryonation of Toxocara eggs in soil (20–30 °C) is more favorable in countries located in lower latitudes, comparable to colder countries at higher latitudes. Furthermore, personal and environmental hygiene, as well as public health education, are fewer practices in these countries [4–7].

Toxocara canis infection in dogs has rates of worldwide distribution ranging from 0 to 99.4%, with disease prevalence rates in dogs and humans in Latin America that vary from 2.5 to 63.2% (with seroprevalence rates ranging from 1.8 to 66.6%). In dogs, infection rates tend to decrease with age, being very high at birth (near 100%), falling significantly after 6 months of life (up to 50%) [8, 9].

Exposure to soil, having or contact with animal sources of toxocariasis and contact with contaminated soil with Toxocara eggs, geophagia, contact with dogs or ownership of dogs or cats as well as consuming raw/undercooked meat are among the risk factor of Ocular toxocariasis [3].

OT was more prevalent in males than females, due to the possible susceptibility and/or more curiosity of male individuals [3]. Age is a differentiating factor between OT and retinoblastoma, while about 90% of the cases of retinoblastoma were reported before 5 years [10], the age range of 11–20 years was the most prevalent age ranges of OT [3]. In the United States, OT usually affects children in the age group of 2–14 years [11, 12]. In Japan [13] and South Korea [14], the mean age of onset was >20 years. In these countries, ocular toxocariasis affects adults as they usually eat raw food.

Pathophysiology

Toxocariasis is a parasitic infection caused by invading the tissues by larval stages of Toxocara canis or Toxocara cati. The adult worms of these nematodes parasitize the small intestines of dogs and cats, respectively [15]. The human disease occurs by ingesting the viable Toxocara embryonated eggs, commonly from contaminated raw vegetables or from polluted water sources as well as from contact with domestic dogs and cats, especially puppies and kittens, which harbor eggs in their fur, and the contact with contamination soil and geophagia (especially in children population) [16].

Ocular toxocariasis is caused by the migration of Toxocara larvae into the posterior segment of the eye. Based on studies executed in animal models, the migration route of Toxocara larvae may follow several pathways. The most common one is via the brain to the cerebrospinal fluid and then to the choroid. The other possible pathways are via the brain to the optic nerve or via the arteries from the internal carotid artery to the ophthalmic artery, retinal central artery, or ciliary artery [17].

Migrated larvae secrete enzymes, waste products, and cuticular components, which cause tissue damage, necrosis, and marked inflammatory reaction, with eosinophils as the most component. These eosinophils release toxic proteins which contribute to the pathology and symptomatology of toxocariasis. The typical pathological finding in ocular toxocariasis is eosinophilic granulomas with central necrosis and remnants of Toxocara larva surrounded by a mixed inflammatory infiltrate with numerous eosinophils [15]. Ocular toxocariasis is usually due to a single Toxocara larva invading the eye. This results in a low-level immune response which is insufficiently activated to kill the larva and allows its persistence in the eye for years. During this long period, it can migrate through ocular tissues causing mechanical and immunopathological damage [18]. Thus, the pathogenesis of ocular toxocariasis in the human depends on the inflammatory reactions activated by the existence of larva in the eye, the host immune response, the number of the larvae present in the eye, the incidence of reinfection, and the host sensitization to the secreted or excreted products by the larvae [19].

Clinical Manifestations

Clinical manifestations and severity of ocular toxocariasis rely on the primary anatomical site implicated, the number of the larvae existing in the eye, and the immune reaction of the host [20]. The most common symptoms of ocular toxocariasis include photophobia, floaters, leukocoria, strabismus, white pupillary reflex, conjunctival hyperemia, mild ocular pain, vitreous inflammation, and blindness of one eye which is recorded in about 80% of cases and is permanent in the most patients. In young children, the eye infection may not be observed until they fail a school vision screening test [21].

There exist three essential clinical types of human toxocariasis: Visceral larva migrans syndrome is due to severe systemic infestation leading to fever, hepatosplenomegaly, pneumonitis, and convulsions. Serum IgE may be elevated, the blood exhibits substantial eosinophilia and leukocytosis, and it affects primarily 1- to 5-year-old children [22].

Ocular larva migrans syndrome is most commonly seen in otherwise healthy patients, manifesting into three clinical types that were classified by Wilkinson and Welch: peripheral inflammatory mass type, posterior pole granuloma type, and diffuse nematode endophthalmitis [11, 13, 22, 23]. Ocular larva migrans syndrome generally occurs in children older than 8 years. These patients have a normal white blood count, normal serum IgE, and no eosinophilia [22].

Covert toxocariasis has been diagnosed in patients who do not fall into the visceral larva migrans syndrome or ocular larva migrans syndrome categories but instead reveal vague symptomatology. Raised levels of Toxocara antibodies have been implicated in signs and symptoms, such as hepatomegaly, cough, sleep disturbances, abdominal pain, headaches, and behavioral changes [22].

Regarding the 3 major findings of OT:

1. Chronic endophthalmitis: observed in 25% of cases, between 2 and 8 years-old, presenting with leukocoria, strabismus, and hypopyon and in the fundus there are granulomatous vitritis, cyclitic membranes and retinal detachment, that can be confirmed by diagnostic imaging. Main differential diagnosis for this is the retinoblastoma [24].
2. Posterior granuloma: It represents 25–46% of cases in ages between 4 and 14 years-old, with a white pseudogliomatous mass at the posterior pole seen on fundus, retinal folds, hemorrhagic perilesional retinal detachment, intralesional neovascularization and subretinal hemorrhages [24].

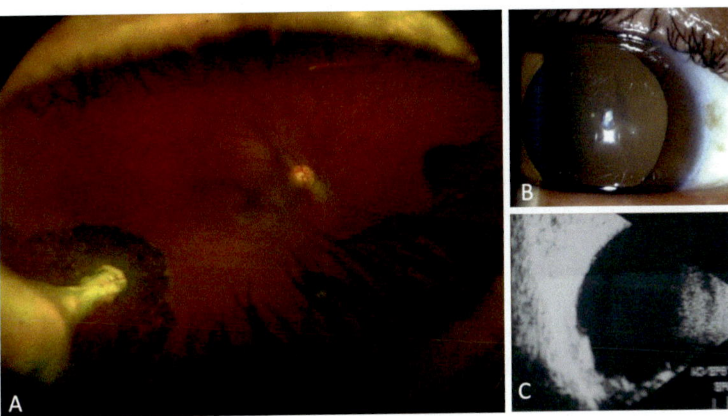

Fig. 52.1 16 years old male patient referred to our ophthalmology clinic to rule out the possibility of an intraocular tumor later diagnosed as ocular toxocariasis. Ultra-wide field fundus photo of the right eye (**A**) showing a large yellow-white mass associated with peripheral retinal fold of a fibroexudative character, extending anteriorly to pars plana surrounded by a hyperpigmented area associated with RPE alterations. In the examination performed with Goldmann three mirrors, a white cyclic membranous structure extending in the pars plana region was observed. Mild vitreous haze was also present. The anterior segment photography (**B**) showed mild posterior subcapsular cataract. The ocular B-scan ultrasonography (**C**) was in line with fundus findings and showed a peripheral mass. In laboratory tests, T.Canis ELISA IgG was positive, eryhthrocyte sedimentation and serum total IGE were also found to be high (39 mm/hour and 815 UI/ml, respectively)

3. Peripheral granuloma: It is observed 20–40% of cases between 6 and 40 years-old, in the fundus the findings are: granuloma anterior to the equator (90% temporally), retinal folds with vitreous tractive membranes, macular and optic nerve diversion and retinal detachment [24] (Fig. 52.1).

There are reports of OT with uveitis, and these represent 1–2% of cases of uveitis in children [24]. Sometimes, OT represents with atypical manifestations such as bullous retinal detachment [25], subacute unilateral neuroretinitis [26], multifocal granuloma [27], cataract formation [28], and bilateral scleritis [29].

OT produces loss of visual acuity by the following mechanisms: severe vitritis (62.6%), cystoid macular edema (47.4%) and tractional retinal detachment (36.8%); these produce definitive loss vision on the affected eye, that is the main complication of the ocular disease [24].

Diagnosis

Diagnosis of OT is based on the identification of clinical signs consistent with disease on ophthalmologic examination, supported by testing for antibodies against T. canis [28].

Fundoscopic examination is a significant tool either for direct observation of a movable larva beneath the retina [18] or for recognition of typical features of ocular toxocariasis such as peripheral chorioretinal granuloma, posterior pole granuloma, endophthalmitis, and pars planitis [26]. Clinical suspicion should be confirmed by the detection of Toxocara antibodies in serum and/or intraocular fluids using immunodiagnostic techniques [18].

The choice of serodiagnostic methods are ELISA-IgG against Toxocara excreted-secreted (TES) antigen as a screening test and confirm the positive samples by western blot test. Immunoblot analysis is usually used in research for separation and identification of proteins. Western blot using crude antigen prepared from Toxocara canis larvae revealed antigenic proteins of typical seven bands (24, 28, 30, 35, 132, 147, 200 kDa). The high specificity of this assay is related to its ability to discriminate between high molecular weight bands (not specific and suggestive of cross-reactions with other helminths) and low molecular weight bands (24–35 kDa), which have a high level of specificity [30].

For visceral larva migrans syndrome and some forms of covert toxocariasis, the sensitivity and specificity of the Toxocara ELISA is estimated at 78% and 92%, respectively, at a titer of 1:32 [31]. However, the sensitivity of the ELISA for ocular larva migrans syndrome is considerably less. The larvae may remain alive within the host for months, and host antibody levels may remain strongly positive for 2 or 3 years or more [31]. Therefore, in the Centers for Disease Control and Prevention, the presence of antibody titers greater than 1:32 may be considered reflective of active infection [31].

Another important immune-ophthalmological method is the Goldmann-Witmer coefficient. This is an effective way to assess the intraocular production of antibodies against Toxocara. A cutoff value of 3.0 is considered suggestive of ocular toxocariasis [32, 33].

Imaging studies such as ophthalmic ultrasound, OCT and fluorescein angiography (FA) may be useful for supporting diagnosis and making differential diagnosis with other ocular diseases, especially with retinoblastoma [1]. Ultrasonographic findings include: a solid, highly reflective peripheral mass, a vitreous membrane extending between the posterior pole, the mass itself and tractional retinal detachment or fold from the posterior pole of the mass.

OCT can be used to look for chorioretinal lesions. The retinal findings at OCT are subretinal extension and idiopathic choroidal neo-vascularization in the active stage (in the case of granuloma due to toxocariasis), peripapillary serous retinal detachment and a well-demarcated cystic lesion [32].

Medical Treatment

Corticosteroids are the mainstay medical treatment for ocular toxocariasis as they can decrease the release of local mediators of inflammation leading to the suppression of inflammation, induce cell membranes stabilization, and prevent vitreous opacification and tractional retinal detachment. In spite of that, corticosteroids have limited efficiency to deal with structural complications in the retina. The inflammation treated with corticosteroids is either topically or periocularly [34]. Oral prednisolone is also used as an anti-inflammatory with a dosage of 1 mg/kg/day for 1 month and then tapered [18]. Cycloplegic agents are used in the presence of an anterior segment inflammation to prevent posterior synechia. Regarding antiparasitic therapy, some authors recommend it only with the concomitant use of steroids, others prefer to use anthelmintic agents when the response to steroids is inadequate [1]. Albendazole (10 mg/kg daily per 1–2 weeks), a broad-spectrum drug, is effective against the larval and it crosses the blood brain barrier [1, 10, 20]. Other anthelmintic agents that could be used are thiabendazole (25–50 mg/kg/day for 5–7 days) and mebendazole (20–25 mg/kg/day for 3 weeks), as well as ivermectin, diethylcarbamazine, levamisole and tinidazole [1, 10, 20, 32].

Surgical Treatment

Retinal detachment, epiretinal membrane, and persistent vitreous opacity are common surgical indications for vitreoretinal surgery performed in eyes with OT. PPV is the most common surgical procedure for OT and used to patients that are refractory to medical treatment and for the abovementioned complications [28, 34] (Figs. 52.2, 52.3 and 52.4).

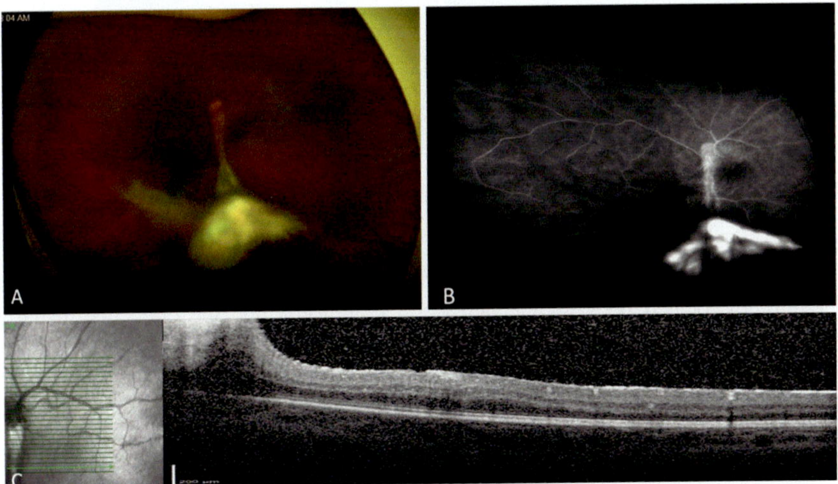

Fig. 52.2 Ultra-wide field photo of the left eye **A** showing peripheral granuloma and tractional retinal detachment at 6 o'clock position with fibrous membranes extending to the optic disc. Fundus fluorescein angiography **B** showing staining and leakage from the retinal folds and from the all the retinal vessels signifying the presence of inflammation. Optical coherence tomography of macula **C** shows dragging of macula to the inferior with loss of the foveal pit and contour

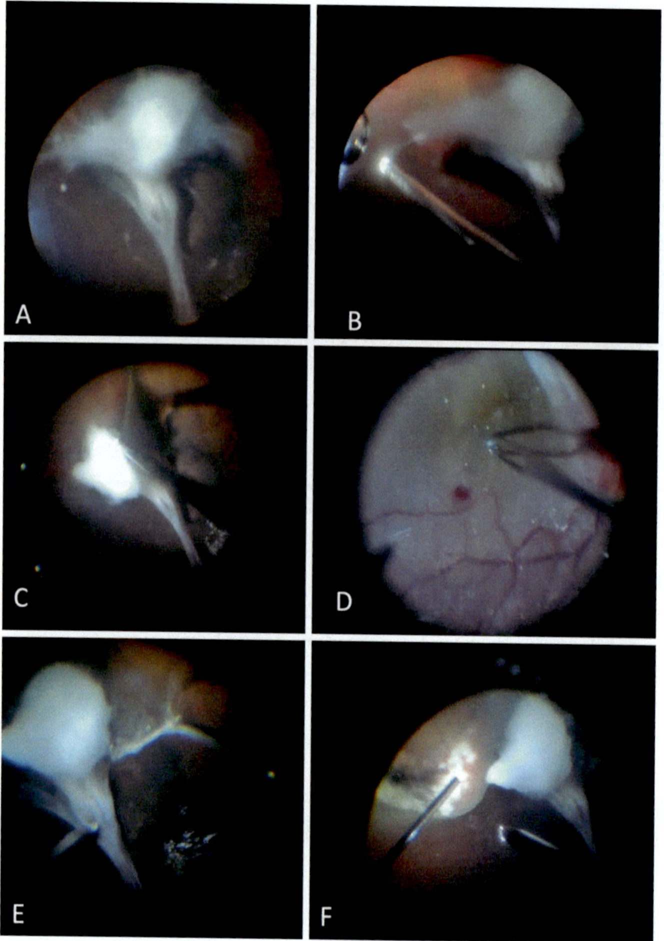

Fig. 52.3 (A–F) Principal steps of the vitreoretinal surgery for toxocara peripheral granuloma

There are few things that is needed to be kept in mind. First, the fibrous membranes located between the peripheral granuloma and the optic disc usually have extensions into the underlying retina and need to be carefully lifted off from the retinal surface before they can be severed. These membranes usually remain tightly adherent to the optic disc and the peripheral granuloma. They often need to be circumcised rather than delaminated or peeled. Granulomas are also problematic since they are in the parts of the retina; therefore, attempts to extirpate the retinal granuloma usually are unsuccessful and may cause undesirable complications so the granulomas are left in place [1, 35–38].

Delicate manipulation of the eye during surgery is also essential, and the surgical incision site should be carefully chosen due to presence of multiple peripheral granulomas in majority of affected eyes [38]. In earlier studies that used UBM

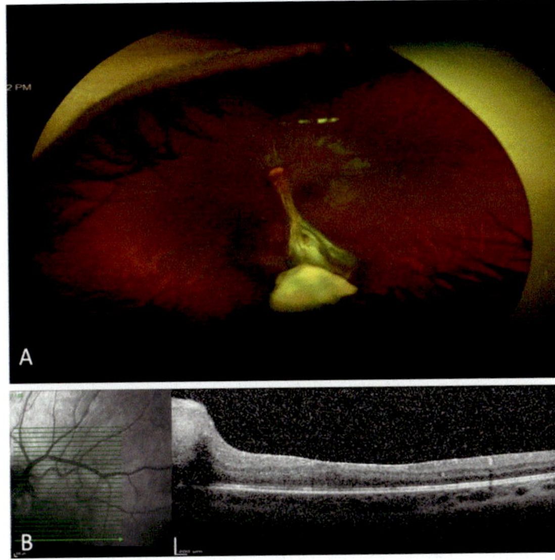

Fig. 52.4 Postoperative ultra-wide field (**A**) and optical coherence tomography (**B**) images of the patient shown on Fig. 52.3. Note that fundus view is clearer with better-formed fovea free of epiretinal membranes

imaging, more than three-quarters of peripheral granulomas were adjacent to the nasal or temporal side of the horizontal meridian [38, 39]. Therefore, the incision site should be carefully chosen based on UBM imaging and scleral indentation to avoid peripheral granulomas or TRD. For these reasons, corneal incisions were preferred in eyes with multiple peripheral granulomas [38].

The results of modern vitrectomy techniques in which epiretinal and subretinal components of the granuloma are removed by PPV and retinotomy techniques are reported to provide achievement of macular or complete retinal reattachment at high rates. Additionally, visual improvement after PPV was obtained in 50–70% of cases in some reports [37, 38]. Preoperative VA was associated with final VA and macular involvement was associated with a final VA of <20/70 and no other factors were associated with this VA [37, 38].

One of complications of surgery was recurrence of RD, but due to the introduction of small- gauge vitrectomy the number of iatrogenic damages decrease and thus reducing the risk of recurrence [38]. Scleral buckling can be used in combination with vitrectomy where it may weakens the peripheral—posterior traction and reduces RD [37]. Another complication of surgical management is the recurrence of vitreous inflammation most probably due to the granuloma but could be managed with topical or systemic steroids [1].

Laser photocoagulation is recommended when Toxocara larva is directly visualized inside the eye. This procedure may induce an inflammatory reaction; therefore, it needs to be given with steroid therapy [28]. Cryotherapy is used to treat ocular granulomas. It is applied directly to exudation parts at the pars plana by using a double freeze–thaw procedure followed by steroid therapy administration and it preferred with both general and periocular anesthesia in children to reduce post-operative pain and discomfort [1].

Case presentation 1: An 8-year-old girl was referred to our clinic with redness in her left eye (LE) for the last few days. She had strabismus in her LE for the last 2 years. She was coming from a rural area in the southeast part of Turkey. Examination of the right eye (RE) was unremarkable with full vision. Examination of the LE revealed; a visual acuity of counting fingers from 3 m. There was hypertropia and exotropia in primary position, 1(+) cells in the anterior chamber, 2–3(+) cells in the vitreous. Fundus examination revealed a retinal fold extending from the optic nerve head to the inferior periphery to attach to the back of the lens pulling the surrounding peripheral retina anteriorly with inflammatory membranes. There was a whitish mass resembling a granuloma in the inferior periphery (Fig. 52.2). Macula was ectopic towards inferior. Fluorescein angiography showed staining of the optic disc and leakage from the retinal fold and all of the retinal capillaries signifying the presence of inflammation. OCT shows epiretinal membrane with dragging of macula to the inferior and loss of the foveal pit and contour. Serum IgE and Toxocora IgM/IgG were ordered and the patient was consulted to the pediatric infectious disease department and systemic albendazole treatment together with topical steroids and cycloplegics were started. A lens sparing vitrectomy could be performed one week later (Fig. 52.3, **see the video**). After insertion of trocars a vitreous sample was obtained under air to avoid dilution of the vitreous first. Core vitrectomy was followed by relieving the membranous vitreous strands from the peripheral granuloma and retinal fold to the back of the lens, pars plana and optic nerve head with the vitrectomy probe (Fig. 52.3A–C). ILM peeling is also performed to relieve the additional tractional forces and to prevent further epiretinal membrane formation (Fig. 52.3D). Residual membranes adherent to peripheral retina are relieved (Fig. 52.3E) and the endolaser is done to avascular retinal areas around the granuloma (Fig. 52.3F). Eye was filled with air only and inferior posterior subtenon triamcinolone injection was done at the end of the surgery. Serum and vitreous samples were negative for ELISA test. Retina stayed attached, vitreous inflammation disappeared, and vision improved to 20/120 within 4 months follow up (Fig. 52.4).

Case presentation 2: A 13-year-old girl who noticed blurred vision in her left eye was referred to our clinic. Examination of the right eye (RE) was unremarkable with full vision. Examination of the LE revealed, a visual acuity of hand motions, exotropia in primary gaze, a quiet anterior chamber. There was 2–3(+) cells in the vitreous, macula was totally covered with white thick membranes giving strands to the vitreous, some vascular sheathing around some of the retinal vessels, a peripheral thin granuloma in the extreme superior periphery (Fig. 52.5A, B). We have put OT in the differential diagnosis and asked about cat/dog exposure. The family informed us that they have adapted a kitten and she has many scratches in her body. Serum IgE and Toxocora IgM/IgG were ordered which were found to be normal/negative and the patient was consulted to the pediatric infectious disease department and systemic albendazole treatment. An encircling band (2.5 mm, 240S style) with lens sparing vitrectomy could be performed one week later where the epiretinal membrane could be peeled completely from the macular area together

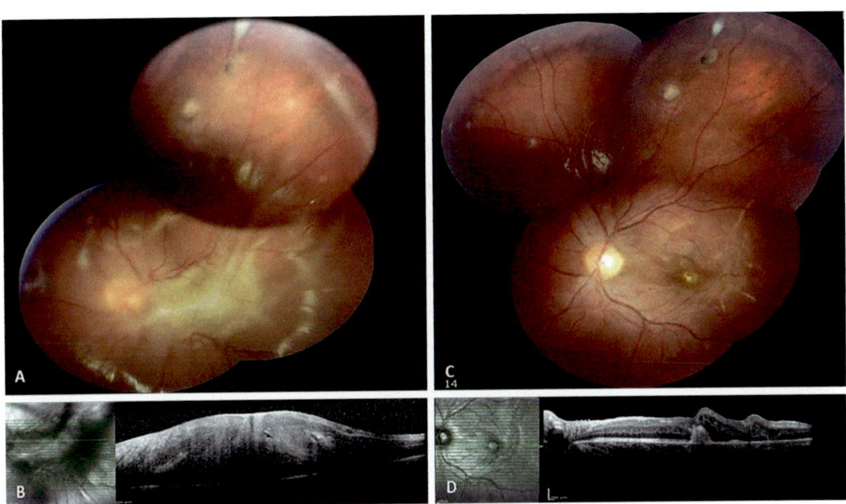

Fig. 52.5 Fundus collage image of the left eye **A** showing a thick epiretinal membrane that is causing macular dragging towards the peripheral granuloma located at the superotemporal periphery. Note the vascular sheathing around the retinal vessels. Optical coherence tomography **B** image shows the thick hyperreflective epiretinal membrane with back shadowing on the retinal layers. Fundus collage image of the left eye after vitrectomy and encircling band **C** showing central foveal scarring and absence of the epiretinal membrane and the buckle effect on the peripheral granuloma. Optical coherence tomography **D** image showing distorting of the foveal contour, and central foveal scarring

with ILM. Peripheral granuloma was supported with the encircling band. 1 mg/kg p.o prednisolone was tapered within 6 weeks. Vision improved to only counting fingers level because of the central foveal scarring with significant recovery of the retinal anatomy in postoperative 2nd month follow-up (Fig. 52.5C, D).

Conclusion

Ocular toxocariasis is a zoonotic infection that is related to toxocara canis and toxocara cati. It is caused by ingestion of toxocara embryonated eggs that contaminate the soil. Children are typically affected, and a child may present with uniocular vision loss and advanced ocular affection due to delay in diagnosis; thus routine screening for pediatric population in areas that toxocarasis is highly prevalent such as warm countries, and areas with poor hygiene and low standards of living is recommended.

Ocular toxocariasis is typically a unilateral disease and the typical ocular manifestations are: chronic endophthalmitis, peripheral granuloma, and central granuloma. Diagnosis is done mainly on clinical findings supported by laboratory exams, serology and ocular imaging.

Steroids are typically used as medical treatment to decrease the inflammation and prevent structural complication. The role of anthelminthic medication is not adequately established, but few studies showed favorable results when used with steroids.

Besides medical treatment, surgical intervention is aimed to treat the structural complications of ocular toxocariasis such as persistent vitreous opacities, retinal detachment and epiretinal membrane. Early intervention is sometimes favorable in cases refractory to medical treatment and to avoid complications. Preoperative visual acuity and macular macular involvement are prognostic indicators for post-operative VA. The advances in the surgical techniques in vitrectomy has led to decrease in perioperative complications and a more favorable outcome.

Review Questions

1. The organism *most* commonly responsible for ocular toxocarasis is:

a. Toxocara vitulorum
b. Toxocara cani
c. Toxocara cati
d. Toxocara leonine

2. Contact with toxocariasis is by ingestion of soil contaminated with:

a. Round worms
b. Embryonated eggs
c. Unembryonated eggs
d. First stage larvae

3. Which is not a risk factor for toxocariasis infection.

a. Cold climate
b. Low socioeconomic status
c. Geophagia
d. Contact with puppies

4. The *definitive diagnosis* for ocular toxocariasis:

a. Histopathological diagnosis
b. Demonstration of toxocara eggs in human host stools
c. Clinical findings supported by serological and ocular imaging
d. Detecting eosinophilia in blood

5. The typical pathological findings in ocular toxocariasis:

a. Eosinophilic granulomas with central necrosis and remnants of Toxocara larva surrounded by a mixed inflammatory infiltrate

b. Non eosnophilc granulomas with central necrosis and remnants of Toxocara larva surrounded by a mixed inflammatory infiltrate

c. Eosinophilic granulomas without central necrosis and remnants of Toxocara larva surrounded by a mixed inflammatory infiltrate

d. Granulomas with central necrosis and remnants of Toxocara larva surrounded by macrophages

6. Which is not related to Wilkinson and Welch classification for ocular toxocariasis clinical manifestations:

a. Chronic endophthalmitis
b. Optic neuritis
c. Posterior Pole granuloma
d. Peripheral granuloma

7. Retinoblastoma is a main differential diagnosis in which type of ocular toxocariasis:

a. Chronic endophthalmitis
b. Atypical type
c. Posterior Pole granuloma
d. Peripheral granuloma

8. The antigens used in the different immunoassays for diagnosis of toxocariasis:

a. Toxocara excreted-secreted (TES) antigen
b. Toxocara egg somatic extracts
c. Toxocara adult worm somatic extracts
d. All of the above

9. According to the Centers for Disease Control and Prevention, the presence of antibody titers greater than what value may be considered reflective of active infection in Ocular toxocariasis:

a. 1:100
b. 1:32
c. 1:8
d. 1:24

10. The mainstay of medical treatment for toxocariasis:

a. Corticosteroids
b. Anthelminthic antibiotic
c. Observation
d. None of above

11. Which is not an indication for surgical intervention for ocular toxocariasis:

a. Persistent vitreous opacity
b. Tractional RD with macular affection

c. Peripheral granuloma with no retinal traction
d. Severe inflammation refractory to medical treatment

12. The rationale in adoption of preoperative UBM in ocular toxocariasis:

a. Detection of lens subluxation before surgery
b. Assessing the anterior chamber angle
c. Guidance of trocar insertion to avoid peripheral retinal pathology
d. None of the above

Answers

1. B
2. B
3. A
4. A
5. A
6. B
7. A
8. D
9. B
10. A
11. C
12. C

References

1. Arevalo JF, Espinoza JV, Arevalo FA. Ocular toxocariasis. J Pediatr Ophthalmol Strabismus. 2013;50(2):76–86.
2. Badri M, Eslahi AV, Olfatifar M, et al. Keys to unlock the enigma of ocular toxocariasis: a systematic review and meta-analysis. Ocul Immunol Inflamm. 2021;29(7–8):1265–76.
3. Rostami A, Riahi SM, Holland CV, et al. Seroprevalence estimates for toxocariasis in people worldwide: a systematic review and meta-analysis. PLoS Negl Trop Dis. 2019;13(12): e0007809. (Published 2019 Dec 19).
4. McMichael AJ. The urban environment and health in a world of increasing globalization: issues for developing countries. Bull World Health Organ. 2000;78(9):1117–26.
5. Aiello AE, Larson EL. What is the evidence for a causal link between hygiene and infections? Lancet Infect Dis. 2002;2(2):103–10.
6. Gamboa MI. Effects of temperature and humidity on the development of eggs of Toxocara canis under laboratory conditions. J Helminthol. 2005;79(4):327–31.
7. Azam D, Ukpai OM, Said A, Abd-Allah GA, Morgan ER. Temperature and the development and survival of infective Toxocara canis larvae. Parasitol Res. 2012;110(2):649–56.
8. Delgado O, Rodriguez-Morales AJ. Aspectos clínicoepidemiológicos de la toxocariasis: Una enfermedad desatendida en Venezuela y América Latina. Bol Malar Salud Ambient. 2009;49:1–34.
9. Despommier D. Toxocariasis: Clinical aspects, epidemiology, medical ecology, and molecular aspects. Clin Microbiol Rev. 2003;16:265–72.

10. Fan C-K, Holland CV, Loxton K, Barghouth U. Cerebral toxocariasis: silent progression to neurodegenerative disorders? Clin Microbiol Rev. 2015;28(3):663–86. https://doi.org/10.1128/CMR.00106-14.

11. Wilkinson CP, Welch RB. Intraocular toxocara. Am J Ophthalmol. 1971;71(4):921–30. https://doi.org/10.1016/0002-9394(71)90267-4.

12. Good B, Holland CV, Taylor MR, Larragy J, Moriarty P, O'Regan M. Ocular toxocariasis in schoolchildren. Clin Infect Dis. 2004;39(2):173–8.

13. Yokoi K, Goto H, Sakai J, Usui M. Clinical features of ocular toxocariasis in Japan. Ocul Immunol Inflamm. 2003;11(4):269–75.

14. Kwon SI, Lee JP, Park SP, Lee EK, Huh S, Park IW. Ocular toxocariasis in Korea. Jpn J Ophthalmol. 2011;55(2):143–7.

15. Fillaux J, Magnaval JF. Laboratory diagnosis of human toxocariasis. Vet Parasitol. 2013;193 (4):327–36.

16. Holland CV. Knowledge gaps in the epidemiology of Toxocara: the enigma remains. Parasitology. 2017;144(1):81–94.

17. Hayashi E, Akao N, Fujita K. Evidence for the involvement of the optic nerve as a migration route for larvae in ocular toxocariasis of Mongolian gerbils. J Helminthol. 2003;77(4):311–5. https://doi.org/10.1079/joh2003186.

18. Magnaval JF, Glickman LT, Dorchies P, Morassin B. Highlights of human toxocariasis. Korean J Parasitol. 2001;39(1):1–11.

19. Fan CK, Liao CW, Cheng YC. Factors affecting disease manifestation of toxocarosis in humans: genetics and environment. Vet Parasitol. 2013;193(4):342–52.

20. Azira NM, Zeehaida M. A case report of ocular toxocariasis. Asian Pac J Trop Biomed. 2011;1(2):164–5.

21. Rubinsky-Elefant G, Hirata CE, Yamamoto JH, Ferreira MU. Human toxocariasis: diagnosis, worldwide seroprevalences and clinical expression of the systemic and ocular forms. Ann Trop Med Parasitol. 2010;104(1):3–23.

22. Barisani-Asenbauer T, Maca SM, Hauff W, et al. Treatment of ocular toxocariasis with albendazole. J Ocul Pharmacol Ther. 2001;17(3):287–94.

23. do Lago A, Andrade R, Muccioli C, Belfort R Jr. Optical coherence tomography in presumed subretinal Toxocara granuloma: case report. Arq Bras Oftalmol. 2006;69(3):403–5.

24. Pivetti-Pezzi P. Ocular toxocariasis. Int J Med Sci. 2009;6:129–30.

25. Tou N, Ibi K, Tawara A, Nakamura F, Hadeyama T. Nippon Ganka Gakkai Zasshi. 2006;110 (5):415–20.

26. Cortez RT, Ramirez G, Collet L, Giuliari GP. Ocular parasitic diseases: a review on toxocariasis and diffuse unilateral subacute neuroretinitis. J Pediatr Ophthalmol Strabismus. 2011;48(4):204–12.

27. Kuniyal L, Biswas J. Multifocal granulomata in presumed Toxocara canis infection in adult. World J Ophthalmol. 2013;3(4):38–40.

28. Woodhall D, Starr MC, Montgomery SP, et al. Ocular toxocariasis: epidemiologic, anatomic, and therapeutic variations based on a survey of ophthalmic subspecialists. Ophthalmology. 2012;119(6):1211–7.

29. Pak KY, Park SW, Byon IS, Lee JE. Ocular toxocariasis presenting as bilateral scleritis with suspect retinal granuloma in the nerve fiber layer: a case report. BMC Infect Dis. 2016;16 (1):426. (Published 2016 Aug 18).

30. Magnaval JF, Malard L, Morassin B, Fabre R. Immunodiagnosis of ocular toxocariasis using Western-blot for the detection of specific anti-Toxocara IgG and CAP for the measurement of specific anti-Toxocara IgE. J Helminthol. 2002;76(4):335–9.

31. Hotez PJ, Wilkins PP. Toxocariasis: America's most common neglected infection of poverty and a helminthiasis of global importance?. PLoS Negl Trop Dis. 2009;3(3):e400.

32. Martínez-Pulgarín DF, Muñoz-Urbano M, Gomez-Suta LD, Delgado OM, Rodriguez-Morales AJ. Ocular toxocariasis: new diagnostic and therapeutic perspectives. Recent Pat Antiinfect Drug Discov. 2015;10(1):35–41.

33. de Visser L, Rothova A, de Boer JH, et al. Diagnosis of ocular toxocariasis by establishing intraocular antibody production. Am J Ophthalmol. 2008;145(2):369–74.
34. Ahn SJ, Ryoo NK, Woo SJ. Ocular toxocariasis: clinical features, diagnosis, treatment, and prevention. Asia Pac Allergy. 2014;4(3):134–41.
35. Arevalo JF, Garcia-Amaris RA. The role of vitreo-retinal surgery in children with uveitis. Int Ophthalmol Clin. 2008;48(3):153–72.
36. Erb MH, Kuppermann BD. Surgical approaches to uveitis. In: Hartnett ME, Trese M, Capone A Jr, Bronya JBK, Scott MS, eds. Pediatric Retina. Philadephia: Lippincott, Williams & Wilkins;2005. p. 445–466.
37. Zhang T, Guo D, Xu G, Jiang R. Ocular toxocariasis: long-term follow-up and prognosis of patients following vitrectomy. Ocul Immunol Inflamm. 2020;28(3):517–23.
38. Giuliari GP, Ramirez G, Cortez RT. Surgical treatment of ocular toxocariasis: anatomic and functional results in 45patients. Eur J Ophthalmol. 2011;21(4):490–4.
39. Chen Q, Gu J, Jiang R, Zhou M, Chang Q. Role of ultrasound biomicroscopy in diagnosis of ocular toxocariasis. Br J Ophthalmol. 2018;102(5):642–6.

Pars Planitis in Children

53

Lisa J. Faia

Abstract

Pars planitis is a diagnostic term that defines a subset of idiopathic intermediate uveitis where there is snowbank or snowball formation in the absence of infectious or systemic disease. It predominantly affects children and adolescents. Most cases are bilateral, with more severe disease seen in those with earlier onset. Most pediatric cases are relatively asymptomatic and found on routine examination. Testing should include ruling out both infectious and non-infectious etiologies of intermediate uveitis. Systemic associations are rarely seen in children. Treatment ranges from local medical therapy to systemic immunomodulation and surgical interventions for both control of the inflammation as well as repair of complications seen with pars planitis. Complications include cataract, macular edema, retinal neovascularization, vitreous hemorrhage, and retinal detachment. Adequate control of inflammation and prompt detection of associated complications are essential in improving the overall prognosis of the pediatric uveitis patient.

Keywords

Uveitis · Pars planitis · Immunosuppression · Pediatric · Vitrectomy · Macular edema · Cataract · Complications · Snowbank · Snowball

Supplementary Information The online version contains supplementary material available at https://doi.org/10.1007/978-3-031-14506-3_53.

L. J. Faia (✉)
Ophthalmology, Oakland University William Beaumont School of Medicine, 3555 W. 13 Mile Road, LL-20, Royal Oak, MI 48073, USA
e-mail: lfaia@arcpc.net

Introduction

Pars planitis is a diagnostic term that defines a subset of idiopathic intermediate uveitis where there is snowbank or snowball formation in the absence of infectious or systemic disease [1]. Intermediate uveitis has been reported in 16–33% of all uveitis cases presenting among children [2]. Pars planitis predominantly affects children and adolescents [3–5]. Cases presenting at an earlier age tend to be more severe than those presenting later. Although the majority of cases are asymmetric, 70–90% of cases are bilateral [6]. Treatment is based on disease severity and may require systemic immunomodulation. Complications such as cataract, macular edema, retinal neovascularization, vitreous hemorrhage, and retinal detachment can be seen if this entity is not controlled. The association of intermediate uveitis with a systemic disease is exceedingly rare in children.

Young children with pars planitis are usually asymptomatic and diagnosed during a routine ophthalmologic examination. Some children are diagnosed only after significant visual impairment or the development of complications that cause leukocoria or strabismus. Typical clinical findings include mild to moderate anterior segment inflammation, diffuse vitreous cells and haze, and snowballs and snowbanks located inferiorly. Band keratopathy, peripheral corneal endotheliopathy, and posterior synechiae may be seen in childhood pars planitis but are rare in adults. Cataracts and cystoid macular edema are the most frequent complications. Neovascularization of the optic disc or associated with snowbanks may cause vitreous hemorrhage and is more common in children than adults with pars planitis.

Epidemiology

Pars planitis accounts for 5–30% of pediatric uveitis in different series [5, 7, 8]. Although sufficient data is available, it is difficult to compare the frequency of idiopathic pars planitis among previously published series since, in some series, cases with pars planitis have been considered as idiopathic uveitis, while in others, it has been reported as a distinct entity. The occurrence of pars planitis has been reported to be highest among children 6–10 years of age [5, 9, 10]. Gender distribution may be affected by age as several reports have found a male predominance but there are a few in which a female predominance has been seen [10–12]. Though cases may be asymmetrical, the majority of studies have reported bilateral involvement [6]. The majority of patients do not need systemic therapies for treatment, though a small percentage do require steroid sparing systemic immunomodulation [4].

Associations between pars planitis and HLA-DR2, -DR15, -B51 and -DRB1*0802 haplotypes have been described but are not definitive for the diagnosis [12–14]. Those with HLA-DR15 positivity were reported to have systemic findings of other HLA-DR15 related disorders such as multiple sclerosis, optic neuritis, and narcolepsy, suggesting a common genetic background [13, 14]. In Mexican

Mestizos, more severe inflammation was seen in HLA-B51 associated female patients and HLA-DRB1*0802 associated male patients [13]. Smith et al. reported race and ethnicity to be associated with predisposition to different patterns of uveitis, as well as pars planitis [8]. They found that in their pediatric population, the prevalence of pars planitis was significantly lower in Hispanic children as compared to non-Hispanics (9.6 vs. 19.2%) [8].

Signs and Symptoms—Clinical Presentation

Patients often present with minimal symptoms, such as floaters and blurred vision, but very rarely present with pain, photophobia, or redness of the eye. A mild anterior chamber reaction may or may not be present. Posterior subcapsular cataracts are the most common anterior segment complication, ranging from 15 to 60%, with a surprisingly low incidence of glaucoma [11, 13].

Posteriorly, vitreous cells are the most characteristic sign for pars planitis, ranging from mild to severe. Large gray-white or yellow exudative aggregates, called snowballs, may be present during active pars planitis (Fig. 53.1).

White collagen bands at the pars plana may be seen chronically in some patients, even during periods of quiescence, called snowbanks. Vitreous inflammation tends to be mild early in the course of disease, but the vitreous can later become organized and opacified [15, 16]. Peripheral retinal neovascularization may occur, resulting in vitreous hemorrhage. Cystoid macular edema is the most common cause of permanent visual loss, and it may occur in 30–67% of patients [15]. Serous, tractional, rhegmatogenous, and combined retinal detachments occur in 5% of eyes (Fig. 53.2). Optic disc edema is common.

The clinical course of pars planitis may range from a mild course with complete remission to a relentlessly progressive course with severe exudation, neovascularization, and resistance to local therapies, more often in children. Brockhurst and

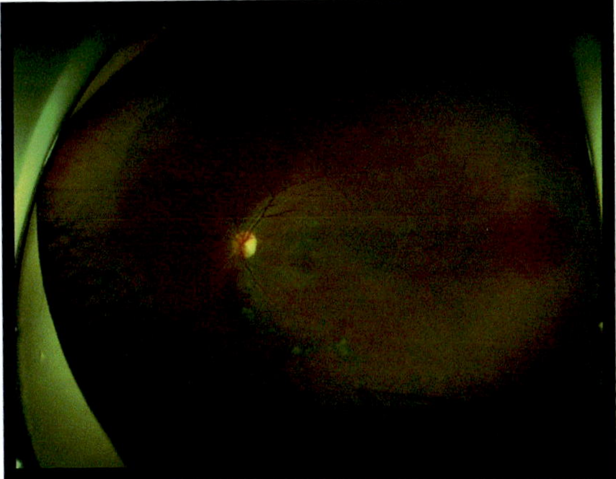

Fig. 53.1 10-year-old Hispanic female with active pars planitis OS with prominent snowballs inferiorly

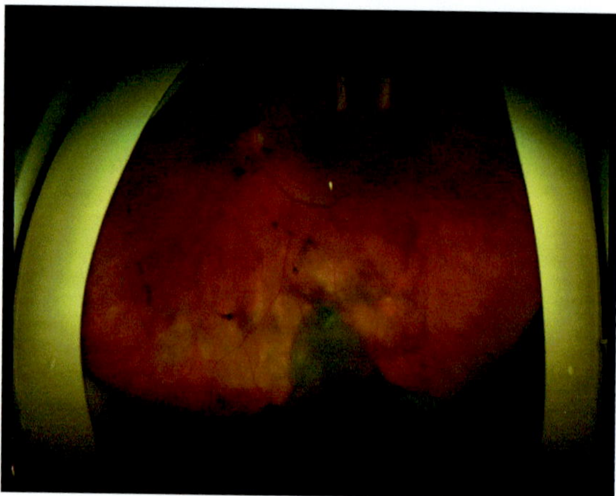

Fig. 53.2 14-year-old Caucasian male who presented with uncontrolled inflammation secondary to pars planitis. Despite systemic immunosuppression, he developed an inferior tractional retinal detachment that required surgical repair with a scleral buckle and cryotherapy

Schepens described four different groups as defined by their clinical course [17]. A mild course with complete remission was seen in 31% of patients, a mild chronic course in 49%, a severe chronic course in 15%, and a relentlessly progressive course in 5%. Others found 19% to have mild inflammation, 42% moderate inflammation, and 39% severe inflammation in their group of patients with 10-year follow up [18].

Diagnosis

The diagnosis is based on clinical findings. Though there are HLA haplotype associations, there is no direct laboratory testing for pars planitis. When intermediate uveitis is seen, infectious as well as non-infectious causes must be ruled out, even in the presence of snowbanks or snowballs.

Possible infectious etiologies that must be rules out include Lyme disease, toxocariasis, Whipple disease, tuberculosis, syphilis, human T cell leukemia virus type 1, Epstein-Barr virus, and Cat Scratch disease. Equally important is the exclusion of possible systemic autoimmune diseases, such as sarcoidosis, Behçet's disease, multiple sclerosis, retinoblastoma, familial juvenile systemic granulomatous, or intraocular leukemia/lymphoma. Initial laboratory screening should include a complete blood count with differential, angiotensin converting enzyme, chest x-ray film, tuberculin skin test with anergy panel or QuantiFERON Gold testing or equivalent, microhemagglutinin *Treponema pallidum* or fluorescent treponemal antibody absorption test, ANA, Lyme, Toxoplasma, and Toxocara antibody testing [19].

Management

Medical

Currently, the presence of macular edema, visually significant vitreous opacities, band keratopathy, cataract, retinoschisis, vasculitis or a severe infiltration of the pars plana are indications for treatment irrespective of the level of visual acuity.

Treatment is based on the severity of the disease. Topical steroids are usually the first line though most are effective for the anterior uveitic component only. Newer topical therapies, such as difluprednate, may have more posterior penetration. If this is not effective, then one may try periocular or intravitreal steroids, though cataract formation and glaucoma tend to be more difficult to treat in the pediatric population. Topical NSAIDs may be used for the CME component of pars planitis. If inflammation persists, oral steroids are the next step. Unlike in adults, long term steroid therapy, even at low doses, is not recommended in children due to long term deleterious effects. Steroid-sparing immunomodulation is necessary if long-term oral steroids are needed for control.

Methotrexate, mycophenolate mofetil, azathioprine, and cyclosporine may be used alone or in combination. With the advent of newer immunosuppressive therapies that are better tolerated, the use of immunosuppression for treatment is now started sooner to prevent vision loss and reduce steroid load. Methotrexate is the most widely used first-line immunosuppressive agent in children with chronic non-infectious uveitis because of its long-term safety record and well tolerance. It is important to remember that these agents need 4–8 weeks to become effective and that local or systemic steroids may still be needed during this time. Due to serious potential side effects, alkylating agents, such as cyclophosphamide and chlorambucil, should be avoided in children.

Anti-tumor necrosis factor-α (Anti-TNF-α) agents may be used successfully if the patient is not responding to more conventional therapies. Both infliximab and adalimumab have shown to be efficacious in pediatric uveitis including pars planitis [20–23]. Though studies comparing the two have shown a similar effect in terms of controlling inflammation, adalimumab was superior when it came to preventing attacks and maintaining remission (Fig. 53.3). Use of adalimumab as the first-line anti-TNF-α agent was more effective as compared to its use in cases of infliximab failure [24, 25]. As pars planitis is associated with an increased risk for MS development and anti-TNF-α agents may potentiate demyelinating disease, extreme

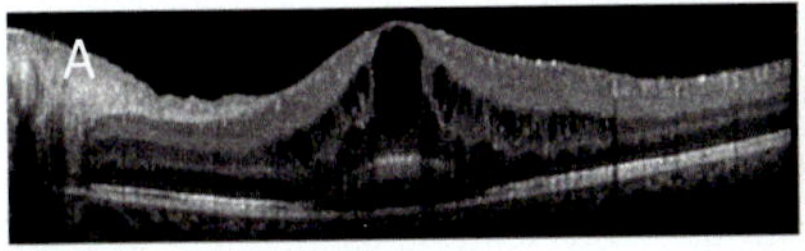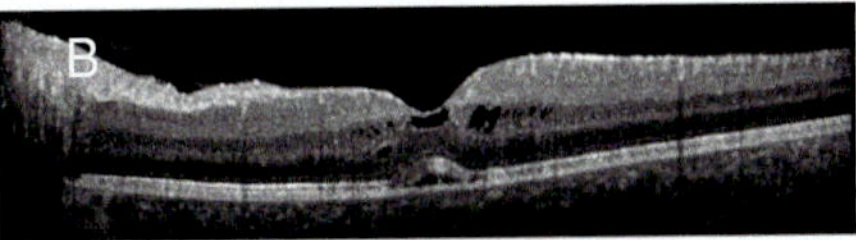

Fig. 53.3 12-year-old Caucasian female presented with macular edema secondary to pars planitis. She was on methotrexate at the time with a vision of 20/50 (Panel A). After the initiation of adalimumab, her edema improved, and her vision improved to 20/30 (Panel B)

caution is needed before starting such therapy in patients with pars planitis. Interferon (IFN) alpha had previously been shown to improve macular edema due to non-infectious uveitis in 24 patients, of which 18 subjects had intermediate uveitis [26].

Surgical

The rationale for performing cryotherapy and laser photocoagulation before immunosuppression was used to induce regression of vitreous base neovascularization and consequently stabilize the inflammation. Although favorable results with cryotherapy have been previously reported, it is believed that cryotherapy aggravates blood-ocular barrier disruption and possibly accelerates the rate of retinal detachment by inducing vitreous contraction [27–29]. Compared to cryotherapy, laser photocoagulation is an easier and safer method with fewer ocular complications. It has been shown to be effective for treatment of peripheral retinal neovascularization. Pulido and associates hypothesized that laser photocoagulation helped to diminish inflammation in pars planitis by decreasing the release of angiogenic factors [30, 31]. Again, with the advent of better and more tolerable immunotherapies, laser photocoagulation should not be considered as a treatment step alone but instead as an adjunctive treatment, especially in cases associated with peripheral neovascularization, retinal traction, or retinoschisis.

Pars plana vitrectomy (PPV) is typically used to treat the complications of pars planitis, such as vitreous condensation, vitreous hemorrhage, retinal detachment, and epiretinal membranes causing retinal traction. PPV has also been shown to be effective in patients with active inflammation and cystoid macular edema refractory to medical treatment [32–35].

Advantages of PPV include mechanical clearance of inflammatory mediators and debris, anatomical correction of retinal pathology such as vitreoretinal traction, opportunity to obtain vitreous samples for adjunctive diagnostic purposes, and reduction of post-operative anti-inflammatory medication [33, 35] (**see the video**).

Video: *Pars plana vitrectomy for the removal of a vitreous hemorrhage obscuring the posterior pole and impeding vision.*

The video shows a surgical case of a vitreous hemorrhage in an 11-year-old female with pars planitis and retinal neovascularization. The patient initially presented with a vitreous hemorrhage in the context of a history of trauma, though the child could not recall a distinct traumatic event. Early vitrectomy was performed, and the patient continued to have prominent intraocular inflammation, which was controlled with methotrexate as well as topical and systemic steroids. The video displays first the dense vitreous hemorrhage with shaving with the vitrector. Along the retina, there are areas of blood clots and granulomatous—like lesions associated with the retina. Due to the ischemia caused by the uveitis, the patient developed neovascularization of the disc, which one can see being delaminated during the procedure.

Endolaser photocoagulation was applied due to the presence of the neovascularization. Due to the risk of hypotony associated with uveitis patients after surgery, the incisions were closed with 7-0 Vicryl sutures.

Complications

Complications may be a result of the disease as well as the treatment. The most frequent complications encounter with pars planitis are cataract, band keratopathy, cystoid macular edema, epiretinal membrane, retinal neovascularization, vitreous hemorrhage, visually obscuring vitreous opacities, retinoschisis, and retinal detachments. The longer the disease remains uncontrolled, the more likely for the above complications to occur. As with any complication in uveitis that may require surgical intervention, waiting until the eye has been quiet for at least 3 months is recommended as well as aggressive treatment of peri-operative and post-operative inflammation. In order to avoid further complications after surgery, escalation of the current inflammatory treatment regimen may be required.

Cataract

Cataract formation is a complication encountered by these individuals, whether from the inflammation itself or consequential treatments. Cataract extraction may be achieved through a limbal approach with phacoemulsification or through a pars plana approach with lensectomy in combination with a pars plana vitrectomy. In the pediatric population, if control was difficult to obtain, lens placement may be deferred to a second surgery, placed 6 months or more later as long as the eye remains quiet. A peripheral iridectomy may need to be made at the time of surgery if recurrent or chronic inflammation is anticipated. As with most uveitic patients and ocular surgery, the eye should be quiet for at least 3 months or longer if surgery can be deferred. As an effort to avoid severe reactivation of inflammation, pre-operative escalation of immunomodulation, whether topically or systemically, should be considered. Peri-operative inflammation must be rigorously controlled and can be done through topical, periocular, or systemic means. Maximum control of inflammation pre-operatively, intra-operatively, and post-operatively allows the greatest chance for a successful surgical result.

Cataract surgery using phacoemulsification and intraocular lens implantation has been reported to be safe in cases with pars planitis [36, 37]. After pre-operative control of inflammation for three months, visual acuity of $\geq 20/40$ could be achieved in 88% of patients following cataract surgery [37]. As in all uveitis cases, adequate pre-operative control of inflammation, a meticulous surgical technique, a foldable hydrophobic acrylic intraocular lens implanted in the capsular bag, and good post-operative inflammatory control are crucial for successful cataract surgery in pars planitis patients.

Macular Edema

Cystoid macular edema has been reported to be the leading cause of visual morbidity in children with pars planitis, with an incidence between 44 and 67% [38, 39]. It is related to disease chronicity, with a reported interval of 5.7 years between disease onset and the development of cystoid macular edema [4]. Treatments as outlined above with more aggressive progression needed with more severe disease as macular edema can be very difficult to treat. Vitrectomy may potentially reduce cystoid macular edema either by eliminating the contact between an inflamed vitreous body and the macula or by allowing better penetration or distribution of corticosteroids [40].

Epiretinal Membrane

Donaldson et al. reported a rate of 39.6% of epiretinal membrane formation in pars planitis patients with development 6.5–7.0 years after onset [4]. Dev et al. demonstrated that pars plana vitrectomy with epiretinal membrane peel showed overall improvement from baseline visual acuity to those who underwent surgery [41].

Peripheral Neovascularization

Patients with pars planitis, especially chronic, may develop thick ropy neovascularization in the far periphery extending over the ora serrata, which often is obscured from visualization by pars plana exudation and vitritis. In patients with unremitting chronic pars planitis that is recalcitrant to steroid or NSAID therapy, children are put on systemic immunosuppression before cryotherapy is done to reduce some of the inflammation this procedure may cause. Regression of snow-banking and neovascularization may occur with aggressive systemic immunosuppression [42].

Cryotherapy is thought to reduce inflammation by eliminating the inflammation stimulus in the peripheral retinal tissue. Reduction in neovascularization may be caused by direct vessel ablation or by destruction of ischemic retinal tissue [43–45].

Vitreous Hemorrhage and Visually Obscuring Vitreous Opacities

In patients with vitreous opacities impairing vision, causing amblyopia, or obscuring the ophthalmologist's view of the periphery, pars plana vitrectomy is an effective treatment for visual rehabilitation as well as attenuation of inflammation. Pars plana vitrectomy with or without pars plana lensectomy is used to treat certain complications of intermediate uveitis, such as vitreous opacification, tractional retinal detachment, vitreous hemorrhage, and epiretinal membrane. In cases of vitreous inflammation refractory to medical therapy, pars plana vitrectomy clears the visual axis by removal of media opacities and vitreous debris. Vitrectomy also may alter the course of inflammation and result in stabilization of the disease by removing immunocompetent cells and inflammatory mediators from the vitreous cavity [32–34].

Retinoschisis

Inferior peripheral retinoschisis is another complication that develops almost exclusively in children. Malalis et al. reported retinoschsis in 19% of the eyes in their population, with over half being bilateral [46]. They also reported that it may progress despite good inflammatory control. In these patients, a scleral buckle is recommended to relieve any possible tractional component, with laser barricade of the schisis cavity if possible and cryotherapy to the pars plana to ensure no small holes are missed and neovascularization, which may be a component of the traction, is treated.

Retinal Detachment

The occurrence of retinal detachment in pars planitis is anywhere from 4.2 to 10% [5, 47, 48]. Kim et al. showed that repair with encircling scleral buckle resulted in 78% of primary re-attachment, with final re-attachment rate of 96.8% after pars plana vitrectomy for those who failed a primary buckle [49].

Prognosis

Because of the insidious nature of pars planitis, it should be considered as a potentially blinding disease. Risk factors include age of onset, severity of inflammation, duration of inflammation, and male gender. Smith et al. reported that 10% of patients had a self-limited course, whereas 59% had a prolonged course with exacerbations and 31% had a chronic smoldering course with few episodes of exacerbations [50]. Up to 70% of patients will develop complications leading to visual loss [33].

One of the most important factors in determining prognosis appears to be age. With a younger age of onset, it appears the course may be more aggressive. Kalinina Ayuso et al. have shown that children with disease onset at 7 years of age or younger were more prone to development of complications and had worse visual prognosis as compared to older children [51]. Another important risk factor is severity and duration of inflammation. Eyes with more severe inflammation are more prone to develop macular edema while those with vitreous strands may sustain retinal traction and detachment [52].

Adequate control of inflammation and prompt detection of associated complications are essential in improving the overall prognosis of the pediatric uveitis patient. Children and their treatment regimens warrant a treatment strategy that includes regular evaluations and aggressive control. Because of its insidious nature, children may present with permanent vision loss. As compared to adults, children have a more severe course and poorer visual prognosis. Delayed diagnosis and inadequate treatment may result in severe visual loss and amblyopia. Early and aggressive treatment is effective in terms of preserving visual function, rather than waiting until visual acuity is decreased.

Review Questions

1. The most common complication responsible for vision loss in pediatric patients with pars planitis is:

a. CME
b. RD
c. Glaucoma
d. VH

2. Common immunosuppressive therapies used to treat pars planitis in children include all except:

a. Adalimumab
b. Methotrexate
c. Cyclophosphamide
d. Cyclosporine

3. Prognosis for worse visual acuity includes all except:

a. Young age at disease onset
b. Female gender
c. Failure to respond to local therapies
d. Numerous complications

Answers

1. (**A**) CME. Cataract and CME are the most common cause of vision loss, with the occurrence of cataract up to 60% of patients and CME up to 67% of patients.
2. (**C**) Cyclophosphamide. Methotrexate and cyclosporine are more conventional immunomodulatory therapies on which children are started and well tolerated. If these therapies are not enough to induce regression, biological medications, such as

adalimumab, have also been shown to control inflammation. Cyclophosphamide, due to it malignancy associations, is not ideal for the pediatric population.

3. (**B**) Female gender. Risk factors include age of onset, severity of inflammation, duration of inflammation, and male gender.

References

1. Jabs DA, Nussenblatt RB, Rosenbaum JT. Standardization of Uveitis Nomenclature (SUN) Working Group. Standardization of uveitis nomenclature for reporting clinical data. Results of the First International Workshop. Am J Ophthalmol. 2005;140:509–16.
2. Kump LI, et al. Analysis of pediatric uveitis cases at a tertiary referral center. Ophthalmology. 2005;112(7):1287–92.
3. Tugal-Tutkun I. Pediatric uveitis. J Ophthalmic Vis Res. 2011;6:259–69.
4. Donaldson MJ, Pulido JS, Herman DC, Diehl N, Hodge D. Pars planitis: a 20-year study of incidence, clinical features, and outcomes. Am J Ophthalmol. 2007;144:812–7.
5. Nikkhah H, Ramezani A, Ahmadieh H, Soheilian M, Azarmina M, Dehghan MH, et al. Childhood pars planitis; clinical features and outcomes. J Ophthalmic Vis Res. 2011;6: 249–54.
6. Thorne JE, Daniel A, Jabs DA, Kedhar SR, Peters GB, Dunn JP. Smoking as a risk factor for cystoid macular edema complicating intermediate uveitis. Am Ophthalmol. 2008;145:841–6.
7. Soylu M, Ozdemir G, Anli A. Pediatric uveitis in Southern Turkey. Ocul Immunol Inflamm. 1997;5:197–202.
8. Smith JA, Mackensen F, Sen HN, Leigh JF, Watkins AS, Pyatetsky D, et al. Epidemiology and course of disease in childhood uveitis. Ophthalmology. 2009;116:1544–51.
9. Rosenberg KD, Feuer WJ, Davis JL. Ocular complications of pediatric uveitis. Ophthalmology. 2004;111:2299–306.
10. Paroli MP, Spinucci G, Monte R, Pesci FR, Abicca I, Pivetti PP. Intermediate uveitis in a pediatric Italian population. Ocul Immunol Inflamm. 2011;19:321–6.
11. Romero R, Peralta J, Sendagorta E, Abelairas J. Pars planitis in children: epidemiologic, clinical, and therapeutic characteristics. J Pediatr Ophthalmol Strabismus. 2007;44:288–93.
12. Raja SC, Jabs DA, Dunn JP, Fekrat S, Machan CH, Marsh MJ, et al. Pars planitis: clinical features and class II HLA associations. Ophthalmology. 1999;106:594–9.
13. Arellanes-García L, Navarro-López P, Concha-Del Río LE, Unzueta-Medina JA. Idiopathic intermediate uveitis in childhood. Int Ophthalmol Clin. 2008;48:61–74.
14. Tang WM, Pulido JS, Eckels DD, Han DP, Mieler WF, Pierce K. The association of HLA-DR15 and intermediate uveitis. Am J Ophthalmol. 1997;123:70–5.
15. de Boer J, Berendschot TT, van der Does P, Rothova A. Long-term follow-up of intermediate uveitis in children. Am J Ophthalmol. 2006;141:616–21.
16. Lauer AK, Smith JR, Robertson JE, Rosenbaum JT. Vitreous hemorrhage is a common complication of pediatric pars planitis. Ophthalmology. 2002;109:95–8.
17. Brockhurst RJ, Schepens CL. Peripheral uveitis. The complication of retinal detachment. Arch Ophthalmol. 1968;80: 747.
18. Deane JS, Rosenthal AR. Course and complications of intermediate uveitis. Acta Ophthalmol Scand. 1997;75:82–4.
19. Holland GN, Stiehm ER. Special considerations in the evaluation and management of uveitis in children. Am J Ophthalmol. 2003;135:867–78.
20. Tugal-Tutkun I, Ayranci O, Kasapcopur O, Kir N. Retrospective analysis of children with uveitis treated with infliximab. J AAPOS. 2008;12:611–3.
21. Ardoin SP, Kredich D, Rabinovich E, Schanberg LE, Jaffe GJ. Infliximab to treat chronic noninfectious uveitis in children: retrospective case series with long-term follow-up. Am J Ophthalmol. 2007;144:844–9.

22. Biester S, Deuter C, Michels H, Haefner R, Kuemmerle-Deschner J, Doycheva D, et al. Adalimumab in the therapy of uveitis in childhood. Br J Ophthalmol. 2007;91:319–24.
23. Gallagher M, Quinones K, Cervantes-Castañeda RA, Yilmaz T, Foster CS. Biological response modifier therapy for refractory childhood uveitis. Br J Ophthalmol. 2007;91:1341–4.
24. Simonini G, Taddio A, Cattalini M, Caputo R, De Libero C, Naviglio S, et al. Prevention of flare recurrences in childhood-refractory chronic uveitis: an open-label comparative study of adalimumab versus infliximab. Arthritis Care Res (Hoboken). 2011;63:612–8.
25. Simonini G, Taddio A, Cattalini M, Caputo R, de Libero C, Parentin F, et al. Superior efficacy of Adalimumab in treating childhood refractory chronic uveitis when used as first biologic modifier drug: Adalimumab as starting anti-TNF-α therapy in childhood chronic uveitis. Pediatr Rheumatol Online J. 2013;11:16.
26. Deuter CM, Kötter I, Günaydin I, Stübiger N, Doycheva DG, Zierhut M. Efficacy and tolerability of interferon alpha treatment in patients with chronic cystoid macular oedema due to non-infectious uveitis. Br J Ophthalmol. 2009;93:906–13.
27. Aaberg TM, Cesarz TJ, Flickinger RR. Jr Treatment of pars planitis I. Cryotherapy. Surv Ophthalmol. 1977;22:120–5.
28. Devenyi RG, Mieler WF, Lambrou FH, Will BR, Aaberg TM. Cryopexy of the vitreous base in the management of peripheral uveitis. Am J Ophthalmol. 1988;106:135–8.
29. Mieler WF, Aaberg TM. Further observations on cryotherapy of the vitreous base in the management of peripheral uveitis. Dev Ophthalmol. 1992;23:190–5.
30. Park SE, Mieler WF, Pulido JS. Peripheral scatter photocoagulation for neovascularization associated with pars planitis. Arch Ophthalmol. 1995;113:1277–80.
31. Pulido JS, Mieler WF, Walton D, Kuhn E, Postel E, Hartz A, et al. Results of peripheral laser photocoagulation in pars planitis. Trans Am Ophthalmol Soc. 1998;96:127–37.
32. Heiligenhaus A, Bornfeld N, Foerster MH, Wessing A. Long-term results of pars plana vitrectomy in the management of complicated uveitis. Br J Ophthalmol. 1994;78:549–54.
33. Quinones K, Choi JY, Yilmaz T, Kafkala C, Letko E, Foster CS. Pars plana vitrectomy versus immunomodulatory therapy for intermediate uveitis: a prospective, randomized pilot study. Ocul Immunol Inflamm. 2010;18:411–7.
34. Trittibach P, Koerner F, Sarra GM, Garweg JG. Vitrectomy for juvenile uveitis: prognostic factors for the long-term functional outcome. Eye (Lond). 2006;20:184–90.
35. Stavrou P, Baltatzis S, Letko E, Samson CM, Christen W, Foster CS. Pars plana vitrectomy in patients with intermediate uveitis. Ocul Immunol Inflamm. 2001;9:141–51.
36. Ganesh SK, Babu K, Biswas J. Phacoemulsification with intraocular lens implantation in cases of pars planitis. J Cataract Refract Surg. 2004;30:2072–6.
37. Kaufman AH, Foster CS. Cataract extraction in patients with pars planitis. Ophthalmology. 1993;100:1210–7.
38. Capone A, T.M.A., Intermediate uveitis. In: Albert DM, Jakobiec FA. Editors. Principles and practice of ophthalmology. Philadelphia: WB Saunders Company;1994. p. 423–2.
39. Michelson JB, Friedlaender MH, Nozik RA. Lens implant surgery in pars planitis. Ophthalmology. 1990;97(8):1023–6.
40. Wiechens B, Nolle B, Reichelt JA. Pars plana vitrectomy in cystoid macular edema associated with intermediate uveitis. Graefes Arch Clin Exp Ophthalmol. 2001;239(7):474–81.
41. Dev S, Mieler WF, Pulido JS, Mittra RA. Visual outcomes after pars plana vitrectomy for epiretinal membranes associated with pars planitis. Ophthalmology. 1999;106:1086–90.
42. Kump L, Vitale AT, Foster CS. Pediatric uveitis. In: Foster CS, Vitale AT, editors. Diagnosis and treatment of uveitis. New Delhi, India: Highlights Medical Publishers; 2013. p. 1223–5.
43. Tugal-Tutkun I, Güney-Tefekli E, Kamaci-Duman F, Corum I. A cross-sectional and longitudinal study of Fuchs uveitis syndrome in Turkish patients. Am J Ophthalmol. 2009;148:510-5.e1.
44. Davis JL. Diagnosis of intraocular lymphoma. Ocul Immunol Inflamm. 2004;12:7–16.

45. Forrester JV, Okada AA, Ben Ezra D, Ohno S, editors. Posterior segment intraocular inflammation: guidelines. The Hague, Netherlands: Kugler Publications;1998. Pars planitis. p. 93–7.
46. Malalis JF, Bhat P, Shaprio M, Goldstein DA. Retinoschisis in pars planitis. Ocul Immunol Inflamm. 2017;25(3):344–8.
47. Romero R, Peralta J, Sendagorta E, Abelairas J. Pars planitis in children: epidemiologic, clinical and therapeutic characteristics. J Pediatr Ophthalmol Strabismus. 2007;44:288–93.
48. Malinowski SM, Pulido JS, Folk JC. Long term visual outcome and complications associated with pars planitis. Ophthalmology. 1993;100:818–25.
49. Kim Y-K, Yoon W, Ahn JK, Park SP. Scleral buckling for rhegmatogenous retinal detachment associated with pars planitis. J Ophthalmol. 2016; Article ID 4538193, 5 p.
50. Smith RE, Godfrey WA, Kimura SJ. Chronic cyclitis. I. Course and visual prognosis. Trans Am Acad Ophthalmol Otolaryngol. 1973;77:OP760–8.
51. Kalinina Ayuso V, ten Cate HA, van den Does P, Rothova A, de Boer JH. Young age as a risk factor for complicated course and visual outcome in intermediate uveitis in children. Br J Ophthalmol. 2011;95:646–51.
52. Zierhut M, Doycheva D, Biester S, Stübiger N, Kümmerle-Deschner J, Deuter C. Therapy of uveitis in children. Int Ophthalmol Clin. 2008;48:131–52.

Other Inflammatory Disorders in Children

54

Stephanie M. Llop and Lucia Sobrin

Abstract

Management and treatment of vitreoretinal inflammatory disorders in children, mainly uveitis, is different from adults requiring special considerations for this population. Based on limited data on surgical interventions in children with uveitis, the most important aspect of treatment is achieving control of the inflammation prior to surgery. Pars plana vitrectomy remains a useful tool in the treatment of patients with posterior and panuveitis, especially treating its complications including epiretinal membrane, cataract, posterior capsular opacification, vitreous hemorrhage, retinal detachment, hypotony, among others.

Keywords

Pediatric uveitis · Posterior uveitis · Panuveitis · Uveitis complications · Epiretinal membrane · Hypotony · Posterior capsule opacification

Supplementary Information The online version contains supplementary material available at https://doi.org/10.1007/978-3-031-14506-3_54.

S. M. Llop (✉)
Clinical Ophthalmology, Bascom Palmer Eye Institute, University of Miami, Miami, FL, USA
e-mail: sxl1789@med.miami.edu

L. Sobrin
Charles Edward Whitten Professor of Ophthalmology, Harvard Medical School, Mass Eye and Ear, Boston, MA, USA
e-mail: lucia_sobrin@meei.harvard.edu

Ş. Özdek et al. (eds.), *Pediatric Vitreoretinal Surgery*,
https://doi.org/10.1007/978-3-031-14506-3_54

Pediatric Uveitis: Posterior and Panuveitis

Uveitis in children is not as common as in adults but it deserves special consideration because of its unique diagnostic and therapeutic challenges. Children comprise between 2.2 to 13.8% of patients in uveitis clinics. Childhood uveitis is often chronic and difficult to treat as many patients are asymptomatic, uncooperative, or preverbal. Also, the risk of poor visual outcomes is higher than in the adult population due to common delays in treatment, insidious onset, and risk of amblyopia [1].

Posterior uveitis refers to inflammation of the choroid, retina, or both. The differential diagnosis for posterior uveitis is shown in the table below.

Differential diagnosis for posterior uveitis in children

Infectious	Non-infectious
Toxocariasis	Tubulointerstitial nephritis and uveitis
Toxoplasmosis	Vogt-Koyanagi-Harada syndrome
Tuberculosis	Sarcoidosis
Rubella	Multiple sclerosis
Syphilis	Behcet's disease
Cytomegalovirus retinitis	White dot syndromes
Acute retinal necrosis (HSV, VZV)	Systemic lupus erythematosus
Diffuse subacute unilateral neuroretinitis	Inflammatory bowel disease
Presumed ocular histoplasmosis syndrome	Familial juvenile systemic granulomatosis (Blau syndrome)
Lyme disease	Neonatal-onset multisystem inflammatory disease (NOMID)

Panuveitis is defined as inflammation in all parts of the uvea (iris, ciliary body, and choroid) and may include involvement of the optic nerve, the retina or retinal vessels.

Differential diagnosis for panuveitis in children

Infectious	Non-infectious
Tuberculosis	Behcet's disease
Cat-scratch disease	Sympathetic ophthalmia
Toxoplasmosis	Vogt-Koyanagi-Harada syndrome
Syphilis	Sarcoidosis
Lyme	Tubulointerstitial nephritis and uveitis

Depending on whether the etiology is infectious or non-infectious, the first line treatment for posterior and panuveitis is antimicrobial therapy or corticosteroids, respectively. For some infectious etiologies, corticosteroids are used alongside antimicrobial therapy to dampen the inflammatory response after the infection has shown some improvement on antimicrobial therapy. One example is Tuberculosis-related uveitis.

Tubercular (TB) uveitis can be seen in children and the incidence in TB endemic countries is estimated to be around 4.9–7.4% in comparison to 6.9–10.5% in adults [2]. The most common type of TB uveitis is posterior uveitis followed by panuveitis and clinical findings include vasculitis (which can be occlusive), choroiditis, snow banking, granulomatous keratic precipitates, iris nodules and less frequently choroidal granulomas and disc edema. All patients must have a positive Mantoux test and/or a positive interferon gamma release assay [2]. The recommended treatment is standard four-drug anti-tubercular therapy (ATT) with oral prednisone (1 mg/kg). If no response or partial response to treatment is seen after 3 months, adding immunosuppressive therapy needs to be considered as children tend to have higher levels of inflammatory response that require a more aggressive approach when compared to adults. Complications that may require surgical intervention include vitreous hemorrhage due to retinal neovascularization in areas of occlusive vasculitis, cataracts, glaucoma, and retinal detachment [2].

Cat-scratch disease (CSD) is a benign and often self-limiting disease that commonly occurs in children and is caused by *Bartonella species,* including *Bartonella henselae* and *Bartonella quintana* [3, 4]. Ocular involvement occurs in about 5–10% of patient with CSD and the classic ocular manifestation is neuroretinitis associated with a macular star (exudates) or papillitis [4]. Other posterior findings may include intraretinal infiltrates, retinal edema, retinal infarcts, choroidal infiltrates, intermediate uveitis, acute endophthalmitis and intraretinal hemorrhages [3, 4]. The mainstay of laboratory diagnosis of CSD is serology: anti-*B. henselae* or *B. quintana* IgM and IgG antibodies [5]. The use of antibiotic therapy is controversial and there is no consensus in the literature about the preferred agent or addition of systemic corticosteroids [3]. Doxycycline, rifampicin, and azithromycin are antibiotics of choice, but fluoroquinolones, intravenous aminoglycosides and trimethoprim- sulfamethoxazole have all been used with success [4]. In a case report by Kalogeropoulos et al. of 13 patients (age 10–77) with ocular bartonellosis, retinal complications included epiretinal membranes, retinal neovascularization, macular hole, macula scars and cataract [4].

Syphilis, caused by *Treponema pallidum,* is a sexually communicated disease that can be seen in neonates due to transplacental transmission or adolescents who have high risk sexual behaviors [6]. Ocular findings of congenital syphilis include chorioretinitis, cataracts and glaucoma, so every child evaluated for congenital syphilis, should have an eye examination [6]. Treatment for acquired syphilis is benzathine penicillin G 50,000 U/kg intramuscular with a maximum of 2.4 million units in a single dose. If there is late latent infection or infection of unknown duration, the treatment should be done weekly for 3 weeks. However, for any case of ocular syphilis, the patient should be treated with aqueous crystalline penicillin G 18–24 million U/d. Congenital syphilis (proven, probable, or possible) is also treated with aqueous crystalline penicillin G, given every 12 h for the first 7 days of life and every 8 h thereafter for 10 days [6].

Cytomegalovirus is another entity that can be seen in children (approximately 6% of children with acquired immunodeficiency syndrome) and causes a necrotizing retinitis [7]. Treatment consists of intravenous ganciclovir (induction dose 5 mg/kg twice daily) or foscarnet (60 mg/kg three times daily) for 2–5 weeks [7]. Delayed diagnosis in the pediatric population contributes to worse prognosis and visual outcomes with often bilateral involvement, extending to the fovea [7].

Lyme Disease is caused by the tick-borne *Borrelia burgdorferi* infection and ocular involvement can rarely be seen in children in either the early stages (follicular conjunctivitis) or late stages (anterior uveitis, intermediate uveitis and keratitis) [8]. The recommended treatment is intravenous ceftriaxone [8].

For noninfectious uveitis, when corticosteroids cannot be tapered without worsening of inflammation, immunomodulatory therapy is often required. Sarcoidosis, although not common in children, frequently has ocular manifestations, only second to pulmonary abnormalities [9]. Most reported cases are in pre-adolescents and adolescents but young children under 5 years of age have also been reported [9]. Anterior segment inflammation (granulomatous uveitis) is most commonly seen (>80%); posterior segment involvement includes periphlebitis, focal or multifocal chorioretinitis, chorioretinal nodules and could be associated with central nervous system involvement (papilledema, papillitis, optic neuritis) [9]. Treatment with corticosteroids is usually effective but some case progress to blindness despite treatment and immunosuppressive therapy should be considered early.

Behcet's disease (BD) is a multisystemic inflammatory disease which is not common in children. Two hallmarks of the diagnosis are the presence of oral and/or genital ulcers [10]. Ocular involvement is common and can cause significant vision loss. The overall frequency of ocular involvement in juvenile BD is similar to that in adults, and the most common manifestation is posterior uveitis with retinal vasculitis, followed by anterior uveitis [10, 11]. It is important to mention that uveitis can be the presenting symptom in 10% of cases and common complications include cystoid macular edema and cataracts [11].

Tubulointerstitial nephritis and uveitis syndrome (TINU) is characterized by the presence of interstitial nephritis and uveitis, most commonly bilateral acute anterior uveitis [12]. The uveitis commonly presents between 2 months prior to and 12 months after the onset of the systemic symptoms and urine B2-microglobulin has been shown to be a marker of disease [12]. In a case series of 17 patients with TINU, 100% had anterior uveitis and posterior findings were seen in 65% of patients, including chorioretinal lesions, choroidal neovascular membranes (CNVM), vitreous hemorrhage secondary to optic disc neovascularization, macular edema and retinal vasculitis [12]. Uveitis tends to become chronic and while initially it is treated with corticosteroids, it often requires immunosuppressive therapy.

There are specific instances in which, in addition to systemic treatment, surgery is indicated for the management of uveitis. Pars plana vitrectomy (PPV) is an important treatment option, especially in patients with complications induced by inflammation including macular edema, vitreous hemorrhage, vitreous opacities, epiretinal membrane and retinal detachment. Also, it can be considered in patients with recalcitrant disease that does not respond to immunomodulatory therapy [13].

Soheilian et al. published a series of ten patients with pediatric VKH in which surgical intervention was required in 9 of the 20 eyes for significant cataract, extensive posterior synechiae, peripheral anterior synechiae and/or high intraocular pressure. In all their cases a 4 mm infusion cannula was anchored to the sclera 3 mm posterior to the limbus and pars-plana lensectomy, posterior capsulectomy and vitrectomy were performed. In eyes with glaucoma and extensive synechiae, goniosynechiolysis was also performed. Intraocular lenses were not implanted. Intraocular dexamethasone 400 µg was injected at the end of each case followed by closure of the conjunctiva and injection of antibiotic and corticosteroid subconjunctivally. Visual acuity improved more than 2 Snellen lines in all eyes. In six eyes with glaucoma, goniosynechiolysis was performed at the time of the vitrectomy, and in all six eyes, intraocular pressure (IOP) was controlled postoperatively with timolol alone. Is important to clarify that all these patients had surgery after immunomodulatory therapy was initiated and inflammation was controlled, which most likely contributed to the good visual outcomes, lack of post-operative complications, and lack of worsening of inflammation [14].

Giuiari et al. also published their experience with pars-plana vitrectomy in 28 eyes of 20 pediatric patients of which 8 eyes (29%) had idiopathic panuveitis. In their series, all patients had active uveitis at the time of the PPV with or without medical therapy and at the last follow up visit 27/28 eyes (96%) had no sign of active uveitis following PPV with or without medical therapy. Their approach was using 20-G instruments in 68% of the study eyes and 7% (2 eyes) developed retinal tears, which were treated intra-operatively. One of these eyes developed a rhegmatogenous retinal detachment one week after PPV that required repair with a scleral buckle. Of the eyes that underwent surgery with 25-G instruments (32%), none developed any intra- or postoperative complications, favoring the use of smaller gauge vitrectomy for these cases. The only eye in this series that had persistent inflammation after PPV had panuveitis with retinal vasculitis that was treated with chlorambucil prior to PPV and then required a switch to infliximab to achieve better control. Most of the cases that had retinal vasculitis that required steroid-sparing immunomodulatory therapy to control the inflammation, but PPV might have helped with control since all patients were active prior to surgery and all but one were quiet at the end of the study [15].

Management of Complications from Uveitis

Epiretinal Membrane

Epiretinal membranes (ERM) can be seen as wrinkling or distortion of the retinal surface, especially the macula, caused by retinal cell proliferation. They are most common in older patients (>50 years of age) but less frequently present in the pediatric population in the setting of ocular inflammation, tumors or following trauma. A retrospective study looking into ERM in the pediatric population of

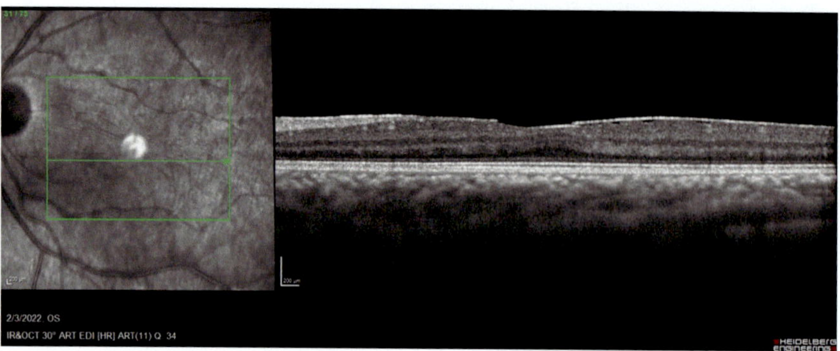

Fig. 54.1 Epiretinal membrane in a 14 y/o with intermediate uveitis

Olmsted County, Minnesota found 44 new cases in children in a period of 30 years out of a population of about 100,000 and among those only 9 (20.5%) occurred in the setting of uveitis [16]. Of these, premacular fibrosis type was the most frequently diagnosed type of ERM, while the cellophane macular reflex type comprised the remaining cases. Most cases were managed with observation (54.5%) while 8 cases (18.2%) underwent PPV. Of those who had surgery, pre-op visual acuity ranged from 20/40 to 20/400, and there was a mean improvement of 3.8 lines during a mean follow up of 33 months. Out of the 9 eyes that had PPV, only 1 reported a recurrent ERM within 3 months as a complication and one developed a cataract (follow up of 97 months) [16]. Based on this report and a few other studies, it can be said that membrane peeling can be safely performed with improvement in visual acuity (Fig. 54.1).

Hypotony

Hypotony has been reported to occur in about 19% of patients with juvenile idiopathic arthritis (JIA)-associated uveitis which is a higher rate than in pediatric patients with other types of uveitis [17]. Hypotony occurs due to decreased aqueous production during active inflammation in addition to increased uveoscleral outflow. Chronic hypotony can result from formation of cyclitic membranes which produces traction on the ciliary body and results in cyclodialysis that increases uveoscleral outflow. Damage to the ciliary epithelium can also cause a decrease in aqueous production [17]. This can lead to vision loss secondary to anterior chamber collapse, vitreous haze, retinal or macular edema, choroidal detachment, and corneal complications that could eventually result in loss of function (phthisis bulbi).

A study by Yu et al. looked at patients that had surgery for hypotony (defined at IOP <5 mmHg). In all patients (two adults and two children), the ocular inflammation was controlled prior to surgery. They all had a standard three-port vitrectomy with identification of ciliary membranes that were dissected and removed using and MVR blade and forceps or intraocular scissors. An assistant was needed to depress the sclera near the ciliary body with a cotton-tip applicator to help with visualization, and removal. If the membranes could not be completely dissected, four cuts were made to decrease circumferential traction on the ciliary body. After vitrectomy was completed, sclerostomies were closed and dexamethasone 400 μg was injected to the posterior chamber. All eyes had low IOP on the first postoperative day, and at one week, one pediatric patient had an increase in IOP from 0 to 18 mmHg. At one month, both pediatric patients had IOP in the teens and the adult patients remained hypotonous. Of note, during surgery both adults were noticed to have atrophy ciliary processes as compared to children who had normal ciliary processes.

Based on clinical experience and limited case reports, it is recommended that when these patients with uveitis, especially those with JIA-associated uveitis, undergo cataract surgery, there should be complete removal of the lens, the capsule and anterior vitreous to prevent membrane formation. Pre-operative ultrasound biomicroscopy (UBM) is recommended to look for the presence of membranes; this will help distinguish whether the cause of hypotony is decreased aqueous production from a dysfunctional ciliary body which would not benefit from surgery [17].

Posterior Capsule Opacification

The development of posterior capsule opacification (PCO) is the most common complication following pediatric cataract surgery (discussed in the following section). The incidence is as high as 100% in infants if the posterior capsule is left intact [18]. The main treatment for PCO is Nd:YAG laser capsulotomy but young or uncooperative children are often unable to stay still for the procedure. In these patients, surgical membranectomy can be performed with anterior vitrectomy via a limbal or pars plana approach. A study by Xie et al. evaluated the outcome of a pars plana approach capsulotomy with anterior vitrectomy, and all patients had the central capsule removed without complications [19].

Clinical Case Scenario

An 8-year-old girl presented with bilateral idiopathic panuveitis. Initial presenting visual acuity was 20/40 OU with exam significant for 1–2+ anterior chamber cell OU and 3+ vitreous cell OD and 2+ vitreous cell OS (Figs. 54.2, 54.3, 54.4, 54.5, 54.6 and 54.7). She was started on oral prednisone 20 mg. Methotrexate was later initiated for a corticosteroid-sparing effect followed by adalimumab. Adalimumab was discontinued by the mother after a few months due to a local injection site reaction. The patient developed worsening of her panuveitis and her vision decreased to HM OD and 20/200 OS with progressive cataracts, posterior synechiae and dense vitritis (Figs. 54.8 and 54.9). Intervention was required to clear the visual axis. Lensectomy and vitrectomy were performed with endolaser applied to the

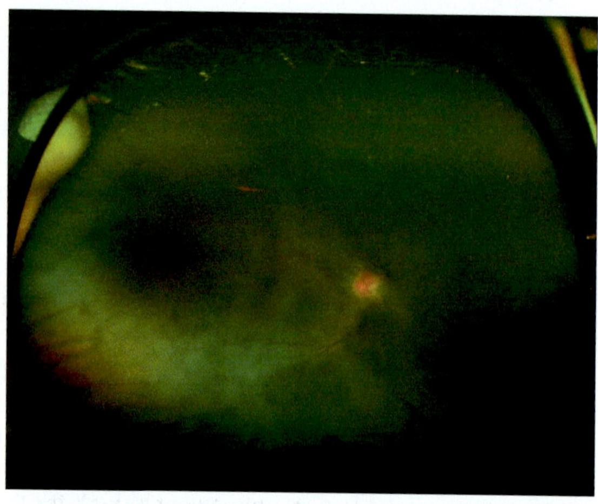

Fig. 54.2 Fundus photo right eye on presentation

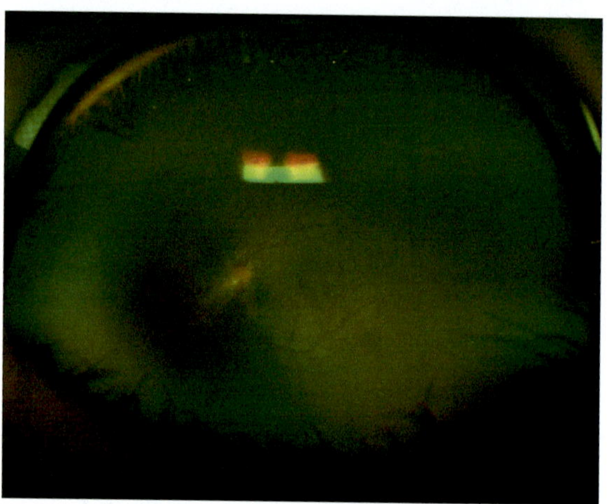

Fig. 54.3 Fundus photo left eye on presentation

areas of prior noted angiographic leakage. The postoperative visual acuities were 20/40 in the right eye and 20/20 in the left eye with aphakic contact lens correction (Figs. 54.10 and 54.11; **video**). The patient is currently suppressed on methotrexate 15 mg weekly and adalimumab 40 mg every 14 days.

In summary, uveitis is a challenging disease to diagnose and treat. In the pediatric population there are additional challenges including poor cooperation with the examination and late diagnosis/referrals due to lack of symptoms. The first line of treatment is usually topical, local or systemic corticosteroids for noninfectious etiologies, with the use antimicrobial therapy for infectious etiologies. Immuno-suppressive therapy plays an important role in the management of non-infectious uveitis, but surgical intervention may be needed to treat inflammation or

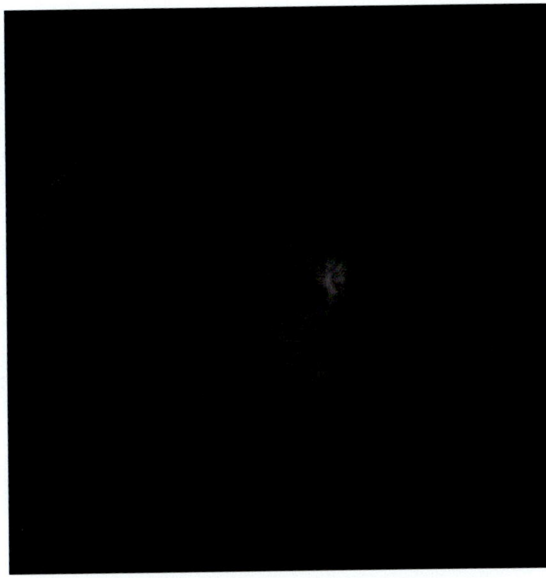

Fig. 54.4 Fluorescein angiography right eye at 10 min (initial presentation)

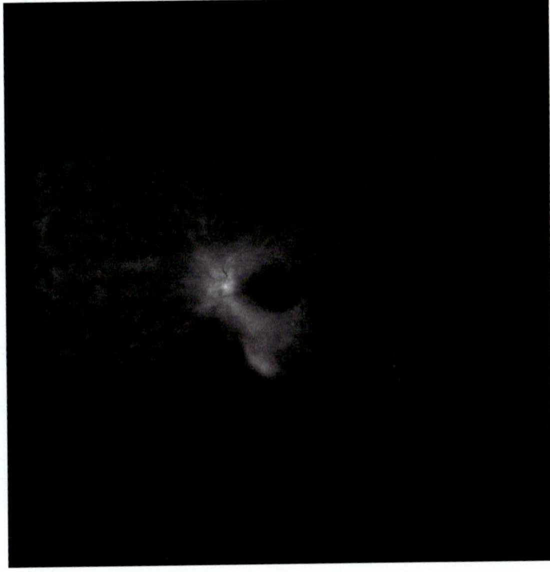

Fig. 54.5 Fluorescein angiography left eye at 10 min (initial presentation)

complications that arise secondary to uveitis. Although the data is scarce, the general consensus is that patients should have adequate control of the inflammatory process prior to surgery to have the best outcomes. Surgery remains as an important tool in the management of uveitis.

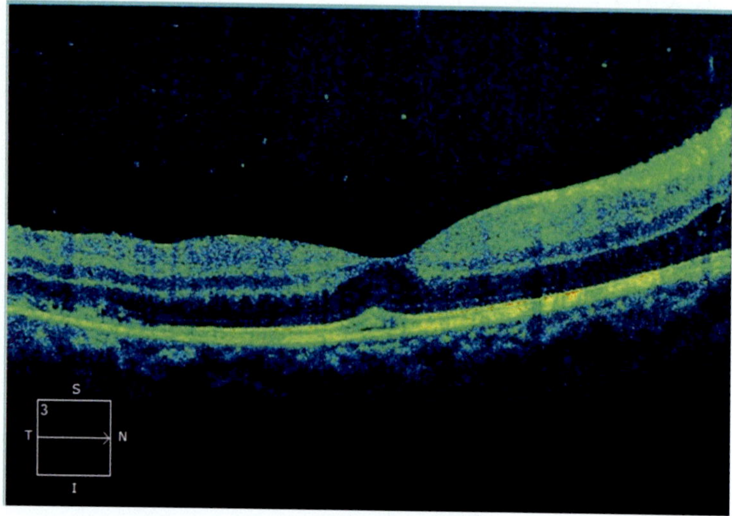

Fig. 54.6 OCT macula right eye (on presentation)

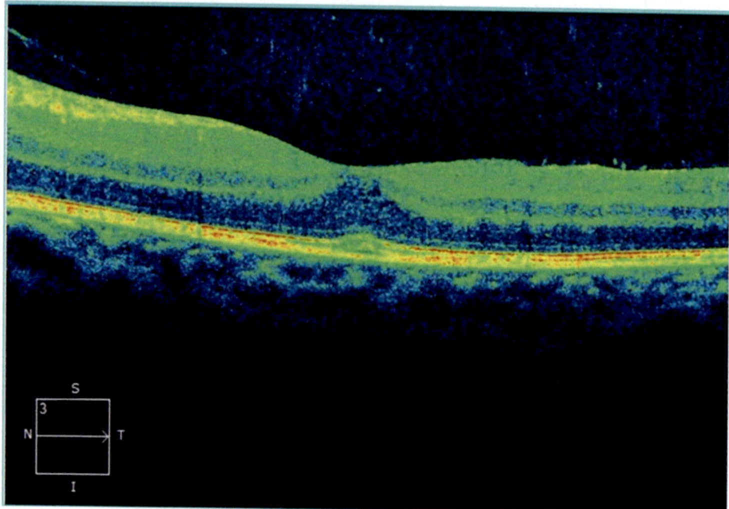

Fig. 54.7 OCT macula left eye (on presentation)

Fig. 54.8 B-scan right eye

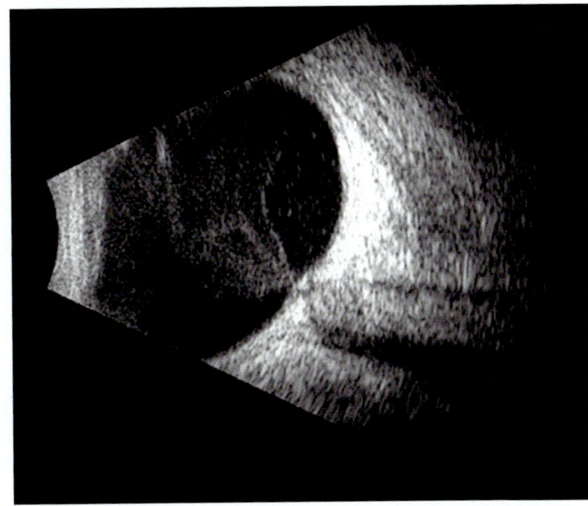

Fig. 54.9 Bscan left eye

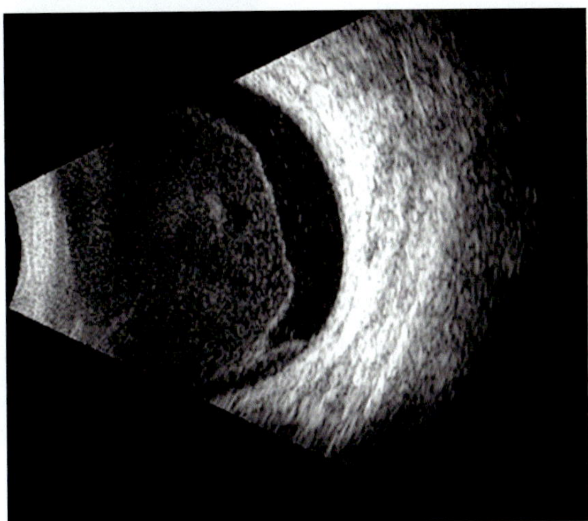

Review Questions

1. Which of the following is not an indication for pars plana vitrectomy in patients with posterior uveitis?

a. Macular edema
b. Vitreous hemorrhage
c. Optic nerve head edema
d. Epiretinal membrane

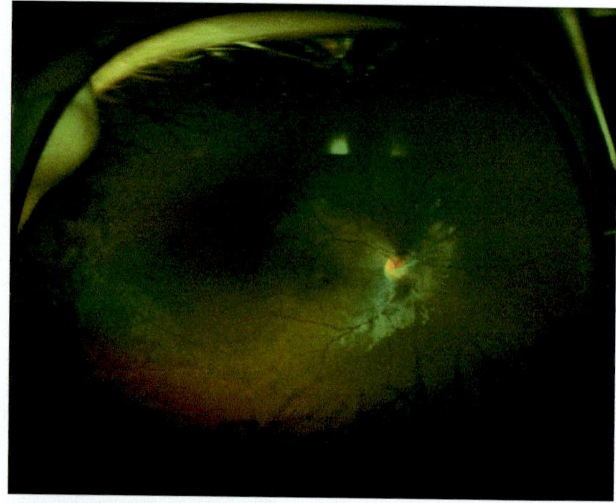

Fig. 54.10 Fundus photo right eye after vitrectomy/lensectomy and endolaser

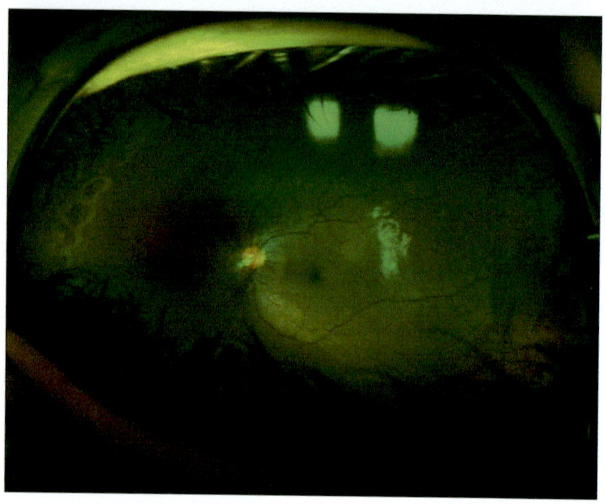

Fig. 54.11 Fundus photo left eye after vitrectomy/lensectomy and endolaser

2. Which type of epiretinal membrane is the most frequently diagnosed in the pediatric uveitis population?

a. Premacular fibrosis
b. Cellophane macular reflex
c. Extramacular fibrosis
d. Vitreomacular traction

3. In cases of hypotony, which of the following is recommended preoperatively?

a. MRI-orbit to look for posterior scleral thickening
b. Ultrasound biomicroscopy to look for the presence of membranes
c. Pilocarpine for ciliary muscle contraction

d. OCT macula to look for retinal folds

Answers

1. (**C**) Optic nerve head edema

Pars plana vitrectomy (PPV) is an important treatment option, especially in patients with complications induced by inflammation including macular edema, vitreous hemorrhage, vitreous opacities, epiretinal membrane and retinal detachment. Also, it can be considered in patients with recalcitrant disease that does not respond to immunomodulatory therapy.

2. (**A**) Premacular fibrosis

A retrospective study looking into ERM in the pediatric population of Olmsted County, Minnesota found 44 new cases in children in a period of 30 years out of a population of about 100,000 and among those only 9 (20.5%) occurred in the setting of uveitis. Of these, premacular fibrosis type was the most frequently diagnosed type of ERM, while the cellophane macular reflex type comprised the remaining cases. Most cases were managed with observation (54.5%) while 8 cases (18.2%) underwent PPV.

3. (**B**) Ultrasound biomicroscopy to look for the presence of membranes

Pre-operative ultrasound biomicroscopy (UBM) is recommended to look for the presence of membranes; this will help distinguish whether the cause of hypotony is decreased aqueous production from a dysfunctional ciliary body which would not benefit from surgery.

References

1. Wentworth BA, Freitas-Neto CA, Foster CS. Management of pediatric uveitis. F1000Prime Reports. 2014;6. https://doi.org/10.12703/P6-41.
2. Kaur S, Aggarwal K, Agarwal A, et al. Clinical course and outcomes of pediatric tubercular uveitis in North India. Ocul Immunol Inflamm. 2018;26(6):859–64. https://doi.org/10.1080/09273948.2017.1296579.
3. Ormerod LD, Skolnick KA, Menosky MM, Pavan PR, Pon DM. Retinal and choroidal manifestations of cat-scratch disease. Ophthalmology. 19986;105(6):1024–31. https://doi.org/10.1016/S0161-6420(98)96003-1.
4. Kalogeropoulos D, Asproudis I, Stefaniotou M, et al. Bartonella henselae- and quintana-associated uveitis: a case series and approach of a potentially severe disease with a broad spectrum of ocular manifestations. Int Ophthalmol. 2019;39(11):2505–15. https://doi.org/10.1007/s10792-019-01096-7.
5. Habot-Wilner Z, Trivizki O, Goldstein M, et al. Cat-scratch disease: ocular manifestations and treatment outcome. Acta ophthalmologica. 2018;96(4):e524–32. https://doi.org/10.1111/aos.13684.
6. Heston S, Arnold S. Syphilis in children. Infect Dis Clin North Am. 2018;32(1):129–44. https://doi.org/10.1016/j.idc.2017.11.007.
7. Baumal CR, Levin AV, Read SE. Cytomegalovirus retinitis in immunosuppressed children;1999.

8. Huppertz HI, Münchmeier D, Lieb W. Ocular manifestations in children and adolescents with Lyme arthritis. Br J Ophthalmol. 1999;83(10):1149–52. https://doi.org/10.1136/bjo.83.10.1149.
9. Kataria S, Trevathan GE, Holland JE, Kataria YP. Ocular presentation of sarcoidosis in children. Clin Pediatr (Phila). 1983;22(12):793–7. https://doi.org/10.1177/000992288302201201.
10. Turk MA, Hayworth JL, Nevskaya T, Pope JE. Ocular manifestations of Behçet's disease in children and adults: a systematic review and meta-analysis. Clin Exp Rheumatol. 39 Suppl 132(5):94–101. https://doi.org/10.55563/clinexprheumatol/pt60bc.
11. Koné-Paut I. Behçet's disease in children, an overview. Pediatric Rheumatol Online J. 2016;14(1): 10.https://doi.org/10.1186/s12969-016-0070-z.
12. Koreishi AF, Zhou M, Goldstein DA. Tubulointerstitial Nephritis and Uveitis syndrome: characterization of clinical features. Ocul Immunol Inflamm. 2021;29(7–8):1312–7. https://doi.org/10.1080/09273948.2020.1736311.
13. Trittibach P, Koerner F, Sarra GM, Garweg JG. Vitrectomy for juvenile uveitis: prognostic factors for the long-term functional outcome. Eye. 2006;20(2):184–90. https://doi.org/10.1038/sj.eye.6701845.
14. Soheilian M, Aletaha M, Yazdani S, Dehghan MH, Peyman GA. Management of pediatric Vogt-Koyanagi-Harada (VKH)-associated panuveitis. Ocul Immunol Inflamm. 2006;14(2):91–8. https://doi.org/10.1080/09273940600557001.
15. Giuliari GP, Chang PY, Thakuria P, Hinkle DM, Foster CS. Pars plana vitrectomy in the management of paediatric uveitis: the Massachusetts eye research and surgery Institution experience. Eye. 2010;24(1):7–13. https://doi.org/10.1038/eye.2009.294.
16. Khaja HA, McCannel CA, Diehl NN, Mohney BG. Incidence and clinical characteristics of epiretinal membranes in children. Arch Ophthalmol. 2008;126(5):632–6. https://doi.org/10.1001/archopht.126.5.632.
17. Yu EN, Paredes I, Foster CS. Surgery for hypotony in patients with juvenile idiopathic arthritis-associated uveitis. Ocul Immunol Inflamm. 2007;15(1):11–7. https://doi.org/10.1080/09273940601147729.
18. Mohan A, Kumar A, Sen P, Shah C, Jain E, Sen A. Outcome of surgical membranectomy with a vitrector via limbal approach for posterior capsular opacity in children. J Pediatr Ophthalmol Strabismus. 2020;57(1):33–8. https://doi.org/10.3928/01913913-20191112-01.
19. Xie LX, Zhang WB, Huang YS. The surgical treatment for posterior capsule opacification in children with pseudophakic eyes. Zhonghua Yan Ke Za Zhi. 2005;41(6):511–4.

Part IX

Approach to Cataract and the Crystalline Lens in Pediatric Retinal Surgery

To Preserve or Not to Preserve the Crystalline Lens

55

Hailey Robles-Holmes and Eric Nudleman

Abstract

Removal of the pediatric crystalline lens may be necessary due to lens opacity or for safe surgical access to the posterior pole. The major disadvantages of lensectomy include aphakic glaucoma and amblyopia. Therefore, it is recommended that the lens is preserved whenever possible. The most common circumstances for the pediatric retina specialist to consider lensectomy include advanced retinopathy of prematurity, persistent fetal vascular syndrome, and pediatric rhegmatogenous retinal detachments. Surgical techniques to preserve the lens, and to remove the lens when required, are reviewed.

Keywords

Lensectomy · Lens-sparing vitrectomy · Retinopathy of prematurity · Persistent fetal vascular syndrome · Pediatric rhegmatogenous retinal detachment

H. Robles-Holmes
University of Miami Miller School of Medicine, Miami, FL, USA
e-mail: hkr4@med.miami.edu

E. Nudleman (✉)
Shiley Eye Institute, Rady Children's Hospital, University of California, San Diego, La Jolla, CA, USA
e-mail: enudleman@health.ucsd.edu

Ş. Özdek et al. (eds.), *Pediatric Vitreoretinal Surgery*,
https://doi.org/10.1007/978-3-031-14506-3_55

Introduction

Removal of the pediatric crystalline may be required for two main reasons: (1) lens opacity or dislocation that obstructs vision, or (2) safe surgical access to the retina without causing iatrogenic retinal tears. Whenever possible, preservation of the lens is preferred. Advantages of preserving the lens include the avoidance of lensectomy complications such as aphakic glaucoma, amblyopia, monocular aphakia, and the need for additional surgery. On average, 15% of infants who undergo lensectomy develop aphakic glaucoma within five years of surgery [1, 2] and 51–83% of patients develop amblyopia within a year [3, 4]. Although good visual outcomes following lensectomy are possible, visual prognosis is often poor, especially in patients where the fellow eye remains phakic [3]. Conserving vision is dependent on timely screening and diagnosis which is difficult given the challenges of evaluating young children [5, 6]. In addition, aphakic glaucoma, amblyopia, and monocular aphakia are complications that may require surgery or lifelong medical management. Here we will review common circumstances relevant to the pediatric retina surgeon where preservation of the crystalline lens is favorable and where lensectomy is required.

Retinopathy of Prematurity

Advanced Retinopathy of Prematurity (ROP) is characterized by complete (Stage 5) or incomplete (Stage 4) retinal detachment that require incisional surgery for repair. Surgical options include lensectomy vitrectomy (LV), and lens-conserving procedures such as scleral buckling (SB) and lens-sparing vitrectomy (LSV). In general, surgical access to the posterior pole is possible with LSV for most stage 4A, some stage 4B, and rare stage 5 [7–11].

The primary goal of LSV to treat late-stage ROP is to eliminate tractional forces on the retina that result in retinal detachment. Successful anatomical outcomes of LSV when compared to alternatives such as SB and LV have been well established [12, 13]. Reattachment rates following LSV for stage 4 range from 74%–91% for Stage 4A [8, 12, 13], 62–92% for stage 4B [9, 14, 15], and 22–48% for stage 5 detachments [11, 16, 17]. Visual outcomes after LSV for Stage 4 ROP can be excellent, with letter reading vision reported in approximately 80% of Stage 4A eyes and 60% of Stage 4B eyes following LSV [8, 15, 18, 19]. Earlier surgery tends to improve anatomic outcomes for Stage 5, but functional expectations should remain guarded, with vision rarely achieving letter reading (for review, see Kychenthal and Dorta [20]).

The surgical approach for a LSV begins with entering the eye at the pars plicata, approximately 0.5 mm posterior to the limbus. Due to the proximity to the lens, attention to the vector of trocar insertion is critical to avoid lens trauma. The insertion of the trocar should be perpendicular to the iris plane, rather than pointed toward the center of the eye [10]. If using a trocar system, the cannula may be too

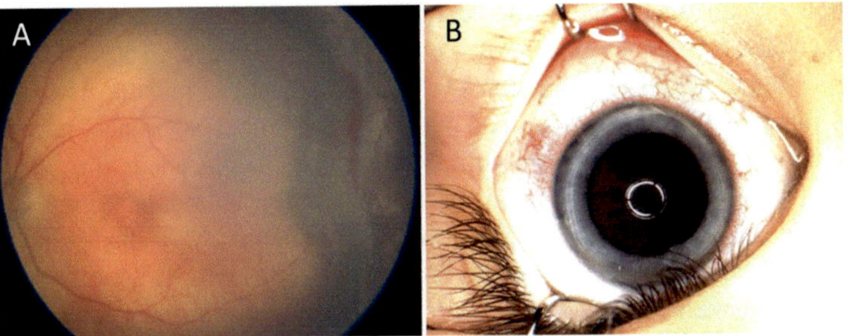

Fig. 55.1 Lens opacity following LSV. **A** Infant with Stage 4A ROP prior to 3-port LSV. **B** Two years after surgery, a mild posterior capsular opacity is evident temporally in the area where the trocars were placed, and the dissection was focused. The opacity was not in the visual axis, and the patient was observed

long to allow access to the far periphery in order to segment the peripheral fibrosis. Therefore, it may be helpful to either insert the instruments directly through the sclerotomies or to partially withdraw the cannulas for peripheral maneuvers. During the procedure, the attention is directed to segmenting vectors of traction. The location of the sclerotomies and the potential need for maneuvers in the anterior periphery creates significant risk of causing trauma to the peripheral lens. Unlike vitrectomy in adults, wherein cataract formation occurs due to the exposure of the lens to high levels of oxygen after surgery [21–23], the vitrectomy in infants is focused on relieving traction and the removal of vitreous is typically incomplete. Therefore, rather than the vitrectomy itself resulting in cataract formation, iatrogenic trauma as a consequence of operating in this tight space is the most common cause (Fig. 55.1).

Post-operative cataract following LSV occurs in up to 33% of infants and tends to occur within a year of surgery [24]. A severe cataract can be detrimental to the development of the infantile visual axis and therefore requires urgent attention. In general, lensectomy is recommended within 6 weeks of identified opacity that occludes the visual axis. This guideline is based on data from full-term infants with a unilateral congenital cataract, where there is no difference in the visual outcome when cataract surgery was performed within this latent period [25, 26].

The timing of cataract surgery must consider the risk of aphakic glaucoma, which is reduced with time. In the Infant Aphakia Treatment Study (IATS), the risk of glaucoma one year after surgery was reduced by 50% by delaying cataract surgery from 4 to 8 weeks of age [27]. The incidence of glaucoma was shown to be threefold higher if cataract surgery was performed when an infant was 4–6 weeks of age compared to 7 weeks–6 months of age [28]. This is particularly relevant for infants with ROP that develop lens opacity following LSV, since these opacities often develop eccentrically and slowly (Fig. 55.1). Similar to congenital cataract, lensectomy in eyes with a history of ROP increases the risk of glaucoma [29]. Hence, if a clear view of the posterior pole remains, it is preferable to continue to observe.

In cases of advanced retinal detachment or a poor view posterior to the lens, including stage 5 ROP, surgical space is limited and there is high risk of creating an iatrogenic break when entering the eye through the pars plicata. Therefore, the surgery must be performed though an anterior (translimbal) approach, necessitating a lensectomy. An inferotemporal infusion cannula is placed at the limbus and additional limbal incisions are made superonasally and superotemporally for instruments. The crystalline lens first incised with an MVR blade and is then aspirated with the vitrector. Once the nucleus and cortex have been removed, the attention is directed to the lens capsule. Preserving capsular support for potential secondary intraocular lens implantation in the future is not recommended, since residual capsule can serve as a scaffold for preretinal proliferation, circumferential vitreoretinal contraction, and hypotony. Even if the retina is detached to the level of the posterior lens capsule, stripping the capsule in its entirety can be done without significant risk to the underlying retina. The anterior capsule is grasped with forceps inserted through the paracentesis 180° away and pulled to release from the zonule. Once free, the forceps are inserted through the opposite side, released, and the capsule is removed in a single sheet through the paracentesis (Fig. 55.2). The surgeon may then proceed with anterior dissection of preretinal proliferative tissue.

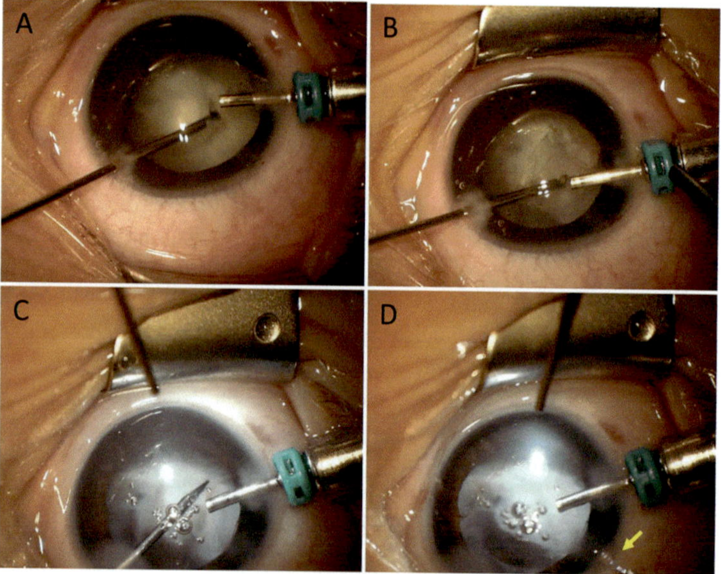

Fig. 55.2 Lensectomy in Stage 5 FEVR. **A** Following opening of the anterior capsule with an MVR blade, the vitrector is placed in the nucleus and **B** aspiration is used to perform the lensectomy. **C** Once the lens is removed, MaxGrip forceps are used to grasp the anterior capsule and release the capsule from the zonule. External illumination with the light pipe aids in visualization. **D** The capsule is released from the opposite side and removed through the sideport incision (arrow)

Persistent Fetal Vasculature Syndrome

Persistent Fetal Vasculature Syndrome (PFVS) is a developmental disease caused by the failed involution of the primary hyaloidal vasculature system during the second trimester. PFVS can result in tractional forces on the retina, ciliary body, and lens with highly variable visual morbidity. Clinical findings may include microphthalmos, shallow anterior chamber, hypotony, and tractional retinal detachment. The degree of and location of abnormal involution impacts the variability of the disease. Management is typically dependent on extent of disease. Broadly, PFVS can be categorized as anterior, posterior, or combined [30–33]. The goal of surgical intervention is to clear the visual axis and to release anterior–posterior traction. Earlier surgery has been reported to provide improved functional and cosmetic outcomes [34–36].

Mostly posterior PFVS with opacification that does not block the visual axis can be managed successfully with LSV [32, 35]. In such cases, it is critical to carefully examine the pars plana prior to insertion of the trocars, since there can be abnormalities of the anterior retina including traction from anterior branches of the stalk. Once a location for safe entry is confirmed, a standard 3-port setup is used. The goal of the vitrectomy is to segment the stalk posterior to the lens. The stalk is often vascularized, and the risk of bleeding increases the more posterior the stalk is transected. Once the stalk is freed, the anterior tip is cauterized with diathermy to prevent postoperative hemorrhage. A limited vitrectomy is then performed around the stalk to free any additional adhesions. Over time, the stalk often retracts with reduced traction on the retina (Fig. 55.3). If the lens is opacified within the visual axis, or there is any concern for a location to safely place the trocars, a translimbal approach is preferred. The strategy is similar to the LV for advanced ROP described above. In cases where the lens is clear, but the stalk is within the visual axis, it is possible to leave the peripheral anterior capsule to allow for the placement of a sulcus intraocular lens, especially in older children. Mostly anterior PFVS, however, can have a highly abnormal anterior segment including a shallow anterior chamber, posterior synechiae, and a dense fibrous membrane posterior to the lens

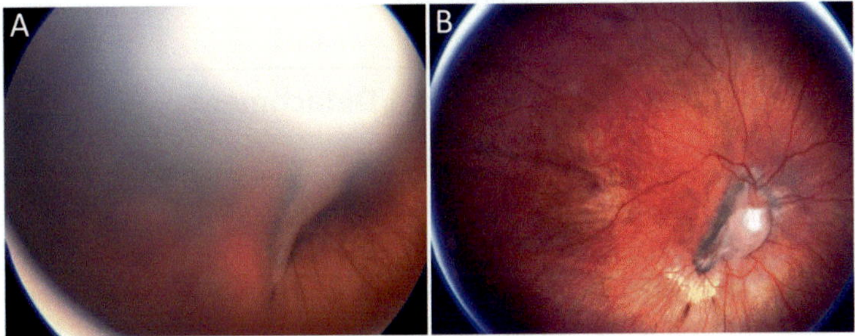

Fig. 55.3 Posterior PFVS. **A** Stalk with eccentric insertion into the posterior lens capsule. **B** One year following LSV and transection of the stalk anteriorly, the stalk retracted

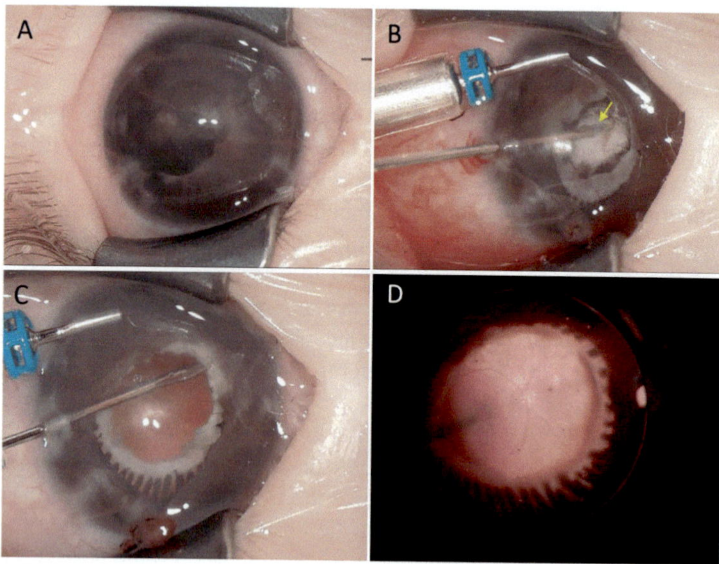

Fig. 55.4 Anterior PFVS. **A** This eye had a small cornea, shallow anterior chamber, secluded pupil, and a dense retrolental membrane. There was no stalk evident on B-scan ultrasonography. The fellow eye was normal. **B** After the iris was opened, the lens and capsule were removed, and the dense fibrous membrane was incised and extended with the vitrector (arrowhead). **C** Once the central plaque was cleared, the fibrosis was trimmed from the ciliary processes using horizontal scissors. **D** Following dissection, a limited vitrectomy was performed. The posterior pole had normal anatomy with only a small remnant of a stalk

capsule and adherent to the ciliary processes (Fig. 55.4). In these cases, once the iris is opened and the lens, capsule, and fibrous plaque are removed, there may be only a small remnant of a stalk from the optic nerve. With appropriate patching and fitting of an aphakic contact lens, anterior PFVS typically has better visual potential than mostly posterior PFVS [35, 36]. Very severe cases with combined anterior and posterior dysgenesis have a poor prognosis. In these cases, and in mild cases with no opacification distorting the visual axis, observation is appropriate.

Pediatric Rhegmatogenous Retinal Detachment

Pediatric rhegmatogenous retinal detachments occur most commonly due to inherited dystrophies (including Stickler syndrome), myopia, trauma, developmental anomalies, and previous intraocular surgery [37–40]. Unlike adult rhegmatogenous retinal detachments, children often present with chronic detachments, and the risk of proliferative vitreoretinopathy postoperatively is high. As a result, success rates are considerably lower than adults, with approximately 50% single surgery success, and 75% final reattachment rate [37, 38, 40–42]. It is not uncommon for patients to require multiple procedures to achieve successful reattachment. Additionally, functional outcomes are often poor, with most having final visual acuity worse than 20/200.

Surgical approach for these complex cases is often staged. In cases where a scleral buckle alone is possible, this is the ideal procedure [40, 43]. If a vitrectomy is necessary, either as an initial procedure or as a second procedure, silicone oil tamponade is often used due to the inability for children to reliably position. Silicone oil associated cataracts form in approximately 50–75% of eyes within 2 years after surgery [44]. If the retina remains attached after silicone oil removal, lensectomy can then be performed with placement of an intraocular lens. However, if repair of the retinal detachment is hindered by the presence of the crystalline lens due to anterior PVR, lensectomy and removal of the capsule may be necessary.

Case Scenario

A child was born at gestational age of 26 3/7 weeks, with a birthweight of 935 g. She had developed stage 3 ROP in zone 2 with plus disease and underwent ablative laser at a postmenstrual age of 40 4/7 weeks to both eyes. She had intravenous methylprednisolone during the procedure to prevent serous retinal detachment. Approximately 2000 spots were delivered to her left eye, and 5000 spots were delivered to the right eye. Postoperatively, she was using topical prednisolone acetate four times daily in both eyes. She was seen one week following the procedure. Her left eye had a clear view with regressing disease. In her right eye, the cornea was edematous, the anterior chamber was shallow, the lens was opacified, and there was a small hyphema. There was no view of the posterior pole. A B-scan ultrasound demonstrated an attached retina. The steroid drops were increased to hourly in the right eye, and the child was referred to a pediatric retina specialist with a diagnosis of anterior segment ischemia (Fig. 55.5). After 3 more weeks of frequent topical steroids, the cornea had cleared but the lens remained completely

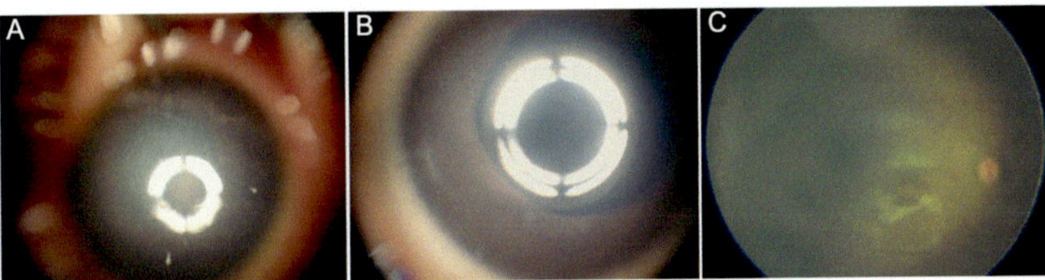

Fig. 55.5 Complete opacification of the lens. This child underwent laser for the treatment of type 1 ROP and developed anterior segment ischemia. The cornea is edematous, the anterior chamber is shallow, there is posterior synechiae, and there is no view of the posterior pole (**A**). Following 1 month of topical steroids, the cornea cleared but the lens remained unchanged. Lensectomy was performed with removal of the capsule (**B**). The retina was attached (**C**)

opacified. The decision was made to perform a lensectomy to clear the visual axis. At the time of the surgery, the anterior chamber was shallow and there was 360° of posterior synechiae. The lens and capsule were removed in their entirety, and an anterior vitrectomy was performed. During the surgery, the retina was attached with complete lasering of the avascular retina. Postoperatively, the cornea remained clear, the anterior chamber was formed, the iris was round and the retina attached. The child is now wearing an aphakic contact lens with undergoing patching therapy. Her intraocular pressure has remained normal, and she has developed normal visual behavior with her right eye.

Conclusion

Removing the pediatric lens can result in serious and irreversible sight-threatening complications. Whenever possible, it is ideal to use techniques to preserve the lens, including scleral buckle and lens sparing vitrectomy. When lensectomy is required due to opacity or for surgical access, most cases benefit from removing the lens and the capsule in their entirety. The pediatric retina surgeon must be prepared to work closely with an interdisciplinary team, including pediatric ophthalmologists and pediatric glaucoma specialists to manage common sequalae and to optimize the chances of a successful outcome.

Review Questions

1. The incidence of aphakic glaucoma following pediatric lensectomy within 5 years is:

A. 5%
B. 15%
C. 50%
D. 75%

2. It is recommended that a lens opacity that occludes the visual axis is removed within:

A. 1 week
B. 6 weeks
C. 3 months
D. 6 months

3. When removing the lens in an infant to safely access the posterior pole, the lens capsule should be:

A. Removed completely
B. Preserved, with placement of an IOL
C. Preserved to allow for potential subsequent placement of an IOL
D. Persevered to maintain a two chamber eye

Answers

1. B
2. B
3. A

References

1. Stech M, et al. Risk of aphakic glaucoma after pars plana-lensectomy with and without removal of the peripheral lens capsule. Eye. 2019;33:1472–7.
2. Chen TC, Walton DS, Bhatia LS. Aphakic Glaucoma after congenital cataract surgery. Arch Ophthalmol-chic. 2004;122:1819–25.
3. Repka MX, et al. Visual acuity and ophthalmic outcomes 5 years after cataract surgery among children younger than 13 years. Jama Ophthalmol. 2022;140:269–76.
4. Writing Committee for the PEDIG., et al. Visual acuity and ophthalmic outcomes in the year after cataract surgery among children younger than 13 years. Jama Ophthalmol. 2019;137:817–24.
5. Rabiah PK. Frequency and predictors of glaucoma after pediatric cataract surgery. Am J Ophthalmol. 2004;137:30–7.
6. Magnusson G, Abrahamsson M, Sjöstrand J. Glaucoma following congenital cataract surgery: an 18-year longitudinal follow-up. Acta Ophthalmol Scan. 2000;78:65–70.
7. Capone A, Trese MT. Lens-sparing vitreous surgery for tractional stage 4A retinopathy of prematurity retinal detachments. Ophthalmology. 2001;108:2068–70.
8. Hubbard GB, Cherwick DH, Burian G. Lens-sparing vitrectomy for stage 4 retinopathy of prematurity. Ophthalmology. 2004;111:2274–7.
9. Lakhanpal RR, Sun RL, Albini TA, Holz ER. Anatomic success rate after 3-port lens-sparing vitrectomy in stage 4A or 4B retinopathy of prematurity. Ophthalmology. 2005;112:1569–73.
10. Maguire AM, Trese MT. Lens-sparing vitreoretinal surgery in infants. Arch Ophthalmol. 1992;110:284–6.
11. Lakhanpal RR, Sun RL, Albini TA, Holz ER. Anatomical success rate after primary three-port lens-sparing vitrectomy in stage 5 retinopathy of prematurity. Retina. 2006;26:724–8.
12. Moshfeghi AA, Awner S, Salam GA, Ferrone PJ. Excellent visual outcome and reversal of dragging after lens sparing vitrectomy for progressive tractional stage 4a retinopathy of prematurity retinal detachment. Retina (Philadelphia, PA). 2004;24:615–6.
13. Bhende P, Gopal L, Sharma T, Verma A, Biswas RK. Functional and anatomical outcomes after primary lens-sparing pars plana vitrectomy for Stage 4 retinopathy of prematurity. Indian J Ophthalmol. 2009;57:267–71.
14. Choi J, Kim JH, Kim S-J, Yu YS. Long-term results of lens-sparing vitrectomy for stages 4B and 5 retinopathy of prematurity. Korean J Ophthalmol: KJO. 2011;25:305–10.
15. Rayes ENE, Vinekar A, Capone A. Three-year anatomic and visual outcomes after vitrectomy for stage 4B retinopathy of prematurity. Retina (Philadelphia, PA). 2008;28:568–72.

16. Cusick M, et al. Anatomical and visual results of vitreoretinal surgery for stage 5 retinopathy of prematurity. Retina. 2006;26:729–35.
17. Trese MT, Droste PJ. Long-term postoperative results of a consecutive series of stages 4 and 5 retinopathy of prematurity. Ophthalmology. 1998;105:992–7.
18. Lakhanpal RR, et al. Visual outcomes after 3-port lens-sparing vitrectomy in stage 4 retinopathy of prematurity. Arch Ophthalmol. 2006;124:675–9.
19. Prenner JL, Capone A, Trese MT. Visual outcomes after lens-sparing vitrectomy for stage 4A retinopathy of prematurity. Ophthalmology. 2004;111:2271–3.
20. Kychenthal A, Dorta P. A quick guide to pediatric retina. 2021. p. 91–8. https://doi.org/10.1007/978-981-15-6552-6_12.
21. Holekamp NM, Shui Y-B, Beebe DC. Vitrectomy surgery increases oxygen exposure to the lens: a possible mechanism for nuclear cataract formation. Am J Ophthalmol. 2005;139:302–10.
22. Shui Y-B, et al. The gel state of the vitreous and ascorbate-dependent oxygen consumption: relationship to the etiology of nuclear cataracts. Arch Ophthalmol. 2009;127:475–82.
23. Filas BA, Shui Y-B, Beebe DC. Computational model for oxygen transport and consumption in human vitreous. Invest Opthalmol Vis Sci. 2013;54:6549.
24. Nudleman E, et al. Long-term outcomes on lens clarity after lens-sparing vitrectomy for retinopathy of prematurity. Ophthalmology. 2015;122:755–9.
25. Birch EE, Stager DR. The critical period for surgical treatment of dense congenital unilateral cataract. Invest Ophth Vis Sci. 1996;37:1532–8.
26. Hartmann EE, Lynn MJ, Lambert SR, Infant Aphakia Treatment Study Group. Baseline characteristics of the infant aphakia treatment study population: predicting recognition acuity at 4.5 years of age. Invest Ophth Vis Sci. 2014;56:388–95.
27. Beck AD, et al. Glaucoma-related adverse events in the infant aphakia treatment study: 1-year results. Arch Ophthalmol-Chic. 2012;130:300–5.
28. Freedman SF, et al. Glaucoma-related adverse events in the first 5 years after unilateral cataract removal in the infant aphakia treatment study. Jama Ophthalmol. 2015;133:907–14.
29. Nudleman E, et al. Glaucoma after lens-sparing vitrectomy for advanced retinopathy of prematurity. Ophthalmology. 2017. https://doi.org/10.1016/j.ophtha.2017.11.009.
30. Walsh MK, Drenser KA, Capone A, Trese MT. Early vitrectomy effective for bilateral combined anterior and posterior persistent fetal vasculature syndrome. Retina (Philadelphia, PA). 2010;30:S2-8.
31. Zeydanlı EÖ, Tefon AB, Atalay HT, Özdek Ş. Pseudo-hyaloidal stalk in anterior persistent fetal vasculature: a report of two cases. Turkish J Ophthalmol. 2021;51:407–11.
32. Shaikh S, Trese MT. Lens-sparing vitrectomy in predominantly posterior persistent fetal vasculature syndrome in eyes with nonaxial lens opacification. Retina (Philadelphia, PA). 2003;23:330–4.
33. Hu A, et al. Combined persistent fetal vasculature: a classification based on high-resolution b-mode ultrasound and color doppler imaging. Ophthalmology. 2015. https://doi.org/10.1016/j.ophtha.2015.09.001.
34. Bosjolie A, Ferrone P. Visual outcome in early vitrectomy for posterior persistent fetal vasculature associated with traction retinal detachment. Retin. 2015;35:570–6.
35. Sisk RA, Berrocal AM, Feuer WJ, Murray TG. Visual and anatomic outcomes with or without surgery in persistent fetal vasculature. Ophthalmology. 2010;117:2178-83.e2.
36. Bata BM, et al. Long-term visual and anatomic outcomes following early surgery for persistent fetal vasculature: a single-center, 20-year review. J Am Assoc Pediatric Ophthalmol Strabismus. 2019;23(327):e1-327.e5.
37. Fivgas GD, Capone A. Pediatric rhegmatogenous retinal detachment. Retina. 2001;21:101–6.
38. Gonzales CR, et al. Pediatric rhegmatogenous retinal detachment: clinical features and surgical outcomes. Retina. 2008;28:847–52.

39. Weinberg DV, Lyon AT, Greenwald MJ, Mets MB. Rhegmatogenous retinal detachments in children: risk factors and surgical outcomes. Ophthalmology. 2003;110:1708–13.
40. Smith JM, et al. Rhegmatogenous retinal detachment in children clinical factors predictive of successful surgical repair. Ophthalmology. 2019;126:1263–70.
41. Soheilian M., et al. Clinical features and surgical outcomes of pediatric rhegmatogenous retinal detachment. Retina. 2009;29:545–51.
42. Read SP, et al. Retinal detachment surgery in a pediatric population. Retina. 2018;38:1393–402.
43. Errera M-H, Liyanage SE, Moya R, Wong SC, Ezra E. Primary scleral buckling for pediatric rhegmatogenous retinal detachment. Retina. 2015;35:1441–9.
44. Scott IU, et al. Silicone oil in the repair of pediatric complex retinal detachments: a prospective, observational, multicenter study. None of the authors has a financial or proprietary interest in SILIKON 1000. Ophthalmology. 1999;106:1399–408.

General Guidelines for Lens Surgery at Pediatric Age

56

Serena Wang and Nallely Morales-Mancillas

Abstract

Timing is everything in congenital cataract treatment. Timely surgery, refractive correction, and amblyopia management are the critical aspects to minimize vision loss and maximize vision gain in childhood cataract management. Individualized surgical design, minimal invasive technique, proper intraocular lens selection, and reduction of complications are important intraoperative considerations. Postoperative care and long-term visual rehabilitation are important follow up to surgery to achieve best visual outcomes. Understanding "critical periods" of developmental biology for vision, as understood from experimental basic science, is essential in the management off treatable and preventable vision, loss diseases in children.

Keywords

Childhood cataract · Cortical periods, lensectomy, aphakia, intraocular lens · Surgical planning · Visual rehabilitation

Supplementary Information The online version contains supplementary material available at https://doi.org/10.1007/978-3-031-14506-3_56.

S. Wang (✉) · N. Morales-Mancillas
UT Southwestern Medical Center, Dallas, TX, USA
e-mail: serena.wang@utsouthwestern.edu

Introduction

Childhood cataract is one of the leading treatable causes of visual impairment in children worldwide [1, 2]. Children are different from adults. They are a unique population, have different anatomical structure, physiology, psychology, and even differ among age groups. In short, the visual deficit caused by cataracts in children occurs in the context of developmental biology, while cataracts in adults occur in senescent biology. Further because of this partially understood developmental biology, unilateral congenital cataracts have different consequences for vision than bilateral congenital cataracts. Cataract surgery in an adult, for example, will restore reduced visual acuity, but in a child it may mean restoring vision in an older child, allowing a normal visual (brain) development in a child younger than five, or having a chance to be able to see in a newborn.

A cataract blurs the image received by the retina and disrupts the development of the visual pathways in the central nervous system in a young child, and the younger the child the more the potential impact. The timing of surgery is very important and even critical in infant cataract to give the child a chance to develop normal vision. The surgical technique, the choice of aphakic, pseudophakia, refractive correction, and amblyopia management are of utmost importance in achieving good and long-lasting results [3].

Critical Periods

As mentioned, one of the fundamental concepts in the management of pediatric pathologies and treatment is the necessity of understanding developmental biology as the scaffold on which optimal outcomes depend. Management of congenital cataract is a classic example of this benefit. Adaption of therapies informed by developmental biology has transformed the pathology of congenital cataract from an irremediable cause of lifelong blindness into a preventable cause of visional impairment.

In the 1960s work on the postnatal feline visual cortex by David Hubel and Torsten Wiesel beget the idea of an early critical period, or time threshold, in the development of vision that was demonstrated by simultaneous structural changes in the visual cortex. This seminal work and subsequent clinical application have led to general hypotheses of the development of vision.

- First, there is a short period of time that is critical for connections to the visual cortex from the eye to develop. Structurally normal visual cortex is represented as some connections from each eye separately as well as a predominance of bilateral (binocular) cells. This critical period is both progressive and limited to about the first couple of months. If visual image is deprived to an eye, these connections are decreased or absent. Correction of profound deficit after the critical period produces no improvement of visual effect or connections. Early experience is critical in neurodevelopment.

- Second, competition between eyes and representative visual cortex occurs from or near the start of the critical time for light perception. If only one eye is deprived, the critical time for visual development for that eye is shortened as both eyes compete for dominance. The deprived eye's cortical structure and functionality is limited by both the deprivation of developmental stimulation and the fellow eye competition.
- Third, the competition between the visual cortex for dominance of vision starts in and continues beyond the critical time of establishment of visual connections between the eye and cortex. Forced use of the less developed eye by deprivation of the better eye can reverse the competitive loss of connections and vision of the partially deprived eye. This time period for rehabilitation starts but extends beyond the critical period for initial connections for light perception likely into early childhood.

Due to the above overlay of multiple factors of normal visual development it is difficult, but not impossible, to completely restore to normal vision in the pediatric patient. Unlike in the adult population where removal of a cataract and correction of refraction produces a likelihood of normal vision, in congenital cataracts management there are many causes of hysteresis or lag in correction. None the less an understanding of these developmental insights has propelled modern congenital cataract management into the arena of preventable visual impairment (Table 56.1).

Table 56.1 Critical periods for visual development [4, 5]

1 **Visual deprivation**	**2** **Interocular competition**	**3** **Visual Rehabilitation**
• Short period of time that is critical for to **connections to the visual cortex from the eye** to develop. • Progressive and limited to the **first couple of months**. • If visual image is deprived an eye, these connections are decreased or absent.	• Occurs from or near the **start of the critical time for light perception.** • The deprived eye's cortical structure and functionality is limited by both the deprivation of developmental stimulation and the fellow eye competition.	• Forced use of the less developed eye by deprivation of the better eye **can reverse the competitive loss of connections and vision of the partially deprived eye.** • Extends beyond the critical period into **early childhood**.

Indeed, it was only in early 1980s when Creig Hoyt and Elwin Marg showed that early removal (1–41 days) of dense unilateral cataract in a series of eight infants could lead to near normal or normal vision [6]. Shortly afterward Richard Held described further recovery of large visual deficit with rehabilitation by occlusion of the fellow eye after unilateral early cataract removal [7].

A decade and a half later Eileen Birch and David Stager collaborated in Dallas to show a composite of reported results that help define the expectations of current surgery for congenital cataract. Their main findings are presented graphically [8, 9].

In Fig. 56.1, though there is a wide scatter, near normal (0.3 logMAR) vision can be achieved anytime within the first 6 weeks of age by removal of dense unilateral cataract. Delay of surgery precipitates a doubling of the eventual visual deprivation for every doubling of age per six weeks. The decline in vision is steep if surgery is delayed such that by 1-year little improvement can expected. They describe this curve as Bilinear/Early Window in that plotted in log coordinates shows an initial "early window" in which a flat or stable favorable window of time result from surgery after which there is rapid visual loss linearly [9].

In contrast for bilateral congenital cataracts the log visual acuity verse age of surgery (Fig. 56.2) falls linearly from near normal at birth to about 0.6 logMAR at about 14 weeks where visual acuity "plateaus" even if further delay in surgery [11].

Incidentally at about 6 weeks or end of the critical and early window, the average visual acuity from early surgery for bilateral congenital cataracts passes through the same visual acuity (0.3 logMAR) of the flat portion of the unilateral cataract curve. This suggests that similar causal effects are happening initially to the immediate post-natal inexperienced eye whether the initial experience is unilateral [8, 9] or bilateral [11].

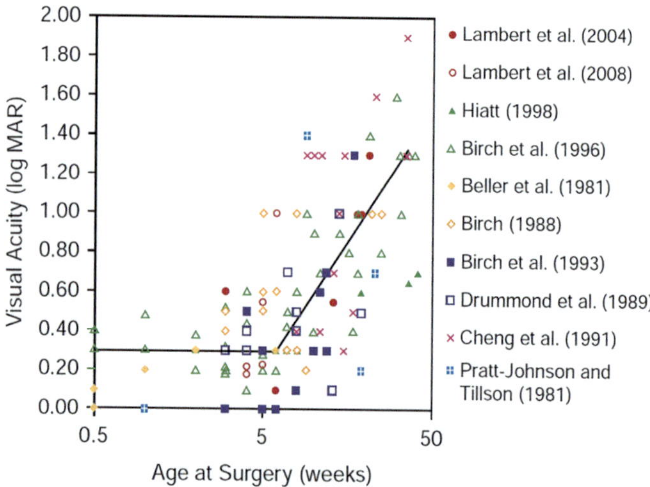

Fig. 56.1 Best-fit model of the critical period for development with visual deprivation due to congenital unilateral cataract based on the data from Birch and Stager [10]. (Wilson ME, Trivedi RH. Pediatric Cataract Surgery: Techniques, Complications and Management. Lippincott Williams & Wilkins, Chap. 6, page 49; 2014)

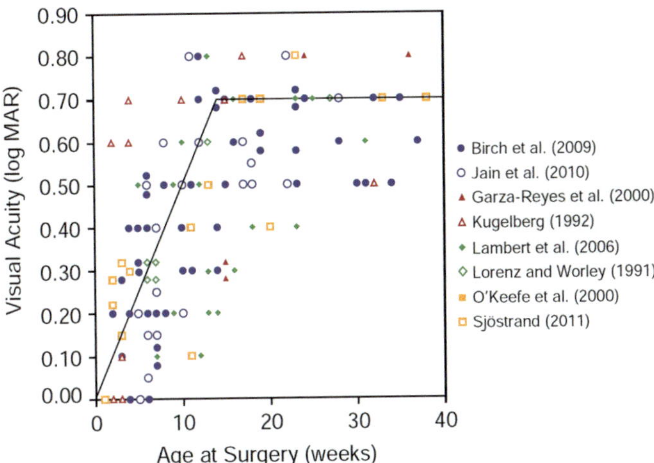

Fig. 56.2 Best-fit model of the critical period for development with visual deprivation due to congenital bilateral cataract based on the data from Birch et al. [10]. (Wilson ME, Trivedi RH. Pediatric Cataract Surgery: Techniques, Complications and Management. Lippincott Williams & Wilkins, Chap. 6, page 50; 2014)

However, soon or by six weeks the deprived eye in unilateral cataract also suffers not only the initial deprivation, but the superior competition of the normal fellow eye which prevents further development of the surgically restored eye. Published data confirms that measured visual acuity in both unilateral and bilateral cataract eyes are similar for early surgery but diverge worsening for the unilateral cataract eye with delay. This intraocular competition effect also provides a ready explanation for the salutary effects of the dominate fellow eye occlusion for rehabilitation of the surgically restored but still "weak" eye. If surgery for unilateral dense cataract is done early enough to allow for some input in the early window time frame for the surgically treated eye, then contra lateral occlusion of the fellow eye allows for improved development of the surgical eye by inhibition of the competition from the fellow eye.

Amblyopia

Amblyopia should always be considered in the management of children with a condition that vision is affected. Preventing and actively treating amblyopia are the principal essential elements to successful visual outcomes in the management of pediatric cataracts [12]. Even with technically successful surgery without a prompt initiation of optical correction and treatment of amblyopia, the visual outcome may be dismal, especially in very young unilateral cases. As described by Leinfelder a condition of "congenital amblyopia" in children with congenital cataracts and poor

Table 56.2 Types of amblyopia in pediatric cataract

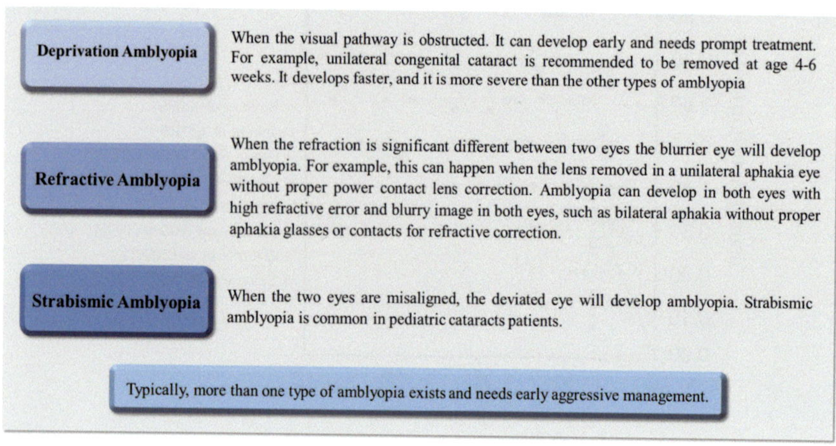

vision results after lens removal [13]. It was once even debatable if surgical management of unilateral congenital cataracts was advisable [14].

Amblyopia caused by congenital or acquired cataracts or any visual pathway obstruction in amblyogenic age can cause a complex of amblyopia. Table 56.2 [12, 15, 16].

Amblyopia therapy remains critical in the rehabilitation of unilateral cataract patients. Occlusion of the sound eye remains the main treatment [17]. Optical blur and atropine penalization is less effective in this type of amblyopia. Unilateral cataracts require a substantial amount of occlusion to obtain a good visual outcome. A randomized clinical trial (IATS 2A) found that 6 hours of occlusion achieves the same visual outcome as the occlusion of all but 1 waking hour when treating severe amblyopia (20/100 to 201/400) in patients under seven years of age [18].

New binocular amblyopia treatments have been described, such as pieoptic training, perceptual learning, binocular dichoptic training, and contrast-rebalanced binocular games. It has been described that contrast-rebalanced binocular games may improve visual acuity in patients with amblyopia. Birch et al. recently published a pilot randomized trial testing the contrasted-binocular iPad game in children with unilateral deprivation amblyopia. They found a visual acuity improvement after 8 weeks of treatment, suggesting that some binocular connections are intact in patients who had unilateral deprivation [19].

In summary, for children, especially very young children with visually significant cataract, it is important to promptly remove the visual obstructing pathology and to begin immediate optical refraction with amblyopia treatment to achieve successful visual outcomes. Successful cataract surgery should be followed by adequate adherence to amblyopia therapy. Parents should be counseled, even before surgery, on the importance of amblyopia treatment (Table 56.3).

Table 56.3 Amblyopia summary

- Remove the cause of visual obstruction.
- Early correction of refractive error and continue monitoring the refractive changes with the appropriate adjustment of glasses and/or contact lenses.
- Early initiation of patch treatment.

Surgery Planning

Pediatric cataract surgery planning is a complex issue. Surgery itself is just a first step on the long journey to establish the ability to see and to continue growth with good visual function to eventually achieve good vision. Considerable and continued effort throughout childhood, especially in very young children, mirrors the time frame of the development of normal visual acuity. There are many factors to consider when planning surgery. These factors are: when to operate, what type of surgery, with or without intraocular lens placement, with or without posterior capsulotomy, and anterior vitrectomy. Immediate post operative optical refractive correction and amblyopia management plan requires long term commitments of patient, family and surgeon. There isn't one plan that will fit every child, and continual modification is often required. Generally, patient age, laterality of the cataract, and resource of rehabilitation after surgery are the important factors to consider in surgical planning [1, 3, 20].

When to Do Surgery?

For congenital visually significant cataract, prompt cataract removal is critical. Generally, the younger the child and denser the cataract, the earlier removal of the cataract is necessary. For unilateral congenital cataract removal is recommended at 4–6 weeks [8, 9, 21]. For bilateral congenital cataracts up to 10 weeks is acceptable.

Surgery time between two eyes should be within 1–2 weeks if not done under the same anesthetic [11, 22, 23].

Lens opacity of size >3 mm is considered visually significant; however, it is also affected by the type of cataract and location of the opacity. Typically, the more posterior location and the more central of the opacity, the more visually significant and more amblyogenic the cataract is [24]. It can be difficult to decide if the cataract has caused significant visual obstruction in young and nonverbal children. In addition to slit lamp examination, red reflexes in the un-dilated pupil with retinoscopy and the distortion of the streak on retinoscopy are very important tools to help assess if the cataract is visually significant. It is important to keep in mind to not sacrifice normal youthful accommodation by too aggressive timing unless the visual disturbance is significant. In pediatric patients, especially of amblyogenic age, decision-making can be critical to avoid unnecessary iatrogenic risk of lifelong visual impairment by removal of less significant cataracts. This must be balanced with the conservative approach of not removing a cataract that is significant to visual acuity development. There isn't one recommendation that can fit all. Indeed, it is often not clear what any individual patient most needs. It is a very individual-based decision and plan for each child. The lifelong visual development needs to be carefully considered, especially in the amblyogenic age up to 5 [10].

For older children less likely to develop amblyopia, it is important to evaluate if the child's vision acuity is impaired and their visual needs. Generally, cataract surgery is recommended if Snellen visual acuity (VA) is 20/50 or worse [10].

If a partial cataract is being treated conservatively, it is important to carefully follow these children. Not all cataracts in childhood required surgical intervention either immediately or ever. Sometimes the use of mydriatic drops may be kept in reserve for eyes with slowly progressive cataracts or paracentral cataracts <3 mm, especially, in patients for whom cataract surgery needs to be deferred for any reasons, such as, medical (high risk for anesthesia), social, or economical. There is little reason to recommend long term mydriatic therapy [10, 15, 20, 25].

What Type of Surgery?

Even though intraocular lens (IOL) implant in children is still labeled as an "off-label" use by Food and Drug Administration (FDA), IOL is widely used or considered "standard care" for children older than 2 years. For infants younger than 7 months generally no intraocular lens (IOL) is recommended, according to IATS study [26]. The Infant Aphakia Treatment Study (IATS) is a randomized, multi-center, clinical trial to compare the use of IOL versus contact lenses in patients with congenital unilateral cataract aged between 1–6 months. Cataract extraction with anterior vitrectomy is the preferred surgery in patients with bilateral congenital cataract. For unilateral cataract, however, dependent on other management factors (such as the availability of aphakia contact lens, readily access to continuing care, family support, etc.), some surgeons may choose an IOL placement. Cataract extraction with or without IOL, posterior capsulotomy, and anterior vitrectomy is recommended for children younger than 5 years [26–31].

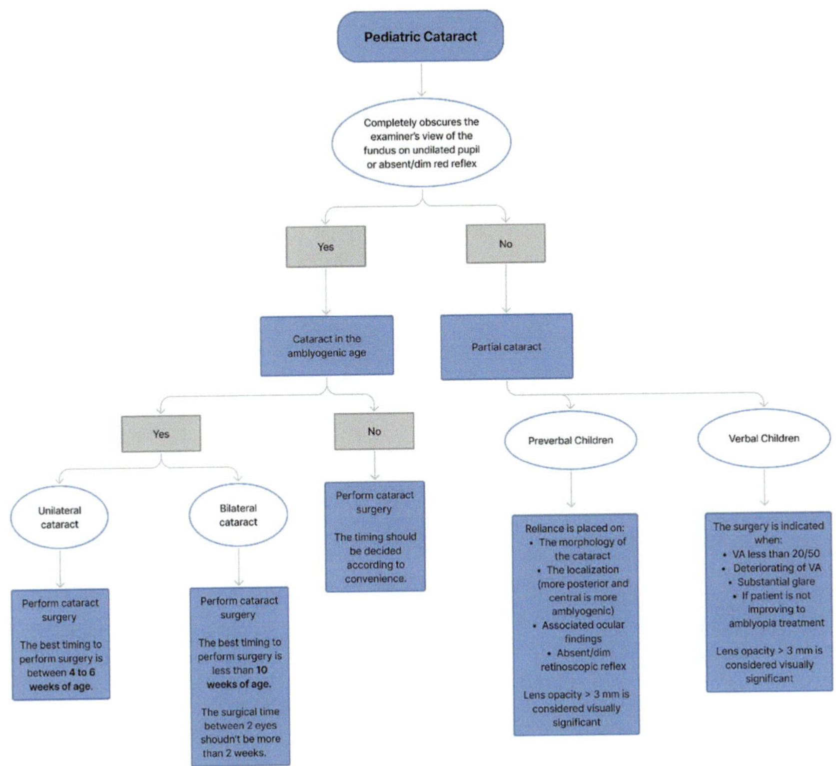

Flowchart 1 When to perform pediatric cataract surgery?

The use of IOL in pediatric cataract surgery has appropriately lagged that of adults as the device needs to last a lifetime. Surgeons cannot tell in the short and intermediate term what problems may accrue over a three or four score time frame. Older children seem to respond to IOL much as do adults, but younger children and particularly infants have proved less receptive to the devices. IOL in infants are technically more difficult to perform, and subsequent complications are more common. This has improved with both modified techniques and implants. However, with infants and younger children visual axis opacification (VAO) is higher in the pseudophakic eye than the aphakic eye. Reoperations are significantly more common in the pseudophakic group mostly for reproliferation and pupillary membranes in the visual axis [26].

Nonetheless IOL, especially in the unilateral cataract, offers some compelling advantages for visual rehabilitation in the infant. In many patients, corrective refraction by contact lens or glasses are either poorly tolerated or logistically difficult for infant caregivers. IOL offers the expectation of some partial AND continuous refraction compared to an aphakic eye. The pseudophakic eye, therefore, is likely less amblyogenic than an aphakic one. Most surgeons venture into IOL insertion in a subset of their unilateral cataract patients by age 6 months and some

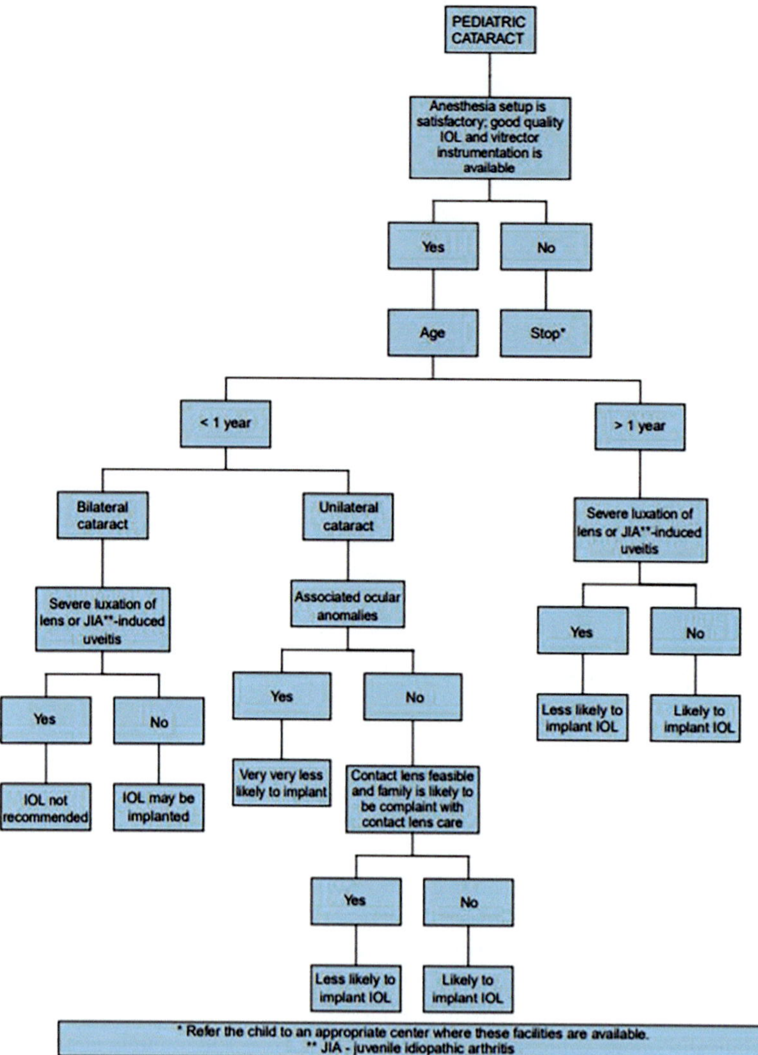

Figure 25.5. Flow diagram of our current considerations when determining whether or not to offer an IOL as treatment for a child with a cataract.

Flowchart 2 chart from the book by Wilson ME, Trivedi RH "*Pediatric Cataract Surgery: Techniques, Complications and Management*". Page 164. Current considerations when determining whether or not to offer an IOL as treatment for a child with a cataract [10]

do so earlier. In bilateral cataract patients, because both eyes have largely the same limitations and competition from the fellow eye is much less likely, the potential advantages of earlier IOL implantation may be less enticing than the potential complications also present in the younger cohorts [23].

How to Do Surgery?

I. Examination under anesthesia

General anesthesia is required for pediatric cataract surgery. While under general anesthesia the first step is a thorough examination of both eyes:

(1) Check intraocular pressure (IOP) during the induction of anesthesia. Anesthetic agents may lower IOP [32].
(2) Slit lamp examination of anterior segment, measure the cornea diameter
(3) Detailed fundus examination
(4) Biometry (keratometry and contact or immersion A-scan ultrasonography) IOL or contact lens power calculations
(5) Refraction if it is needed.
    In older children biometry can be obtained pre-operatively using non-contact biometry (e.g. IOL Master) if it is available [33, 34] (Fig. 56.3).

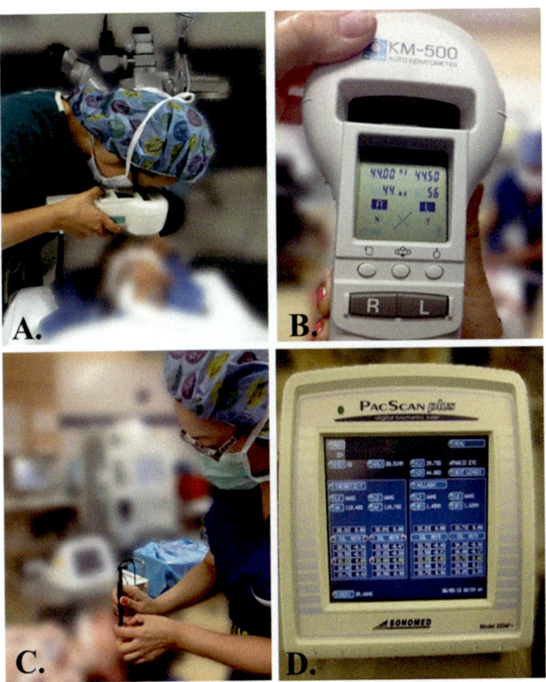

Fig. 56.3 **A** and **B**. Handheld automated keratometer (Nidek Km-500) **C** and **D**. A-Scan ultrasonography (PacScan Plus)

II. Surgical technique

    A. Cataract extraction without Intraocular Lens Implantation
       Bimanual technique is the most common used when IOL is not implanted. Using two small corneal/limbal incisions with 20-, 23-, or 25 gauge blades, make sure the incision size is the same as the vitrector and irrigation tip to ensure tight fitting wounds. Anterior capsular opening can be done with a manual capsulorrhexis, or with a vitrectomy cutter, a vitrectorhexis technique. This is followed by irrigation and aspiration to sweep clean the lens material and followed by posterior capsulotomy and anterior vitrectomy. Posterior capsulotomy size should be slightly smaller than the anterior capsulotomy for better fusion of the capsular edges to block the rejuvenated lens material from reaching the visual center. Anterior vitrectomy should be "generous" to help prevent secondary membrane formation [35] (Figs. 56.4, 56.5, 56.6 and 56.7).

    B. Cataract extraction with Intraocular Lens Implantation
       If IOL implantation is planned, either bimanual or single incision techniques can be used. Although vitrectorrhexis is preferred by some surgeons for very young children, manual anterior capsulorrhexis is the usual technique for the anterior capsular management [36, 37]. When removing the cortical material it is very important to carefully "polish" the lens capsule to minimize lens epithelial cell re-proliferation [38, 39]. A 23g vitrectomy is now commonly used, and 25g used by some, enabling aspiration of adherent lens matter through smaller incisions [40]. However, 20g vitrectomy cutters are still used by some pediatric surgeons for its efficiency, especially in cases with very dense cataracts or capsular plaques. In a single incision technique, a 2.5 mm Keratome is used for the cornea/limbal incision. An infusion sleeve is placed on the 20g vitrector for irrigation and anterior chamber stabilization.
       It is essential to remove the central posterior capsule (PC) and anterior vitrectomy in young children up to 5 years and optional for children 5-8

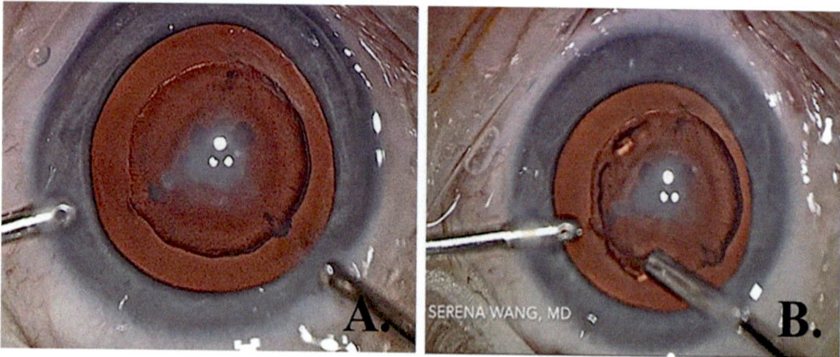

Fig. 56.4 **A.** Bimanual technique separate irrigation and aspiration port. **B.** Anterior capsular vitreorhexis

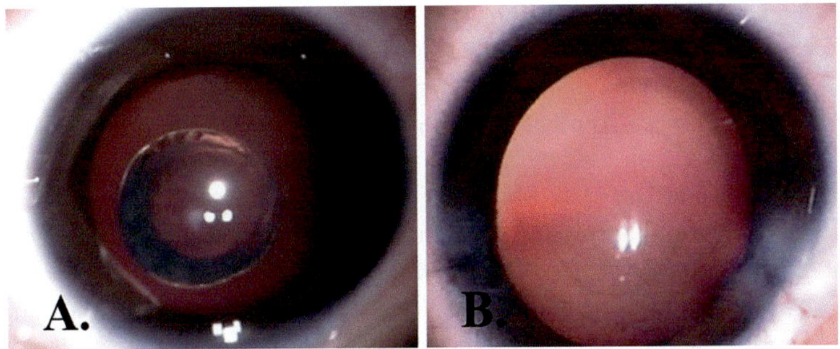

Fig. 56.5 6-month-old with posterior lenticonus. Before (**A**) and After (**B**) lensectomy and anterior vitrectomy

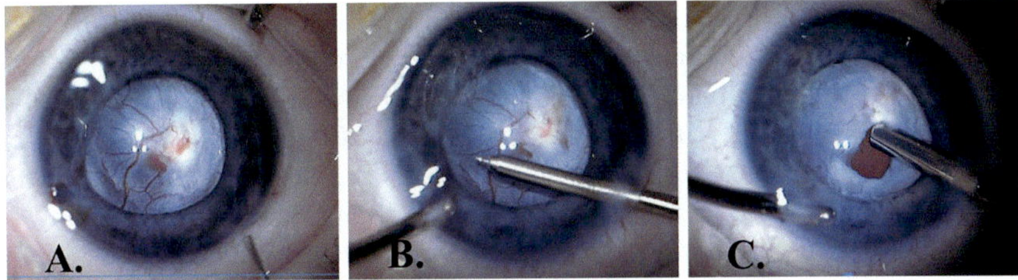

Fig. 56.6 **A**. Bimanual technique for PFV cataract removal. **B**. Cauterize the blood vessels on the posterior capsule. **C**. Posterior capsulotomy with a vitrector

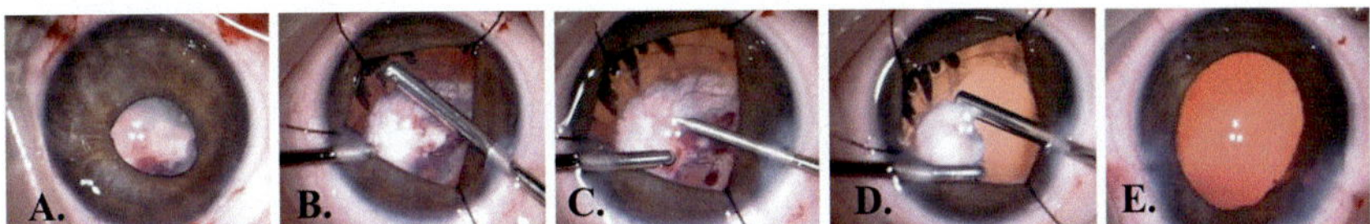

Fig. 56.7 Bimanual technique for PFV cataract removal **A** and **B**. Lens material removal. **C**. Cauterize the blood vessels on the posterior capsule. **D**. Removal of the fibrovascular membrane with a vitrector. **E**. After PFV removal

years due to the significant risk of re-opacification. This should also be considered in older children with developmental delay, poor cooperation, and where outpatient Nd:YAG capsulotomy may not be feasible [41–43].

   i. Cataract extraction with Intraocular Lens Implantation, posterior capsulotomy and anterior vitrectomy
With a bimanual technique, the corneal wound is enlarged to 2.5 mm prior to insertion of the foldable one-piece IOL or 3.5 mm for a 3-piece foldable IOL using an injection or folding technique.

A commonly used approach in the USA, as in the IATS study [26], is an IOL implanted into the intact bag. The corneal wounds are closed, and then pars plana posterior capsulotomy and anterior vitrectomy are performed. Another common approach is manual posterior capsulorrhexis, followed by anterior vitrectomy and insertion of IOL into the capsular bag [10]. My (SW) preferred technique is vitrector automated posterior capsulotomy, anterior vitrectomy, and injection of an IOL in the capsular bag. Other techniques include prior in the bag IOL insertion immediately after lensectomy, followed by lifting up of the IOL and automated posterior capsulotomy and anterior vitrectomy.

The amount of vitreous needed to be removed cannot be measured. Sufficient vitreous should be removed centrally so that the vitreous face cannot be used by the lens epithelial cells as a scaffolding to create VAO [10] Any vitreous above the plane of the posterior capsulectomy needs to be removed. Intracameral triamcinolone [44, 45] can be used to visualize vitreous strands. Optic capture, a positioning of the IOL optic through the posterior capsulotomy, is preferred by some surgeons as it provides great stability and reduces PC opacification [10, 46, 47]. Optic capture, especially in cases such as traumatic cataract when the integrity of the anterior and/or posterior capsulorrhexis/capsulotomy is compromised, may be useful [48, 49] (Figs. 56.8 and 56.9).

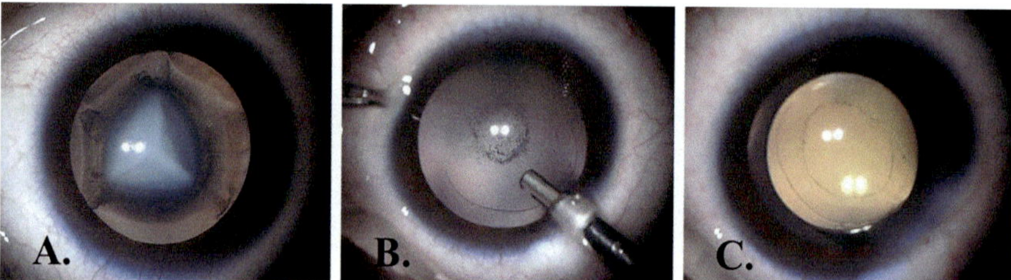

Fig. 56.8 **A.** Central fetal nuclear cataract. **B.** Posterior capsular defect noticed after lens material removal. **C.** IOL in the bag after posterior capsulotomy and anterior vitrectomy

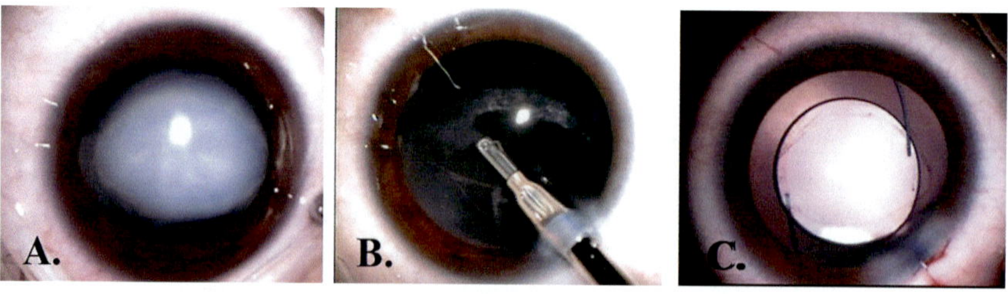

Fig. 56.9 **A.** Posterior lentiglobus with a large posterior capsular defect. **B.** Posterior capsule defect. **C.** 3-piece IOL placed in sulcus

ii. Cataract extraction with Intraocular Lens Implantation, without posterior capsulotomy and anterior vitrectomy

For older children (age 5–8) who are cooperative without complex medical conditions and when Nd:YAG laser is available, posterior capsulotomy can be safely performed in an office setting. It is unnecessary to open the posterior capsular during the IOL implantation.

In all cases a less traumatic surgical technique is especially important to reduce postoperative intraocular inflammation. Near tight-fitting instrumentation matching the size of surgical incisions helps maintain a stable anterior chamber in which to work. Limiting the entries and exits into the anterior chamber to the least necessary further reduces surgical trauma. These are some of the important keys to modern minimally invasive eye surgery (Fig. 56.10).

C. Most commonly used IOL in children

According to a worldwide survey of 329 pediatric cataract surgeons conducted in 2007 AcrySof hydrophobic acrylic IOL (Alcon Laboratories, Inc.) were the preferred IOLs. A 1-piece AcrySof IOL was preferred for in-the-bag implantation, and 3-piece for sulcus fixation [50].

Currently the cutting-edge premium or multifocal IOLs are rarely used in children because the refractive shift that occurs in growing eyes makes this impossible to predict precise refractive outcomes.

D. Wound closure

It is necessary to suture close all the wounds for pediatric cataract surgery. Typically using 10/0 polyglactin (Vicryl) [51], a self-absorbing suture is

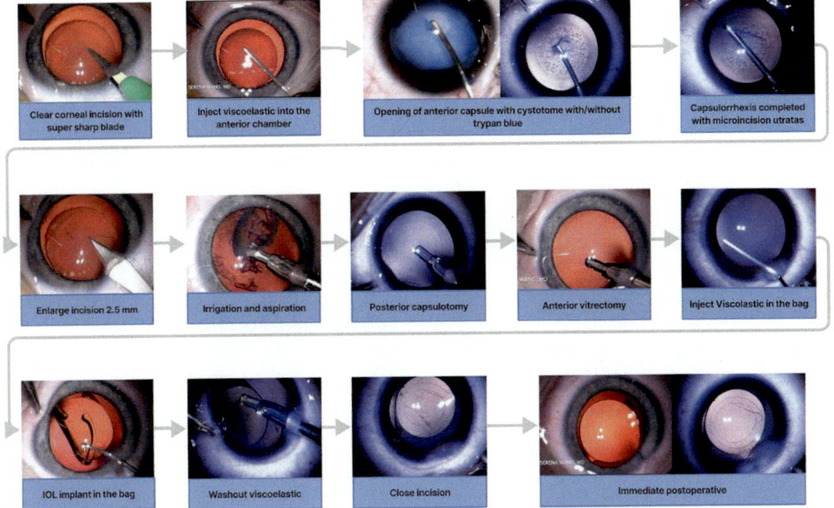

Fig. 56.10 Step by step single incision cataract extraction with Intraocular Lens Implantation, posterior capsulotomy anterior vitrectomy

used, to avoid removal. Closure is followed by subconjunctival injection of antibiotics and steroids. Some surgeons prefer intracameral injection of cefuroxime [52] and either subconjunctival or intracameral steroids.

Surgical summary

There are different effective techniques in pediatric cataract surgery. Surgeons should understand the importance of the essential steps. Variations of techniques and patient presentation can affect the outcome significantly despite common themes. Surgeons should be comfortable with a variety of techniques and choose the way in which surgery is managed for each patient based on the multiple factors unique to each patient. This also prepares the surgeon to devise the most efficient plan for the patient and patient's caregivers.

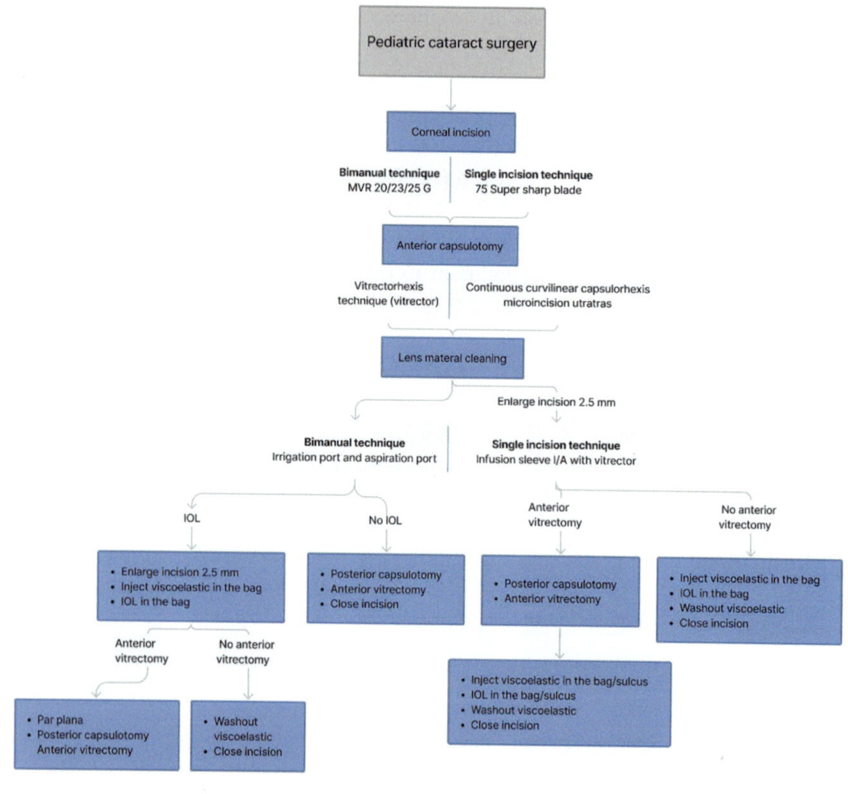

Flowchart 3 How to perform pediatric cataract surgery?

IOL Power Selection

The correct power IOL to implant into a growing changing eye can be a challenging decision, especially in very young children and in unilateral cases. This decision, too, depends particularly on the developmental understanding of interocular competition. Another important factor is the trend of myopic shift in aphakia and pseudophakic eyes. When targeting postoperative refractive condition close to emmetropic at the time of surgery, due to this myopic drift the child may have high myopia later but will have less amblyopia due to more equal interocular competition initially. If on the other hand, cataract surgery leaves the child with significant anisometropia, high or even low, the induced refractive amblyopia may be very difficult to treat.

In bilateral cataracts with similar visual acuity targeting mild, moderate, or even a marked amount of hypermetropia is reasonable, especially in very young children as both eyes are equal competitively. In bilateral implants there is more room for error for higher post surgical myopia that is part of normal growth which is accelerated by removal of the highly accommodative native early childhood lens. There are several nomograms have been published in the literature to assist with the selection of IOL power. Nevertheless, strict reliance on such nomograms is not advised as it is very important to make decision individually on each patient's particular condition based on many variables factors such as age, laterality [one eye or both], amblyopia status [dense or mild], resource availability to the patient (accessibility to eye care) the compliance with glasses, and family history of high myopia among other peculiar factors of each patient. It is better to error toward better vision with less amblyopia at younger age even if later the patient may have high myopia or need IOL exchange. Visual acuity, and its corrective options, is usually better later when myopia occurs, rather than having planned for a later small refractive error but forced to deal with a dense refractive amblyopia earlier [53, 59].

In theory, minimal refractive error at the time of surgery and maintenance of a minimal refractive error later on would be ideal. This may more often require IOL exchange later on and multiple procedures may needed. For this reason, most surgeons defer IOL implant if cataract removal is required in the very young patient. More surgeons pursue earlier IOL implantation for the unilateral cataract patient after lensectomy, but institutional and practitioner biases complicate any general recommendation (Table 56.4).

Parent Counseling

It is extremely important to have good patent counseling for pediatric cataract surgery. Lengthy discussions between the parents/caregivers and the surgeon are usually necessary. The better the parents/caregivers understand the nature of the problem and the needs for dedicated long term efforts, the more committed they partner for better visual outcomes. This process will also help surgeons make

Table 56.4 Initial target refraction: Published Refractive Goals of Cataract Surgery with Intraocular Lens Implantation [60–65]

Postoperative coal (D)						
Age at surgery (yr)	Dahan 1997 % of undercorrection	Enyedi 1998	Plager 2002	Crouch 2002	Trivedi and Wilson 2009	Personal preferences
<1	20%				+7	+7
1	20%	+6		+4	+6	+6
2	100%	+5		+3.5	+5	+5
3		+4	+5	+2.5		+5
4		+3	+4	+2.5	+4	+4
5		+2	+3	+2	+3	+2-3
6		+1	+2.25	+2	+2	+1-2
7		Plano	+1.5	+1	+1.5	+1-2
8		−1 to −2	+1	+1	+1	+0.5
10			+0.5	Plano	+0.5	
>1					Plano	Plano

decisions on surgical plans, for future optical correction choices, and amblyopia treatment strategy. Parents need preparation to face the challenge of tedious patient care to help maintain compliance with medications, glasses, contact lenses, and occlusion therapy. After all, most of the vision rehabilitation work, especially the most challenging amblyopia management work, is done at home with the patients. Every child with a good visual outcome child has a dedicated parent(s) along with a dedicated team—pediatric ophthalmologist, orthoptist, pediatrician, etc. Procedures need to not only achieve good anatomical structure, which is a necessary precondition, but also lifelong good vision function which is separate and ongoing from the proper anatomical structure that surgery provides [10, 66].

One step that is different in such counseling and distinct from adult cataract practice is that examination under anesthesia (EUA) is necessary for most children undergoing cataract surgery. It is important to obtain accurate biometric information and help make choices on surgical plan and thus partner with parents to make decisions on future management strategy [20].

Immediate Postoperative Care

Immediate proper postoperative care is crucial for a successful surgical outcome and reduces the risk of long-term complication. An uneventful successful operation is only the first step toward achieving the main goals of good vision outcomes in pediatric patients.

1. **Postoperative Medications**

Pediatric patients, especially very young children, can have intensive inflammatory reactions to cataract surgical procedures. Early postoperative complications such as serious inflammation, fibrinous membrane formation, pupillary block, pigmentary and cellular deposits on the intraocular lens (IOL), and posterior synechia, are encountered more frequently in pediatric cataract surgery than in adults.

Proper use of anti-inflammation medication and antibiotics for infection prevention are extremely important. Children, especially small children, and infants, depend on their parents or a caretaker for the administration of medications; it is very important to make sure the parents and care givers understand the importance and comply with the instructions.
The postoperative regimens should be tailored individually, although there are general guidelines.

I. Antibiotics

Currently most common used antibiotics are fourth generation fluoroquinolones such as gatifloxacin and moxifloxacin. They offer a broader spectrum of coverage. These potent topical bactericidal agents have greater antibacterial properties against gram positive organisms and atypical mycobacteria.

Studies showed that fourth-generation fluoroquinolones achieved great aqueous humor concentration with four times a day regimen [67–70].

Intracameral antibiotics safety has been described in cataract surgery. Most of the reports on reducing endophthalmitis are for intracameral Moxifloxacin in adults [71–73]. It has been demonstrated that intracameral Moxifloxacin (250 µg) has an equivalent safety compared to subconjunctival antibiotics in pediatric cataract [74].

II. Steroids

Again, since inflammatory response following cataract surgery is more intense in children, frequent administration of topical steroids is needed to reduce the risk of complications. In very young children or infants steroids may be used every 2–3 hours the first week postop and then depending on the inflammation can taper off the following 3–4 weeks. The most commonly used topical steroid is 1% prednisolone acetate eye drops for routine use [47, 75–77]; 0.1% betamethasone is an acceptable alternative as is Difluprednate 0.05% [78].

Intracameral injection of preservative free triamcinolone acetonide (Triessence, Alcon Labs, and Fort Worth) improves visualization through the vitreous, ensuring a complete anterior vitrectomy without adverse postoperative effects during pediatric cataract surgery [79]. It was also used by some surgeons to reduce the dependence on topical steroids use.

The insertion of steroids into the tear duct has also been investigated to reduce the need or dependence of topical drops. Dextenza (Ocular Therapeutix Inc, Bedford, MA; https://www.ocutx.com/products/dextenza/) an intracanalicular sustained-released dexamethasone, is FDA approved in adults. Triveli and Wilson, recently published about the use for postoperative intraocular inflammation in pediatric cataract. The implant releases 0.4 mg dexamethasone for 30 days. They concluded that this device may help decrease the need for postoperative drops [80].

III. Nonsteroidal Anti-Inflammatory Drugs (NSAIDS)

This class of medications reduces inflammation through inhibition of prostaglandin synthesis. A possible advantage of these medications is the potential for reduction of steroid related complications such as increased IOP, risk of infections, cystic macular edema (CME), to promote rapid visual recovery. Since CME is a rare complication in children and steroids are well tolerated, NSAIDS are rarely part of the routine postoperative regimen after pediatric cataract surgery [81, 82].

IV. Cycloplegics and Mydriatics

Mydriatics and cycloplegics relax ciliary spasm, stabilize the blood aqueous barrier, and dilate the pupil. They can reduce pain, inflammation, and the risk of pupillary block caused by synechia or fibrinous membranes.

There is no uniformity in the postoperative use of cycloplegics in pediatric cataract surgery. Some surgeons prescribe these medications routinely for infants (once per day for 4 weeks) but not older children, some for all patients one to three times daily for 1 to 4 weeks; others avoid the routine use of these drugs altogether [10, 83].

We generally don't use cycloplegic agents in eyes with IOL implants unless we see significant inflammation and risk of pupillary membrane forming. In the young aphakic eye (infants and children less than the 2 years of age) we typically use 1% atropine once at bedtime to reduce the risk of synechia formation, lessen photophobia, and help postoperative examination and refraction (Table 56.5).

2. Follow-up

Frequent postop follow up is important to pediatric cataract surgery. We follow up patients at day 1, week 1 and week 4 postoperatively. At each visit we carefully evaluate patient vision, use slit lamp examination, and check IOP if possible. In infants and young children optical correction or contact lens and initiation of amblyopia treatment begins at postop day 1. At each visit it is necessary to recheck and adjust medication treatment as needed. Again, and it cannot be stressed enough, communication with parents and caregivers is extremely important to ensure the best complaint of the care. (Table 56.6).

Table 56.5 Postoperative medications

- ***Antibiotic***
  - Fourth-generation fluoroquinolones
    - 4 times a day for 1 week

- ***Steroid***
  - 1% prednisolone acetate eye drops
    - First week (Every 2-4 hours)
    - Week 2-4 (Taper off)

- ***Combined steroid and antibiotic ointment***
  - At bedtime 1-4 weeks

- ***Cycloplegics and Mydriatics***
  - 1% atropine
    - At bedtime 4 weeks*in aphakic patients

Table 56.6 Postoperative follow-up

- 1st day, 1st week and 4th week.
  - Slit lamp examination
  - IOP check
  - 1st postoperative visit:
    - Start optical correction-fitting contact lens
    - Start amblyopia treatment
- Subsequent visits
  - Recheck and adjust treatment as needed

Long Term Care

Regular frequent follow up is necessary for long term care of pediatric cataract patients.

It is important to monitor refractive changes, amblyopia treatment, and possible long-term complications. It is well established that aphakia and pseudophakic eyes refraction changes faster and has a high myopic shift. It is important to refract patients every visit and change prescription as indicated. Amblyopia management also requires frequent evaluation and reinforcement. Long term complications of pediatric cataract surgery such as secondary cataracts, opacification of the visual axis, glaucoma, and less commonly, detached retina can occur at any time postoperatively even after many years post-surgery.

I. Complications

    a. Visual Axis Opacification

    Visual axis opacification (VAO) may occur as a result of many factors including corneal opacity, pupillary membrane, anterior capsular phimosis or closure, IOL surface opacification, posterior capsular opacification (PCO), lens reproliferation into the visual axis, and reticular fibrosis after cataract surgery in children [84, 85]. It may occur anytime postoperatively, even many years later.

    b. Glaucoma

    The reported incidence of glaucoma following pediatric cataract surgery ranges widely between 5 and 41% [86–91]. Glaucoma is a life-long risk. It too, may occur any time after cataract surgery, in the early or late postoperative period, even many years later. Most common is open-angle glaucoma, however angle-closure glaucoma is also a rare possibility. Ophthalmologists must always be vigilant about evaluating for glaucoma even with long-term follow-up.

    c. IOL-related complications

    IOL Decentration/Dislocation/Opacification can occur with capsular fibrosis or constriction, if the IOL was asymmetrically implanted, or in cases with zonular weakness and/or inadequate capsular support [92–94].

    d. Retinal detachment

    Retinal detachment is a serious but uncommon complication in pediatric cataract surgery with current surgical techniques. However, children with lens subluxation (such as Marfan's), ectopia lentis, Stickler syndrome; and traumatic cataract are at higher risk for the development of this complication. Retinal detachment also, may develop many years after surgery, so long-term follow-up again is very important [94, 95].

In summary, a successful outcome in pediatric cataract surgery depends on continuous and periodic reevaluation with the meticulous attention of the pediatric ophthalmologist, and the parents or caretaker for long term aphakia and pseudophakic management and amblyopia treatment.

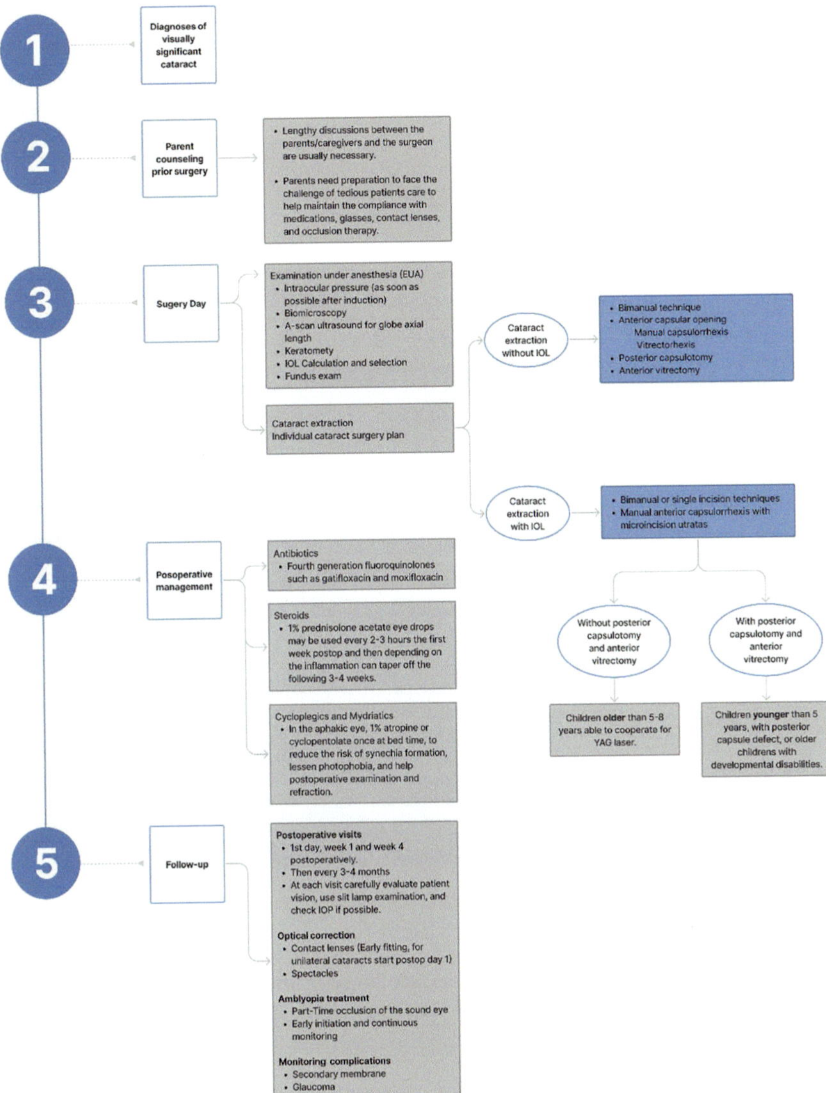

Flowchart 4 Timeline of pediatric cataract surgery

Case Scenario

A 2 y.o. generally healthy boy failed vision screening at pediatrician's office and was referred for additional evaluation. There was no family history of cataract or eye diseases.

Examination:

	Preoperative visit	
	Right eye	**Left eye**
Uncorrected Visual Acuity	CSUM	CSM
Red reflex	Dim red reflex	Normal red reflex
Cornea	Clear	Clear
Anterior Chamber	Deep and quiet	Deep and quiet
Iris	Round and reactive	Round and reactive
Lens	Cortical lens opacity	Clear
Vitreous	Normal	Normal
Fundus exam	Blurry fundus exam	Normal
Cycloplegic refraction	Unable	+2.0 D
IOP	12 mmHg	12 mmHg

Diagnosis: visually significant cataract Right Eye.

Discuss cataract treatment including cataract surgery, intraocular lens implantation, risks, benefits, alternative of surgery, postoperative care including glasses, and amblyopia treatment with parents.

Scheduled for Examination Under Anesthesia (EUA)/Intraocular Lens (IOL) power calculation/lensectomy, anterior vitrectomy, and IOL implant.

Surgery Day:

EUA:

	EUA	
	Right eye	**Left eye**
Cornea	Clear Diameter 10 x 10.5 mm	Clear Diameter 10 x 10.5 mm
Anterior Chamber	Deep and quiet	Deep and quiet
Iris	Round and reactive	Round and reactive
Lens	**Cortical lens opacity**	Clear
Vitreous	Normal	Normal
Fundus exam	**Blurry fundus exam**	Normal
IOP	14 mmHg	15 mmHg

Keratometry to measure the cornea curvature, and A-type Ultrasound to measure axial length.

IOL calculation: Target postop refraction +5.0D (his left eye is +2.0 D, no more than 3D different between two eyes for better amblyopia management)

Patient then prep-draped for surgery
Please see video 2

Post operative care:

Day one: Exam the eye, check vision, check IOP if possible.
Also start medications: steroids, antibiotic eye drops, steroids and antibiotic combination ointment for night.
Start patch treatment, patch left eye at least 2 hours per day.

Week 1: Exam the eye, check vision, check IOP if possible.
Start taper steroids if no significant inflammation to taper off in 4 weeks. Continue patch amblyopia treatment. Prescribe glasses if no significant astigmatism induced by suture.

Week 4: Exam the eye, check vision, check IOP if possible.
Taper off all medication if no inflammation.
Prescribe glasses, continue amblyopia treatment.

Month 3, and every 3–4 months thereafter: Exam the eye, check vision, check IOP

Refraction frequently since aphakia pseudophakic eye has refraction changes more rapidly. Update prescription for glasses if necessary. Continue amblyopia treatment. Monitor long term complications such as visual axis opacification or glaucoma.

Review Questions

1. What is the optimum time to operate on a child with bilateral congenital cataracts?

A. Less than 10 weeks of age, with surgical time between 2 eyes of less than 2 weeks.
B. Before 4 weeks of age, with surgical time between 2 eyes of less than 1 month.
C. Between 4 to 6 months of age, with surgical time between 2 eyes of less than 2 weeks.
D. Between 4 to 6 weeks of age, with surgical time between 2 eyes of more than 1 month.

2. What is the optimum time to operate on a child with unilateral congenital cataracts?

A. Less than 10 weeks of age
B. Before 4 weeks of age
C. Between 4 to 6 months of age
D. Between 4 to 6 weeks of age

3. After unilateral congenital cataract surgery, when is the best time to start optical correction?

A. First day postoperative within one week
B. After 3 months
C. After 2 weeks
D. After 6 months

4. Which of the following surgeries is the preferred treatment for unilateral congenital cataract in a 1-month-old baby?

A. Lensectomy, anterior vitrectomy; and IOL implantation
B. Lensectomy and anterior vitrectomy
C. Phacoemulsification, anterior vitrectomy; and IOL implantation
D. Lensectomy without anterior vitrectomy

5. When selecting an IOL for a 5-year-old with bilateral cataract, what would be your initial target refraction?

A. −2 or −3 D
B. −5 D
C. +2 or +3 D
D. +7 D

6. For cataract extraction with IOL placement at what age would you consider leaving the posterior capsule intact?

A. Less than 1 year old
B. Older than 18 years old
C. Older than 5 years old
D. Less than 6 months old

Answers

1. A
2. D
3. A
4. B
5. C
6. C

Videos

Video 1. *Cataract extraction, posterior capsulotomy, and anterior vitrectomy in a 6-week-old patient.*

Video 2. *Single-incision cataract extraction, posterior capsulotomy, anterior vitrectomy, and IOL implant in a 2-year-old patient.*

Video 3. *Single incision cataract extraction, posterior capsulotomy, anterior vitrectomy, and IOL implant in a 13-month-old patient.*

Video 4. *Cataract extraction in a 9-month-old patient with persistent fetal vasculature. Removal of the fibrovascular membrane and anterior vitrectomy.*

References

1. Bremond-Gignac D, Daruich A, Robert MP, Valleix S. Recent developments in the management of congenital cataract. Ann Transl Med [Internet]. 2020;8(22):1545. https://pubmed.ncbi.nlm.nih.gov/33313290.
2. Sheeladevi S, Lawrenson JG, Fielder AR, Suttle CM. Global prevalence of childhood cataract: a systematic review. Eye (Lond). 2016;30(9):1160–9.
3. Chan WH, Biswas S, Ashworth JL, Lloyd IC. Congenital and infantile cataract: aetiology and management. Eur J Pediatr. 2012;171(4):625–30.
4. Hubel DH. Exploration of the primary visual cortex, 1955–78. Nature. 1982;299(5883):515–24.

5. Wiesel TN. Postnatal development of the visual cortex and the influence of environment. Nature. 1982;299(5884):583–91.

6. Beller R, Hoyt CS, Marg E, Odom JV. Good visual function after neonatal surgery for congenital monocular cataracts. Am J Ophthalmol. 1981;91(5):559–65.

7. Jacobson SG, Mohindra I, Held R. Development of visual acuity in infants with congenital cataracts. Br J Ophthalmol. 1981;65(10):727–35.

8. Birch EE, Stager DR. Prevalence of good visual acuity following surgery for congenital unilateral cataract. Arch Ophthalmol (Chicago, Ill 1960). 1988;106(1):40–3.

9. Birch EE, Stager DR. The critical period for surgical treatment of dense congenital unilateral cataract. Invest Ophthalmol Vis Sci. 1996;37(8):1532–8.

10. Wilson ME, Trivedi RH. Pediatric cataract surgery: techniques, complications and management. Lippincott Williams & Wilkins; 2014.

11. Birch EE, Cheng C, Stager DRJ, Weakley DRJ, Stager DRS. The critical period for surgical treatment of dense congenital bilateral cataracts. J AAPOS Off Publ Am Assoc Pediatr Ophthalmol Strabismus. 2009;13(1):67–71.

12. Wu C, Hunter DG. Amblyopia: diagnostic and therapeutic options. Am J Ophthalmol. 2006;141(1):175–84.

13. Leinfelder PJ. Amblyopia associated with congenital cataract. Trans Am Ophthalmol Soc. 1962;60:236–42.

14. Costenbader FD, Albert DG. Conservatism in the management of congenital cataract. AMA Arch Ophthalmol. 1957;58(3):426–30.

15. Hered RW, Archer SW, Braveman RS, Khan AO, Lee KA, Lueder GT, O'Hara MA. KT-H. 2021–2022 Basic and Clinical Science Course, Section 06: Pediatric ophthalmology and strabismus. 2021. 497 p.

16. Medsinge A, Nischal KK. Pediatric cataract: challenges and future directions. Clin Ophthalmol [Internet]. 2015;9:77–90. https://pubmed.ncbi.nlm.nih.gov/25609909

17. Yu T, Dahan E. Bilateral uneven cataracts in children: amblyopia management by sequential intraocular lens implantation. Eye (Lond). 2009;23(6):1451–5.

18. Holmes JM, Kraker RT, Beck RW, Birch EE, Cotter SA, Everett DF, et al. A randomized trial of prescribed patching regimens for treatment of severe amblyopia in children. Ophthalmology. 2003;110(11):2075–87.

19. Birch EE, Jost RM, Wang SX, Kelly KR. A pilot randomized trial of contrast-rebalanced binocular treatment for deprivation amblyopia. J AAPOS Off Publ Am Assoc Pediatr Ophthalmol Strabismus. 2020;24(6):344.e1-344.e5.

20. Khokhar SK, Pillay G, Dhull C, Agarwal E, Mahabir M, Aggarwal P. Pediatric cataract. Indian J Ophthalmol [Internet]. 2017;65(12):1340–9. https://pubmed.ncbi.nlm.nih.gov/29208814

21. Wilson MEJ, Trivedi RH, Hoxie JP, Bartholomew LR. Treatment outcomes of congenital monocular cataracts: the effects of surgical timing and patching compliance. J Pediatr Ophthalmol Strabismus. 2003;40(6):323–4.

22. Lambert SR, Lynn MJ, Reeves R, Plager DA, Buckley EG, Wilson ME. Is there a latent period for the surgical treatment of children with dense bilateral congenital cataracts? J AAPOS Off Publ Am Assoc Pediatr Ophthalmol Strabismus. 2006;10(1):30–6.

23. Kim D-H, Kim JH, Kim S-J, Yu YS. Long-term results of bilateral congenital cataract treated with early cataract surgery, aphakic glasses and secondary IOL implantation. Acta Ophthalmol. 2012;90(3):231–6.

24. Traboulsi EI, Utz VM. Practical management of pediatric ocular disorders and strabismus. Springer; 2016.

25. Vasavada AR, Nihalani BR. Pediatric cataract surgery. Curr Opin Ophthalmol. 2006;17(1):54–61.

26. Lambert SR, Lynn MJ, Hartmann EE, DuBois L, Drews-Botsch C, Freedman SF, et al. Comparison of contact lens and intraocular lens correction of monocular aphakia during

infancy: a randomized clinical trial of HOTV optotype acuity at age 4.5 years and clinical findings at age 5 years. JAMA Ophthalmol. 2014;132(6):676–82.

27. Wang M, Xiao W. Congenital cataract: progress in surgical treatment and postoperative recovery of visual function. Eye Sci. 2015;30(1):38–47.

28. Chen J, Chen Y, Zhong Y, Li J. Comparison of visual acuity and complications between primary IOL implantation and aphakia in patients with congenital cataract younger than 2 years: a meta-analysis. J Cataract Refract Surg. 2020;46(3):465–73.

29. Vasavada AR, Vasavada V. Current status of IOL implantation in pediatric eyes: an update. Expert Rev Med Devices. 2017;1–9.

30. Solebo AL, Russell-Eggitt I, Cumberland PM, Rahi JS. Risks and outcomes associated with primary intraocular lens implantation in children under 2 years of age: the IoLunder2 cohort study. Br J Ophthalmol. 2015;99(11):1471–6.

31. Kumar P, Lambert SR. Evaluating the evidence for and against the use of IOLs in infants and young children. Expert Rev Med Devices. 2016;13(4):381–9.

32. Termühlen J, Gottschalk A, Eter N, Hoffmann EM, Van Aken H, Grenzebach U, et al. Does general anesthesia have a clinical impact on intraocular pressure in children? Paediatr Anaesth. 2016;26(9):936–41.

33. Trivedi RH, Wilson ME. Selection of an initial contact lens power for infantile cataract surgery without primary intraocular lens implantation. Ophthalmology. 2013;120(10): 1973–6.

34. Trivedi RH, Lambert SR, Lynn MJ, Wilson ME. The role of preoperative biometry in selecting initial contact lens power in the Infant Aphakia Treatment Study. J AAPOS Off Publ Am Assoc Pediatr Ophthalmol Strabismus. 2014;18(3):251–4.

35. Self JE, Taylor R, Solebo AL, Biswas S, Parulekar M, Dev Borman A, et al. Cataract management in children: a review of the literature and current practice across five large UK centres. Eye (Lond). 2020;34(12):2197–218.

36. Wilson MEJ, Trivedi RH, Bartholomew LR, Pershing S. Comparison of anterior vitrectorhexis and continuous curvilinear capsulorhexis in pediatric cataract and intraocular lens implantation surgery: a 10-year analysis. J AAPOS Off Publ Am Assoc Pediatr Ophthalmol Strabismus. 2007;11(5):443–6.

37. Bartholomew LR, Wilson MEJ, Trivedi RH. Pediatric anterior capsulotomy preferences of cataract surgeons worldwide: comparison of 1993, 2001, and 2003 surveys. J Cataract Refract Surg. 2007;33(5):893–900.

38. Baile R, Sahasrabuddhe M, Nadkarni S, Karira V, Kelkar J. Effect of anterior capsular polishing on the rate of posterior capsule opacification: a retrospective analytical study. Saudi J Ophthalmol Off J Saudi Ophthalmol Soc. 2012;26(1):101–4.

39. Luft N, Kreutzer TC, Dirisamer M, Priglinger CS, Burger J, Findl O, et al. Evaluation of laser capsule polishing for prevention of posterior capsule opacification in a human ex vivo model. J Cataract Refract Surg. 2015;41(12):2739–45.

40. Rastogi A, Mishra M, Goel Y, Thacker P, Kamlesh. Comparative study of 25- versus 20-gauge pars plana capsulotomy and vitrectomy in pediatric cataract surgery. Int Ophthalmol. 2018;38(1):157–61.

41. Choi SH, Kim YD, Yu YS, Kim MK, Choi HJ. Long-term outcome of Nd:YAG laser posterior capsulotomy in children: procedural strategies and visual outcome. Am J Ophthalmol. 2019;197:121–7.

42. Buckley EG, Klombers LA, Seaber JH, Scalise-Gordy A, Minzter R. Management of the posterior capsule during pediatric intraocular lens implantation. Am J Ophthalmol. 1993;115 (6):722–8.

43. Vasavada AR, Praveen MR, Tassignon M-J, Shah SK, Vasavada VA, Vasavada VA, et al. Posterior capsule management in congenital cataract surgery. J Cataract Refract Surg. 2011;37(1):173–93.

44. Gupta R, Ram J, Sukhija J, Singh R. Outcome of paediatric cataract surgery with primary posterior capsulotomy and anterior vitrectomy using intra-operative preservative-free triamcinolone acetonide. Acta Ophthalmol. 2014;92(5):e358–61.
45. Ventura MC, Ventura BV, Ventura CV, Ventura LO, Arantes TE, Nosé W. Outcomes of congenital cataract surgery: intraoperative intracameral triamcinolone injection versus postoperative oral prednisolone. J Cataract Refract Surg. 2014;40(4):601–8.
46. Vasavada AR, Trivedi RH. Role of optic capture in congenital cataract and intraocular lens surgery in children. J Cataract Refract Surg. 2000;26(6):824–31.
47. Vasavada AR, Trivedi RH, Singh R. Necessity of vitrectomy when optic capture is performed in children older than 5 years. J Cataract Refract Surg. 2001;27(8):1185–93.
48. Vasavada AR, Vasavada V, Shah SK, Trivedi RH, Vasavada VA, Vasavada SA, et al. Postoperative outcomes of intraocular lens implantation in the bag versus posterior optic capture in pediatric cataract surgery. J Cataract Refract Surg. 2017;43(9):1177–83.
49. Zhou H-W, Zhou F. A Meta-analysis on the clinical efficacy and safety of optic capture in pediatric cataract surgery. Int J Ophthalmol. 2016;9(4):590–6.
50. Wilson ME, Trivedi RH. Choice of intraocular lens for pediatric cataract surgery: survey of AAPOS members. Vol. 33, Journal of cataract and refractive surgery. United States; 2007. p. 1666–8.
51. Matalia J, Panmand P, Ghalla P. Comparative analysis of non-absorbable 10–0 nylon sutures with absorbable 10–0 Vicryl sutures in pediatric cataract surgery. Indian J Ophthalmol. 2018;66(5):661–4.
52. George NK, Stewart MW. The routine use of intracameral antibiotics to prevent endophthalmitis after cataract surgery: how good is the evidence? Ophthalmol Ther. 2018;7(2):233–45.
53. Mohammadpour M, Shaabani A, Sahraian A, Momenaei B, Tayebi F, Bayat R, et al. Updates on managements of pediatric cataract. J Curr Ophthalmol [Internet]. 2018;31(2):118–26. https://pubmed.ncbi.nlm.nih.gov/31317088.
54. Lim ME, Buckley EG, Prakalapakorn SG. Update on congenital cataract surgery management. Curr Opin Ophthalmol. 2017;28(1):87–92.
55. Wilson MEJ, Bartholomew LR, Trivedi RH. Pediatric cataract surgery and intraocular lens implantation: practice styles and preferences of the 2001 ASCRS and AAPOS memberships. J Cataract Refract Surg. 2003;29(9):1811–20.
56. Lambert SR, Buckley EG, Drews-Botsch C, DuBois L, Hartmann EE, Lynn MJ, et al. A randomized clinical trial comparing contact lens with intraocular lens correction of monocular aphakia during infancy: grating acuity and adverse events at age 1 year. Arch Ophthalmol (Chicago, Ill 1960). 2010;128(7):810–8.
57. Lambert SR, Lynn M, Drews-Botsch C, Loupe D, Plager DA, Medow NB, et al. A comparison of grating visual acuity, strabismus, and reoperation outcomes among children with aphakia and pseudophakia after unilateral cataract surgery during the first six months of life. J AAPOS Off Publ Am Assoc Pediatr Ophthalmol Strabismus. 2001;5(2):70–5.
58. Trivedi RH, Wilson MEJ, Bartholomew LR, Lal G, Peterseim MM. Opacification of the visual axis after cataract surgery and single acrylic intraocular lens implantation in the first year of life. J AAPOS Off Publ Am Assoc Pediatr Ophthalmol Strabismus. 2004;8(2):156–64.
59. Birch EE, Cheng C, Stager DRJ, Felius J. Visual acuity development after the implantation of unilateral intraocular lenses in infants and young children. J AAPOS Off Publ Am Assoc Pediatr Ophthalmol Strabismus. 2005;9(6):527–32.
60. Dahan E, Drusedau MU. Choice of lens and dioptric power in pediatric pseudophakia. J Cataract Refract Surg. 1997;23(Suppl 1):618–23.
61. Enyedi LB, Peterseim MW, Freedman SF, Buckley EG. Refractive changes after pediatric intraocular lens implantation. Am J Ophthalmol. 1998;126(6):772–81.
62. Plager DA, Kipfer H, Sprunger DT, Sondhi N, Neely DE. Refractive change in pediatric pseudophakia: 6-year follow-up. J Cataract Refract Surg. 2002;28(5):810–5.

63. Crouch ER, Crouch ERJ, Pressman SH. Prospective analysis of pediatric pseudophakia: myopic shift and postoperative outcomes. J AAPOS Off Publ Am Assoc Pediatr Ophthalmol Strabismus. 2002;6(5):277–82.

64. Pandey SK, Wilson ME, Trivedi RH, Izak AM, Macky TA, Werner L, et al. Pediatric cataract surgery and intraocular lens implantation: current techniques, complications, and management. Int Ophthalmol Clin. 2001;41(3):175–96.

65. Trivedi RH WM. Selecting intraocular lens power in children. Eyenet Pearls [online]. www.aao.org/publications/eyenet/200601/ pearls.cfm. Accessed on December 17, 2011. Eyenet Pearls [online] [Internet]. www.aao.org/publications/eyenet/200601/%0Apearls.cfm. Accessed on December 15, 2021.

66. Erraguntla V, De la Huerta I, Vohra S, Abdolell M, Levin AV. Parental comprehension following informed consent for pediatric cataract surgery. Can J Ophthalmol. 2012;47(2):107–12.

67. Solomon R, Donnenfeld ED, Perry HD, Snyder RW, Nedrud C, Stein J, et al. Penetration of topically applied gatifloxacin 0.3%, moxifloxacin 0.5%, and ciprofloxacin 0.3% into the aqueous humor. Ophthalmology. 2005;112(3):466–9.

68. McCulley JP, Caudle D, Aronowicz JD, Shine WE. Fourth-generation fluoroquinolone penetration into the aqueous humor in humans. Ophthalmology. 2006;113(6):955–9.

69. Kim DH, Stark WJ, O'Brien TP, Dick JD. Aqueous penetration and biological activity of moxifloxacin 0.5% ophthalmic solution and gatifloxacin 0.3% solution in cataract surgery patients. Ophthalmology. 2005;112(11):1992–6.

70. Watanabe R, Nakazawa T, Yokokura S, Kubota A, Kubota H, Nishida K. Fluoroquinolone antibacterial eye drops: effects on normal human corneal epithelium, stroma, and endothelium. Clin Ophthalmol. 2010;4:1181–7.

71. Haripriya A, Chang DF, Ravindran RD. Endophthalmitis reduction with intracameral moxifloxacin prophylaxis: analysis of 600 000 surgeries. Ophthalmology. 2017;124(6):768–75.

72. Haripriya A, Chang DF, Ravindran RD. Endophthalmitis reduction with intracameral moxifloxacin in eyes with and without surgical complications: results from 2 million consecutive cataract surgeries. J Cataract Refract Surg. 2019;45(9):1226–33.

73. Matsuura K, Miyoshi T, Suto C, Akura J, Inoue Y. Efficacy and safety of prophylactic intracameral moxifloxacin injection in Japan. J Cataract Refract Surg. 2013;39(11):1702–6.

74. Khalili S, Imtirat A, Williams S, Ali A, Tehrani N, Mireskandari K. Safety of intracameral moxifloxacin in the pediatric population: an equivalence study. J Cataract Refract Surg. 2020;46(2):228–34.

75. Awner S, Buckley EG, DeVaro JM, Seaber JH. Unilateral pseudophakia in children under 4 years. J Pediatr Ophthalmol Strabismus. 1996;33(4):230–6.

76. Jensen AA, Basti S, Greenwald MJ, Mets MB. When may the posterior capsule be preserved in pediatric intraocular lens surgery? Ophthalmology. 2002;109(2):324–7; discussion 328.

77. Alexandrakis G, Peterseim MM, Wilson ME. Clinical outcomes of pars plana capsulotomy with anterior vitrectomy in pediatric cataract surgery. J AAPOS Off Publ Am Assoc Pediatr Ophthalmol Strabismus. 2002;6(3):163–7.

78. Ahmadieh H, Javadi MA, Ahmady M, Karimian F, Einollahi B, Zare M, et al. Primary capsulectomy, anterior vitrectomy, lensectomy, and posterior chamber lens implantation in children: limbal versus pars plana. J Cataract Refract Surg. 1999;25(6):768–75.

79. Praveen MR, Shah SK, Vasavada VA, Dixit NV, Vasavada AR, Garg VS, et al. Triamcinolone-assisted vitrectomy in pediatric cataract surgery: intraoperative effectiveness and postoperative outcome. J AAPOS Off Publ Am Assoc Pediatr Ophthalmol Strabismus. 2010;14(4):340–4.

80. Trivedi RH, Wilson ME. A sustained-release intracanalicular dexamethasone insert (Dextenza) for pediatric cataract surgery. J AAPOS Off Publ Am Assoc Pediatr Ophthalmol Strabismus. 2021;25(1):43–5.

81. Miyake K, Ota I, Miyake G, Numaga J. Nepafenac 0.1% versus fluorometholone 0.1% for preventing cystoid macular edema after cataract surgery. J Cataract Refract Surg. 2011;37 (9):1581–8.
82. Kim SJ, Flach AJ, Jampol LM. Nonsteroidal anti-inflammatory drugs in ophthalmology. Surv Ophthalmol. 2010;55(2):108–33.
83. Khokhar SK, Pillay G, Agarwal E, Mahabir M. Innovations in pediatric cataract surgery. Indian J Ophthalmol. 2017;65(3):210–6.
84. Trivedi RH, Wilson ME, Vasavada AR, Shah SK, Vasavada V, Vasavada VA. Visual axis opacification after cataract surgery and hydrophobic acrylic intraocular lens implantation in the first year of life. J Cataract Refract Surg. 2011;37(1):83–7.
85. Shrestha UD, Shrestha MK. Visual axis opacification in children following paediatric cataract surgery. JNMA J Nepal Med Assoc. 2014;52(196):1024–30.
86. Asrani SG, Wilensky JT. Glaucoma after congenital cataract surgery. Ophthalmology. 1995;102(6):863–7.
87. Chrousos GA, Parks MM, O'Neill JF. Incidence of chronic glaucoma, retinal detachment and secondary membrane surgery in pediatric aphakic patients. Ophthalmology. 1984;91 (10):1238–41.
88. Francois J. Late results of congenital cataract surgery. Ophthalmology. 1979;86(9):1586–98.
89. Mills MD, Robb RM. Glaucoma following childhood cataract surgery. J Pediatr Ophthalmol Strabismus. 1994;31(6):355–60; discussion 361.
90. Simon JW, Mehta N, Simmons ST, Catalano RA, Lininger LL. Glaucoma after pediatric lensectomy/vitrectomy. Ophthalmology. 1991;98(5):670–4.
91. Walton DS. Pediatric aphakic glaucoma: a study of 65 patients. Trans Am Ophthalmol Soc. 1995;93:403–20.
92. Struck MC. Long-term results of pediatric cataract surgery and primary intraocular lens implantation from 7 to 22 months of life. JAMA Ophthalmol. 2015;133(10):1180–3.
93. Cheung CS, VanderVeen DK. Intraocular lens techniques in pediatric eyes with insufficient capsular support: complications and outcomes. Semin Ophthalmol. 2019;34(4):293–302.
94. Whitman MC, Vanderveen DK. Complications of pediatric cataract surgery. Semin Ophthalmol. 2014;29(5–6):414–20.
95. Haargaard B, Andersen EW, Oudin A, Poulsen G, Wohlfahrt J, la Cour M, et al. Risk of retinal detachment after pediatric cataract surgery. Invest Ophthalmol Vis Sci. 2014;55 (5):2947–51.

Complications of Lens Surgery at Pediatric Age

57

Marcela Raposo Vieira de Oliveira, H. Tuba Atalay, and Camila V. Ventura

Abstract

Despite the notorious advances in pediatric lens surgery and significant improvement of surgical results, children are at higher risk of developing lens complications during and after surgery compared to adults given their structural differences and exacerbated inflammatory response. The present chapter brings awareness to surgeons of the intraoperative and postoperative complications secondary to pediatric lens surgery to help reduce complication rates and promote early detection and better management of these adverse events.

Keywords

Lens complications · Pediatric lens surgery · Posterior capsule rupture · Dislocated lens · Secondary opacification of visual axis

Supplementary Information The online version contains supplementary material available at https://doi.org/10.1007/978-3-031-14506-3_57.

M. R. V. de Oliveira · C. V. Ventura (✉)
Altino Ventura Foundation, Recife, Brazil
e-mail: camilaventuramd@gmail.com

H. T. Atalay
School of Medicine, Ophthalmology Department, Gazi University, Ankara, Turkey

C. V. Ventura
HOPE Eye Hospital, Recife, Brazil

Introduction

Lens surgery performed in the pediatric population is not the same as in adults given the small sizes of the ocular structures, more elastic anterior capsule, increased vitreous pressure, thinner sclera, smaller pupils, and restricted working space [1]. These additional challenges related to lens surgery in children impose a higher risk of intraoperative complications, which can be devastating and have meaningful impact on visual prognosis and quality of life of children [2]. In addition, pediatric lens surgery is fraught with more robust inflammatory response, high tendency for lens cortex reproliferation and visual axis opacification, and greater chance of wound leakage if not sutured properly [3].

Epidemiology

Despite the reduction of serious complications following childhood cataract surgery since 1960 with the introduction of the aspiration technique, its occurrence was not completely eliminated, which directly affects visual prognosis of operated eyes [4]. Current studies show that the incidence of complications and adverse events following lens surgery varies according to the studied population age and the chosen surgical technique [5–7]. These complications are classified as intraoperative or postoperative according to the moment that they occur [5–7].

The Infant Aphakia Treatment Study (IATS), a multi-center clinical trial, as well as the British Isles Congenital Cataract Interest Group (BICCIG), a prospective cohort study, reported higher intraoperative complication rate in eyes that underwent primary intraocular lens (IOL) implantation (21% of eyes and 16%, respectively) compared to those eyes that were left aphakic (11% and 6%, respectively) [5, 6]. In these two studies children were under 1 year and 2 years of age, respectively. In contrast, the Pediatric Eye Disease Investigator Group (PEDIG) performed a 5-year longitudinal study that included children who underwent lensectomy from birth to less than 13 years of age from 61 centers in Canada, Unites States, and the United Kingdom and they reported a similar incidence of complications in eyes with and without IOL implantation [5–7]. In their study, intraoperative complications were present in 5% of the total eyes and postoperative complications in 16% [7].

- The intraoperative complications of lens surgery include iris prolapse, iris damage, hyphema, posterior capsule rupture (PCR), retained cortex, and lens fragment in vitreous [5].
- Postoperative complications include acute intraocular pressure elevation, corneal edema, uveitis, visual axis opacities, pupillary deformities, retinal hemorrhages, retinal detachment, endophthalmitis, and phthisis bulbi [7].

Intraoperative Complications

Iris Prolapse and Damage

Iris damage is a complication that can be identified in up to 2.6% of eyes and are most commonly related to IOL positioning [6]. Iris prolapse, on the other hand, is the most common intraoperative complication reported in the IATS study and BICCIG study in 5% and 11% of eyes, respectively [5, 6]. Iris prolapse occurs when the forces pulling on the iris toward the wound exceed the ability of the iris' tone to maintain its position in the anterior chamber and iris damage [6, 8]. Factors that contribute to iris prolapse include posterior incision position, enlarged incision, large leak from wound, shallow anterior chamber, high irrigating velocity, and atonic iris [6, 8]. In eyes that undergo IOL implantation, iris prolapse usually occurs after enlargement of the superior wound before IOL placement [6]. To avoid iridodialysis, hyphema, and later sectorial iris atrophy, the iris prolapse must be resolved by repositioning the iris gently [9]. In some cases, an additional incision can be the best management approach to prevent additional complications [10].

Bleeding

Bleeding in cataract surgery ranges from simple subconjunctival hemorrhage, to significant intraocular hemorrhages [1, 11–14]. Anterior chamber hemorrhage during surgery is usually related to iris injury including cyclodialysis and iris prolapse [5, 6]. Hyphema has been reported in 3.1% of eyes and commonly resolves spontaneously with no further complications [11, 12]. However, in cases of recurrent hyphema following lens surgery in children, physicians may need to rule out Swan Syndrome and Uveitis-Glaucoma-Hyphema (UGH) Syndrome [15, 16].

Swan Syndrome is a rare disorder and has been described after intracapsular and extracapsular cataract extraction, including clear corneal incisions [15]. To confirm the diagnosis, abnormal ingrowth of episcleral vessels on the wound site is visualized during gonioscopy [15].

The UGH Syndrome is also a rare entity that has been described following congenital cataract surgery and is caused by the dislocation of the posterior chamber intraocular lens to the anterior chamber [16]. In these cases, explantation of the posterior chamber IOL may be required to control the intraocular inflammation and hyphema [16].

Vitreous hemorrhages, on the other hand, has been reported in up to 10% of eyes and range from mild to severe [12, 13]. Flame-shaped retinal hemorrhages and small vitreous hemorrhage can occur in the first postoperative days after lens surgery, which resolves spontaneously within the first postoperative month [14]. No correlation has been identified between the occurrence of retinal hemorrhages and factors such as patient's age, race, sex, or duration of surgery [14]. However, it has been strongly associated with persistence of fetal vasculature [12]. Therefore, dilated fundus evaluation is strongly recommended in these eyes during initial follow-ups [14].

Posterior Capsule Rupture

One of the most common intraoperative complications among pediatric eyes that undergo lens surgery with or without IOL implantation is the PCR [5–7]. In the PEDIG study, PCR was reported in 1% of eyes [7]. Although PCR may occur at any step of the lens surgery, eyes with history of trauma, vitrectomy, and preexisting congenital defects such as polar cataracts, posterior lenticonus, persistent fetal vasculature are at higher risk of having this complication [5, 17].

Whenever PCR occurs, prompt detection is essential to avoid additional complications associated including anterior displacement of the vitreous to the anterior segment and lens fragment dislocation to the posterior cavity [17].

Retained Cortex and Lens Fragment in the Vitreous

Small amount of retained cortex usually have no lasting effect and causes no postoperative complications [5]. However, if significant lens cortex is retained, eyes can progress with opacification of visual axis, increased IOP, and inflammation that require additional surgical intervention [3].

The dislocation of fragments of the crystalline lens into the vitreous cavity can produce corneal edema, glaucoma, uveitis, and vitreous opacification that results in decreased vision [17, 18]. Anterior and posterior vitrectomy are effective and frequently needed to remove vitreous from the anterior chamber and lens fragments from the vitreous cavity [17, 18].

Postoperative Complications

Ocular Hypertension and Glaucoma

During the postoperative period the IOP commonly fluctuates given that children are more susceptible to steroid-induced ocular hypertension [2, 19, 20]. The incidence of ocular hypertension during first postoperative year varies between 2 and 17% and may occur in both aphakic and IOL eyes [7, 19]. This intermittent complication usually happens at 1 to 2.5-month follow-up and has a mean duration of 30 days [19]. Although ocular hypertension is managed with antiglaucomatous drops, closely monitoring the IOP as well as the optic disc cupping is essential due to high risk early and late onset glaucoma [3, 19].

With the advance of surgical techniques and the introduction of vitrectomy instruments for childhood cataract surgery, the incidence of angle-closure glaucoma with pupillary blockage after lensectomy had decreased [20]. However, postoperative chronic open angle glaucoma is yet considered the most common and most important visually disabling complication following pediatric lens surgery [1, 3, 4, 19–24]. Its incidence ranges from 6 to 58.7% depending on the population studied, surgical technique, and length of follow-up [23]. Studies show that this complication can develop many years after surgery with a higher frequency after 6 years of follow-up [21–23].

Treatment of secondary glaucoma in these pediatric eyes is challenging [21, 23–24]. Antiglaucoma drops usually temporizes measures, but surgery and laser treatments are usually required [21, 23–24]. In the IATS, 4.4% of patients requires surgical management for glaucoma within the first postoperative year, and 7% during the first 5 postoperative years [5]. This gradual increase in number of cases requiring surgical intervention suggests that pediatric patients are at continuous risk of developing glaucoma after cataract surgery and consigned to frequent and indefinite follow-ups, and often multiple surgical interventions [3, 21–24]. Unfortunately, the outcomes of surgical interventions in these cases are often disappointing long-term [17, 23, 24].

The precise etiology of postoperative glaucoma in pediatric lens surgery is incompletely understood [1, 20]. However, studies show that eyes with other coexisting anomalies, retained lens cortex, and those that need secondary membrane surgery increase the risk of developing chronic glaucoma [21, 24]. Other factors such as young age at cataract surgery and aphakia or pseudophakia, remain controversial according to studies [1, 2, 4, 20–27].

Persistent Corneal Edema

Corneal edema is a rare and transient postoperative complication in children [5, 28]. The main underlying condition that can increase the risk for developing corneal edema is the intraocular inflammation that often follows surgery [28]. This complication can last for 2 weeks and resolves with intensified topical steroids [28].

With regards to endothelial cells loss secondary to lens surgery in the pediatric population, a long-term follow-up study showed a low rate of 9.2% endothelial cells loss 12 years after surgery [12].

Secondary Opacification of Visual Axis: Capsular Opacity, Lens re-Proliferation and Pupillary Membranes

Visual axis opacification (VAO) can be caused by posterior capsular opacity, lens re-proliferation, and/or pupillary membrane formation [1, 4]. The proliferation of residual epithelial cells on the posterior capsule leads to the posterior capsular opacity (Fig. 57.1) [1]. The lens re-proliferation in aphakic eyes results in the

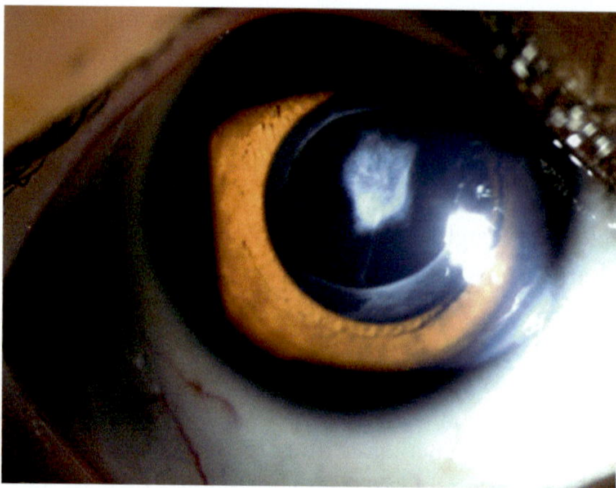

Fig. 57.1 Dense posterior capsular opacification observed in a pediatric eye submitted to congenital cataract surgery with no posterior capsulotomy

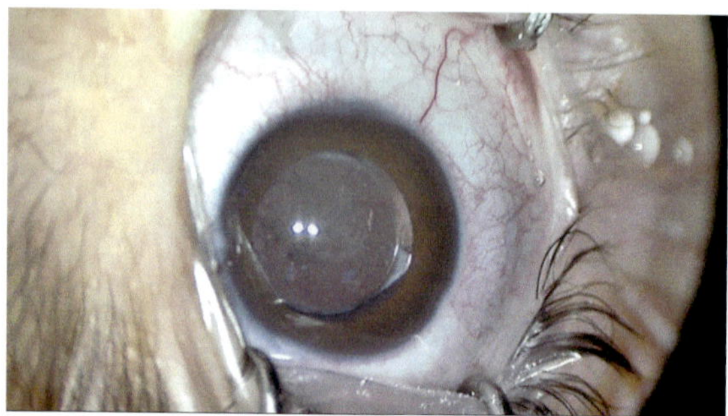

Fig. 57.2 Visual opacification caused by lens re-proliferation (Elschnig pearls) in a pediatric eye submitted to congenital cataract surgery with no posterior capsulotomy

formation of the Sommering's ring behind the iris. Whereas, in pseudophakic eyes the re-proliferation results in Elschnig pearls present outside the capsular leaflets (Fig. 57.2) [1]. Pupillary membrane, on the other hand, typically occludes the pupil and causes posterior synechiae because of the inflammatory response (Fig. 57.3) [1].

Clinically VAOs are identified by the absence or alteration of the red reflex (Fig. 57.4). All causes of VAO are considered amblyogenic given that they reduce visual acuity and hamper optimal refractive correction by limiting retinoscopy [4]. As a consequence, this postoperative complication frequently need to be addressed surgically [1, 3].

Studies report high rates of reoperation to resolve VAOs following pediatric lens surgery [3, 5, 6]. In the Infant Aphakia Treatment Study (IATS), 47% of infant eyes required surgical removal of a visual axis opacity during the first postoperative year

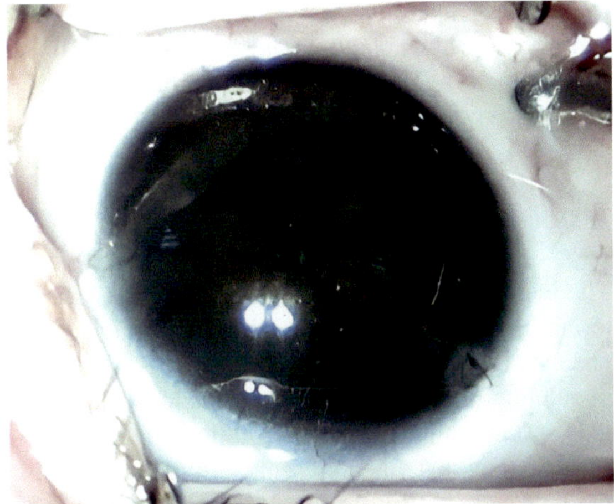

Fig. 57.3 A 2-month-old baby presenting a pupillary blockage and bombé iris 1-week after being submitted to lensectomy and anterior vitrectomy. Intraocular pressure was 30 mmHg in that eye

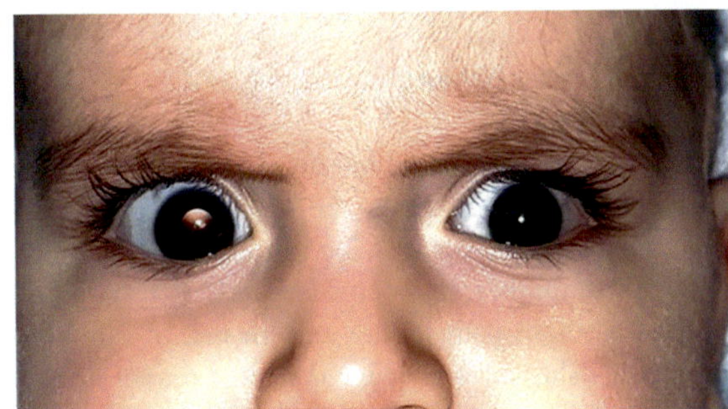

Fig. 57.4 Absence of red reflex in the left eye of a child caused by visual axis opacification

[5]. To corroborate with this finding, Jackson et al. [3] suggest that VAOs are more likely to occur within the first 3 postoperative months [3].

Unfortunately, these additional surgical interventions are directly related to chronic glaucoma and retinal detachment in pediatric eyes, as previously mentioned [4]. Thus, by confectioning a wide posterior capsulotomy and performing a thorough anterior vitrectomy during the primary procedure, as well as intensifying steroid therapy postoperatively when doing lens surgery in children especially under 5 years old may reduce the incidence of VAOs and additional surgery [1, 4, 6].

Pupil Abnormalities

Although most postoperative pupil abnormalities such as corectopia occur as a direct damage to the iris when manipulating instruments in the eye, they can also be related to IOL mispositioning and subluxation and synechial sequelae [29].

Pupil abnormalities may have an impact on cosmetics, but most importantly, these alterations may influence visual development in children [29]. After surgery, the pupillary aperture must be centered to avoid amblyopia as well as other visual symptoms such as photophobia and glare [29]. In some cases of pupillary aperture displacement additional surgical approaches such as membranectomy or a pupilloplasty may be needed [30].

Dislocated Lens

The incidence of dislocated lens in pediatric lens surgery is lower when compared to adults. The PEDIG study reported an incidence of 0.1% of lens dislocation in pediatric eyes (Fig. 57.5) [7]. Whereas, Lee et al. reported in a nationwide population-based cohort study an incidence of 0.7% of IOL dislocation in adults [31]. Although lens dislocation following pediatric lens surgery is considered rare, studies show that when present, additional surgical intervention is needed to center the lens and avoid vision loss and amblyopia [7, 32].

Retinal Detachment

Although prognosis of retinal detachments in the pediatric population has improved in the past decades given the advances in pediatric retinal detachment surgery including wide angle viewing systems, faster cutting speed vitrectors, and better surgical techniques, it is considered a serious complication of pediatric lens surgery given that these patients are at high risk of blindness [33–35].

Studies show a higher incidence of retinal detachment in children submitted to lens surgery compared to adults and its incidence varies according to the chosen technique given and follow-up time [33, 36]. Retinal detachments in aphakic pediatric patients have been estimated at 1.5% in a 5-year follow-up study [4].

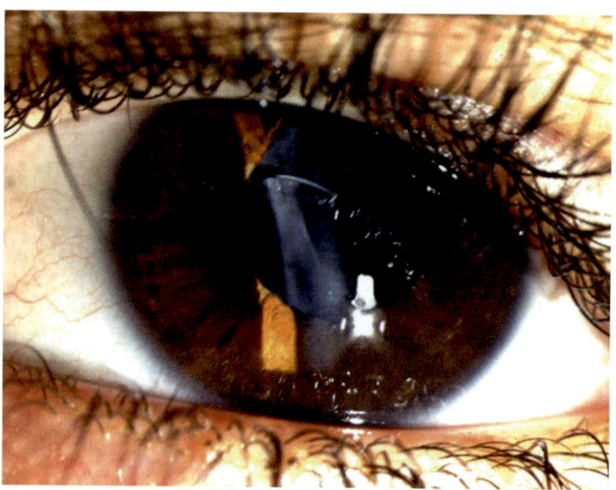

Fig. 57.5 Intraocular lens dislocated inferiorly and posterior capsule opacification in a child submitted to lens surgery

Whereas previous studies on groups of at least 100 eyes without IOL implantation have identified a retinal detachment frequency ranging from 0.6 to 5% [34, 36–38].

Although retinal detachments in children does occur during the first postoperative year, they usually tend to have a late onset [4, 33, 36]. Studies estimate that the mean interval between cataract surgery and retinal detachment is approximately 30 years [33]. However, retinal detachments tend to occur in a shorter time frame—approximately 8 years—in eyes submitted to lensectomy [33].

It appears that chronic vitreoretinal traction in the anterior vitreous caused by lens removal is the major factor in the pathogenesis of retinal detachment after congenital cataract surgery [39]. The chronic vitreoretinal traction may cause undetected retinal breaks commonly identified in the upper nasal quadrant near the ora serrata that progress to regmatogenous retinal detachments [33, 39].

Most retinal detachments have been identified in the male population [33]. However, it is not clear whether males have an increased risk of congenital cataract, or an increased risk of retinal detachment following lens surgery [33, 36]. To date, the risk factors identified in previous studies that are associated with retinal detachment include myopia, aphakia refraction, and wound dehiscence [1, 34, 36]. Studies show that vitreous disturbance plays an important role in the pathophysiology of retinal detachment [4, 36]. Myopia's association with peripheral retinal degenerations and retinal breaks may explain its relationship to retinal detachment in this population [36]. Aphakia and wound dehiscence, on the other hand, may predispose retinal detachments due to the disturbance of the vitreous that leading to vitreoretinal traction and breaks formation [36]. Moreover, children that present additional ocular abnormalities such as persistent fetal vasculature and retinopathy of prematurity have a higher risk of retinal detachment [4, 12, 36].

To manage this complication, studies have shown that an internal approach improves the likelihood of anatomical success as it allows a thorough inspection of the peripheral retina and identification of retinal breaks [34, 40, 41]. The primary reattachment rate in these eyes vary between 59.3 and 82%, and with additional surgery between 81.4 and 93.3% [33].

Endophthalmitis

The estimated incidence of endophthalmitis in children submitted to lens surgery is 7 cases per 10,000 operations [1, 42, 43]. Cases of pediatric endophthalmitis are mostly related to nasolacrimal duct obstruction or upper respiratory infection at the time of lens extraction [1]. The signs of endophthalmitis are usually present by the third postoperative day and gram positive microorganisms are the most common associated agents to these cases [1, 42, 43]. Despite being considered a rare event, it is usually a dramatic complication usually associated with poor visual outcomes [1, 42].

Phthisis Bulbi

Phthisis bulbi is an extremely rare complication of pediatric lens surgery that leads to permanent visual loss. This complication is mostly related to multiple surgical interventions in the same eye [5]. In the IATS cohort, the sole phthisis bulbi was related to an eye that progressed with retinal detachment [5]. Additionally, patients with retinopathy of prematurity that undergo aggressive laser photocoagulation treatment may develop anterior segment ischemia and are specifically under high risk of developing phthisis bulbi secondary to ischemia after cataract surgery [44].

Video Case

We present the case of a 14-month-old male patient, presented visual axis opacification due to capsular phimosis, Soemmerring ring formation, and epithelial proliferation noted 1 year after phacoaspiration surgery with no IOL implantation in the right eye. The patient was submitted to anterior vitrectomy and surgical removal of the fibrotic tissue and visual axis clearance was again obtained.

Conclusions

Over the years, pediatric lens surgery made substantial leaps that resulted in better visual and functional prognosis for children. However, their small and complex ocular structure increase the risk of intraoperative and postoperative complications. The incidence of intraoperative complications when performing pediatric lens surgery varies between 5 and 21%, whereas postoperative complications are reported in 16% of eyes. Surgeons should be aware that iris prolapse, hyphema, and posterior capsule rupture are the most common intraoperative complications, and that open angle glaucoma and visual axis opacification are the most frequent postoperative complications identified in these eyes. In addition, unlike adults, children are most likely to have late onset retinal detachments. Therefore, close monitoring of pediatric eyes submitted to lens surgery is essential for early detection and prompt surgical intervention of this serious postoperative complication.

Review Questions

1. When performing a pediatric lens surgery, what is the most likely intraoperative complication that you might encounter?

a. Hyphema
b. Iris prolapse

c. Cloudy cornea

d. Posterior capsule rupture

2. You are performing an exam under anesthesia of a 3-yo female child that was submitted to lens surgery one year ago. What is the most common post-operative complication that you might encounter?

a. Retinal detachment

b. Uveitis

c. Glaucoma

d. Lens dislocation

3. What is the most common cause of additional surgical interventions in children submitted to lens surgery?

a. Retained cortex

b. Visual axis opacification

c. Ocular hypertension

d. Retinal detachment

4. About retinal detachment following pediatric lens surgery:

a. Occurs most commonly in the first postoperative year.

b. Occurs less frequently than in adults.

c. Mostly caused by severe ocular inflammation.

d. Mostly related to myopia.

5. When examining a 4-year-old child who underwent lens surgery at the age of 2, you notice no red reflex. What is the most probable complication this patient might have?

a. Posterior capsule opacity

b. Dislocated IOL

c. Posterior capsule rupture

d. Retinal detachment

Answers

1. (**B**) Although hyphema, and posterior capsule rupture are common intraoperative complications of pediatric lens surgery, iris prolapse is the most frequently intra-operative complication reported in the IATS and BICCIG studies.

2. (**C**) Postoperative chronic open angle glaucoma is considered the most common complication following pediatric lens surgery and can develop many years after surgery.

3. (**B**) Studies have shown that visual axis opacification caused by capsular opacity, lens re-proliferation, and pupillary membranes is the major complication that leads pediatric patients to additional surgical interventions.

4. (**D**) Retinal detachment secondary to lens surgery occurs most frequently in pediatric population and tend to have a late onset. The risk factors associated with retinal detachment in the pediatric population submitted to lens surgery include myopia, aphakia refraction, and wound dehiscence. Retinal detachment in these cases is related to vitreoretinal traction that is a precursor of retinal breaks.

5. (**A**) Although retinal detachment may also course with red reflex loss, this complication usually has a late onset in the pediatric population. Posterior capsule opacity, on the other hand, develops due to the proliferation of residual lens epithelial cells on the posterior capsule and has an earlier onset. To avoid this complication, posterior capsulotomy and anterior vitrectomy should be performed as part of the initial surgical intervention.

References

1. Whitman MC, Vanderveen DK. Complications of pediatric cataract surgery. Semin Ophthalmol. 2014;29(5–6):414–20. https://doi.org/10.3109/08820538.2014.959192. PMID: 25325868.
2. Pena CRK, Jorge PA, Kara-Junior N. Intraocular lenses and clinical treatment in paediatric cataract. Rev Bras Oftalmol. 2015;74(3):189–93.
3. Jackson CM, Bickford M, Trivedi RH, Wilson ME. Unplanned returns to the operating room within three months of pediatric cataract-related intraocular surgery: indications and risk factors. J AAPOS. 2019;23(4):224.e1–224.e4. https://doi.org/10.1016/j.jaapos.2019.05.007 Epub 2019 Jun 21. PMID: 31229608.
4. Chrousos GA, Parks MM, O'Neill JF. Incidence of chronic glaucoma, retinal detachment and secondary membrane surgery in pediatric aphakic patients. Ophthalmology. 1984;91: 1238–41.
5. Plager DA, Lynn MJ, Buckley EG, Wilson ME, Lambert SR. Infant Aphakia Treatment Study Group. Complications, adverse events, and additional intraocular surgery 1 year after cataract surgery in the infant Aphakia Treatment Study. Ophthalmology. 2011118(12):2330–4. https://doi.org/10.1016/j.ophtha.2011.06.017. Epub 2011 Sep 16. PMID: 21925737; PMCID: PMC3230731.
6. Solebo AL, Russell-Eggitt I, Cumberland PM, Rahi JS. British Isles Congenital Cataract Interest Group. Risks and outcomes associated with primary intraocular lens implantation in children under 2 years of age: the IoLunder2 cohort study. Br J Ophthalmol. 2015;99 (11):1471–6. https://doi.org/10.1136/bjophthalmol-2014-306394. Epub 2015 May 6. PMID: 25947553.
7. Repka MX, Dean TW, Lazar EL, Yen KG, Lenhart PD, Freedman SF, et al. Pediatric eye disease investigator group. Cataract surgery in children from birth to less than 13 years of age: baseline characteristics of the cohort. Ophthalmology. 2016;123(12):2462–73. https://doi.org/10.1016/j.ophtha.2016.09.003. Epub 2016 Oct 18. PMID: 27769584; PMCID: PMC5121052.
8. Allan BDS. Mechanism of iris prolapse: a qualitative analysis and implications for surgical technique. J Cataract Refract Surg. 1995;21:182–6.
9. Kraff CR, Kraff MC. Cataract surgery. In: Krupin T, Kolker A, editors. Atlas of complications in ophthalmic surgery. London: Mosby-Year Book Europe; 1993. p. 4.2–4.26.

10. Yap EY, Aung T, Fan RF. Pupil abnormalities on the first postoperative day after cataract surgery. Int Ophthalmol. 1996–1997;20(4):187–92. https://doi.org/10.1007/BF00175258. PMID: 9112185.

11. Carrasquillo AM, Gupta BK, Wilensky JT. Recurrent hyphema in an aphakic child: swan syndrome. J AAPOS. 2001;5(1):55–7. https://doi.org/10.1067/mpa.2001.112437 PMID: 11182676.

12. Kuhli-Hattenbach C, Lüchtenberg M, Kohnen T, Hattenbach LO. Risk factors for complications after congenital cataract surgery without intraocular lens implantation in the first 18 months of life. Am J Ophthalmol. 2008;146(1):1–7.https://doi.org/10.1016/j.ajo.2008. 02.014Epub 2008 Apr 14. PMID: 18407241.

13. Chen TC, Bhatia LS, Walton DS. Complications of pediatric lensectomy in 193 eyes. Ophthalmic Surg Lasers Imaging. 2005;36(1):6–13. PMID: 15688966.

14. Christiansen SP, Muñoz M, Capó H. Retinal hemorrhage following lensectomy and anterior vitrectomy in children. J Pediatr Ophthalmol Strabismus. 1993;30(1):24–7. PMID: 8455121.

15. Lin CJ, Tan CY, Lin SY, Jou JR. Uveitis-glaucoma-hyphema syndrome caused by posterior chamber intraocular lens–a rare complication in pediatric cataract surgery. Ann Ophthalmol (Skokie). 2008 Fall-Winter;40(3–4):183–4. PMID: 19230361.

16. Vajpayee RB, Sharma N, Dada T, Gupta V, Kumar A, Dada VK. Management of posterior capsule tears. Surv Ophthalmol. 2001;45(6):473–88. https://doi.org/10.1016/s0039-6257(01) 00195-3. PMID: 11425354.

17. Gilliland GD, Hutton WL, Fuller DG. Retained intravitreal lens fragments after cataract surgery. Ophthalmology. 1992;99(8):1263–7; discussion 1268–9. https://doi.org/10.1016/ s0161-6420(92)31814-7. PMID: 1513581.

18. Lin H, Chen W, Luo L, Zhang X, Chen J, Lin Z, et al. Study Group of CCPMOH. Ocular hypertension after pediatric cataract surgery: baseline characteristics and first-year report. PLoS One. 2013;8(7):e69867. https://doi.org/10.1371/journal.pone.0069867. PMID: 23922832; PMCID: PMC3726742.

19. Chen TC, Walton DS, Bhatia LS. Aphakic glaucoma after congenital cataract surgery. Arch Ophthalmol. 2004;122(12):1819–25.

20. Mandal AK, Netland PA. Glaucoma in aphakia and pseudophakia after congenital cataract surgery. Indian J Ophthalmol. 2004;52(3):185–98 PMID: 15510457.

21. Rabiah PK. Frequency and predictors of glaucoma after pediatric cataract surgery. Am J Ophthalmol. 2004;137:30–7.

22. Chak M, Rahi JS. Incidence of and factors associated with glaucoma after surgery for congenital cataract: findings from the British Congenital Cataract Study. Ophthalmology. 2008;115:1013–8.

23. Papadopoulos M, Khaw PT. Meeting the challenge of glaucoma after paediatric cataract surgery. Eye. 2003;17:1–2.

24. Asrani S, Freedman S, Hasselblad V, et al. Does primary intraocular lens implantation prevent "aphakic" glaucoma in children? JAAPOS. 2000;4:33–9.

25. Trivedi RH, Wilson ME Jr, Golub RL. Incidence and risk factors for glaucoma after pediatric cataract surgery with and without intraocular lens implantation. J AAPOS. 2006;10:117–23.

26. Egbert JE, Christiansen SP, Wright MM, et al. The natural history of glaucoma and ocular hypertension after pediatric cataract surgery. J AAPOS. 2006;10:54–7.

27. Simon JW, Miter D, Zobal-Ratner J, Hodgetts D, Belin MW. Corneal edema after pediatric cataract surgery. J AAPOS. 1997;1(2):102–4.https://doi.org/10.1016/s1091-8531(97)90007-0 PMID: 10875086.

28. Borghol Kassar R, Menezo Rozalen JL, Harto Castano MA, Desco Esteban MC. Long-term follow-up of the corneal endothelium after pediatric cataract surgery. Cornea 2012;31(5): 529–532.

29. Yap EY, Aung T, Fan RF. Pupil abnormalities on the first postoperative day after cataract surgery. Int Ophthalmol. 1996–1997;20(4):187–92. https://doi.org/10.1007/BF00175258. PMID: 9112185.

30. Waiswol M, Ejzenbaum F, Wu DC, Kagohara E, Reggi JR. Congenital fibrovascular pupillary membrane. Einstein (Sao Paulo). 2015;13(1):163–4. https://doi.org/10.1590/S1679-45082015AI2850. Epub 2015 Mar 3. PMID: 25993083; PMCID: PMC4946823.

31. Lee GI, Lim DH, Chi SA, Kim SW, Shin DW, Chung TY. Risk factors for intraocular lens dislocation after phacoemulsification: a nationwide population-based cohort study. Am J Ophthalmol. 2020;214:86–96.https://doi.org/10.1016/j.ajo.2020.03.012Epub 2020 Mar 21. PMID: 32209346.

32. Struck MC. Long-term results of pediatric cataract surgery and primary intraocular lens implantation from 7 to 22 months of life. JAMA Ophthalmol. 2015;133(10):1180–3. https://doi.org/10.1001/jamaophthalmol.2015.2062 PMID: 26111188.

33. Yorston D, Yang YF, Sullivan PM. Retinal detachment following surgery for congenital cataract: presentation and outcomes. Eye (Lond). 2005;19(3):317–21. https://doi.org/10.1038/sj.eye.6701463 PMID: 15258607.

34. Eckstein M, Vijayalakshmi P, Gilbert C, Foster A. Randomised clinical trial of lensectomy versus lens aspiration and primary capsulotomy for children with bilateral cataract in south India. Br J Ophthalmol. 1999;83:524–9.

35. Kanski JJ, Elkington AR, Daniel R. Retinal detachment after congenital cataract surgery. Br J Ophthalmol. 1974;58(2):92–5. https://doi.org/10.1136/bjo.58.2.92.PMID:4820989;PMCID: PMC1017316.

36. Rabiah PK, Du H, Hahn EA. Frequency and predictors of retinal detachment after pediatric cataract surgery without primary intraocular lens implantation. J AAPOS. 2005;9(2):152–9. https://doi.org/10.1016/j.jaapos.2004.12.013 PMID: 15838443.

37. Keech RV, Tongue AC, Scott WE. Complications after surgery for congenital and infantile cataracts. Am J Ophthalmol. 1989;108:136–41.

38. Hing S, Speedwell L, Taylor D. Lens surgery in infancy and childhood. Br J Ophthalmol. 1990;74:73–7.

39. Toyofuku H, Hirose T, Schepens CL. Retinal detachment following congenital cataract surgery. I. Preoperative findings in 114 eyes. Arch Ophthalmol. 1980;98(4):669–75. https://doi.org/10.1001/archopht.1980.01020030663003. PMID: 7369901.

40. Jagger JD, Cooling RJ, Fison LG, Leaver PK, McLeod D. Management of retinal detachment following congenital cataract surgery. Trans Ophthalmol Soc UK. 1983;103:103–7.

41. Bonnet M, Delage S. Retinal detachment after surgery of congenital cataract. J Fr Ophtalmol 1994;17:580–4.

42. Wheeler DT, Stager DR, Weakley DR Jr. Endophthalmitis following pediatric intraocular surgery for congenital cataracts and congenital glaucoma. J Pediatr Ophthalmol Strabismus. 1992;29(3):139–41.

43. Good WV, Hing S, Irvine AR, Hoyt CS, Taylor DS. Postoperative endophthalmitis in children following cataract surgery. J Pediatr Ophthalmol Strabismus. 1990;27(6):283–5. PMID: 2086742.

44. Lambert SR, Capone A Jr, Cingle KA, Drack AV. Cataract and phthisis bulbi after laser photoablation for threshold retinopathy of prematurity. Am J Ophthalmol. 2000;129(5): 585–91. https://doi.org/10.1016/s0002-9394(99)00475-4.Erratum.In:AmJOphthalmol2000Dec; 130(6):908 PMID: 10844048.

Secondary IOL Implantation at Pediatric Age

58

Parveen Sen, Shobhit Varma, Kavitha Kalaivani Natarajan, and Gayathri J. Panicker

Abstract

This chapter aims to cover the various management options for pediatric aphakia with main stress on the surgical approach. The pre-operative assessment and IOL power calculation is an important consideration before planning surgery. Surgical approach and IOL options depend on presence or absence of capsular support. Special emphasis has been made in discussion of various techniques of scleral fixated IOLs in absence of capsular support. Sutured and sutureless fixation of scleral fixation have been elaborated in simplistic way in order to make the reader understand the surgical technique.

Keywords

Secondary IOL in children · Pediatric SFIOL · Pediatric Aphakia · Iris fixated IOL · Scleral fixated IOL · Glued IOL · Pediatric vision rehabilitation

Supplementary Information The online version contains supplementary material available at https://doi.org/10.1007/978-3-031-14506-3_58.

P. Sen (✉) · S. Varma
Shri Bhagwan Mahaveer Department of Vitreoretinal Services, Sankara Nethralaya, Chennai, India
e-mail: parveensen@gmail.com

K. K. Natarajan · G. J. Panicker
Department of Pediatric Ophthalmology and Strabismus, Sankara Nethralaya, Chennai, India
e-mail: drkkv@snmail.org

Introduction

Cataract surgery with intraocular lens (IOL) implantation is a common surgical procedure performed in children. In a systematic review conducted in 2016 using data from articles published from five different regions across the globe, the overall prevalence of childhood cataract and congenital cataract was reported to be 0.32 to 22.9/10000 children (median = 1.03) and 0.63 to 9.74/10000 (median = 1.71), respectively [1]. The most desirable location for an Intraocular lens (IOL) in the eye after cataract surgery is within the capsular bag and this is best done during cataract extraction. While implanting a primary IOL for children above 2 years is usually done, implantation of the same in children younger than 2 years is controversial as these eyes can develop intense inflammation and have increased rates of posterior capsular opacification (PCO) [2]. These eyes are sometimes left aphakic during the primary surgery. Loss of capsular support can also happen during surgery or due to trauma or congenital conditions (Table 58.1) (Fig. 58.1).

After the primary cataract surgery, challenge lies in the early and effective management of paediatric aphakia. It is difficult to expect that the refractive needs of an aphakic child can be adequately met with contact lenses or spectacles in the long term. Various methods have been used for correction of aphakia in children are tabulated in Table 58.2.

Problems arising out of aphakic glasses include:

1. Optical aberrations,
2. Field restriction
3. Poor cosmesis

Problems associated with contact lenses include:

1. Wearing compliance,
2. Corneal surface disease,
3. Fitting challenges

Table 58.1 Table enumerates common causes of aphakia in children

S no	Causes of Aphakia
1	Loss or rupture of the posterior capsule during primary cataract extraction surgery
2	Aphakia after planned lensectomy for congenital cataract in very young babies
3	Traumatic cataract with zonular dehiscence
4	Primary congenital ectopia lentis
5	Ectopia lentis associated with congenital disorders with complete dislocation (luxated) or partial dislocation (subluxated) of crystalline lens like Marfan's Syndrome, Homocystinuria, Weil-Marchesani's syndrome, Sulphite oxidase deficiency, Hyperlysinemia, Ehlers-Danlos syndrome, Sticklers syndrome and Congenital Aniridia
6	Occasionally, IOLs which have opacified with time or got damaged (pitting during Nd Yag capsulotomy), decentered, induced high myopia or refractive error or have become an optical hindrance may need removal and replacement with a secondary IOL

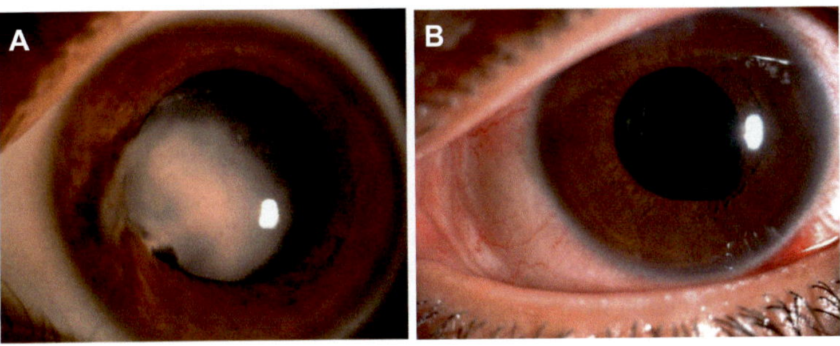

Fig. 58.1 **A** Left eye 7 year old boy showing traumatic cataract and adherent leukoma; **B** Surgical aphakia post cataract surgery in a 6 year old

Table 58.2 Various methods used for correction of aphakia in children

Serial no	Type of correction
1	Aphakic glasses
2	Contact lenses
3	Anterior chamber IOL(ACIOL)
4	Iris Claw Lens
5	"In-the-bag" secondary IOL
6	In the sulcus secondary IOL
7	Scleral Fixated IOL (SFIOL) which may be a. Sutureless SFIOL with Intrascleral fixation of IOL c. Sutured SFIOL (SSFIOL)

These problems with glasses and contact lenses result in poor compliance and therefore interfere with normal visual development and functioning. Need for better functional vision for school going age children may also necessitate alternate methods of aphakic correction [3]. Due to these limitations with aphakic glasses and CL, a secondary IOL implantation is commonly preferred as a treatment option [4].

Timing of Surgery

Over the last decade, various studies on secondary IOLs in children have reported different average age for secondary IOL implantation from as early as 2 years of age [5–7] to even as late as 8yrs [8, 9]. Though best corrected visual acuity (BCVA) of as good as 20/55 over long term in children who have had secondary IOL around 2 years of age has been reported, [4] the recent landmark Infant Aphakia Treatment Study (IATS) suggested that delaying implantation of secondary IOL in children to after 5 years of age may help to reduce the "IOL surprises" that may occur due to axial length elongation seen between infancy and 5 years [10]. This allows a more predictable refractive outcome.

Early surgery, glaucoma and secondary opacities in addition may result in increased rates of axial elongation and high myopic shift. When elective implantation of secondary IOL is planned and done by an experienced surgeon after age 5 years, the complications encountered are less with lower rates of adverse events than when performed in infancy [10]. While this criterion of age may be appropriate for bilateral aphakes, the age at secondary IOL implantation is recommended to be as early as 2 years or younger in unilateral aphakes to allow adequate management of associated problems of unilateral aphakia [11]. Early successful secondary IOL implantation especially in unilateral aphakia resulting in clear visual axis and optimal refractive correction allows:

1. Good visual maturation
2. Management of anisometropia
3. Management and even reversal of amblyopia in some children
4. Management of Strabismus.

A large case series of 220 eyes of 148 patients who underwent surgery for pediatric cataract was reported by Sefi-Yurdakul et al. [12]. They reported an incidence of strabismus in 23% of eyes undergoing primary IOL as against 30% of eyes undergoing secondary IOL implantation.

Preoperative Considerations

Careful preoperative planning and patient selection helps in optimization of results and improved surgical and functional outcome. A complete clinical examination, under general anesthesia when needed, must be done to look for any corneal pathology, glaucoma, presence or absence of adequate capsular support and retinal status before deciding on secondary IOL implantation.

Preoperative assessment must include the following:

(1) Assessment of Best corrected visual acuity (BCVA)
(2) Assessment of preexisting refractive error
(3) Anterior segment evaluation to assess the cornea (diameter, thickness and any associated corneal degeneration/dystrophy)
(4) Presence or absence of iris tissue.
(5) Associated anterior segment distortion due to prior trauma, congenital defects or previous surgeries.
(6) Presence or absence of capsular support. The planning for a secondary IOL is best begun during primary cataract surgery. This is especially important in babies that are operated for cataract without an IOL implantation in the first year of life. A 4–5 mm anterior and posterior capsulotomy during this procedure allows a clear visual axis as well as leave an adequate 360-degree rim support for subsequent secondary in the bag or sulcus IOL.
UBM is a useful tool to assess the capsule and zonular support and the presence and extent of posterior peripheral synechiae, which may interfere with pupil dilatation and sulcus implantation of IOL (Fig. 58.2). Thus preoperative UBM may help to formulate an appropriate surgical strategy [13].

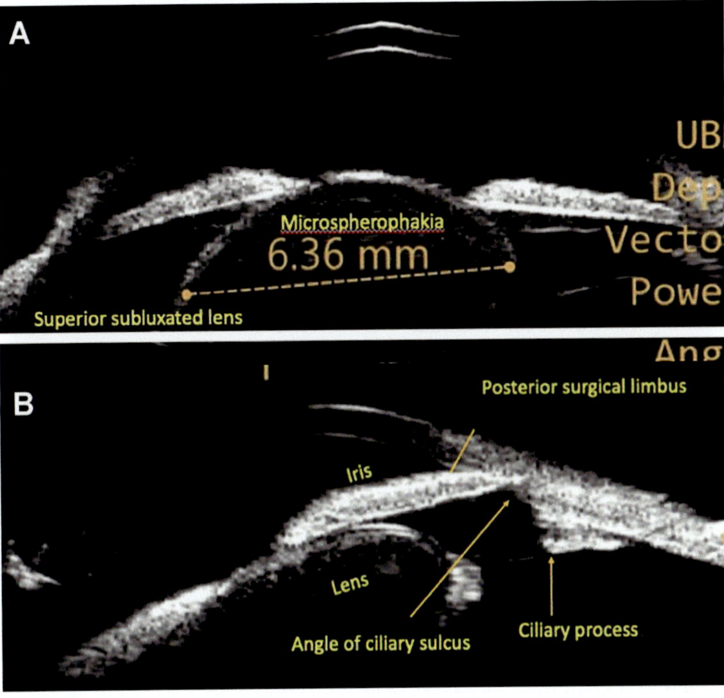

Fig. 58.2 A UBM of 14-year-old having microspherophakia with superior subluxated lens. **B** UBM shows the scanty zonules with normal ciliary processes and ciliary body

(7) Any associated scleral scarring due to previous surgeries or trauma should be noted especially when planning a SFIOL.

(8) Intraocular pressure (IOP) measurement is vital. Associated glaucoma must be managed and must be well under control before surgery.

(9) Any intraocular inflammation will need proper management prior to surgery.

(10) Any associated posterior segment pathologies like retinal detachment or preexisting peripheral retinal lesions like retinal holes or lattice degeneration are best taken care of prior to planning secondary IOL

(11) Choice of IOLs depending on the individual case.

(12) A note of the associated systemic issues which may be particularly relevant for safe anaesthesia for surgery

Contraindications

It is important for the paediatric ophthalmologist to identify cases in whom a secondary IOL surgery is to be deferred.

1. Uncontrolled glaucoma: Risk of postoperative IOP spikes and associated risk of axial elongation and high myopia are reasons for avoiding secondary IOL in children with uncontrolled glaucoma.
2. Acute, chronic and recurrent uveitic conditions can exacerbate with any surgical procedure and in presence of active ocular inflammation surgical procedures for secondary IOL are best avoided.
3. Anterior segment structural congenital anomalies like microcornea and microphthalmos may also preclude secondary IOL implantation [14].

IOL Power Calculation in Children

One of the key advantages of operating at about 5 years of age is the ability of the child to cooperate for keratometry and axial length measurements needed for IOL power calculation. In case the child is uncooperative, then these measurements must be done under sedation or general anaesthesia prior to surgery.

Most IOL calculation methods depend on accurate measurement of axial length. Various techniques employed for IOL calculation include applanation methods like the ultrasound A scan or optical biometers like the IOL master. Few authors recommend performing IOL power calculations using IOL master in cooperative children for more predictable post-operative refractive outcomes [7]. Errors in measurements of axial length using applanation techniques are largely due to lack of a lens spike in aphakic patients, causing inability to ascertain the correct visual axis. Also, inadvertent increase in corneal compression during applanation techniques can result in incorrect estimation of axial length [15]. Another issue with IOL calculation in paediatric eyes is that they have shorter axial lengths in younger age that increases as the eye ball grows with age. This may necessitate insertion of higher IOL powers (>23D) reducing the predictability of postoperative refractive error as the child grows older [7]. Though literature suggests that most of the IOL power calculation formulae can give a fairly accurate IOL power in paediatric eyes, the SRK II formula has been found most suitable [16, 17]. It can be used for a wide range of axial lengths but is sometimes less predictable with axial length of less than 22 mm for which Holladay 2 formula may be used preferably [7, 18]. Existing cycloplegic refraction and the final refractive goal (whether any under correction is required) for the eye to be operated is to be considered. Also, refraction of the fellow eye must always be taken into consideration to avoid any iatrogenic anisometropia which may be result in amblyopia [19].

Surgical Techniques

When Capsular Support is Adequate

In most cases of surgical paediatric aphakia, the presence of a pre-existing good capsular support aids in placement of secondary IOL in the ciliary sulcus or in the capsular bag. Surgically, placing the IOL in the ciliary sulcus is easier as compared to in the bag placement of secondary IOL. The key steps in implanting a secondary IOL in ciliary sulcus involve releasing all posterior synechiae in 360° from 2 side ports at 3 and 9 o clock positions followed by adequate viscoelastic injection into the sulcus space. The foldable three piece IOL is then carefully injected into the ciliary sulcus via a main 12 o clock incision. Viscoleastic material is thoroughly cleared and AC formed with saline after suturing all wounds with 10–0 vicryl (**Video** 1). The main hindrance to surgical ease of sulcus placement of IOL is the presence of the Soemmering ring in some eyes which forms in between the remnants of anterior and posterior capsule leaflets after primary cataract extraction and posterior capsulorrhexis procedure [10]. This Soemmering ring may result in IOL tilt, decentration, pupillary capture or pseudophakic pupillary block glaucoma [20]. Also it may result in change of the effective lens position during sulcus placement. Placing an IOL in the ciliary sulcus also carries a higher risk of iris chafing, chronic inflammation, pigment dispersion, glaucoma, and late IOL dislocation as compared to in the bag IOL implantation [10].

At the time of primary cataract surgery if a central round approximately 4.5 mm anterior and posterior capsulotomy is made, then in-the-bag secondary IOL implantation technique can be used. If the capsulotomy is too large or irregular, IOL implantation will have to be in the sulcus. The technique of use of vitrector probe for in-the-bag secondary implantation in children was described by Wilson et al. [21]. The point of fusion of anterior and posterior capsules can be trimmed and separated with the vitrector and then remove the Soemmerring ring material. In another technique a cystotome was used for opening the bag and the Soemmerring ring was then aspirated using a manual Simcoe cannula. Once the capsular leaflets are adequately opened up, the IOL is carefully dialled and inserted in the bag [22]. Care must be taken to prevent partial or complete dislocation of Soemmerring ring into the vitreous cavity, risk of which is lower with ocular viscoelastic devices (OVD) use as described by Grewal and Basti [20]

Though visual outcomes of Secondary IOLs in sulcus are comparable to those of secondary in the bag IOL implantation, in the bag IOL implantation has lesser risk of postoperative inflammation and corneal degeneration [8]. On the other hand advantage of sulcus IOLs is that they rarely form adhesions in place and if deemed necessary can easily be rotated, and/or exchanged even several years after being implanted [23].

Poor pupillary dilation, a common problem in secondary IOL implantation for congenital cataracts can be managed by:

1. Non-mechanical enlargement (using pharmacological agents)
2. Mechanical enlargement using various mechanical devices [24].

Inflammatory adhesions after cataract surgery make pharmacological pupil dilatation less effective in some eyes [25]. Reduced intraoperative risks with mechanical pupil expanders have been reported [26]. This can be achieved effectively with iris hooks or the new XpandNT iris speculum which creates a near circular opening of around 6.7 mm during secondary IOL implantation [27].

When Capsular Support is Insufficient

Anterior Chamber IOLs

With better alternatives such as iris fixated IOLs and scleral fixated IOLs, there is virtually little role for ACIOL implantation for pediatric aphakia without capsular support in modern surgical practice inspite of ease of surgery [28].

Common complications associated with ACIOLs include:

1. Pseudophakic bullous keratopathy due to endothelial cell loss
2. Pigment dispersion
3. Uveitis glaucoma hyphema syndrome

Wilson et al. [29] reported 31 eyes of 18 children in whom angle supported IOLs were placed. Though they did not report corneal decompensation in the limited follow up, in 7 eyes (22.6%) ACIOL had to be removed within 3 to 5 years and in 4 eyes (12.9%) IOL repositioning was required. In some of these cases ACIOL showed rotation with the growth of the eyeball with age resulting in a reoperation rate of 35.5% [30].

Iris Fixated IOLs

Iris fixated IOLs have also been used in the absence of adequate sulcus support. Worst Fechner claw lens or Artisan lens developed by Worst et al. [30, 31] for iris fixation is a 5.4 mm biconvex PMMA lens. It has a vaulted lens design which allows sufficient clearance between the iris and the IOL allowing adequate aqueous flow. The lens haptic is enclavated at mid periphery of iris and is at contact with iris in only that portion thus theoretically reducing iris contact. This allows less pigment dispersion with minimal interference with normal physiological functioning of the iris. Surgical PI is mandatory in these cases in order to prevent pupillary block. Though studies have shown acceptable visual outcomes and less postoperative complications with minimal postoperative increase in IOP while using these lenses for pediatric aphakia, long term effect on children however need to be seen [32].

Common complications associated with Iris claw lens include:

1. Endothelial cell loss
2. Pupillary block
3. De-enclavation of IOL
4. Pigment dispersion
5. Cystoid macular edema

Posterior iris fixation using 10–0 polypropylene suture has also been described [33]. Due to high incidence of IOL dislocation of iris fixated IOL in children (upto 41%) it should be placed with extreme caution [34].

Sutured or Sutureless Scleral Fixated IOL

Sutured Scleral fixated IOL(SSFIOL) and sutureless Scleral fixated IOL(SLSFIOL) have both been described in children. Wong et al. [34] published a major systematic review on scleral fixated IOL where they analyzed data of 421 pediatric patients with a mean age of 9.90 ± 4.86 years. Majority patients had undergone SSFIOL in the study and while only 2 out of the 7 studies had glued SFIOL data.

Basic Principles of the Surgery

Surgery for SFIOLs has been described both by the anterior as well as posterior route [35].

Complete pars plana vitrectomy (PPV) reduces the long-term risk of development of rhegmatogenous retinal detachment (RRD) [36]. Removal of capsular remnants and peripheral vitreous especially in the area of lens anchorage, reduces risk of suture entanglement as well as reduced chances of suture lysis because of reduced metabolic activity and inflammation surrounding it.

Intraoperative Steps of Sutured SFIOL

(a) Construction of flap
(b) Sclerocorneal tunnel
(c) Tucking of the 9–0 or 10–0 prolene suture needle into 26 gauge needle
(d) Passing the suture through eyelet of the IOL
(e) Suture needle being passed under the scleral flap
(f) Tightening of sutures ensuring correct IOL positioning

2 Point Fixation Versus 4 Point Fixation

2-point fixation (scleral fixation at only 2 points) has been described using a 10–0 polypropylene suture with the needle spanning from 3 to 9 o'clock meridian [37]. The suture is brought out in the middle through the corneo-scleral section and cut in the middle; the cut ends are tied on to the haptic on each side of the IOL. The sutures are tied on either side under the flaps after inserting the IOL into the eye.

The 4-point fixation technique commonly used has described by Lewis et al. [38] and Rao et al. [36]. It involves the insertion of the 9/0 or 10/0 polypropylene suture needle into the eye under the flaps and brought out from the corneo-scleral insertion via a rail road technique. Both suture ends are then tied into a knot which is then rotated and buried internally. A 4-point fixation allows a better stability of IOL with less chances of IOL tilt and reduced risk of knot exposure.

The salient steps of the surgery are as described in Fig. 58.3a–h: Radial keratotomy marker is used for accurate positioning (Fig. 58.4) of 3 mm X 2 mm scleral flaps at 3 and 9 o'clock positions along the horizontal meridian. Scleral flaps are of 50% thickness. 6.5 mm scleral tunnel is made. 9/0 or 10/0 polypropylene suture (Ethicon Inc) is used. A rail road technique is used for threading the sutures through a 26 gauge, 16 mm long hollow straight needle. The direction of passage of suture is changed in opposite eyelets to neutralize the torque on the IOL. The traction on the sutures is gently balanced as the IOL is introduced and fixated at the sulcus. Knots are rotated inside the globe and covered by the scleral flaps. The partial thickness scleral flaps are closed with suture or glue. The intraoperative steps are shown in Fig. 58.5.

SFIOL fixation can be combined with macular hole surgery in cases of traumatic cataract with macular hole (**Video** 2).

Types of Suture Commonly used for SSFIOL

(a) 10–0 polypropylene fixation
(b) 9–0 polypropylene fixation
(c) Gore-tex fixation

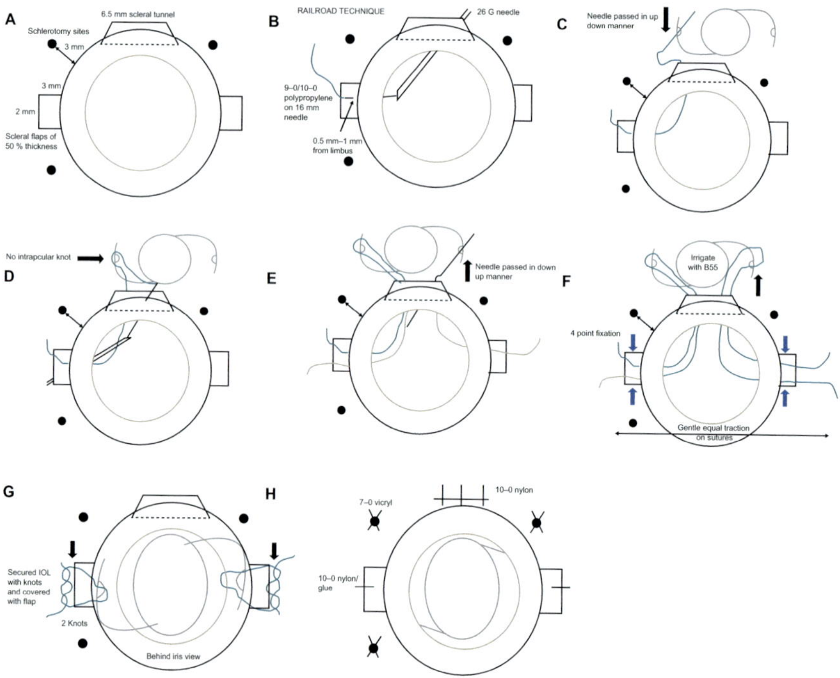

Fig. 58.3 A–H: Surgical steps of sutured scleral fixated IOL

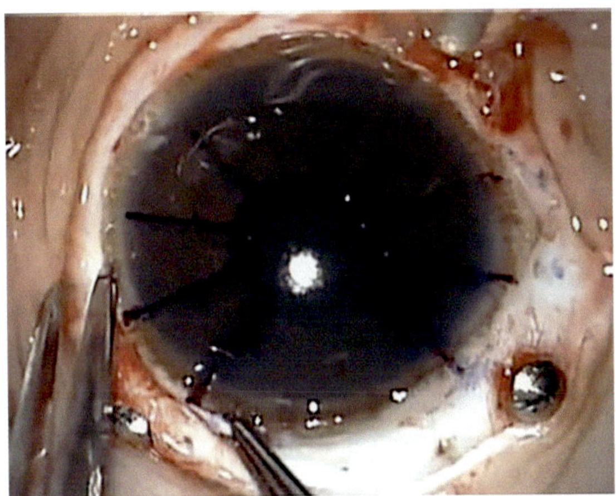

Fig. 58.4 Marking the cornea for correct incision location

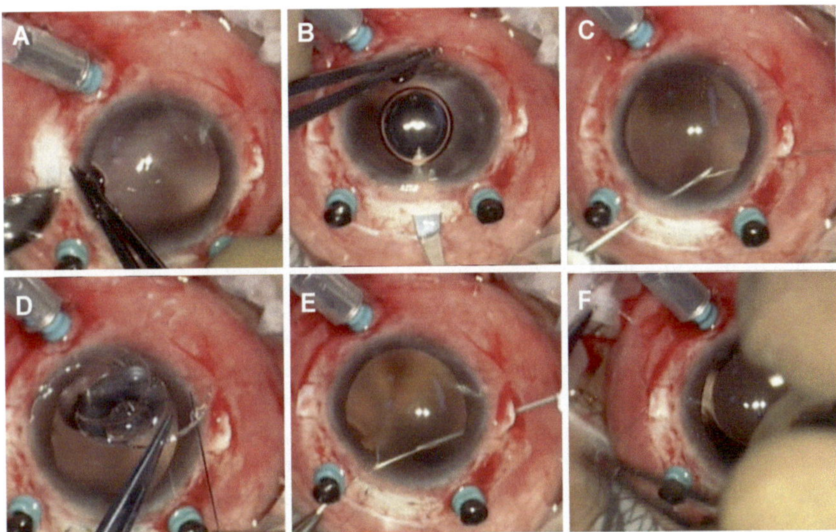

Fig. 58.5 Showing intraoperative steps of Sutured SFIOL

Polypropylene suture (a monofilament suture) has been the most common suture technique used for scleral fixation of IOL. Polypropylene suture doesn't cause fibrosis. Suture degradation is a natural course over a long period of time which may lead to dislocation of the IOL. Additional risks of suture breakage in pediatric cases are due to increasing axial length of the globe and trauma associated risk factors that increase risk of IOL dislocation.

Gore-tex suture has been recently used for SSFIOL. It is also a monofilament suture that is made of expanded polytetrafluoroethylene and has a high tensile strength. It is white colored with minimal memory and easy to manipulate intraoperatively. They too cause minimal inflammatory response. Khan et al. [39] in their series of SFIOL fixation using Gore-tex suture found that the suture knots integrate with the sclera in long term thus preventing any suture erosion or exposure. The post-operative complications were found to be comparable to other techniques of SSFIOL.

Intraocular lenses used for SFIOL

Most commonly used IOL for SSFIOL is the rigid, nonfoldable, polymethylmethacrylate (PMMA), single piece lens with eyelet in the haptic and 6 mm optic and overall diameter of 13.5 mm. Akreos AO60 IOL (Bausch & Lomb, Rochester, NY) a hydrophilic acrylic foldable IOL with a modified four-haptic design has been used recently for 4-point fixation [40].

Sutureless Intrascleral Fixation (SL-SFIOL)

Sutureless fixation techniques have been developed to overcome the concerns regarding the suture related complications of SSFIOL especially the long-term degradation of sutures seen leading to IOL dislocation. Though many sutureless techniques have been described in the adults, very few and small case series with limited follow up only have been reported for pediatric eyes. Kumar et al. & Kannan et al. [30] reported a series of pediatric eyes undergoing SL-SFIOL using fibrin glue. Figure 58.6a–f demonstrates the surgical steps of sutureless scleral fixated IOL. After a complete three ports PPV, lamellar scleral flaps are performed similar to the SSFIOL. The corneal tunnel required is about 2–3 mm if a foldable IOL is used. Sclerotomies are made 1–2 mm from the limbus under the scleral flaps. Foldable three piece IOL is loaded in injector and inserted into the anterior chamber while using intraocular forceps to hold the leading haptic. The tip of the leading haptic is exteriorized under the scleral flap. The trailing haptic is also held with the 23G forceps and using hand shake technique, it is also exteriorized under the flap. The haptics of 3-piece IOL are then covered under partial thickness scleral flaps which are then apposed with fibrin glue. The surgical steps are shown in Fig. 58.7. IOL subluxation has been reported with SL-SFIOL as well [41].

The technique of Flanged haptic SL-SFIOL has been described by Yamane et al. [42] in adults which is termed as transconjunctival sutureless, flapless, glueless method of SFIOL. In this procedure foldable 3-piece IOL is injected into the anterior chamber. Two 30-gauge needles are inserted trans conjunctivally 2 mm from the limbus on each side and the haptics are externalized with the help of these needles. The tip of the externalized haptic is then cauterized at the tip which creates a bulbous flange whose diameter is larger than the haptic thickness. This flange is then pushed inside the substance of sclera and then covered with conjunctiva. Sternfeld et al. in a small case series of 12 cases described the Yamane technique in pediatric eyes with a short mean follow up of 8 ± 5 months [43]. There aren't many large studies with long term experience with Yamane's in pediatric eyes.

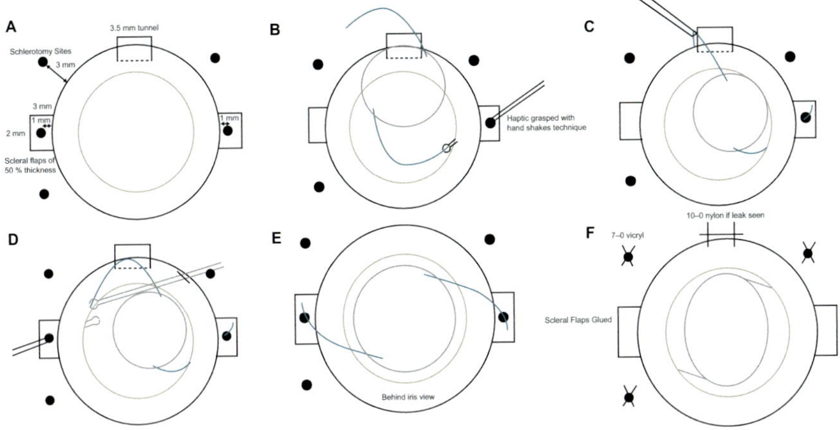

Fig. 58.6 **A–F**: Surgical steps of sutureless scleral fixated IOL

This technique has some benefits as compared to other methods as it avoids conjunctival opening, scleral flaps or pockets thus making the process less complicated, less traumatic and potentially faster. However, narrow orbital space can be a limitation for this technique in young children. Also, low scleral rigidity of children can lead to scleral collapse during insertion of second instrument which makes the technique more difficult.

Though intermediate visual outcomes of SL-SFIOL are comparable to those of SSFIOL, there is lack of consensus regarding their use in pediatric eyes.

Surgical Steps of Glued IOL

(a) Inserting three piece IOL through the main wound
(b) Insertion of lower haptic in the needle

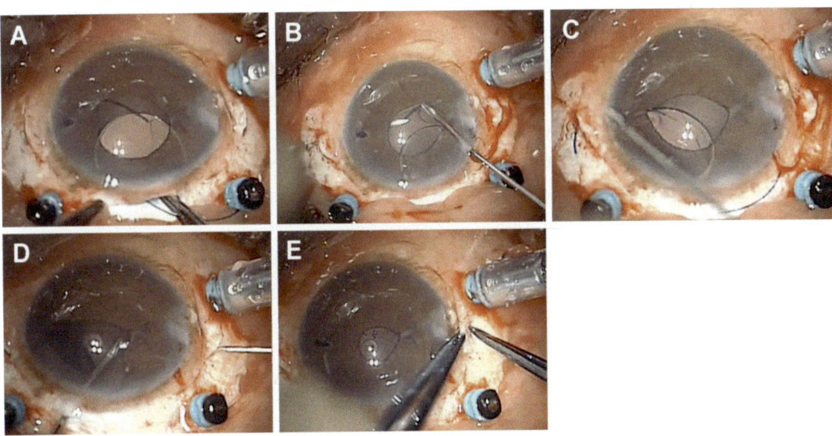

Fig. 58.7 **A–E**: Surgical steps of Glued IOL

(c) Extrusion of haptic under the scleral flap
(d) Similar step is repeated on other side
(e) Tucking of haptic in sclera followed by glue

Complications of Secondary IOLs

Some complications (36) associated with sulcus or in the bag secondary IOL include:

1. Visual axis opacification (VAO)
2. Glaucoma
3. Dislocation/decentration of IOL
4. Pupillary capture
5. Endophthalmitis

Post-operative secondary glaucoma is a significant complication seen after pediatric cataract surgery [9]. Angle structures in infants are not fully developed and aphakia at an early age leads to inflammation and subsequently maldevelopment of the structures of the angle thus making child prone for open angle glaucoma [44].

Risk factors for development of glaucoma are:

1. Early age at time of cataract extraction
2. Sulcus implantation of IOL
3. Severe postoperative inflammation
4. Mechanical absence of lens itself [45] is known to increase risk of glaucoma.

In the bag IOL after cataract surgery has lower rates of glaucoma as compared to sulcus IOL. Early postoperative acute rise in IOP was noted in higher proportion of eyes (27.3%) with pre-existing aphakic glaucoma as compared to 2.7% eyes without glaucoma [46]. Meticulous viscoelastic wash at the end of surgery and probably use of prophylactic topical anti glaucoma medication during the early postoperative period can reduce the risk of post-operative secondary glaucoma [47].

Almost 5.4% eyes may need repeat surgery to clear the visual axis [4]. The risk for Visual axis opacification (VAO) appears to be higher in cases of in the bag secondary IOL which may be due to reopening of the capsule leaflets and allowing potential space for re-proliferation of lens epithelial cells. However risk of IOL dislocations/ decentrations, endophthalmitis and refractive surprise is more with sulcus IOLs [3].

Intraoperative complications seen with suspension of a SFIOL include:
Early postoperative complications:

1. Vitreous hemorrhage
2. Choroidal detachment due to hypotony and suprachoroidal haemorrhage.
3. Rhegmatogenous retinal detachment (RRD)
4. IOL tilt,

5. IOL decentration
6. Optic capture.

Late postoperative complications are:

1. Suture erosion through conjunctiva,
2. Suture breakage,
3. Late endophthalmitis,
4. IOL dislocation
5. Macular edema.

Incidence of suture erosion as reported in literature is between 0 to 28.5%. Suture exposure over a period of time provides a communication between intraocular and extraocular environment which may potentially lead to 'suture wick' endophthalmitis [30]. Incidence of suture breakage is reportedly high especially with 10–0 polypropylene suture. Microscopic examination of the suture material removed in dislocated IOL revealed presence of cracked suture and not untied knots [47]. Constant rubbing of the edges of the eylets on the haptics through which the suture passes may also contribute to the suture erosion [47]. Sen et al. reported mean time of IOL dislocation period being 9.2 years [36]. The various complications of SFIOL reported from different studies are presented in (Table 58.3).

RRD seen in pediatric age group after surgery for secondary IOL can be a cause of profound visual loss and deserves special mention. Eyes undergoing surgery for SFIOL in conditions like ectopia lentis and Marfan's syndrome or trauma may be associated with an increased risk of RRD. While early intervention can help in a successful outcome, delay in surgery can lead to rapid development of PVR with the risk of permanent visual loss. Parents need to be counselled regarding the same and a regular follow up is essential to look for RRD. Sen et al. have reported an incidence of 5.73% of retinal detachment in a series of 279 pediatric patient [36]. The incidence of retinal detachment is between 0–5.73% according to various studies on pediatric SFIOL [36, 55].

Traumatic cataracts especially following penetrating injuries are also usually associated with traumatic partial or complete aniridia or iridodialysis (Fig. 58.8). Treatment options that can be done along with cataract extraction and SSFIOL include iridoplasty or using IOLs with iris prosthesis. The latter has the advantage of correcting the iris defect and managing aphakia at the same sitting. Long term clinical outcomes of the Artisan iris reconstruction IOL in traumatic pediatric aniridia and aphakia show promising results [56]. Vanderveen and Dean et al. demonstrated improved overall visual performance and a stable or improved BCVA in 90.9% of eyes after secondary IOL implantation [57].

To conclude, the technique, relative safety and efficacy of secondary IOL implantation in paediatric eyes has been widely reported. Good results can be obtained with meticulous planning and a careful surgery. Involvement of parents and/or guardians can help to improve follow up as well as management of postoperative complications.

Table 58.3 Sutured SFIOL comparative data for complications

Author	Year	Eyes (N)	Mean Age At SFIOL (Years)	IOL dislocation	Retinal Detachment	Raised IOP	Vitreous hemorrhage	Choroidal detachment	Endophthalmitis	Suture exposure
Buckley [48]	2007	33	9.7	9%(3)	0	6%(2)	3%(1)	0	0	0
Asadi and kheirkhah [49]	2008	25	6.6	24% (6)	4% (1)	0	52% (13)	8%(2)	4(1)	0
Burcu et al. [50]	2014	24	11.5	0	0	12.5% (3)	0	0	0	4.2%(1)
Sen et al. [36]	2015	279	10.8	4.65%(13)	5.73%(16)	12.54% (35)	2.86%(8)	2.86%(8)	0.72% (2)	0
Abdulaziz et al. [51]	2017	18	3.5	5.5%(1)	0	5.5% (1)	0	0	0	0
Byrd et al. [52]	2018	67	7.25	4.4%(3)	0	1.5% (1)	0	0	0	0
Sen et al. [53]	2020	73	11.2	6.8%(5)	4.1%(3)	4.1% (3)	1.3%(1)	1.3%(1)	0	0
Meng et al. [54]	2021	47	61.6	9%(4)	0	0	0	9%(1)	0	9%(1)

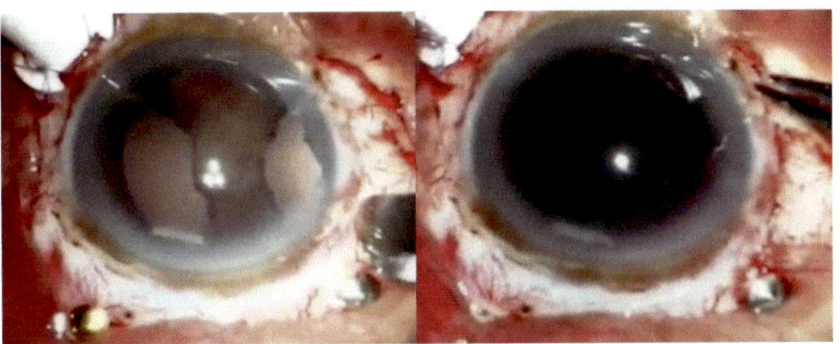

Fig. 58.8 Iridodialysis repair in a 9 year old boy

Review Questions

1. A 4 year old girl is brought by parents with history of both eye cataract surgery done during infancy. Following the surgery child was advised spectacles and regular follow up. O/E Her BCVA OU with +12DS and +3D add is 6/9, N6 and OU aphakia noted. Which is the best management option for this child?

a. Continue aphakic glasses
b. Contact lenses
c. Secondary IOL implantation
d. All of the above

2. Reasons given by IATS for delaying secondary IOL implantation in children

a. Better cooperation for biometry
b. Less risk for glaucoma
c. More predictable refractive outcomes
d. All of the above

3. A child planned for secondary IOL implantation has very poorly dilating 2 mm pupils which of the following is NOT a necessary step in management

a. Preoperative assessment of capsular support using UBM
b. Using iris hooks/mechanical pupil expansion rings during surgery
c. US B scan for posterior segment pathologies preoperatively
d. Use of viscoelastic materials to dilate pupils intraoperatively

4. Which is true regarding contraindications for secondary IOL implantation in children

a. If glaucoma is well controlled with medications a secondary IOL may be implanted
b. Uveitis may not be exacerbated

c. Customised IOLs may be implanted in microcornea/microphthalmos
d. All of the above

5. Best method to calculate IOL power in children

a. A-scan Ultrasound biometry, SRK II
b. IOL Master, SRK II
c. A-scan Ultrasound biometry, SRK T
d. IOL Master, SRK T

6. Advantage of Sulcus placement of IOL over in the bag placement are all except

a. Less risk of glaucoma
b. Technically easier
c. Less risk for syncehiae formation and IOL adhesions
d. Less risk of postoperative Visual axis opacification

7. Technique of using OVD for in the bag IOL placement was described by

a. Wilson
b. Gimbel and Venkatramanan
c. Grewal and Basti
d. None of the above

8. Which of these complications is not associated with Anterior chamber IOL:

a. Formation of peripheral anterior synechiae
b. Suture wick endophthalmitis
c. Pseudophakic bullous keratopathy
d. Pupillary block

9. Rail road technique of suture placement is used in which secondary IOL:

a. 2 point fixated SFIOL
b. 4 point fixated SFIOL
c. Yamane technique of SFIOL
d. None of these

10. Which of these statements is incorrect regarding iris fixated IOL:

a. IOL is enclavated in the peripheral iris area
b. Surgical PI is mandatory for preventing pupillary block
c. Artisan lens is used which is biconvex vaulted PMMA lens
d. Endothelial cell loss is an associated complication

11. Which of these statements is incorrect regarding SFIOL:

a. Complete PPV reduces long term risk of retinal detachment
b. 6–0 polypropylene suture is commonly used for SFIOL fixation
c. Removal of capsular remnants prevents suture entanglement and suture lysis.
d. 4 point fixation gives better IOL stability than 2 point fixation.

12. Which of these statement is correct for SFIOL and glaucoma:

a. Secondary angle closure glaucoma is seen in pediatric aphakia
b. SFIOL Postoperative IOP spike has no association with pre-existing glaucoma in pediatric aphakia
c. Aphakia in early age doesn't cause abnormal development of angle structures.
d. In the bag IOL has lower incidence of glaucoma than sulcus fixated IOL

13. Which of these statements is not correct for Gore-tex suture:

a. It is made of polytetrafluoroethylene.
b. High tensile strength and multifilament suture
c. Easy to manipulate
d. None of these

Answers

1. C.
2. C.
3. D.
4. A.
5. B.
6. A.
7. C.
8. B.
9. B.
10. A.
11. B.
12. D.
13. B.

References

1. Sheeladevi S, Lawrenson JG, Fielder AR, Suttle CM. Global prevalence of childhood cataract: a systematic review. Eye (Lond). 2016;30(9):1160–9.
2. Wilson ME, et al. Intraocular lens implantation: has it become the standard of care for children? Ophthalmology. 1996;103:1719–20.
3. Wilson ME Jr, Hafez GA, Trivedi RH. Secondary in-the-bag intraocular lens implantation in children who have been aphakic since early infancy. J AAPOS. 2011;15(2):162–6.

4. Wood K, Tadros D, Trivedi R, et al. Secondary intraocular lens implantation following infantile cataract surgery: intraoperative indications, postoperative outcomes. Eye. 2016;30:1182–6.

5. Kim DH, Kim JH, Kim SJ, Yu YS. Long-term results of bilateral congenital cataract treated with early cataract surgery, aphakic glasses and secondary IOL implantation. Acta Ophthalmol. 2012;90(3):231–6.

6. Tadros D, Trivedi RH, Wilson ME. Primary versus secondary IOL implantation following removal of infantile unilateral congenital cataract: outcomes after at least 5 years. J AAPOS. 2016;20(1):25–9.

7. Shenoy BH, Mittal V, Gupta A, Sachdeva V, Kekunnaya R. Refractive outcomes and prediction error following secondary intraocular lens implantation in children: a decade-long analysis. Br J Ophthalmol. 2013;97(12):1516–9.

8. Nihalani BR, VanderVeen DK. Secondary intraocular lens implantation after pediatric aphakia. J AAPOS. 2011;15:435–40.

9. Nihalani BR, VanderVeen DK. Long-term outcomes of secondary intraocular lens implantation in children. Graefes Arch Clin Exp Ophthalmol. 2021 Nov 6.

10. VanderVeen DK, Drews-Botsch CD, Nizam A, Bothun ED, Wilson LB, Wilson ME, Lambert SR; Infant Aphakia Treatment Study. Outcomes of secondary intraocular lens implantation in the Infant Aphakia Treatment Study. J Cataract Refract Surg. 2021;47(2):172–7.

11. Repka MX. Visual rehabilitation in pediatric aphakia. Dev Ophthalmol. 2016;57:49–68.

12. Sefi-Yurdakul N, Berk AT. Primary and secondary intraocular lens implantations in children with pediatric cataract: visual acuity and strabismus at the age of 2 years and older. J Pediatr Ophthalmol Strabismus. 2017;54(2):97–102.

13. Alexander JL, Wei L, Palmer J, Darras A, Levin MR, Berry JL, Ludeman E. A systematic review of ultrasound biomicroscopy use in pediatric ophthalmology. Eye (Lond). 2021;35 (1):265–76.

14. Bremond-Gignac D, Daruich A, Robert MP, Valleix S. Recent developments in the management of congenital cataract. Ann Transl Med. 2020;8(22):1545.

15. Khan AO, AlGaeed A. Paediatric secondary intraocular lens estimation from the aphakic refraction alone: comparison with a standard biometric technique. Br J Ophthalmol. 2006;90 (12):1458–60.

16. Neely DE, Plager DA, Borger SM, Golub RL. Accuracy of intraocular lens calculations in infants and children undergoing cataract surgery. J AAPOS. 2005;9(2):160–5.

17. Kekunnaya R, Gupta A, Sachdeva V, Rao HL, Vaddavalli PK, Om PV. Accuracy of intraocular lens power calculation formulae in children less than two years. Am J Ophthalmol. 2012;154(1):13–9.

18. Holladay JT. Standardizing constants for ultrasonic biometry, keratometry, and intraocular lens power calculations. J Cataract Refract Surg. 1997;23(9):1356–70.

19. Steinert RF. Surgical management of pediatric cataracts and aphakia. Cataract surgery 3rd edition.

20. Grewal, Dilraj S. MD; Basti, Surendra MD* Modified technique for removal of Soemmerring ring and in-the-bag secondary intraocular lens placement in aphakic eyes. J Cataract Refract Surgery. 2012:38(5):739–42.

21. Wilson ME Jr, Englert JA, Greenwald MJ. In-the-bag secondary intraocular lens implantation in children. J AAPOS. 1999;3(6):350–5.

22. Gimbel HV, Venkataraman A. Secondary in-the-bag intraocular lens implantation following removal of Soemmering ring contents. J Cataract Refract Surg. 2008;34:1246–9.

23. Wilson ME, Trivedi RH. Safety of piggyback intraocular lenses (polypseudophakia) in children: long-term outcomes of a 15-year, single-surgeon study. J AAPOS. 2020;24(4):230. e1-230.e4.

24. Grzybowski A, Kanclerz P. Methods of achieving adequate pupil size in cataract surgery. Curr Opin Ophthalmol. 2020;31:33–42.

25. Chang DF. Use of Malyugin pupil expansion device for intraoperative floppy-iris syndrome: results in 30 consecutive cases. J Cataract Refract Surg. 2018;34:835–41.

26. Nderitu P, Ursell P. Iris hooks versus a pupil expansion ring: Operating times, complications, and visual acuity outcomes in small pupil cases. J Cataract Refract Surg. 2019;45(2):167–73.

27. Huang L, Jin H, Zhao P. Application of an iris speculum for removing Soemmerring's ring during secondary intraocular lens implantation in congenital cataract patients with small pupils. J Cataract Refract Surg. 2021;47(11):e1–5.

28. David Epley K, Shainberg MJ, Lueder GT, Tychsen L. Pediatric secondary lens implantation in the absence of capsular support. J AAPOS. 2001;5:301–6.

29. Wilson ME, et al. Long-term outcome of angle-supported anterior chamber intraocular lens implantation for pediatric aphakia. J Am Assoc Pediatric Ophthalmol Strabismus {JAAPOS}, 25(4):e11.

30. Cheung CSY, VanderVeen DK. Intraocular lens techniques in pediatric eyes with insufficient capsular support: complications and outcomes. Seminars Ophthalmol. 2019;34(4):293–302.

31. Barbara R, Rufai SR, Tan N, Self JE. Is an iris claw IOL a good option for correcting surgically induced aphakia in children? A review of the literature and illustrative case study. Eye (Lond). 2016;30(9):1155–9.

32. Gawdat GI, Taher SG, Salama MM, Ali AA. Evaluation of Artisan aphakic intraocular lens in cases of pediatric aphakia with insufficient capsular support. J AAPOS. 2015;19(3):242–6.

33. Dick HB, Augustin AJ. Lens implant selection with absence of capsular support. Curr Opin Ophthalmol. 2001;12(1):47–57.

34. Wong HM, Kam KW, Rapuano CJ, Young AL. A systematic review on three major types of scleral-fixated intraocular lens implantation. Asia Pac J Ophthalmol (Phila). 2021;10(4): 388–96.

35. Shuaib AM, El Sayed Y, Kamal A, El Sanabary Z, Elhilali H. Transscleral sutureless intraocular lens versus retropupillary iris-claw lens fixation for paediatric aphakia without capsular support: a randomized study. Acta Ophthalmol. 2019;97(6):e850–9.

36. Sen P, S VK, Bhende P, Rishi P, Rishi E, Rao C, Ratra D, Susvar P, Kummamuri S, Shaikh S, Gopal L. Surgical outcomes and complications of sutured scleral fixated intraocular lenses in pediatric eyes. Can J Ophthalmol. 2018;53(1):49–55.

37. Stem MS, Todorich B, Woodward MA, Hsu J, Wolfe JD. Scleral-fixated intraocular lenses: past and present. J Vitreoretin Dis. 2017;1(2):144–52.

38. Lewis JS. Ab externo sulcus fixation. Ophthalmic Surg. 1991;22(11):692–5.

39. Khan MA, Gupta OP, Smith RG, Ayres BD, Raber IM, Bailey RS, Hsu J, Spirn MJ. Scleral fixation of intraocular lenses using Gore-Tex suture: clinical outcomes and safety profile. Br J Ophthalmol. 2016;100(5):638–43.

40. Junqueira NB, Chaves LJ, Poli-Neto O, Scott IU, Jorge R. Scleral fixation using a hydrophilic four-haptic lens and polytetrafluoroethylene suture. Sci Rep. 2021;11(1):15793.

41. Nb K, Kohli P, Pangtey BPS, Ramasamy K. Evaluation of sutureless, glueless, flapless, intrascleral fixated posterior chamber intraocular lens in children with ectopia lentis. J Ophthalmol. 2018;29(2018):3212740.

42. Yamane S, Sato S, Maruyama-Inoue M, Kadonosono K. Flanged intrascleral intraocular lens fixation with double-needle technique. Ophthalmology. 2017;124(8):1136–42.

43. Sternfeld A, Taranum Basith SS, Kurup SP, Basti S. Secondary intraocular lens implantation using the flanged intrascleral fixation technique in pediatric aphakia: case series and review of literature. J AAPOS. 2020;24(5):286.e1-286.e6.

44. Kirwan C, O'Keefe M. Paediatric aphakic glaucoma. Acta Ophthalmol Scand. 2006;84 (6):734–9.

45. Sahin A, Caça I, Cingü AK, Türkcü FM, Yüksel H, Sahin M, Cinar Y, Ari S. Secondary glaucoma after pediatric cataract surgery. Int J Ophthalmol. 2013;6(2):216–20.

46. Asrani S, Freedman S, Hasselblad V, Buckley EG, Egbert J, Dahan E, Gimbel H, Johnson D, McClatchey S, Parks M, Plager D, Maselli E. Does primary intraocular lens implantation prevent "aphakic" glaucoma in children? J AAPOS. 2000;4(1):33–9.

47. Boden JH, Mickler C, Trivedi RL, Wilson ME. Intraocular pressure spike after secondary IOL implantation in aphakic glaucoma. J AAPOS. 2011;15(1): e14.
48. Buckley EG. Hanging by a thread: the long-term efficacy and safety of transscleral sutured intraocular lenses in children (an American Ophthalmological Society thesis). Trans Am Ophthalmol Soc. 2007;105:294–311.
49. Asadi R, Kheirkhah A. Long-term results of scleral fixation of posterior chamber intraocular lenses in children. Ophthalmology. 2008;115(1):67–72.
50. Burcu A, Yalniz-Akkaya Z, Abay I, Acar MA, Ornek F. Scleral-fixated posterior chamber intraocular lens implantation in pediatric and adult patients. Semin Ophthalmol. 2014;29 (1):39–44.
51. Al Somali AI, Al-Dossari FN, Emara KE, Al Habash A. Outcomes of Scleral-fixated Intraocular-lens in Children with Idiopathic Ectopia Lentis. Middle East Afr J Ophthalmol. 2017;24(4):167–70.
52. Byrd JM, Young MP, Liu W, Zhang Y, Tate DB, Crandall AS, Owen LA. Long-term outcomes for pediatric patients having transscleral fixation of the capsular bag with intraocular lens for ectopia lentis. J Cataract Refract Surg. 2018;44(5):603–9.
53. Sen P, Attiku Y, Bhende P, Rishi E, Ratra D, Sreelakshmi K. Outcome of sutured scleral fixated intraocular lens in Marfan syndrome in pediatric eyes. Int Ophthalmol. 2020;40 (6):1531–8.
54. Meng X, Cao X, Jia Y, Pan J, Du Y, Li X. Sutured scleral fixation of posterior chamber intraocular lens in children under the age of 9 with congenital ectopia lentis. Ophthalmic Res. 2021;64(5):837–43.
55. Price MO, Price FW Jr, Werner L, Berlie C, Mamalis N. Late dislocation of scleral-sutured posterior chamber intraocular lenses. J Cataract Refract Surg. 2005;31(7):1320–6.
56. Sminia ML, Odenthal MT, Gortzak-Moorstein N, Wenniger-Prick LJ, Völker-Dieben HJ. Implantation of the Artisan iris reconstruction intraocular lens in 5 children with aphakia and partial aniridia caused by perforating ocular trauma. J AAPOS. 2008;12(3):268–72.
57. Vanderveen DK, Dean WH. Visual acuity after secondary intraocular lens implantation in pediatric aphakia. J AAPOS. 2013;17(2):e30–1.

Management of Aphakia at Pediatric Age

59

Huban Atilla

Abstract

Cataracts in infancy and childhood can lead to deprivational amblyopia that has many challenges in diagnosis and treatment with relativley poor prognosis. In sensitive period for visual development cataract itself and the postoperative aphakia have all the amblyogenic risk factors such as deprivation, anisometropia and associated strabismus. Timing of the surgery has great importance in the final visual outcome however aphakia after cataract surgery in this age group also can cause amblyopia. Additionally, the uncooperative child with difficult examinations and measurements makes the conditions more unfavourable. Spectacles can be the first choice for aphakic correction in bilateral aphakia cases and contact lenses are the main option for unilateral cases. IOL implantation has many advantages over aphakic glasses and contact lenses such as better optical resolution however difficulties in obtaining precise measurements of corneal curvature, anterior chamber depth and axial length in uncooperative children with less accurate measurement of IOL power calculation will make the outcome less predictable and optimum. After cataract surgery and correction of aphakia,

Supplementary Information The online version contains supplementary material available at https://doi.org/10.1007/978-3-031-14506-3_59.

H. Atilla (✉)
Prof of Ophthalmology, Faculty of Medicine, Department of Ophthalmology, Ankara University, Ankara, Turkey
e-mail: hatilla@medicine.ankara.edu.tr

amblyopia treatment with patching must be part of the treatment and follow up and these patients must be followed till early adulthood for dynamic refractive changes.

Keywords

Pediatric aphakia · Congenital cataract · Pediatric cataract · Correction of aphakia

Introduction

Congenital and juvenile cataracts are the most common causes of treatable and preventable blindness in childhood and treatment will not end after surgical removal of the opaque lens. Management of congenital and childhood cataracts is more challenging than management of adult cataracts. Main challenges are;

- Cooperation problems prior to surgery make the examination and measurements less reliable
- Smaller eyes have increased intraoperative and postoperative difficulties and complications
- Inflammatory response in the postoperative period is higher
- Growing eye makes the postoperative refraction predictions difficult
- Associated ocular pathologies are more frequent

Management of aphakia correction and accommodation loss after surgery have crucial importance in visual development period and cataract surgery is only the first step in treatment. Visual rehabilitation and follow-up should continue during visual development period and the cooperation of the parents/ caregivers have great importance in this period. Ophthalmologist should inform them that surgery is the first step, but successful visual outcome can only be achieved with parents' effort and cooperation for adequate aphakic correction, amblyopia treatment and frequent follow ups. Frequent visits especially in the early postoperative period is needed due to changing refraction, possible complications such as inflammatory reaction, glaucoma and visual axis opacification. Management of aphakia is the mainstay of rehabilitation or habilitation of visual development after surgery and should be started at the earliest possible time period. Aphakia can be corrected with different methods according to the age of patient, associated ophthalmic conditions and the socioeconomical factors. The easiest and the most common solution is aphakic glasses especially in bilateral cases. Contact lenses and introcular lenses are the other modalities for correction of aphakia.

Aphakic Glasses

Correction of aphakia with glasses has the advantages of easiness and safety however it has disadvantages of optical distortion with high diopters such as induced magnification, visual field restriction, prismatic effect of the spectacles and cosmetic appearance (Fig. 59.1). The power of glasses is within the range of +15 to +23 diopters and this is associated with thick appearance, heavy weight of the glasses and the lower quality of optical correction. These may result in poor compliance of the babies and infants and also the families. Dynamic refractive status of the child will necessitate frequent change of the glasses that can be an economical burden for the family.

Aphakic glasses are the preferred method of aphakic correction in bilateral cases in infancy that cannot have intraocular lens implantation or that are intolerant to contact lenses. In unilateral cases, because of the anisekonia induced by the high diopters and the asymmetric weight and the appearance of glasses, contact lenses are the first choice for aphakia correction but prescription for glasses should also be given in unilateral cases especially for the period of time without contact lenses and during occlusion treatment.

When glasses are prescribed, the ophthalmologist should also give information to the family about the glasses, frames and its use. There are some tips for glasses and frame selection;

- The glasses should have high refractive index so that they will be lighter and thinner.
- The frame should be light and small so that the heavy weight of the glasses can be balanced.
- The visual center should be in the vertical center of the frame so that the glasses will fit the face of baby for optimal vision.
- The bridge of the frame should not be too high so that the glasses will not be lower in the face and the child will not look over it, or not too low so that the child can look through the visual center.
- Cable temples (earpieces) will help to keep heavier glasses in position with support of the ears and spring hinges will absorb the trauma to the glasses especially in toddlers. In infancy earpiece can be replaced by a band so that baby

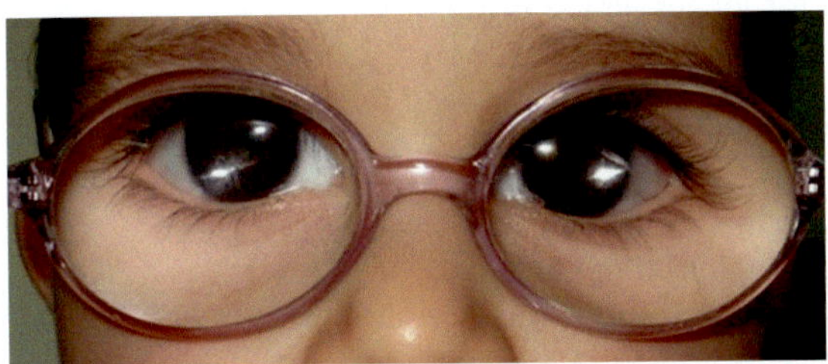

Fig. 59.1 Aphakic correction with glasses in a case of bilateral congenital cataract

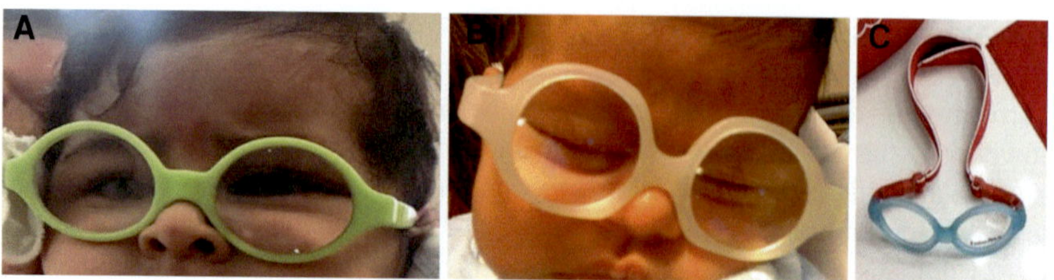

Fig. 59.2 Aphakic correction with glasses in (**A**) and (**B**). Earpieces can be replaced by straps so that baby can keep the glasses while laying down (**C**)

can keep the glasses while laying down and it will be easier to keep the glasses with these straps (Fig. 59.2). If possible child should be involved in selection of the frames so that acception will be easier. Colorful frames may take attention away from the thick lenses [1, 2].

For the lenses of the spectacles there are different types of lenses. The most commonly used ones are;

- Lenticular lenses; have the power at the center of the lens and the center is surrounded by a ring with little or no power. These are not the most preferred lenses but they can be found easily in powers greater than +20 D.
- Aspheric lenticular lenses; have nonspherical (aspheric) central area surrounded by a ring with little or no power. These are better than lenticular lenses optically and can be found in the range of +10 to +20 D.
- Multidrop lenses have a spherical central zone that flattens into an aspheric zone and then is blended into an area of lesser power. The lens resembles the aspheric lenticular lens without a noticable ring and it is better than the other lenses. It can found in +10 to +16 D range [1, 2].

Advantages

- For uncooperative parents or families, correction of aphakia with aphakic glasses is easy
- When we compare with contact lenses, prices of glasses can be lower and glasses can be used for longer period of time.

Disadvantages

- Visual field narrowing to about 30º
- Increase in nystagmus amplitude.
- Aniseconia, disparity in retinal image size of about 30%.
- Anisometropia exceeding 3D in spherical error or 1.5D in cylindrical error causes confusion that can lead to permanent suppression, and amblyopia or

anomalous retinal correspondence may cause development of concomitant strabismus.

– In unilateral aphakia cases optical properties can be an obstacle to binocular vision that may lead to amblyopia.
– The weight and size of the glasses will be difficult to fit in newborns and infants. Small sizes can be difficult to find.
– Thick glasses are cosmetically, visually, and psychologically undesirable (Table 59.1).

Table 59.1 Advantages and disadvantages of glasses for aphakic correction

Advantages	Disadvantages
Cost	Cost
Safe	Induced magnification
Easily changed with changes in refraction	Prismatic effect
Easy to measure and use	Visual field restriction
	Heavy weight
	Cosmetic problems

Another important point that we need to consider is near vision in aphakic and pseudophakic children. Due to loss of accommodation after cataract surgery, near vision should be corrected with bifocals. However, use of bifocals are not easy in toddlers so monofocal glasses are prescribed for near vision till age of 3–4 yrs. As most of the activities are at near (about 1–3 m range) in younger children and toddlers + 2.0/ + 2.5 D is added on the retinoscopic refraction and single vision glasses are prescribed. As the child grows the activity span enlarges and wider range of visual tasks are needed so bifocal glasses with a near addition of +2.5 is prescribed.

Contact Lenses

Contact lenses are also used for aphakic correction after cataract surgery in infancy and childhood. When compared with glasses, contact lenses have the advantages of less magnification, better visual field and better stereopsis. On the other hand, dynamic refraction at infancy and childhood as well as changing corneal curvature will result in frequent need for changing contact lenses and this will cause economical burden to the families. Also, frequent loss of contact lenses due to difficulty in handling may increase the cost. Extended-wear soft or rigid lenses are generally well tolerated, though frequent power changes and lost lenses are significant financial barriers for many families. In developed countries, contact lens use is more common and in developing countries use of contact lenses for pediatric aphakia is less likely to be succesful because of several problems including economical constraints, hygiene problems and poor compliance [1].

Pediatric contact lens fitting is different than adults and for measurements and fitting in uncooperative babies and children, examination under general anesthesia is usually needed (**video**). Even for short term of general anesthesia, requirements like blood tests and operating room admissions will be time consuming and economical burden to the families. Families are needed to be cooperative, willing and enduring for insertion and removal of the contact lenses in a crying, resisting and squeezing baby or child. Extended wear lenses are usually preferred for partially overcoming this problem however intolerance to the lens because of papillary conjunctivitis or corneal vascularisation are other issues that limit use of contact lenses. Extended use of contact lenses may also cause infectious keratitis that may result in vision loss. Eye structures, are developing and growing in children and infants and the conjunctival fornix is shallower and the globe is smaller than the adult eye. The infant cornea is smaller and steeper. The continuously changing refraction in pediatric eyes is primarily related to the increasing axial length but the corneal flattening in the first few years of life also contributes and has more effect on contact lens fitting [2].

There are various types of contact lenses that can be used in pediatric aphakic correction, but three types of contact lenses are utilized more commonly: rigid gas permeable (RGP), silicone elastomer and hydrogel lenses. The most widely used ones are Orbis™ (by Swisslens), Silsoft/Silsoft Super Plus™ (by Bausch and Lomb) and Pediatric Ultravision CLPL (by Ultravision). According to the age of the patient and the availability of the contact lenses, the prescription can be given with the parameters in Fig. 59.3.

Silicone elastomer lenses: have very high oxygen permeability, more than RGP lenses and this property addresses one of the major issues of concern with longterm contact lens use for extended periods, such as corneal endothelial morbidity [1]. Silicone elastomer lenses are preferred as they have lower lens loss rate and easier to handle for parents. Due to the physical properties of silicone elastomer,

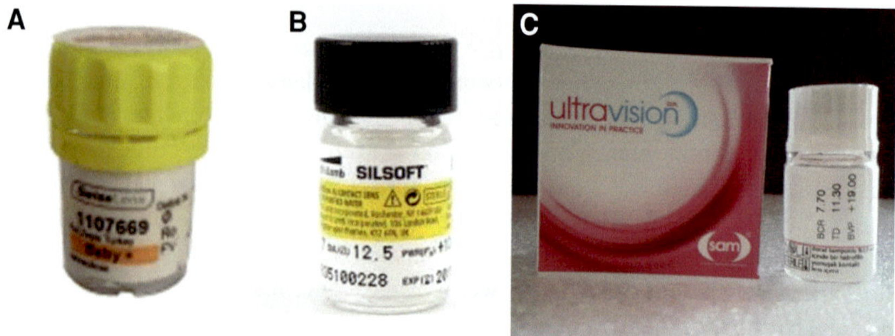

Fig. 59.3 A–C—Contact Lenses that can be given in pediatric aphakia.

lipid-mucin deposits easily accumulate on the surface of such lenses leading to corneal and conjunctival complications, and this may limit extended wear [3].

Hydrogel lenses: in principle, should be used in children over 4 years of age. These lenses are manufactured commercially in selected parameters, which are considered as a disadvantage with the small eyeballs and steep corneas of newborns and infants. In pediatric aphakia, high plus power lenses have a thick central portion which inherently decreases oxygen permeability resulting in several corneal and conjunctival complications such as conjunctivitis, giant papillary conjunctivitis, neovascularization, corneal edema, abrasions, infective keratitis, endothelial polymegathism, and acute red eye reactions so these lenses can cause damage to the developing eye. However, their main advantage is lower cost. This type of lens is used only in exceptional cases. Hydrogel lenses have more comfort with less foreign body sensation however they are associated with more frequent loss and difficulty in manipulation [1, 3].

Rigid Gas Permeable RGP lenses: can be chosen for treatment of pediatric aphakia however special fitting considerations are required in case of microphthalmic eyes which have steep corneas and medium post-operative astigmatism, especially when silicone or hydrogel lenses are not available or suitable. Due to small corneal diameter and narrow lid fissure with tense lids, RGP lenses can be better choice. In comparison with other types of contact lenses, RGP lenses are the healthiest lens for the small developing eye. It requires simple daily care which is of great convenience for parents. However the principal problems of wearing contact lenses are poor compliance with long term use, loss of lenses, and ocular irritation and infection. The smallest lens that does not decenter is chosen and fluorescein can be used for fitting guidance [1, 4–7]. Advantages and disadvantages of contact lens use in pediatric aphakia patients are summarized in Table 59.2.

Table 59.2 Advantages and disadvantages of contact lenses for aphakic correction

Advantages	Disadvantages
Cost	Cost
Parental manipulation	Difficulty in handling
No prismatic effect	Risk for infectious keratitis
	Restrictive power for high powers

Intraocular Lenses (IOL)

Advances in surgical techniques and intraocular design and materials enable surgeons to use intraocular lenses more and earlier than before in pediatric cataracts. After the successful implantation of an IOL in an adult by Ridley in 1949, Epstein implanted an IOL in the eye of a child in 1951 [8]. Choyce performed an anterior chamber IOL in a 10 year old child's eye, in 1955 as first case [9]. The first study on intraocular lens (IOL) implantation in children was published by Hiles [10]. IOL implantation in children did not become common practice until 1990s because of frequent complications caused by the IOL material and design and the enhanced inflammatory response in children [11, 12]. Improvements in surgical techniques, instruments, intraocular lens materials and design increased use of intraocular lenses in infants and children and primary or secondary IOL implantation became common practice after 1990s. They have the main advantage of instant correction of aphakia with better optical properties. IOL implantation in children provides the benefit of reducing dependency on compliance in comparison with other external optical devices (aphakic glasses and contact lenses) providing partial correction [1, 3].

Refinements in surgical techniques like continuous curvilinear capsulorhexis (CCC) with intact capsular bag for safe fixation of in the bag IOL, posterior capsulotomy/capsulorhexis with anterior vitrectomy for a clear optical axis with lesser posterior capsule opacification enable and encourage surgeons for earlier IOL implantation in pediatric cataracts so that IOL are replacing the contact lenses and aphakic glasses for aphakic correction in pediatric cases. In children older than two years of age at the time of cataract surgery, primary intraocular lens implantation has become the standard management method for correction of aphakia. However, there are still disadvantages of IOLs in pediatric age groups such as; accurate calculation of IOL power in rapidly growing eye and unpredictable long term changes such as myopic shift and these factors limit use in children younger than 18–24 months of age. There are also contraindications for IOL implantation in children; microphthalmia, glaucoma, aniridia, recurrent uveitis and inadequate capsular support [1].

Primary intraocular lens implantation is preferred more frequently and at earlier ages however there are still many challenges. IOL power calculation, unpredictability of postoperative refraction and choice of material and design are the main concerns of the surgeons dealing with pediatric cataracts. The uncooperative child or infant is the main obstacle for reliable measurements. Also, dynamic growth period makes the longterm refractive prediction almost impossible. Almost all the IOL power calculation formulas are for adults and not always give the correct result for small, growing eyes. Even with the most reliable calculations, the final refraction status of the child is difficult to predict and still there is need for improvements.

The optimal age for the primary intraocular IOL implantation is still uncertain for unilateral and bilateral cataract cases. There are many studies and case series and the Infant Aphakia Treatment Study (IATS) was conducted about 2 decades ago to find out the visual outcome and risks of unilateral intraocular lens implantation in unilateral cataract surgery prospectively. The results of the aphakic and pseudophakic studies showed statistically similar visual acuity, strabismus and glaucoma outcomes at 5 years of age however pseudophakic infants had higher visual axis opacification, pupillary membrane and reoperations. The Toddler Aphakia and Pseudophakia Study (TAPS) evaluated retrospectively the children with unilateral and bilateral cataracts operated by IATS surgeons between 1 to 24 months of age and the results were published according to the age intervals. When they evaluated the outcomes of unilateral cataracts in infants and toddlers 7 to 24 months of age, they reported that the incidence of complications, reoperations, and glaucoma was low when surgery was performed between 7 and 24 months of age and compared favorably with same IATS data for infants undergoing surgery before 7 months of age. It was concluded that IOL implantation is relatively safe in children older than 6 months and younger than 2 years [13]. Same study group evaluated the bilateral cataract cases that were operated at 1 to 7 months of age and they reported that aphakia management did not affect visual outcome or adverse event incidence, but IOL implantation increased the risk of visual axis opacification and adverse events and glaucoma correlated with a younger age at surgery [14]. When the children that underwent bilateral cataract surgery with and without IOL implantation at age 7 to 24 months were evaluated at 5th year postsurgical follow-up, it was reported that IOL implantation increased the risk of visual axis opacification, irrespective of age at the time of surgery [15].

Secondary IOL implantation is preferred in cases that had surgery at early ages and Infant Aphakia Treatment Study evaluated the outcomes of secondary IOL implantation at 10.5 year of the study. They reported more predictable refractive outcome at long-term but the range of refractive errors was found to be still large and the visual outcome was similar for IOL implantation group and the aphakic group [16].

Intraocular Lens Power Calculation

<u>Preoperative Measurements</u>: Major components of the intraocular power calculation are axial length (AL) and corneal keratometry (K) and followed by corneal diameter of the eye, intraocular pressure and corneal thickness [17]. As these measurements are difficult to get in young children, examination under general anesthesia or sedation can be needed or measured just prior to surgery. Axial length measurement can be done with A mode ultrasound of portable biometry under anesthesia, however during measurement the probe should be directed perpendicularly, toward the macula and relatively soft cornea should not be intended (**video**). Keratometry can be performed with handheld keratometry device also under anesthesia. The same device can be used for contact lens fitting after cataract surgery. If there is no available device for keratometry the keratometric data from study of Trivedi and Wilson can be used [18]. Gordon and Donzis published normative data on axial lenght and keratometry values, by having cross-sectional series of children from different age groups. Refraction of normal eyes changes approximately 1 D from infancy to adulthood however, aphakic eyes become less hyperopic with time and have an average myopic shift of 10 D [19, 20].

Holladay et al. described potential errors in IOL calculations and they suggested that any error in measurement of axial length or keratometry is the main factor resulting in unexpected refractive results. Inaccurate keratometric values cause errors of 0.8–1.3 diopters in both adults and children, on the other hand inaccurate AL measurement can account for 3–4 diopters of error for each millimeter difference in IOL power in adults and 4–14 diopters or higher in pediatric eyes [17, 21]. Also all instruments are designed and calibrated for adults, not for children so this may be source of error. Surgeon should repeat the measurement when the axial length or keratometry are outside the expected average range, or when there is significant asymmetry between eyes and when the calculated IOL power is outside the expected value [17]. Main sources of inaccurate measurements for the patients are short eyes, steep cornea, shallow anterior chamber depth, short axial length, dense cataracts that may affect the final measurement to a greater extent in shorter eyes and denser vitreous that can reduce ultrasound transmission.

Pediatric IOL calculator is a computer program using the Holladay 1 algorithm and pediatric normative data for AL and keratometry readings as established by Gordon and Donzis [19]. It aims to calculate the postoperative pseudophakic refraction of a child during the immediate postoperative period and later to predict the refractive change as the child grows. For secondary intraocular lens implantation, lens power can be calculated by using the aphakic refraction.

<u>IOL Power Calculation Formulas:</u> Since their origin in the 1950s, formulae for IOL power calculation have been subject to constant evolution. There are two basic types of formulae: *theoretical,* determined by application of geometrical optics to the schematic and reduced eyes using various constants, and *regression*, using the actual postoperative results of implant power as a function of the variables of corneal power and AL or formulae which include a combination of both of the above. Various parameters, such as corneal power, AL, effective lens position, and vertex distance, are involved in the determination of implant power and expected postoperative refraction. Theoretical formulas (real, theoretical, physical) are based on geometric optic principles. In theoretical formulas, values such as corneal refraction, cornea-lens distance, lens-retina distance, aqueous refractive index, corneal refractive index, postoperative anterior chamber depth are used. Calculations in theoretical formulas are basically based on subtracting the vergence effect created by the lens from the vergence effect created by the cornea. The biggest problem encountered in the theoretical formulas is the difficulty in determining the postoperative predicted anterior chamber depth. The complexity of the formulas is another disadvantage.

Regression formulas were created from pre- and postoperative retrospective analyzes of eyes with uncomplicated IOL implantation. The most appropriate equation was tried to be found by comparing the postoperative results, axial length, keratometry and emmetropic intraocular lens power. There are various formulas used for calculation and in pediatric patients data derived from adult eyes is used, and this may be impractical to use in the eyes of children. There is constant evolution of these formulas parallel to the changing technology. The most known is the SRK formula, defined by Retzlaff, Sanders, and Kraff in 1980 and is the "First Generation Regression Formulas". There are many other new generation theoretical and regression formulas however they give reliable results in 22.0 – 24.5 mm normal range eyes but have lower reliability in longer and shorter eyes. This will result in post-operative hyperopia in short eyes and myopia in long eyes. It is well known that fourth-generation IOL power calculation formulas have verified their accuracy in adults, while the third-generation formulas are the most common formulas applied in pediatric eyes. Controversy still exists regarding the optimal IOL calculation formula for pediatric cataract patients. To date, the comparisons of the predictability of the IOL calculation formulas for pediatric cataract patients have yielded inconsistent results. A comprehensive meta-analysis evaluated 12 studies including 1,647 eyes with pediatric cataracts [22]. Based on this meta-analysis, the SRK/T formula exhibited a significantly smaller postoperative refractive error than the Hoffer Q in patients younger than 24 months. Among patients aged 24–60 months, both the SRK/T and Hoffer Q formulas were superior to Holladay 2, and SRK II outperformed Holladay 1. For patients with AL < 22 mm, SRK/T and Holladay 1 showed a smaller postoperative refractive error than SRK II (22). Chang P et al. reported that in patients younger than 2 years of age or with AL 21 mm, the SRK/T formulas were relatively accurate, while the Barrett and Haigis formulas were better in patients older than 2 years or with AL > 21 mm [23].

Target Refraction: Another problem encountered with intraocular lens implantation in infants and children is the target refraction after surgery. In children considering the myopic shift related to axial growth, surgeons usually target hypermetropia after intraocular lens implantation in infants and children till 7 years of age. However, in IATS despite targeting about 6–8 D of hypermetropia postoperatively, the mean refractive error after 5 year follow up was about 2.25 D of myopia. The axial length changes from an average of 17 mm at birth to 23 mm in adulthood and parallel to this growth corneal power decreases from 51 D to 43.5 D in adulthood and there is less hypermetropia with growth of the child. This change is also different in aphakic children and their eyes become less hypermetropic, aka more myopic with time and there can be an average of 10 D myopic shift from infancy to adulthood. According to the experience and practice of the surgeon, target refractive error can be decided and this must be discussed with the parents.

- If surgeon decides emmetropia as the target refraction postoperatively, these children will not need glasses for distance however they will need near glasses or bifocals for compensation of loss of accommodation. In adulthood, the myopic shift will result in moderate to high myopia. Early emmetropia may be better for amblyopia but near vision should be considered in young children.
- When we consider the growth of child and aim hypermetropia at younger patients (less than 7 years of age) the final refraction at adulthood will be low to moderate myopia. However, these patients will need hypermetropic glasses for distance and near after surgery and this may be disadvantage for amblyopia treatment and visual develeopment. Frequent follow-up visits for refractive measurement are needed in these patients. Our preference is to aim low to moderate hypermetropia according to the age of child (about 4-5 D hypermetropia for 2–4 years of age and 2–3 D hypermetropia for 5–7 years of age).
- If myopia is the target refraction postoperatively, this may have the advantage of better near vision however patient will need glasses for distance. These patients may have better response to amblyopia treatment as they have better near vision but in adulthood they will have high myopic refractive error.
- Associated astigmatic refractive error may be related to the structure of the eye as in microcornea and microphthalmia or may be related to surgery. This should be corrected accordingly to have better visual outcome and prevent amblyopia (Table 59.3).

Table 59.3 Advantages and disadvantages of target refraction

Initial refraction	Advantage	Disadvantage
Emmetropia	Better vision initially	Myopic shift
	Good for amblyopia	Myopia in adulthood
	No need for distance glasses	
Hypermetropia	Less myopic shift	Glasses for distance and Amblyopia
	Emmetropia or low myopia in adulthood	
Myopia	Near vision can be better	Large myopic shift
	No need for near glasses	High myopia in adulthood

Case Scenarios

Case 1: A 5 months old baby boy was seen with a complaint of white color change in the pupillary area of both eyes. Mother noticed this change about 1 week ago while she was breast feeding. Ophthalmic examination revealed poor fixation reflex in both eyes with normal biomicroscopic findings except nuclear cataracts. Dilated fundus examination with indirect ophthalmoscopy was normal but retinoscopy could not be performed. Family history was negative with normal ophthalmic examinations of the parents and the pediatric evaluation was normal without any systemic disease or laboratory findings. Cataract surgery was performed in both eyes one day apart. On second postoperative day, retinoscopy was +16.0 D OD / + 15.0 D OS and eyeglasses +19.0 D OD, +18.0 D OS was prescribed for near vision and the baby was followed on monthly intervals. He adapted to the glasses easily and he had an uncomplicated postoperative period with normal intraocular pressure and clear visual axis till 3 years of age. Secondary intraocular lens implantation was scheduled at the age of 3. His visual acuity with LEA symbols was 0.5 OD and 0.4 OS preoperatively. Biometric measurements were performed under general anesthesia prior to surgery and for the postoperative period +3 D of hyperopia was aimed however postoperative refraction was +2.25(+0.5 110) and +1.75 (+0.75 95). Bifocal glasses was prescribed to compensate accommodation loss and as he was orthophoric with latent nystagmus, no patching was given. At last follow up visit, at 12 years of age, his visual acuities were 0.8/0.8 and 0.9 binocularly with correction [−1.75 (−1.0 axis 5) OD and −2.25 (−1.75 axis 170)]. He is still under followup for myopic shift.

Case 2: Two weeks old baby girl was noticed to have a smaller left eye by the pediatrician and referred for ophthalmic evaluation. She was a healthy baby without any systemic disease and the parents also had normal ophthalmic findings. She was operated with the diagnosis of left persistent fetal vasculature (PFV) at 5th weeks of age and preoperative measurements under anesthesia revealed 19 mm of axial length of the right and 17.3 mm left eye with normal IOP, and ultrasonography was normal. She had an uneventful cataract surgery with iridectomy and anterior

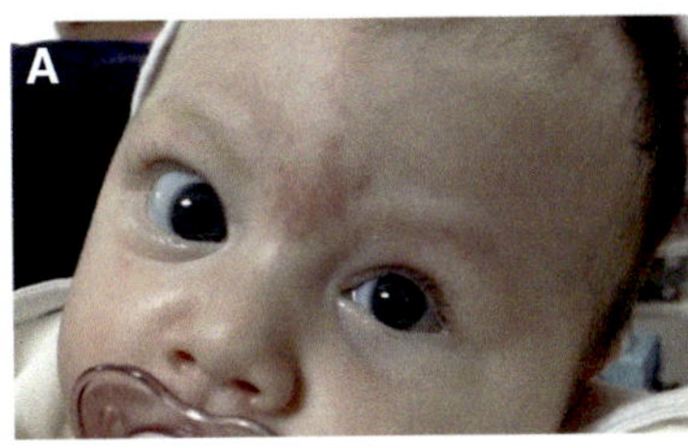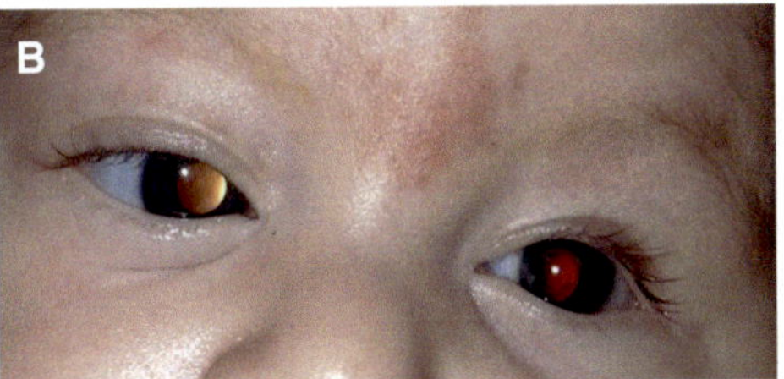

Fig. 59.4 A, B: Unilateral aphakia due to persistent fetal vasculature (**A**) before contact lens correction and (**B**) after contact lens correction.

vitrectomy. She was given eyeglasses (plano/ + 21.0 D) on 2nd postoperative day and at 10 weeks of age +31 D of contact lens and patching were prescribed (Fig. 59.4). As she had 9 mm of corneal diameter in the left eye, intraocular lens implantation cannot be performed at the age of 18 months and she was followed with contact lens. Her visual acuity at the last follow up (5 years of age) was 0.8 in the right eye (with +3.75 hypermetropia) and 0.05 in the left eye with contact lens and she had 12 PD of left esotropia and she was still doing daily patching of 2 h per day.

Conclusions

Our aim in pediatric cataracts is to have good visual acuity and to prevent deprivational amblyopia however loss of accommodation, the aphakia itself and anisometropia after surgery, and associated strabismus, all have adverse effects on visual development. We need to perform surgery at optimal age with minimum calculation errors and complications, and perfect follow-up for successful amblyopia treatment with cooperative patient and family. Frequent follow-up visits and checking for refractive changes are mandatory to prevent and treat complications and to correct the dynamic refractive errors and to combat with amblyopia.

IOL implantation has many advantages over aphakic glasses and contact lenses however difficulties in obtaining precise measurements of corneal curvature, anterior chamber depth and axial length in uncooperative children with less accurate instrumentation of IOL power calculation will make the outcome less predictable and optimum. This is further confounded by the fact that IOL power prediction formula in common use today is based on the theoretical models or regression from normative data from adult eyes. Refractive surprises can occur early in the postoperative period due to inaccurate IOL power measurement and calculation and later from myopic shift. The refraction of the other eye whether phakic or pseudophakic should be considered also. However even with the very careful measurements and calculations the final refraction is difficult to predict and achieve.

Review Questions

1. What are the amblyogenic risk factors in congenital cataract patients?

a. Deprivation
b. Anisometropia
c. Strabismic
d. All of them
e. None of them

2. Which one of the followings is a disadvantage for aphakic correction with glasses (spectacles)?

a. Safety
b. Easy to measure and access
c. Prismatic effect
d. Parental convenience
e. No risk for infection

3. Which one of the followings is correct for intraocular lens implantation in children?

a. It is easy to measure and calculate for intraocular lens power
b. Myopic shift with development is predictable and desirable
c. Refraction in the early postoperative period is not important in visual development
d. There is no need for spectacles after intraocular lens implantation
e. Unilateral intraocular lenses have the least amount of induced aniseconia in comparison to glasses and contact lenses

Answers:

1. D
2. C
3. E

Video: *Retinoscopy and follow up measurements can be performed in awake babies or under general anesthesia.*

References

1. Ram J, Brar GS. Options in the management of pediatric aphakia (chapter 5). In Eds Ram J, Brar GS, editors. Pediatric cataract surgery. Jaypee Brothers Medical Publishers Ltd New Delhi; 2007. p. 47–59.
2. Trivedi RH, Wilson ME. Correction of Aphakia: Glasses and contact lens (chapter 45). In: Wilson ME, Trivedi RH, editors. Pediatric cataract surgery. Techniques, complications and management. 2nd edition. Wolters Kluwer Health. Philadelphia; 2014, p. 306–15.

3. Baradaran-Rafii A, Shirzadeh E, Eslani M, Akbari M. Optical correction of aphakia in children. J Ophthalmic Vis Res. 2014;9(1):71–82.

4. Baker JD. Visual rehabilitation of aphakic children. II. Contact lenses. Surv Ophthalmol. 1990;34:366–71.

5. Jacobs DS. The best contact lens for baby? Int Ophthalmol Clin. 1991;31:173–9.

6. McQuaid K, Young TL. Rigid gas permeable contact lens changes in the aphakic infant. CLAO J. 1998;24:36–40.

7. Pratt-Johnson JA, Tillson G. Hard contact lenses in the management of congenital cataracts. J Pediatr Ophthalmol Strabismus. 1985;22:94–6.

8. Letocha CE, Pavlin CJ. Follow up of 3 patients with Ridley intraocular len simplanttaion. J Cataract Refract Surg. 1999;25:587–91.

9. Choyce DP. Correction of uni-ocular aphakia by means of anterior chamber acrylic implants. Trans Ophthalmol Soc UK. 1958;78:459–70.

10. Hiles D. Intraocular lenses in children. Int Ophthalmol Clin. 1977;17:221–42.

11. Nishi O. Fibrinous membrane formation on the posterior chamber lens during early postoperative period. J Cataract Refract Surg. 1988;14:74–7.

12. Vasavada A, Chauhan H. Intraocular lens implantation in infants with congenital cataract. J Cataract Refract Surg. 1994;20:592–8.

13. Bothun ED, Wilson ME, Traboulsi EI, et al. Outcomes of unilateral cataracts in infants and toddlers age 7–24 months: toddler Aphakia and Pseudophakia Study (TAPS). Ophthalmology. 2019;126:1189–95.

14. Bothun ED, Wilson ME, VanderVeen DK, et al. Outcomes of bilateral cataracts removed in infants 1 to age 7 months of age using Toddler Aphakia and Pseudophakia Study Registry. Ophthalmology. 2020;127:501–10.

15. Bothun ED, Wilson ME, Yen KG, et al. Outcomes of Bilateral Cataract Surgery in infants 7–24 months of age using the Toddler Aphakia and Pseudophakia Study Registry. Ophthalmology. 2021;128:302–8.

16. VanderVeenDK, Drews-Botsch CD, Nizam A, et al. Outcomes of secondary iontraocular lens implantation in the Infant Aphakia Treatment Study. J Cataract Refract Surg. 2021;47:172–7.

17. McClatchey SK, Hofmeister EM. Introcular lens power calculation for children. Chapter 7. In Wilson ME, Trivedi RH, Pandey SK, editors. Pediatric cataract surgery. Techniques, complications and management. Philadelphia: Lippincott Williams & Wilkins; 2005. p. 30–7.

18. Keratometry in pediatric eyes with cataract. Trivedi RH. Wilson ME. Arch Ophthalmol. 2008;126:38–42.

19. Gordon RA, Donzis PB. Refractive development of the human eye. Arch Ophthalmol. 1985;103:785–9.

20. McClatchey SK, Parks MM. Myopic shift after cataract removal in childhood. J Pediatr Ophthalmol Strabismus. 1997;34:88–95.

21. Eibschitz-Tsimhoni M, Tsimhoni O, Archer SM, DelMonte MA. Effect of axial length and keratometry measurement error on intraocular lens implant power prediction formulas in pediatric patients. J AAPOS. 2008;12:173–6.

22. Zhong Y, et.al. Accuracy of intraocular lens power calculation formulas in pediatric cataract patients: a systematic review and meta-analysis. Front Med (Lausanne). 2021;8.

23. Chang P, et al. Accuracy of 8 intraocular lens power calculation formulas in pediatric cataract patients. Graefes Arch Clin Exp Ophthalmol. 2020;258(5):1123–31.

24. McClatchey SK, Hofmeister EM. Chapter 7 Intraocular lens power calculation for children Wilson ME, Trivedi RH, Pandey SK. Pediatric cataract surgery, Techniques, complications and management. Lippincott Williams & Wilkins. A Wolters Kluwer Company. Philadelphia; 2005. p 30–7.

Part X
Retinoblastoma

Genetic Counseling

60

Deborah Im, Shreya Sirivolu, Sona Shah, and Jesse L. Berry

Abstract

Retinoblastoma, the most common pediatric intraocular cancer, can occur in both heritable and non-heritable forms. As the heritable form also confers an additional cancer predisposition syndrome, all providers must be aware of the additional implications of this diagnosis. Thus, genetic testing and counseling is an essential component in the management of newly diagnosed retinoblastoma patients, even in the absence of family history or unilateral disease. In addition to

Disclosures: Dr. Berry has filed a patent application entitled, Aqueous Humor Cell Free DNA for Diagnostic and Prognostic Evaluation of Ophthalmic Disease. Otherwise, the authors declare no potential conflicts of interest.

D. Im · S. Sirivolu · S. Shah · J. L. Berry (✉)
The Vision Center at Children's Hospital Los Angeles, Los Angeles, CA, USA
e-mail: jesse.berry@med.usc.edu

D. Im
e-mail: deborahi@usc.edu

S. Sirivolu
e-mail: sirivolu@usc.edu

S. Shah
e-mail: Sona.Shah@med.usc.edu

D. Im · S. Sirivolu · S. Shah · J. L. Berry
USC Roski Eye Institute, Keck School of Medicine of the University of Southern California, Los Angeles, CA, USA

J. L. Berry
Norris Comprehensive Cancer Center, Keck School of Medicine, University of Southern California, Los Angeles, CA, USA

The Saban Research Institute, Children's Hospital Los Angeles, Los Angeles, CA, USA

© The Author(s), under exclusive license to Springer Nature Switzerland AG 2023
Ş. Özdek et al. (eds.), *Pediatric Vitreoretinal Surgery*,
https://doi.org/10.1007/978-3-031-14506-3_60

the management of the primary tumor, the hereditary status of a retinoblastoma patient determines the length and frequency of follow-up to monitor for new intraocular tumors or secondary cancer development. This chapter outlines the differences between hereditary and non-hereditary retinoblastoma genetics, recommendations for genetic counseling and follow-up schedules, and provides two clinical cases to demonstrate different presentations and management of retinoblastoma patients.

Keywords

Retinoblastoma · Genetic counseling · Genetic testing

Introduction

Retinoblastoma (Rb) represents 3.0% of all childhood cancers and is the most common primary pediatric intraocular carcinoma. Retinoblastoma is diagnosed in approximately 8,000 children and infants each year worldwide [1–3]. Two-thirds of patients are diagnosed prior to the age of two and 95% prior to the age of five [4], with presenting signs typically including leukocoria or strabismus [5]. Diagnosis of Rb is made by an ophthalmologist on the basis of fundus examination and ultrasonography, with magnetic resonance imaging (MRI) providing further assessment of disease extension along the optic nerve or the presence of CNS disease [6]. Rb occurs in both heritable and non-heritable, or somatic, forms. As 40% of Rb cases are heritable and part of a broader cancer predisposition syndrome, patients and often relatives, must undergo genetic testing to understand the genetic risks of the disease in addition to a new cancer diagnosis. Patient survival of the disease is >95% in high income countries but <30% globally [3], as it is a highly fatal condition if left untreated. Children who survive may demonstrate long-term visual field deficits, blindness [7], and may even require surgical removal of the eye (enucleation) to prevent extraocular tumor spread. This chapter will focus on the genetic counseling aspect of the disease; the differential diagnosis and treatment modalities for Rb will be discussed in the following chapters.

Retinoblastoma Genetics

The vast majority of germline and somatic cases of Rb are initiated by biallelic inactivation of the retinoblastoma tumor suppressor gene (*RB1*) in a developing retinal cell [8, 9]. The *RB1* gene on chromosome 13q was the first cloned tumor suppressor gene [10–12]. The molecular role of the *RB1* gene and its protein product (pRB) has been widely studied; it is involved in the cell cycle, cell senescence, growth arrest, apoptosis, and differentiation [13]. Therefore, it not only plays a role in Rb, but also in other human cancers including small cell lung cancer, osteosarcoma, pancreatic cancer, and breast cancer. It was through studying the difference of age at diagnosis between unilateral and bilateral Rb in 1971 that Knudson developed the "two-hit" tumorigeneses hypothesis [14]. After evaluating the rate, age, and timing of tumor onset of 48 Rb cases, he concluded that two separate mutational events, or "hits," were required for oncogenesis in Rb. His findings continue to serve as the foundation for understanding the role and implications of mutations in recessive tumor suppressor genes.

Hereditary Versus Non-hereditary RB

The discovery and characterization of *RB1* as the first tumor suppressor gene demonstrated the first genetic basis for cancer development. Rb can be hereditary (40% of cases) wherein the mutation is present in the germline (or a majority of germline cells). These patients often present with bilateral and or multifocal ocular tumors, although some patients do have unilateral disease only. The majority of cases of Rb are nonhereditary with a localized somatic *RB1* mutation in the tumor only—these patients only develop unilateral disease. Knudson's "two-hit" model was further explained by Comings in that the two "hits," or mutational events (termed M1 and M2) consisted of losses of both alleles of a single gene and thus were the initiating steps of carcinogenesis [15]. Both mutational events in tumor suppressor gene *RB1* are necessary for tumor initiation. In heritable Rb, the first mutational event (M1) is a germline mutation, and the second (M2) is the subsequent somatic mutation usually in retinal progenitor cells that results in either unilateral or bilateral Rb. The first germline mutation may have been inherited from a parent or may have occurred spontaneously during embryonic development. In nonheritable Rb, there is no germline mutation, and both somatic mutations occur in a single somatic retinal cell, thus causing unilateral Rb.

Bilateral cases are always hereditary (by definition) and arise from inherited or from de novo mutation in the *RB1* gene [16]. Bilateral Rb patients frequently present with multifocal lesions due to a "second hit" in multiple somatic cells [17]. As all cells (in both eyes) contain a germline mutation, only one subsequent sporadic mutation is needed to initiate new cancer growth. Although most unilateral cases are nonhereditary, 15% of unilateral patients without a positive family history may still harbor the hereditary, germline mutation [17]. Furthermore, patients may present with incomplete penetrance as well as mutational mosaicism in which mosaicism is associated with delayed retinoblastoma onset [18]. Though late and unilateral presentation typically indicates nonhereditary status, these characteristics are not sufficient to rule out heritable disease. Patients as old as 10 years of age with hereditary Rb have been detected due to atypical presentations with germline mutations [19]. **Thus, it is of utmost importance for patients to undergo genetic testing even in the absence of family history and unilateral tumor presentation.**

As heritable Rb has additional ramifications beyond ocular Rb tumor formation, it is important for the physician to identify the hereditary status of these patients. This is the single most important take home point from this chapter. Sadly, still in 2022 unilateral patients without any family history of Rb are advised that they do not need genetic testing and then go on to have children of their own with retinoblastoma having been inappropriately counselled on this risk of passing on this mutation. To underscore the genetic emphasis of this cancer, The American Joint Committee on Cancer (AJCC) 8th edition includes hereditary trait "H" in the staging of retinoblastoma [20]. By this system, retinoblastoma patients are placed in one of three categories: (1) those who carry the *RB1* pathogenic variant (H1), (2) those with normal *RB1* alleles (H0), and (3) those with an unknown *RB1* status (HX). A fourth category, H0*, has also been proposed to describe patients with <1% residual risk of a *RB1* pathogenic variant due to undetectable mosaicism [9].

MYCN as a Genetic Cause of Non-hereditary Retinoblastoma

Although a loss of function mutation in the *RB1* gene is the primary cause of most cases (98%) of Rb, other genes have been implicated in tumorigenesis. In 1986, it was thought that the oncogene *MYCN*, which is commonly amplified and over-expressed in neuroectodermal tumors such as neuroblastoma and Rb, was not essential to tumor initiation but likely involved in tumor progression [21]. Of all Rb tumors, 3% harbored *MYCN* amplification, and *MYCN* gain has been implicated as a later mutational event after tumorigenesis [22]. However, in 2013, Rushlow et al. identified a rare and genetically distinct form of non-hereditary Rb in which the *RB1* gene is normal and there is a copy number amplification in the *MYCN* oncogene ($RB1^{+/+}MYCN^A$) [23]. Interestingly, *MYCN* retinoblastomas are less likely to display characteristic somatic copy number alterations of Rb (1q and 6p gain, 16q loss) and instead present with variations similar to neuroblastoma (17q gain, 11q loss) [23].

This unique form of non-hereditary Rb presents in 1% of children with unilateral Rb. These patients are generally diagnosed at a significantly younger age than those with traditional biallelic loss of *RB1* ($RB1^{-/-}$) tumors at a median age of 4.5 months compared to 12 months for hereditary and 24 months for non-hereditary cases [23–25]. Histologically, primary MYCN amplified ($RB1^{+/+}MYCN^A$) tumors have distinct features similar to neuroblastoma (round nuclei with prominent large multiple nucleoli) and present with large and invasive tumors. Due the aggressive nature of these tumors, it is recommended that most patients are treated promptly with enucleation. However, because direct tissue biopsy is not done for diagnosis of Rb, it is not easy to identify these tumors by clinical features alone leading to initial attempts to salvage the eye. Unfortunately, two cases of metastatic and fatal $RB1^{+/+}MYCN^A$ tumors have been reported in two children diagnosed at 17 and 30 months [26]. The two patients presented with orbital and cervical lymph node involvement and rapidly progressed to fatal disease due to chemoresistance. A recent report of conservative management of one $RB1^{+/+}MYCN^A$ case in a 6 month old boy demonstrated that even with multiple chemotherapy treatments secondary enucleation was unavoidable due to the highly aggressive and resistant nature of the tumor [27]. Recent work on liquid biopsy approaches for Rb have demonstrated the ability to diagnosis and evaluate retinoblastoma on a molecular level in the absence of tumor tissue [28]; hopefully in the future this will facilitate the detection and characterization of these MYCN driven tumors at diagnosis in order to prevent potentially dangerous attempts to salvage these eyes.

Secondary Chromosomal Alterations that Cause Tumorigenesis

While biallelic inactivation of *RB1* is necessary for the initiation of Rb in a vast majority of cases, additional secondary chromosomal alterations can further drive tumorigenesis [29, 30]. These subsequent changes are crucial for tumor progression in not only Rb, but in many other cancers as well [29]. Rb tumors analyzed after enucleation have shown recurrent somatic copy number alterations (SCNAs), such as highly recurrent chromosomal gains on 1q, 2p, and 6p, and losses on 13q and 16q [22, 29, 31–33]. A clinically important aim of studying the role of SCNAs in tumorigenesis is the determination of whether certain SCNAs portend a more aggressive disease course. One study showed that 1q and 6p gain and 16q loss are associated with a more invasive pattern of tumor growth [34]. Another study showed that 6p gain is associated with less differentiated tumors with higher rates of optic nerve invasion [35]. These studies, however, were performed on tumor samples taken from advanced, enucleated eyes, which limits their clinical application. As mentioned, this is because invasive tissue biopsies in Rb are prohibited due to risks of extraocular tumor spread [36, 37].

In an effort to overcome this limitation, Berry et al. has shown that the aqueous humor is a source of tumor-derived cell-free DNA (cfDNA) [8]. Because the aqueous humor can be safely extracted from eyes undergoing therapy [38], genomic findings have a greater potential in direct clinical utility. For instance, SCNAs have the potential to serve as prognostic biomarkers in predicting the eye's response to treatment. In a study correlating SCNAs in the aqueous humor with clinical outcomes, Berry and colleagues demonstrated that chromosome 6p gain is associated with a nearly tenfold increased odds of enucleation [39, 40]. Further prospective research across multiple treatment centers will hopefully allow for the shift towards using SCNAs to predict clinical outcomes at diagnosis.

Genetic Testing for Retinoblastoma: Current and Future Applications

Identifying the genetic etiology of Rb is important not only for planning disease management but also for determining the risk of disease carried by family members. Molecular diagnostic testing analyzes both germline DNA, using either a peripheral blood or saliva sample, and tumor DNA when available [24]. Genetic testing for Rb can detect approximately 95% of *RB1* mutations [24]. Although children with bilateral disease can be presumed to have a germline mutation, 15% of patients with unilateral disease without positive family history have a detectable mutation in the peripheral blood [19]. It is further important to determine whether the detected mutation is a true germline mutation or a mosaic mutation, as family members do not require screening in the case of mosaicism [18], and the degree of mosaicism can determine the risk of additional tumors in the patient [41].

The Impact of Hereditary Retinoblastoma: Tumor Predisposition Syndrome and Increased Risk for Secondary Cancers

Unfortunately, heritable Rb (i.e. presence of a germline *RB1* mutation) also constitutes *RB1* cancer syndrome, a syndrome which confers lifelong cancer risk beyond Rb tumorigenesis. Even after successful management of the primary tumor, *RB1* cancer syndrome puts the patient and offspring at risk of Rb and non-ocular tumor development. Patients with a germline mutation are at a slightly higher risk of secondary cancer compared to a de novo germline mutation, with osteosarcoma (37%), cutaneous melanoma (7.4%), soft tissue sarcomas (6.9%) and brain tumors (4.5%) being the most common [42, 43]. Leiomyosarcoma was the most frequent subtype of the soft tissue sarcomas found among heritable Rb patients, with most patients being diagnosed 30 years after diagnosis of Rb [44]. This risk has been attributed to genetic susceptibility and past radiotherapy or chemotherapy treatment [42, 45–48]. Patients with a germline mutation are additionally at increased risk for midline tumors, named "trilateral retinoblastoma," with a risk of 4–10% [49, 50]. Even beyond the conferred secondary cancer risk with a germline mutation, common Rb therapies such as external beam radiotherapy and chemotherapy add additional cancer risk. Young patients have been seen to develop midface hypoplasia with increased risk of osteosarcomas, soft tissue sarcomas and brain tumors after undergoing radiotherapy [47, 51]. Risks are also associated with systemic intravenous chemotherapy, which often utilizes carboplatin, etoposide and vincristine. Development of secondary acute myeloid leukemias is associated with the use of etoposide, however the benefits are often considered to outweigh risks in the case of systemic chemotherapy [52]. Thus, it is important to discuss the associated *RB1* cancer syndrome in hereditary Rb patients and the risks of certain therapies with the patient's family.

Unilateral Hereditary Clinical Case

A 10-month-old boy with no significant past medical history was referred for leukocoria in the right eye. His mother had a history of unilateral retinoblastoma for which she underwent enucleation at the age of 2. Unfortunately, she had been incorrectly counselled that due to the unilaterality of her disease she could not carry a germline mutation. Anterior examination was unremarkable. On dilated examination of the right eye there was a large tumor involving most of the macula. There was also a second tumor at 1:00 anterior to the equator and was approximately 5 disc diameters in size. There were no vitreous seeds or subretinal fluid present. The left eye was normal without tumor formation. B scan ultrasonography revealed macular tumor at posterior pole 5.9 mm × 10 mm without subretinal fluid in the right eye. MRI of the brain and orbit with contrast revealed a 4 mm (transverse) × 10 mm (apical) lesion in the right globe. There was no involvement of the optic nerves.

The patient was determined to have unilateral sporadic multifocal Group B disease in the right eye. Serum genetic testing was positive for a germline *RB1* mutation. He was treated with systemic chemotherapy with carboplatin, vincristine and etoposide. Following therapy, posterior segment examination revealed significant regression of both tumors involving the inferior macula and remaining tumor from the fovea inferiorly and laser consolidation was initiated (Fig. 60.1).

The patient will undergo examinations initially monthly from the time of diagnosis to monitor for appropriate tumor regression and surveillance for new tumors to prevent progression of disease. Due to the hereditary nature of the disease, the patient will undergo repeat MRI of brain and orbits every 6 months until

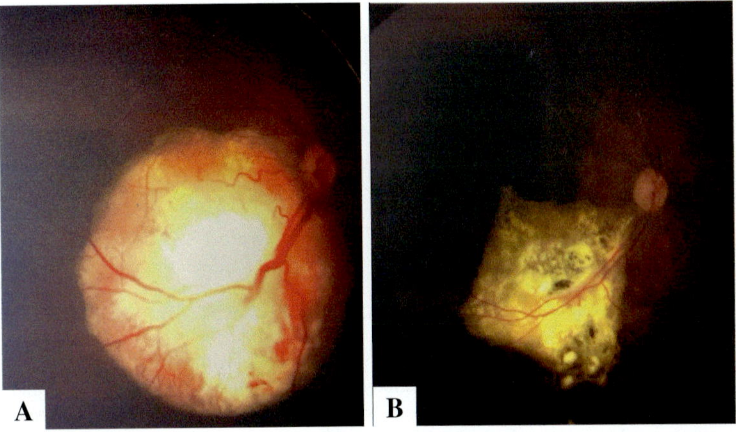

Fig. 60.1 Fundus photograph. **A** Endophytic retinoblastoma tumor formation under the nerve, International Intraocular Retinoblastoma Classification (IIRC) Group B/AJCC CT1b. **B** Same patient after treatment with chemotherapy

the age of 3 to monitor for pinealoblastoma surveillance. The patient will require lifelong surveillance for secondary tumor formation as well as genetic counselling as there is a 50% risk of passing the *RB1* mutation to future offspring.

Bilateral Hereditary Clinical Case

A 21-month-old female with no significant past medical history presented with leukocoria and strabismus. During screening examination she was diagnosed with bilateral retinoblastoma International Intraocular Retinoblastoma Classification (IIRC) Group D in the right eye and Group D in the left eye. The patient had no family history of retinoblastoma. Dilated examination of the right eye revealed a large endophytic retinal tumor in the superonasal fundus measuring 11.2 mm (transverse) × 8.2 mm (apical). A second tumor was present in the superior aspect of the macula. There were hundreds of thick confluent vitreous seeds involving all of the quadrants, with the heaviest concentration in the posterior pole and inferior mid-periphery. Dilated examination of the left eye revealed a large endophytic tumor in the inferior mid-periphery with the posterior margin just at the inferior vascular arcade measuring 6.3 mm (transverse) × 9.9 mm (apical). There were scattered inferior vitreous seeds.

Serum genetic testing was positive for a germline *RB1* mutation with 30% mosaicism. Mosaicism is by definition consistent with a new germline mutation that is not inherited from the parents. The patient underwent a total of 6 cycles of systemic chemotherapy with carboplatin, etoposide and vincristine with concomitant intravitreal injections in the right eye for cycles 4–6. Additional local consolidation therapy of bilateral tumors was required and the patient was treated with cryotherapy and laser therapy in both eyes (Fig. 60.2). Due to continued

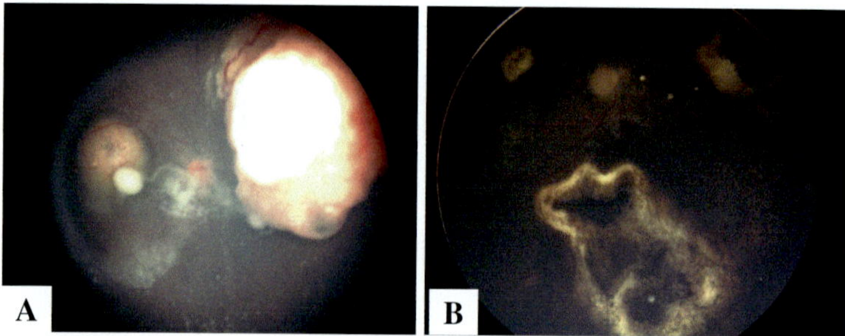

Fig. 60.2 Fundus photograph. An example of a patient with IIRC Group D multifocal retinoblastoma in the right eye. **A** large endophytic retinal tumor in the superonasal fundus, with the posterior margin near to but not contiguous with the optic nerve. There is a second tumor in the superior aspect of the macula which is smaller and also endophytic. There are hundreds of vitreous seeds involving all quadrants with the heaviest concentration in the posterior pole and inferior mid-periphery; there is a cloud of active vitreous seeding in the inferior vitreous. The retina is attached throughout the fundus. **B** Fundus photograph of the same patient after therapy, demonstrating stable, regressed retinoblastoma with residual scarring. This eye went on to eventual enucleation due to retinal recurrence of tumor

seeding the patient underwent a total of 10 intravitreal melphalan injections in the right eye. Due to massive tumor recurrence overlying the optic nerve and associated seeding in the right eye, the patient underwent enucleation of the right eye at 3.5 years of age.

Following therapy, the left eye was cured with a visual acuity in the left eye of 20/40. Posterior segment examination of the left eye revealed a large partially regressed endophytic retinoblastoma tumor located in the inferior mid-periphery with the posterior margin just at the inferior vascular arcade. There was stable, fibrous regressed retinoblastoma centrally without evidence of recurrence. There were scattered inferior seeds which appear calcified and no evidence of active seeding. There was a slight elevation of the nerve fiber layer inferior to the optic nerve that had not changed compared to multiple previous photographs.

The patient was followed by ophthalmology monthly during active treatment, and now undergoes examination under anesthesia every 3–4 months for appropriate tumor regression and surveillance for new tumors. Additionally, due to the hereditary nature of the disease the patient underwent repeat MRI of brain and orbits every 6 months until the age of 3 to monitor for pinealoblastoma development and her MRIs remained normal. The patient will require lifelong surveillance for secondary tumor formation as well as genetic counselling as there is a 50% risk of passing the *RB1* mutation to future offspring.

In summary, hereditary Rb patients require closer follow up with ophthalmology and oncology for life due to a higher risk of new Rb tumors in either eye and development of secondary cancers; however any child with Rb undergoing attempts to salvage the eye with treatment needs to be monitored closely for local tumor recurrence. The status of the eye and treatment needs dictate the intervals. However, patients with a known *RB1* mutation (usually tested because of family history) generally undergo monthly examinations under anesthesia by ophthalmology in the first year of life as surveillance for ocular tumor formation. Nonhereditary Rb patients may be followed by ophthalmology and oncology closely during active treatment but may have visits extended to longer intervals sooner than hereditary patients. Additionally, MRIs of the brain and orbits should be monitored every 6 months until the age of 3 to screen for pinealoblastoma development in hereditary Rb patients, while nonhereditary patients do not require this surveillance. While there are many effective therapies for the primary Rb tumor, follow-up frequency is dependent on the response of the tumor to therapy. Additionally, patients' families must receive appropriate counseling on their risk as well, as it relates to themselves and to future children.

Counselling for Families with Retinoblastoma

For a newly-diagnosed retinoblastoma patient & their family.

Due to the cancer syndrome that is associated with a germline mutation in heritable Rb and the risk of passing on the pathologic *RB1* variant to offspring, all newly-diagnosed Rb patients should be evaluated by a genetic counselor.

Table 60.1 Reference [56]

Family history	Retinoblastoma presentation			Probability that an RB1 germline pathogenic variant is present (%)
	Unilateral		Bilateral	
	Multifocal	Unifocal		
Positive[a]		+		100
	+			100
			+	100
Negative[b]			+	Close to 100[c]
	+			14–95
		+		~14

Note (1) If neither *RB1* pathogenic variant identified in tumor tissue is found in the DNA of constitutional DNA, the affected individual has a low probability of having an *RB1* germline pathogenic variant. (2) Because blood mosaicism as low as 20% can usually be detected by conventional molecular analysis such as sequencing, the failure to detect an *RB1* pathogenic variant in constitutional DNA reduces but cannot eliminate the probability that the individual has a germline *RB1* pathogenic variant. Table reprinted with permission from the University of Washington, Seattle. Lohmann DR, Gallie BL. Retinoblastoma. 2000 Jul 18 [Updated 2018 Nov 21]. In: Adam MP, Ardinger HH, Pagon RA, et al., editors. GeneReviews® [Internet]. Seattle (WA): University of Washington, Seattle; 1993–2021. Available from: https://www.ncbi.nlm.nih.gov/books/NBK1452/

[a] Positive = more than one affected family member (10% of retinoblastoma)

[b] Negative = only one affected individual in the family (90% of retinoblastoma)

[c] *RB1* pathogenic variants are identified by conventional molecular testing in 90–97% of simplex cases with bilateral involvement; the remaining 5% may have translocations, deep intronic splice variants, or low-level mosaic pathogenic variants that may or may not be in the germline

Table 60.1 shows the possibility of a patient possessing the heritable *RB1* trait based on laterality, focality and tumor size—while these clinical features are helpful, the most important information to make the determination of heritability is serum blood testing which is especially important for unilateral patients. Bilateral Rb patients always possess the heritable *RB1* trait and can be followed as such, however, ~15% of unilateral Rb patients also possess a germline mutation which dramatically changes their management. Thus, genetic evaluation **must** be based on more than phenotypic presentation. As such, all newly-diagnosed Rb patients are followed as if possessing a heritable Rb trait until proven otherwise.

Additionally, all first-degree relatives should undergo a single dilated ophthalmic examination if possible. An undiagnosed retinoma or regressed retinoblastoma in a relative may be discovered, indicating a heritable *RB1* trait in the family. The pretest risk of a mutant allele in a relative of an affected child without family history of retinoblastoma is presented in Table 60.2. For example, a parent of a bilateral proband has a pretest risk of 5%, while a unilateral proband's parents has a risk less than 1% [53]. A patient with heritable Rb (assuming germline mosaicism is not present), has a 45% risk of having a child with RB (45% is due to a 50% chance of passing along the pathogenic variant allele and overall penetrance of the allele of 90%) [54]. Furthermore, parents of the proband who are considering subsequent

Table 60.2 Reference [53] Pretest risk for relatives to carry the mutant *RB1* allele of the proband

	Pretest risk for mutant allele (%)	
Relative of proband	Bilateral proband (100)	Unilateral proband (15)
Offspring (infant)	50	7.5
Parent	5	0.8
Sibling	2.5	0.4
Niece/nephew	1.3	0.2
Aunt/uncle	0.1	0.007[a]
First cousin	0.05	0.007[a]
General population	0.007	0.007

Pretest risk for *RB1* mutation in family members of an affected child with retinoblastoma. Risk for *RB1* mutant allele is shown as a percentage for unilateral and bilateral probands without family history of retinoblastoma.

[a] Third- and fourth-degree relatives of unilateral probands have calculated risks of 0.003% and 0.001%, respectively, which are less than the normal population risk of 0.007% (1 in 15 000 live births); therefore, the risk is stated at 0.007%. Reprinted with permission from Elsevier. Skalet AH, Gombos DS, Gallie BL, et al. Screening Children at Risk for Retinoblastoma: Consensus Report from the American Association of Ophthalmic Oncologists and Pathologists. *Ophthalmology*. 2018;125(3):453–458. https://doi.org/10.1016/j.ophtha.2017.09.001

pregnancies should be followed by a genetic counselor and be offered prenatal genetic testing as well as discussion of fertility options including pre-implantation genetic diagnosis.

Genetic testing should be conducted by a Clinical Laboratory Improvement Amendments certified laboratory with retinoblastoma experience, as laboratory genetic testing sensitivities may vary and post-test risk of a pathogenic *RB1* variant must be calculated based on sensitivity. Of probands with a germline *RB1* pathogenic variant, ~5% will have a parent with the same variant [53]. However, most probands with heritable Rb have the pathogenic variant due to a de novo germline mutation. Counseling based on genetic tests must be done carefully, especially in the case of an adult survivor of Rb. A non-diagnostic test, for example, may be secondary to an undetectable mutation leading to a normal result; as mentioned earlier, improvements in liquid biopsy testing that allow for identification of the tumor-derived mutation(s) may lower this risk in the future.

Secondary malignancies are the most common cause of mortality in patients who survive after initial diagnosis of bilateral retinoblastoma [48]. A recent review for adult survivors of Rb strongly recommends an annual skin examination, and moderately recommends an annual history and physical examination with attention to bone structures [55]. Some institutions survey adult survivors of Rb with routine head, neck, or whole-body magnetic resonance imaging (MRI), but there is no evidence of diagnostic benefit and in fact some concern for increasing psychological distress and unnecessary testing due to false-positive results [55]. However, standard monitoring of trilateral retinoblastoma, or midline primitive neuroectodermal tumors in heritable Rb patients, is established at most centers. Standard of care consists of surveillance with MRI every 6 months until the age of 3 years (up to 7 years at some centers). Surveillance protocols for other non-ocular tumors have not been established and vary by center.

For at-risk children

While rare, it is possible that a patient with a heritable germline mutation may never develop Rb due to mosaicism or lack of subsequent mutational events after the first initiating *RB1* mutation (M1). Thus, recent guidelines released by the American Association of Ophthalmic Oncologists and Pathologists recommend that all at-risk children undergo serum genetic testing [53]. Children are considered to be "at-risk" if they have a **family history of Rb in a parent, sibling, or first- or second-degree relative.** In addition to genetic testing, at-risk children should undergo clinical examinations as listed below.

Recommendations for at-risk children:

(1) At-risk children should undergo serial dilated screening fundus examinations by an ophthalmologist with specific experience in retinoblastoma up until 7-years of age. At-risk infants should undergo examination shortly after birth and frequently thereafter (every 2–4 weeks).
(2) After 7-years of screening, asymptomatic children no longer require screening examinations **unless individuals carry a known pathogenic *RB1* mutation.** In the case of *RB1* carriers, patients should undergo screening every year.

Follow-up frequency is determined based on the age of the child and pre-test risk. Recommended examination schedule is shown in Fig. 60.3 for patients who are at risk of Rb but have not been diagnosed with Rb. Of note, cases of unilateral disease that subsequently were found to have retinoblastoma in the other eye have also been described [57]. Such cases highlight the need for continued monitoring of both eyes until the patient's *RB1* hereditary status is known.

Conclusion

The discovery of the *RB1* retinoblastoma tumor suppressor gene has laid the groundwork for molecular genetics associated with cancer tumorigenesis. This has led to improved screening and early detection in affected patients. Genetic testing, and lifelong counseling is the standard of care for all families with retinoblastoma and understanding the genetics of this disease is critical for physicians involved in the care of patients with Rb. This includes primary care doctors, fertility specialists, and genetic counsellors as the inappropriate counselling of an adult patient with unilateral Rb who never had testing to determine whether or not a germline mutation is present can lead to devastating consequences for their future children. Continued advancements in non-invasive genetic testing and surveillance will hopefully lead to further reductions in patient morbidity and mortality.

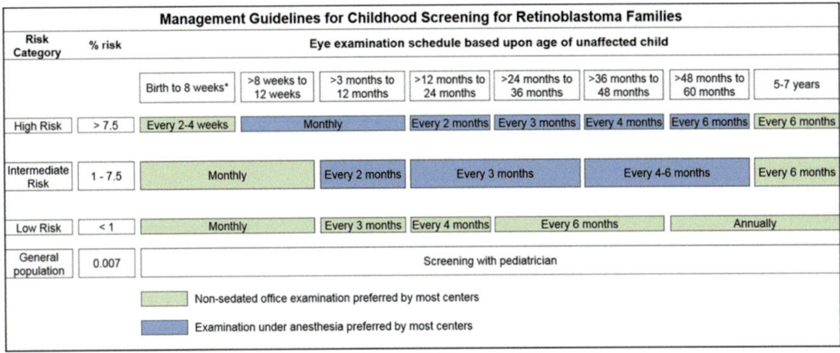

Fig. 60.3 Reference [53] Management guidelines for childhood screening for retinoblastoma. The presented schedules are general guidelines and reflect a schedule for examinations in which no lesions of concern are noted. It may be appropriate to examine some children more frequently. Decisions regarding examination method, examination under anesthesia (EUA) versus non-sedated examination in the office, are complex and best decided by the clinician in discussion with the patient's family. The preference of the majority of the clinical centers involved in the creation of this consensus statement is reflected, but individual centers may make policy decisions based on available resources and expert clinician preference. Examination under anesthesia will be strongly considered for any child who is unable to participate in an office examination sufficiently to allow thorough examination of the retina. *A minority of clinical centers also prefer EUA for high- and intermediate-risk children (calculated risk >1%) from birth to 8 weeks of age. Figure reprinted with permission from Elsevier. Skalet AH, Gombos DS, Gallie BL, et al. Screening Children at Risk for Retinoblastoma: Consensus Report from the American Association of Ophthalmic Oncologists and Pathologists. *Ophthalmology*. 2018;125(3):453–458. https://doi.org/10.1016/j.ophtha.2017.09.001

Review Questions

1. An 8-month old infant presents with bilateral retinoblastoma lesions, after primary treatment how long must the patient be followed by ophthalmology?

a. No more follow-up is necessary
b. Follow-up for life
c. Follow-up is dependent on the results of genetic testing
d. Follow-up until 6 years of age

2. A patient should undergo early screening for retinoblastoma if:

a. They have a first-degree relative with a history of sarcoma
b. All patients are "at-risk" for retinoblastoma and require a dilated fundus examination by an ophthalmologist
c. They have a first or second-degree relative with a history of retinoblastoma
d. No patients require early screening

3. Who should undergo genetic testing?

a. All patients with retinoblastoma
b. Patients with bilateral retinoblastoma
c. Patients who presented with retinoblastoma before the age of 1
d. All of the above

Answers

1. (**B**) This patient has bilateral retinoblastoma lesions, which is by definition hereditary retinoblastoma. Hereditary Rb patients constitutes *RB1* cancer syndrome which confers lifelong risk for intraocular recurrence of Rb and secondary cancers later in life. Patients with an inherited germline mutation are at a higher risk of secondary cancers with osteosarcoma, cutaneous melanoma and soft tissue sarcomas being the most common. These patients must be followed by ophthalmology and oncology to survey for future tumorigenesis.

2. (**C**) Children are considered to be "at-risk" and require early eye examinations if they have a family history of Rb in a parent, sibling, or first- or second-degree relative. In addition to genetic testing to determine the presence of a germline RB1 mutation, at-risk children should undergo clinical examinations as listed below.

Recommendations for at-risk children:

(1) At-risk children should undergo serial dilated fundus examinations by an ophthalmologist with experience with Rb up until 7-years of age. At-risk infants should undergo examination early and frequently.
(2) After 7-years of screening, asymptomatic children no longer require screening examinations unless individuals carry a known pathogenic *RB1* mutation. In the case of *RB1* carriers, patients should undergo screening every year.

3. (**D**) Hereditary Rb patients may present later in life or may present with unilateral lesions. Although commonly hereditary Rb patients will present with a positive family history, present early and with bilateral lesions, the lack of these signs does not rule-out hereditary Rb. 15% of patients with unilateral disease without a positive family history have a detectable mutation in the peripheral blood. It is further important to determine whether the detected mutation is a true germline mutation or a mosaic mutation, as family members do not require screening in the case of mosaicism, and the degree of mosaicism can determine the risk of additional tumors in the patient. Genetic testing, and lifelong counseling is the standard of care for all families with hereditary retinoblastoma, and understanding the genetics of this disease is critical for physicians involved in the care of patients with Rb.

References

1. Rao R, Honavar SG. Retinoblastoma. Indian J Pediatr. 2017;84(12):937–44. https://doi.org/10.1007/s12098-017-2395-0.

2. Mendoza PR, Grossniklaus HE. The biology of retinoblastoma. Prog Mol Biol Transl Sci. 2015;134:503–16. https://doi.org/10.1016/bs.pmbts.2015.06.012.

3. Dimaras H, Corson TW, Cobrinik D, et al. Retinoblastoma. Nat Rev Dis Primer. 2015;1:15021. https://doi.org/10.1038/nrdp.2015.21.

4. Rodriguez-Galindo C, Orbach DB, VanderVeen D. Retinoblastoma. Pediatr Clin North Am. 2015;62(1):201–23. https://doi.org/10.1016/j.pcl.2014.09.014.

5. Ortiz MV, Dunkel IJ. Retinoblastoma. J Child Neurol. 2016;31(2):227–36. https://doi.org/10.1177/0883073815587943.

6. de Graaf P, Göricke S, Rodjan F, et al. Guidelines for imaging retinoblastoma: imaging principles and MRI standardization. Pediatr Radiol. 2012;42(1):2–14. https://doi.org/10.1007/s00247-011-2201-5.

7. Abramson DH, Melson MR, Servodidio C. Visual fields in retinoblastoma survivors. *Arch Ophthalmol Chic Ill 1960*. 2004;122(9):1324–1330. doi:https://doi.org/10.1001/archopht.122.9.1324

8. Berry JL, Xu L, Murphree AL, et al. Potential of aqueous humor as a surrogate tumor biopsy for retinoblastoma. JAMA Ophthalmol. 2017;135(11):1221–30. https://doi.org/10.1001/jamaophthalmol.2017.4097.

9. Soliman SE, Racher H, Zhang C, MacDonald H, Gallie BL. Genetics and molecular diagnostics in retinoblastoma–an update. Asia-Pac J Ophthalmol Phila Pa. 2017;6(2):197–207. https://doi.org/10.22608/APO.201711.

10. Friend SH, Bernards R, Rogelj S, et al. A human DNA segment with properties of the gene that predisposes to retinoblastoma and osteosarcoma. Nature. 1986;323(6089):643–6. https://doi.org/10.1038/323643a0.

11. Lee WH, Bookstein R, Hong F, Young LJ, Shew JY, Lee EY. Human retinoblastoma susceptibility gene: cloning, identification, and sequence. Science. 1987;235(4794):1394–9. https://doi.org/10.1126/science.3823889.

12. Fung YK, Murphree AL, T'Ang A, Qian J, Hinrichs SH, Benedict WF. Structural evidence for the authenticity of the human retinoblastoma gene. Science. 1987;236(4809):1657–61. https://doi.org/10.1126/science.2885916.

13. Yun J, Li Y, Xu C-T, Pan B-R. Epidemiology and Rb1 gene of retinoblastoma. Int J Ophthalmol. 2011;4(1):103–9. https://doi.org/10.3980/j.issn.2222-3959.2011.01.24.

14. Knudson AG. Mutation and cancer: statistical study of retinoblastoma. Proc Natl Acad Sci U S A. 1971;68(4):820–3.

15. Comings DE. A general theory of carcinogenesis. Proc Natl Acad Sci U S A. 1973;70(12):3324–8. https://doi.org/10.1073/pnas.70.12.3324.

16. Richter S, Vandezande K, Chen N, et al. Sensitive and efficient detection of RB1 gene mutations enhances care for families with retinoblastoma. Am J Hum Genet. 2003;72(2):253–69. https://doi.org/10.1086/345651.

17. Dimaras H, Corson TW. Retinoblastoma, the visible CNS tumor: a review. J Neurosci Res. 2019;97(1):29–44. https://doi.org/10.1002/jnr.24213.

18. Rodríguez-Martín C, Robledo C, Gómez-Mariano G, et al. Frequency of low-level and high-level mosaicism in sporadic retinoblastoma: genotype-phenotype relationships. J Hum Genet. 2020;65(2):165–74. https://doi.org/10.1038/s10038-019-0696-z.

19. Berry JL, Lewis L, Zolfaghari E, et al. Lack of correlation between age at diagnosis and RB1 mutations for unilateral retinoblastoma: the importance of genetic testing. Ophthalmic Genet. 2018;39(3):407–9. https://doi.org/10.1080/13816810.2017.1420807.

20. Amin MB, Greene FL, Edge SB, et al. The eighth edition AJCC cancer staging manual: continuing to build a bridge from a population-based to a more "personalized" approach to cancer staging. CA Cancer J Clin. 2017;67(2):93–9. https://doi.org/10.3322/caac.21388.

21. Squire J, Goddard AD, Canton M, Becker A, Phillips RA, Gallie BL. Tumour induction by the retinoblastoma mutation is independent of N-myc expression. Nature. 1986;322 (6079):555–7. https://doi.org/10.1038/322555a0.

22. Bowles E, Corson TW, Bayani J, et al. Profiling genomic copy number changes in retinoblastoma beyond loss of RB1. Genes Chromosomes Cancer. 2007;46(2):118–29. https://doi.org/10.1002/gcc.20383.

23. Rushlow DE, Mol BM, Kennett JY, et al. Characterisation of retinoblastomas without RB1 mutations: genomic, gene expression, and clinical studies. Lancet Oncol. 2013;14(4):327–34. https://doi.org/10.1016/S1470-2045(13)70045-7.

24. Mallipatna A, Marino M, Singh AD. Genetics of Retinoblastoma. Asia Pac J Ophthalmol (Phila). 2016;5(4):260–4. https://doi.org/10.1097/APO.0000000000000219.

25. Thériault BL, Dimaras H, Gallie BL, Corson TW. The genomic landscape of retinoblastoma: a review. Clin Exp Ophthalmol. 2014;42(1):33–52. https://doi.org/10.1111/ceo.12132.

26. Zugbi S, Ganiewich D, Bhattacharyya A, et al. Clinical, genomic, and pharmacological study of *MYCN*-amplified *RB1* wild-type metastatic retinoblastoma. Cancers (Basel). 2020;12 (9):2714. Published 2020 Sep 22. https://doi.org/10.3390/cancers12092714.

27. Moulin AP, Stathopoulos C, Marcelli F, Schoumans Pouw J, Beck-Popovic M, Munier FL. Secondary enucleated retinoblastoma with MYCN amplification. Ophthalmic Genet. 2021;42 (3):354–9. https://doi.org/10.1080/13816810.2021.1897847.

28. Xu L, Kim ME, Polski A, et al. Establishing the clinical utility of ctDNA analysis for diagnosis, prognosis, and treatment monitoring of retinoblastoma: the aqueous humor liquid biopsy. Cancers (Basel). 2021;13(6):1282. Published 2021 Mar 13. https://doi.org/10.3390/cancers13061282.

29. Corson TW, Gallie BL. One hit, two hits, three hits, more? Genomic changes in the development of retinoblastoma. Genes Chromosomes Cancer. 2007;46(7):617–34. https://doi.org/10.1002/gcc.20457.

30. Dimaras H, Khetan V, Halliday W, et al. Loss of RB1 induces non-proliferative retinoma: increasing genomic instability correlates with progression to retinoblastoma. Hum Mol Genet. 2008;17(10):1363–72. https://doi.org/10.1093/hmg/ddn024.

31. Kooi IE, Mol BM, Massink MP, et al. Somatic genomic alterations in retinoblastoma beyond RB1 are rare and limited to copy number changes. Sci Rep. 2016;6:25264. Published 2016 Apr 29. https://doi.org/10.1038/srep25264.

32. Kooi IE, Mol BM, Massink MP, et al. A meta-analysis of retinoblastoma copy numbers refines the list of possible driver genes involved in tumor progression. PLoS One. 2016;11(4): e0153323. Published 2016 Apr 26. https://doi.org/10.1371/journal.pone.0153323.

33. Grasemann C, Gratias S, Stephan H, et al. Gains and overexpression identify DEK and E2F3 as targets of chromosome 6p gains in retinoblastoma. Oncogene. 2005;24(42):6441–9. https://doi.org/10.1038/sj.onc.1208792.

34. Kapatai G, Brundler MA, Jenkinson H, et al. Gene expression profiling identifies different sub-types of retinoblastoma. Br J Cancer. 2013;109(2):512–25. https://doi.org/10.1038/bjc.2013.283.

35. Cano J, Oliveros O, Yunis E. Phenotype variants, malignancy, and additional copies of 6p in retinoblastoma. Cancer Genet Cytogenet. 1994;76(2):112–5. https://doi.org/10.1016/0165-4608(94)90459-6.

36. Karcioglu ZA. Fine needle aspiration biopsy (FNAB) for retinoblastoma. Retina. 2002;22 (6):707–10. https://doi.org/10.1097/00006982-200212000-00004.

37. Karcioglu ZA, Gordon RA, Karcioglu GL. Tumor seeding in ocular fine needle aspiration biopsy. Ophthalmology. 1985;92(12):1763–7. https://doi.org/10.1016/s0161-6420(85)34105-2.

38. Francis JH, Abramson DH, Ji X, et al. Risk of extraocular extension in eyes with retinoblastoma receiving intravitreous chemotherapy. JAMA Ophthalmol. 2017;135 (12):1426–9. https://doi.org/10.1001/jamaophthalmol.2017.4600.

39. Berry JL, Xu L, Kooi I, et al. Genomic cfDNA analysis of aqueous humor in retinoblastoma predicts eye salvage: the surrogate tumor biopsy for retinoblastoma. Mol Cancer Res. 2018;16 (11):1701–12. https://doi.org/10.1158/1541-7786.MCR-18-0369.

40. Xu L, Polski A, Prabakar RK, et al. Chromosome 6p amplification in aqueous humor cell-free DNA is a prognostic biomarker for retinoblastoma ocular survival. Mol Cancer Res. 2020;18 (8):1166–75. https://doi.org/10.1158/1541-7786.MCR-19-1262.

41. Xu L, Shen L, Polski A, et al. Simultaneous identification of clinically relevant *RB1* mutations and copy number alterations in aqueous humor of retinoblastoma eyes. Ophthalmic Genet. 2020;41(6):526–32. https://doi.org/10.1080/13816810.2020.1799417.

42. Kleinerman RA, Yu CL, Little MP, et al. Variation of second cancer risk by family history of retinoblastoma among long-term survivors. J Clin Oncol. 2012;30(9):950–7. https://doi.org/ 10.1200/JCO.2011.37.0239.

43. Moll AC, Imhof SM, Bouter LM, Tan KE. Second primary tumors in patients with retinoblastoma. A review of the literature. Ophthalmic Genet. 1997;18(1):27–34. https://doi. org/10.3109/13816819709057880.

44. Kleinerman RA, Tucker MA, Abramson DH, Seddon JM, Tarone RE, Fraumeni JF Jr. Risk of soft tissue sarcomas by individual subtype in survivors of hereditary retinoblastoma. J Natl Cancer Inst. 2007;99(1):24–31. https://doi.org/10.1093/jnci/djk002.

45. Draper GJ, Sanders BM, Kingston JE. Second primary neoplasms in patients with retinoblastoma. Br J Cancer. 1986;53(5):661–71. https://doi.org/10.1038/bjc.1986.110.

46. Wong FL, Boice JD Jr, Abramson DH, et al. Cancer incidence after retinoblastoma. Radiation dose and sarcoma risk. JAMA. 1997;278(15):1262–7. https://doi.org/10.1001/jama.278.15.1262.

47. Kleinerman RA, Schonfeld SJ, Sigel BS, et al. Bone and soft-tissue sarcoma risk in long-term survivors of hereditary retinoblastoma treated with radiation. J Clin Oncol. 2019;37 (35):3436–45. https://doi.org/10.1200/JCO.19.01096.

48. Shinohara ET, DeWees T, Perkins SM. Subsequent malignancies and their effect on survival in patients with retinoblastoma. Pediatr Blood Cancer. 2014;61(1):116–9. https://doi.org/10. 1002/pbc.24714.

49. Kingston JE, Plowman PN, Hungerford JL. Ectopic intracranial retinoblastoma in childhood. Br J Ophthalmol. 1985;69(10):742–8. https://doi.org/10.1136/bjo.69.10.742.

50. Blach LE, McCormick B, Abramson DH, Ellsworth RM. Trilateral retinoblastoma–incidence and outcome: a decade of experience. Int J Radiat Oncol Biol Phys. 1994;29(4):729–33. https://doi.org/10.1016/0360-3016(94)90560-6.

51. Messmer EP, Fritze H, Mohr C, et al. Long-term treatment effects in patients with bilateral retinoblastoma: ocular and mid-facial findings. Graefes Arch Clin Exp Ophthalmol. 1991;229 (4):309–14. https://doi.org/10.1007/BF00170686.

52. Gombos DS, Hungerford J, Abramson DH, et al. Secondary acute myelogenous leukemia in patients with retinoblastoma: is chemotherapy a factor? Ophthalmology. 2007;114(7):1378–83. https://doi.org/10.1016/j.ophtha.2007.03.074.

53. Skalet AH, Gombos DS, Gallie BL, et al. Screening children at risk for retinoblastoma: consensus report from the american association of ophthalmic oncologists and pathologists. Ophthalmology. 2018;125(3):453–8.https://doi.org/10.1016/j.ophtha.2017.09.001.

54. Draper GJ, Sanders BM, Brownbill PA, Hawkins MM. Patterns of risk of hereditary retinoblastoma and applications to genetic counselling. Br J Cancer. 1992;66(1):211–9. https://doi.org/10.1038/bjc.1992.244.

55. Tonorezos ES, Friedman DN, Barnea D, et al. Recommendations for long-term follow-up of adults with heritable retinoblastoma. Ophthalmology. 2020;127(11):1549–57. https://doi.org/ 10.1016/j.ophtha.2020.05.024.

56. Lohmann DR, Gallie BL. Retinoblastoma. In: Adam MP, Ardinger HH, Pagon RA, et al., eds. *GeneReviews*®. Seattle (WA): University of Washington, Seattle; July 18, 2000.

57. Berry JL, Cobrinik D, Kim JW. Detection and intraretinal localization of an 'Invisible' retinoblastoma using optical coherence tomography. Ocul Oncol Pathol. 2016;2(3):148–52. https://doi.org/10.1159/000442167.

Differential Diagnosis of Retinoblastoma

61

İrem Koç and Hayyam Kiratli

Abstract

Retinoblastoma is the most common intraocular malignancy of childhood. The diagnosis is almost exlusively based on clinical findings and imaging studies, hence it is compulsory to be familiar with the entities which lie in the differential diagnosis. In the literature in up to nearly half of the cases of retinoblastoma suspects, simulating conditions have been reported. Herein we aim to cover the most clinically prevalent of these entities, namely, Coats' Disease, persistent fetal vasculature, familial exudative vitreoretinopathy, astrocytic hamartoma, medulloepithelioma and ocular toxocariasis, focusing on their differentiating properties from retinoblastoma. In each disease careful clinical observation together with conventional and contemporary multimodal imaging plays a crucial role.

Keywords

Retinoblastoma · Differential diagnosis · Coats' disease · Persistent fetal vasculature · Familial exudative vitreoretinopathy

İ. Koç · H. Kiratli (✉)
Ocular and Periocular Oncology Unit, Department of Ophthalmology, Hacettepe University School of Medicine, Ankara, Turkey
e-mail: hkiratli@hacettepe.edu.tr

© The Author(s), under exclusive license to Springer Nature Switzerland AG 2023
Ş. Özdek et al. (eds.), *Pediatric Vitreoretinal Surgery*,
https://doi.org/10.1007/978-3-031-14506-3_61

911

Introduction

Retinoblastoma is the most common primary intraocular malignant tumor in children with an incidence of 1 in 16.000 live births [1]. In contrast to many other cancers where surgical tissue biopsy is the rule for the definitive confirmation, the diagnosis of retinoblastoma is established mainly based on clinical tumor features supported by certain magnetic resonance imaging (MRI) and ocular ultrasonographic characteristics. Despite technical advances and significant experience accumulated over decades in retinoblastoma centers worldwide, a great variety of ocular diseases may still occasionally cause diagnostic uncertainties (Table 61.1). Several reports have shown that between 16 to 53% of patients referred as retinoblastoma had other simulating conditions designated as pseudoretinoblastoma [3–5]. On the whole, the three most common conditions simulating retinoblastoma included Coats' disease (40%), persistent fetal vasculature (PFV) (28%), and vitreous hemorrhage (5%) according to a large series [4]. If age is considered as a criterion, PFV (49%), Coats' disease (20%), and vitreous hemorrhage (7%) respectively were more common in infants under 1 year of age [4]. In children between 2 to 5 years of age, Coats' disease (61%), toxocariasis (8%), and PFV (7%) were more common, whereas in children older than 5 years Coats' disease (57%), toxocariasis (8%), and familial exudative vitreoretinopathy (FEVR) (6%) were more frequently encountered [4].

This chapter will selectively focus on Coats' disease, PFV, medulloepithelioma, FEVR, and retinal astrocytic hamartoma. Other relevant topics are covered in greater depths in appropriate parts of the book.

Table 61.1 Differential diagnosis of retinoblastoma

A. Congenital malformations	B. Inflammatory diseases
Persistent fetal vasculature	Congenital toxoplasmosis
Cataract	Ocular toxocariasis
Myelinated nerve fibers	Endophthalmitis
Choroidal coloboma	Cytomegalovirus retinitis
Norrie' disease	Herpes simplex retinitis
Retinal folds	
Retinal dysplasia	
Morning glory syndrome	
Incontinentia pigmenti	
C. Vascular diseases	D. Tumors
Coats' disease	Medulloblastoma
Familial exudative vitreoretinopathy	Retinal astrocytic hamartoma
Retinopathy of prematurity	Combined hamartoma
	Choroidal osteoma
	Vasoproliferative tumor

Adopted and modified from Kim and Singh [2]

Coats' Disease

Coats' disease is an idiopathic, unilateral exudative retinal vascular abnormality characterized by telangiectasia and aneurysmal dilatations of the retinal capillary network, particularly in the temporal macula and mid-periphery [6]. The clinical severity may range from isolated vascular abnormalities in one quadrant to massive exudation leading to total retinal exudative detachment and phythisis bulbi [7, 8]. The traditional assumption that Coats' disease is almost always unilateral has recently been challenged by ultra-widefield imaging findings [9]. The demonstration of capillary bed abnormalities in 77.8% and microaneurysms in 22.2% of fellow eyes suggested that Coats' disease might in fact be an asymmetric bilateral disease [9]. Several clinical and imaging features may help to distinguish Coats' disease from retinoblastoma (Table 61.2) (Fig. 61.1).

Table 61.2 Selected suggestive distinguishing features of retinoblastoma and Coats' disease

Feature	Retinoblastoma	Coats' disease
Mean age at presentation (years)	1.5	5
Sex predilection	None	Male
Laterality	Unilateral: 60% Bilateral: 40%	Unilateral: > 90%
Pupillary reflex	Leukocoria	Xanthocoria
Globe size	Variable	Not microphthalmic but usually small
Retinal vasculature	Tortous, uniformly dilated, runs into the tumor, dips in	Irregularly dilated, bulbous endings, sheating
Calcification	Frequent, randomly distributed	Rare, curvilinear if osseous metaplasia is present
Intraretinal macrocyst	None	38%
Shape of retinal detachment	Sharp V	Wide V
Autofluorescence [13, 14]	Hyperautofluorescence of calcified tumors, variable elsewhere	Hyperautofluorescence of retinal exudates
Genetics	*RB1* mutations on chromosome 13q14	Somatic mutation in *NDP* gene on chromosome Xp11
Ultrasonography	Retinal detachment, presence of vitreous seeds, internal calcification of the mass	Retinal detachment, subretinal cholesterol deposits
Computerized tomography	Retinal detachment, retinal mass containing calcification	Retinal detachment
Magnetic resonance imaging	Retinal detachment, enhancing retinal mass with limited diffusion	Retinal detachment, hyperintense, homogenous subretinal fluid without enhancement

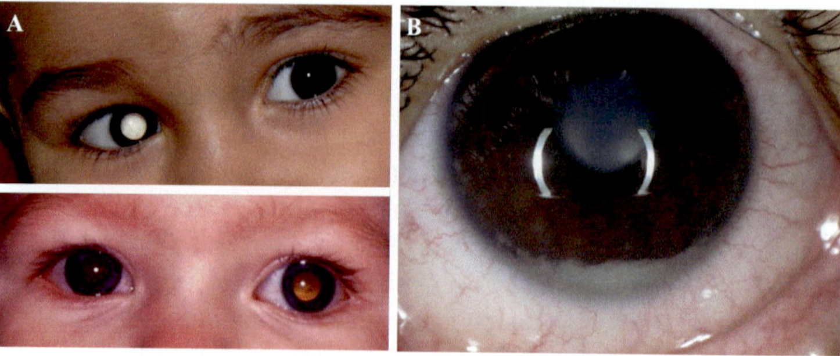

Fig. 61.1 Clinical features aiding in the diagnosis of retinoblastoma, **A:** Leukocoria in retinoblastoma (top image) versus xanthocoria in an eye with Coats' disease (bottom image). **B:** Pseudohypopyon indicating tumor cells in the anterior chamber in a patient with retinoblastoma

In the early stages (1 or 2A) there may be light bulb-like telangiectatic retinal vessels, subretinal exudation, and peripheral non-perfusion best demonstrated with fluorescein angiography [6–8]. Optical coherence tomography may be of limited utility by documenting exudates in all retinal layers but particularly in the outer nuclear layer and small preretinal hyperreflective dots probably representing inflammatory or red blood cells [10]. These features are unlikely to be seen in retinoblastoma. Stage 2B2 with a subfoveal fibrotic nodule may more closely resemble a retinoblastoma (Fig. 61.2) however it is at stage 3B and 4 with the presence of total exudative retinal detachment when most diagnostic difficulties arise. In these advanced cases other imaging studies may be of help. Ocular ultrasonography in Coats' disease may show a clear subretinal fluid and multiple small faint opacities in the vitreous corresponding to cholesterolosis [7]. In Coats'

Fig. 61.2 Subfoveal fibrotic nodule with exudation typically associated with Coats' disease

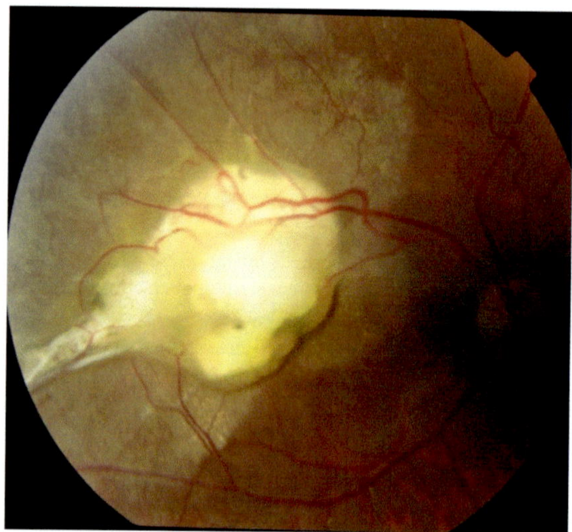

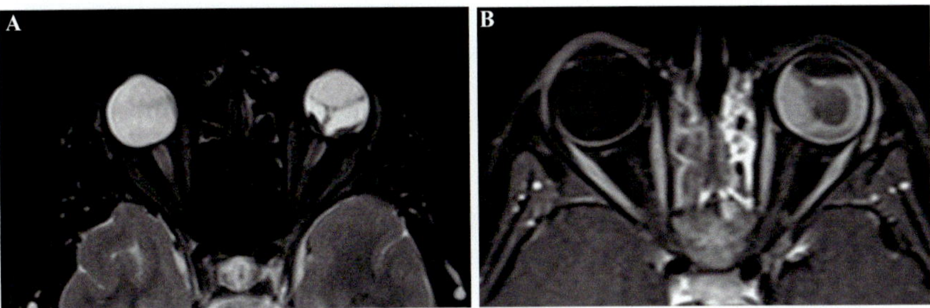

Fig. 61.3 MRI studies of 2 patients with Coats' disease, **A:** Axial T2-weighted scan shows wide V-shaped retinal detachment, hyperintense subretinal fluid and hypointense subretinal nodules, typical for this disease, and **B:** Axial contrast-enhanced T1-weighted image demonstrating the retinal macrocyst

disease magnetic resonance imaging studies usually demonstrate hyperintense subretinal fluid both on T1 and T2 sequences, non-enhancing subretinal fibrotic nodules (Fig. 61.3A), and intraretinal macrocysts (Fig. 61.3B) [11].

In contrast to retinoblastoma, intraretinal macrocysts are common in Coats' disease which develop in chronically detached retinas [12]. In advanced Coats' disease, glistening yellow cholesterol crystals can be observed in the anterior chamber whereas a white pseudohypopyon (Fig. 61.1B) or multiple white iris nodules can be found in group E or very advanced retinoblastoma. On rare occasions, the distinction can only be made by histopathological examination following enucleation.

Persistent Fetal Vasculature (PFV)

Formerly known as persistent hyperplastic primary vitreous, PFV is a congenital ocular malformation which may present with leukocoria usually in association with microphthalmia and strabismus [15]. The fetal intraocular vascular system is composed of capsulopupillary artery, tunica vasculosa lentis, and vasa hyaloidea propria from anterior to posterior. Failure of these vessels to regress after 20th week of intrauterine life results in PFV and the clinical manifestations and severity of the anomaly are determined by the vascular component that persists [15, 16]. Fourteen hub genes are so far identified that may lead to PFV development and these are mostly related to VEGF rceptor signaling pathways, ocular morphogenesis, apotosis, and cancer [17]. The most typical anterior segment signs include a shallow anterior chamber, engorged iris vessels, cataract, a white retrolental membrane, and elongated ciliary processes [15, 16]. In the posterior segment, Bergmeister papilla, inferotemporal retinal folds, hyaloidal stalk, retinal dysplasia and detachment, and optic nerve hypolasia can be observed [15, 16]. Although unilateral involvement is the rule, bilateral cases may rarely be diagnosed [18]. However, recent

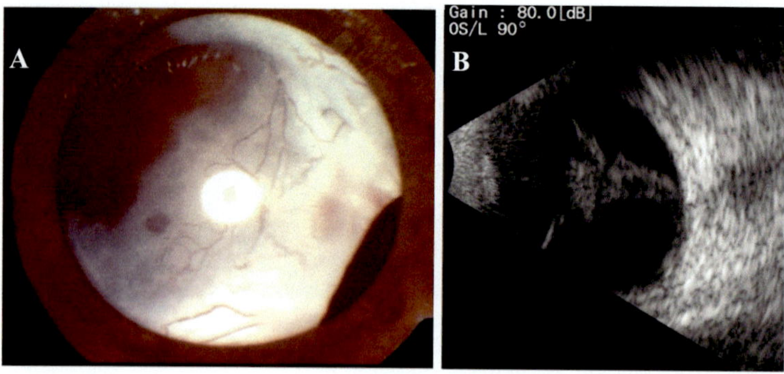

Fig. 61.4 **A:** Color anterior segment photography of a 12-month-old girl revealing white, fibrotic membrane behind the lens. Note the vessels of normal calibre. **B:** Ocular B-mode ultrasonogram of a 15-month-old child with PFV shows a funnel-shaped total retinal detachment. The axial lenght of the eye was 15.3 mm. There was no calcification.

investigations using widefield fluorescein angiography demonstrated vascular abnormalities in 75.6% of the fellow eyes of patients with PFV suggesting that the disease might be a bilateral asymmetric process, similar to Coats' disease [19].

Retinoblastoma may be in the differential diagnosis if there is a white retrolental membrane causing leukocoria or a total retinal detachment in an infant (Fig. 61.4 A). In these selected cases imaging studies can provide clues for the proper diagnosis. Ocular ultasonography may typically show a shortened axial length and an echogenic band extending between the optic disc and posterior lens capsule (Fig. 61.4B) [20].

This band may ve I, Y, inverted Y or X shaped with or without ciliary body traction [20]. These features definitely are not in favor of retinoblastoma. Color doppler flow imaging may demonstrate high resistive index and low-end diastolic velocity strongly suggesting PFV as these vessels do not supply any functioning tissue [21]. The inverse is true for a retinal detachment not associated with PFV [21]. MR imaging may provide important information in eyes suspected to have PFV and for its differential diagnosis. Eyes with PFV tend to be smaller compared to eyes having Coats' disease or retinoblastoma [11]. MRI shows lens swelling, deformations of the ciliary body, intraocular hemorrhage, and vitreous membranes in PFV (Fig. 61.5A) [11]. Other typical finding include optic nerve atrophy and a Y-shaped retinal detachment (Martini glass sign) without any signs of calcification (Fig. 61.5B) [11]. Bilateral PFV (Fig. 61.6) is the second most common cause of bilateral leukocoria after retinoblastoma and prompt diagnosis is essential to save at least one eye with functional vision since any delay will increase the risks and extent of PFV-related complications [16, 18].

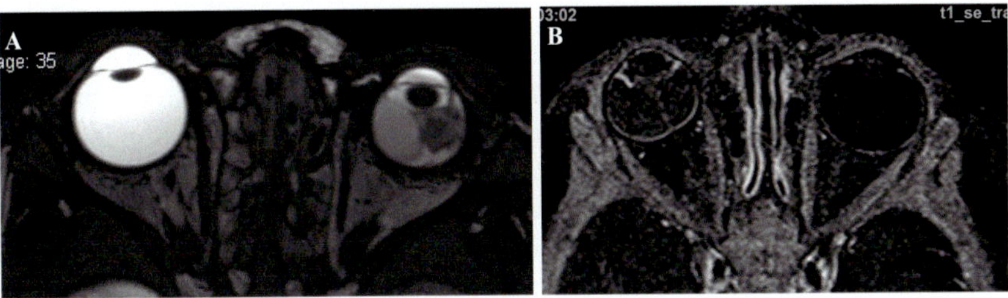

Fig. 61.5 A: Axial T2-weighted orbital MR scan of a 7-month-old infant revealed left microphthalmia with lens and ciliary body deformation, retinal detachment, and vitreal and subretinal hemorrhages favoring the diagnosis of PFV, **B**: This axial orbital MRI scan demonstrates optic nerve atrophy and a stalk between the optik disc and the posterior lens forming a Martini glass appearance

Fig. 61.6 Axial T2-weighted orbital MR scan of a 22-month-old baby with bilateral PFV

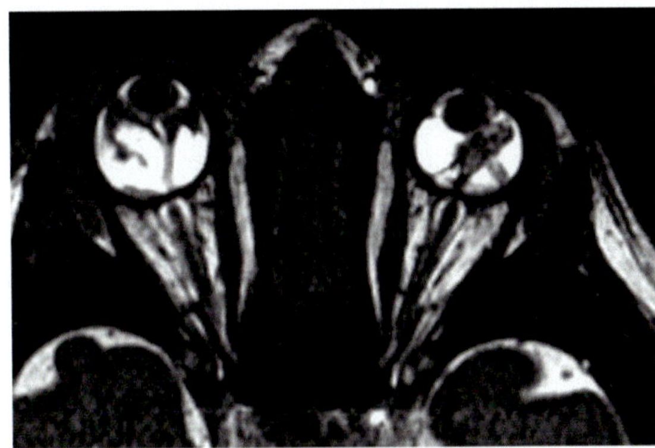

Familial Exudative Vitreoretinopathy

Familial exudative vitreoretinopathy (FEVR) is a hereditary condition which is characterized by abnormal retinal vascularization. Avascular peripheral retina is the key clinical feature of the disease and it is most commonly observed in the temporal quadrant. FEVR is exclusively bilateral, albeit asymmetric findings in most of the cases. Even though clinical features of FEVR resemble retinopathy of prematurity (ROP) more it does retinoblastoma, FEVR can constitute 1–6% of cases which require differentiation from retinoblastoma [4]. The likelihood of FEVR to be encountered among retinoblastoma-simulating conditions increases with patient age, and the prevalance of FEVR reaches 6% in patients with a lesion simulating retinoblastoma [4]. FEVR is a heterogenous disease in terms of mode of inheritance and pattern of gene expression, in consequence it can present with a wide variety of features ranging from asymptomatic peripheral vascularization to severe tractional retinal detachment. Inheritance pattern is most commonly autosomal dominant, followed by autosomal dominant and X-linked recessive patterns [22]. As of today, the most commonly identified genes in the FEVR spectrum are defined to be: *FZD4, LRP5, NDP, TSPAN12, KIF11* and *ZNF408* [23]. Biologically the first 4 of these genes function in the Wnt and Norrin signaling pathways which are responsible in cell proliferation, differentiation and migration all aiding in normal retinal vascular formation. The latter 2 have roles in mitotic spindle establishment and Zinc finger protein formation which is functional in DNA binding [24, 25].

Ophthalmologically, apart from peripheral retinal avascularity, preretinal neovascularization and fibrosis at the junction of normal and avascular retina can lead to fibrosis and tractions in moderate to severe cases [26]. In more severe cases these tractions can result in retinal folds, tractional retinal detachment or ectopic fovea. Retinal exudation and epiretinal membranes may accompany secondarily [26]. Fundus fluorescein angiography (FFA) assists in diagnosis of FEVR by visualizing avascular zones of the retina and additionally aids in screening of asymptomatic cases by displaying retinal vasculature in wide periphery with wide-field FFA. In addition, leakage on FFA is presumed to be a marker of active disease and a precursor of retinal exudate [22]. There are several proposed classification schemes for FEVR and some are based on clinical findings alone [27, 28], while others incorporate FFA findings into disease stratification [29, 30]. Presence of neovascularization or retinal detachment are critical landmarks in disease classification [27–30]. The mainstay of treatment is laser photocoagulation to avascular retina and anti-VEGF treatment may play an adjunct role in decreasing the VEGF burden keeping in mind that intravitreal anti-VEGF injections can paradoxically increase vitreoretinal tractions. Surgery for retinal detachment may include scleral buckling or vitrectomy in order to relieve tractions exerted on the retina.

Astrocytic Hamartoma

Retinal astrocytic hamartomas are relatively rare tumors of the retina. They are primarily glial tumors which mainly arise from inner retinal layers, particularly the nerve fiber layer. The tumor may occur sporadically or in association with phakomatoses such as tuberous sclerosis and neurofibromatosis. Even though histopathologically retinal astrocytic hamartoma and retinoblastoma are distinct entities, the clinical appearance may resemble each other and differential diagnosis is based on clinical and imaging features in almost all patients. Retinal astrocytic hamartoma constitutes 1–5% of all pseudoretinoblastoma cases [4]. Clinically it may have a grayish translucent color and may appear whiter if the calcium deposits are more prominent. The calcified white retinal astrocytic hamartoma displays a rather glistening white-yellow look rather than the dull chalky-white reflex of a calcified retinoblastoma [31]. Retinal astrocytic hamartoma is more likely to be non-related to a phakomatosis if it is single, juxtapapillary in location and does not contain giant astrocytes upon histopathology (Fig. 61.7) [32].

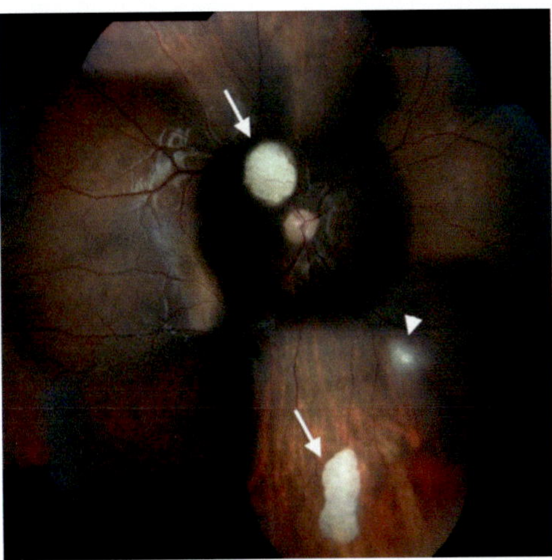

Fig. 61.7 12-year-old patient with the diagnosis of tuberous sclerosis presented with multiple white retinal lesions corresponding to retinal astrocytoma. The classical mulberry pattern is seen in the larger, more peripherally located two retinal lesions (arrows) while inferonasally the tumor is more translucent, less calcified and has more indistinct borders (arrowhead)

In general, retinal astrocytic hamartoma is a white-yellow retinal mass, which can be multilobulated in mulberry shape in larger tumors. The feeder vessels, if present, are not as prominent as those expected in retinoblastoma. Upon FFA, retinal astrocytic hamartomas may display a fine capillary intrinsic network in the early venous phase which is superseded by a prominent late staining in the late venous phase whereas retinoblastoma is generally expected to display a rapid filling [33]. In cases where the fine capillary network cannot be displayed, FFA characteristics such as blockage of fluorescence in the early phases and late staining in an area larger than the clinically visible lesion, which are both not exclusive to retinal astrocytic hamartoma, would be generally expected [34].

In optical coherence tomography (OCT) imaging, retinal astrocytic hamartomas lie in a spectrum from a translucent, flat lesion confined in the nerve fiber layer to a more elevated tumor extending to full thickness in the retina. Mild to moderate retinal traction can be shown in some cases. There are several proposals of classification based on OCT appearances of retinal astrocytic hamartoma and among those Pichi et al. [35] defines 4 morphological types of the tumor based on spectral-domain OCT as: type 1 (translucent, flat tumor), type 2 (tumor with slight retinal elevation and evidence of retinal traction), type 3 (tumor with 'moth-eaten' appearance of optically void areas corresponding to intrinsic calcification) and type 4 (tumor with intralesional degenerative cavities). Additionally, vitreous changes and vitreous seeding are also reported as common OCT findings in retinal astrocytic hamartoma [36].

Retinal astrocytic hamartoma can be managed with clinical observation as the lesion rarely grows. If there is evidence of exudative retinal detachment or neovascular glaucoma, palliative measures targeting the secondary intraocular changes should be taken. Watching for tumor growth should be warranted if the diagnosis is uncertain.

Medulloepithelioma

Medulloepithelioma is a congenital tumor arising from non-pigmented ciliary epithelium. Because of its origin, it is in most part anteriorly located rather than in posterior fundus. It is a tumor of childhood and it is seen unilaterally in most of the cases. Clinical presentation is usually with leukocoria, pain, raised intraocular pressure, reduced vision or angle-closure depending on the location of the tumor. Clinically the tumor is a vascularised, grey-salmon mass which can contain cystic components which can later become free-floating in the aqueous humor or the vitreous. In MRI, the tumor tissue is denser and appears less vascular, and calcifications, if present, appear larger than in retinoblastoma [37]. Although the tumor is slowly-growing, there is a malignant potential in almost half of the cases which can be revealed by presence of undifferentiated neuroblastic cells in histopathology [38]. Overall survival is chiefly dependent on the presence of extraocular extension or lack thereof.

Ocular Toxocariasis

Ocular toxocariasis is a parasitic infestation with roundworm *Toxocara canis*. The definitive hosts are dogs and cats and humans may become affected after ingestion of soil contaminated with the ova. The presentation is mostly unilateral and includes leukocoria, strabismus, floaters and reduced vision. The form of inflammatory reaction to the larva may either occur as a granuloma or secondary endophytic inflammatory response (Fig. 61.8). The granuloma which shows contrast enhancement in MRI may be located in the posterior pole or in the periphery. Intraocular inflammation may be seen in the form of endophthalmitis causing severe retinal traction, which is the key feature in differentiating from retinoblastoma. The size and the extent of traction in most of the toxocariasis cases is more aggravated than that expected in untreated retinoblastoma. The mainstay of treatment is ocular and systemic corticosteroids to effectively suppress inflammation.

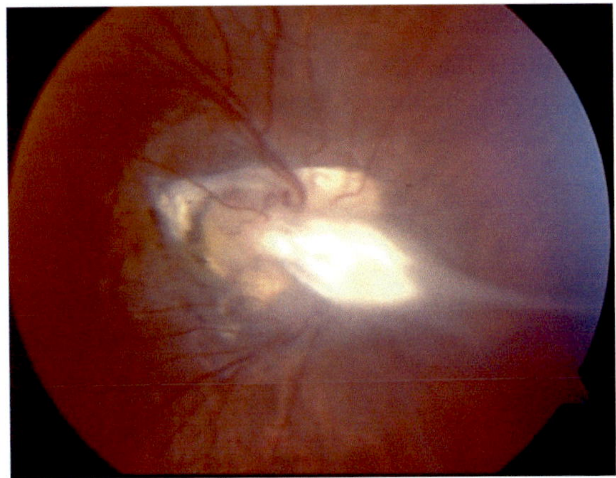

Fig. 61.8 Right eye of an 8-year-old boy with ocular toxocariasis exhibiting a falciform retinal fold extending to the right optic disc

Review Question

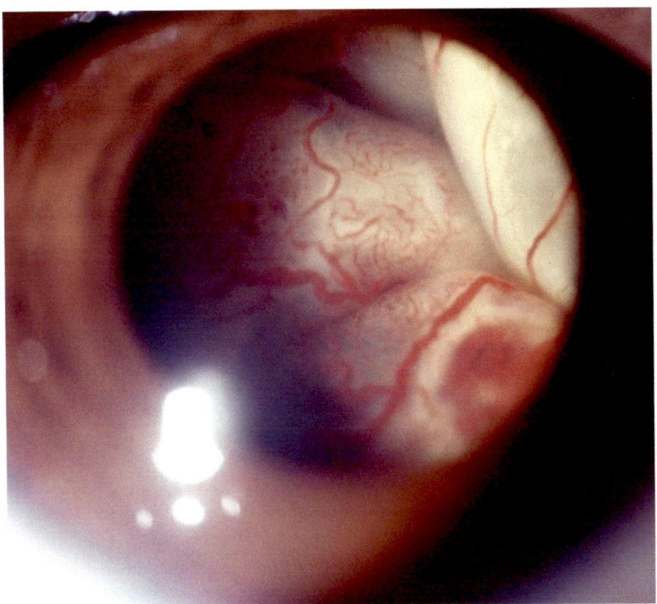

1. This 18-month-old male baby was consulted for exotropia and "color change" in the right eye, first noted by the parents 3 months earlier. The fellow eye was within normal limits. Based on the clinical photograph of his right eye, which diagnosis is most likely?

A. Congenital cataract
B. Uveal coloboma
C. Coats' disease
D. Retinoblastoma
E. Retinal astrocytic hamartoma

Answer

1. (**C**) There are typical features that would favor Coats' disease including yellow exudation, clear vitreous without any evidence of seeding, and most impostantly irregularly dilated retinal vessels on the totally detached retina.

References

1. Dimaras H, Corson TW. Retinoblastoma, the visible CNS tumor: a review. J Neurosci Res. 2019;97:29–44.
2. Kim JW, Singh AD. Differential diagnosis of leukocoria. In: Singh AD, Murphree AL, Damato BE, editors. Clinical ophthalmic oncology: retinoblastoma. Berlin Heidelberg: Springer-Verlag; 2015. p. 13–27.
3. Vahedi A, Lumbroso-Le Rouic C, Levy Gabriel C, et al. Diagnotic différentiel du rétinoblastome: étude rétrospective de 486 cas. J Fr Ophtalmol. 2008;31:165–72.
4. Shields CL, Schoenberg E, Kocher K, et al. Lesions simulating retinoblastoma (pseudoretinoblastoma) in 604 cases. Results based on age at presentation. Ophthalmology 2013;120: 311–6.
5. Maki JL, Marr BP, Abramson DH. Diagnosis of retinoblastoma: how good are referring physicians? Ophthalmic Genet. 2009;30:199–205.
6. Yang X, Wang C, Su G. Recent advances in the diagnosis and treatment of Coats' disease. Int Ophthalmol. 2019;39:957–70.
7. Sen M, Shields CL, Honavar SG, Shields JA. Coats' disease: an overview of classification, management and outcomes. Indian J Ophthalmol. 2019;67:763–71.
8. Shields CL, Udyaver S, Dalvin LA, et al. Coats disease in 351 eyes: analysis of features and outcomes over 45 years (by decade) at a single center. Indian J Ophthalmol. 2019;67:772–83.
9. Rabiolo A, Marchese A, Sacconi R, et al. Refining Coats' disease by ultra-wide field imaging and optical coherence tomography angiography. Graefes Arch Clin Exp Ophthalmol. 2017;255:1881–90.
10. Ong SS, Cummings TJ, Vazjovic L, et al. Comparison of optical coherence tomography with fundus photographs, fluorescein angiography and histopathological analysis in assessing Coats' disease. JAMA Ophthalmol. 2019;137:176–83.
11. Jansen RW, de Bloeme CM, Brisse HJ, et al. MR imaging features to differentiate retinoblastoma from Coats' disease and persistent fetal vasculature. Cancers. 2020;2 (12):3592. https://doi.org/10.3390/cancers12123592.
12. Liu J-H, Deng G, Ma J, et al. Clinical characteristics of pediatric Coats' disease with retinal cyst using wide-angle fluorescein angiography. Front Med. 2021;8: 709522. https://doi.org/10.3389/fmed.2021.709522.

13. Ramasubramanian A, Shields CL, Mellen PL, et al. Autofluorescence of treated retinoblastoma JAAPOS. 2011;15:167–72.
14. Goel S, Saurabh K, Roy R. Blue light fundus autofluorescence in Coats' disease. Retina. 2019;39:e34–5.
15. Chen C, Xiao H, Ding X. Persistent fetal vasculature. Asia Pac J Ophthalmol. 2019;8:86–95.
16. Prakhunhungsit S, Berrocal AM. Diagnostic and management strategies in patients with persistent fetal vasculature: current insights. Clin Ophthalmol. 2020;14:4325–35.
17. Thomas DM, Kannabiran C, Balasubramanian D. Identification of key genes and pathways in persistent hyperplastic primary vitreous of the eye using bioinformatic analysis. Front Med 2021;8:690594. https://doi.org/10.3389/fmed.2021.690594. eCollection 2021.
18. Maqsood H, Younus S, Fatima M, et al. Bilateral persistant hyperplastic primary vitreous: a case report and review of the literature. Cureus. 2021;13(2): e13105. https://doi.org/10.7759/cureus.13105.
19. Laura DM, Staropoli PC, Patel NA, et al. Widefield fluorescein angiography in the fellow eyes of patients with presumed persistent fetal vasculature. Ophthalmol Retina. 2021;5:301–7.
20. Hu A, Pei X, Ding X, et al. Combined persistent fetal vasculature. Classification based on a high-resolution B-mode ultrasound and color doppler imaging. Ophthalmology 2016;123: 19–25.
21. Chiaroni PM, Chapron T, Purcell Y, et al. Diagnostic accuracy of quantitative color doppler flow imaging in distinguishing persistent fetal vasculature from retinal detachment. Acta Ophthalmol Scand 2021. https://doi.org/10.1111/aos.14793.
22. Tauqeer Z, Yonekawa Y. Familial exudative vitreoretinopathy: pathophysiology, diagnosis, and management. Asia Pac J Ophthalmol (Phila). 2018;7(3):176–82. Epub 2018/04/11. https://doi.org/10.22608/APO.201855. PubMed PMID: 29633588.
23. Tao T, Xu N, Li J, Li H, Qu J, Yin H, et al. Ocular features and mutation spectrum of patients with familial exudative vitreoretinopathy. Invest Ophthalmol Vis Sci. 2021;62(15):4. Epub 2021/12/04. https://doi.org/10.1167/iovs.62.15.4. PubMed PMID: 34860240; PubMed Central PMCID: PMCPMC8648064.
24. Wojcik EJ, Buckley RS, Richard J, Liu L, Huckaba TM, Kim S. Kinesin-5: cross-bridging mechanism to targeted clinical therapy. Gene. 2013;531(2):133–49. Epub 2013/08/21. https://doi.org/10.1016/j.gene.2013.08.004. PubMed PMID: 23954229; PubMed Central PMCID: PMCPMC3801170.
25. ZNF408 GIBNLoMU, National Center for Biotechnology Information; 2004 – [cited 2022 01 01]. https://www.ncbi.nlm.nih.gov/gene/79797#reference-sequences.
26. Gilmour DF. Familial exudative vitreoretinopathy and related retinopathies. Eye (Lond). 2015;29(1):1–14. Epub 2014/10/18. https://doi.org/10.1038/eye.2014.70. PubMed PMID: 25323851; PubMed Central PMCID: PMCPMC4289842.
27. Pendergast SD, Trese MT. Familial exudative vitreoretinopathy. Results of surgical management. Ophthalmology. 1998;105(6):1015–23. Epub 1998/06/17. https://doi.org/10.1016/S0161-6420(98)96002-X. PubMed PMID: 9627651.
28. Canny CL, Oliver GL. Fluorescein angiographic findings in familial exudative vitreoretinopathy. Arch Ophthalmol. 1976;94(7):1114–20. Epub 1976/07/01. https://doi.org/10.1001/archopht.1976.03910040034006. PubMed PMID: 947162.
29. Miyakubo H, Hashimoto K, Miyakubo S. Retinal vascular pattern in familial exudative vitreoretinopathy. Ophthalmology. 1984;91(12):1524–30. Epub 1984/12/01. https://doi.org/10.1016/s0161-6420(84)34119-7. PubMed PMID: 6084219.
30. Kashani AH, Brown KT, Chang E, Drenser KA, Capone A, Trese MT. Diversity of retinal vascular anomalies in patients with familial exudative vitreoretinopathy. Ophthalmology. 2014;121(11):2220–7. Epub 2014/07/10. https://doi.org/10.1016/j.ophtha.2014.05.029. PubMed PMID: 25005911.
31. Shields JA, Shields CL, Parsons HM. Differential diagnosis of retinoblastoma. Retina. 1991;11(2):232–43 Epub 1991/01/01 PubMed PMID: 1925090.

32. Ulbright TM, Fulling KH, Helveston EM. Astrocytic tumors of the retina. Differentiation of sporadic tumors from phakomatosis-associated tumors. Arch Pathol Lab Med. 1984;108 (2):160–3. Epub 1984/02/01. PubMed PMID: 6421263.
33. Margo CE, Barletta JP, Staman JA. Giant cell astrocytoma of the retina in tuberous sclerosis. Retina. 1993;13(2):155–9. Epub 1993/01/01. https://doi.org/10.1097/00006982-199313020-00013. PubMed PMID: 8337500.
34. Mennel S, Meyer CH, Eggarter F, Peter S. Autofluorescence and angiographic findings of retinal astrocytic hamartomas in tuberous sclerosis. Ophthalmologica. 2005;219(6):350–6. Epub 2005/11/16. https://doi.org/10.1159/000088377. PubMed PMID: 16286794.
35. Pichi F, Massaro D, Serafino M, Carrai P, Giuliari GP, Shields CL, et al. Retinal astrocytic hamartoma: optical coherence tomography classification and correlation with tuberous sclerosis complex. Retina. 2016;36(6):1199–208. Epub 2015/12/01. https://doi.org/10.1097/IAE.0000000000000829. PubMed PMID: 26618803.
36. Kato A, Obana A, Gohto Y, Seto T, Sasano H. Optic coherence tomography appearances of retinal astrocytic hamartoma and systemic features in tuberous sclerosis of Japanese patients. Eur J Ophthalmol. 2019;29(3):330–7. Epub 2018/07/12. https://doi.org/10.1177/1120672118787441. PubMed PMID: 29991284.
37. Apushkin MA, Apushkin MA, Shapiro MJ, Mafee MF. Retinoblastoma and simulating lesions: role of imaging. Neuroimaging Clin N Am. 2005;15(1):49–67. Epub 2005/06/02. https://doi.org/10.1016/j.nic.2005.02.003. PubMed PMID: 15927860.
38. Saunders T, Margo CE. Intraocular medulloepithelioma. Arch Pathol Lab Med. 2012;136 (2):212–6. Epub 2012/02/01. https://doi.org/10.5858/arpa.2010-0669-RS. PubMed PMID: 22288972.

Treatment Modalities and Enucleation

62

Linnet Rodriguez, Maura Di Nicola, Jared J. Ebert,
and Basil K. Williams

Abstract

Retinoblastoma is the most common pediatric primary intraocular malignancy. The current available treatments include focal treatment (cryotherapy and transpupillary thermotherapy), chemotherapy (intravenous, intra-arterial, intravitreal, and intracameral), radiation (plaque and external beam), and enucleation. The International Classification of Retinoblastoma was developed to identify outcomes and response to treatment by grouping tumors into categories based on tumor size, location, exudative retinal detachment, associated subretinal and/or vitreous seeding, and other signs of advanced disease. Additionally, laterality, extent of disease, presence of a germline mutation, parental and physician preference and availability of treatment options also play a role in treatment choice. While treatment options have evolved, the main goal remains to save the patient's life first, and then to salvage the globe and maximize vision when possible.

Keywords

Cryotherapy · Enucleation · External beam radiotherapy · International Classification of Intraocular Retinoblastoma · Intra-arterial chemotherapy · Intravitreal chemotherapy · Plaque brachytherapy · Retinoblastoma · Systemic chemotherapy · Transpupillary thermotherapy

L. Rodriguez (✉)
Virginia Commonwealth University, Richmond, VA, USA
e-mail: Linnet.Rodriguez@vcuhealth.org

M. Di Nicola · J. J. Ebert · B. K. Williams
Department of Ophthalmology, University of Cincinnati College of Medicine, Cincinnati, OH, USA

© The Author(s), under exclusive license to Springer Nature Switzerland AG 2023
Ş. Özdek et al. (eds.), *Pediatric Vitreoretinal Surgery*,
https://doi.org/10.1007/978-3-031-14506-3_62

925

Introduction

Retinoblastoma is the most common pediatric primary intraocular malignancy. While treatment protocols for retinoblastoma primarily depend on disease classification (Table 62.1), additional factors including disease laterality, presence of germline mutations, available institutional resources, treating physician preferences, as well as family, social, and economic factors contribute to treatment paradigms [1]. Ongoing efforts to maintain or improve efficacy while minimizing side effects have broadened treatment alternatives with the ultimate goal of providing individualized and targeted treatment to preserve life, preserve the globe and maximize visual potential.

Historically, enucleation was the most common primary treatment for retinoblastoma until external beam radiotherapy (EBRT) was introduced as a globe-sparing option. The increased risk of secondary malignancies and facial deformities resulting from EBRT sparked the need for additional therapies for globe salvage, which have been implemented over the last three decades. Intravenous chemotherapy (IVC) was introduced in the 1990s, resulted in good tumor control when used with local therapy causing it to replace EBRT as first line globe-sparing treatment despite some systemic side effects. More recently, intra-arterial chemotherapy (IAC) was introduced to provide a higher concentration of chemotherapy in the eye and to limit systemic side effects. Currently, a wide arsenal of treatment options exists for management of retinoblastoma including IVC, IAC, intravitreal chemotherapy (IvitC), intracameral chemotherapy, cryotherapy, transpupillary thermotherapy (TTT), plaque radiotherapy, external beam radiotherapy (EBRT), and enucleation [1, 2].

A thorough history, complete ophthalmic examination most commonly performed under anesthesia, and magnetic resonance imaging (MRI) of the brain and orbits are all critically important in staging disease and guiding therapeutic decisions.

Treatment Modalities

Focal Treatment Modalities

Transpupillary Thermotherapy

TTT is a focal treatment option commonly used as primary treatment of Group A tumors and Group B tumors sparing the macula and/or papilla [3]. TTT can also be used as adjunctive treatment with IVC or IAC. TTT was first used for the treatment of retinoblastoma in 1982 with a 2450 MHz microwave applicator, and it is now performed using an 810-nm diode laser with an indirect ophthalmoscope or operating room microscope [3, 4]. Spot size and power settings can be adjusted and these parameters vary by center [5]. Treatment is performed with continuous laser

Table 62.1 International classification of retinoblastoma

Group	International Classification of Retinoblastoma (Philadelphia)[a]	International Classification of Retinoblastoma (Children's Hospital of Los Angeles)[b]
Group A	Retinoblastoma ≤ 3 mm in basal diameter or thickness	All tumors are 3 mm or smaller, confined to the retina and at least 3 mm from the foveola and 1.5 mm from the optic nerve. No vitreous or subretinal seeding is allowed
Group B	Retinoblastoma >3 mm in basal diameter or thickness or • tumor location ≤ 3 mm from foveola • tumor location ≤ 1.5 mm from optic disc • tumor-associated subretinal fluid ≤ 3 mm from tumor margin	Eyes with no vitreous or subretinal seeding and discrete retinal tumor of any size or location. Retinal tumors may be of any size or location not in group A. Small cuff of subretinal fluid extending ≤ 5 mm from the base of the tumor is allowed
Group C	Retinoblastoma with: • subretinal seeds ≤ 3 mm from the tumor • vitreous seeds ≤ 3 mm from tumor • both subretinal and vitreous seeds ≤ 3 mm from tumor	Eyes with focal vitreous or subretinal seeding and discrete retinal tumors of any size and location. Any seeding must be local, fine, and limited so as to be theoretically treatable with a radioactive plaque. Up to one quadrant of subretinal fluid may be present
Group D	Retinoblastoma with: • subretinal seeds >3 mm from tumor • vitreous seeds >3 mm from tumor • both subretinal and vitreous seeds >3 mm from tumor	Eyes with diffuse vitreous or subretinal seeding and/or massive, nondiscrete endophytic or exophytic disease. Eyes with more extensive seeding than Group C. Massive and/or diffuse intraocular disseminated disease may consist of 'greasy' vitreous seeding or avascular masses. Subretinal seeding may be plaque-like, includes exophytic disease and >1 quadrant of retinal detachment
Group E	Retinoblastoma occupying >50% of the globe or • neovascular glaucoma • opaque media from hemorrhage in subretinal space, vitreous, or anterior chamber • invasion of postlaminar optic nerve, choroid (>2 mm), sclera, orbit, anterior chamber	Eyes that have been destroyed anatomically or functionally with one or more of the following: Irreversible neovascular glaucoma, massive intraocular hemorrhage, aseptic orbital cellulitis, tumor anterior to anterior vitreous face, tumor touching the lens, diffuse infiltrating retinoblastoma, phthisis or pre-phthisis

[a] *Adopted from Shields CL, Mashayekhi A, Au AK, Czyz C, Leahey A, Meadows AT, Shields JA. The International Classification of Retinoblastoma predicts chemoreduction success. Ophthalmology. 2006 Dec;113(12):2276–80*
[b] Adopted from: Linn Murphree A. Intraocular retinoblastoma: the case for a new group classification. Ophthalmol Clin North Am. 2005 Mar;18(1):41–53, viii

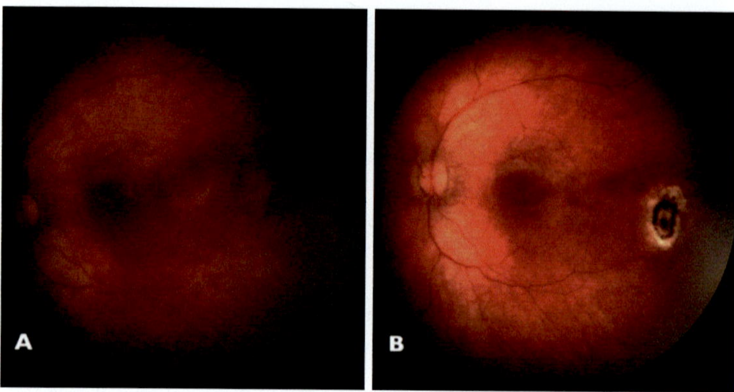

Fig. 62.1 A 9-month old female with Group A retinoblastoma in the left eye (**A**) was treated with 3 sessions of transpupillary thermotherapy, the last 2 of which were enhanced by indocyanine green. The lesion regressed to a flat scar (**B**)

to cause graying/whitening to the entirety of the lesion being treated. In general, tumors located posterior to the equator can be easily treated with TTT.

TTT has been found to be an effective primary treatment for smaller tumors [5]. Male gender, increasing age at diagnosis, and tumors with larger basal dimensions requiring more energy for treatment have been associated with a higher risk of local recurrence [5].

Indocyanine green (ICG)-enhanced TTT can be used for cases resistant to traditional TTT, including larger sized tumors by basal diameter or thickness and well-differentiated tumors [6]. ICG-enhanced TTT can help achieve significant tumor regression without additional ocular side effects [6].

Complications of TTT include focal cataract, iris atrophy, and retinal hemorrhages [7]. More rare complications include retinal vein occlusions, vitreoretinal traction, and retinal detachments [1] (Fig. 62.1).

Cryotherapy

Similar to TTT, cryotherapy is often used for primary treatment of Group A and non-macula/papilla involving Group B tumors and can also be performed as adjuvant therapy with IAC or IVC. Cryotherapy is performed using a triple freeze–thaw cycle technique until the entirety of tumor and margins of adjacent retina have been treated under direct visualization using indirect ophthalmoscopy [8]. In general, tumors located anterior to the equator are easier to reach with cryotherapy as opposed to laser therapy. Cryotherapy has a low rate of complications including intraocular inflammation and more rarely vitreous hemorrhage, exudative retinal detachment, and rhegmatogenous retinal detachment [1, 8].

Chemotherapy

Intravenous Chemotherapy (IVC)

While previously used in the second half of the twentieth century for extraocular or metastatic disease, intravenous chemotherapy was introduced in the 1990s as the mainstay of primary retinoblastoma treatment for chemoreduction with adjuvant focal treatment [9]. Intravenous chemotherapy is frequently used for the treatment of unilateral or bilateral disease, bridge therapy for patients <3 months old and/or weighing <5 kg, and in centers without access to IAC [1, 3, 9]. Additionally, it is commonly used as adjuvant treatment following enucleation when high-risk pathologic risk features are noted including residual tumor at the optic nerve margin or sclera, massive choroidal invasion, post-laminar optic nerve invasion [3].

Intravenous chemotherapy is typically administered monthly using a 6-cycle protocol that includes vincristine, etoposide and carboplatin. [10] Treatment coincides with examinations under anesthesia, where concurrent focal therapy is often performed, which has been shown to significantly increase the rates of local control and globe salvage [11, 12] (Fig. 62.2). Systemic side effects of IVC include neutropenia, neutropenic fever, alopecia, opportunistic infections, ototoxicity, neuropathy, and secondary malignancies [1, 9, 10, 13].

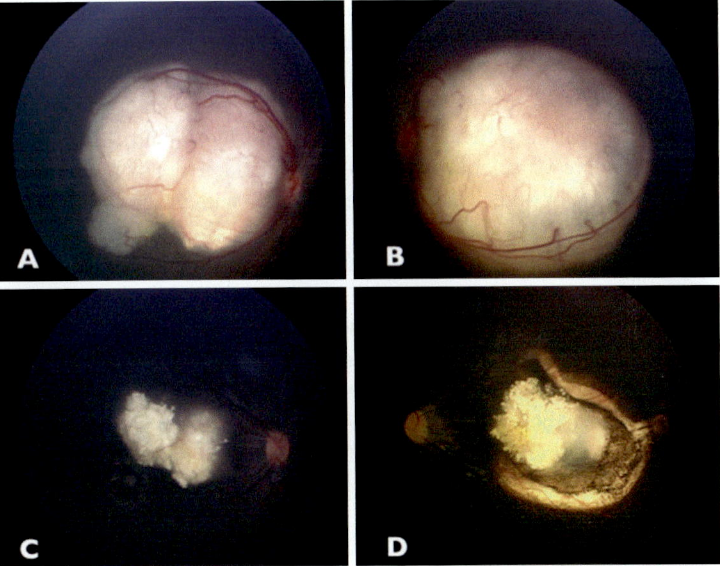

Fig. 62.2 A 16-month old male without a family history presented with bilateral multifocal retinoblastoma (**A**, **B**). He underwent 6 sessions of systemic chemotherapy with vincristine, etoposide, and carboplatin combined with focal transpupillary thermotherapy, and achieved complete regression (**C**, **D**)

Intra-Arterial Chemotherapy (IAC)

Pioneered in the 1990s in Japan, intra-arterial chemotherapy is now a mainstay for treatment of retinoblastoma in developed countries, especially in cases of unilateral disease [9] (Fig. 62.3). Current indications for IAC include primary treatment of patients with unilateral group B (with macular involvement), C, or D disease [9]. IAC is also used as secondary globe-salvage therapy for recurrent or persistent disease after previous IAC or failure of other treatment modalities [14]. In the case of bilateral disease, some centers use perform simultaneous bilateral IAC whereas other centers prefer the use of IVC [3, 14].

IAC is performed using selective microcatheterization of the ophthalmic artery via a fluoroscopy-guided femoral artery approach by an experienced neurosurgeon or interventional neuroradiologist to deliver high doses of chemotherapy to the eye with reduced systemic toxicity [9]. Since its introduction, the rate of technical success has been reported to be as high as 97% [15]. Multiple chemotherapy regimens for IAC exist ranging from single agent melphalan to combinations of 2 or 3-drugs, most commonly including melphalan, topotecan, and carboplatin [16]. Cycles of IAC are repeated every 3–4 weeks for 3–6 cycles depending on tumor response [1, 14].

Use of IAC is limited by vascular access, institutional resources and experience. Most neurosurgeons or interventional neuroradiologists wait until at least 3 months of age and a weight of >5 kg to allow for vasculature maturation amendable to IAC [9]. For patient's diagnosed prior to 3 months of age that are candidates for IAC, bridge therapy with IVC can be initiated until IAC can be safely performed. IAC is commonly used for unilateral group B, C, and D disease in the United States, but it is less widely available in lower-income countries. Contraindications to primary IAC include eyes with significant disease requiring more than local therapy (evidence of optic nerve or scleral extension, extraocular extension, central nervous system involvement, or other systemic disease), eyes with group E disease and poor tumor visualization [1, 14].

Transient complications of IAC include periocular and forehead hyperemia, eyelid edema and ptosis [14]. More severe ocular complications include ophthalmic and retinal artery occlusion, vitreous hemorrhage, and retinal detachments, which can all have visually devastating consequences [1, 17]. The incidence of ophthalmic vascular complications following IAC has decrease over time, presumably secondary to increased experience performing the procedure [18]. The most commonly reported systemic side effect following intra-arterial melphalan is neutropenia, and additional systemic side effects include bronchospasm and autonomic reactions [9, 14].

Intravitreal Chemotherapy (IVitC)

Following the introduction of IVC and IAC for treatment of retinoblastoma, rates of ocular survival have dramatically improved over the last three decades. However, persistent vitreous seeding is a common cause of treatment failure given the lack of blood supply to the vitreous limiting the penetration of chemotherapy [19]. The presence of vitreous seeding was associated with an increased risk of recurrence

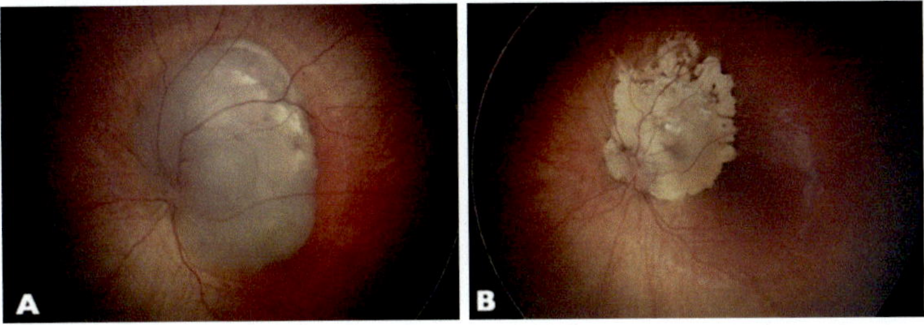

Fig. 62.3 A 10-month old female with a sporadic retinoblastoma mutation was diagnosed with Group C disease in the left eye (**A**). She underwent 3 cycles of intra-arterial chemotherapy resulting in complete regression of her disease

prior to the availability of intravitreal chemotherapy, but since its introduction, rates of progression-free survival and recurrence-free survival have increased [20]. Intravitreal chemotherapy is not used as solo therapy alone and is most commonly used as adjuvant treatment with IAC and/or IVC for control of vitreous seeding [1]. However, recent studies have suggested that it may be a helpful adjunct for persistent subretinal seeding or recurrent retinal disease also [21].

Intravitreal injection of chemotherapy for retinoblastoma was not widely adopted secondary to concerns of possible tumor dissemination through the needle tract [22], until 2012 when a modified "anti-reflux" technique for intravitreal injection in patients with retinoblastoma was introduced [23]. The technique consists of using a small gauge needle for an anterior chamber paracentesis, followed by the intravitreal chemotherapy injection. At the time of needle withdrawal, cryotherapy is performed at the injection site using a triple freeze–thaw technique. The eye is shaken using forceps to distribute the chemotherapeutic throughout the vitreous cavity [23]. Several large series have reported no injection-related extraocular spread, confirming the safety of this procedure [23, 24]. Intravitreal chemotherapy is most commonly performed using melphalan and/or topotecan and repeated at intervals ranging from one week to one month until the vitreous seeding resolves [1, 25, 26].

Complications arising from intravitreal chemotherapy include focal cataract, hypotony, vitreous hemorrhage, subretinal hemorrhage, pigmentary retinopathy, anterior segment toxicity, optic neuropathy, and retinal toxicity [1, 19, 26, 27].

Intracameral Chemotherapy

Anterior chamber seeding has traditionally been regarded as an indication for enucleation. More recently, intracameral chemotherapy has been used to control anterior chamber seeding in patients with group E disease to attempt globe-salvage [28]. Intracameral injection involves aqueous suppression by intravenous administration of acetazolamide, complete aspiration of the aqueous humor from both the anterior and posterior chamber, syringe exchange and injection of 1/3 volume of melphalan into the anterior chamber, perforation of the iris at a tumor free margin (as previously determined by ultrasound biomicroscopy), and transiridal injection of the remaining 2/3 volume of melphalan into the posterior chamber. Triple freeze–thaw cryotherapy is then performed at the entry site [28].

The experience with intracameral melphalan has been reported in small series of patients with anterior chamber seeding whose parents refused enucleation [29]. Initial aqueous seed regression has been observed in some cases, but enucleation is still required for persistent or recurrent disease [29].

Complications with this technique include cataract formation and heterochromia [29]. As with all invasive treatment modalities for retinoblastoma, the risk of extraocular spread must be weighed against the visual potential of the treated eye, the ability to control intraocular disease, and the status of the contralateral eye.

Radiotherapy

Plaque Brachytherapy

Plaque brachytherapy may be used for primary treatment of group A and B tumors (Fig. 62.1), or as secondary treatment of persistent or recurrent retinal disease [1, 30]. Iodine-125 is the most common isotope currently used in the United States, but Ruthenium-106 is also used (Fig. 62.4). Plaque brachytherapy is performed using a radiation dose of 3500–4000 cGy to the tumor apex with treatment extending to a 2 mm safety margin beyond the margins of the tumor [31]. Plaque brachytherapy has also been described for diffuse anterior chamber involvement of retinoblastoma [32].

Complications from plaque brachytherapy include plaque malposition, scleral perforation, extraocular muscle damage, diplopia, and radiation-induced side effects including cataract, neovascular glaucoma, retinopathy and maculopathy, vitreous hemorrhage, and optic neuropathy [1, 30, 33].

External Beam Radiotherapy

Prior to the introduction of IVC for chemoreduction, external beam radiotherapy was used throughout the twentieth century for globe salvage in patients with

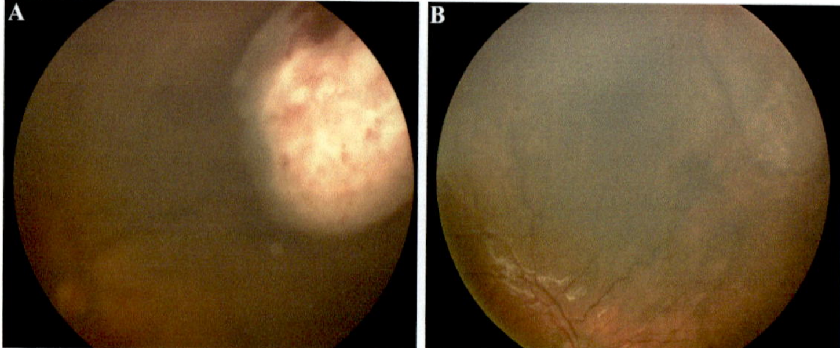

Fig. 62.4 Fundus photograph of a superonasal retinoblastoma lesion in the right eye (**A**) of a patient with bilateral retinoblastoma. After Ru-106 plaque radiotherapy the lesion regressed to a flat scar (**B**)

retinoblastoma [34]. With the introduction of IVC and IAC, EBRT is now very rarely used for globe-salvaging therapy in high-income countries, mainly because of the side effect profile. However, EBRT retains a role in the treatment of extraocular extension, orbital disease, or in patients with a positive optic nerve margin following enucleation [1, 3].

The most important complication of EBRT is the development of secondary malignancies, most commonly sarcomas in the field of radiation, in patients with a germline mutation [8, 34, 35]. Facial deformities following EBRT for retinoblastoma are also common [1]. Ocular side effects of EBRT include dry eye, radiation-induced cataract, radiation retinopathy and maculopathy, vitreous hemorrhage, glaucoma, retinal detachment, and optic neuropathy, among others [8, 34, 36].

Enucleation

Despite the advances in current treatments for retinoblastoma, enucleation remains a treatment option for eyes with group E and occasionally group D tumors with poor tumor visualization, buphthalmos, pthisis bulbi, extraocular extension, neovascular glaucoma, anterior chamber seeding, and diffuse infiltrating retinoblastoma as well as for persistent or recurrent disease that has failed globe-salvaging management [1, 3].

The technique for enucleation for retinoblastoma is similar to the standard enucleation technique with a few exceptions. Special care must be taken to avoid globe perforation given the risk of extraocular extension, and the longest possible stump of the optic nerve should be obtained [8]. If histopathology demonstrates high-risk disease, postlaminar optic nerve involvement, residual disease at the cut end of the optic nerve, extraocular extension, massive choroidal invasion, and scleral invasion, most centers will recommend systemic chemotherapy [3] (Fig. 62.5).

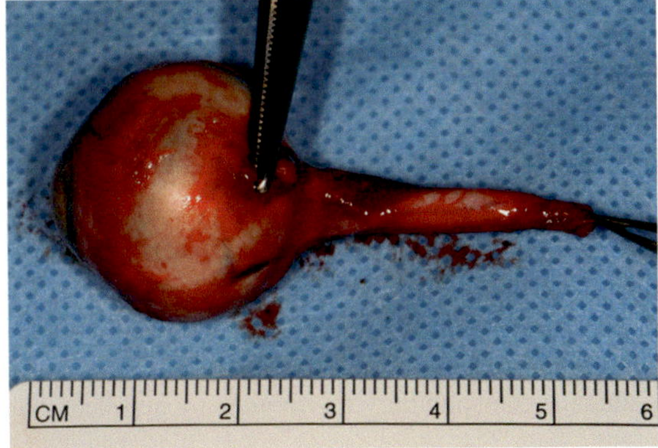

Fig. 62.5 Enucleated globe in a child with advanced unilateral retinoblastoma demonstrating a long stump of the optic nerve to reduce the risk of leaving residual disease at the cut margin

Conclusion

Treatment of retinoblastoma has become more sophisticated and targeted in the last few decades. The introduction of IAC and has allowed for delivery of high doses of chemotherapeutic agents directly to the eye, reducing the systemic side effects of chemotherapy, and IVitC has improved the prognosis of patients with vitreous involvement. Traditional treatment modalities remain vital options. Systemic chemotherapy is often still used as primary treatment for bilateral disease in many centers, and TTT and cryotherapy are employed as primary treatment for select group A and B eyes or adjuvant treatment in combination with IVC and IAC. Plaque brachytherapy is used for select group A or B eyes and in cases of small or medium-sized retinal tumor recurrence, and enucleation is employed for advanced cases. The goal for ocular oncologists treating retinoblastoma remains to save the patient's life first, and then to salvage the globe and maximize vision when possible. Future advancements in retinoblastoma care will allow for an even more personalized treatment of this disease.

Clinical Case Scenario

A 14-month old female presented with a diagnosis of presumed retinoblastoma. Two months prior to presentation, she was noted to have drifting of the right eye (OD) by her mother, who thought it was due to a lazy eye because of a paternal family history of strabismus. Over the 3 weeks prior, the mother also appreciated white reflex, which prompted an appointment with their pediatrician. The pediatrician confirmed the presence of leukocoria and strabismus and referred the patient with concern for retinoblastoma. The patient was born full-term by C-section without complications and had no other medical conditions or surgeries.

At presentation, the patient had leukocoria OD and a 30-prism diopter right exotropia by Hirschberg testing. She was able to fix and follow with binocular assessment. Examination under anesthesia revealed a normal external and anterior segment examination in both eyes. Fundus examination OD showed a prominent white exophytic retinal tumor involving the entire macula with a small second lesion noted at the inferior margin of the larger lesion (Fig. 62.6A). There was an associated exudative detachment inferiorly with subretinal seeds extending from the tumor margin to the inferior and nasal periphery. B-scan ultrasonography of the macular tumor demonstrated a large heterogenous mass with intrinsic calcifications and posterior shadowing (Fig. 62.6B). The left eye was normal.

The patient was diagnosed with unilateral Group D retinoblastoma OD. An MRI of the brain and orbits with and without contrast did not demonstrate any evidence of optic nerve or brain involvement. Genetic testing revealed a germline mutation. The patient was treated with three-drug intraarterial chemotherapy using 3 mg of Melphalan, 0.3 mg of Topotecan and 30 mg of Carboplatin. She underwent supplemental transpupillary thermotherapy and demonstrated an excellent response to

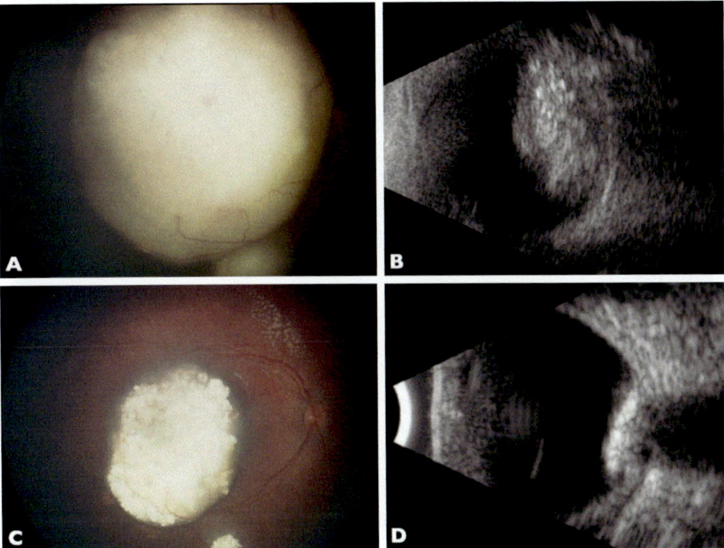

Fig. 62.6 A large macular retinoblastoma lesion abuts the optic nerve in the right eye and a smaller lesion is noted at the inferior margin (**A**). B-scan ultrasound shows the intralesional calcifications and posterior shadowing of the macular lesion (**B**). Excellent regression and near complete calcification of bot lesions is noted after treatment (**C**). Subretinal exudation is noted superior to the optic nerve highlighting the previous presence of an exudative retinal detachment. B-scan ultrasound shows significant regression of the macular lesion with prominent calcification and posterior shadowing (**D**)

treatment with complete clinical regression after 4 cycles administered 4 weeks apart (Fig. 62.6C, D). Two years after completion of therapy, the patient remained in remission with no evidence of tumor recurrence OD, and no tumor developed OS.

Review Questions

1. The following are treatment modalities for retinoblastoma EXCEPT:

a. Intra-arterial chemotherapy
b. Intravenous chemotherapy
c. Cryotherapy
d. Intravitreal aflibercept

2. Which of the following chemotherapeutic agents is not used for intravenous chemotherapy?

a. Vincristine
b. Carboplatin
c. Doxorubicin
d. Etoposide

3. Intra-arterial chemotherapy technique consists in delivering chemotherapy directly to the?

a. Internal carotid artery
b. Ophthalmic artery
c. Central retinal artery
d. Posterior communicating artery

Answers

1. (**D**) Intravitreal aflibercept is not directly used for treatment of retinoblastoma.
2. (**C**) Doxorubicin
3. (**B**) Ophthalmic artery

References

1. Ancona-Lezama D, Dalvin LA, Shields CL. Modern treatment of retinoblastoma: a 2020 review. Indian J Ophthalmol. 2020;68(11):2356–65.
2. Gudiseva HV, Berry JL, Polski A, Tummina SJ, O'Brien JM. Next-generation technologies and strategies for the management of Retinoblastoma. Genes (Basel). 2019;10(12).
3. Abramson DH, Shields CL, Munier FL, Chantada GL. Treatment of Retinoblastoma in 2015: agreement and disagreement. JAMA Ophthalmol. 2015;133(11):1341–7.
4. Lagendijk JJ. A microwave heating technique for the hyperthermic treatment of tumours in the eye, especially retinoblastoma. Phys Med Biol. 1982;27(11):1313–24.
5. Abramson DH, Schefler AC. Transpupillary thermotherapy as initial treatment for small intraocular retinoblastoma: technique and predictors of success. Ophthalmology. 2004;111 (5):984–91.
6. Francis JH, Abramson DH, Brodie SE, Marr BP. Indocyanine green enhanced transpupillary thermotherapy in combination with ophthalmic artery chemosurgery for retinoblastoma. Br J Ophthalmol. 2013;97(2):164–8.
7. Hasanreisoglu M, Saktanasate J, Schwendeman R, Shields JA, Shields CL. Indocyanine Green-Enhanced Transpupillary thermotherapy for Retinoblastoma: analysis of 42 Tumors. J Pediatr Ophthalmol Strabismus. 2015;52(6):348–54.
8. Shields JA, Augsburger JJ. Current approaches to the diagnosis and management of retinoblastoma. Surv Ophthalmol. 1981;25(6):347–72.
9. Munier FL, Beck-Popovic M, Chantada GL, et al. Conservative management of retinoblastoma: Challenging orthodoxy without compromising the state of metastatic grace. "Alive, with good vision and no comorbidity". Prog Retin Eye Res. 2019;73:100764.
10. Shields CL, Bas Z, Tadepalli S, et al. Long-term (20-year) real-world outcomes of intravenous chemotherapy (chemoreduction) for retinoblastoma in 964 eyes of 554 patients at a single centre. Br J Ophthalmol. 2020;104(11):1548–55.

11. Wilson MW, Rodriguez-Galindo C, Haik BG, Moshfeghi DM, Merchant TE, Pratt CB. Multiagent chemotherapy as neoadjuvant treatment for multifocal intraocular retinoblastoma. Ophthalmology. 2001;108(11):2106–2114; discussion 2114–2105.

12. Shields CL, Mashayekhi A, Cater J, Shelil A, Meadows AT, Shields JA. Chemoreduction for retinoblastoma. Analysis of tumor control and risks for recurrence in 457 tumors. Am J Ophthalmol. 2004;138(3):329–337.

13. Raval V, Bowen RC, Soto H, Singh A. Intravenous chemotherapy for Retinoblastoma in the Era of intravitreal chemotherapy: a systematic review. Ocul Oncol Pathol. 2021;7(2):142–8.

14. Manjandavida FP, Stathopoulos C, Zhang J, Honavar SG, Shields CL. Intra-arterial chemotherapy in retinoblastoma—a paradigm change. Indian J Ophthalmol. 2019;67(6): 740–54.

15. Yamane T, Kaneko A, Mohri M. The technique of ophthalmic arterial infusion therapy for patients with intraocular retinoblastoma. Int J Clin Oncol. 2004;9(2):69–73.

16. Chen M, Jiang H, Zhang J, et al. Outcome of intra-arterial chemotherapy for retinoblastoma and its influencing factors: a retrospective study. Acta Ophthalmol. 2017;95(6):613–8.

17. Wang L, Han M, Zhao J, et al. Intra-arterial chemotherapy for unilateral advanced intraocular retinoblastoma: Results and short-term complications. Medicine (Baltimore). 2018;97(42): e12676.

18. Dalvin LA, Ancona-Lezama D, Lucio-Alvarez JA, Masoomian B, Jabbour P, Shields CL. Ophthalmic vascular events after primary unilateral intra-arterial chemotherapy for retinoblastoma in early and recent eras. Ophthalmology. 2018;125(11):1803–11.

19. Francis JH, Schaiquevich P, Buitrago E, et al. Local and systemic toxicity of intravitreal melphalan for vitreous seeding in retinoblastoma: a preclinical and clinical study. Ophthalmology. 2014;121(9):1810–7.

20. Francis JH, Levin AM, Zabor EC, Gobin YP, Abramson DH. Ten-year experience with ophthalmic artery chemosurgery: ocular and recurrence-free survival. PLoS ONE. 2018;13(5): e0197081.

21. Abramson DH, Ji X, Francis JH, Catalanotti F, Brodie SE, Habib L. Intravitreal chemotherapy in retinoblastoma: expanded use beyond intravitreal seeds. Br J Ophthalmol. 2019;103 (4):488–93.

22. Kaneko A, Suzuki S. Eye-preservation treatment of retinoblastoma with vitreous seeding. Jpn J Clin Oncol. 2003;33(12):601–7.

23. Munier FL, Soliman S, Moulin AP, Gaillard MC, Balmer A, Beck-Popovic M. Profiling safety of intravitreal injections for retinoblastoma using an anti-reflux procedure and sterilisation of the needle track. Br J Ophthalmol. 2012;96(8):1084–7.

24. Francis JH, Abramson DH, Ji X, et al. Risk of extraocular extension in eyes with Retinoblastoma Receiving Intravitreous chemotherapy. JAMA Ophthalmol. 2017;135 (12):1426–9.

25. Munier FL, Gaillard MC, Balmer A, et al. Intravitreal chemotherapy for vitreous disease in retinoblastoma revisited: from prohibition to conditional indications. Br J Ophthalmol. 2012;96(8):1078–83.

26. Shields CL, Manjandavida FP, Arepalli S, Kaliki S, Lally SE, Shields JA. Intravitreal melphalan for persistent or recurrent retinoblastoma vitreous seeds: preliminary results. JAMA Ophthalmol. 2014;132(3):319–25.

27. Berry JL, Kim ME, Pefkianaki M, et al. Intravitreal Melphalan for Retinoblastoma: the impact of toxicity on recurrence and ultimate globe salvage. Ocul Oncol Pathol. 2020;6(6):388–94.

28. Munier FL, Gaillard MC, Decembrini S, Bongiovanni M, Beck-Popovic M. Intracameral Chemotherapy (Melphalan) for aqueous seeding in retinoblastoma: bicameral injection technique and related toxicity in a pilot case study. Ocul Oncol Pathol. 2017;3(2):149–55.

29. Munier FL, Moulin A, Gaillard MC, et al. Intracameral chemotherapy for globe salvage in retinoblastoma with secondary anterior chamber invasion. Ophthalmology. 2018;125(4): 615–7.

30. Shields CL, Shields JA, Cater J, Othmane I, Singh AD, Micaily B. Plaque radiotherapy for retinoblastoma: long-term tumor control and treatment complications in 208 tumors. Ophthalmology. 2001;108(11):2116–21.
31. Shields CL, Mashayekhi A, Sun H, et al. Iodine 125 plaque radiotherapy as salvage treatment for retinoblastoma recurrence after chemoreduction in 84 tumors. Ophthalmology. 2006;113 (11):2087–92.
32. Shields CL, Lally SE, Manjandavida FP, Leahey AM, Shields JA. Diffuse anterior retinoblastoma with globe salvage and visual preservation in 3 consecutive cases. Ophthalmology. 2016;123(2):378–84.
33. Sener EC, Kiratli H, Gedik S, Sanac AS. Ocular motility disturbances after episcleral plaque brachytherapy for uveal melanoma. J aapos. 2004;8(1):38–45.
34. Abramson DH, Jereb B, Ellsworth RM. External beam radiation for retinoblastoma. Bull N Y Acad Med. 1981;57(9):787–803.
35. Abramson DH, Frank CM. Second nonocular tumors in survivors of bilateral retinoblastoma: a possible age effect on radiation-related risk. Ophthalmology. 1998;105(4):573–579; discussion 579–580.
36. Pradhan DG, Sandridge AL, Mullaney P, et al. Radiation therapy for retinoblastoma: a retrospective review of 120 patients. Int J Radiat Oncol Biol Phys. 1997;39(1):3–13.

Part XI
Miscellaneous

Pediatric Choroidal Neovascularization

63

Ethan K. Sobol and G. Baker Hubbard

Abstract

Pediatric choroidal neovascularization is a rare but significant cause of vision loss in children. Pediatric CNV tends to differ from adult CNV in its epidemiology, etiology, and response to treatment. This chapter outlines the characteristics, causes, imaging features, and provides an overview of treatment strategies in this unique population.

Keywords

Choroidal neovascularization · Pediatrics · Anti-VEGF · Intravitreal injection · Inflammatory CNV · Best disease · Type 2 CNV · Traumatic CNV

Introduction

Choroidal neovascularization (CNV) is a significant cause of central vision loss in children and adolescents. However, unlike adult CNV, pediatric CNV differs in frequency of occurrence, underlying etiology, as well as response to treatment. In

E. K. Sobol · G. B. Hubbard (✉)
Emory Eye Center, Emory University School of Medicine, Atlanta, GA, USA
e-mail: Ghubba2@emory.edu

E. K. Sobol
e-mail: ethan.k.sobol@emory.edu

E. K. Sobol · G. B. Hubbard
Children's Hospital of Atlanta, 1365 Clifton Road, Clinic Building B, Atlanta, GA 30322, USA

© The Author(s), under exclusive license to Springer Nature Switzerland AG 2023
Ş. Özdek et al. (eds.), *Pediatric Vitreoretinal Surgery*,
https://doi.org/10.1007/978-3-031-14506-3_63

adults, the most common cause of CNV is age-related macular degeneration (AMD), while in younger patients, CNV is often secondary to acquired or inherited conditions, high myopia, trauma, or deemed idiopathic. This chapter reviews the common causes, characteristics, and management of CNV in the pediatric population.

Epidemiology

In the largest study to date on pediatric CNV, which retrospectively analyzed the records of 4,883,839 patients under 18 years of age in the IRIS registry over a 5-year study period, 2353 eyes of 1920 patients (0.04%) carried a diagnosis of CNV [1]. Many patients present with bilateral involvement, ranging from 13% [2] to 22% [1], although unilateral occurrence is far more common [2, 3]. No consensus exists regarding a gender predilection, as some studies note a majority of cases in males [2, 3], while others have reported a female predominance [4, 5]. Given that the CNV location is subfoveal in more than half of all cases [2, 3], presentation tends to be visually significant.

Etiology

Inflammatory CNV

While studies differ, post-inflammatory CNV has been reported as one of the most common causes of pediatric CNV. In the study by Rishi et al., 38% of all cases were due to a post-inflammatory etiology, with unclassified choroiditis being the most common (19%) within this group [3]. Studies by Kozak et al. and Ranjan et al. also observed a post-inflammatory etiology as the most common cause [2, 5]. This can perhaps be explained by inflammation leading to a breach in the RPE-Bruch's membrane complex, after which inflammatory mediators further potentiate the development of CNV [2].

CNV can occur in different stages of inflammatory activity, commonly appearing at the border of a pigmented chorioretinal scar [3, 6]. In one series, 40% of all eyes with inflammatory CNV had active inflammation at the time of diagnosis [7] compared with 70% in another study [6], highlighting the need for concurrent control of uveitic inflammation. Corticosteroids are the first line treatment for rapid control of non-infectious inflammation but are also known to suppress CNV growth and abnormal vascular permeability [6]. After initial control of inflammation, corticosteroid sparing immunosuppressive agents can be added to achieve long term suppression. These patients must have long-term follow up, as both the secondary CNV or the primary uveitic inflammation may recur.

Etiologies of Inflammatory CNV

Presumed Ocular Histoplasmosis Syndrome (POHS)

CNV may result from presumed ocular histoplasmosis syndrome (POHS). Although most reports indicate an onset of CNV related POHS in adulthood, a subset of CNVs in POHS develop in patients less than 20 years old, which commonly manifests at subfoveal and peripapillary locations [2, 8].

Toxoplasmosis

Toxoplasma chorioretinitis associated CNV can occur due to chorioretinal scarring or in the setting of active infection [2]. At a mean age of 10.6 years, toxoplasmosis accounted for 12% of all CNV cases in one series [3]. When active, the underlying infectious process should be treated, in addition to managing the secondary CNV [6].

Other Infectious or Inflammatory

Although rare, pediatric CNV has also been reported in tuberculosis, rubella retinopathy, sarcoidosis, toxocara canis, VKH, as well as other forms of chronic uveitis [2, 3, 6–8]. Certain etiologies such as tuberculosis-associated uveitis are far more common in endemic countries. This may explain the higher incidence of ocular tuberculosis, which accounted for 40% of inflammatory CNV cases in the cohort study in India by D'Souza et al. [7].

Optic Nerve Head Abnormalities

Although rare, optic nerve head drusen can result in CNV. This etiology accounted for 4% of cases in the study by Rishi and associates [3]. Even though the CNV is in the peripapillary area, it may still result in subfoveal extension [9]. CNV has also been reported in other abnormalities such as optic nerve coloboma, optic nerve pit, morning glory disc anomaly, chronic papilledema, and malignant hypertension [3, 8].

Post Traumatic

After choroidal rupture, secondary CNV may result in significant vision loss. Foveal proximity and longer rupture length are risk factors for CNV development [8]. In the study by Rishi et al., post traumatic cases accounted for 16% of all pediatric CNV, with a mean age of 11.4 years [3]. In these cases, 13 of 18 eyes had an identifiable choroidal rupture [3]. Patients should be regularly monitored after trauma, as CNV development may occur years after the initial injury (Fig. 63.1).

Retinal Dystrophies

A number of retinal dystrophies may lead to CNV, such as Best disease [10], Stargardt disease, North Carolina macular dystrophy [5], and choroideremia [8]. In the case series by Padhi et al., 33% of all CNV cases resulted from Best disease, which differs from other studies that found uveitis or inflammatory causes to be more common [4]. Rishi et al. observed CNV associated with Best disease in 12%

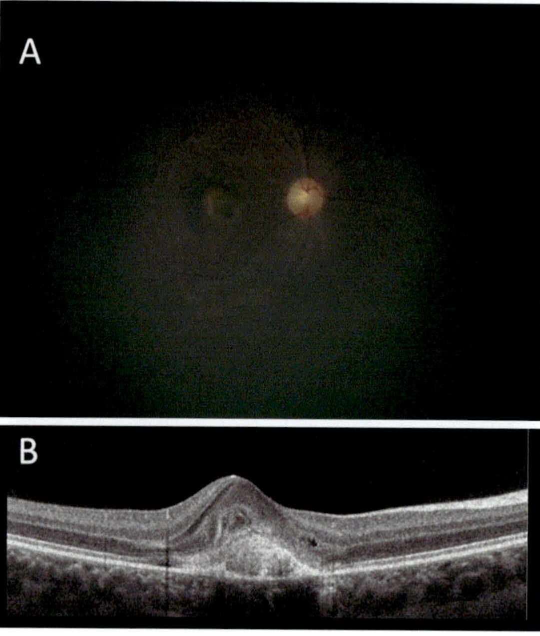

Fig. 63.1 Retcam fundus photograph (**A**) and OCT through the fovea (**B**) of the right eye in an 11-year-old girl who presented with 20/100 vision and CNV several years after blunt ocular trauma. Prior to presentation, vision had been 20/20. The patient was diagnosed with post-traumatic CNV and was given intravitreal bevacizumab. CNV remained inactive after one injection, although vision did not improve due to central macular scarring

of all cases, with a mean presenting age of 10.3 years. Nearly half of those reported were bilateral [3]. Other retinal dystrophies less frequently result in CNV [3]. CNV associated with retinal dystrophies tends to occur in younger patients when compared with uveitic or idiopathic CNV [5].

Myopia

In the series by Rishi et al., all cases of myopic CNV were unilateral [3]. In the recent study by Finn et al., myopic CNV was relatively common, accounting for 18% of all cases [1]. Myopic CNV tends to occur in a subfoveal location [11]. With the increasing prevalence of myopia worldwide, myopic CNV may have a more widespread impact on visual morbidity in years to come.

Choroidal Osteoma

Secondary CNV was found in approximately 2% of cases by two different case series [1, 3]. In one small study, CNV from choroidal osteoma made up 30% of pediatric CNV cases [12].

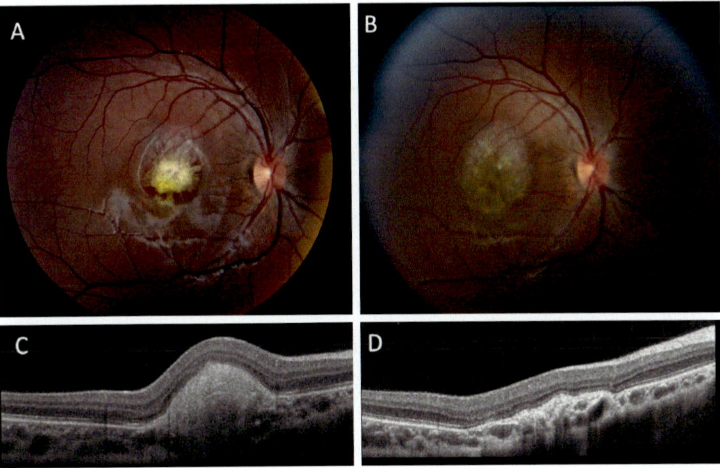

Fig. 63.2 An 11-year-old girl presented with 20/100 vision in the right eye and subretinal hemorrhage associated with idiopathic CNV (**A**). Over the course of a 6-year period, the patient underwent 8 intravitreal injections of bevacizumab, with 20/20 vision at final follow up. A residual chorioretinal scar is observed in the location of prior hemorrhage and CNV (**B**). OCT images are shown before (**C**) and after (**D**) treatment. The CNV remains inactive, and the patient continues to be followed with plans for additional intravitreal injections on an as-needed basis

Angioid Streaks

Angioid streaks, commonly observed in patients with pseudoxanthoma elasticum as well as other systemic conditions, may result in CNV due to a breach in Bruch's membrane [12].

Idiopathic

When no underlying cause can be identified, the CNV is deemed idiopathic. These cases tend to present in a unilateral fashion [8] (Fig. 63.2). Studies vary in the reported incidence, ranging from 11 to 38% [1, 3, 5, 13]. The variability in frequency of occurrence could be accounted for by inconsistencies in what is classified as "idiopathic," especially since many uveitic or post-inflammatory causes are in essence idiopathic without a known or identifiable underlying cause.

CNV Characteristics

CNV most commonly presents in a subfoveal location (in more than half of all cases), accounting for the visually significant nature of this condition [2, 4]. Peripapillary and extrafoveal lesion location are less common. Type 1 (sub-RPE) and type 2 (sub-retinal) CNV may occur, although type 2 lesions are observed more frequently [2, 4].

Imaging Features

The gold standard for the diagnosis of CNV is dye leakage as demonstrated on fluorescein angiography (**Example Case**: Fig. 63.3A–D).

Due to the generally healthy RPE and Bruch's membrane seen in children, lesions tend to be type 2 (sub-retinal) with a classic appearance (as opposed to occult or minimally classic) on fluorescein angiography [12]. Optical coherence tomography (OCT) characteristics such as subretinal hyperreflective material and the presence of subretinal fluid may also play a role in diagnosis (**Example Case:** Fig. 63.3E–H), as well as in assessing response to treatment (**Example Case:** Fig. 63.3I–J).

A recent study suggests that OCT angiography (OCT-A) may demonstrate features that differ between active and quiescent CNV, thereby obviating the need for the more invasive measures (i.e., general anesthesia) typically necessary to obtain FA images in pediatric patients [14]. Ong et al. describe the appearance of active CNV on OCT-A as the presence of dense, fine capillaries with frequent anastomoses and vascular loops. These features were noted to resolve after treatment. In contrast, quiescent CNV was reported to appear as larger caliber, mature vessels with lower capillary density, and without the anastomoses and vascular loops seen in active CNV [14]. In Best disease, it can be difficult to visualize a CNV complex using traditional fluorescein angiography or indocyanine green angiography, on account of late hyperfluorescence from subretinal vitelliform material that may mask vascular flow [10]. As an alternative, Elbany et al. describe the use of OCT-A to diagnose an associated neovascular membrane in Best disease [10]. After treatment with anti-VEGF agents, OCT-A showed a reduction in size of the CNV, while multimodal imaging demonstrated a reduction in subretinal fluid and other angiographic features. In Best disease as well as other causes of CNV, OCT-A may serve as a useful imaging modality for diagnosis as well as monitoring response to treatment [10, 14].

Management

Treatment of CNV in the pediatric population poses significant challenges due to a relative paucity of information on the natural history as well as the absence of prospective data and clinical trials. As is the case in many pediatric conditions, presentation may occur later compared to adults. Management options may include observation, thermal laser photocoagulation, submacular surgery, photodynamic therapy, and intravitreal injections of anti-VEGF agents. Given the rarity of pediatric CNV, the exact timing and frequency of treatment has not been established.

Observation

Although there is limited data on the natural untreated course of CNV in children, studies have suggested a more favorable natural course when compared with adults. Goshorn et al. reported spontaneous involution in 11 of 19 cases (58%) of subretinal neovascular membranes [15] while Rishi et al. reported spontaneous regression in 36% of eyes [3]. The higher incidence of spontaneous regression in pediatric CNV has been explained by the relatively well-preserved RPE-Bruch's membrane complex integrity [2]. Variable outcomes have been reported depending on the underlying cause [8]. Other studies have shown improved visual outcomes in treated eyes than in those that underwent spontaneous regression [6, 13].

In the recent study by Rishi et al., although spontaneous regression was noted to occur, eyes that received treatment tended to have better visual outcomes, suggesting against observation especially when the CNV location is subfoveal [3]. These results highlight the importance of early diagnosis and management, most commonly with the use of intravitreal anti-VEGF alone or in combination with other modalities.

Photocoagulation

Prior to the anti-VEGF era, thermal laser photocoagulation served as a viable option for select patients with extrafoveal or juxtafoveal CNV [13]. However, treatment risks scarring and thermal injury.

Photodynamic Therapy

Photodynamic therapy (PDT) with verteporfin has been successfully used in children and was shown to be well tolerated without significant side effects [16–18]. In the study by Giansanti et al., CNV leakage was absent at 12 months in 4 of 5 cases, while vision improved in 3 of 5 subjects at final follow up of 12 to 18 months. Although no adverse events were reported, atrophic changes in the retinal pigment epithelium were observed in a halo around regressed CNV [16]. Mimouni et al. reported successful treatment in 3 cases of pediatric subfoveal CNV, with resultant stable or improved vision, as well as cessation or reduction of leakage from CNV at final follow up [17]. In this series, all three patients underwent second sessions after 10–14 weeks, while one patient received a third. Vision was either improved or stable at final follow up of 7 to 12 months. Like adults, dosing was calculated based on body surface area (6 mg/m^2 of verteporfin) activated with a light dose of 50 J/cm^2 using a 689 nm diode laser over an 83 s duration [17]. Ozdek et al. reported the use of a single session of PDT in five eyes of four patients with CNV associated with Best disease. All eyes responded to one treatment session, with visual acuity improvement in four of five eyes, with stability through final follow up at a mean of 25 months [18]. In addition to primary therapy, PDT has been described as a useful adjunctive procedure in patients who previously received anti-VEGF injections [19]. Other series have noted successful use of anti-VEGF injections in patients whose initially underwent PDT [3, 12]. No large trials or series exist in the pediatric population, necessitating extrapolation from adult CNV data as well as the small studies mentioned above. Although no adverse events unique to children have been observed, the informed consent process should address our relatively limited knowledge of the risks and benefits of this intervention.

Surgery

In children, CNV usually occurs in the subretinal rather than sub-RPE space and is more likely to have a single ingrowth location, compared to patients with AMD where CNV typically grows within the Bruch membrane/RPE complex. These features allow for increased success with surgical management. Described techniques involve creation of a retinotomy adjacent to or on top of the choroidal neovascular membrane after which a localized retinal detachment is induced with balanced salt solution, followed by removal with subretinal forceps [20, 21]. Good outcomes have been reported in select patients, with post-operative visual acuity improvements comparing favorably to the natural history of untreated membranes [20–22]. Uemura and Thomas reported that 70% of pediatric patients with subfoveal CNV who underwent surgery had a final visual acuity improvement of 2 or more Snellen lines, while nearly half of all patients achieved a final vision of 20/40 of better [22]. These results did not differ based on the underlying etiology of CNV. Mateo et al. describe successful surgical excision in eyes with peripapillary CNV associated with optic disc drusen [9]. However, there are reports of prolonged and additional treatments being required even after surgery [4]. Even with successful surgical removal, reported recurrences were present in 33% of patients in the series by Sears et al. [20] compared with 37% in the study by Uemura and Thomas [22]. In the anti-VEGF era, less invasive measures are typically preferred over surgical intervention, especially as first line treatments. However, surgical excision of CNV may be of benefit, albeit in a select subset of patients who have failed other therapies.

Intravitreal Anti-VEGF

In recent years, the off-label use of intravitreal anti-VEGF has largely supplanted older modalities, with multiple studies demonstrating its benefit. A summary of the major studies can be found in Table 63.1.

Not only has anti-VEGF been the most successful therapy for CNV, but it is also the least destructive to the retina and RPE when compared with other treatment options. Given the rarity of pediatric CNV and its varied etiologies, there are inherit barriers to conducting randomized trials to analyze outcomes based on treatment regimens. Although no standardized protocols have been established, a common treatment approach consists of monthly anti-VEGF injections on a *pro re* nata (PRN) basis until CNV resolution has been achieved [2, 4, 23]. When retrospectively compared with PRN anti-VEGF dosing, a loading dose of three-monthly injections did not appear to confer any additional benefit in terms of visual acuity gains [4].

Unlike CNV associated with other conditions such as age-related macular degeneration, fewer anti-VEGF injections are typically required to achieve quiescence. In a single-center series of 26 eyes of 23 patients, Ranjan et al. reported that in 19 eyes with active CNV, an average of 2 (±1.1) injections (of bevacizumab or ranibizumab monotherapy) were needed to achieve complete CNV regression [2].

Table 63.1 A summary of several major retrospective studies on pediatric choroidal neovascularization

Study	No. of Eyes (Patients)	Average age (years) at diagnosis	Follow-up	Most common etiologies	Eyes treated with anti-VEGF	Average no. of injections to achieve initial suppression	BCVA* (logMAR)	
							Initial	Final
Finn [1]	2353	12.9	Up to 2 years	Idiopathic (38.2%) Inflammatory (19.4%) Myopia (18.4%)	925	68.4% received <3 injections	0.62	0.39
Ranjan [2]	26 (23)	11.7	Average: 28.1 months	Inflammatory (61.5%) Idiopathic (19.2%)	19	2	0.4 gained	
Rishi [3]	111 (96)	11.4	Average: 17 months	Inflammatory (38%) Trauma (16%)	13	NA	1.02	0.87
Padhi [4]	43 (35)	11.2	Range: 6 months to 7 years	Best disease (32.5%) Idiopathic (27.9%)	30	2.11	0.44 gained when subfoveal	
Kozak [5]	45 (39)	12 (median)	Average: 14.1 months	Inflammatory, retinal dystrophy, idiopathic	45	2.2	0.87	0.7

Abbreviations: No. = number; VEGF = vascular endothelial growth factor; logMAR = logarithm of the minimum; anlge of resolution; NA = not available
*BCVA of treated eyes

Similarly, Padhi et al. found that an average of 2.11 anti-VEGF injections were needed for CNV regression [4]. In this study, 20% of eyes stabilized after a single anti-VEGF injection [4]. Most cases in Kozak et al. responded to a single anti-VEGF injection, while only 20% required repeated injections [5].

With anti-VEGF monotherapy, the series by Padhi et al. reported stabilization without recurrence in 63% of eyes [4]. Due to the small sample size, there was a clinically but not statistically significant improvement in vision after treatment [4]. The series by Kozak et al., patients treated with 1.25 mg of bevacizumab or 0.5 mg of ranibizumab achieved a statistically significant improvement in BCVA at a mean final follow up of 12.8 months. Forty-eight percent of eyes in this study gained 3 or more lines of vision, 60% achieved a final vision of 20/50 or better, while only 20% did not improve and had final vision of 20/200 or worse [5]. In the study by Henry et al., 86% of eyes treated with intravitreal bevacizumab achieved stabilization or improvement in vision [19]. At final follow up in the study by Ranjan et al. (mean 28.1 months), there was an improvement in BCVA (mean of 20/125 at presentation to 20/50 at final follow up) in the treated patients corresponding to an equivalence of 20 EDTRS letters, and a reduction in mean central macular thickness, both of which were statistically significant. None of these eyes experienced any systemic or intraocular complications due to anti-VEGF therapy [2]. Much like the reported visual outcomes, anatomic outcomes as measured by central macular thickness have been shown to significantly reduce after anti-VEGF treatment [7, 19, 23].

With a recurrence rate as low as 5%, it has been hypothesized that this is due to an intact surrounding RPE and the focal nature of most CNV in pediatric patients [2]. In other studies, such as D'Souza et al., CNV recurrence occurred in nearly 27% of patients. Yet, regression was achieved in each of these recurrent cases after a single repeat injection of bevacizumab or ranibizumab, further highlighting the effectiveness or PRN anti-VEGF dosing [7]. In some eyes, subretinal fibrosis may occur after CNV suppression, thereby limiting the final visual acuity, especially when located at or near the fovea [7, 12].

In addition to anti-VEGF monotherapy, adjunctive therapies have also been reported as beneficial. The study by Henry et al. reported successful use of adjunctive intravitreal triamcinolone, subtenon's triamcinolone, PPV with membrane peel, argon laser, and photodynamic therapy [19]. When CNV is present in patients with concurrent ocular inflammation, local or systemic steroids and/or anti-infective treatments are employed to achieve uveitic suppression along with anti-VEGF therapy [7].

Although existing data appear to support both the safety and efficacy of anti-VEGF in children [23], future questions remain. Limited data exist to compare whether there are any differences between anti-VEGF agents for pediatric CNV. However, aflibercept has been used as a second-line agent when other agents fail [12]. Decreased systemic VEGF levels have been reported in infants treated with anti-VEGF for retinopathy of prematurity. Yet, little is known regarding the long-term effects and serum levels of anti-VEGF in pediatric patients with CNV, who tend to be older children and adolescents. All the studies cited in this chapter used the typical adult dosing of anti-VEGF medications. At the time of writing, no dose–response relationship or comparative efficacy studies appear to have addressed these questions. Given the rarity of pediatric CNV, randomized controlled trials are unlikely to occur, which poses a significant challenge in further elucidating these unanswered questions. Overall, compared with the other treatments described above, anti-VEGF monotherapy, usually on a PRN dosing schedule, appears to have a more favorable side effect profile as well as superior visual and anatomic outcomes.

Conclusion

Pediatric CNV is a rare but important cause of vision loss. Its broad scope of underlying etiologies highlights the need for regular follow-up in at-risk patients. Especially since most cases tend to be unilateral, children may compensate with the fellow eye, and are therefore less likely to present early in the disease course. While fluorescein angiography remains as the gold standard in diagnosis, the use of less invasive imaging modalities has proven useful in both diagnosis as well as for assessing treatment response and detecting recurrences. In the setting of active uveitic inflammation, the underlying cause as well as the secondary CNV must be addressed. Intravitreal anti-VEGF shows promise as a safe and effective treatment. Yet, older therapies may still play a role in select scenarios or as adjuvant treatments.

Example Case

A 4-year-old female presented with 20/25 and 20/125 vision in the right and left eyes, respectively. Exam under anesthesia was performed, and a diagnosis of Best disease was made. Retcam fundus photos (A,B) and early fluorescein angiography images (C,D) confirmed the presence of CNV in the left eye. Hypofluorescence due to blockage (*) is present in both eyes (C,D), while a CNV membrane has resulted in early hyperfluorescence due to leakage (white arrow) in the left eye (D) 21 s after intravenous dye injection. The patient was treated with a series of intravitreal bevacizumab injections, which resulted in subsequent stability over several years.

Six years later, the now 10-year-old female with Best disease presented with a decline in vision in the right eye. Vision was 20/80 in the right eye and 20/40 in the left eye. Examination of the right eye revealed grayish subretinal fibrotic material with an adjacent crescent of subretinal hemorrhage (E). In the left eye, a fibrotic subfoveal scar with a cuff of subretinal fluid was present, which had remained stable over a several year period (F). OCT of the right eye through the fovea (white dotted line) revealed subretinal hyperreflective material corresponding to subretinal hemorrhage, with an overlying focus of subretinal fluid (G). In the left eye, a subfoveal pillar of fibrosis with adjacent subretinal fluid was present and unchanged from

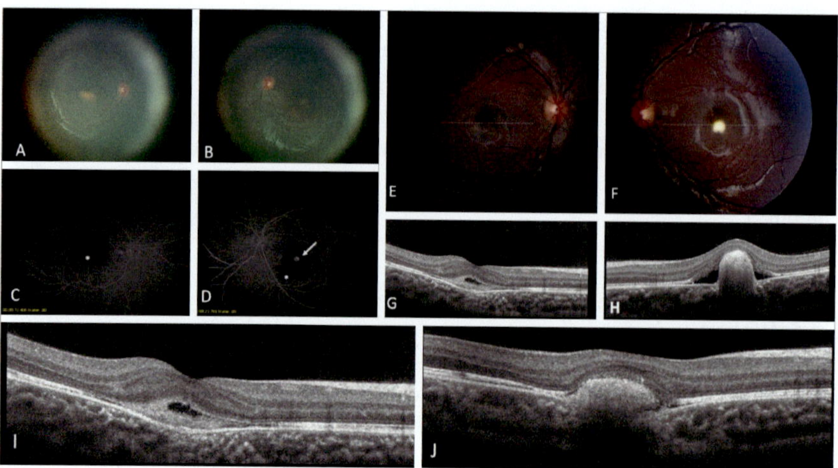

Fig. 63.3 Example case

prior serial exams (H). The decision was made to treat the right eye with a series of intravitreal bevacizumab until suppression of the newly diagnosed CNV was achieved.

After a series of monthly intravitreal bevacizumab injections, subretinal hemorrhage resolved, subretinal fluid improved, and the subretinal hyperreflective material became more fibrotic appearing. A comparison before and after treatment is seen in Fig. 63.3I (an enlarged image of 3G) with notable improvement depicted in Fig. 63.3J. Vision improved to 20/20–2 in the right eye and remained stable at 20/40 in the left eye. The CNV membrane remained inactive over the next several years, with plans to treat on an as needed basis.

Review Questions

1. True or false. Choroidal neovascular membranes in the pediatric population tend to be type I lesions, beneath the retinal pigment epithelium.

2. True or false. Inflammatory CNV only occurs only when the underlying inflammatory process is active.

3. True or False. Pediatric CNV typically requires fewer injections than adult CNV secondary to exudative macular degeneration.

Answers

1. False. Lesions tend to be type II, located beneath the retina but above the RPE.

2. False. Secondary CNV may occur in the setting of both active and quiescent uveitic inflammation.

3. True. Pediatric CNV typically regresses after fewer injections when compared with AMD, and often can be treated on an as-needed basis once initial suppression is achieved.

References

1. Finn AP, Fujino D, Lum F, Rao P. Etiology, treatment patterns, and outcomes for choroidal neovascularization in the pediatric population: an intelligent research in sight (IRIS®) registry study. Ophthalmol Retina. 2021;S2468–6530(21):00176–7.
2. Ranjan R, Salian R, Verghese S, et al. Pediatric choroidal neovascularization: etiology and treatment outcomes with anti-vascular endothelial growth factors. Eur J Ophthalmol. 2021;7:11206721211048800.
3. Rishi P, Bharat RPK, Rishi E, et al. Choroidal neovascularization in 111 eyes of children and adolescents. Int Ophthalmol. 2021. https://doi.org/10.1007/s10792-021-02018-2.
4. Padhi TR, Anderson BJ, Abbey AM, et al. Choroidal neovascular membrane in paediatric patients: clinical characteristics and outcomes. Br J Ophthalmol. 2018;102(9):1232–7.
5. Kozak I, Mansour A, Diaz RI, et al. Outcomes of treatment of pediatric choroidal neovascularization with intravitreal antiangiogenic agents. Retina. 2014;34(10):2044–52.
6. Ganesh SK, Ahmed AS. Pediatric inflammatory CNV: a case series from a tertiary referral centre. Ocul Immunol Inflamm. 2020;28(1):26e32.
7. D'souza P, Ranjan R, Babu U, Kanakath AV, Saravanan VR. Inflammatory choroidal neovascular membrane: long-term visual and anatomical outcomes after intravitreal anti-vascular endothelial growth factor therapy. Retina. 2018;38(7):1307–1315.
8. Sivaprasad S, Moore AT. Choroidal neovascularisation in children. Br J Ophthalmol. 2008;92(4):451–4.
9. Mateo C, Moreno JG, Lechuga M, Adan A, Corcostegui B. Surgical removal of peripapillary choroidal neovascularization associated with optic nerve drusen. Retina. 2004;24(5):739–45.
10. Elbany S, Kodjikian L, Boucher S, Loria O, Burillon C, Mathis T. Neovascularized Best disease in child: contribution of optical coherence tomography angiography. Ophthalmic Surg Lasers Imaging. Retina. 2019;50(9):597e601.
11. Cohen SY, Laroche A, Leguen Y, Soubrane G, Coscas GJ. Etiology of choroidal neovascularization in young patients. Ophthalmology. 1996;103(8):1241–4.
12. Barth T, Zeman F, Helbig H, Oberacher-Velten I. Etiology and treatment of choroidal neovascularization in pediatric patients. Eur J Ophthalmol. 2016;26(5):388–93.
13. Rishi P, Gupta A, Rishi E, Shah BJ. Choroidal neovascularization in 36 eyes of children and adolescents. Eye (Lond). 2013;27(10):1158–68.
14. Ong SS, Hsu ST, Grewal D, et al. Appearance of pediatric choroidal neovascular membranes on optical coherence tomography angiography. Graefes Arch Clin Exp Ophthalmol. 2020;258(1):89–98.
15. Goshorn EB, Hoover DL, Eller AW, Friberg TR, Jarrett WH, Sorr EM. Subretinal neovascularization in children and adolescents. J Pediatr Ophthalmol Strabismus May-Jun. 1995;32(3):178–82.
16. Giansanti F, Virgili G, Varano M, et al. Photodynamic therapy for choroidal neovascularization in pediatric patients. Retina. 2005;25:590–6.
17. Mimouni KF, Bressler SB, Bressler NM. Photodynamic therapy with verteporfin for subfoveal choroidal neovascularization in children. Am J Ophthalmol. 2003;135(6):900–2.
18. Ozdek S, Ozmen MC, Tufan HA, Gurelik G, Hasanreisoglu B. Photodynamic therapy for best disease complicated by choroidal neovascularization in children. J Pediatr Ophthalmol Strabismus. 2012;49(4):216–21.
19. Henry CR, Sisk RA, Tzu JH, et al. Long-term follow-up of intravitreal bevacizumab for the treatment of pediatric retinal and choroidal diseases. J AAPOS. 2015;19(6):541–8.

20. Sears J, Capone A Jr, Aaberg T Sr, et al. Surgical management of subfoveal neovascularization in children. Ophthalmology. 1999;106(5):920–4.
21. Jain K, Shafiq AE, Devenyi RG. Surgical outcome for removal of subfoveal choroidal neovascular membranes in children. Retina. 2002;22(4):412–7.
22. Uemura A, Thomas MA. Visual outcome after surgical removal of choroidal neovascularization in pediatric patients. Arch Ophthalmol. 2000;118:1373–8.
23. Hykin P, Staurenghi G, Wiedemann P, et al. MINERVA study group. Ranibizumab 0.5 mg treatment in adolescents with choroidal neovascularization: subgroup analysis data from the MINERVA study. Retin Cases Br Rep. 2021;15(4):348–355.

Nanophthalmos in Children

64

Sumita Agarkar, Muthumeena Muthumalai, Debahuti Midya, and Şengül Özdek

Abstract

Nanophthalmos is a rare ocular developmental disorder which is characterised by short axial length accompanied by thickened sclera. Diagnostic criteria include high hyperopia, axial length of 20.0 mm or less, high corneal curvature, shallow anterior chamber, high ratio of lens-to-eye volume, posterior wall thickening of more than 1.7 mm. Non-contact biometry remains the gold standard to diagnose nanophthalmos by measuring axial length, corneal diameter and curvature, anterior chamber depth, lens thickness and scleral thickness. Posterior segment associations include; crowded optic discs (pseudopapiledema appearance), macular striae/folds, foveal aplasia, foveal schisis,, retinitis pigmentosa like phenotype, choroidal effusion and exudative retinal detachment most of which can be picked up on ocular coherence tomography. Management includes full correction of refractive errors with spectacles, bifocals, or contact lenses. This is especially important in children to prevent amblyopia and strabismus. With increase in lens size with age, anterior chamber may become progressively shallow, leading to a risk of acute angle closure glaucoma. Regular monitoring with gonioscopy and early prophylactic laser iridotomy is recommended. Any intraocular procedure including lasers must be taken up with care due to risk of spontaneous effusion. Several surgical techniques of scleral window surgery that allow egress of suprachoroidal fluid have been described

Supplementary Information The online version contains supplementary material available at https://doi.org/10.1007/978-3-031-14506-3_64.

S. Agarkar (✉) · M. Muthumalai · D. Midya
Department of Pediatric Opthalmology and Adult Strabismus, Medical Research Foundation, Chennai, India
e-mail: drsar@snmail.org

Ş. Özdek
School of Medicine, Gazi University, Ankara, Turkey

for treatment of nanophthalmos related uveal effusion. Discovery of many new genes and pathways have advanced our understanding of the pathogenesis and opened up possibility of potential markers for genetic diagnosis and gene therapy for this entity.

Keywords

Nanophthalmos · Microphthalmos · Exudative retinal detachment · Thick sclera · Scleral window surgery · Vortex vein decompression · High hypermetropia · Expulsive choroidal hemorrhage · Macular fold · Angle closure glaucoma · Pseudopapiledema

Introduction

Nanophthalmos is a rare ocular developmental disorder. Conceptually nanophthalmos is considered to be a pure form of microphthalmos in which the anterior and posterior segments of the eyeball do not develop into a normal size in the absence of other major ocular or systemic anomalies. It includes a spectrum of disorders with a phenotypically small but structurally normal eye [1, 2].

Epidemiology: It has a prevalence of <1% in most populations. Most cases are bilateral and sporadic. Both sexes are equally affected [2].

Terminology: Nanophthalmos is derived from Greek word-Nanos meaning dwarf eye [3]. Small eye phenotypes include microphthalmos, nanophthalmos, posterior microphthalmos and cornea plana. Microphthalmos is defined as an axial length of at least two standard deviations below the average for the patient's age. It is categorized as simple and when accompanied by other ocular abnormalities, complex. Nanophthalmos is a clinical phenotype of simple microphthalmos [2–4].

Clinical phenotypes of small eye	Clinical features
Simple microphthalmos	Short axial length due to global eye reduction and no other anomalies
Complex microphthalmos	Short axial length due to global eye reduction and associated ocular malformations (eg., colobomas, persistent fetal vasculature, retinal dysplasia)
Nanophthalmos	Short axial length caused by shortening of the anterior and posterior segments, accompanied by thickened sclera
Relative anterior microphthalmos	Short axial length caused by shortening of the anterior segment, with a normal-sized posterior segment and without scleral thickening
Posterior microphthalmos	Short axial length caused by shortening of the posterior segment, with a normal-sized anterior segment and thickened sclera

Nanophthalmos Versus Posterior Microphthalmos: Some reports consider nanophthalmos and posterior microphthalmos as manifestations of the spectrum of hyperopia, rather than two completely distinct entities [5]. The fact that mutations in the same genes may cause both posterior microphthalmos and nanophthalmos supports this concept. However, many other studies have noted several clinical and structural differences with respect to corneal size and curvature, anterior chamber depth, lens thickness, angle characteristics, and propensity for complications between the two conditions [6, 7].

- Although both conditions are characterized by shortened axial lengths and high hyperopia, in nanophthalmos anterior chamber dimensions are decreased whereas in posterior microphthalmos the anterior segment is of normal (or slightly subnormal) size.
- In a study by Relhan et al. which biometrically analyzed eyes of 38 patients with high hyperopia (defined in the study as greater than + 7.00 D), they defined patients with corneal diameters less than 11.0 mm as nanophthalmos and those with corneal diameters greater than or equal to 11.0 mm as posterior microphthalmos [6].
- They noted that nanophthalmic eyes tend to have shallow anterior chamber depth, thicker lens, and steeper cornea, compared to eyes with posterior microphthalmos.
- They also found that the incidence of angle-closure glaucoma was 69.23% in the nanophthalmos group compared to 0% in the posterior microphthalmos group [6].

Pathophysiology: Nanophthalmos develops as a result of arrested growth of the eye in the early stages of embryogenesis [7, 8]. The eye develops normally till the embryonic fissure is closed, but thereafter grows very slowly in all dimensions.

- Nanophthalmic eyes have abnormal collagen fibrils in each of the three layers of the sclera [7]. These abnormal fibers are thought to be the cause for the increased scleral thickness.
- The sclera is thicker than that of a normal eye and its collagen lamellae disorganized, with variable sizes, decreased amounts of GAGs and elevated fibronectin content.
- The combination of these factors also contributes to its inelasticity, which impairs vortex venous drainage and reduces transcleral flow of proteins.
- These histopathological features and anatomical factors may be responsible for higher incidence of angle closure glaucoma as well as uveal effusion syndrome and retinal detachment in nanophthalmic eyes [8, 9]. However, it is not clear whether the abnormal scleral structure is a primary or a secondary effect of the genetic changes that induce nanophthalmos as many of the genes implicated in this condition are also expressed in retina and retinal pigment epithelium.

Inheritance and genetics: Nanophthalmos can occur either as a sporadic condition or as a familial disorder with autosomal-dominant or recessive transmission [9]. Sporadic forms may be due to environmental factors or new mutations that result in the arrest of ocular growth. There are many reported familial cases with autosomal-dominant and recessive forms of inheritance. Five genes and two loci have been reported to be associated with familial nanophthalmos [9]. NNOS2 is connected to mutations in the membrane frizzled-related protein, or *MFRP*, gene [10]. This gene appears to have a central function in ocular development as a regulator of ocular dimension. Velez et al. found that introducing a normal copy of the *MFRP* gene through adenoviral-based gene therapy may reverse some of these pathogenic changes-like- rescue of photoreceptor death, normalization of retinal function, and regulation of eye length in *MFRP rd6/rd6* in adult mice [11]. These findings suggest that gene therapy may be a viable option for this disease. Several cases of *MFRP* mutations leading to reduced eye axial length have been reported [11–13]. Wasmann et al. reported a case of two sisters who presented with low visual acuity, high hyperopia, macular retinal folds, with the older sibling also having thickened sclera, and optic nerve head drusen with confirmed *MFRP* mutations [14]. The mutations in the *MFRP* gene have also been linked to the autosomal-recessive syndrome of posterior microphthalmos, retinitis pigmentosa, foveoschisis, and optic disc drusen [13].

Two additional genes, Crumbs homologue gene *CRB1* and Bestrophin 1 *BEST1* (*VMD2*), have been implicated in nanophthalmos and have profound roles in photoreceptor and retinal pigment epithelial (RPE) function, respectively [15].

Crumbs homologue gene is located in chromosome 1, in the interval 1q31.2-1q32.1, and its mutations are classically associated with various heritable retinal dystrophies, including Leber's Congenital Amaurosis. Furthermore, some recent reports showed association of mutation in *CRB1* with nanophthalmos and retinitis pigmentosa [16, 17].

Bestrophin 1 (BEST1/VMD2)-gene is located on chromosome 11q12. It encodes an integral membrane protein, bestrophin 1, localized predominantly in the baso-lateral plasma membrane of the RPE and most prominently near the macula. *BEST1* mutations are classically associated with Best vitelliform macular dystrophy (BVMD) but also has also been reported to be in association with other widespread ocular abnormalities, such as autosomal-dominant vitreoretinochoroidopathy (ADVIRC) and autosomal-recessive bestrophinopathy (ARB), which are both associated with nanophthalmos [17, 18].

The autosomal-dominant nanophthalmos NNO1 is caused by a defect on chromosome 11. This region may also be associated with more severe angle-closure glaucoma manifestations [19]. The precise genetic change at this locus has yet to be confirmed, though coding and regulatory mutations in BEST1 have been excluded as a cause. Another form of autosomal-dominant disease, NNO3 was described in a family with simple microphthalmia, microcornea, and high hyperopia, and it was reported to be linked to chromosome 2q11-14 [20].

Transmembrane Protein 98 Gene (*TMEM98*) gene encodes a transmembrane protein that is universally expressed in the human body, including in the ocular tissues, such as iris, choroid, retinal pigment epithelium, and sclera [21]. In a large pedigree, Awadalla and coworkers found a missense mutation in the *TMEM98* (A193P) that may be associated with autosomal-dominant nanophthalmos [21].

Protease Serine 56 (PRSS56)-is located in the chromosome 2q37.1 and encodes a protein which functions as a serine protease. There are reports of its association with nanophthalmos and posterior microphthalmos cases [22].

Table showing genes involved in pathogenesis of nanophthalmos:

Gene (locus)	Location	Inheritance	Gene expression (localization)	Gene function	Phenotypic characteristics of mutations
MFRP (NNO2)	11q23.3	AR	RPE/CB (transmembrane)	Wnt signalling pathway effector	(i) Nanopthalmos, high hyperopia, and angle-closure glaucoma (ii) Retinitis pigmentosa, foveoschisis, and optic disc drusen syndrome
TMEM98 (NNO4)	17q11.2	AD	RPE/CB/sclera (transmembrane)	Unknown	High hyperopia, angle-closure glaucoma, and increased optic disc drusen
PRSS56 (MCOP6)	2q37.1	AR	Retina/sclera (cytoplasmic)	Serine protease	(i) Nanophthalmos, angle-closure glaucoma, and high hyperopia (ii) Posterior microphthalmia
CRB1	1q31.3	AR	Retina (transmembrane)	Controls cell polarity	(i) Nanophthalmos and retinitis pigmentosa (ii) Leber congenital amaurosis (iii) Pigmented paravenous chorioretinal atrophy (iv) Retinitis pigmentosa
Best1/VMD2	11q12	AD or AR	RPE/CB (transmembrane)	Chloride channel	(i) ADVIRC: autosomal-dominant vitreoretinochoroidopathy with nanophthalmos (ii) ARB: autosomal-recessive bestrophinopathy (iii) BVMD: best vitelliform macular dystrophy
Unknown (NNO3)	2q11-q14	AD	Unknown (NNO3)		Microphthalmia, microcornea, and high hyperopia

Syndromes associated with nanophthalmos:

Nanophthalmos is usually an isolated entity but can also be a part of a syndrome:

- Nanophthalmos-retinitis pigmentosa-foveoschisis-optic disc drusen syndrome-It is rare AR disorder caused by biallelic variants in the *MFRP* gene [23].
- Oculodentodigital syndrome: Oculodentodigital dysplasia (ODDD) is a rare inherited disorder affecting the development of the face, eyes, teeth, and limbs [24].
- Autosomal dominant vitreoretinochoroidopathy with nanophthalmos (ADVIRC)- ADVIRC is a rare condition characterized by a peripheral circumferential hyperpigmented band with punctate white opacities in the retina, chorioretinal atrophy in the midperipheral or peripapillary retina, and vitreous fibrillary condensations. There are reports of association of this condition with nanophthalmos and a higher incidence of angle-closure glaucoma [18].
- Kenny syndrome characterised by low birth weight, dwarfism due to hypocalcemia, delayed closure of anterior fontanelle [25].
- Cryptorchidism has been reported once in association with nanophthalmos [26]

Diagnosis: Currently there is a lack of consensus regarding the diagnostic criteria for nanophthalmos. Widely different criteria for the diagnosis of nanophthalmos have been used. The most commonly followed diagnostic criteria include high hyperopia, axial length of 20.0 mm or less, high corneal curvature shallow anterior chamber, high ratio of lens-to-eye volume, posterior wall thickening of more than 1.7 mm [27]. Wu et al. have proposed shallow anterior chamber, high hyperopia, axial length up to 21 mm, and posterior wall thickness greater than 1.7 mm as criteria to define nanophthalmos [28]. Similarly, Yalvac et al. have modified it by reducing axial length as less than 20.5 mm and have also added the high lens/eye volume ratio as an additional criteria [29]. Nanophthalmos diagnosis mainly relies on clinical examination, biometry and imaging.

Clinical features:

- Small eye without any ocular malformations
- Highly hyperopic eye deeply set in orbit
- Shallow anterior chamber
- Axial length <21 mm
- Thickened sclera
- Normal to large lens with high lens eye volume ratio
- Smaller corneal diameter with topographically high curvature with or without astigmatism.
- Increased retinochoroidal scleral thickness >1.7 mm
- Narrow palpebral fissures

Posterior segment findings

Recent literature review suggests that patients with high axial hyperopia associated with retinal abnormalities should be included in nanophthalmos spectrum [30]. Posterior segment associations of nanophthalmos can be explained by disparity in growth between neurosensory retina and outer layers of eye. Smaller internal area causes crowding of the retina, folding of the choroid around the macula, an abnormal fovea and crowded disc (Serrano et al. 1998) [30]. Other posterior segment anomalies include; (Fig. 64.1).

- Crowded optic discs (pseudopapiledema appearance)
- Papillomacular striae/folds due to the redundancy of retinal tissue as a result of the disparity between the normal growth of the retina and the halted growth of the sclera (Figs. 64.1, 64.2, 64.5, 64.6, 64.7).
- Foveal aplasia and an absent /rudimentary foveal avascular zone (FAZ) [31]. Foveal schisis has also been described in association with nanophthalmos (Figs. 64.1, 64.2) [32].
- Yellowish deposits similar to flecks which appear as dark spots with autofluorscence imaging with RPE mottling and atrophy (Fig. 64.6).
- Retinitis pigmentosa like phenotype is seen occasionally [57] (Fig. 64.7).
- Choroidal effusion and exudative retinal detachment (Figs. 64.4, 64.5, 64.7).
- Exudative retinal detachment secondary to uveal effusion syndrome can occur following sudden decompression of the globe during any intraocular surgery, including laser iridotomy in nanophthalmic eyes [27].

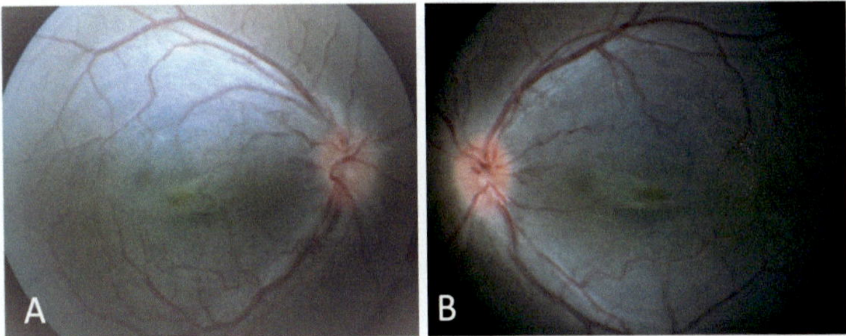

Fig. 64.1 Color fundus image of the right eye of a 14 year old male patient with nanophthalmos showing the papillomacular fold and cystic changes in the foveal region in the right (**A**) and left (**B**) eyes. Also note the pseudopapilledema appearance in both eyes

- **Investigations**

Non-contact biometry: It remains the gold standard to diagnose nanophthalmos. Biometry includes measurements of axial length, corneal diameter and curvature, anterior chamber depth, lens thickness and scleral thickness.

In the absence of gonioscopy, which may not be feasible in young children without anesthesia, noncontact biometry may be used to identify children at risk of developing occludable angles in nanophthalmic eyes. As it is suggested by the previous study done by Agarkar et al., that the probability of occludable angles increases five-fold if the anterior chamber depth is <3.02 mm (OR = 4.46) [32]. Similarly, children with lens thickness of >4 mm have a five times higher risk of angle closure (OR = 5.14). With an anterior chamber depth of <3 mm and lens thickness of >4 mm, the risk of occludable angles increases up to six times (OR = 6.03) [32].

Optical coherence tomography (OCT): Imaging techniques such as OCT have improved our knowledge of posterior segment anomalies associated with nanophthalmos. OCT features described in association with nanophthalmos include absence of the foveal pit,

Macular thickening, macular schisis, foveal cyst, and retinal and choroidal folds (Fig. 64.2) [33, 34].

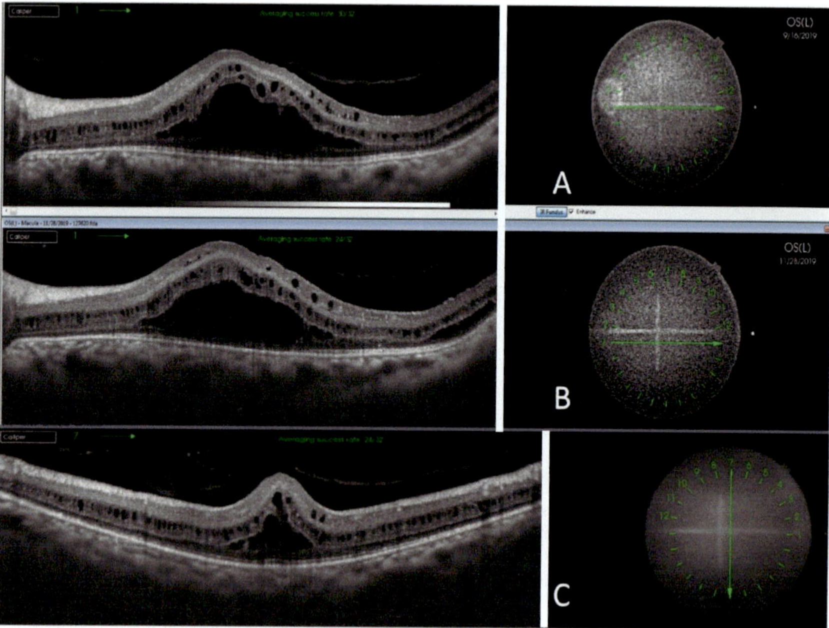

Fig. 64.2 Horizontal line scan images (**A**, **B**) of macula obtained on Swept source OCT in a nanophthalmos patient showing foveal elevation with schitic changes in the retinal layers. C shows the vertical line scan in the same eye showing the macular fold more prominently

Ultrasound Biomicroscopy

The most common associations of nanophthalmos noted on UBM include.

- Anteriorly placed ciliary body
- Reduced ciliary sulcus and
- Plateau iris like configuration [35]

Management:

Management of patients with nanophthalmic eyes can pose significant challenges because of the inherent characteristics of these eyes, such as high hyperopia, short axial length, and structural abnormalities of the sclera. Early diagnosis and management is vital.

- Refractive errors: Refractive errors should be fully corrected with spectacles, bifocals, or contact lenses. This is especially important in children to prevent amblyopia and strabismus. Bifocal lenses results in better performance of near activities in younger children. In children with amblyopia, patching is preferable in asymmetrical cases. If the axial hyperopia is not corrected in early childhood, it may lead to irreversible amblyopia and visual impairment. Ametropic amblyopia is the leading cause of visual impairment in these children.
- Strabismus: It usually manifests as partially refractive or non-accommodative esotropia. High hypermetropia secondary to short axial length leads to esotropia. In the study by Sener et al., non-accommodative and partially accommodative refractive esotropia were the common types of strabismus noted in nanophthalmos [36]. They noted persistent amblyopia in several of their subjects despite close monitoring. Authors do not recommend modification in the surgical plan owing to shorter axial length in case strabismus surgery is contemplated. These children are also likely to have poor binocular function due to higher incidence of amblyopia, relatively delayed surgical intervention and poor optical quality of vision due to high refractive error.

Glaucoma in nanophthalmos:

In childhood the anterior chamber may be deep but with increase in lens size with age, it may become progressively shallow, leading to a risk of acute angle closure glaucoma. A high ratio of lens-to-eye volume may result in a shallow anterior chamber, high iris convexity, and a narrow or closed angle with peripheral anterior synechiae (PAS) [37]. Laser iridotomy may be beneficial in early stages before the development of PAS. Once PAS develops, intraocular surgery may be required. Surgery for glaucoma in these eyes is often considered as a last resort due to high risk of complications. This is due to sudden decompression of the globe during surgery which may trigger the development of massive uveal effusion, leading to secondary retinal detachment, intraocular haemorrhage and malignant glaucoma with loss of vision. In nanophthalmos even relatively younger patients are at a risk of developing occludable angle requiring intervention. In a retrospective study by Agarkar et al. which retrospectively analysed 75 children with nanophthalmos, 17 (23%) had occludable angles of which 14 (19%) underwent prophylactic peripheral iridotomy. The mean age of patients who underwent peripheral iridotomy was 16 years. This underlines the importance of serial biometric measurements and gonioscopy during follow up. LT/AXL ratio along with anterior chamber depth and lens thickness is an important marker to detect potentially occludable angles in children with nanophthalmos [32].

Exudative Retinal detachment in nanophthalmos

Treatment for nanophthalmus related uveal effusion can be challenging and usually does not respond to corticosteroids, immune modulating agents, laser therapy, or routine surgical techniques for retinal detachment repair [38–40]. Other medical therapies such as topical non-steroid anti-inflammatory drugs, topical prostaglandin analogs, and systemic carbonic anhydrase inhibitors are reported but have not found much use clinically [41, 42].

Several surgical procedures have been reported for treatment of uveal effusion with the surgical goal being to create a durable, low-resistance pathway for choroidal fluid to exit. Surgical decompression of the vortex veins where they exit the sclera was first described by Brockhurst which combines sclerectomy to unroof the vortex veins with small sclerotomies in the scleral dissection bed to drain the suprachoroidal fluid [43]. Another approach popularised by Johnson and Gass is to create full-thickness equatorial sclerectomies to facilitate the egress of suprachoroidal fluid. The average time to reattachment was 2 to 3 months, with recurrence in 23% of eyes [40].

Faulborn and Kölli reported an anterior sclerotomy technique, where they created 2 by 8 mm scleral windows without sclerectomy, 4 mm posterior to the limbus. They showed that the equatorial location of scleral surgery may not be as critical as previously thought [44].

Uyama et al. described a modified subscleral sclerectomy technique in which scleral flaps measuring 4 mm by 5 mm were made in the inferotemporal and inferonasal quadrants. Beneath each flap, the remaining sclera was excised to expose the choroid and edges of the scleral wounds were cauterized before the flap was loosely sutured. Additional sclerectomies were performed in the upper quadrants if needed. Mannitol and acetazolamide was administered postoperatively to hasten the resolution of fluid. Their surgical approach resulted in resolution of subretinal fluid and choroidal thickening in nanopthalmic eyes and normal-sized eyes with scleral thickening but not in eyes with normal axial length and scleral thickness [45].

Mansour et al. described an extensive circumferential partial-thickness scleral excision technique, which resulted in quick resolution of effusion in 8 nanophthalmic eyes [46].

Ozdek et al. compared the visual and anatomic outcomes between the 4 and 2 quadrants sclerectomy with sclerotomy techniques. They found the 4-quadrant extensive sclerectomy technique to be superior, but suggested that 2-quadrant surgery may be used in mild cases with glaucoma to preserve the superior quadrants for future glaucoma surgeries [47]. Figure 64.3 shows the surgical technique and Figs. 64.4 and 64.5 are example cases for this treatment.

Ghazi et al. described a modified ultrasound guided surgical technique to identify areas of maximal scleral choroidal thickening in each involved quadrant, which were chosen for sclerostomy placement using a Kelly punch. They reported complete resolution of choroidal thickening and subretinal fluid in five of six eyes using this technique [48].

Many adjuncts and modifications have been described along with scleral thinning procedures to increase their efficacy. Studies have shown topical application of MMC at sclerectomy sites might prevent episcleral and scleral scarring that can lead to postoperative closure of the scleral windows [49–51]. Yepez and Aravalo used Ex-Press Glaucoma Filtration Device (Alcon) shunts to maintain patency of the sclerotomies [52]. Intravitreal anti-VEGF injections have been tried to increase the efficacy of partial thickness sclerectomy surgery in intractable cases [53].

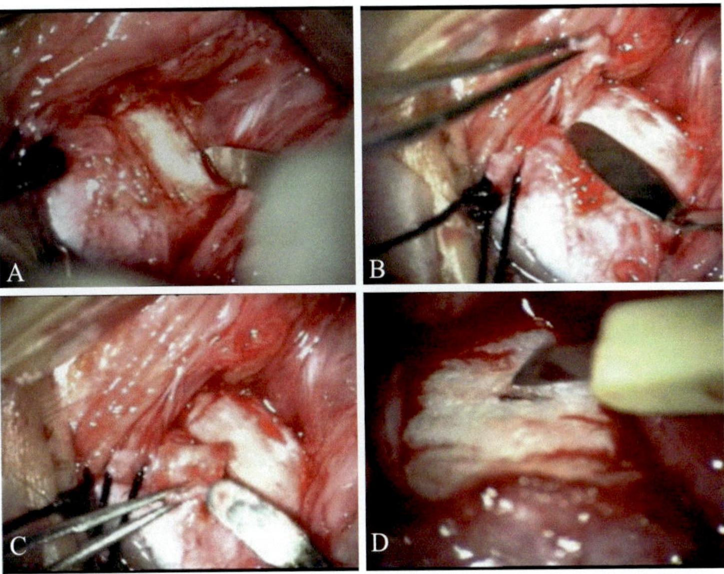

Fig. 64.3 The technique of scleral window surgery. Rectangular partial scleral excision is performed from 4 quadrants. Anterior border is just posterior to the insertion of the rectus muscles, posterior border is limited by the vortex vein ampulla (Courtesy of Şengül Özdek). See the central full thickness linear sclerotomy (d) which does not aim to drain the subretinal fluid but only to see the thickness of the sclera left

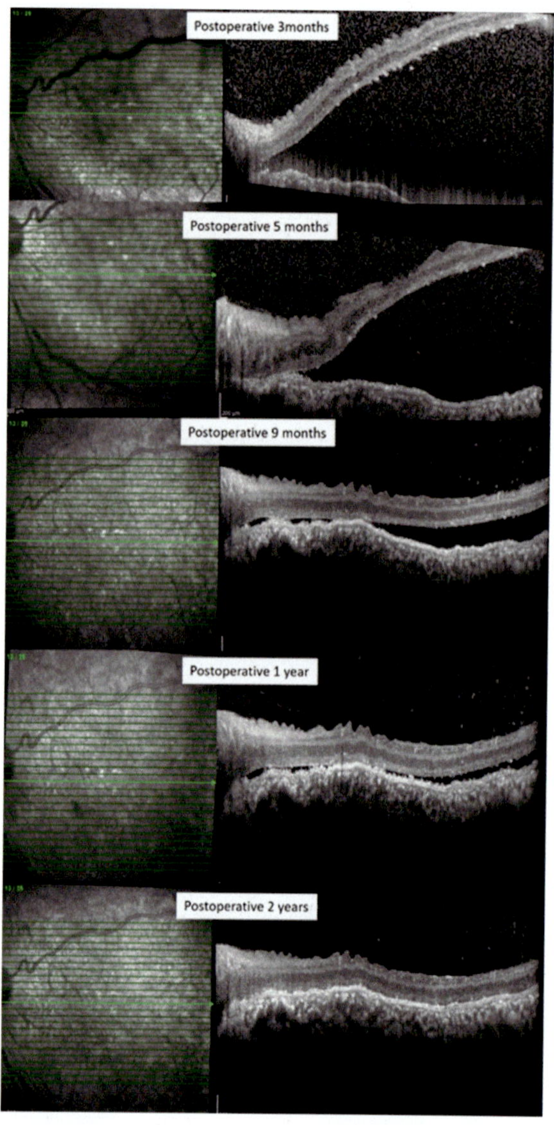

Fig. 64.4 Slow resolution of exudative RD in a series of OCT pictures following 4-quadrant scleral window surgery within 2 years period in a nanophthalmos case with superior bullous retinal detachment involving macula. Image and video courtesy of Şengül Özdek (**see the video**)

Intraocular surgery in nanophthalmos

These eyes are more prone to complications that can occur spontaneously or following ocular intervention such as peripheral laser iridotomy, cataract surgery or filtering procedure [54].

The most frequently seen complications include [55, 56]

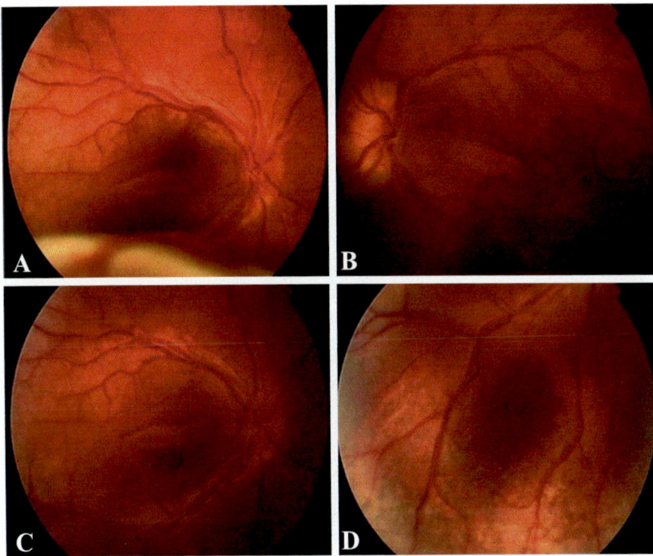

Fig. 64.5 **A** RE: Inferior bullous exudative RD. **B** LE: Macular fold. **C** RE following scleral window surgery. **D** Note the inferior RD is resorbed and retina is attached leaving only a macular fold. (Image courtesy of Dr. Şengül Özdek)

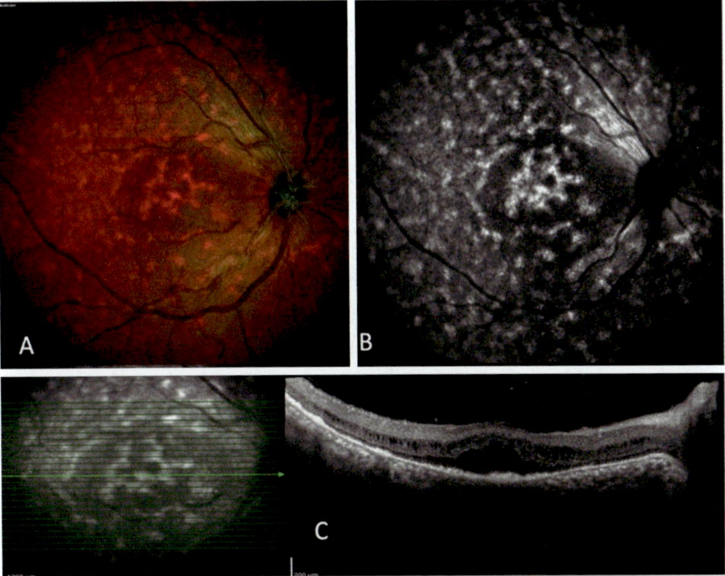

Fig. 64.6 Postoperative pictures of a case with nanophthalmos associated exudative retinal detachment treated with 4-quadrant scleral window surgery. Note the yellowish deposits similar to flecks (**A**) which appear hyperautofluorescent in autofluorscence imaging (**B**). There is still some edema in the fovea but exudative retinal detachment has totally resolved (**C**). (Image courtesy of Dr. Şengül Özdek)

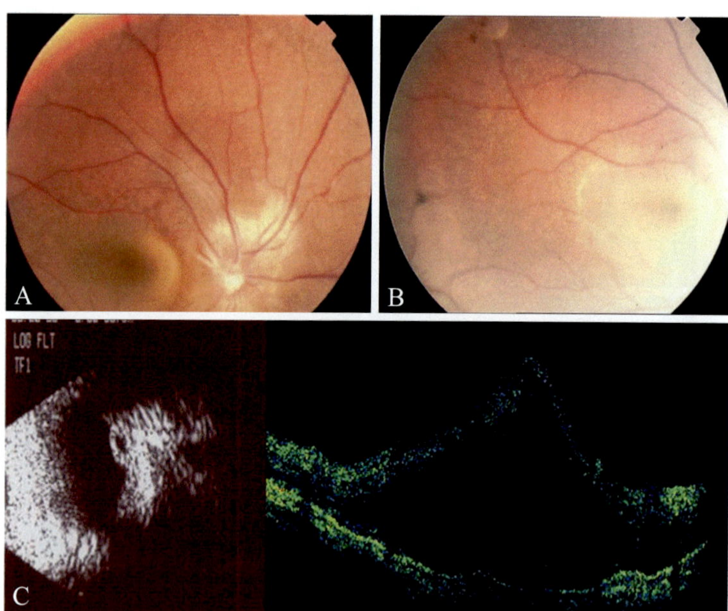

Fig. 64.7 A 15 y old boy with bilateral macular detachment associated with nanophthalmos (**A**). There is also pigmentary retinopathy in the peripheral retina (**B**). Note the macular detachment seen in B scan (**C**) and in OCT (**D**). (Image courtesy of Dr. Şengül Özdek)

- Choroidal effusion
- Exudative retinal detachment
- Malignant glaucoma
- Pupillary block
- Expulsive suprachoroidal hemorrhage

Some surgeons may prefer to perform a scleral window surgery as an aid to decrease the risk of expulsive suprachoroidal haemorrhage during cataract surgery in nanophthalmus eyes. However this is not a scientifically proven prophylaxis.

Uveal effusion which is more common in adults with nanophthalmos is very rarely noted in children. Sclera in children is relatively less rigid and thinner, thereby compression on vortex veins is not significant enough to cause effusion.

Case Presentations

Case 1: A five year old boy reported with diminished vision in both eyes and difficulty in dim illumination. On examination, his BCVA was 6/38 (Lea symbols) for distance and near vision was 6/18 (reduced snellens chart) in both eyes. Refraction showed a hypermetropia of + 16 D in both eyes. Intraocular pressure and anterior segment examination was within normal limits. Fundus evaluation showed hyperemic crowded discs with blurred margins along with heaped up retina at the macula. Optical coherence tomography (OCT) revealed cystoid macular edema with increased retinal thickening with macular schisis involving the inner retinal layers. Biometry showed axial length of 15.39 and 15.38 mm in right and left eye respectively. He was diagnosed as a case of nanophthalmos. He was prescribed glasses and regular follow up. In 2017, at age 10, during follow up visit gonioscopy revealed appositional angle closure. He underwent Nd yag laser iridotomy in both eyes. Post iridotomy, angles were open and IOP was normal without any anti glaucoma medications. ERG showed reduced scotopic response with normal photopic responses suggestive of RP variant. By the age of 12 years mid peripheral RPE mottling was also seen in both eyes. Child was treated with topical dorzox eye drops for chronic macular edema associated with RP variant and follow up OCT scans showed reduction in cystoid spaces and retinal thickness. He continues to be under follow up.

Video 1: *describes scleral window surgery with subretinal fluid drainage in a case of very highly bullous exudative retinal detachment associated with nanophthalmos with light perception only vision which improved to 0.2 level after surgery. (video courtesy of Şengül Özdek).*

To summarize, nanophthalmos is a rare developmental anomaly. High hyperopia with resultant amblyopia and strabismus are important ophthalmic considerations in pediatric patients. Ophthalmologists should routinely include complete evaluation for glaucoma especially gonioscopy during follow up in children with high hyperopia. With advanced imaging and surgical techniques there has been significant progress in the diagnosis and management of this rare condition leading to better outcomes. Also new discoveries in the genetics have led to the discovery of many new genes and pathways to understand the pathogenesis. These advances will ultimately improve our understanding of this entity and provide novel avenues for treatment, including potential markers for genetic diagnosis and possibility of gene therapy.

Review Questions

1. Which of the following is false regarding nanophthalmos

A. Shortened anterior segment
B. Shortened posterior segment
C. No ocular malformations
D. Thin sclera

2. Please indicate the correct sentences related to clinics of nanophthalmos below:

A. Macular fold is one of the most common findings associated with nanophthalmos
B. Exudative retinal detachment is usually secondary to increased vascular permeability

C. Massive bullous exudative retinal detachment can be treated surgically with scleral window surgery
D. Glaucoma type in nanophthalmos is usually an open angle glaucoma
E. Expulsive choroidal haemorrhage rate is higher than usual during anterior segment surgeries in these eyes.

Answers

1. (**D**) Nanophthalmos is accompanied by thickened sclera which is due to abnormal scleral collagen arrangement and responsible for most of the complications including angle closure, uveal effusion and retinal detachment.
2. **A, C, E**

References

1. Duke-Elder S. Anomalies in the size of the eye. In: Duke-Elder S, ed. System of Ophthalmology. St. Louis, MO: Mosby–Year Book, 1963;3(pt 2):488–95.
2. Warburg M. Classification of microphthalmos and coloboma. J Med Genet. 1993;30:664–9.
3. O'Grady RB. Nanophthalmos. Am J Ophthalmol. 1971;71:1251–3.
4. Warburg M. Genetics of microphthalmos. Int Ophthalmol. 1981;4(1–2):45–65.
5. Nowilaty SR, Khan AO, Aldahmesh MA, Tabbara KF, Al-Amri A, Alkuraya FS. Biometric and molecular characterization of clinically diagnosed posterior microphthalmos. 2013;155(2):361–72.
6. Relhan N, Jalali S, Pehre N, Rao HL, Manusani U, Bodduluri L. High-hyperopia database, part I: clinical characterisation including morphometric (biometric) differentiation of posterior microphthalmos from nanophthalmos. Eye (Lond). 2016;30(1):120.
7. Khan AO. Posterior microphthalmos versus nanophthalmos. 2008;29(4)
8. Yamani A, Wood I, Sugino I, Wanner M, Zarbin MA. Abnormal collagen fibrils in nanophthalmos: a clinical and histologic study. Am J Ophthalmol. 1999;127(1):106–8.
9. Carricondo PC et al. Nanophthalmos: a review of the clinical spectrum and genetics. J Ophthalmol. 2018.
10. Katoh M. Molecular cloning and characterization of MFRP, a novel gene encoding a membrane-type frizzled-related protein. 2001;282(1):116–123.
11. Velez G, Tsang SH, Tsai YT, et al. Gene therapy restores Mfrp and corrects axial eye length. 2017;7(1):16151. https://doi.org/10.1038/s41598-017-16275-8.
12. Crespí J, Buil JA, Bassaganyas F et al. A novel mutation confirms MFRP as the gene causing the syndrome of nanophthalmos–renititis pigmentosa–foveoschisis–optic disk drusen. 2008;146(2):323–328.
13. Zacharias LC, Susanna R, Sundin O, Finzi S, Susanna BN, Takahashi WY. Efficacy of topical dorzolamide therapy for cystoid macular edema in a patient with MFRP-related nanophthalmos–retinitis pigmentosa–foveoschisis–optic disk drusen syndrome. 2015;9(1):61–63.
14. Wasmann RA, Wassink-Ruiter JS, Sundin OH, Morales E, Verheij JB, Pott JW. Novel membrane frizzled-related protein gene mutation as cause of posterior microphthalmia resulting in high hyperopia with macular folds. 2014;92(3):276–81.
15. Lotery AJ, Jacobson SG, Fishman GA, et al. Mutations in the CRB1 gene cause Leber congenital amaurosis. 2001;119(3):415–420.
16. Paun CC, Pijl BJ, Siemiatkowska AM, et al. A novel crumbs homolog 1 mutation in a family with retinitis pigmentosa, nanophthalmos, and optic disc drusen.
17. Boon CJ, Klevering BJ, Leroy BP, Hoyng CB, Keunen JE, den Hollander AI. The spectrum of ocular phenotypes caused by mutations in the BEST1 gene. 2009;28(3):187–205.

18. Yardley J, Leroy BP, Hart-Holden N, et al. Mutations of VMD2 splicing regulators cause nanophthalmos and autosomal dominant vitreoretinochoroidopathy (ADVIRC). 2004;45 (10):3683–3689.
19. Othman MI, Sullivan SA, Skuta GL et al. Autosomal dominant nanophthalmos (NNO1) with high hyperopia and angle-closure glaucoma maps to chromosome 11. 1998;63(5):1411–1418.
20. Li H, Wang JX, Wang CY, et al. Localization of a novel gene for congenital nonsyndromic simple microphthalmia to chromosome 2q11–14. 2008;122(6):589–593.
21. Awadalla MS, Burdon KP, Souzeau E, et al. Mutation in TMEM98 in a large white kindred with autosomal dominant nanophthalmos linked to 17p12-q12. 2014;132(8):970–977.
22. Gal A, Rau I, El Matri L, et al. Autosomal-recessive posterior microphthalmos is caused by mutations in PRSS56, a gene encoding a trypsin-like serine protease. 2011;88(3):382–390.
23. Ayala-Ramirez R, Graue-Wiechers F, Robredo V, Amato-Almanza M, Horta-Diez H, Zenteno JC. A new autosomal recessive syndrome consisting of posterior microphthalmos, retinitis pigmentosa, foveoschisis, and optic disc drusen is caused by a MFRP gene mutation. Mol Vis. 2006;12:1483–9.
24. Sugar HS, Thompson JP, Davis JD. The oculo-dento-digital dysplasia syndrome. Am J Ophthalmol. 1966;61(6):1448–51.
25. Bergada I, Schiffrin A, Abu Srair H, et al. Kenny syndrome: description of additional abnormalities and molecular studies. Hum Genet. 1988;80:39–42.
26. Barad RF, Nelson LB, Cowchock FS, Spaeth GL. Nanophthalmos associated with cryptorchidism. Ann Ophthalmol. 1985;17(5):284–8.
27. Singh OS, Simmons RJ, Brockhurst RJ, Trempe CL. Nanophthalmos: a perspective on identification and therapy. 1982;89(9):1006–1012.
28. Wu W, Dawson DG, Sugar A, et al. Cataract surgery in patients with nanophthalmos: results and complications. 2004;30(3):584–90.
29. Yalvac IS, Satana B, Ozkan G, Eksioglu U, Duman S. Management of glaucoma in patients with nanophthalmos. 2008;22(6):838–43.
30. Serrano JC, Hodgkins PR, Taylor DSI, et al. The nanophthalmic macula. British J Ophthalmol. 1998;82:276–279.
31. Walsh MK, Goldberg MF. Abnormal foveal avascular zone in nanophthalmos. 2007;143 (6):1067–8.
32. Agarkar S, Koladiya N, Kumar M, Vijaya L, Raman R. Nanophthalmos in children: morphometric and clinical characterization. J AAPOS. 2020;24(1):27.e1-27.e5. https://doi. org/10.1016/j.jaapos.2019.11.010.
33. Jackson T, Yang Y, Shun-Shin G. Spectral domain optical coherence tomography findings in retinal folds associated with posterior microphthalmos. J AAPOS. 2012;16(4):389–91.
34. Rao A, Padhi TR, Jena S, Mandal S, Das T. Atypical features of nanophthalmic macula–a spectral domain OCT study. BMC Ophthalmol. 2012;12:12.
35. Ishikawa H, Liebmann JM, Ritch R. Quantitative assessment of the anterior segment using ultrasound biomicroscopy. Curr Opin Ophthalmol. 2000;11:133–9.
36. Sener EC, Mocan MC, Sarac OI, Gedik S, Sanac AS. Management of strabismus in nanophthalmic patients: a long-term follow-up report. Ophthalmology. 2003;110:1230–6.
37. Sharan S, Grigg J, Higgins R. Nanophthalmos: ultrasound biomicroscopy and Pentacam assessment of angle structures before and after cataract surgery. J Cataract Refractive Surg. 2006;32(6):1052–5.
38. Gass JD, Jallow S. Idiopathic serous detachment of the choroid, ciliary body, and retina (uveal effusion syndrome). Ophthalmology. 1982;89(9):1018–32.
39. Gass JD. Uveal effusion syndrome: a new hypothesis concerning pathogenesis and technique of surgical treatment. 1983. Retina. 2003;23(6 Suppl):159–163.
40. Johnson MW, Gass JD. Surgical management of the idiopathic uveal effusion syndrome. Ophthalmology. 1990;97(6):778–85.

41. Kerstetter JR, Brubaker RF, Wilson SE, Kullerstrand LJ. Prostaglandin F2 alpha-1-isopropylester lowers intraocular pressure without decreasing aqueous humor flow. Am J Ophthalmol. 1988;105(1):30–4.

42. Andrijević Derk B, Benčić G, Corluka V, et al. Medical therapy for uveal effusion syndrome. Eye (Lond). 2014;28(8):1028–31.

43. Brockhurst RJ. Vortex vein decompression for nanophthalmic uveal effusion. Arch Ophthalmol. 1980;98(11):1987–2190.

44. Faulborn J, Kolli H. Sclerotomy in uveal effusion syndrome. Retina. 1999;19:504–7.

45. Uyama M, Takahashi K, Kozaki J, et al. Uveal effusion syndrome: clinical features, surgical treatment, histologic examination of the sclera, and pathophysiology. Ophthalmology. 2000;107(3):441–9.

46. Mansour A, Stewart MW, Shields CL, Hamam R, Fattah MA, Sheheitli H, Mehanna C-J, Yassine S, Chahine H, Keaik M. Extensive circumferential partial- thickness sclerectomy in eyes with extreme nanophthalmos and spontaneous uveal effusion. Br J Ophthalmol. 2019;103:1862–7.

47. Ozdek S, Yalinbas Y, Hasanreisoglu M, Ozmen MC. Treatment of Nanophthalmos Related Uveal Effusion with Two vs. Turkish J Ophthalmology: Four Quadrant Partial Thickness Sclerectomy and Sclerotomy Surgery. In press; 2022.

48. Ghazi NG, Richards CP, Abazari A. A modified ultrasound-guided surgical technique for the management of the uveal effusion syndrome in patients with normal axial length and scleral thickness. Retina. 2013;33(6):1211–9.

49. Akduman L, Adelberg DA, Del Priore LV. Nanophthalmic uveal effusion managed with scleral windows and topical mitomycin-C. Ophthalmic Surg Lasers. 1997;28(4):325–7.

50. Suzuki Y, Nishina S, Azuma N. Scleral window surgery and topical mitomycin C for nanophthalmic uveal effusion complicated by renal failure: case report. Graefes Arch Clin Exp Ophthalmol. 2007;245(5):755–7.

51. Sabrosa NA, Smith HB, MacLaren RE. Scleral punch method with topical mitomycin C for safe revision of failed deep sclerectomy in nanophthalmic uveal effusion syndrome. Graefes Arch Clin Exp Ophthalmol. 2009;247(7):999–1001.

52. Yepez JB, Arevalo JF. Ex-Press shunt for choroidal fluid drainage in uveal effusion syndrome type 2: a potentially novel technique. JAMA Ophthalmol. 2015;133(4):470–1.

53. Guo J, Cao X, Li X. Partial thickness sclerectomy and intravitreal anti-VEGF therapy for intractable uveal effusion syndrome. Int Ophthalmol. 2019;39:1885–90.

54. Faucher A, Hausanee K, Rootman DS. Phacoemulsification and intraocular lens implantation in nanophthalmic eyes: report of a medium-sized series. J Cataract Refract Surg. 2002;28:837–42.

55. Hoffman RS, Vasavada AR, Allen QB, et al. Cataract surgery in the small eye. J Cataract Refract Surg. 2015;41:2565–75.

56. Neelakantan A, Venkataramakrishnan P, Rao BS, Krishnan N, Vijaya L, John S, Kar B. Familial nanophthalmos: Management and complications. Indian J Ophthalmol. 1994;42:139–43.

57. Urgancioglu B, Ozdek S, Hasanreisoglu B. Coats'-like retinitis pigmentosa variant and nanophthalmos. Can J Ophthalmol. 2007;42(6):877–8. https://doi.org/10.3129/i07-170 PMID: 18059514.

Management of Deformed Blind Eye

65

Onur Konuk

Abstract

The management of the pediatric anophthalmic and microphthalmic socket is different from adults as socket and facial development is dependent on orbital growth. The main aim of the reconstruction in microphtalmic and anophthalmic socket in a pediatric case is to encourage socket growth. In this text surgical decisions, choice of orbital implants, various techniques of socket expansion, and socket reconstructions are discussed.

Keywords

Anophthalmia · Microphthalmia · Conformers · Enucleation · Evisceration · Orbital expanders · Dermis fat graft · Orbital implants · Orbit reconstruction · Sympathetic ophthalmia

Introduction

Management of blind eye in pediatric cases usually has some controversies and difficulties as ophthalmologists should deal with functional, cosmetic, socioeconomic, and psychological facts. The main aim in the blind and phthisic eye is to restore the volume loss in the socket to promote orbital and facial development. Initially, the proposal of eye removal may be difficult in children, and conservative use of conformers or ocular prosthesis on an unpainful phthisic eye can be a simple

O. Konuk (✉)

Gazi University Medical School Department of Ophthalmology, Oculoplastic and Orbital Unit, Beşevler Ankara, Turkey

e-mail: dronurkonuk@yahoo.com

© The Author(s), under exclusive license to Springer Nature Switzerland AG 2023

Ş. Özdek et al. (eds.), *Pediatric Vitreoretinal Surgery*,

https://doi.org/10.1007/978-3-031-14506-3_65

option, however, eye removal may be necessary for recalcitrant intraocular malignancies, severe ocular trauma, intraocular and extraocular infections, blind and painful eyes, as well as for cosmetic management of a disfigured eyes.

The etiology of anophthalmic socket in pediatric patients can be either congenital or acquired. Congenital anophthalmia and microphthalmia are the causes of an early embryonic developmental defect of the optic vesicle and are not in the scope of this chapter. Even though their incidences are decreasing, ocular trauma and intraocular tumors especially retinoblastoma is still the leading cause of eye removal in pediatric cases. Primary persistent hyperplastic vitreous, recalcitrant endophthalmitis, and blind painful eyes are the other reasons for surgical removal of the eye [1–3].

Examination of Microphthalmic Eye: The Oculoplastic Surgery Perspective

The initial examination of a pediatric case with a blind deformed eye has difficulties as the families usually have anxiety and despondency regarding the causes of blindness. They usually seek for clues about a physical sign indicating a potential vision and have little or no idea about the course of the treatment and its long-term cosmetic outcomes. Thus, the initial thing to do is to raise awareness and gain the trust of the family and organize an appropriate treatment plan. Vision should be the first thing to examine to finalize the expectancy for sight. The next steps should include evaluation of adnexal deformities, eyelid length and position, conjunctival cul-de-sac problems, lacrimal patency, and maxillofacial development. The decrease of malar eminence, the size of the anterior orbit may show the presence of facial asymmetry and may be helpful to emphasize the urgency of management of microphthalmic socket [4].

Management of Microphthalmic Blind Eye

The indications for surgical treatment in a deformed blind eye include;

1. Management of pain due to trauma or previous surgical procedures.
2. Treatment of recalcitrant infection of the eye or socket.
3. Treatment of severe ocular trauma and decrease of the potential risk regarding sympathetic endophthalmitis.
4. Treatment of intraocular tumor.
5. Management of the asymmetry between healthy and disfigured eyes and improvement of the cosmetic outcome.

The removal of the eye in pediatric patients can be performed by evisceration or enucleation. The surgical choice usually depends on the underlying disease, clinical features, the surgeon's preferred technique. Additionally, the surgical outcome will also be influenced by the continuing orbital growth [5]. The argument over enucleation versus evisceration has persisted in the ophthalmic literature for years. From a clinical and surgical view, evisceration is technically easier and often has better cosmetic outcomes than enucleation, however, it can be complicated by the dissemination of unanticipated intraocular tumors and the possibility of sympathetic ophthalmia [6–8]. Additionally, enucleation can be the preferred procedure in the pediatric population because in some cases it permits the placement of a larger implant [9]. However, current evisceration techniques provide larger orbital implantation similar to enucleation [10–11]. Thus, several factors must be considered in choosing the most appropriate procedure.

Anophthalmia, Microphtlamia, and Orbital Growth

Facial maturation is significantly related to orbital growth. A microphthalmic eye can cause severe consequences on overall orbital and facial development. The terminology of microphtalmia includes eyes with corneal diameter less than 10 mm or axial length less than 20 mm thus follow-up of these patients in oculoplastic services is mandatory. The normal infant globe is approximately 70% of its adult size and grows rapidly in the first year of age [12]. At 3 months of age, the face is only approximately 40% the size of the adult face, and by 2 years of age, the face reaches 70% of the adult size. Farkas et al. determined age-related orbital growth patterns and demonstrated that approximately 90% of orbital growth occurs by the age of 5 years [13–14]. In clinical practice, the management of anophthalmic or microphthalmic socket in a pediatric case younger than 5 years usually needs an implant that can increase in size like dermis fat draft or expandible orbital implants.

Intraocular Tumor

The presence or suspicion of an intraocular tumor is the most important contraindication for evisceration surgery. Examination of the fundus or evaluating the globe using an appropriate radiological technique in cases with opaque media is mandatory. There have been reports about inadvertent intraocular surgery in unsuspected retinoblastoma cases [15]. Thus, an intraocular malignancy should be ruled out before evisceration is recommended.

Endophthalmitis

In the presence of endophthalmitis, either evisceration or enucleation can be selected [9]. The author prefers evisceration over enucleation to reduce the exposition of subarachnoid fluid to the infective area. Additionally, these patients usually had orbital inflammation or underwent several intraocular surgeries including scleral buckling that makes evisceration surgery more versatile. Placement of an implant after evisceration or enucleation in an endophthalmitis case is under discussion. Some authors primarily perform eye removal for the management of endophthalmitis and do orbital implantation as a secondary procedure when socket inflammation heals. On the other hand, in cases with endophthalmitis orbital implantation related risks are relatively lower in the antibiotic era and can also be performed with eye removal in one session [16]. Ideally, surgery can be delayed until the eye is phthisic and the orbital inflammation is healed with systemic antibiotics and anti-inflammatory treatment at which time eye removal and orbital implantation can be performed at the same session.

Sympathetic Ophthalmia

Sympathetic ophthalmia (SO) is a rare, bilateral, granulomatous panuveitis that occurs following accidental or surgical penetrating eye trauma [17]. The main hypothesis for sympathetic ophthalmia is the CD4 helper T-cell and late CD8 cytotoxic T-cell induced responses to newly exposed antigens from the photoreceptor layer and choroidal melanocytes [18–19]. Additionally, HLA-DRB1*04 and DQA1*03 genotypes haplotypes are reported for increased susceptibility to the severity of sympathetic ophthalmia [20–21]. The shortest time interval from trauma to the occurrence of sympathetic ophthalmia was reported as 10 days, but there have been cases reported decades after injury [22, 23]. A prospective surveillance study reported the incidence of SO at 0.03 per 100,000 while other incidence estimates range from 0.2% to 0.5% following injury and 0.01% after intraocular surgery [19, 24]. In recent years, ocular surgery, especially vitrectomy, has become an increasingly prevalent risk factor for SO. History for vitrectomy was reported in about 31.4% of patients, and transscleral cyclophotocoagulation in 15.8% of patients [18]. One possible cause of this difference could be early and more sophisticated and standardized treatment after ocular trauma reduced the incidence of SO. Another possible reason is that the number of ocular surgeries has increased with the promotion and popularization of many types of ocular surgeries. There has been a myth that evisceration may cause or does not prevent SO. A careful review of the literature does not allow one to come to a definitive conclusion regarding the risk of sympathetic ophthalmia after evisceration [25]. It is, however, interesting to note that in several retrospective studies involving over 3000 eviscerations, no cases of sympathetic ophthalmia were identified [26, 27]. In conclusion was that evisceration is a safe and effective procedure with little risk of sympathetic ophthalmia.

Implant Selection

The main purpose of orbital implantation after evisceration or enucleation is to achieve the most acceptable cosmetic outcome after losing an eye with vision. The options to be discussed for orbital implantation are the size and type of the implant. The implant should be big enough to replace the volume loss of the orbit after eye removal, but also should not induce size-related complications. On the other hand, the implant should be compatible with the growing orbit in a pediatric case. The most used implant choices are silicone or polymethyl methacrylate (PMMA) synthetic spheres, coralline hydroxyapatite, synthetic hydroxyapatite, porous polyethylene, and dermis fat grafts [28, 29].

The non-integrated solid implants like polymethyl methacrylate and silicone are still popular as they can easily be inserted, have low complication rates, and are relatively cheaper than integrated porous implants. As these implants are not integrated into the orbital tissues they have the risk of implant migration after implantation. On the other hand, these implants can easily be replaced or removed especially in cases with severe trauma that may necessitate multiple socket surgeries (Fig. 65.1).

The porous orbital implants have become popular because of the potential fibrovascular ingrowth of orbital fibrovascular tissue into the hydroxyapatite and porous polyethylene implants (Fig. 65.2). In theory, fibrovascular ingrowth protects against migration, infection, and extrusion. However, it is shown that the hydroxyapatite and porous polyethylene implants have much higher rates of extrusion than the smooth acrylic and silicone implants [30, 31]. Attaching the extraocular muscles to the implant allows for near-normal movement of the implant. It is reported that there is no difference in implant or prosthetic movement between sclera-covered

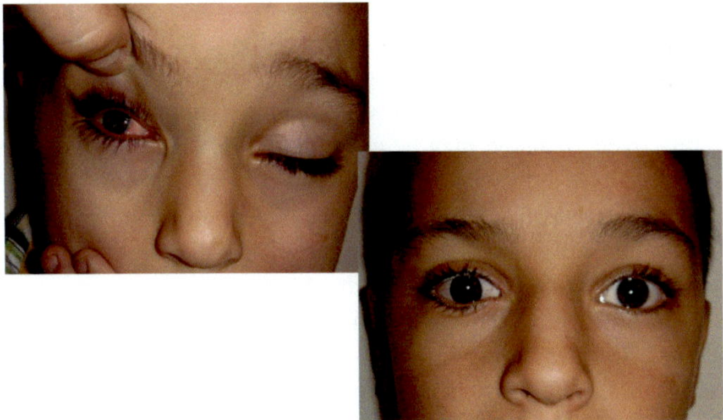

Fig. 65.1 Evisceration and orbital implantation give favorable results when optimal implant size is selected. In this case, a modified evisceration technique with scleral flaps is used and a 20 mm silicone sphere is introduced into the orbit. A thin prosthesis on the socket gives acceptable cosmetic results

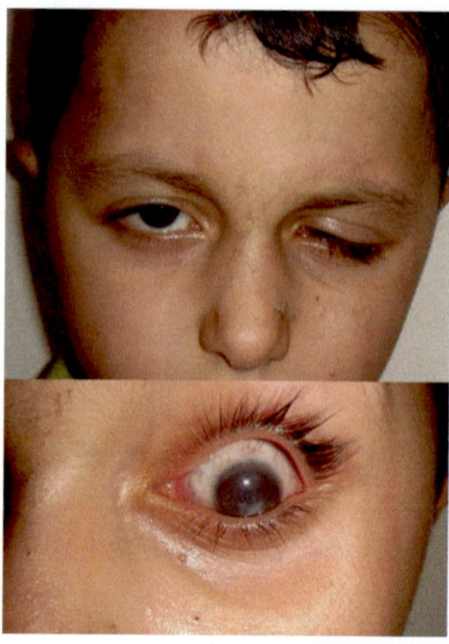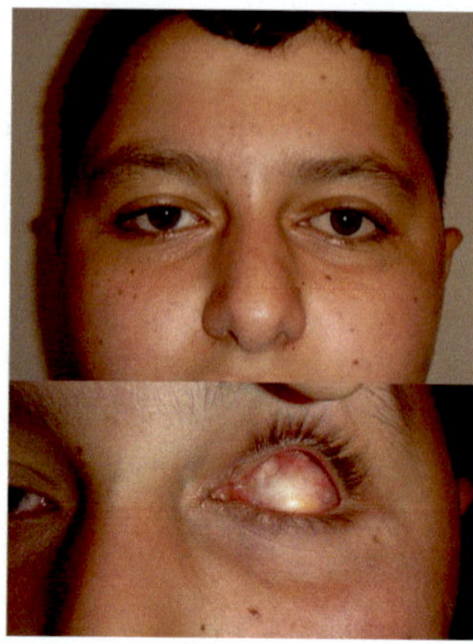

Fig 65.2 Modified evisceration technique with scleral flaps and 20 mm hydroxyapatite sphere is introduced in this 5-year-old boy. A thin prosthesis on the socket gives acceptable cosmetic results in 8 years of follow-up

nonpegged hydroxyapatite porous implants and sclera-covered spherical acrylic implants [32, 33]. The main potential advantage of porous implants is they allow for secondary pegging. The aim of pegging is to couple the prosthesis to the implant with a motility peg and increase the moving range of the prosthesis. However, many surgeons do not place pegs, and many patients refuse them due to peg-related complications [34–36].

Dermis fat grafts (DFG) can be used alternatively as an autogenous implant for volume augmentation after eye removal (Figs. 65.3 and 65.4). There are several advantages of DFG. It shows good integration with no possibility of extrusion, it may provide deeper fornices in contracted sockets, and its usage reduces the cost when compared with alloplastic implants [37]. The DFG is an ideal implant for children younger than 5 years old as it can expand with the growing pediatric orbit [38]. The use of DFG also has some disadvantages. It is time-consuming as it needs an additional surgical site. It can show contraction due to insufficient vascular support. Rarely overexpansion may be encountered that may necessitate resection, and surgical site may need revisions due to infection or scar [5, 28–29, 37–38].

Tissue expanders are usually used for congenital anophthalmia or severe microphtalmia where conformers cannot be introduced due to severe volume deficit and socket contracture or when planned orbital bony growth cannot be achieved by aggressive expansion with conformers (Fig. 65.5). There are two kinds of orbital expanders. First, self-expanding hydrogel expanders are designed in hemispheric and spheric shapes. The hemispheric hydrogel expanders are used for socket expansion, and spheric ones are placed intraconally for orbital expansion (Fig. 65.6). Even though implantation of hydrogel expanders is an easy and one-stage procedure, their quick and uncontrolled fashion of expansion brings out complications as implant exposure or extrusion [39–41]. The second type of

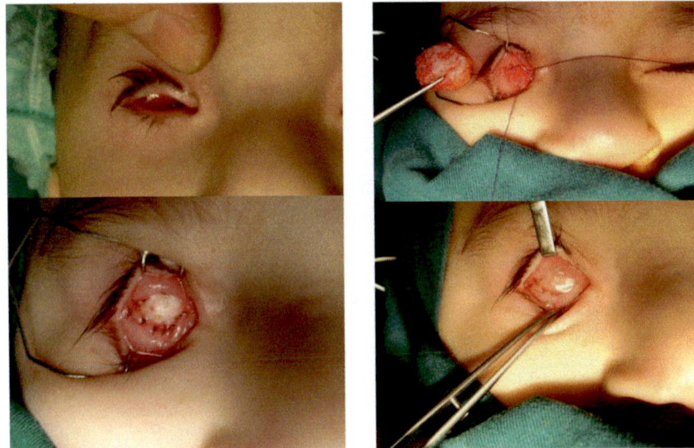

Fig. 65.3 Dermis fat grafting is an ideal technique for pediatric cases that have a potential for self-expansion with the growing orbit

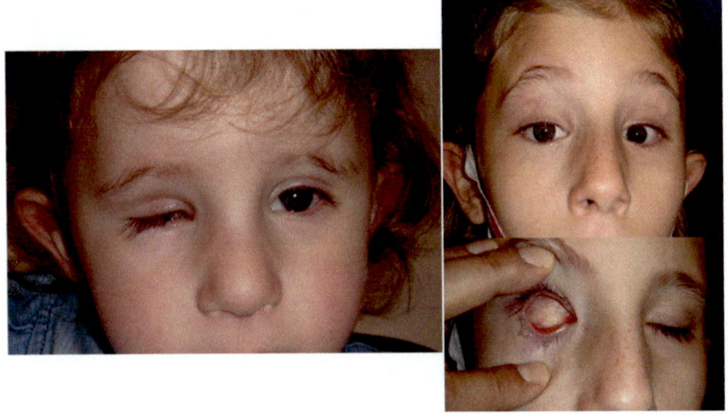

Fig. 65.4 A 4-year-old girl presented with blind painful eye due to open globe injury. Enucleation surgery is performed, and a dermis fat graft is preferred for orbital volume augmentation since these grafts have the potential to enlarge with growing bony orbit in pediatric cases. 5 years later the graft worked successfully and treated the volume loss and the patient did not need additional orbital surgery

expander is the silicone expander in which saline is injected gradually over time into a port in the parietal region that is connected to the tissue expander. It provides a gradual increase in size with a target inflation period of over 20 to 36 weeks to decrease the risk of expander extrusion [42]. The main disadvantage of the procedure is recurrent injections and clinical visits that may irritate the child and the family during the follow-up period.

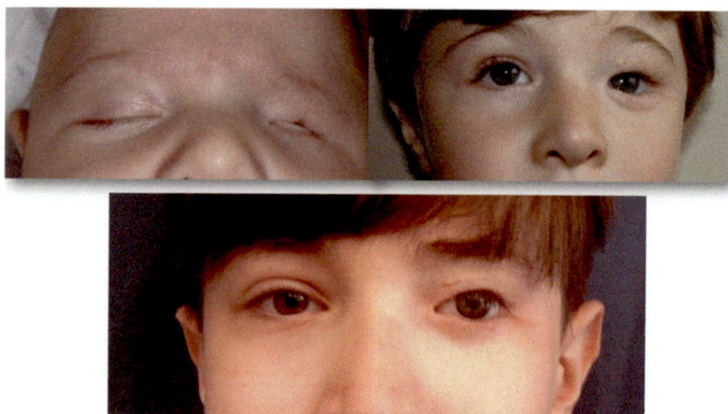

Fig. 65.5 Hydrogel self-expanders are alternative treatment options for congenital anophthalmia or severe microphthalmia if the socket is too shallow for placement of conformers. This 2 month of age patient received spherical and hemispherical self-expanders for orbit and socket respectively. The expansion of socket and orbit give an acceptable result after 3 and 11 years

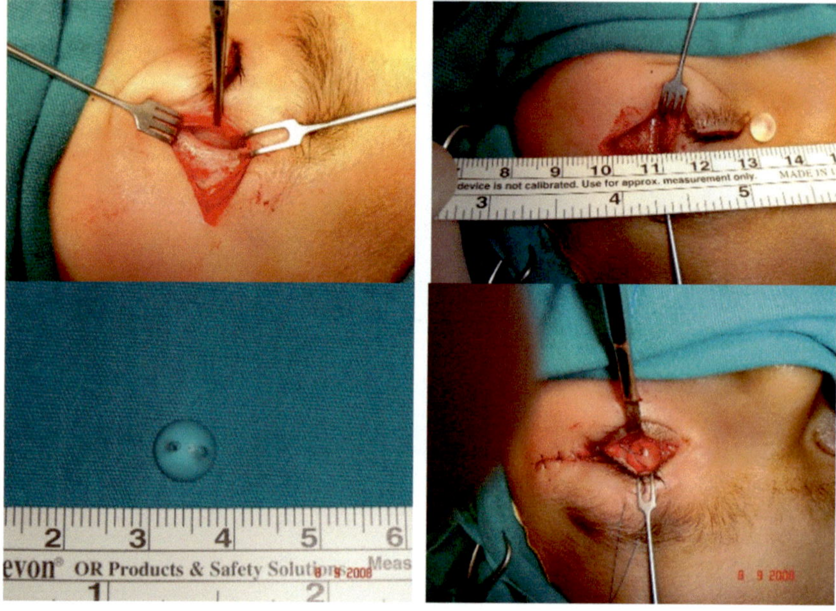

Fig. 65.6 Hydrogel self-expanders for socket and orbit. Note that spherical implant is introduced to the orbit where the hemispheric implant is inserted to the socket

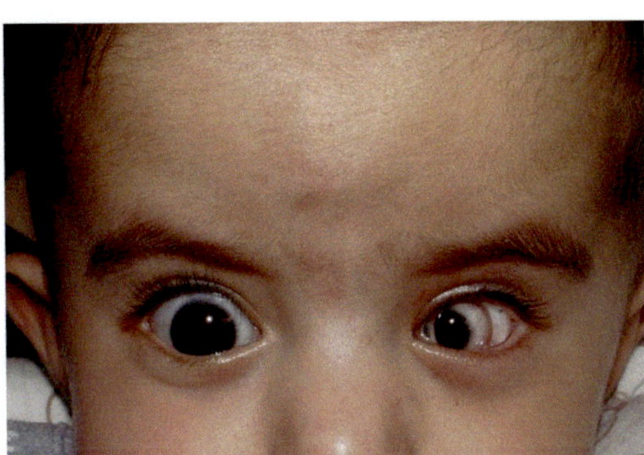

Fig. 65.7 Presence of microphthalmic eye with relatively acceptable volume in a pediatric patient, the use of ring conformers can be an option. If the patient feels comfortable without any ocular irritation ocular prosthesis can be used over the phthisic eye as a next step. However close monitoring with an experienced ocularist is necessary for optimal socket rehabilitation

Conformers can be used as primary treatment before the removal of the blind eye if the globe is not severely phthisic or not painful or if there are some conflicts for surgical removal of the eye due to the expectations of the family at the first visit (Fig. 65.7).

An experienced ocularist using monthly progressive conformer expansion can achieve growth of both soft tissue and bone [5–40]. Occasionally, oral mucous membrane grafts are needed to reconstruct the conjunctival cul-de-sac to accommodate larger conformers. Conjunctival flaps and, mucous membrane or amniotic membrane grafts can also be used to cover the cornea in cases of corneal irritation. The application of the conformers or prosthesis on the small eye does not need surgical intervention and it seems practical for both physician and the family. However, a large prosthesis over a small phthisic eye may cause orbital volume deficiency and facial asymmetry, and eyelid malposition as well. Thus, close collaboration between the ocularist and the ophthalmologist is necessary to achieve the optimal outcome (Fig. 65.8).

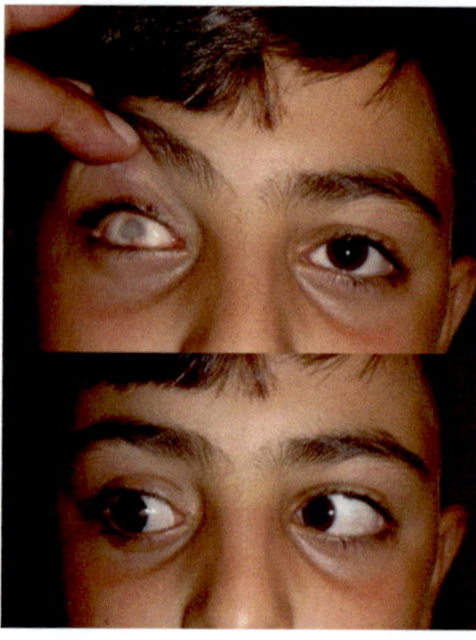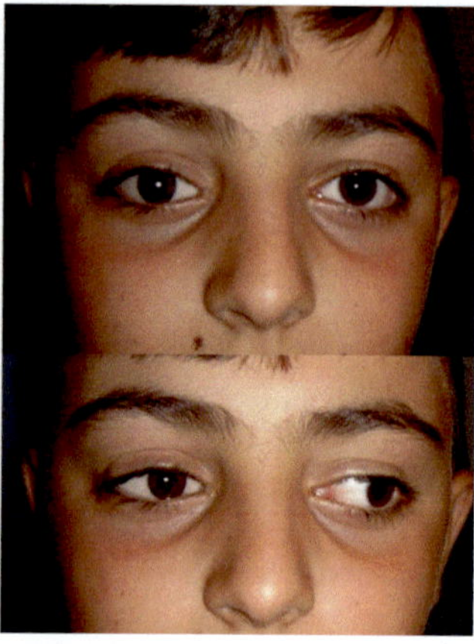

Fig. 65.8 9 years old boy presented with phthisis bulbi on the right eye after vitrectomy surgery due to penetrating eye injury. He has considerable globe volume without any pain or ocular symptoms. He received an ocular prosthesis over his phthisic eye with an acceptable cosmetic result

Conclusions

1. The management of anophthalmic or microphthalmic socket in a pediatric case younger than 5 years usually needs an implant that can increase in size like dermis fat draft or expandible orbital implants.
2. The presence or suspicion of an intraocular tumor is the most important contraindication for evisceration surgery. In the presence of endophthalmitis, either evisceration or enucleation can be selected Ideally, surgery can be delayed until the eye is phthisic and the orbital inflammation is healed with systemic antibiotics and anti-inflammatory treatment at which time eye removal and orbital implantation can be performed at the same session.
3. A careful review of the literature does not allow one to come to a definitive conclusion regarding the risk of sympathetic ophthalmia after evisceration. Evisceration is a safe and effective procedure with little risk of sympathetic ophthalmia.
4. The most used implant choices are silicone or polymethyl methacrylate (PMMA) synthetic spheres, coralline hydroxyapatite, synthetic hydroxyapatite, porous polyethylene, and dermis fat grafts. it is shown that the hydroxyapatite and porous polyethylene implants have much higher rates of extrusion than the smooth acrylic and silicone implants. there is no difference in implant or prosthetic movement between sclera-covered nonpegged hydroxyapatite porous implants and sclera-covered spherical acrylic implants.
5. Dermis fat graft shows good integration with no possibility of extrusion, it may provide deeper fornices in contracted sockets, and its usage reduces the cost when compared with alloplastic implants. The dermis-fat graft is an ideal

implant for children younger than 5 years old as it can expand with the growing pediatric orbit.

6. Conformers can be used as primary treatment before the removal of the blind eye if the globe is not severely phthisic or not painful or if there are some conflicts for surgical removal of the eye due to the expectations of the family at the first visit.

Review Questions

1. Which of the following implants will be more appropriate for orbital volume replacement after eye removal in a 3 years old patient?

a. Acrylic implant
b. Dermis fat graft
c. Fascia lata graft
d. Hydroxyapatite implant
e. Silicone implant

2. Which of the following materials cannot be used as an implant for orbital volume augmentation after eye removal?

a. Silicone
b. Dermis fat
c. Fascia lata
d. Glass
e. PMMA

3. Which statement is true for evisceration surgery?

a. It increases the risk for symphatetic ophthalmia
b. It can be preferred to enucleation for management of recalcitrant enophthalmitis
c. Only small implants can be used in phthisic globes
d. Surgeons need additional wrapping material for implantation during evisceration
e. Only hydroxyapatite materials can be used for implantation during evisceration procedure

Answers

1. B
2. C
3. B

References

1. Dunn ES, Jaeger EA, Jeffers JB, et al. The epidemiology of ruptured globes. Ann Ophthalmol. 1992;24(11):405–10.
2. Spraul C, Grossniklaus H. Analysis of 24,444 surgical specimens accessioned over 55 years in an ophthalmic pathology laboratory. Int J Ophthalmol. 1997–1998;21(5):283–304.
3. Wong TY, Seet MB, Ang CL. Eye injuries in twentieth century warfare: a historical perspective. Surv Ophthalmol. 1997;41(6):433–59.
4. Kennedy RE. The effect of early enucleation on the orbit in animals and humans. Adv Ophthalmic Plast Reconstr Surg. 1992;9:1–39.
5. Chen D, Heher K. Management of the anophthalmic socket in pediatric patients. Curr Opin Ophthalmol. 2004;15(5):449–53.
6. Timothy NH, Freilich DE, Linberg JV. Evisceration versus enucleation from the Ocularist's perspective. Ophthal Plast Reconstr Surg. 2003;19(6):417–20.
7. Dortzbach RK, Wog JJ. Choice of procedure: enucleation, evisceration, or prosthetic fitting over globe. Ophthalmol. 1985;92(9):1249–55.
8. Walter WL. Update on enucleation and evisceration surgery. Ophthal Plast Reconstr Surg. 1985;1(4):243–52.
9. O'Donnell BA, Kersten R, McNab A, Rose G, Rosser P. Enucleation versus evisceration. Clin Exp Ophthalmol. 2005;33(1):5–9.
10. Long JA, Tann TM, Girkin CA. Evisceration: a new technique of trans-scleral implant placement. Ophthal Plast Reconstr Surg. 2000;16(5):322–5.
11. Massry GG, Holds JB. Evisceration with scleral modification. Ophthal Plast Reconstr Surg. 2001;17(1):42–7.
12. Isenberg SJ, Editor, The eye in infancy. Chicago: Year Book Medical Publishers. 1989:31–6.
13. Farkas LG, Posnick JC, Hreczko TM, et al. Growth patterns in the orbital region: a morphometric study. Cleft Palate-Craniofac J. 1992;29(4):315–8.
14. Bentley RP, Sgouros S, Natarajan K, et al. Normal changes in orbital volume during childhood. J Neurosurg. 2002;96(4):742–6.
15. Kaliki S, Taneja S, Palkonda VAR. Inadvertent intraocular surgery in children with unsuspected retinoblastoma: a study of 14 cases. Retina. 2019;39(9):1794–2180.
16. Dresner SC, Karesh JW. Primary implant placement with evisceration in patients with endophthalmitis. Ophthalmology. 2000;107(9):1661–4.
17. Chaithanyaa N, Devireddy SK, Kishore RVK, et al. Sympathetic ophthalmia: a review of literature. Oral Surg Oral Med Oral Pathol Oral Radiol. 2012;113(2):172–6.
18. Yang J, Li Y, Xie R, et al. Sympathetic ophthalmia: report of a case series and comprehensive review of the literature. Eur J Ophthalmol. 2021;31(6):3099–109.
19. Chu XK, Chan C-C. Sympathetic ophthalmia: to the twenty-first century and beyond. J Ophthalmic Inflamm Infect. 2013;3(1):49.
20. Kilmartin DJ, Wilson D, Liversidge J, et al. Immunogenetics and clinical phenotype of sympathetic ophthalmia in British and Irish Patients. Br J Ophthalmol. 2001;85(3):281–6.
21. Zhong Z, Su G, Kijlstra A, et al. Activation of the interleukin-23/interleukin- 17 signalling pathway in autoinflammatory and autoimmune uveitis. Prog Retin Eye Res. 2021;80: 100866.
22. Stafford WR. Sympathetic ophthalmia: report of a case occurring ten and one-half days after injury. Arch Ophthalmol. 1965;74(4):521–4.
23. Karpinski H, Laszczyk WA. Sympathetic ophthalmia 30 years after evisceration. Klin Oczna. 1969;39(2):333–6.
24. Kilmartin DJ, Dick AD, Forrester JV. Prospective surveillance of sympathetic ophthalmia in the UK and Republic of Ireland. Br J Ophthalmol. 2000;84(3):259–63.
25. Bilyk JR. Enucleation, evisceration, and sympathetic ophthalmia. Curr Opin Ophthalmol. 2000;11(5):372–86.

26. Hansen AB, Petersen C, Heegaard S, et al. Review of 1028 bulbar eviscerations and enucleations: changes in etiology and frequency over a 20-year period. Acta Ophthalmol Scand. 1999;77(3):331–5.

27. Levine MR, Pou CR, Lash RH. The 1998 Wendell Hughes lecture. Evisceration: is sympathetic ophthalmia a concern in the new millennium? Ophthal Plast Reconstr Surg. 1999;15(1):4–8.

28. Migliori ME. Enucleation versus evisceration. Curr Opin Ophthalmol. 2002;13(5):298–302.

29. Quaranta-Leoni FM, Fiorino MG, Quaranta-Leoni F, et al. Anophthalmic socket syndrome: prevalence impact and management strategies. Clin Ophthalmol. 2021;15:3267–81.

30. Nunery WR, Heinz GW, Bonnin JM, et al. Exposure rate of hydroxyapatite spheres in the anophthalmic socket: histopathologic correlation and comparison with silicone sphere implants. Ophthal Plast Reconstr Surg. 1993;9(2):96–104.

31. Li T, Shen J, Duffy MT. Exposure rates of wrapped and unwrapped orbital implants following enucleation. Ophthal Plast Reconstr Surg. 2001;17(6):431–5.

32. Wladis EJ, Aakalu VK, Sobel RK, et al. Orbital implants in enucleation surgery: a report by the American Academy of Ophthalmology. Ophthalmol. 2018;125(2):311–7.

33. Colen TP, Paridaens DA, Lemij HG, et al. Comparison of artificial eye amplitudes with acrylic and hydroxyapatite spherical enucleation implants. Ophthalmology. 2000;107(10):1889–94.

34. Jordan DR, Stoica B, Klapper SR. Current indications for pegging in the anophthalmic socket: are there any? Curr Opin Ophthalmol. 2016;27(5):465–73.

35. Lin CW, Liao SL. Long-term complications of different porous orbital implants: a 21-year review. Br J Ophthalmol. 2017;101(5):681–5.

36. Viswanathan P, Sagoo MS, Olver JM. UK national survey of enucleation, evisceration and orbital implant trends. Br J Ophthalmol. 2007;91(5):616–9.

37. Jovanovic N, Carniciu AL, Russell WW, et al. Reconstruction of the orbit and Anophthalmic socket using the dermis fat graft: a major review. Ophthalmic Plast Reconstr Surg. 2020;36(6):529–39.

38. Modugno AC, Resti AG, Mazzone G, et al. Long-term outcomes after cosmetic customized prostheses and dermis fat graft in congenital anophthalmia: a retrospective multicentre study. Eye (Lond). 2018;32(12):1803–10.

39. Schittkowski MP, Guthoff RF. Injectable self-inflating hydrogel pellet expanders for the treatment of orbital volume deficiency in congenital microphthalmos: preliminary results with a new therapeutic approach. Br J Ophthalmol. 2006;90(9):1173–7.

40. Quaranta-Leoni FM. Congenital anophthalmia: current concepts in management. Curr Opin Ophthalmol. 2011;22(5):380–4.

41. Tao JP, LeBoyer RM, Hetzler K, et al. Inferolateral migration of hydrogel orbital implants in microphthalmia. Ophthal Plast Reconstr Surg. 2010;26(1):14–7.

42. Grossman MD, Mohay J, Roberts DM. Expansion of the human microphthalmic orbit. Ophthalmology. 1999;106(10):2005–9.

Management of Combined Hamartoma of the Retina and Retinal Pigment Epithelium in Children

66

Sofía M. Muns, Victor M. Villegas, and Timothy G. Murray

Abstract

Combined hamartoma of the retina and the retinal pigment epithelium (CHRRPE) is a congenital benign proliferation of the retinal pigment epithelium, neurosensory retina, retinal vasculature, and adjacent vitreous. CHRRPE usually presents as a unilateral slightly elevated and variably pigmented mass with vascular tortuosity and epiretinal membrane (ERM) formation in a pediatric patient. Lesions may be classified based on fundus location, structural retinal components and optical coherence tomography findings using the CHRRPE classification system. This system may be a valuable tool for quantifying severity and guiding management. In general, macular lesions are more likely to cause poor visual acuity and progressive visual loss. Close follow-up is

S. M. Muns · V. M. Villegas
Department of Ophthalmology, University of Puerto Rico, San Juan, Puerto Rico, USA
e-mail: sofia.muns@upr.edu

V. M. Villegas
e-mail: v.villegas@villegasmd.com

V. M. Villegas
Bascom Palmer Eye Institute, University of Miami Miller School of Medicine, Miami, FL, USA

T. G. Murray (✉)
Miami Ocular Oncology and Retina, Miami, FL, USA
e-mail: tmurray@murraymd.com

© The Author(s), under exclusive license to Springer Nature Switzerland AG 2023
Ş. Özdek et al. (eds.), *Pediatric Vitreoretinal Surgery*,
https://doi.org/10.1007/978-3-031-14506-3_66

987

recommended to monitor disease progression including exudation, subretinal neovascularization and ERM progression. Pars plana vitrectomy with membrane peeling may be considered in select cases.

Keywords

Combined hamartoma of the retina and retinal pigment epithelium · Vitreoretinal surgery · Optical coherence tomography · Fluorescein angiography · Epiretinal membrane

Introduction

Background

Combined hamartoma of the retina and the retinal pigment epithelium (CHRRPE) is an uncommon benign proliferation of the retinal pigment epithelium (RPE), neurosensory retina, retinal vasculature, and adjacent vitreous [1–6]. The acronym "CHRRPE" was first coined by Gass et al. in 1973 after histopathological studies [5, 6]. Decreased visual acuity (VA) may be present at initial diagnosis depending on the location of the lesion [2, 3]. It usually presents as a unilateral lesion located on or adjacent to the optic disc, at the macula, or in the peripheral retina [1, 2]. Common characteristics of these tumors include vascular tortuosity, variable pigmentation, slight elevation, and epiretinal membrane (ERM) formation [1, 4–7].

Pathophysiology

CHRRPE appears to be a congenital lesion, but its pathogenesis remains unknown [2, 7, 8]. Pujari and colleagues [8] hypothesized that the tumor may arise from inner layer progenitor cells that differentiate into RPE like cells. These ectopic RPE cells may be unable to undergo further differentiation into mature RPE because of lack of necessary local homeostatic factors [8]. This arrest in development may lead to hyperplasia and fibrosis that results in an intra-retinal mass consisting of glial cells, vascular tissue, and sheets of pigment epithelial cells [7, 8].

Clinical Features

Painless vision loss is the most common presenting symptom of CHRRPE [2, 5, 7, 9, 10]. Amblyopia and strabismus are also frequently present [2, 7–10]. Less prevalent findings include floaters, afferent pupillary defect, ocular pain, leukocoria, and intraocular inflammation [2, 7].

CHRRPE lesions are slightly elevated and variably pigmented, usually gray in color [2, 3, 7]. These lesions are frequently unilateral and are commonly found in the macula but may also be present in the peripapillary and peripheral regions [2, 9]. Retinal vascular tortuosity is a prominent feature of CHRRPE [2] (Fig. 66.1). Other

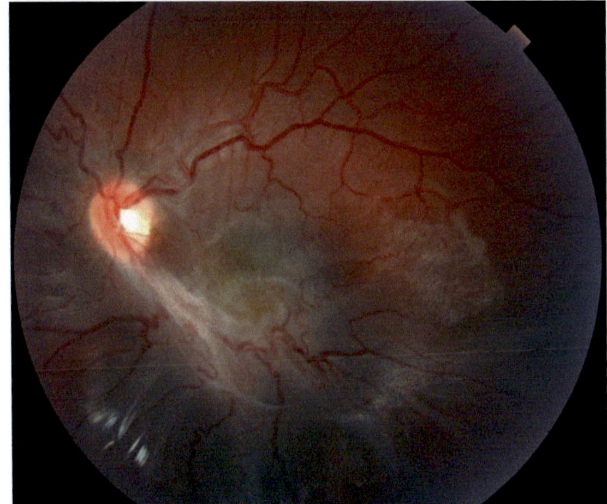

Fig. 66.1 Color fundus photograph of CHRRPE showing classical grayish color, preretinal fibrosis, and vascular tortuosity along the inferotemporal arcade

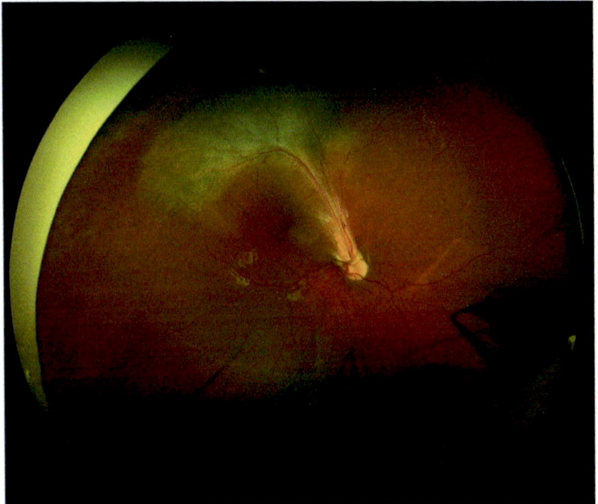

Fig. 66.2 Infrared pseudocolor photograph of CHRRPE showing vascular dragging of the superotemporal arcade in a 4-year-old boy with 20/20 visual acuity

fundus characteristics include retinal exudation, traction, fibrosis/gliosis, retinal detachment, vitreous hemorrhage, macular edema, choroidal neovascularization, and foveal dragging [2, 7, 10] (Fig. 66.2).

Lesions may be classified based on fundus location, structural retinal components and optical coherence tomography (OCT) findings (Table 66.1) [3]. Patients with macular and peripapillary lesions (Zone 1) are at greater risk of developing vision loss secondary to amblyopia and/or macular detachment. Lesions with no retinal traction (Stage 1) are associated with the best visual prognosis. Lesions with an epiretinal component only (A) have better visual prognosis and are less likely to have macular detachment. Patients with lesions that have retinal detachment and complete retinal and RPE involvement (Stage 3C) have the highest risk of vision loss.

Table 66.1 Classification system for combined hamartoma of the retina and retinal pigment epithelium lesions developed by Dedania and colleagues [3]

Fundus location of lesion	Structural status of retina	Anatomy of lesion
Zone 1: macular/peripapillary lesion	Stage 1: lesion with no retinal traction	A: lesion with an epiretinal component only
		B: lesion with partial retinal involvement
		C: lesion with complete retinal and RPE involvement
	Stage 2: lesion with retinal traction or retinoschisis	A: lesion with an epiretinal component only
		B: lesion with partial retinal involvement
		C: lesion with complete retinal and RPE involvement
	Stage 3: lesion with detached retina	A: lesion with an epiretinal component only
		B: lesion with partial retinal involvement
		C: lesion with complete retinal and RPE involvement
Zone 2: lesion at mid-periphery	Stage 1: lesion with no retinal traction	A: lesion with an epiretinal component only
		B: lesion with partial retinal involvement
		C: lesion with complete retinal and RPE involvement
	Stage 2: lesion with retinal traction or retinoschisis	A: lesion with an epiretinal component only
		B: lesion with partial retinal involvement
		C: lesion with complete retinal and RPE involvement
	Stage 3: lesion with detached retina	A: lesion with an epiretinal component only
		B: lesion with partial retinal involvement
		C: lesion with complete retinal and RPE involvement

(continued)

Table 66.1 (continued)

Fundus location of lesion	Structural status of retina	Anatomy of lesion
Zone 3: lesion at far periphery	Stage 1: lesion with no retinal traction	A: lesion with an epiretinal component only
		B: lesion with partial retinal involvement
		C: lesion with complete retinal and RPE involvement
	Stage 2: lesion with retinal traction or retinoschisis	A: lesion with an epiretinal component only
		B: lesion with partial retinal involvement
		C: lesion with complete retinal and RPE involvement
	Stage 3: lesion with detached retina	A: lesion with an epiretinal component only
		B: lesion with partial retinal involvement
		C: lesion with complete retinal and RPE involvement

Fluorescein angiography (FA), OCT and ultrasound are also useful in describing CHRRPE lesions. OCT usually shows a thickened retinal mass with hyperreflective surface, deep shadowing, ERM associated with retinal folds, striae, and full-thickness retinal disorganization [6] (Fig. 66.3). FA typically shows lesions with vascular tortuosity, abnormal retinal capillaries, and leakage from anomalous retinal vessels within the lesion [2]. Ultrasound commonly shows a hyperechoic epiretinal mass (Fig. 66.4) that may also be associated to tractional changes [11].

Non-surgical Management

The main goal of treatment for patients with CHRRPE is to preserve visual function. Small peripheral asymptomatic lesions may be observed. However, children in the amblyogenic age range with macular involvement and visual prognosis should be treated promptly to improve or preserve foveal function and start amblyopia therapy. Although evidence is limited, amblyopia therapy has been associated with improvement in VA even in eyes with historically poor prognosis [2, 3].

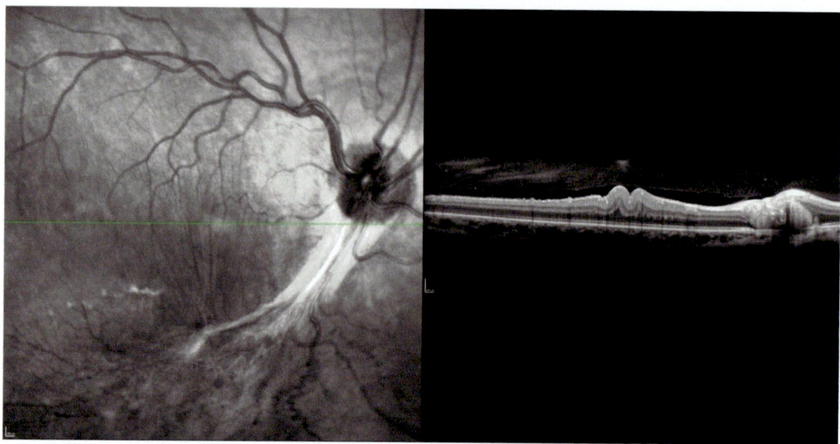

Fig. 66.3 Macular spectral domain OCT showing retinal thickening, retinal folds, and loss of retinal architecture

Fig. 66.4 Ultrasonography shows a juxtapapillary epiretinal hyperechoic mass with posterior shadowing

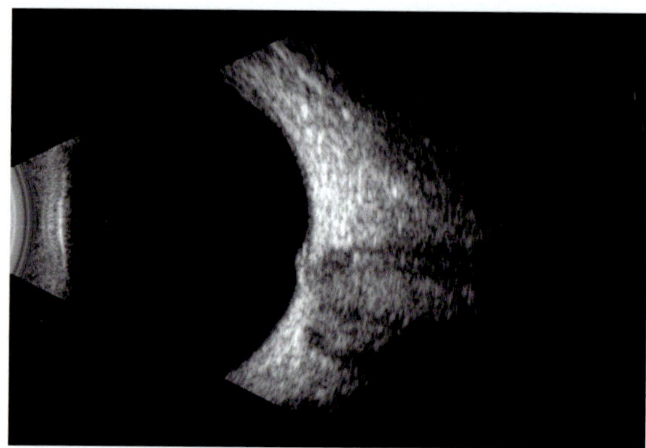

Patients with CHRRPE should undergo a complete ophthalmological examination and periodic follow-up evaluation, including OCT characterization [3]. Patients should be monitored for ERM progression, exudation, tractional retinal detachment, vitreous hemorrhage, choroidal neovascularization and visual decline [2, 7, 10]. Intravitreal antiangiogenic agents may be considered if exudative changes are present.

The classification system developed by Dedania et al. [3] is a useful tool to guide follow-up in patients with CHRRPE. Patients with macular and peripapillary lesions (Zone 1) may benefit from routine evaluation at least every 2 to 4 months. Patients with lesions in the midperiphery (Zone 2) and retinal traction or retinoschisis (Stage 2) may be followed every 3 to 4 months. Patients with lesions in the midperiphery (Zone 2) and no retinal traction (Stage 1) may be followed every 6 months. Patients with lesions in the far periphery (Stage 3) may be followed every 6 or 12 months, depending on the stage of lesion.

Patients with bilateral CHRRPE lesions may benefit from genetic testing due to its frequent association with neurofibromatosis Type 1 and 2 [3].

Surgical Management

Literature regarding the utility of surgery in pediatric patients with CHRRPE remains limited and results are controversial. Varying degrees of VA improvement have been observed after pars plana vitrectomy (PPV) with membrane peeling among patients with CHRRPE [2, 7]. However, some recent reports have shown encouraging results.

Pediatric patients with VA loss, CHRRPE and associated ERM formation may benefit from PPV with membrane peeling [1, 12–15]. This surgery has been associated with post-operative improvements in VA and retinal anatomy [1, 12–15]. Some studies have reported post-operative improvement in retinal thickness and disorganization in OCT [1, 15, 16]. Decrease in retinal vascular tortuosity has also been observed post-operatively among these patients [13, 15, 16]. Patients should be monitored for recurrence of ERM after surgery [12, 14]. Future prospective studies may elucidate the risks and benefits of surgery to remove the ERM in patients with CHRRPE [7].

Conclusion

CHRRPE is a congenital benign hamartomatous lesion that may be associated to permanent visual loss. The classical presentation includes a unilateral slightly elevated and variably pigmented mass with vascular tortuosity and ERM formation in a pediatric patient. The CHRRPE classification system may be a valuable tool for quantifying severity and guiding management. In general, macular lesions are more likely to cause poor VA and progressive visual loss. Close follow-up is recommended to monitor disease progression including exudation, subretinal neovascularization and ERM progression. PPV with membrane peeling may be considered in select cases.

Review Questions

1. A 7-year-old boy with progressive vision loss is diagnosed with combined hamartoma of the retina and the retinal pigment epithelium (CHRRPE). What is the most accurate statement regarding the surgical management of pediatric patients with CHRRPE?

A. Pars plana vitrectomy (PPV) with membrane peeling in pediatric patients with loss of VA, CHRRPE and associated ERM formation has been consistently associated with worsening VA post-operatively.
B. PPV with membrane peeling in pediatric patients with loss of VA, CHRRPE and associated ERM formation is associated with increased vascular tortuosity post-operatively.
C. PPV with membrane peeling in pediatric patients with loss of VA, CHRRPE and associated ERM formation is contraindicated.
D. Pediatric patients with loss of VA, CHRRPE, and associated ERM formation may benefit from PPV with membrane peeling. This surgery has been associated with post-operative improvements in VA and retinal anatomy.

2. A 6 year-old girl is evaluated at your clinic. Fundus findings show a lesion with grayish color, preretinal fibrosis, and vascular tortuosity along the inferotemporal arcade. OCT shows retinal thickening, retinal folds, and loss of retinal architecture. What is true about the visual prognosis of these lesions?

A. Lesions with no retinal traction are associated with poor visual prognosis.
B. Lesions with an epiretinal component only have worse visual prognosis and are more likely to have macular detachment.
C. Patients with macular and peripapillary lesions are at greater risk of developing vision loss secondary to amblyopia and/or macular detachment.
D. Patients with lesions that have retinal detachment and complete retinal and retinal pigment epithelium (RPE) involvement have a low risk of vision loss.

3. A 9 year-old girl is referred for ophthalmic evaluation due to vision loss and suspected CHRRPE. What would you expect to see on fundus autofluorescence (FA)?

A. A lesion with vascular tortuosity, abnormal retinal capillaries, and leakage from anomalous retinal vessels at the peripheral margin of the lesion.
B. A lesion with vascular tortuosity, abnormal retinal capillaries, and leakage from anomalous retinal vessels within the lesion.
C. A lesion with vascular tortuosity, normal retinal capillaries, and leakage from anomalous retinal vessels within the lesion.
D. A lesion without vascular tortuosity, abnormal retinal capillaries, and leakage from anomalous retinal vessels within the lesion.

Answers

1. (**D**) Literature regarding the utility of surgery in pediatric patients with CHRRPE remains limited and results are controversial. Varying degrees of VA improvement have been observed after PPV with membrane peeling among patients with CHRRPE. However, some recent reports have shown encouraging results. Pediatric patients with loss of VA, CHRRPE and associated ERM formation may benefit from PPV with membrane peeling. This surgery has been associated with post-operative improvements in VA and retinal anatomy. Some studies have

reported post-operative improvement in retinal thickness and disorganization in optical coherence tomography (OCT). Decrease in retinal vascular tortuosity has also been observed post-operatively among these patients.

2. (**C**) CHRRPE lesions may be classified based on fundus location, structural retinal components and OCT findings. Patients with macular and peripapillary lesions (Zone 1) are at greater risk of developing vision loss secondary to amblyopia and/or macular detachment. Lesions with no retinal traction (Stage 1) are associated with the best visual prognosis. Lesions with an epiretinal component only (A) have better visual prognosis and are less likely to have macular detachment. Patients with lesions that have retinal detachment and complete retinal and RPE involvement (Stage 3C) have the highest risk of vision loss.

3. (**B**) FA may be useful in describing CHRRPE lesions. FA usually shows lesions with vascular tortuosity, .abnormal retinal capillaries, and leakage from anomalous retinal vessels within the lesion.

References

1. Sun LS, Raouf S, Rhee D, Ferrone PJ. Surgical outcomes of Epiretinal membrane removal due to combined hamartoma of the retina and RPE. 2020;51:546–54.
2. Schachat AP, Shields JA, Fine SL, Sanborn GE, Weingeist TA, Valenzuela RE, Brucker AJ. Combined hamartomas of the retina and retinal pigment epithelium. 1984;91:1609–15.
3. Dedania VS, Ozgonul C, Zacks DN, Besirli CG. Novel classification system for combined hamartoma of the retina and retinal pigment epithelium. 2018;38:12–9.
4. McDonald HR, Abrams GW, Burke JM, Neuwirth J. Clinicopathologic results of vitreous surgery for epiretinal membranes in patients with combined retinal and retinal pigment epithelial hamartomas. 1985;100:806–13.
5. Gass JD. An unusual hamartoma of the pigment epithelium and retina simulating choroidal melanoma and retinoblastoma. 1973;71:171–83.
6. Arrigo A, Corbelli E, Aragona E, Manitto MP, Martina E, Bandello F, Parodi MB. Optical coherence tomography and optical coherence tomography angiography evaluation of combined hamartoma of the retina and retinal pigment epithelium. 2019;39:1009–15.
7. Shields CL, Thangappan A, Hartzell K, Valente P, Pirondini C, Shields JA. Combined hamartoma of the retina and retinal pigment epithelium in 77 consecutive patients visual outcome based on macular versus extramacular tumor location. 2008;115:2246–2252.
8. Pujari A, Agarwal D, Chawla R, Todi V, Kumar A. Congenital simple hamartoma of the retinal pigment epithelium: what is the probable cause? 2019;123:79–80.
9. Ledesma-Gil G, Essilfie J, Gupta R, Fung AT, Lupidi M, Pappuru RR, Nayak S, Sahoo NK, Kaliki S, Yannuzzi LA, Reid K, Lim L, Sacconi R, Dave V, Singh SR, Ayachit A, Gabrielle PH, Cai S, Lima LH, Querques G, Arevalo JF, Freund KB, Shields CL, Chhablani J. Presumed natural history of combined hamartoma of the retina and retinal pigment epithelium. 2021;5:1156–63.
10. Font RL, Moura RA, Shetlar DJ, Martinez JA, McPherson AR. Combined hamartoma of sensory retina and retinal pigment epithelium. 1989;9:302–11.
11. Shields CL, Mashayekhi A, Dai VV, Materin MA, Shields JA. Optical coherence tomographic findings of combined hamartoma of the retina and retinal pigment epithelium in 11 patients. 2005;123:1746–50.

12. Cohn AD, Quiram PA, Drenser KA, Trese MT, Capone A Jr. Surgical outcomes of epiretinal membranes associated with combined hamartoma of the retina and retinal pigment epithelium. 2009;29:825–30.
13. Sappenfield DL, Gitter KA. Surgical intervention for combined retinal-retinal pigment epithelial hamartoma. 1990;10:119–24.
14. Benhamou N, Massin P, Spolaore R, Paques M, Gaudric A. Surgical management of epiretinal membrane in young patients. 2002;133:358–64.
15. Konstantinidis L, Chamot L, Zografos L, Wolfensberger TJ. Pars plana vitrectomy and epiretinal membrane peeling for vitreoretinal traction associated with combined hamartoma of the retina and retinal pigment epithelium (CHRRPE). 2007;224:356–9.
16. Zhang X, Dong F, Dai R, Yu W. Surgical management of epiretinal membrane in combined hamartomas of the retina and retinal pigment epithelium. 2010;30:305–9.

Telemedicine for Pediatric Retinal Disorders: Retinopathy of Prematurity Screening Programs

67

Amy E. Pohodich, Michael F. Chiang, and Allison R. Loh

Abstract

Retinopathy of prematurity (ROP) stems from abnormal vascular development within the retina of premature infants. As the rates of both premature births and survival of premature babies increases, the demand for ROP screening has increased. In order to improve access to care, the number of telemedicine programs that provide remote ROP screening of premature infants has increased. Telemedicine programs for ROP have proven cost-effective and safe. The key components of a telemedicine program include well-trained personnel, robust communication networks, adequate equipment and data storage.

Keywords

Retinopathy of prematurity · Premature infant · Telemedicine · Screening program

A. E. Pohodich (✉) · A. R. Loh
Department of Ophthalmology, Oregon Health and Science University, Portland, USA
e-mail: pohodich@ohsu.edu

A. R. Loh
e-mail: loha@ohsu.edu

M. F. Chiang
National Eye Institute, National Institutes of Health, Bethesda, USA
e-mail: Michael.chiang@nih.gov

Ş. Özdek et al. (eds.), *Pediatric Vitreoretinal Surgery*,
https://doi.org/10.1007/978-3-031-14506-3_67

997

Introduction

Telemedicine harnesses telecommunications technology to provide healthcare remotely, and has the potential benefits of expanding access to healthcare, decreasing costs, and improving health outcomes. There are two main methods of telemedicine: real-time which is the synchronous interaction of healthcare provider and patient (e.g., teleconferencing virtual visit), and store-and-forward where data is collected and transmitted for future evaluation (e.g., interpretation of lab results or images by a specialist from a different institution) [1]. Within the scope of pediatric retina, the primary application of telemedicine is in the context of screening and diagnosis of retinopathy of prematurity (ROP) using the store-and-forward method.

ROP results from abnormal retinal vasculature development in premature infants, with the highest incidence of ROP (68%) in babies with birth weight less than 1251 g [2]. ROP is an appropriate disease for screening because the disease prevalence is high in the target population, abnormal exam findings can be seen before symptom onset, and there are effective treatments that can reduce morbidity [3]. Historically, the gold standard for ROP screening has been in person indirect ophthalmoscopy by a pediatric ophthalmologist or a retina specialist while the baby is in the neonatal intensive care unit (NICU). Interest in developing ways to expand ROP screening care has grown as the number of premature infants requiring screening rises due to increasing rates of premature births and enhanced survival of premature infants [4–6]. Numerous studies over the last two decades have evaluated the use of remote screening for ROP, and have shown high accuracy and validity of retinal photography for detecting clinically significant ROP, and evaluation of wide-field images by trained reviewers has been shown to be as effective as indirect ophthalmoscopy for patient screening [7–13]. Further, telemedicine screening programs for ROP have been shown to be safe, cost-effective, and improve access to care [14–17].

Background

Per current guidelines from the American Academy of Pediatrics, American Academy of Ophthalmology, and the American Association for Pediatric Ophthalmology and Strabismus, screening for ROP should be performed for infants that have a birth weight $\leq$ 1500 g, gestational age (GA) $\leq$ 30 weeks, or selected high-risk infants (prolonged supplemental oxygen support, oxygen supplementation without blood saturation monitoring, or hypotensive requiring inotropes) with a birth weight between 1500 and 2000 g or GA of > 30 weeks [18]. Timing of the initial screening exam depends on the infant's GA at birth (Table 67.1) [18].

Table 67.1 Timing of initial screening exam based on gestational age at birth

Gestational age at birth (weeks)	Age at initial exam (weeks)	
	Postmenstrual age	Chronologic age
22	31	9
23	31	8
24	31	7
25	31	6
26	31	5
27	31	4
28	32	4
29	33	4
30	34	4
High risk for ROP	–	4

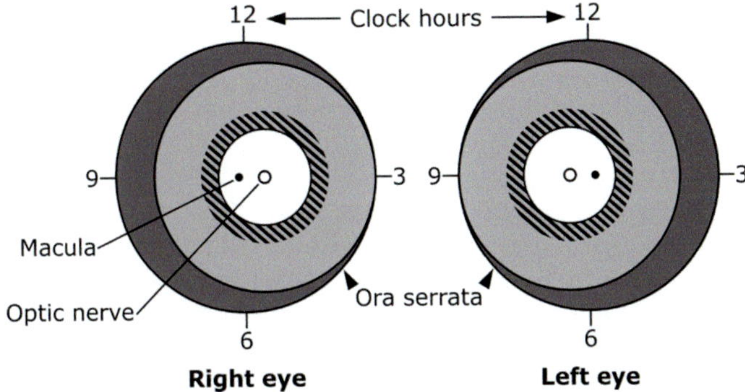

Fig. 67.1 Retina schematic showing ROP zones. White circle: Zone I. Light grey circle: Zone II. Dark grey circle: Zone III. Shaded area represents posterior Zone II. Adapted from [19]

ROP is described and classified based on its location (Fig. 67.1), extent, stage and the presence or absence of plus disease. A brief outline of this classification system is provided in Table 67.2. Please see the original article from the International Committee for the Classification of Retinopathy of Prematurity (ICROP) for additional details and images [19].

Approach to Screening

Step 1. Creating a telemedicine screening program for ROP. Important considerations for establishing a telemedicine program include obtaining the necessary equipment, determining the means of communication and data storage, and training personnel [1]. For telemedicine in ROP, remote digital fundus imaging should be

Table 67.2 International Committee for the Classification of Retinopathy of Prematurity guidelines. Adapted from [19]. Classification should include zone, stage, plus disease and extent

ICROP classification system	
Location	All zones are circles centered on the optic disc
Zone I	The radius is two times the distance from the center of the optic disc to the center of the macula
Zone II	The radius is the distance from the center of the optic disc to the nasal ora serrata
Posterior Zone II	Starts at the junction of Zones I and II and extends two disc diameters into Zone II
Zone III	The remaining portion of retina anterior to Zone II
Extent	Logged as clock-hours
Stage of acute disease	
Stage 1	Demarcation line separating avascular (anterior) and vascularized retina (posterior)
Stage 2	Formation of a ridge (has height and width) in the area of the demarcation line. May have "popcorn", which are small areas of neovascular tissue posterior to ridge
Stage 3	Extension of fibrovascular proliferation from ridge to vitreous. Graded as mild, moderate or severe
Retinal detachment	
Stage 4	Partial retinal detachment Stage 4A: extrafoveal. Stage 4B: foveal
Stage 5	Total retinal detachment Stage 5A: optic disc visible on ophthalmoscopy. Stage 5B: Optic disc not visible (due to closed funnel detachment or obstructing retrolental fibrovascular tissue). Stage 5C: Stage 5B+anterior segment changes (e.g., corneal opacification, anterior chamber shallowing, iridocorneolenticular adhesions)
Plus disease	Arteriolar tortuosity and venous dilation of posterior pole retinal vessels in Zone I. Denoted by (+) after ROP stage
Pre-plus disease	Vascular changes in Zone I that do not meet criteria for plus disease
Aggressive ROP	Quickly progressive form of ROP that does not advance through the typical stages of ROP. Characterized by rapid development of severe plus disease and neovascularization
Regression	Either spontaneous or after treatment. Can be complete or incomplete. Must be documented with the location and extent of peripheral avascular retina
Reactivation	Occurs after ROP treatment and includes new ROP lesions or vascular abnormalities. Documented as "reactivated stage #"
Long-term sequelae	Numerous ocular abnormalities have been documented in patients who were born prematurely, including late retinal detachments, retinoschisis, macular abnormalities, persistent avascular retina, glaucoma, and persistent retinal vascular changes

obtained with a digital, color, wide-field camera. There are numerous wide-field mydriatic fundus cameras available (e.g., RetCam, Phoenix ICON, Visunex PanoCam, 3Nethra Neo). The remote facility must have imaging software, a secure storage medium, and internet access in order to process, log and transmit the images. Similarly, at the receiving institution, a robust information technology (IT) infrastructure must also be in place to ensure images are received and handled according to security and privacy guidelines and tracked to ensure prompt evaluation. The receiving institution should also have appropriately high-resolution monitors for viewing and grading the images.

A key feature of a successful telemedicine program is open and ready communication. Timing of image acquisition, including time of day and day of week, should be coordinated between the two institutions. Images should be sent with a notification to the receiving provider(s), and receipt should be acknowledged by the provider(s) [20]. Upon receipt, images should be analyzed and results reported back to the remote NICU promptly, commonly within 24 hours [20]. Communication of patient details and imaging grading should also be standardized to eliminate error due to variability, and a system should be set in place to ensure repeat imaging, if necessary, is obtained and reviewed.

Finally, to produce meaningful results, a telemedicine program must have trained personnel. The remote NICU team should be well versed in camera use, infant dilation, and post-dilation monitoring. When learning to use the camera, images should initially be compared with bedside indirect ophthalmoscopy until reliable imaging is obtained [20]. Image graders should also undergo training and oversight to ensure consistency and accuracy of grading. Multiple institutions have created their own training program overseen by a reading center, with multiple stages for certification [21, 22]. It is important to note that there should be multiple individuals able to obtain photographs and multiple graders to review images. Lastly, administrators also play a critical role in facilitating, maintaining and following up on communications between institutions.

Step 2. Image acquisition. The neonate should have his or her eyes dilated and wide-field photographs taken of both eyes. Typically, photos are taken of the posterior pole including the nerve and macula and the superior, temporal, inferior and nasal regions. Iris photos can also be taken to document dilation, which may be helpful in determining whether operator error or poor dilation could be causing poor image quality [20].

> Tip: care should be taken to not distort the globe when taking the image. Increased pressure can lead to impaired blood flow and incorrect interpretation of images [23].

Step 3. Image storage. The software used to store images and associated patient information should be secure. There should be back-ups of the data. If images need to be compressed, it should be done using a loss-less compression format.

Step 4. Image transfer. Should be performed using a secure method, with notifications between institutions when the image is sent and received.

Step 5. Reviewing an image.

- Set up: image grading should be done in a dark room on a computer with a big and bright monitor.

  Tip: Viewing images in a dark room can help with detection of subtle ROP changes (see Fig. 67.2).

- Is the image of good quality? Prior to grading, assess the photo for clarity and appropriate field of view.

  Tip: If the image is blurry, consider repeat imaging sooner vs immediate reimaging depending on patient age and risk assessment.

- Be systematic when grading. Establishing a standardized protocol for all reviewers improves accuracy and consistency amongst reviewers.

  Tip: Incorporate the protocol into the training module and imaging reporting system (see [24] for a training module example).

- Consider comparing image grading among different reviewers and adjust final reading as necessary to reach consensus, especially when establishing a program.

  Tip: Although small, there is a significant increase in both specificity and sensitivity for determining referral warranted ROP when comparing double adjudicated grading to single-reader grading [25].

Step 6. Referral for NICU transfer.

- A neonate should be transferred to a NICU for indirect ophthalmoscopy if there is 1. Plus disease in Zone I, 2. Stage 3 disease in Zone I, or 3. Stage 2–3 disease in Zone II with plus disease (see Fig. 67.1 and Table 67.2) [20, 26].

  Tip. Also consider transfer if there is rapid disease progression on serial imaging, a high concern for plus disease, or if imaging reveals other ocular concerns (e.g., cataract, buphthalmos, aniridia, etc.) (Fig. 67.3).

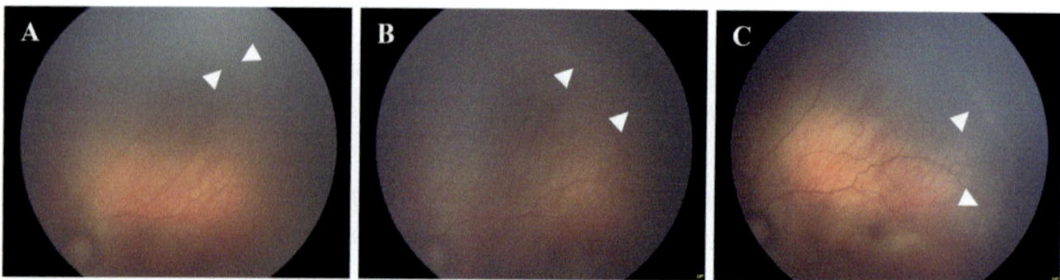

Fig. 67.2 Example of subtle ROP findings. **A.** Initial imaging showing faint demarcation line (between arrow heads). **B.** Image taken one week later showing progression to stage 2 disease (ridge indicated by arrows). **C.** Image obtained 10 days after (B) that more clearly shows stage 2 disease

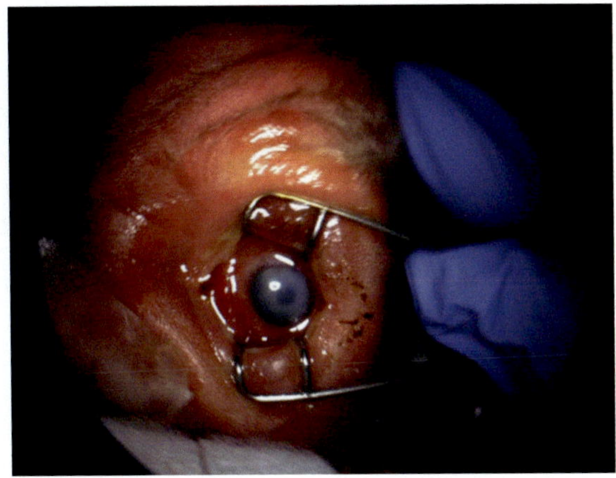

Fig. 67.3 Example of an ocular abnormality sent for review that was captured along with ROP screening images. This photo prompted urgent transfer to a tertiary medical center where the infant was diagnosed with Peter's anomaly

Case Presentation

History: The patient is a female (B.G.) born at 24 4/7 weeks gestational age with birth weight of 810 g. She has a history of bronchopulmonary dysplasia requiring temporary intubation, periventricular leukomalacia, perinatal intraventricular hemorrhage, and a patent ductus arteriosus requiring coiling.

Screening events:

- Postmenstrual age (PMA) 31 6/7 weeks: Initial ROP screening photos (Fig. 67.4A and B). Image quality limited interpretation, and B.G. was diagnosed as having Stage 1–2 disease in Zone I or posterior Zone II in both eyes.
- PMA 32 6/7 weeks: Because the initial imaging was insufficient to allow for definitive staging, she had repeat imaging performed 1 week later that showed bilateral Stage 2 ROP in Zone I or posterior Zone II (Fig. 67.4C and D).
- PMA 33 3/7 weeks: The presence of Stage 1–2 ROP in Zone I is an indication for follow-up in one week or less, and B.G. had repeat imaging performed 4 days after her prior exam (Fig. 67.4E and F). Her photographs showed stable Stage 2 ROP in Zone I or posterior Zone II in both eyes.
- PMA 34 2/7 weeks: One-week follow up imaging revealed bilateral Zone II, Stage 2 ROP with a few small areas of "popcorn" in the temporal retina of the left eye (Fig. 67.4G and H).
- PMA 35 2/7 weeks: B.G. had photographs taken 1 week after her prior imaging. Right eye grading remained stable (Fig. 67.4I). However, there was notable progression in the left eye to Stage 3 ROP in Zone II with Pre-plus disease (Fig. 67.4J).

Fig. 67.4 ROP screening photos of BG. **A** and **B**. Initial screening photo of B.G.'s **A** right eye and **B** left eye at PMA 31 6/7 weeks. **C** and **D**. One week follow up imaging of **C** right eye and **D** left eye. **E** and **F**. Imaging at postmenstrual age 33 3/7 weeks of **E** right eye and **F** left eye. **G** and **H** Imaging at postmenstrual age 34 2/7 weeks of **G** right eye and **H** left eye, which also has small areas of "popcorn" (arrows). **I** and **J** Imaging done at postmenstrual age 35 2/7 weeks of **I** right eye and **J** left eye. **K** and **L** Imaging done at postmenstrual age 35 2/7 weeks of **K** right eye and **L** left eye

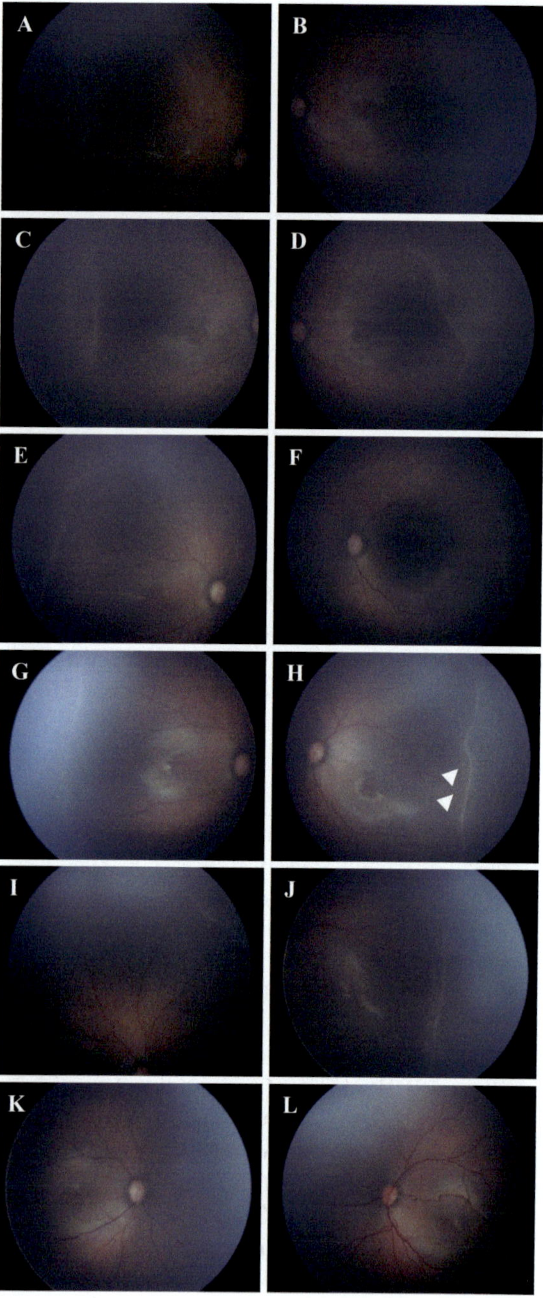

- <u>PMA 35 5/7 weeks</u>: Due to worsening disease OS with the presence of pre-plus disease, repeat imaging was obtained 3 days after last exam. Photographs showed disease progression in both eyes. Her right eye was graded as Zone II, Stage 2 ROP with pre-plus disease (Fig. 67.4K). Her left eye now had Zone II, Stage 3 ROP with plus disease (Fig. 67.4L), warranting her immediate transfer for indirect ophthalmoscopy.

After NICU transfer:

- <u>PMA 35 6/7 weeks</u>: B.G. evaluated at bedside and found to have plus disease in both eyes.
- <u>PMA 36 0/7 weeks</u>: Laser photocoagulation of the peripheral avascular retina was performed in both eyes.
- <u>PMA 36 4/7 weeks</u>: Repeat bedside indirect ophthalmoscopy showed good laser scars bilaterally with improved posterior vasculature in her right eye (Zone II, Stage 2 with pre-plus disease) and persistent plus disease in B.G.'s left eye (Zone II, Stage 3+).
- <u>PMA 37 4/7 weeks</u>: Both eyes showed significant improvement and disease regression. Her right eye had Stage 1 ROP with normal posterior vasculature, and her left eye had very thin Stage 3 remnants with normal posterior vasculature.
- <u>PMA 37 5/7 weeks</u>: B.G. was transferred back to her original NICU.

Ongoing follow-up:

- After returning to her original NICU, B.G. was followed remotely with weekly retinal imaging while she remained inpatient. Imaging showed regressed ROP with normal posterior vasculature in both eyes (Fig. 67.5A and B).
- B.G.'s retinal exam remained stable on office visits at 4.5 months of age and 7 months of age, and her appointments were spaced to yearly office visits.

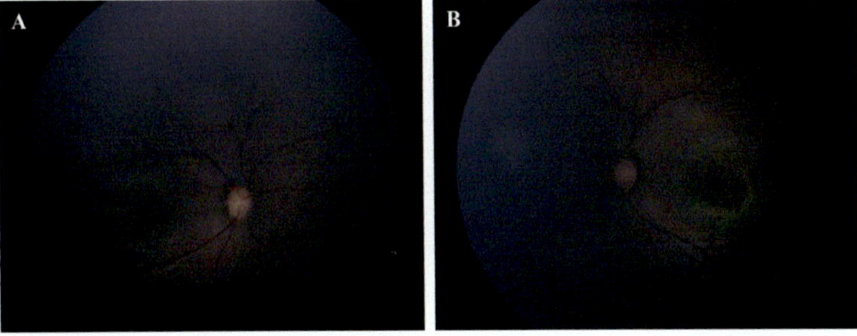

Fig. 67.5 Follow-up imaging of B.G. at 4 months of age showing regressed disease. **A** Right eye. **B** Left eye

Future Applications

As telemedicine screening becomes more widespread, it is likely that these programs could expand to include evaluation of multiple other pediatric eye concerns. Recent studies have shown retinal digital wide field imaging of all newborns to be superior to traditional red reflex testing in detecting ocular abnormalities [27, 28]. These results suggest that newborn retinal screening with imaging may supplant red reflex testing as telemedicine programs become more prevalent. It could also be added to a standard 1-year old well child exam or preschool screening to establish a baseline or detect an otherwise unnoticed congenital abnormality. Further, as with diabetic adults, fundus photography could be used to screen teenagers with diabetes.

Conclusion

The use of telemedicine in screening for ROP has expanded access to care, improved cost, and, anecdotally, helped with the detection and diagnosis of other ocular abnormalities. As the uses and benefits of eye screening via telemedicine increase, more programs will be required to meet these growing needs. Key considerations when establishing these screening programs are infrastructure, personnel and training. Clear and ready communication between collaborating institutions standardized screening approaches are also essential for a successful program.

Review Questions

1. The following are reasons to consider a telemedicine program for ROP screening except:

a. Improved access to trained retina specialists
b. Longer intervals between eye exams
c. Potential improvement in efficient use of resources
d. Improved documentation of exams with photography

2. What ROP stage is this eye?

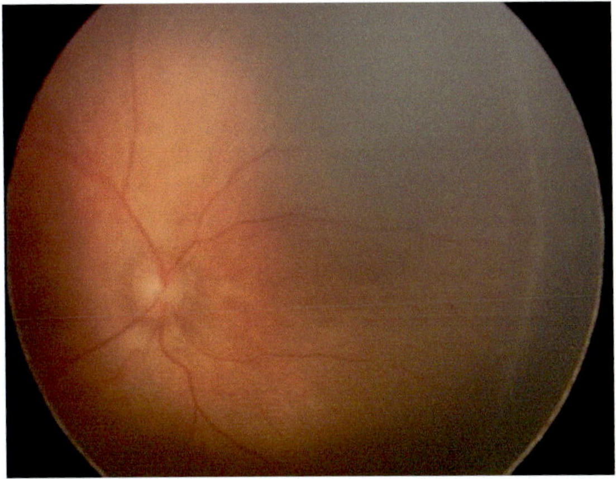

a. Stage 1
b. Stage 2
c. Stage 3

3. The following are requirements of an ROP telemedicine program except:

a. Availability of trained image readers
b. Robust communication and data storage program
c. Mydriatic wide-field fundus camera
d. Certification by a national accreditation body

Answers

1. B
2. B
3. D

References

1. Harnett B. Telemedicine systems and telecommunications. J Telemed Telecare. 2006;12 (1):4–15.
2. Good WV, Hardy RJ, Dobson V, Palmer EA, Phelps DL, Quintos M, et al. The incidence and course of retinopathy of prematurity: findings from the early treatment for retinopathy of prematurity study. Pediatrics. 2005;116(1):15–23.
3. Herman CR, Gill HK, Eng J, Fajardo LL. Screening for preclinical disease: test and disease characteristics. AJR Am J Roentgenol. 2002;179(4):825–31.
4. Blencowe H, Cousens S, Oestergaard MZ, Chou D, Moller A-B, Narwal R, et al. National, regional, and worldwide estimates of preterm birth rates in the year 2010 with time trends

since 1990 for selected countries: a systematic analysis and implications. The Lancet. 2012;379(9832):2162–72.

5. Zhu Z, Yuan L, Wang J, Li Q, Yang C, Gao X, et al. Mortality and morbidity of infants born extremely preterm at tertiary medical centers in China from 2010 to 2019. JAMA Netw Open. 2021;4(5): e219382.

6. Norman M, Hallberg B, Abrahamsson T, Bjorklund LJ, Domellof M, Farooqi A, et al. Association between year of birth and 1-year survival among extremely preterm infants in Sweden during 2004–2007 and 2014–2016. JAMA. 2019;321(12):1188–99.

7. Chiang MF, Keenan JD, Starren J, Du YE, Schiff WM, Barile GR, et al. Accuracy and reliability of remote retinopathy of prematurity diagnosis. Arch Ophthalmol. 2006;124 (3):322–7.

8. Chiang MF, Wang L, Busuioc M, Du YE, Chan P, Kane SA, et al. Telemedical retinopathy of prematurity diagnosis: accuracy, reliability, and image quality. Arch Ophthalmol. 2007;125 (11):1531–8.

9. Lorenz B, Spasovska K, Elflein H, Schneider N. Wide-field digital imaging based telemedicine for screening for acute retinopathy of prematurity (ROP). Six-year results of a multicentre field study. Graefes Arch Clin Exp Ophthalmol. 2009;247(9):1251–62.

10. Scott KE, Kim DY, Wang L, Kane SA, Coki O, Starren J, et al. Telemedical diagnosis of retinopathy of prematurity intraphysician agreement between ophthalmoscopic examination and image-based interpretation. Ophthalmology. 2008;115(7):1222–8 e3.

11. Quinn GE, Ying GS, Daniel E, Hildebrand PL, Ells A, Baumritter A, et al. Validity of a telemedicine system for the evaluation of acute-phase retinopathy of prematurity. JAMA Ophthalmol. 2014;132(10):1178–84.

12. Photographic Screening for Retinopathy of Prematurity Cooperative G. The photographic screening for retinopathy of prematurity study (photo-ROP). Primary outcomes. Retina. 2008;28(3 Suppl):S47–54.

13. Dai S, Chow K, Vincent A. Efficacy of wide-field digital retinal imaging for retinopathy of prematurity screening. Clin Exp Ophthalmol. 2011;39(1):23–9.

14. Wade KC, Pistilli M, Baumritter A, Karp K, Gong A, Kemper AR, et al. Safety of Retinopathy of Prematurity Examination and Imaging in Premature Infants. J Pediatr. 2015;167(5):994–1000 e2.

15. Jackson KM, Scott KE, Graff Zivin J, Bateman DA, Flynn JT, Keenan JD, et al. Cost-utility analysis of telemedicine and ophthalmoscopy for retinopathy of prematurity management. Arch Ophthalmol. 2008;126(4):493–9.

16. Isaac M, Isaranuwatchai W, Tehrani N. Cost analysis of remote telemedicine screening for retinopathy of prematurity. Can J Ophthalmol. 2018;53(2):162–7.

17. Vinekar A, Gilbert C, Dogra M, Kurian M, Shainesh G, Shetty B, et al. The KIDROP model of combining strategies for providing retinopathy of prematurity screening in underserved areas in India using wide-field imaging, tele-medicine, non-physician graders and smart phone reporting. Indian J Ophthalmol. 2014;62(1):41–9.

18. Fierson WM, Ophthalmology AAOPSo, American Academy Of O, American Association For Pediatric O, Strabismus, American Association Of Certified O. Screening examination of premature infants for retinopathy of prematurity. Pediatrics. 2018;142(6):e20183061.

19. Chiang MF, Quinn GE, Fielder AR, Ostmo SR, Paul Chan RV, Berrocal A, et al. International classification of retinopathy of prematurity, third edition. Ophthalmology. 2021;128(10): e51-e68

20. Fierson WM, Capone A, Jr. American Academy of Pediatrics Section on O, American Academy of Ophthalmology AAoCO. Telemedicine for evaluation of retinopathy of prematurity. Pediatrics. 2015;135(1):e238–54.

21. Daniel E, Quinn GE, Hildebrand PL, Ells A, Hubbard GB 3rd, Capone A Jr, et al. Validated system for centralized grading of retinopathy of prematurity: telemedicine approaches to evaluating acute-phase retinopathy of prematurity (e-ROP) study. JAMA Ophthalmol. 2015;133(6):675–82.

22. Vinekar A, Bhende P. Innovations in technology and service delivery to improve retinopathy of prematurity care. Community Eye Health. 2018;31:S20–2.
23. Koreen S, Lopez R, Jokl DH, Flynn JT, Chiang MF. Variation in appearance of severe zone 1 retinopathy of prematurity during wide-angle contact photography. Arch Ophthalmol. 2008;126(5):736–7.
24. Chan RV, Patel SN, Ryan MC, Jonas KE, Ostmo S, Port AD, et al. The global education network for retinopathy of prematurity (Gen-Rop): development, implementation, and evaluation of a novel tele-education system (An American ophthalmological society thesis). Trans Am Ophthalmol Soc. 2015;113:T2.
25. Daniel E, Pan W, Quinn GE, Smith E, Baumritter A, Ying GS, et al. Single grading vs double grading with adjudication in the telemedicine approaches to evaluating acute-phase retinopathy of prematurity (e-ROP) study. J AAPOS. 2018;22(1):32–7.
26. Good WV. Early Treatment for Retinopathy of Prematurity Cooperative G. Final results of the Early Treatment for Retinopathy of Prematurity (ETROP) randomized trial. Trans Am Ophthalmol Soc. 2004;102:233–48; discussion 48–50.
27. da Cunha LP, Cavalcante Costa MAA, de Miranda HA, 2nd, Reis Guimaraes J, Aihara T, Ludwig CA, et al. Comparison between wide-field digital imaging system and the red reflex test for universal newborn eye screening in Brazil. Acta Ophthalmol. 2021;99(7):e1198–205.
28. Ludwig CA, Callaway NF, Blumenkranz MS, Fredrick DR, Moshfeghi DM. Validity of the red reflex exam in the newborn eye screening test cohort. Ophthalmic Surg Lasers Imaging Retina. 2018;49(2):103–10.

Artificial Intelligence for Pediatric Retinal Diseases

68

Luis Acaba-Berrocal, Aaron Coyner, Michael F. Chiang, J. Peter Campbell, and R. V. Paul Chan

Abstract

Artificial intelligence (AI) is an evolving field within medicine in general and specifically in ophthalmology. Ophthalmologic research and development of AI platforms for pediatric retinal disease have largely focused on retinopathy of prematurity (ROP) screening, diagnosis, and patient follow-up. Platforms such as the Imaging and Informatics in ROP Deep Learning (i-ROP DL) algorithm have demonstrated both high sensitivity and specificity for the diagnosis of plus disease. In addition, the i-ROP DL vascular severity score has been shown to be helpful not only in diagnosing ROP disease severity, but also in tracking disease progression and diagnosing treatment requiring-ROP. Therefore, AI has shown promise in helping limit screening on low-risk infants and directing resources to eyes at highest risk for treatment-requiring ROP, increasing the efficiency of ROP screenings and identifying patients likely to need treatment. AI has also

L. Acaba-Berrocal · R. V. Paul Chan (✉)
Illinois Eye and Ear Infirmary, University of Illinois at Chicago, Chicago, IL, USA
e-mail: rvpchan@uic.edu

L. Acaba-Berrocal
e-mail: lacaba2@uic.edu

A. Coyner · J. P. Campbell
Casey Eye Institute, Oregon Health and Science University, Portland, OR, USA
e-mail: coyner@ohsu.edu

M. F. Chiang
National Eye Institute, National Institutes of Health, Bethesda, MD, USA
e-mail: michael.chiang@nih.gov

© The Author(s), under exclusive license to Springer Nature Switzerland AG 2023
Ş. Özdek et al. (eds.), *Pediatric Vitreoretinal Surgery*,
https://doi.org/10.1007/978-3-031-14506-3_68

1011

shown potential in assisting real-time in surgeries. However, barriers including costs, generalizability, and medicolegal interpretations remain and need to be addressed before the algorithms become common place in clinical practice.

Keywords

Artificial intelligence · Retinopathy of prematurity · Retina · Deep learning

Introduction

One of the new evolving frontiers for the field of retina is the use of artificial intelligence (AI) for diagnosis, telemedicine, teaching, and to aid in treatment of various conditions. Artificial intelligence in its basic definition involves the "study of intelligence and its computational manifestations within machines" [1]. Machine learning is the largest subset of AI and involves learning models from presented data [1]. Meanwhile, Deep Learning (DL) is a subset of machine learning that involves training modules with varying levels of processing. Usually, they require large datasets of thousands of examples depending on the complexity of the task [1]. Convolutional neural networks (CNNs) are a type of DL which are fully integrated systems that utilize standardized images as input data, allowing the system to later recognize certain "learned" patterns in new images [1, 2]. Today, the majority of AI systems in retina utilize AI with both DL and CNNs.

AI in Pediatric Retina

In ophthalmology, one goal of AI and DL is to improve accuracy and efficiency of diagnosis, as well as allow for monitoring of disease and risk stratification [3, 4]. Thus, AI has the potential to improve care, specifically in remote areas with limited healthcare access. AI also offers advantages over traditional human diagnosis, as computerized systems may be less likely to demonstrate human biases that could affect diagnosis and do not suffer from fatigue and errors encountered as a response [2]. Specifically in ophthalmology, AI research has mostly focused on the diagnosis of glaucoma, diabetic retinopathy, age-related macular degeneration, and retinopathy of prematurity (ROP); ROP presents a unique opportunity for AI. While ROP has defined criteria for diagnosis, many of those criteria are subjective and it can be a challenging diagnosis to make [1]. Meanwhile, it is a worldwide problem with an increasing prevalence and significant screening burden for countries without robust healthcare systems and a lack of trained physicians. It is estimated that on average, 55 infants need to be screened for every 1 that is treated for ROP [5]. Thus, there is a need for improvement in diagnosis and increase in screening for ROP, and AI presents one solution.

Beginnings of AI for ROP

Initial image-based analysis for ROP, such as the ROPTool, focused on plus disease by measuring posterior pole vascular changes. These systems used fundus photography and algorithms to quantify the level of vessel dilation and tortuosisty [2]. However, machine learning was not involved and these systems required at least one manual step from clinicians [1]. At the time, it was generally felt that the accuracy for detecting plus disease was too low [3] and required too much manual input for the system to be useful in clinical practice [2].

AI for ROP Today

Newer systems have since been developed which utilize CNNs and as such, are independent from clinicians and require no manual input [1]. One of the first fully automated DL systems to demonstrate significant accuracy in plus disease diagnosis and classification is the Imaging and Informatics in ROP deep learning (i-ROP DL) system [2, 3, 6]. Studies have demonstrated a sensitivity and specificity towards plus disease diagnosis of 93 and 94% respectively [3, 6]. The I-ROP DL also utilizes a linear formula to provide an ROP severity score based on the system's prediction probabilities that can be used to classify ROP. Specifically, the algorithm assigns a vascular severity score from 1 to 9 with 1 being the most normal and 9 the most severe (severe plus disease). Recent work has demonstrated that the vascular severity score correlated well with the international classification of ROP (ICROP) disease severity. The algorithm also proved to be effective in following ROP severity over time [7, 8]. Similarly, the rate of change in the severity score was found to be associated with disease progression. Taken together, early work has demonstrated the utility of an AI vascular severity score to not only diagnose ROP but to track the clinical progression of ROP along subsequent visits [7]. This is another advantage of the system that allows for an objective way to measure disease severity and potentially allow for standardization of diagnosis [1, 6]. Recently, the i-ROP DL was externally validated in patients with ROP in multiple NICUs in India, with a specificity and sensitivity of 78% and 100% respectively for detection of treatment requiring ROP [9]. Multiple other studies have demonstrated the potential use of the i-ROP DL system for ROP screening, and monitoring progression and regression [2, 10–12]. Another CNN based system, DeepROP, focusses on ROP screening, specifically in detecting the presence or absence of ROP and grading ROP as severe or minor [2, 13, 14]. The system achieved a sensitivity of 96.6% and specificity of 99% for ROP detection [13, 14].

AI and specifically risk prediction models can also be used to improve screening guidelines in ROP by increasing the specificity and therefore decreasing the number of potential unnecessary screening visits for low-risk infants. Current screening guidelines in the US, based on demographic data, allow for on average 3–8 ROP examinations with <10% of those patients requiring ROP treatment [15]. In response, the i-ROP-DL algorithm was utilized to develop a predictive risk model for incident treatment requiring ROP by adding AI biometric data to already established models based on demographic values [15]. Specifically, the model utilized the vascular severity score and gestational age as variables. When evaluated against an independent dataset, the model identified all patients that eventually required treatment on average 3.5 weeks before treatment was performed (sensitivity 100%) and achieved a specificity of 81%, effectively ruling out a significant portion of the low-risk patients. Although further validation is needed with diverse populations, the model effectively demonstrated that AI could significantly improve screening guidelines for ROP by reducing the amount of screening visits for ROP and could successfully identify treatment requiring infants multiple weeks before treatment is conventionally utilized [15].

Future of AI: Retinal Surgery

Although much of the work regarding AI and ophthalmology has focused on diagnosis of disease, significant effort is also underway to implement AI algorithms in ophthalmic surgery. AI for surgery involves real-time processing of images that are constantly changing with the surgical field. Using phacoemulsification as an example, a CNN was developed to track the pupil and surgical phase and provide real time feedback and guidance to the surgeon [16]. The system was able to accurately track the pupil and provide real time feedback on erratic tool movement and turbulent flow conditions, as well as provide guidance on capsulorrhexis size and how to enhance visualization. In the initial pilot study, 72% of cataract surgeons were mostly or extremely likely to use the system during surgery [16]. In the near future, we can imagine AI as an integral part of retinal surgery not only in providing real time guidance but also by providing insight on potential complications and location of these before they occur. Specifically for pediatric retinal surgery and ROP surgery, AI may have the potential to both improve surgical outcomes and increase the number of trained surgeons for these challenging surgical cases.

Barriers to Implementation

Although current available AI systems show great promise in the field of ROP, none have yet been implemented in routine clinical practice as several barriers remain [2]. First, more work is needed to elucidate how generalizable the system is to different populations. Specifically, data from validation studies using varying settings, populations, and camera systems is needed to see how well the results can be reproduced in the real world [2]. Second, the total cost of the system for a clinical practice has yet to be elucidated and might represent a significant barrier for many practices, especially in low-income countries, as camara systems need to be implemented [2]. Third, workflows for implementations of the system in clinical practice have not been well established [2]. This is imperative, as implementation of the system cannot compromise efficiency in busy retina and pediatric practices. Finally, the medicolegal language needs to be established by regulatory agencies [3].

Conclusion

AI has come a long way in the healthcare setting and ophthalmology is at the forefront. In pediatric retina, the major focus of AI design and implementation has been ROP. Although no system has yet to be a part of clinical practice, multiple systems such as the i-ROP DL have been shown to be effective in identifying and classifying ROP. As new studies continue to externally validate these AI systems against varying populations, AI will become an integral part of ROP diagnosis and follow-up in the clinical realm, especially in rural and areas with limited healthcare (Table 68.1).

Table 68.1 AI algorithms for retinopathy of prematurity

Type of AI algorithm	Measured category	Sensitivity (%)	Specificity (%)
ROPTool [1, 2]	Plus disease	95	78
IROP-DL [3, 6]	Plus disease	93	94
DeepROP [13, 14]	Presence of ROP	96.6	99
RISA [17]	Plus disease	94	94
MiGraph [18]	Presence of ROP	99	95
CNN + Bayes [19]	Plus disease	83	98

Review Question

1. What are two CNN based AI systems that have shown potential for ROP screening and diagnosis?

(a) i-ROP DL, ROPTool
(b) Vessel Map, DeepROP
(c) i-ROP DL, DeepROP
(d) None of the above

Answer

1. (**C**) Both i-ROP DL and DeepROP have high specificity and sensitivity for ROP diagnosis and have demonstrated potential for ROP screening in clinical practice.

References

1. Reid JE, Eaton E. Artificial intelligence for pediatric ophthalmology. Curr Opin Ophthalmol. 2019;30(5):337–46. https://doi.org/10.1097/ICU.0000000000000593 PMID: 31261187.
2. Gensure RH, Chiang MF, Campbell JP. Artificial intelligence for retinopathy of prematurity. Curr Opin Ophthalmol. 2020;31(5):312–7. https://doi.org/10.1097/ICU.0000000000000680.
3. Scruggs BA, Chan RVP, Kalpathy-Cramer J, Chiang MF, Campbell JP. Artificial intelligence in retinopathy of prematurity diagnosis. Transl Vis Sci Technol. 2020;9(2):5. Published 2020 Feb 10. https://doi.org/10.1167/tvst.9.2.5.
4. Valikodath N, Cole E, Chiang MF, Campbell JP, Chan RVP. Imaging in retinopathy of prematurity. Asia Pac J Ophthalmol (Phila). 2019;8:178–86.
5. Haines L, Fielder AR, Scrivener R, et al. Retinopathy of prematurity in the UK I: the organisation of services for screening and treatment. Eye (Lond). 2002;16:33–8.
6. Brown JM, Campbell JP, Beers A, Chang K, Ostmo S, Chan RVP, Dy J, Erdogmus D, Ioannidis S, Kalpathy-Cramer J, Chiang MF. Imaging and informatics in retinopathy of prematurity (i-ROP) research consortium. JAMA Ophthalmol. 2018;136(7):803–10.
7. Taylor S, Brown JM, Gupta K, et al. Monitoring disease progression with a quantitative severity scale for retinopathy of prematurity using deep learning [published online ahead of print, 2019 July 3]. JAMA Ophthalmol. 2019;137(9):1022–8. https://doi.org/10.1001/jamaophthalmol.2019.2433.
8. Redd TK, Campbell JP, Brown JM, et al. Evaluation of a deep learning image assessment system for detecting severe retinopathy of prematurity [published online ahead of print, 2018 Nov 23]. Br J Ophthalmol. 2018;bjophthalmol-2018-313156. https://doi.org/10.1136/bjophthalmol-2018-313156.
9. Campbell JP, Singh P, Redd TK, Brown JM, Shah PK, Subramanian P, Rajan R, Valikodath N, Cole E, Ostmo S, Chan RVP, Venkatapathy N, Chiang MF, Kalpathy-Cramer J. Applications of artificial intelligence for retinopathy of prematurity screening. Pediatrics. 2021;147(3): e2020016618. https://doi.org/10.1542/peds.2020-016618.
10. Redd TK, Campbell JP, Brown JM, et al. Evaluation of a deep learning image assessment system for detecting severe retinopathy of prematurity. Br J Ophthalmol. 2019;103:580–4.
11. Taylor S, Brown JM, Gupta K, et al. Monitoring disease progression with a quantitative severity scale for retinopathy of prematurity using deep learning. JAMA Ophthalmol. 2019;137:1022–8.

12. Gupta K, Campbell JP, Taylor S, et al. A quantitative severity scale for retinopathy of prematurity using deep learning to monitor disease regression after treatment. JAMA Ophthalmol. 2019;137:1029–36.
13. Wang J, Ju R, Chen Y, et al. Automated retinopathy of prematurity screening using deep neural networks. EBioMedicine. 2018;35:361–8.
14. Hu J, Chen Y, Zhong J, Ju R, Yi Z. Automated analysis for retinopathy of prematurity by deep neural networks. IEEE Trans Med Imaging. 2019;38:269–79.
15. Coyner AS, Chen JS, Singh P, Schelonka RL, Jordan BK, McEvoy CT, Anderson JE, Chan RVP, Sonmez K, Erdogmus D, Chiang MF, Kalpathy-Cramer J, Campbell JP. Single-examination risk prediction of severe retinopathy of prematurity. Pediatrics. 2021;148(6): e2021051772. https://doi.org/10.1542/peds.2021-051772 PMID: 34814160.
16. Garcia Nespolo R, Yi D, Cole E, Valikodath N, Luciano C, Leiderman YI. Evaluation of artificial intelligence-based intraoperative guidance tools for phacoemulsification cataract surgery. JAMA Ophthalmol. 2022. https://doi.org/10.1001/jamaophthalmol.2021.5742. Epub ahead of print. PMID: 35024773.
17. Wallace DK, Zhao Z, Freedman SF. A pilot study using 'ROPtool' to quantify plus disease in retinopathy of prematurity. J Am Assoc Pediatr Ophthalmol Strabismus. 2007;11:381–7.
18. Redd TK, Campbell JP, Brown JM, et al. Evaluation of a deep learning image & assessment system for detecting severe retinopathy of prematurity. Br J Ophthalmol 2018;2018-313156.
19. Brown JM, Campbell JP, Beers A, et al. Automated diagnosis of plus disease in retinopathy of prematurity using deep convolutional neural networks. JAMA Ophthalmol. 2018;136: 803–10.

Part XII
Visual Rehabilitation

Refractive Rehabilitation

69

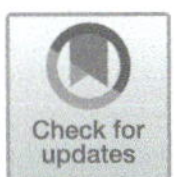

Carla J. Osigian and Kara M. Cavuoto

Abstract

Refractive rehabilitation is a critical aspect of visual rehabilitation following ophthalmic surgery. This is especially important in pediatric patients, as appropriate refractive correction is an essential aspect of optimal visual development. The standard of care to assess refractive errors in children is cycloplegic refraction. Depending on the refractive error present and status of ocular anatomy following ocular surgery, different techniques and options are available to provide appropriate refractive correction and optimize visual acuity and development.

Keywords

Refractive rehabilitation · Cycloplegic refraction · Aphakia · Anisometropia · Myopia · Hyperopia

Introduction

The continuum of eye care extends from the initial evaluation and diagnosis to treatment and visual rehabilitation, with the objective of achieving maximal visual acuity in all patients and providing adequate coping mechanisms for patients with irreversible vision loss [1]. Refractive rehabilitation can be one of the most challenging and yet most critical aspects of visual rehabilitation. This is particularly true for children with retinal pathologies or who have undergone prior vitreoretinal

C. J. Osigian (✉) · K. M. Cavuoto
Bascom Palmer Eye Institute, Pediatric Ophthalmology, University of Miami, Miami, FL, USA
e-mail: cjo39@med.miami.edu

© The Author(s), under exclusive license to Springer Nature Switzerland AG 2023   1021
Ş. Özdek et al. (eds.), *Pediatric Vitreoretinal Surgery*,
https://doi.org/10.1007/978-3-031-14506-3_69

surgery, as they may also have high and/or anisometropic refractive errors and abnormal ocular anatomy. In this section we will review how to assess refractive errors in children with retinal disorders or prior surgeries and the options for correction of refractive error.

How to Check Refractive Error

The standard of care to assess refractive error in the pediatric population is cycloplegic refraction. Cycloplegic refraction allows an assessment of the refractive error by instillation of drops that limit or inhibit accommodation. Children have large accommodative amplitudes which can drastically alter the refraction. Relying on a non-cycloplegic refraction can result in greater myopia than cycloplegic refraction in children and young adults up to 20 years old [2]. This may be complicated by an inability to give a subjective response with manifest refraction. Therefore, performing a cycloplegic refraction in the office or working with a pediatric ophthalmologist to perform a cycloplegic refraction is extremely important.

Cycloplegia may be achieved through a variety of drops including atropine, cyclopentolate and tropicamide. The choice of drop may be determined by the desired duration and potential side effect profile. Cyclopentolate is frequently used due to its effectiveness and shorter duration, as tropicamide alone may not achieve complete cycloplegia. Atropine has a significantly longer duration, but also a higher risk of side effects such as fever, dry mouth, flushing, tachycardia, constipation, and urinary retention [3]. Some clinics will instill a drop that contains a pre-mixed combination of tropicamide, phenylephrine and cyclopentolate to simultaneously maximize both cycloplegia and dilation.

After cycloplegia is achieved, refraction is performed. The gold standard to determine the magnitude and axis of refractive error is retinoscopy. Retinoscopy is an objective technique that relies on the movement of reflected light from the patient's eye, lenses, and a retinoscope to assess for myopia, hyperopia and/or astigmatism. Using an autorefractor may be helpful to provide an approximation of the refractive error in all children as it acquires data rapidly and does not require significant cooperation. This is particularly true for younger children in whom a subjective cycloplegic refraction may not be possible. In children who are able to cooperate, a subjective refraction may be performed at the phoropter or with trial frames.

In some children, adjunctive techniques may be helpful in assessing the refractive correction. Over-refraction is useful in high refractive error, such as high myopia, as the vertex distance is maintained. To perform over-refraction, retinoscopy or manifest refraction is used to determine any residual refractive error while the child is wearing his/her glasses or contact lenses. In patients with lens subluxation, such as children with Marfan syndrome, assessing the refractive error through both the phakic and aphakic spaces is important to provide the optimal correction.

Options for Correction of Refractive Error

The threshold to correct refractive error in children varies by the magnitude of the refractive error, the child's age, and the symptomatology. When appropriate, several options exist for the correction of refractive error in children, which include glasses, contact lenses and laser refractive surgery. These different options may be used alone or in combination. Glasses may be indicated for improving visual acuity, aligning the eyes, treating amblyopia and/or protecting an eye when the contralateral eye has poor vision. It is important to discuss which of the reasons apply to the patient when dispensing a glasses prescription. Contact lenses are an option which may improve tolerance of refractive error correction, particularly for high and/or asymmetric refractive error. Laser refractive surgery has recently been added to the list of potential treatments for refractive error in children. Although it can address myopia, hyperopia or astigmatism, most studies in children have addressed high anisometropic refractive error. Collectively the results of the studies demonstrated a consistent ability to decrease the amount of anisometropia; however, the ability to achieve and maintain a target refraction within one diopter was variable [4–14]. Additionally, many studies found regression of the refractive error over time in both myopia and hyperopic patients [5–8, 10, 11, 13, 14]. Future studies examining the safety and efficacy of these procedures over time will be important in determining its utility.

Refractive Challenges in Children with Retinal Pathologies and/or Prior Vitreoretinal Surgery

1. *High refractive error*

Refractive errors are a leading cause of visual impairment and refractive amblyopia worldwide. If not addressed, their consequences can be particularly harmful for children since vision is developed early in life. Even though many refractive errors can be addressed with eyeglasses, patients with high refractive errors often have specific needs requiring special attention.

Pediatric myopia is a global public health concern and a leading cause of visual impairment, affecting approximately 22.9% of the world population [15]. High myopia is defined as a degree of myopic refractive error of at least −6.00 D. Although most patients with physiologic myopia will retain good vision throughout life if treated early with appropriate optical correction, high myopia is a known life-long risk factor for ophthalmic complications such as retinal detachment, glaucoma, cataract, myopic macular degeneration, choroidal neovascularization and other chorioretinal abnormalities [16]. High myopic refractive errors also tend to be more prevalent in patients with retinal pathologies such as retinopathy of prematurity (ROP), pathologic myopia, and retinal dystrophies and degenerations, as well as systemic conditions such as Marfan syndrome, Sticklers syndrome,

Ehlers-Danlos syndrome, Knobloch syndrome, and ocular albinism. Therefore, high myopia in young children should prompt a detailed review of systems, birth history, complete ocular exam, and a systemic evaluation for associated syndromes.

Most children with bilateral high refractive error take to wearing glasses or contact lenses (CLs) very rapidly given the improved vision provided by optical correction. However, while glasses and/or CLs correct for the refractive error and may enhance visual acuity, patients with high myopia associated with retinal or systemic pathologies may sometimes be unable to correct to 20/20 vision. The anatomical retinal and macular changes (e.g. macular degenerations, colobomas, atrophy, lacquer cracks, macular scars) as well as the increased axial elongation of the eye (e.g. posterior staphyloma) often result in decreased visual potential despite optimal optical correction. In addition, patients with high refractive errors may present with reduced visual acuity despite wearing optimal refractive correction secondary to magnification and minification effects from high prescriptions as well as visual discomfort due to lens thickness. Regardless, the refractive correction that would normally be prescribed using cycloplegic refraction should be attempted. If the patient can tolerate it, the full myopic correction is recommended, as under correction of myopia has been shown to speed up myopia progression and axial elongation over time [17].

2. *Anisometropia*

Patients with unilateral retinal pathologies such as unilateral pathologic myopia or who have undergone unilateral retinal surgeries such as scleral buckling are at increased risk of high anisometropia and amblyopia. Scleral buckling, although an excellent procedure for retinal reattachment, can induce incapacitating refractive errors. The final refractive outcome following a scleral buckling procedure is multifactorial. Postoperative shifts in refraction may be a product of axial elongation induced by the encircling band, forward shift of the lens inducing lenticular myopia, and changes in corneal curvature [18]. These refractive changes alone place the buckled eye at risk of anisometropia and refractive amblyopia irrespective of the outcome of the retinal reattachment procedure.

The myopic shift can be markedly larger in children than in adults, possibly due to the elastic capabilities of a developing eye. A study on refractive changes that occur in infant eyes with ROP retinal detachments that are subjected to scleral buckling demonstrated induced mean anisometropias of up to -9.5 D [19]. To maintain the maximal visual potential in developing eyes it is not only important to achieve retinal reattachment, but also to provide an optically clear image to the retina and stimulate the use of the affected eye. This becomes challenging in presence of high anisometropia, as full correction of anisometropia may equalize image clarity, but will not change the aniseikonia, or difference in image size between the eyes. Significant image size differences between eyes may lead to suppression and abnormal binocular adaptations [20]. Although aniseikonia can sometimes be corrected or reduced by prescribing contact lenses or specially designed spectacle lenses, in some cases it may be impossible to correct fully.

Adherence to glasses in cases of marked aniseikonia becomes particularly challenging in younger children and patients that are unable to tolerate contact lenses.

3. *Irregular astigmatism*

Corneal changes following retinal and vitreous surgeries have been extensively reported. These are more commonly noted following scleral buckle procedures. Scleral buckles indent the sclera, changing the sagittal dimensions of the globe and potentially causing irregular corneal or fundus astigmatism. Although there are many surgical options for treating preexisting or induced corneal astigmatism after retinal surgery for adults—including excimer laser refractive procedures, limbal or corneal relaxing incisions and phakic IOLs—these possibilities are limited in children [21].

In children, spectacles and contact lenses (soft, rigid or scleral) should be tried in an attempt to compensate for corneal irregularities and improve visual potential. However, although they may improve image clarity, they may be not always tolerated and may be often insufficient to obtain a normal visual acuity.

4. *Lenticular issues*

a. Lens subluxation

Lens subluxation or ectopia lentis is one of the most challenging conditions for refractive correction. Lens displacement may occur secondary to congenital conditions such as Marfan syndrome, homocystinuria, Ehlers-Danlos syndrome, hyperlysinemia, sulfite oxidase deficiency, simple ectopia lentis and congenital aniridia, or may be acquired due to trauma [22]. The magnitude of refractive error and decrease in visual acuity will depend on the degree of lens displacement. If the subluxation is mild, the patient will see through the phakic portion of the pupil and refraction should be done over the lens. If the luxation is severe, best refractive correction may be achieved using the aphakic portion of the pupil. In some cases, the edge of the subluxed lens transects the pupil, preventing clear use of the phakic and aphakic portions of the pupil. This may cause decreased visual acuity regardless of refractive correction due to distortion of images and monocular diplopia. In these cases, careful refraction should be done over both the phakic and aphakic portions. If visual acuity cannot be improved with either correction, then lensectomy should be considered.

Case Scenario

A 4 year old female presented for an ophthalmology evaluation due to ectopia lentis. She had no family history of Marfan disease, ectopia lentis or other eye problems. She had been wearing glasses for 2 years with good compliance. Her visual acuity at the initial evaluation was 20/30 in the right eye and 20/400 in the left eye with the following glasses prescription: OD −3.00 + 3.00 × 076 and OS −6.00 + 3.00 × 100.

Slit lamp examination showed mild superior lens displacement in both eyes (Fig. 69.1), with minimal aphakic space visible through undilated pupils. Cycloplegic refraction through the phakic portion of pupil was stable in the right eye, however showed an increase in myopia on the left eye. An updated prescription with the full cycloplegic refraction was prescribed:

$$OD \ -3.00 + 3.00 \times 075: VA \ 20/30$$
$$OS \ -7.25 + 2.75 \times 100: VA \ 20/60$$

Two years later, she presented decreased VA in both eyes with glasses. The visual acuity of the right eye was 20/150 and left eye was 20/300. Slit lamp exam showed progression of superior lens subluxation, with the edge of the lens transecting the pupil in both eyes (Fig. 69.2). Cycloplegic refraction through the phakic portion of the pupil in both eyes showed an increase in myopia and astigmatism with minimal to no improvement in visual acuity of either eye:

$$OD \ -12.00 + 6.50 \times 080: VA \ 20/125$$
$$OS \ -14.00 + 8.00 \times 120: VA \ 20/300$$

Additionally, retinoscopy and refraction through the aphakic portion of the pupil showed no improvement in VA:

$$OD \ +7.50 + 5.50 \times 090: VA \ 20/200$$
$$OS \ +8.00 + 6.00 \times 060: VA \ 20/300$$

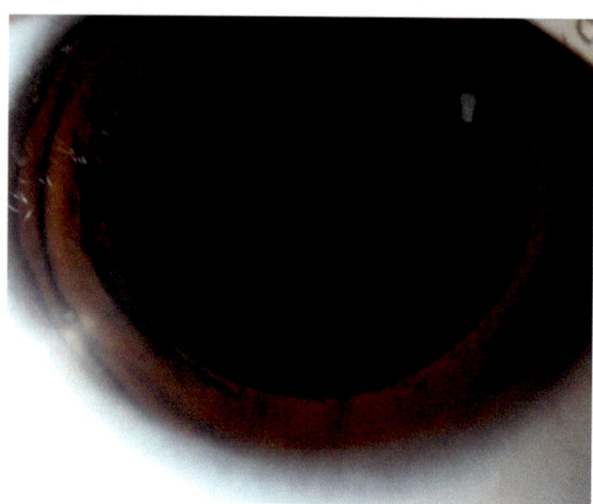

Fig. 69.1 Mild superior lens subluxation in a 4 year old patient

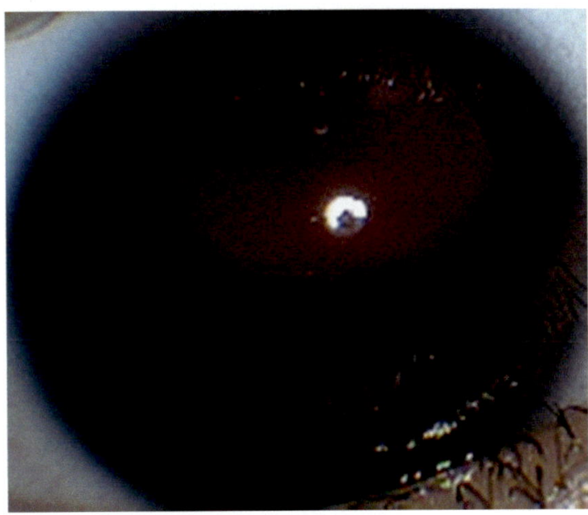

Fig. 69.2 Superior lens subluxation in a 6 year old patient with lens inferior edge transecting the pupil

Given the decrease in visual acuity with no improvement with refraction through either the phakic or aphakic space, surgery was recommended. A pars plana lensectomy with capsulectomy, pars plana vitrectomy, and peripheral endolaser was performed first on the left and then on the right eye. Postoperatively, aphakic contact lenses were fitted and bifocals were provided to wear over the contact lenses as follows:

Contact lenses
OD: +15.50 D
OS: +13.00 D
Glasses
OD: Plano, +3.00 bifocal
OS Plano, +3.00 bifocal
Visual acuity improved to OD 20/30 and OS 20/20 with aphakic correction.

b. Aphakia

Following lens extraction in children, providing a clear retinal image as soon as possible is essential for optimal visual development. Frequent refractions are often needed before the refractive error of the eye stabilizes and optimal optical correction can be determined, usually within the first 2 weeks following surgery.

Aphakia in children younger than 6 months of age is best treated with contact lenses if the patient can tolerate the lens and an accurate fitting can be obtained. Particularly in cases of unilateral aphakia, spectacles are not ideal due to aniseikonia and prismatic imbalance between the eyes. In young infants, an overcorrection by 2.00–3.00 D of the aphakic contact lens is preferred to ensure clear near vision. In patients between ages 2–4 years old, bifocal spectacles can be used over the contact lenses. Aphakic spectacles may be useful in some patients with bilateral aphakia who are contact lens intolerant; however, young infants are often unable to tolerate spectacles with high refractive corrections. High index refraction lenses may be helpful diminishing the weight and size of aphakic spectacle lenses and improving compliance.

c. Pseudophakia

The growth and development of pediatric eyes is regulated by the process of emmetropization. This process becomes altered after pediatric cataract surgery, with a tendency toward axial elongation and a myopic change in refraction. Therefore, many surgeons prefer intentional undercorrection of IOL dioptric power in young children and infants to allow for axial elongation with the corresponding myopic shift, reducing the myopic error when the eye is fully grown. Specialized pediatric IOL calculators have been developed to help predict the myopic shift and lens power to be used depending on the age of the child at the time of IOL implantation. The final refractive status following cessation of axial elongation is aimed at emmetropia or low myopia. The intentional undercorrection in IOL power, however, often leaves the child hypermetropic and early optical correction is necessary to improve visual acuity. The residual refractive error can be corrected with spectacles or contact lenses. Bifocal glasses are preferred in children over 2 years old to improve near acuity. Frequent refractions will be required as the child grows, gradually changes the lens power until the eye reaches full development.

Conclusion

Refractive rehabilitation is a critical component of caring for children who have undergone vitreoretinal surgery. As these children may have complicated issues such as high refractive error, anisometropia, irregular astigmatism, lens subluxation or aphakia, it is particularly important to perform a cycloplegic refraction and optimize the visual acuity with glasses and/or contact lenses. Since refractive errors in children may change over time, assessing the cycloplegic refraction at least once a year is recommended.

Review Questions

1. Which drops may be used to achieve cycloplegia in children?

a. Atropine
b. Cyclopentolate
c. Tropicamide
d. Phenylephrine
e. A, B, C
f. All of the above

2. High myopic refractive errors tend to be more prevalent in patients with what type retinal pathology?

a. Retinopathy of prematurity
b. Retinal dystrophies
c. Marfan syndrome
d. Sticklers syndrome
e. A, C, D
f. All of the above

3. Ectopia lentis may occur in which of the following congenital conditions?

a. Homocystinuria
b. Retinopathy of prematurity
c. Congenital aniridia
d. Marfan syndrome
e. A, C, D
f. All of the above
g. None of the above

Answers

1. (**E**) (A, B, C). Phenylephrine alone is used to dilate the iris without cycloplegia

2. (**F**) (All of the above). High myopic refractive errors also tend to be more prevalent in patients with retinal pathologies such as retinopathy of prematurity (ROP), pathologic myopia, and retinal dystrophies and degenerations, as well as systemic conditions such as Marfan syndrome, Sticklers syndrome, Ehlers-Danlos syndrome, Knobloch syndrome, and ocular albinism.

3. (**E**) (A, C, D). Lens displacement may occur secondary to congenital conditions such as Marfan syndrome, homocystinuria, Ehlers-Danlos syndrome, hyperlysinemia, sulfite oxidase deficiency, simple ectopia lentis and congenital aniridia, or may be acquired due to trauma.

References

1. Fontenot JL, et al. Vision rehabilitation preferred practice pattern[®]. Ophthalmology. 2017;125 (1):228–78.
2. Sanfilippo PG, Chu BS, Bigault O, Kearns LS, Boon MY, Young TL, Hammond CJ, Hewitt AW, Mackey DA. What is the appropriate age cut-off for cycloplegia in refraction? Acta Ophthalmol. 2014;92(6):e458–62.
3. BCSC 2020–2021. Section 6 Pediatric ophthalmology and strabismus. Chapter1: The pediatric eye examination.
4. Autrata R, Rehurek J. Laser-assisted subepithelial keratectomy and photorefractive keratectomy versus conventional treatment of myopic anisometropic amblyopia in children. J Cataract Refract Surg. 2004;30(1):74–84.

5. Paysse EA, Coats DK, Hussein MA, Hamill MB, Koch DD. Long-term outcomes of photorefractive keratectomy for anisometropic amblyopia in children. Ophthalmology. 2006;113(2):169–76.

6. Ghanem AA, Nematallah EH, El-Adawy IT, Anwar GM. Facilitation of amblyopia management by laser in situ keratomileusis in children with myopic anisometropia. Curr Eye Res. 2010;35(4):281–6.

7. Kulikova IL, Pashtaev NP, Batkov YN, Pikusova SM, Terent'eva AE. Femtosecond laser-assisted LASIK in children with hyperopia and anisometropic amblyopia: 7 years of follow-up. J Refract Surg. 2020;36(6):366–73.

8. Lin XM, Yan XH, Wang Z, et al. Long-term efficacy of excimer laser in situ keratomileusis in the management of children with high anisometropic amblyopia. Chin Med J (Engl). 2009;122(7):813–7.

9. Utine CA, Cakir H, Egemenoglu A, Perente I. LASIK in children with hyperopic anisometropic amblyopia. J Refract Surg. 2008;24(5):464–72.

10. Yin ZQ, Wang H, Yu T, Ren Q, Chen L. Facilitation of amblyopia management by laser in situ keratomileusis in high anisometropic hyperopic and myopic children. J AAPOS. 2007;11(6):571–6.

11. Zhang J, Yu KM. Femtosecond laser corneal refractive surgery for the correction of high myopic anisometropic amblyopia in juveniles. Int J Ophthalmol. 2017;10(11):1678–85.

12. Agarwal A, Agarwal A, Agarwal T, Siraj AA, Narang P, Narang S. Results of pediatric laser in situ keratomileusis. J Cataract Refract Surg. 2000;26(5):684–9.

13. Ram R, Kang T, Weikert MP, Kong L, Coats DK, Paysse EA. Corneal indices following photorefractive keratectomy in children at least 5 years after surgery. J AAPOS. 2019;23 (3):149 e141–e143.

14. Tychsen L, Packwood E, Berdy G. Correction of large amblyopiogenic refractive errors in children using the excimer laser. J AAPOS. 2005;9(3):224–33.

15. Holden BA, Fricke TR, Wilson DA, et al. Global prevalence of myopia and high myopia and temporal trends from 2000 through 2050. Ophthalmology. 2016;123(5):1036–42.

16. Pugazhendhi S, Ambati B, Hunter AA. Pathogenesis and prevention of worsening axial elongation in pathological myopia. Clin Ophthalmol. 2020;14:853–73.

17. Chung K, Mohidin N, O'Leary DJ. Undercorrection of myopia enhances rather than inhibits myopia progression. Vision Res. 2002;42(22):2555–9.

18. Rubin ML The induction of refractive errors by retinal detachment surgery. Trans Am Ophthalmol Soc. 1975;73452–90.

19. Chow DR, Ferrone PJ, Trese MT. Refractive changes associated with scleral buckling and division in retinopathy of prematurity. Arch Ophthalmol. 1998;116(11):1446–8.

20. South J, Gao T, Collins A, Turuwhenua J, Robertson K, Black J. Aniseikonia and anisometropia: implications for suppression and amblyopia. Clin Exp Optom. 2019;102 (6):556–65.

21. Kolozsvári BL, Losonczy G, Pásztor D, et al. Correction of irregular and induced regular corneal astigmatism with toric IOL after posterior segment surgery: a case series. BMC Ophthalmol 2017;17(3).

22. Ran D, et al. A rule of astigmatism in pediatric subluxated crystalline lens. J Ophthalmol Vis Res. 2019;1(2).

Amblyopia Management

70

Seyhan B. Özkan

Abstract

Amblyopia is a leading cause of visual loss both in children and adults. Early recognition and timely appropriate management are the key issues both for prevention and treatment. Those who practice anterior or posterior segment surgery in pediatric age group should be familiar with the effect of amblyopia both pre and post operatively. The basics of management are first to eliminate the amblyogenic factor and then to enforce the use of the amblyopic eye. The current treatment methods as well as the promising new treatment options are discussed throughout this chapter.

Keywords

Amblyopia · Refractive amblyopia · Deprivational amblyopia · Organic amblyopia · Strabismic amblyopia · Dynamic retinoscopy · Occlusion · Penalization · Dichoptic treatment · Liquid crystal glasses

Introduction

Amblyopia management is the key issue in pediatric eye diseases for a successful visual outcome. A perfect anterior or posterior segment surgery may become a useless effort by means of improvement of visual acuity unless appropriate amblyopia management is carried out postoperatively. This chapter addresses the management of amblyopia from the clinician's point of view with some pearls and

S. B. Özkan (✉)
Pediatric Ophthalmology and Strabismus, Private Eye Clinic, Aydın, Turkey
e-mail: sbozkan@superonline.com

Ş. Özdek et al. (eds.), *Pediatric Vitreoretinal Surgery*,
https://doi.org/10.1007/978-3-031-14506-3_70

pitfalls about the diagnosis and treatment reflecting the clinical applications of the author under the influence of updated literature information.

General Remarks

Amblyopia is a neurodevelopmental problem of visual cortex that occurs during the early period of life due to abnormal visual stimulation with no demonstrable problem on ocular examination. Amblyopia is a serious social problem with a prevalence of 1–5% as being responsible for loss of vision not only in childhood but also in adulthood because of the high rate of untreated or unrecognized amblyopia [1]. Amblyopia may develop in children under 7 years of age.

The pattern vision deprivation or abnormal binocular interaction is the initiating factor for the visual loss. Amblyopia is not only a simple decrease of visual acuity but runs with contour integration loss, longer reaction time and decreased contract sensitivity as well as some abnormalities in the 'better eye' and it became evident that amblyopia is a binocular dysfunction. The vision of the amblyopic eye is less under binocular conditions than monocular state. When the information coming from one eye is used, the information from the other eye is suppressed which means that the amblyopic eye is not used under binocular conditions. The suppression increases as the amblyopia is deeper indicating that amblyopia is the secondary result of binocular dysfunction. The major mechanism is not the 'lazy' state of one eye but the active inhibition of the amblyopic eye by the better eye that blocks binocularity. The active inhibition by the better eye disrupts the equilibrium between the excitatory and inhibitory signals. The lack of use of amblyopic eye under binocular conditions may most well observed clinically in cases of monofixation syndrome with dynamic retinoscopy. One can easily recognize that while the retinoscopy reflex of amblyopic eye reverses monocularly, it becomes non-reversed under binocular conditions when the occlusion is removed.

The major risk factors for development of amblyopia as for history are; prematurity or low birth weight, cerebral palsy and other neurological impairments, Down syndrome, hydrocephaly, mental retardation, family history of strabismus, amblyopia or childhood cataract, maternal smoking or alcohol intake. On examination the risk factors are; strabismus, monofixation syndrome, refractive errors such as high hypermetropia, myopia, astigmatism and anisometropia, nystagmus, albinism, choroidal coloboma, optic disc hypoplasia, ptosis, opacities of ocular media as cornea, lens and vitreus opacities.

Amblyopia develops during the plasticity period of visual system which is supposed to be first 7–9 years of life. However, the susceptibility of the visual system towards amblyogenic factors is not linear and it is highest during the first 3 months of life, remain high in first 2–3 years of life and decreases towards 6–7 years of age [2]. The effect of treatment is also not linear and consistent with the susceptibility of the visual system.

The amblyogenic factors that affect the visual function during the first months of life cause severe amblyopia. Bilateral stimulus deprivation in first 3 months disrupts the development of fixation reflex and nystagmus appears as a consequence of this. The presence of nystagmus indicates poor visual prognosis, does not disappear after treatment of the primary problem and allows visual acuity of 20/200 even after treatment. The plasticity of visual system is not the same for all of the aspects of visual function and recent studies focus on the possibilities of treatment of adult amblyopia by inducing plasticity of the brain in adulthood.

Classification

Amblyopia may practically be classified as follows:

- Strabismic amblyopia
- Refractive amblyopia:
  - Anisometropic
  - Meridional
  - Bilateral ametropic
- Deprivational amblyopia
- Organic amblyopia
- Idiopathic amblyopia

Strabismic, anisometropic and combined mechanism strabismic-anisometropic amblyopia are the most common types respectively in our clinical practice similar with the previous literature. The overlaps of these groups are commonly seen in clinical practice.

Anisometropic amblyopia is more common in hypermetropia and even 1.0 diopters (D) of difference may cause amblyopia whereas in myopic anisometropia the difference must be at least 2D to cause amblyopia. Astigmatic anisometropia exceeding 1.5D is considered to be amblyogenic. Monofixation syndrome is common in anisometropia as an additional amblyogenic factor that may be responsible for a deeper and more resistant amblyopia [3].

Patients with 'organic amblyopia' who represent the ones with ocular problems such as optic disc hypoplasia, choroidal coloboma, partial lens or corneal opacities deserve special attention for recognition of the coexisting amblyopia [4, 5]. The missed diagnosis of amblyopia in this group may be the reason of very critical changes of the patient's life such as the difference of being educated in visually handicapped or regular schools as they already have a limited capacity for vision.

As a common mistake, many patients in this group are left untreated or over-treated as the decrease of visual acuity is attributed to the associated ocular problem. Most of the time because of the preference of the 'good eye' the visual acuity decreases much less than the primary ocular pathology related decrease. This may cause either a wrong decision of an unnecessary cataract surgery or untreated coexisting amblyopia despite the chance for improvement of visual acuity by treatment of amblyopia. In this group the severity of the ocular problem and the level of visual loss needs to be well analyzed. Infantile partial cataracts should be evaluated carefully both as size and location and fundus illumination. One should not forget that the proximity of the lens opacities to the posterior capsule has a high impact on the severity of visual loss.

Special Remarks on Pediatric Vitreoretinal Problems

Prematurity itself is a well recognized risk factor for amblyopia and those who had laser treatment or vitreoretinal surgery for retinopathy of prematurity (ROP) should certainly be followed for treatment of possible amblyogenic problems. Eyes with previous laser treatment have the tendency of developing high myopic refractive errors and significant anisometropia. Additionally, associated neurological problems may also increase the risks for strabismus and amblyopia. In those where the vitreoretinal problem has settled, the parents should be informed about the necessity of follow up for possible amblyogenic problems.

Pediatric vitreoretinal surgery for any reason, either traumatic problems, ROP or else, requires immediate care for treatment of amblyopia as soon as the post surgical early wound healing is completed. These patients may have combined mechanism amblyopia as deprivational, ametropic, anisometropic and meridional. Appropriate refractive correction is the first step and any pre-existing or new developed amblyogenic factors should be eliminated in combination with aggressive patching regimen both for increasing visual acuity and avoiding further loss of vision because of ongoing amblyogenic factors. Any delay for visual rehabilitation may deepen the amblyopia and reduce the chances for a better visual outcome.

Case presentation—Combined mechanism amblyopia (Fig. 70.1):

- 6 months of age girl, a mass was realized on the right upper eyelid at 2 months of age
- Haemangioma in the right upper eyelid with marked ptosis
- Chin up abnormal head posture with a slight head tilt to the left side indicative of fusion and good capacity of vision in the right eye. Pupillary axis was open on the medial side.
- Eyes were orthophoric and ocular motility was normal
- Refraction: Emmetropia in both eyes
- Fundus examination: R: Morning glory disc L: Normal
- Triamcinolone + betamethasone injection into the upper eyelid lesion
- Left eye occlusion was prescribed as 1 h/day
- 2 months later—follow up visit: Significant decrease of hemangioma

6 months later:
- Good fixation with both eyes, orthophoria with normal ocular motility
- Cycloplegic refraction: Rx: R: $-3.0 \times 180°$ L: Plano
- Left eye occlusion 2 h/day
- The patient did not attend follow up visits

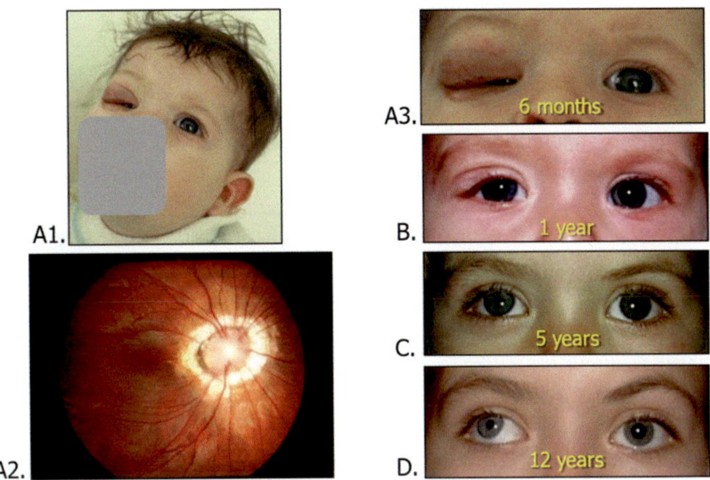

Fig. 70.1 **A1**. Abnormal head posture at first visit in an attempt to stay binocular. **A2**. Morning glory disc in the right eye. **A3**. Haemangioma in the upper eyelid. **B**. After steroid injection ptosis decreased. **C**. Right exo-hypertropia. **D**. Increase of right exo-hypertropia

Examination at age 5:

- No patching, no glasses during the past 4 years
- VA: OD: Counting fingers at 1 m OS: 20/25
- Right eye cannot fixate
- Right exo-hypertropia at near and distance (Krimsky test: 30 PD BI 10 PD BD)
- Cycloplegic refraction: OD: +0.75 × 120° OS: +0.75 × 40°
  - Rx: OD: +0.75 × 120° OS: +0.75 × 40°
- Full time occlusion: Left eye 6 days, Right eye 1 day

Examination at age 6:

- Good compliance with patching
- VA: OD:20/400 OS:20/20 with spectacles
- Right exo-hypertropia
- Bagolini glasses: Suppression in the right eye, TNO: No stereopsis
- Occlusion: Decreased to half day
- The patient did not attend follow up visits

Examination at age 12:

- VA: OD: Counting fingers at 2 m OS: 20/20
- Cannot fixate with the right eye
- CT: Right exo-hypertropia with dissociated vertical deviation (DVD)
- Unsuccessful result despite good capacity of vision as the patient had an abnormal head posture to use the amblyopic eye during infancy.

Evolvement of the ophthalmic findings:

- Morning Glory disc (organic amblyopia)
- Haemangioma related ptosis (Deprivation amblyopia)
- Haemangioma related meridional & anisometropic amblyopia
- Sensory exotropia developed with no clues about the previous deprivational, anisometropic and meridional amblyogenic factors.
- Occlusion would not be considered if the previous medical history was unknown
- The patient would be considered as sensory exotropia related to low visual acuity that would be attributed to the morning glory disc.

Key messages about the case:

- The amblyogenic factors may disappear or change in time and the real cause of amblyopia may no longer exist on examination.
- The patient may have useful vision despite congenital optic disc abnormalities
- In such cases consider treatment of "organic amblyopia".

Case presentation—Amblyopia related to partial cataract (Fig. 70.2):

- 2.5 years old boy
- VA: Fix and follow lights and objects, left fixation preference
- Orthophoric with normal ocular motility
- Slit lamp: Right anterior polar cataract with posterior synechia
- Cycloplegic refraction: OD: −1.50 × 180° OS: +0.25 (−1.50 × 15°)
- Rx: OD: −1.50 × 180° OS: +0.25 (−1.50 × 15°)
- Fundus examination: normal
- Occlusion for left eye 1 h/day

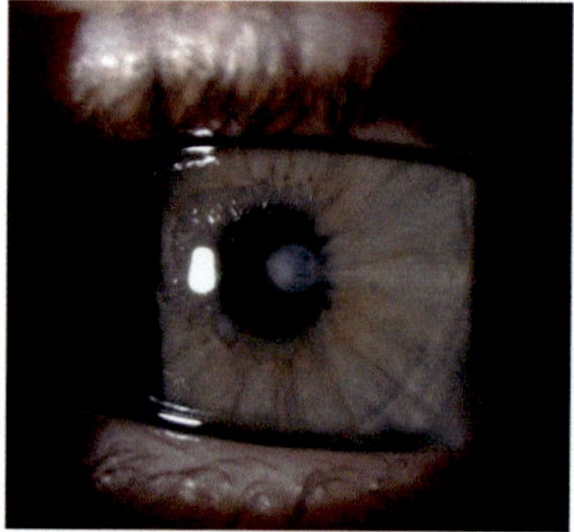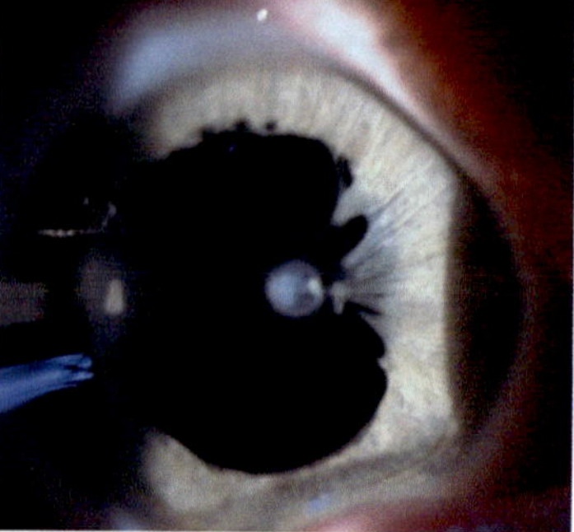

Fig. 70.2 Anterior polar cataract with posterior synechia in the right eye before and after pupillary dilatation

6 months later:

- VA: OD: 20/32 OS: 20/20 (with spectacles)
- Orthophoric at near & distance, ocular motility: normal
- Occlusion 4 h/day

1 year later:

- VA: OD: 20/20 (one letter) OS: 20/20 (with glasses)
- Occlusion 2 h/day

Key messages about the case:

- Anteriorly located lens opacities have a less effect on vision
- Associated ocular abnormalities should not stop treatment
- Consider amblyopia treatment despite the lens opacity depending upon the location and the density of the opacity.

Case Presentation with Infantile Cataract and Bilateral Pseudophakia

- 11 years old child, history of previous cataract surgery at 6th and 7th months of age with one month interval.
- Patching was prescribed but never done.
- VA: OD: Counting fingers at 1.5 m OS: 20/20 with glasses
- Refraction: OD: -5.5 ($1.5 \times 25°$) OS: -3.25 ($-2.50 \times 180°$)
- Slit lamp: Bilateral pseudophakia, in the bag IOL in both eyes with fully clear optical axis
- Fundus examination was within normal range in both eyes.

Key messages about the case:

- The visual outcome of 2 successful surgeries was so different demonstrating the importance of amblyopia therapy in pediatric age group.
- During infancy even the short duration of amblyogenic factors may have a lifelong impact on visual acuity. One month difference in timing of cataract surgery and untreated amblyopia afterwards caused significant loss of vision.

Case Presentation—Amblyopia After ROP Treatment

- 2 years old girl, with left eye squint history, parents think the patient cannot see
- Premature birth at 23th week, 680 g birth weight, 4 months at intensive care unit, laser treatment in both eyes

- Fix and follow with both eyes, 10PD left ET with fusion maldevelopment nystagmus.
- Cycloplegic refraction: RE: −7.0 LE: −9.50 (−1.0 × 180°) Rx: Full correction
- Fundus examination: Laser scars in retinal periphery with no other abnormality

3 months later:

- Fixation preference of right eye
- Part time occlusion: Right eye 2 h a day

3 months later:

- Significant increase in visual performance with no fixation preference
- 10 PD alternating esotropia with glasses
- Occlusion was stopped

3 months later:

- VA: OD: 20/50 OS: 20/200 with glasses
- Part time occlusion: Re-started as 4 h in right eye

3 months later:

- VA: RE: 20/32 LE: 20/50
- Cycloplegic refraction: RE: −6.0 (−2.25 × 180°) LE: −8.0 (−2.75 × 10°) Rx: Full correction
- Occlusion: Increased to 6 h a day in right eye
- 3 months later occlusion was increased to 8 h a day

4 months later:

- VA: OD: 20/25 OS: 20/25 with glasses
- Orthophoric with and without glasses
- Occlusion was decreased to 6 h and 4 h a day with 2 months intervals

Key messages about the case:

- Premature babies who underwent laser treatment may develop high myopia and anisometropia.
- Despite the increase of nystagmus with covering one eye, patching is effective in fusion maldevelopment nystagmus.

- The increase of visual acuity may increase the control of esodeviation despite myopic refractive error.
- If a given amount of patching is not effective despite good compliance, then occlusion time should be increased.

Diagnosis

The diagnosis of amblyopia is not complicated in a child cooperative enough with visual acuity measurement and in a child at any age with strabismus. By definition any difference of visual acuity exceeding 2 lines is accepted as unilateral amblyopia in the presence of an amblyogenic factor. In bilateral amblyopia, visual acuity worse than 20/30 over 5 years of age, worse than 20/40 at 4–5 years of age and 20/50 at 3–4 years of age are required.

The major problem in diagnosis of amblyopia arises at the preverbal period. On examination the interest of the patients on the fixation object, fixation pattern, alternation of fixation in strabismic patients, resistance to closure of one eye, the presence of nystagmus, and the accommodative response on a given near target give important clues about the diagnosis of amblyopia.

A quick retinoscopy gives invaluable information about the fundus reflex, opacities of ocular media and high refractive errors. In preverbal children a near fixation target with movement and sound gives the chance to have a short look enough to evaluate the accommodative response with retinoscopy.

'Dynamic retinoscopy should be among the routine eye examination of any child'.

If the child has strabismus, evaluation of fixation is straightforward. A non-alternating strabismus of any type suggests amblyopia. Alternating fixation is an invaluable tool indicating that there is no significant difference between visual acuity. In the ones with straight eyes 20PD test is very useful. When the child pays attention to an accommodative target, a 20PD vertical prism is hold in front of one eye inducing an artificial vertical deviation. This allows an easy evaluation of the preferred eye for fixation. Besides ocular motility examination, anterior and posterior segment abnormalities must be evaluated carefully.

Cycloplegic refraction is mandatory in evaluation of refractive state and cyclopentolate 1.0%, 3 drops with 5 min intervals, is the most commonly used agent for that purpose. In infants under 10 kg 0.5% needs to be used to reduce side effects. One drop of proparacaine before cyclopentolate both increases permeability and reduces the discomfort of the cyclopentolate and the parents should be advised to press internal cantal area to reduce systemic absorption.

Screening programs are developed and held in most of the countries in an attempt to early diagnosis of amblyopia and there are lots of discussion about timing, screening methods and cost efficiency of those programs.

Challenges in Diagnosis of Amblyopia

Patients in preverbal period without strabismus and the ones with monofixation syndrome at all ages represent the most challenging ones to diagnose. The most commonly missed form of amblyopia by parents is the monofixational and anisometropic amblyopia. Children with unilateral amblyopia have the tendency to consider that it is normal for everyone to see less in one eye and they do not complain about the problem to their parents even in older ages.

Monofixation syndrome may remain unrecognized even by the ophthalmologist if the evaluation is not done properly. The author had seen many adult patients who were sent for brain MRI to search for the etiology of unilateral visual loss while there were typical clinical signs of monofixation syndrome. The observation of fixation reflexes with 4 prism test is not easy even in adults, and in children it is more challenging. It was previously demonstrated that 8PD test also gives the same results but this may also be difficult to observe [6]. The author prefers to start with higher diopters in prism bar to see the fixational reflex better and then decreases it afterwards. This maneuver allows to observe the fixational movements more easily (Fig. 70.3). Monofixation syndrome is frequently accompanied by anisometropia but this is not a rule. When it is accompanied by anisometropia it is a common finding to see the accommodative response monocularly but lack of accommodation in the amblyopic eye when both eyes are open. So, the dynamic retinoscopy response should be evaluated under binocular state.

The other mostly missed group by the ophthalmologists are the ones with lack of accommodation. So, the dynamic retinoscopy response should be assessed regularly especially in risk groups such as the ones with accompanying neurological or developmental problems and Down syndrome. Evaluation of fixation preference is challenging in patients with autism as these children have resistance to eye contact and the examiner should pay attention where the patients fixate.

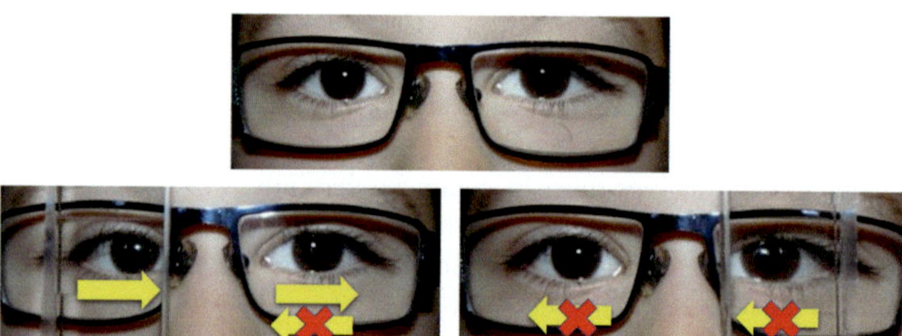

Fig. 70.3 Left monofixation and anisometropia. When base out prism is placed over the right eye, right eye adducts and left eye abducts, the left eye does not make the fusional refixation. When base out prism is placed over the left eye, the image displacement is within the supression scotoma of the left eye and neither left nor right eye moves

Management

Amblyopia management is a race against time! By the time of the diagnosis of amblyopia treatment should be initiated without losing time. This is to achieve prompt response to treatment, to prevent development of secondary deviations, to prevent loss of binocularity and to avoid amblyopia to become more severe. An untreated amblyopia does not show a steady course and as long as the amblyogenic mechanisms work, the visual acuity in the amblyopic eye becomes worse.

Amblyopia is accepted as 'untreatable' in adults, however there are some reports on the increase of visual acuity in the amblyopic eye in case of a loss of sight in the good eye [7].

Management of amblyopia should be built in following steps:

1. Elimination of amblyogenic factors where possible
2. Correction of refractive error
3. Stimulating the use of amblyopic eye
4. Preservation of the level of visual acuity till visual maturation

Elimination of Amblyogenic Factors

That step might be overcome with refractive correction, cataract surgery, ptosis surgery, etc. However, it may not always be possible to eliminate the problem in full. A partial cataract that does not require surgery has a sustained amblyogenic effect and requires close follow up to keep the level of visual acuity achieved by refractive correction and occlusion. Monofixation syndrome is another factor that cannot be eliminated and requires close follow up till visual maturation.

It is a meticulous decision to decide on surgery to eliminate amblyogenic problems as partial cataract. The balance of the potential risks and loss of accommodation with benefits of surgery should be assessed carefully. Some patients may show significant improvement of visual acuity with refractive correction and patching eliminating the need for surgery.

Correction of Refractive Error

The management of amblyopia starts with the correction of refractive error and unfortunately this is the step most prone to many erroneous applications. Management of aphakia and refractive correction is discussed in other separate chapters in this book and only general guidelines in relation with amblyopia will be discussed in this section. A successful amblyopia treatment could not be built without a proper refractive correction, and it is maybe the most important component of amblyopia treatment. There are some guidelines about correction of a refractive errors in children that give some general opinion but *one size does not fit for all* and the decision needs to be individual. The correction of refractive errors in ones with and without strabismus needs to be considered separately.

In a patient with an esodeviation the hypermetropic refractive correction is straightforward as full cycloplegic refraction. However, if the patient has an exodeviation with a hypermetropic refractive error there appears the concern of increasing the deviation. The most common mistake is to leave the child with hypermetropia amblyopic in order to control the exodeviation. As a rule, visual acuity has the priority compared to the control of the exodeviation and decreasing the amount of hypermetropic correction must be arranged depending on the dynamic retinoscopy results. However, some high hyperopes start to accommodate following wearing of glasses that may even facilitate better control of the exodeviation. There may even be cases with exodeviation and high hypermetropia who convert to fully accommodative esotropia after wearing glasses and improvement of visual acuity.

In a non-strabismic patient with hypermetropia, the decision of how much to correct should be based on the accommodative potential of the patient. The evaluation of the accommodative response of the patient has utmost importance in refractive correction of the patient with amblyopia and this evaluation can be done by dynamic retinoscopy. Some ophthalmologists have the tendency to evaluate the accommodative capacity with a non-cycloplegic refraction with a pediatric auto refractometer, but it is not possible to assess the accommodation in binocular state and it is not possible to assess whether the patient is trying to accommodate while looking at the fixation target within the instrument.

Let's consider a preverbal child with +5.0 diopters of hypermetropic refractive error with well aligned eyes. Is it amblyogenic for this child? How much should we correct? We know that if it is left uncorrected some develop amblyopia whereas some others do not. If the child's accommodative effort overcomes +5.0 this child does not need glasses and does not develop amblyopia. However, if the child's accommodative effort is insufficient to overcome full refractive error, then the remaining part needs to be corrected by glasses. So, the decision of the amount of correction that should be prescribed is a case based individual decision. If a reduced correction will be done the reduction must be equal in both eyes and astigmatic correction should not be reduced in presence of amblyopia.

Correction of anisometropia requires full correction of the refraction difference between the eyes. A common mistake in anisometropic amblyopia is not to correct anisometropic difference in full to reduce aniseikonia which represent the size difference in perceived retinal image. Aniseikonia exceeding 5% was demonstrated to cause loss of stereopsis [8]. The alternative methods to correct anisometropia with less aniseikonia are contact lenses or refractive surgery. The use contact lenses in childhood is challenging and many patients give up treatment either because of the costs or contact lens related problems. The effect of aniseikonia is usually overestimated and amblyopia should not be left insufficiently treated with the concern of loss of stereoacuity. It was demonstrated that the level of stereoacuity is close to normal levels with correction of anisometropia with glasses and using glasses is the safest method in childhood anisometropic amblyopia [9]. The reduction of stereoacuity is correlated with the depth of amblyopia more than the level of anisometropia [10]. In high hypermetropia the patient may have no ability to accommodate and with prescription of full cycloplegic refraction and treatment of amblyopia he/she may start to accommodate that may induce an esodeviation. The parents must be warned about this possibility in advance and to be told not to give up wearing the glasses if they start to see an esodeviation. Otherwise, most parents consider glasses as responsible for the esodeviation and may leave treatment with the cost of loss of sight.

In bilateral ametropic amblyopia correction of refractive error properly will eliminate the amblyogenic factor. In those with anisometropic, strabismic and combined mechanism amblyopia, correction of refractive error only may increase visual acuity and may even eliminate the need for other treatments in 25–50% of patients [11–15]. The increase of visual acuity with refractive correction is called as 'refractive adaptation' and it may last 12–18 weeks. So, waiting for the response to refractive correction only is recommended before considering occlusion or other treatment methods. There are 2 advantages of this approach; first any possible increase of visual acuity of the amblyopic eye will reduce the resistance to occlusion therapy; second, the patient may not need any further treatment. On the other hand, there are 2 disadvantages of waiting with refractive correction only; in older children with limited time to obtain any improvement, losing 18 weeks waiting for the response to refractive correction may reduce the chance to improve visual acuity by occlusion. Additionally in ones with strabismus, especially acute acquired deviations that requires surgery, waiting for the effect of glasses on amblyopia and to start occlusion afterwards may reduce the chance for binocular gains after surgery.

In those who had accommodation deficiency despite full correction of refractive error, bifocals are required for a successful amblyopia treatment.

Stimulating the Use of Amblyopic Eye

Occlusion

Occlusion is the golden standard method for amblyopia treatment as an evidence based method to stimulate the use of amblyopic eye and visual cortex. The main rationale of occlusion therapy is to force the visual cortex to use the amblyopic eye and the rule is to achieve the target visual acuity as quick as possible and to give up occlusion; first to increase the chance of recovery, second to decrease the psychological stress on the family and third to increase compliance. Long period of inefficient occlusion decreases the motivation and compliance.

The most major challenge with occlusion therapy is compliance of either children or parents. In preverbal children it is of utmost importance to make the parents understand that it is their responsibility to apply the given treatment and it is not possible to go on further steps such as strabismus surgery in strabismic ones if they do not perform the given treatment. It is also useful to inform the parents about the alternative options with advantages and disadvantages and to let them understand that postponing treatment will mean less response with more treatment hours as the amblyopia will possibly increase and resistance will be more in older ages.

Occlusion was supposed to be effective only during the plasticity of the visual system that means up to 7–8 years of age. However recent evidences suggest that occlusion may be effective in older children as well. The effect of occlusion was found more favorable in those <4 years of age compared to the ones older than

6 years of age and although the success of treatment declines with age, recent evidence suggested that improvement of visual acuity is possible until the age of 18 [16–18]. These findings suggested that it is worth to try for amblyopia treatment in all age groups in children. Even part time occlusion may be beneficial in older ages and the treatment outcome was found more favorable in those without previous patching treatment [19].

How to start occlusion?

Both part time and full time occlusion may be used and the schedule of occlusion is planned considering the severity of amblyopia, age of the patient, coexisting strabismus and the compliance of the patient.

Part time occlusion may be effective in some patients. However, considering the role of active inhibitory signals that originates from the non-amblyopic eye in binocular state, it is expected that the gain with occlusion decrease when both eyes are open. In part time occlusion 2–4–6 or sometimes 8 h of patching may be used and initial duration of part-time occlusion is dependent on the age of the patient and the severity of amblyopia. In a child with mild or moderate amblyopia, part time occlusion of 2–6 h may be prescribed. If no improvement is achieved in 3 months with any type of part time occlusion, the occlusion time needs to be increased without losing time.

In older children at 9 years of age or more with severe amblyopia, starting directly with maximal treatment, which means full time occlusion seems more reasonable because of the decreased time period to achieve successful results and not to waste any time. Below the age of 1 year full time occlusion is not used and maximal treatment is supposed to be 50% of awake hours. Part time occlusion even <2 h may suffice the need in this age group.

The advantage of part time occlusion is the less stress for the patient and the family with less chance for occlusion amblyopia in the better eye. On the other hand, the period to reach the target visual acuity is usually longer and in resistant ones it causes waste of time. In those who do not respond to part time occlusion the motivation of the child and the family decreases. It is known that the longer the duration of the deviation, the less is achieved in binocularity after surgery. Losing a long time for amblyopia treatment is a disadvantage in strabismic patients.

Full time occlusion decreases the time period to reach the target visual acuity, with the cost of more stress and the risk for occlusion amblyopia. In a retrospective unpublished study in our institution, we found that full-time occlusion decreases the period to achieve successful results significantly in strabismic anisometropic amblyopia. The shorter duration of treatment is advantageous in strabismic patients and in old age groups. However, the parents and the child may totally give up treatment as they find full time occlusion inapplicable. It is important not to lose this group of patients and consider alternative part time patching programs. In a child with older age the possibility of occlusion therapy must be discussed both with the patient and the parents and a realistic schedule needs to be prescribed. If a strict full time occlusion is given to a child and if the visual tasks are lower than required for school activities the patient may totally give up treatment. Psychosocial effects of occlusion may be highly disturbing in some school aged children.

Although the role of near activities does not have enough evidence, keeping the child's attention active with the toys and games which attracts them most, seems beneficial either to use accommodation or to keep the child awake. Computer games may be helpful for this purpose and they also help to break the resistance of the child against occlusion. The advice for near activities depends upon the duration of occlusion. It is inapplicable to prescribe near activities in a 3 year old child who is on 4 h patching treatment. In those patients it will be logical to advice near activities for at least 2 h.

These are only general guidelines and on some occasions some individual changes may be considered such as less hours occlusion on school days and more hours of occlusion on weekends. Making the occlusion plan by talking about the daily life conditions with the parents and the child increases adherence to the prescribed treatment. The major problem in occlusion treatment is the compliance which also spoils the outcome for a prescribed treatment. Occlusion dose monitors were used to overcome this problem but even in those studies where the patients were aware of the use of dose monitors, the rate of compliance was around 50% [20].

In order to achieve guidelines for amblyopia treatment, Pediatric Eye Disease Investigator Group (PEDIG) reported a series of multicentric randomized controlled trials and the major results of those amblyopia treatment studies (ATS) about occlusion are summarized below:

- Part time and minimal part time patching for moderate amblyopia gave similar results in moderate amblyopia in 3–6 years of age [21].
- Part time and full time patching for severe amblyopia gave similar results in 3–6 years of age [22].
- In a group of patients with severe amblyopia in 7–12 years of age; optical correction plus occlusion gave better results than optical correction only (23 vs. 5%) [23].
- In a group of patients with moderate amblyopia in 7–12 years of age; optical correction plus occlusion and atropine gave better results that optical correction only (36 vs. 14%) [23].
- In a group of patients with moderate amblyopia in 13–17 years of age, occlusion did not increase success significantly compared to optical correction only (14 vs. 11%) [23].
- In a group of patients with severe amblyopia in 13–17 years of age, optical correction plus occlusion worked to some extent whereas optical correction only did not make any benefit (14 vs. 0%) [23].
- Adding near activities in combination with occlusion give better results in short term, but there is no difference in 8 weeks [24, 25].
- Occlusion and atropine penalization demonstrate similar effect in patients with 7–12 years of age [26].

- Combination of patching and atropine in residual cases with mild amblyopia in 3–6 years of age did not provide improvement [27]
- In those who stopped improvement of visual acuity, increasing the dose of occlusion is beneficial [28]
- Bangerter filters and occlusion have similar effect in moderate amblyopia in 3–9 years of age [29].

It must be emphasized that these results do not compare the 'efficacy' of occlusion hours but they reflect the comparison of 'prescribed' occlusion treatment as they do not include occlusion dose monitors. If a subject in 'prescribed 6 h occlusion' and 'prescribed full time occlusion group' used occlusion for less hours, there might be no difference between the groups by means of real patching time. Finding no difference in results do not indicate that occlusion of more hours will be ineffective in a patient. The major criticisms for those studies are ongoing inhibitory effect of the good eye during the period without patching, the previous clinical experience of the efficiency of full time occlusion, and the absence of occlusion dose monitors in those studies [30–32].

The ATS recommendations mainly demonstrated to avoid overtreatment to achieve a successful result. On the other hand, following all steps as optical correction—part time occlusion—increased occlusion—additional penalization may cause waste of time for those who do not respond part time occlusion and, or optical correction treatment and it may prolong the treatment period. Especially in older age group the time period that is lost for inadequate treatment may lead to loss of the chance for improvement of visual acuity.

In patients with fusion maldevelopment nystagmus syndrome (previously called as manifest latent nystagmus), patching increases the visual acuity in the amblyopic eye despite the increase of nystagmus. Part-time patching has the advantage of allowing the child to have some period with less nystagmus. Penalization may offer a benefit for this group of patients.

The severe amblyopia that develops during the first months of life ending up with nystagmus and the coexistence of eccentric fixation are the main bad prognostic signs. Even in those with inability to fixate, small gains in visual acuity may significantly alter either control or the development of secondary deviations and they should better be treated for amblyopia despite less chance for improvement of visual acuity.

To summarize, in a patient with new diagnosed mild to moderate amblyopia initiation of occlusion should better be part time as 2–4–6 h depending on the age and severity of amblyopia. If the age of the patient is close to limits of plasticity period, starting with higher doses should be considered. If a response could not be observed despite compliance, the occlusion hours should be increased. The most common mistake in clinical practice is to insist on a given schedule of part time occlusion that the patient does not respond.

Inverse occlusion

In an attempt to reformat the inhibitory signals to the amblyopic eye patching the amblyopic eye for a period, thereby interrupting the abnormal binocular interaction is recommended in those with eccentric fixation. The author did not find any improvement with this patient group by that method.

Other use of inverse occlusion is to prevent occlusion amblyopia in ones younger than 7 years of age who are under full time occlusion. As an example, in a 6 years old patient if full time occlusion is used, the amblyopic eye is occluded one day per week as a preventive measure.

Clinical pearls for occlusion therapy:

- Make the parents understand their responsibility.
- Give your time to speak with children in cooperative ages and motivate them.
- Consider that some patients significantly improve just with refractive correction.
- If a surgical treatment is planned, use longer duration of occlusion not to waste time and not to reduce chances for binocular gains after surgery.
- If any part time occlusion treatment does not work despite compliance, then do not insist on the same dose and take the next step by increasing the occlusion time.
- Do not give up treatment in any child unless you prescribed the maximal treatment!

How to follow up?

On follow up visits, fixation preference and fixation pattern, visual acuity, binocularity, ocular motility examination including prism cover test with and without glasses should be checked. The schedule of follow up visits vary depending upon the age of the patient. In infants below 1 year of age, an interval of 4–6 weeks will be reasonable as this age group may demonstrate rapid response to treatment. In older ones with part time occlusion the routine schedule is to see the patient with an interval of 12 weeks. If full time occlusion is prescribed then the interval is the same number of weeks as the age of the patient. For example, if the patient is 5 years old the control visit must be with an interval of 5 weeks. In cooperative children it is useful to show the previous level of visual acuity in visual acuity chart for motivation.

How to stop occlusion?

The aim of amblyopia treatment is ideally to achieve equal and 20/20 visual acuity in both eyes and isoaccommodation with equal fixation preference. These goals especially isoaccommodation may not be achieved in many of the patients. In clinical practice when visual acuity reaches to 20/20 level, the patching treatment should not be stopped abruptly but should better be decreased gradually because of the risk of recurrence of amblyopia. The duration of the decreased occlusion period depends upon the fixation preference of the patient. If there is no fixation preference we decrease the occlusion with 6 weeks intervals, otherwise we decrease the occlusion with 3 months intervals and check visual acuity before decreasing more. In some cases, fixation preference is persistent even though the visual acuity remains stable as 20/20.

In patients with strabismus the amblyopia therapy must be done prior to any surgical intervention as the level of visual acuity influences the deviation. As soon as a successful outcome with amblyopia treatment is achieved, surgical treatment can be done without losing time. The accommodative ability of the amblyopic eye increases with treatment and there may be striking changes in the deviation, even an exotropic patient may convert into an esotropic one or the patient may have a much better control of the exodeviation with the increase of visual acuity.

How to accept a child unresponsive to treatment?

Although there are lots of studies comparing efficacy and how to stop treatment there are no clear guidelines how to accept a child with treatment failure. In order to accept a child unresponsive to amblyopia treatment we prescribe maximal treatment for at least 3 months as recommended by Pratt-Johnson [33]. The maximal treatment means full time occlusion in ones over 1 year of age.

In those with lack of improvement in visual acuity despite the expectance of a good response, missed diagnosis of ocular problems such as optic nerve hypoplasia or subtle macular problems and neurological causes might be considered. Asking for MRI would be logical not to miss any potential neurological problem if no ophthalmological problem could be identified. On the other hand especially in bilateral cases, hysterical visual loss should be considered in differential diagnosis.

Side effects of occlusion

The most serious side effect of occlusion treatment is occlusion amblyopia. If it is unrecognized on time it may dominate over the original problem of the amblyopic eye. Stopping occlusion is usually effective, but occlusion of the previously amblyopic eye may also be required. The importance of attendance to regular control visits should be well informed. Increase of the deviation angle may occur in some cases. The other problem is the psychological stress of the child and the family. The allergic reactions due to the patching material may be troublesome in some patients.

Atropine or Optical Penalization

The rationale is to penalize the good eye to enforce the use of the amblyopic eye. Atropine penalization certainly has a role in treatment of amblyopia and may be an alternative in resistant children. The basic problem with the use of atropine penalization is the excessive UV exposure in areas with sunny climate, photophobia and possible systemic side effects. Optical penalization alone does not seem to be effective in clinical practice as the resistant children will easily eliminate the blurring effect of the glasses. It was previously thought that if the visual acuity of the good eye cannot be decreased less than the amblyopic eye, penalization would not work. However, it was demonstrated that this is not a rule and atropine penalization may be efficient even though the visual acuity could not be decreased less than the good eye [34].

The randomized controlled trials of PEDIG brought useful clinical guidelines of the use of penalization treatment in amblyopia and those results may be summarized as below:

- Patching and atropine penalization have similar effect in both 3–6 and 7–12 years of age [26, 35].
- Daily atropine and weekend atropine have similar effect in 7–12 years of age [36].
- Atropine plus plano lens is more beneficial then atropine only in 3–6 years of age [37].
- Improvement is faster in patching compared to atropine group in patients younger than 7 years of age but the results are similar in 6 months [34].

Alternative Methods

These alternatives may be considered as occlusion alternatives such as liquid crystal glasses and Bangerter filters, stimulation of amblyopic eye without occlusion, dichoptic binocular treatment methods and systemic pharmacological agents.

Bangerter filters

Bangerter filters in different doses, enough to reduce the visual acuity of the good eye 2 lines below the amblyopic eye, may be used but the patients may easily look over the glasses that may reduce its effect. Those filters are mounted on the spectacles and were reported to be effective in mild to moderate amblyopia and may be considered as an alternative for occlusion. Bangerter filters with less density may allow binocular vision, with more acceptable appearance which may be considered as an advantage in mild amblyopia [38–41].

Liquid crystal glasses

Liquid crystal glasses provide a continual occlusion in certain periods in each minute and thus aims to reduce the resistance to occlusion. It may be useful in those who has resistance to standard occlusion methods [42–44]. Some children find those glasses more charming as they look like sunglasses and in our clinical practice, we find them useful as an alternative method. The prescribed glasses are mounted within the glass. The main problem with those glasses is the inability of the liquid crystal glass to become totally transparent. The possible adverse effect of the continuous use of colored glass on the visual acuity of the good eye is not studied. Because of that technical issue it seems more reasonable to recommend the use of those glasses under daylight conditions. Some of the commercially available ones has also colored glasses on the amblyopic eye and it may have a negative influence on the possible increase of the visual acuity of the amblyopic eye (Fig. 70.4). Fully transparent glass over the amblyopic eye should be preferred if liquid crystal glasses will be used.

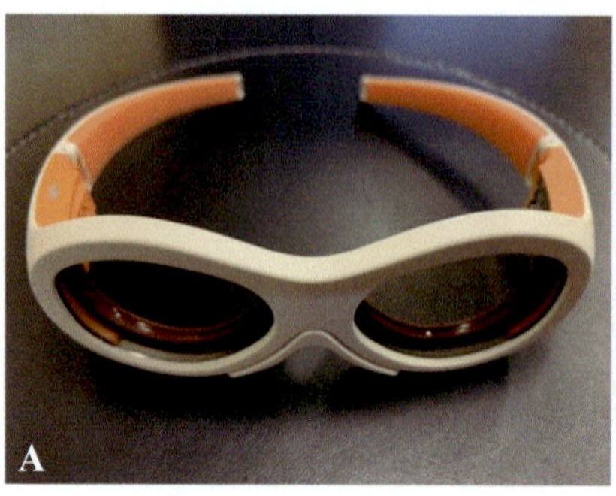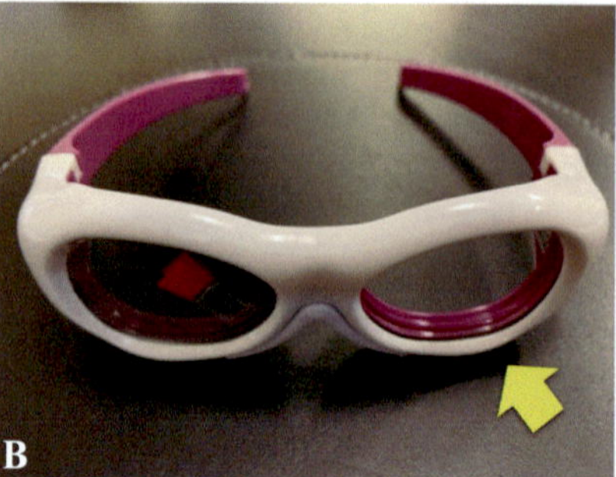

Fig. 70.4 Liquid crystal glasses for intermittent patching. **A.** Both eyes have colored glasses. **B.** Colored liquid crystal glass is on the side of the good eye and the side of the amblyopic eye is transparent (arrow)

Computer games with polarized glasses

Other alternative may be watching videos or computer games with using polarizing glasses. In this equipment only the amblyopic eye sees the computer screen whereas the good eye sees only a white screen (Fig. 70.5). The polarizing film layer of liquid crystal screen is transferred to the polarizing glasses enabling only the amblyopic eye to see image on the i-pad screen. It was reported to have comparable results with patching with a better compliance [45]. Some patients may find it more joyful instead of occlusion and it may increase compliance for amblyopia treatment.

Dichoptic treatment

Dichoptic treatment is another method depending on binocular stimulation of both eyes by sending higher contrast sensitivity signals to the amblyopic eye and less stimulating signals to the good eye. The main purpose is to obtain improvement of visual acuity by stimulating the binocular channels and to improve both visual acuity and the binocularity of the patient depending on the fact that amblyopia is a binocular problem. Encouraging results were reported in limited groups with those methods either as computer games or contrast rebalanced movies [46–50].

Randomized controlled studies of PEDIG demonstrated that part time occlusion was either superior (5–12y, 13–17y) or similar (4–6y) to dichoptic treatment and moreover spectacle only therapy (7–12y) has the same effect [51–55]. The Binocular Treatment of Amblyopia Using Videogames clinical trial group compared the conventional and binocular video games in older children and adults and reported no increase of visual outcomes with binocular games [56].

In a recent review report of American Academy of Ophthalmology it has been stated that binocular treatments do not have enough evidence to replace the standard amblyopia treatment and more research is required [57]. On the other hand, there are encouraging preliminary reports about some variable forms of dichoptic

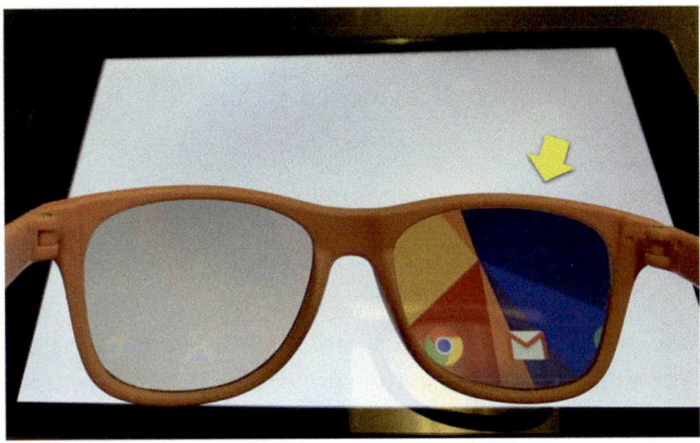

Fig. 70.5 The screen of the digital tablet is seen as white without polarizing glasses. Only the amblyopic eye sees the image (arrow) or video while the good eye sees only the white screen

treatment as passive binocular video viewing and 3D virtual reality either with red green glasses or by head mounted display [58–60].

These binocular stimulation methods require further study results in order to see that they do not induce diplopia similar with anti-suppression exercises that were popular in previous years. Strabismic amblyopes should be regarded with caution for the risk of intractable diplopia. Compliance is also a problem and screen time may be a further concern especially in younger ages. At this stage this method is still under investigation.

Dichoptic treatment methods opened a new window, although not yet as a replacement of occlusion treatment but at least as an alternative or an additional treatment option. However the efficacy, treatment duration, adherence to treatment and side effects are yet to be determined.

Perceptual learning

Perceptual learning is defined on Eleanor Gibson's article as a permanent change in the perception of a stimulus array with practicing this array [61]. The patients are asked to discriminate a variety of visual tasks either monocular or binocular conditions on a computer program. Cambridge visual stimulator (CAM) treatment is a method to stimulate contrast sensitivity by letting the child to color pictures over a rotating contract sensitivity disk with different levels of contrast and it may be accepted as a more simple preliminary form of perceptual learning. This method previously became popular but then demonstrated to have no additional value compared to patching [62–64].

Software based individualized repetitive practice of visual tasks are suggested as beneficial especially in adult amblyopia [65]. However, those studies include small number of patients without long term follow up and is regarded with caution by ophthalmologists. In an unpublished multicentric study in our country the investigators reported no benefit compared to occlusion in childhood amblyopia. The cost of the home-based trainings is another concern of this treatment and we do not consider that there is enough evidence to use this treatment in amblyopic subjects.

Systemic medications in amblyopia treatment

The medications as levodopa-carbidopa combination and citicoline are the possible agents to use in amblyopia [66, 67]. The problems with those agents are transient increase of visual acuity in both eyes and the increase of visual acuity in the non-amblyopic eye that may increase the suppressing signals on the amblyopic eye. In a randomized controlled trial of PEDIG, the use of levodopa in combination with patching was not found beneficial in residual amblyopia [68].

The anti-depressant agent Fluoxetine was recently demonstrated to be beneficial to increase the plasticity period of the visual system in patients 10–40 years old [69].

Although there are some favorable results with those medications it does not yet seem convincing enough for the routine use for treatment of amblyopia [70, 71].

The search for adult amblyopia treatment is ongoing and the promising area is to reopen the plasticity of the visual system in adulthood. Treatment of adulthood amblyopia carries the risk of inducing intractable diplopia and should be regarded with caution especially in strabismic adults.

Conclusions

- Amblyopia is a treatable condition that requires meticulous attention for diagnosis, treatment and follow up.
- Diagnosis of amblyopia may be challenging in preverbal period. Evaluation of fixation preference and dynamic retinoscopy should be within routine eye examination.
- As early as the diagnosis and treatment, as successful as the outcome. However, treatment attempt should be done at all ages in children.
- Appropriate correction of refractive error is the initial step for all types of amblyopia.
- In presence of organic problems of the eye consider accompanying amblyopia.
- Patching of the good eye is currently the golden standard treatment method in unilateral amblyopia.
- Alternative methods have not yet been found superior to patching and they may be considered in case of compliance problems with patching.
- Adult amblyopia treatment is an area under investigation.

Review Questions

1. How do you assess whether a given symmetrical hypermetropic refractive error that is found on cycloplegic refraction is amblyogenic or not in a non strabismic preverbal child?

a. Search for different guidelines in the literature
b. Ask the visual performance of the child to the parents
c. Evaluation of accommodative ability by dynamic retinoscopy
d. Evaluation of fixation preference

2. A 5 years old patient with moderate amblyopia was prescribed for patching with 2 h a day and no improvement was obtained despite good compliance in control visit on 12 weeks. What should be the appropriate choice?

a. Continuing with 2 h patching
b. Increasing the patching hours
c. Accepting the child as unresponsive to treatment
d. Addition of levodopa-carbidopa

3. What should be the correct approach in a 4 years old child who had visual acuity of 20/200 in the right eye and 20/20 in the left eye, with cycloplegic refraction of +1.50D in both eyes and with small right anterior polar cataract that does not affect fundus viewing?

a. Immediate cataract surgery
b. Left eye part time patching
c. No treatment is required
d. Follow up for cataract

Answers

1. (**C**) The accommodative response demonstrates whether the patient can see a clear image or not. If the patient cannot accommodate enough to overcome the hypermetropic refractive error, spectacle correction should be prescribed according to the result of dynamic retinoscopy.

2. (**B**) Duration of patching should be increased if there is no improvement for the prescribed occlusion in 3 months period.

3. (**B**) That patient has a small cataract that possibly will allow a much better vision. Considering organic amblyopia patching should be prescribed in order to overcome the effect of amblyopia.

References

1. Attebo K, Mitchell P, Cumming R, Smith W, Jolly N, Sparkes R. Prevalence and causes of amblyopia in an adult population. Ophthalmology. 1998;105:154–9.
2. Daw N. Critical periods and amblyopia. Arch Ophthalmol. 1998;116(4):502–5.
3. Weakley DR. The association between anisometropia, amblyopia and binocularity in the absence of strabismus. Trans Am Ophthalmol Soc. 1999;48:987–1021.
4. Kushner BJ. Functional amblyopia associated with organic disease. Am J Ophthalmol. 1981;91:39.
5. Kushner BJ. Functional amblyopia associated with the abnormalities of the optic nerve. Arch Ophthalmol. 1984;102:683.
6. Piantanida AC. The 8-diopters base-in test for the diagnosis of microstrabismus in daily practice. In: Transaction of the 32nd ESA meeting. Bergen;2008. p. 27–30.
7. Ellis FD, Schlaegel TF. Unexpected visual recovery: organic amblyopia? Am Orthopt J. 1991;31:7.
8. Campos EC, Enoch JM. Amount of aniseikonia compatible with fine binocular vision: some old and new concepts. J Pediatr Ophthalmol Strabismus. 1980;17:44–7.
9. Lee JY, Seo JY, Baek SU. The effects of glasses for anisometropia on stereopsis. Am J Ophthalmol. 2013;156:1261–6.
10. Tomaç S, Birdal E. Effects of anisometropia on binocularity. J Pediatr Ophthalmol Strabismus. 2001;38:27–33.
11. Chandna A, Gonzales-Martin JA, Norcia AM. Recovery of contour integration in relation to LogMAR visual acuity during treatment of amblyopia in children. Invest Ophthalmol Vis Sci. 2004;45:4016–22.
12. Clarke MP, Wright CM, Hrisos S, Anderson JD, et al. Randomized controlled trial of treatment of unilateral visual impairment detected at preschool vision screening. BMJ 2003;29:327(7426):1251.
13. Cotter SA. Pediatric Eye Disease Investigator Group, Edwards AR, Wallace DK, et al. Treatment of anisometropic amblyopia in children with refractive correction. Ophthalmology. 2006;113(6):895–903.
14. Writing Committee for the Pediatric Eye Disease Investigator Group, Cotter SA, Foster NC, Holmes JM, et al. Optical treatment of strabismic and combined strabismic-anisometropic amblyopia. Ophthalmology. 2012;119(1):150–8.
15. Chen PL, Chen JT, Tai MC, et al. Anisometropic amblyopia treated with spectacle correction alone: possible factors predicting success and time to start patching. Am J Ophthalmol. 2007;143(1):54–60.
16. Stewart CE, Moseley MJ, Stephens DA, et al. Treatment dose-response in amblyopia therapy: the Monitored Occlusion Treatment of Amblyopia Study (MOTAS). Invest Ophthalmol Vis Sci. 2004;45:3048–54.
17. Fronius M, Cirina L, Ackermann H, et al. Efficiency of electronically monitored amblyopia treatment between 5 and 16 years of age: new insight into declining susceptibility of the visual system. Vis Res. 2014;103:11–9.
18. Pediatric Eye Disease Investigator Group. A prospective, pilot study of treatment of amblyopia in children 10 to <18 years old. Am J Ophthalmol. 2004;137:581–3.
19. Scheiman MM, Hertle RW, Beck RW, et al. Randomized trial of treatment of amblyopia in children aged 7 to 17 years. Arch Ophthalmol. 2005;123:437–47.
20. Stewart CE, Moseley MJ, Georgiou P, et al. Occlusion dose monitoring in amblyopia therapy: status, insights, and future directions. J AAPOS. 2017;21(5):402–6.
21. Repka MX, Beck RW, Holmes JM, et al. A randomized trial of patching regimens for treatment of moderate amblyopia in children. Arch Ophthalmol. 2003;121:603–11.
22. Pediatric Eye Disease Investigator Group. A randomized trial of prescribed patching regimens for treatment of severe amblyopia in children. Ophthalmology. 2003;110:2075–87.

23. Pediatric Eye Disease Investigator Group. Randomized trial of treatment of amblyopia in children aged 7 to 17 years. Arch Ophthalmol. 2005;123:437–47.
24. Pediatric Eye Disease Investigator Group. A randomized trial of near versus distance activities while patching for amblyopia in children aged 3 to less than 7 years. Ophthalmology. 2008;115:2071–8.
25. Pediatric Eye Disease Investigator Group. A randomized trial to evaluate 2 hours of daily patching for strabismic and anisometropic amblyopia in children. Ophthalmology. 2006;113:904–12.
26. Pediatric Eye Disease Investigator Group. Patching vs atropine to treat amblyopia in children aged 7 to 12 years: a randomized trial. Arch Ophthalmol. 2008;126:1634–42.
27. Pediatric Eye Disease Investigator Group Writing Committee. Randomized trial to evaluate combined patching and atropine for residual amblyopia. Arch Ophthalmol. 2011;129:960–2.
28. Pediatric Eye Disease Investigator Group. A randomized trial of increasing patching for amblyopia. Ophthalmology. 2013;120:2270–7.
29. Pediatric Eye Disease Investigator Group Writing Committee. A randomized trial comparing Bangerter filters and patching for the treatment of moderate amblyopia in children. Ophthalmology. 2010;117:998–1004.
30. Von Noorden GK, Campos AC. Patching regimens (letter). Ophthalmology. 2004;111:1063.
31. Greenberg MF. Patching regimens (letter). Ophthalmology. 2004;111:1063–4.
32. Kushner BJ. Patching regimen for amblyopia (letter). Ophthalmology. 2005;111:736.
33. Pratt Johnson JA, Tillson G. Management of strabismus and amblyopia: a practical guide. Chap. 7. New York: Thieme Medical Publishers, Inc., 1994. p. 74–90.
34. Pediatric Eye Disease Investigator Group. The course of moderate amblyopia treated with atropine in children: experience of the amblyopia treatment study. Am J Ophthalmol. 2003;136:630–9.
35. Pediatric Eye Disease Investigator Group. Two-year follow-up of a 6-month randomized trial of atropine vs patching for treatment of moderate amblyopia in children. Arch Ophthalmol. 2005;123:49–157.
36. Pediatric Eye Disease Investigator Group. A randomized trial of atropine regimens for treatment of moderate amblyopia in children. Ophthalmology. 2004;111:2076–85.
37. Pediatric Eye Disease Investigator Group. Pharmacological plus optical penalization treatment for amblyopia: results of a randomized trial. Arch Ophthalmol. 2009;127:22–30.
38. Pediatric Eye Disease Investigator Group Writing Committee, Rutstein RP, Quinn GE, Lazar EL, et al. A randomized trial comparing Bangerter filters and patching for the treatment of moderate amblyopia in children. Ophthalmology. 2010;117:998–1004.
39. Laria C, Pinero DP. Characterization of Bangerter filtereffect in mild and moderate amblyopia associated with strabismus. Binocul Vis Strabolog Q. 2012;27:174–86.
40. Iacobucci I, Archer S, Furr B, et al. Bangerter foils in the treatment of moderate amblyopia. Am Orthopt J. 2001;51:84–91.
41. Agervi P. Treatment with Bangerter filters. J AAPOS. 2011;15:121–2.
42. Spierer A, Raz J, Benezra O, et al. Treating amblyopia with liquid crystal glasses: a pilot study. Invest Ophthalmol Vis Sci. 2010;51:3395–8.
43. Wang J, Neely DE, Galli J, et al. A pilot randomized clinical trial of intermittent occlusion therapy liquid crystal glasses versus traditional patching for treatment of moderate unilateral amblyopia. J AAPOS. 2016;19:257–9. Randomized trial using liquid crystal glasses for occlusion therapy.
44. Erbağcı I, Okumuş S, Öner V, et al. Using liquid crystal glasses to treat amblyopia in children. J AAPOS. 2015;19:257–9.
45. Totsuka, S, Handa T, Ishikawa H, et al. Improvement of adherence with occlu-pad therapy for pediatric patients with amblyopia. BioMed Res. Int. 2018; 1–5.
46. Li SL, Reynaud A, Hess RF, et al. Dichoptic movie viewing treats childhood amblyopia. J AAPOS. 2015;19:401–5.

47. Reynaud A, Hess RF, Wang YZ, et al. Dichoptic movie viewing treats childhood amblyopia. J AAPOS. 2015;19:401–5.
48. Birch EE, Li SL, Jost RM, et al. Binocular iPad treatment for amblyopia in preschool children. J AAPOS. 2015;19:6–11.
49. Birch EE, Jost RM, De La Cruz A, et al. Binocular amblyopia treatment with contrast rebalanced movies. J AAPOS. 2019;23:160.e1-e5.
50. Kelly KR, Jost RM, Dao L, et al. Binocular iPad game vs Patching for treatment of amblyopia in children: a randomized clinical trial. JAMA Ophthalmol. 2016;134:1402–8.
51. Holmes JM, Manh VM, Lazar EL, et al. Pediatric eye disease investigator group. effect of a binocular ipad game vs part-time patching in children aged 5 to 12 years with amblyopia: a randomized clinical trial. JAMA Ophthalmol. 2016;134:1391–400.
52. Pediatric Eye Disease Investigator Group, Holmes JM, Manny RE, Lazar EL, et al. A randomized trial of binocular dig rush game treatment for amblyopia in children aged 7 to 12 years. Ophthalmology. 2019;126:456–66
53. Manh VM, Holmes JM, Lazar EL, et al. Pediatric eye disease investigator group. randomized trial of a binocular ipad game versus part-time patching in children aged 13 to 16 years with amblyopia. Am J Ophthalmol. 2018;186:104–15.
54. Holmes JM, Manney RE, Kraker R, et al. RCT of binocular treatment for amblyopia in 4–6 year-olds. Presented at: American Academy of Ophthalmology 2020 annual meeting; 13–15 November 2020. Abstract PO320.
55. The Binocular Treatment of Amblyopia Using Videogames clinical trial group compared the conventional and binocular video games in older children and adults and reported no increase of visual outcomes with binocular games. Effectiveness of a Binocular Video Game vs Placebo Video Game for improving visual functions in older children, teenagers, and adults with amblyopia: a randomized clinical trial. JAMA Ophthalmol. 2018;136(2):172–81.
56. Gao TY, Guo CX, Babu RJ, Black JM, Bobier WR, Chakraborty A, Dai S, Hess RF, Jenkins M, Jiang Y, Kearns LS, Kowal L, Lam CSY, Pang PCK, Parag V, Pieri R, Raveendren RN, South J, Staffieri SE, Wadham A, Walker N, Thompson B. BRAVO study team. JAMA Ophthalmol. 2018;136(2):172–81.
57. Pineles SL, Aakalu VK, Hutchinson AK, et al. Binocular Treatment of amblyopia a report by the American Academy Of Ophthalmology. Ophthalmology. 2020;127:261–72.
58. Xiao S, Gaier ED, Mazow ML, et al. Improved adherence and treatment outcomes with an engaging, personalized digital therapeutic in amblyopia. Sci Rep. 2020;10(1):8328.
59. Žiak P, Holm A, Halička J, et al. Amblyopia treatment of adults with dichoptic training using the virtual reality oculus rift head mounted display: preliminary results. BMC Ophthalmol. 2017;17:105.
60. Xiao S, Angjeli E, Wu HC, et al. Luminopia pivotal trial group. randomized controlled trial of a dichoptic digital therapeutic for amblyopia. Ophthalmology. 2022;129:77–85.
61. Gibson EJ. Perceptual learning. Ann Rev Psychol. 1963;14:29–56.
62. Willshaw HE, Malmheden A, Clarke J, et al. Experience with the CAM vision stimulator: preliminary report. Br J Ophthalmol. 1980;64:339–41.
63. Tytla ME, Labow-Daily LS. Evaluation of the CAM treatment for amblyopia: a controlled study. Invest Ophthalmol Vis Sci. 1981;20:400–6.
64. Nyman KG, Singh G, Rydberg A, et al. Controlled study comparing CAM treatment with occlusion therapy. Br J Ophthalmol. 1983;67:178–80.
65. Levi DM, Li RW. Perceptual learning as a potential treatment for amblyopia: a mini-review. Vis Res. 2009;49:2535–49.
66. Leguire LE, Walson PD, Rogers GL, Bremer DL, McGregor ML. Levodopa/carbidopa treatment for amblyopia in older children. J Pediatr Ophthalmol Strabismus. 1995;32:143–51.
67. Campos EC, Bolzani R, Schiavi C, Baldi A, Porciatti V. Cytidine-5-diphosphocholine enhances the effect of part-time occlusion in amblyopia. Doc Ophthalmol. 1997;93:247–63.

68. Pediatric Eye Disease Investigator Group, Repka MX, Kraker RT, Dean TW, et al. A randomized trial of levodopa as treatment for residual amblyopia in older children. Ophthalmology. 2015;122:874–81.
69. Sharif MH, Talebnejad MR, Rastegar K, et al. Oral fluoxetine in the management of amblyopic patients aged between 10 and 40 years old: a randomized clinical trial. Eye (Lond). 2019;33:1060–7.
70. Pawar PV, Mumbare SS, Patil MS, et al. Effectiveness of the addition of citicoline to patching in the treatment of amblyopia around visual maturity: a randomized controlled trial. Indian J Ophthalmol. 2014;62(2):124–9.
71. Pandey PK, Chaudhuri Z, Kumar M, et al. Effect of levodopa and carbidopa in human amblyopia. J Pediatr Ophthalmol Strabismus. 2002;39(2):81–9.

Low Vision Aids

71

Aysun İdil and Esra Şahli

Abstract

Low vision rehabilitation includes ascertaining patients' needs and requirements, assessing their visual capabilities, training techniques, and prescribing an appropriate low vision aid. Low vision aids can be classified into optical aids (telescopes, magnifiers, high dioptric power eyeglasses), non-optical aids (filters, lighting, typoscopes, reading stands, etc.), electro-optic systems such as closed-circuit television systems; and electronic assistive technologies (specialized computer adaptation, mobile phone and tablet applications). Early intervention with low vision rehabilitation will improve visual function by reducing visual deprivation at an early age. Enhancement of visual function improves the quality of life and strengthens academic performance in visually impaired children.

Keywords

Low vision aid · Low vision rehabilitation · Telescopes · Magnifiers · Electronic vision enhancement systems · Visual habilitation

A. İdil (✉) · E. Şahli
Ophthalmologist, Department of Ophthalmology, School of Medicine, Low Vision Rehabilitation and Research Center, Ankara University, Ankara, Turkey
e-mail: sefayaysunidil@gmail.com

E. Şahli
e-mail: esracansizoglu@gmail.com

Introduction

According to the 11th revision of the World Health Organization International Classification of Diseases, a person has 'low vision or moderate to severe vision impairment' if his/her visual acuity is less than 6/18 (20/63) but equal to or better than 3/60 (20/400). 'Blindness' is defined as visual acuity of less than 3/60. 'Visual impairment' includes both low vision and blindness [1]. Childhood low vision refers to visual impairment in a person under the age of 15 years that cannot be corrected by medical or surgical treatments or conventional eyeglasses or contact lenses and which causes a restriction in the everyday life [2].

Children with low vision have different needs from adults since reduced visual input interferes with the acquisition and development of fundamental developmental skills in early and later childhood [2]. Vision is the most important sense of integration for humans. It enables the child to interact with his/her environment and provides information transfer to other sensory input systems. If there is no or insufficient visual stimulation, the motor, mental, emotional, and social development of children is delayed.

Visual impairment does not affect just the children's life negatively, but also the entire family and the community, and the country at large. Due to the potential life-years ahead, children have a predominant role in public health measures. In terms of the burden of blindness, measured in blind-person-years, childhood blindness is second only to cataracts in the world population [3, 4]. So, childhood has a priority in low vision rehabilitation compared to other age groups. The main goals of low vision rehabilitation for children are to develop visual perception, to maximize the child's current vision with appropriate methods and devices, and to increase the quality of life, for example, to ensure that the child gets the most out of educational opportunities.

Low vision rehabilitation starts with ascertaining patients' needs and requirements as well as assessing their visual capabilities to facilitate a program that may involve prescribing an appropriate device, environmental modification, and/or training techniques. History-taking from children with low vision or their parents differs from that in the routine eye examination. Special attention needs to be given to the children's daily routine including home environment, school, hobbies, and sports. Questions should be asked about which activities they are limited in and wish to continue doing. It should be determined whether they use any methods to help them perform the activities that they have difficulty with. The children's visual complaints, level of independence, support for performing tasks should also be detected. Commonly reported problems in school are in copying information from blackboard/whiteboard, reading books, handwriting, or drawing. Children usually use the strategies for distant tasks like walking up to the blackboard, copying from friends' notebooks, or taking notes from peers or teachers, and copying at home. At near tasks, they usually prefer reading the text very close or they may need a larger print size. It must be kept in mind that patients may have different needs, and each patient should be offered personalized solutions.

The approach to the management of pediatric patients with low vision will vary depending on the child's age and level of visual functions. Children's ability to perform important sight-based tasks is defined as "visual functions". In addition to visual acuity, visual functions should be assessed using parameters such as visual field, contrast sensitivity, electrophysiological tests, adequacy of preferred retinal locus, color vision, binocularity, and stereopsis. Accurately measuring distant and near visual acuity is vital for determining the best-corrected acuity with refraction, monitoring disease progression and the effect of treatment, as well as estimating the dioptric power of optical devices to be tested.

Interventions

The objective of interventions in children is to improve visual functions through optical and non-optical aids, and/or electronic devices. Improving visual functions is done by modifying the retinal image through magnification, filtration, or sometimes minification, and to improve environmental conditions related to visual function. Magnification is the main method in low vision rehabilitation. It can be achieved in four ways, and they can be combined to provide even further magnification in most of the low vision aids (LVA). These ways are increasing the relative size of the object itself, increasing its relative size by reducing its relative distance, angular magnification (telescopic magnification), and amplification by electronic projection [5]. When determining the correct power of a low vision device equivalent viewing distance (EVD) is the most appropriate way to represent magnification. The EVD is the distance at which the object would subtend an angle that is equal to the angle that the image subtends at the eye. Because children can accommodate far better than adults, EVD proves to be the ideal measure for magnification in children [6].

For patients to benefit from LVAs, their visual acuity should be within a range. Patients with visual acuity better than 20/400 have a higher chance of being successful with the use of optical aids and the patients with a corrected visual acuity of around 20/40 can usually perform the daily activities adequately without the need for LVA [5, 7–9].

A low vision aid is any device that enables a person with low vision to improve visual performance. LVAs can be classified into optical aids (telescopes, magnifiers, high dioptric power eyeglasses), non-optical aids (filters, lighting, typoscopes, reading stands, etc.), electro-optic systems such as closed-circuit television systems (CCTV's); and electronic assistive technologies (specialized computer adaptation, mobile phone and tablet applications).

1. Telescopes

The telescope offers advantages to children in many distant and near daily tasks, such as reading what is written on the blackboard, reading street signs or bus numbers, and even reading a book. Telescopes can promote or increase their independence in school and social life.

Telescopes are either Galilean or Keplerian depending on their optical principles. The Galilean telescope consists of two lenses, a plus objective lens, and a minus eyepiece lens, and it gives an upright image. The Keplerian telescope also consists of two lenses, a plus objective lens, and a plus eyepiece lens. The inverted image obtained with Keplerian telescopes is corrected with prisms. Although Galilean telescopes have certain advantages such as being shorter and lighter and having a larger visual field, Keplerian telescopes have better image quality because they use light more efficiently. Keplerian telescopes are more complex with a wider range of focus (Fig. 71.1) [10, 11].

Telescopes can be focusable or fixed focus depending on their focusing characteristics. In focusable telescopes, the patient's spherical error can be corrected, so the addition of a base lens is often not necessary, except in the presence of high

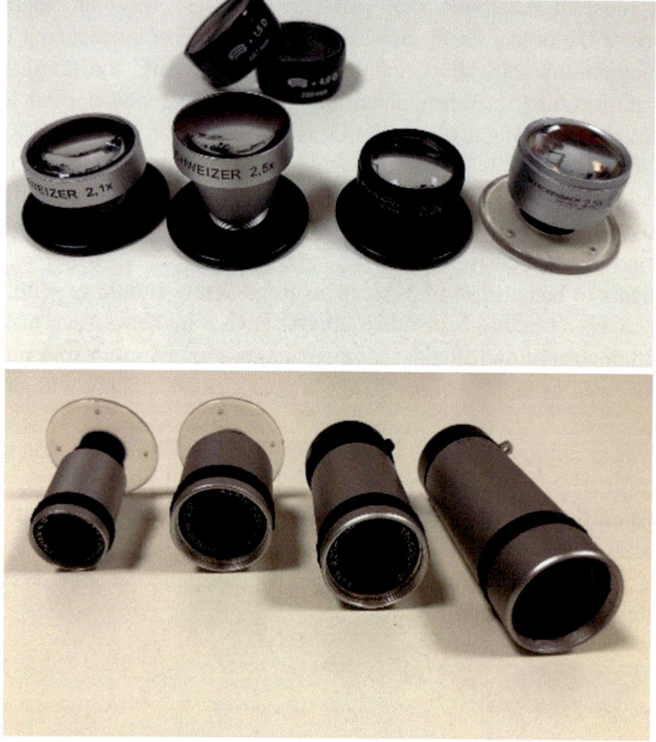

Fig. 71.1 Examples of Galilean and Kepler telescopes

astigmatism. With fixed-focus telescopes, the patient's refractive error (both spherical and cylindrical) should be given as the base lens. Depending on the patient's vision level, telescopes can be prescribed monocularly or binocularly. They can be used hand-held together with apparatus such as a chain worn on the neck or a ring worn on the finger, or they can be fitted custom made eyeglasses and used as hands-free. Hand-held telescopes must be positioned directly in front of the eye. The focusable focus devices are controlled by manually adjusting the distance. Therefore, using focusable telescopes can be challenging for young children. Eyeglass-mounted telescopes require no hand coordination and control [6]. They are mostly used for watching television or looking at the board by school-aged children, whereas a monocular hand telescope is hung around the neck or held in the palm and used only when needed, allowing the user to continue their everyday activities. Binocular telescopes are usually better for children with nystagmus. Because the amplitude and frequency of nystagmus can increase under monocular viewing conditions.

The advantage of telescopes includes being able to magnify an image at a wide working distance. Most focusable models can be focused between 20 cm and infinity. Fixed focus telescopes are for distant vision, a +3.00 to +12.00 D reading cap can be attached for near vision [10]. The major disadvantage of these telescopes is the narrow visual field, caused by the field of fixation that is restricted by the exit pupil of the telescope. Their length increases with their magnifying power, and the visual field narrows as their length increases and their diameter decreases. When moving using a telescope is difficult and dangerous, because of restrictions in the visual field, and difficulty in achieving binocularity. The other handicaps are its expensiveness and aesthetic concerns [6]. Although telescopes are not suitable for use when moving due to the narrowing of the visual field, various special designs have been developed to overcome this limitation. These designs, which are used when performing mobility tasks, are bioptic telescopes. In these telescopes, a compact, low-power magnifying telescope is placed in an area in the patient's visual field, usually the superotemporal region. The patient can see the magnified view from the telescope, when necessary, by adjusting the head or eye position while looking through her glasses. Bioptic telescopes can be used at magnifications of up to 6x (Fig. 71.2) [10]. Problems with manipulating the focus in these telescopic devices resulted in the development of a bioptic telescope with autofocus. With autofocus bioptic telescopes, this process is modified with a motorized focusing system so that the user can easily follow objects at different distances. Although bioptic telescopes are useful for distance viewing, their use is limited by their appearance and the ring scotoma surrounding the magnified image [10, 11].

The use of telescopic systems in visually impaired children should be promoted as early as possible. Fixed focus telescopic systems with low magnification are frequently preferred in pre-school and school-age children due to their ease of manipulation and their large field of vision. The focusable models require good eye-hand coordination. When telescopes are prescribed, children should be trained on how to control focus and search for a target before using telescopic glasses (Fig. 71.3) [5, 12].

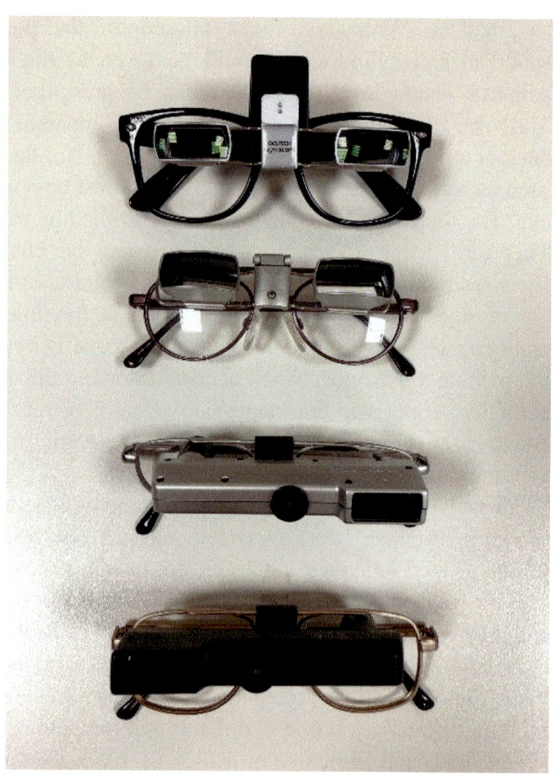

Fig. 71.2 Examples of bioptic telescopes

2. Magnifiers

Children with low vision often move closer and adopt an unnatural body position to view objects and prints in more detail. A larger range of accommodation of the children allows for an enlargement of the retinal image by decreasing the distance between the eye and the object [5]. But, this can cause poor posture over time. These children may benefit from several optical near-vision aids include hand-held magnifiers, stand magnifiers, and dome magnifiers. They can be used to meet the needs of children with low vision when reading and performing tasks requiring near vision. With hand-held magnifiers, the magnification factor can be manipulated by changing the distance between the magnifier and the object, as well as by changing the distance between the eye and the magnifier. The larger the distance between the magnifier and the object (provided it is less than one focal length), the greater the magnification. The magnification power also increases as the distance between the eye and the magnifier decreases [12]. As the magnification power increases, the field of vision decreases, and the effects of this can be solved by reducing the magnifier to eye distance. Children can choose the most suitable and comfortable viewing distance for different activities, depending on the size of the print or the object. Some advantages of hand-held magnifiers are that they are portable, can be used at longer working distances than eyeglasses, and are inexpensive. Some can

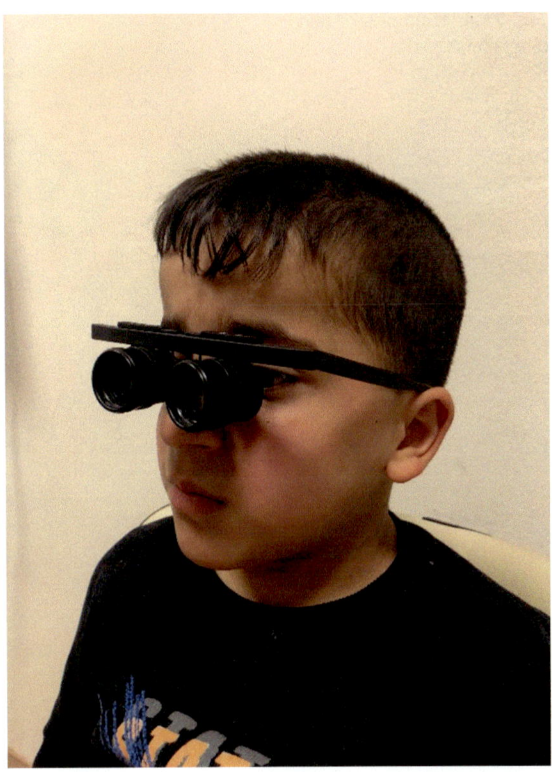

Fig. 71.3 A boy wearing telescopic glasses

have built-in illumination that makes them a good choice for most low-vision children who need more illumination. Aspheric magnifiers provide better image quality. The hand-held magnifiers require steady hands at a fixed working distance and good eye-hand coordination, especially for high-power magnifiers. This limits the usability of these devices for young children [10, 13]. Older children may prefer a small, discrete pocket magnifier as it can be hidden in their hands easily when using it (Fig. 71.4).

Stand, dome and bar magnifiers are also required hand control for nearby vision, but they must be navigated while resting on a fixed, flat surface (Fig. 71.5). So, the magnification power, therefore, is more stable and is only influenced by the eye-to-lens distance.

They usually include a built-in light source. This increases contrast and reduces the amount of magnification needed, thus increasing reading speed. Because the emerging light from a stand magnifier is divergent, it should be used with near eyeglasses of about +3.00 to +3.50 D in elderly patients. Providing the child has sufficient accommodation, a near addition is often not required for use with the stand magnifier. It is also preferred due to its ease of use in children. It may also be preferable for those who cannot use hand-held magnifiers due to poor hand–eye coordination, tremor, paralysis, or arthritis [14]. Stand magnifiers offer the most

Fig. 71.4 Examples of hand magnifiers

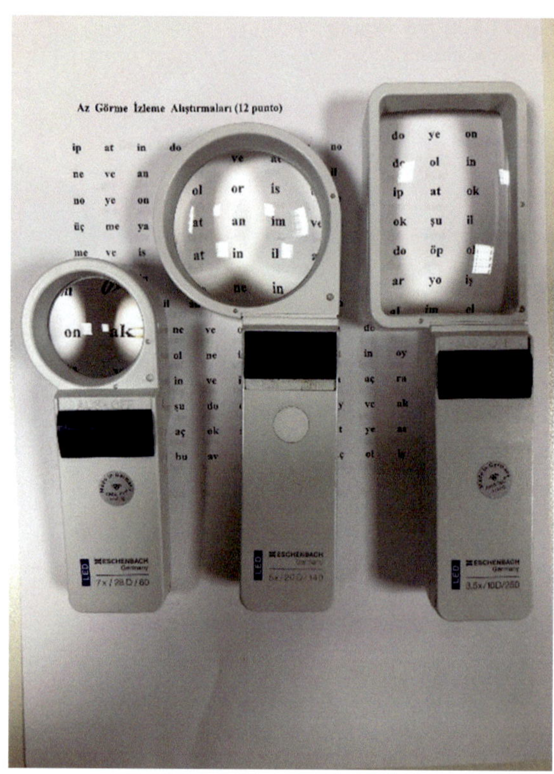

Fig. 71.5 Examples of stand, bar, and dome magnifiers

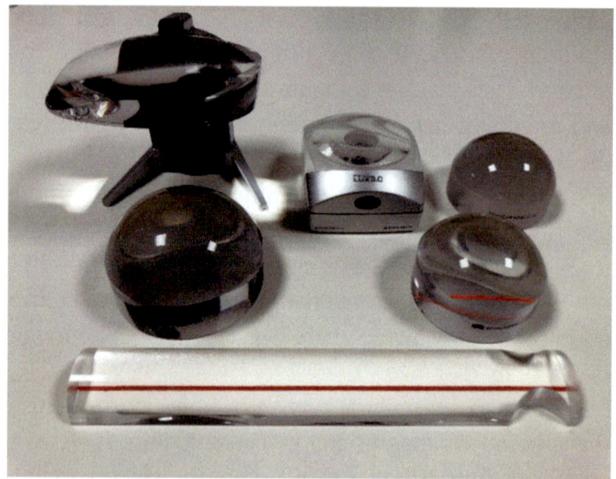

stable image compared to high dioptric power eyeglasses and hand-held magnifiers; this makes them a good choice for beginners, especially those who require high magnification. Dome magnifiers are very easy to use and often liked by children, but the available magnification power is typically only around 2x (Fig. 71.6) [5, 12].

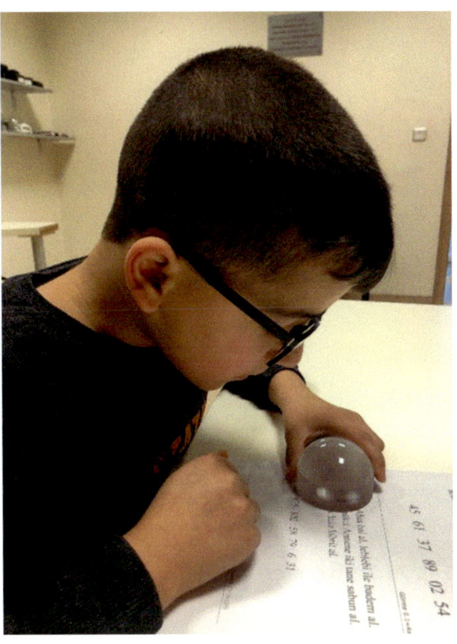

Fig. 71.6 A boy using dome magnifier when reading

3. **High dioptric power eyeglasses**

High dioptric power eyeglasses provide a large field of view, and this prolongs a child's reading time. The other advantages are that it looks good cosmetically and can be used hands-free compared to other devices. The major disadvantage of these glasses, the relatively short working distance, is also not usually a concern, as children with low vision are normally accustomed to reading closely (Fig. 71.7).

There are several ways to estimate the dioptric power of eyeglasses. In Kestenbaum's rule near addition is calculated as the inverse of best-corrected visual acuity. For example, in a patient with a corrected visual acuity of 20/200, the near add is the inverse of visual acuity, 200/20 = 10 diopters, and the reading distance is 1/10 = 10 cm. The addition is gradually increased to the dioptric power that allows the patient to comfortably read a text size of 1 M. Another more accurate and logical way is to estimate the required near addition by measuring near visual acuity using continuous text or words. Using near word or text acuities, equivalent viewing distance was calculated for specified print size, often 1 M print. Near dioptric power providing the calculated equivalent viewing distance is determined and tested [15]. The actual value will be higher than the predicted value in patients with low contrast sensitivity or macular scotoma. For the patients who want to read letters smaller than 1 M, the addition should also be increased. Binocular vision is possible if the addition is up to +10 diopters. As the dioptric power increases, the reading distance is reduced accordingly. It's difficult to tolerate values >10 diopters binocularly (Fig. 71.7) [10, 16].

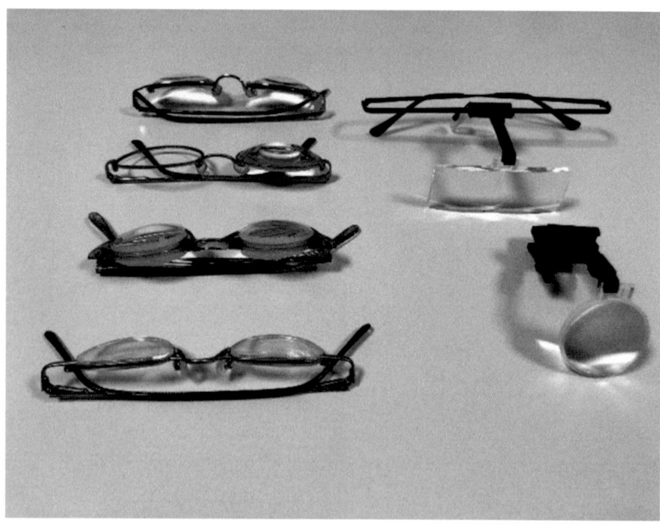

Fig. 71.7 Examples of high dioptric power eyeglasses with and without prisms and attachment magnifiers

In patients whose binocular vision is better than their monocular vision (i.e., with similar visual acuity in both eyes), a base-in prism should be incorporated into the near prescription to facilitate accommodative convergence. Although there are various formulas to calculate prism addition, a base-in prism with a power of 1 diopter more than the dioptric power addition can be added to both eyes. If the patients' reading performance is better when their worse sighted eye is closed (i.e., the patient is functionally monocular), a frosted lens can be prescribed for the worse eye or the patient can be instructed to close the lens in front of the worse eye when reading [16]. High dioptric (greater than +4.5 D) additions in bifocal and progressive lenses are difficult to tolerate binocularly. The problems at intermediate distance and far distance increase in parallel with dioptric power. So the patients with low vision should be recommended to use near glasses separate from the distant glasses, instead of progressive glasses. Moreover, as the use of high dioptric near glasses provides a larger visual field, it will enable eccentric viewing in patients with central scotoma [10].

4. Electro-optic Systems and Electronic Assistive Technologies

Electro-optic devices are called Electronic Vision Enhancement Systems (EVES) or Closed-circuit Television Systems (CCTV's). These systems project a text or image to a screen and enable adjustments such as magnifying, enhancement of brightness and contrast. They can be stand-mounted, head-mounted, hand-held, or mouse-operated. In general, they include a video camera, a monitor, and illumination. There is an additional XY table for placing the text to be read in the stand-mounted EVES. The advantages of electro-optic devices over optic devices are a larger field of view, a more comfortable working distance, and a wider magnification range. Magnification, brightness, contrast, and background color can be changed manually. Autofocus, voice-command controls, text to speech capability, and automatic forwarding have also been added to some systems. With these advantages, they are good options for children with severe visual impairment. Despite their many advantages, they are usually more expensive and larger than optical devices. However, with technological advances, these devices have become portable sizes and less expensive [6, 10].

The stand-mounted EVES is a device that electronically magnifies images and is frequently used for the enhancement of books. The book is placed on a controllable surface and the page is shown on a large screen. Magnification levels can be adjusted as desired. The disadvantages of the device are that it is bulky and relatively difficult to manipulate (Fig. 71.8).

More portable options are the hand-held and mouse-operated EVES, which are designed for bringing the camera to the object to be viewed. The hand-held devices are often on rollers, which makes them easier to move across a flat working surface. A mouse-operated electronic magnifier is a computer mouse with a camera that is moved over the material and records the image, which is shown on a computer screen. It can be connected to most personal computers. Hand-held and mouse-operated devices require good eye-hand coordination and have a limited field of view. However, they are easy to carry and cheaper than stand-mounted devices (Fig. 71.9). In head-mounted EVES, the camera is placed on a headset. The image recorded by the camera is enhanced electronically and projected in front of the eye. In most electro-optic devices, the adjustments such as magnification,

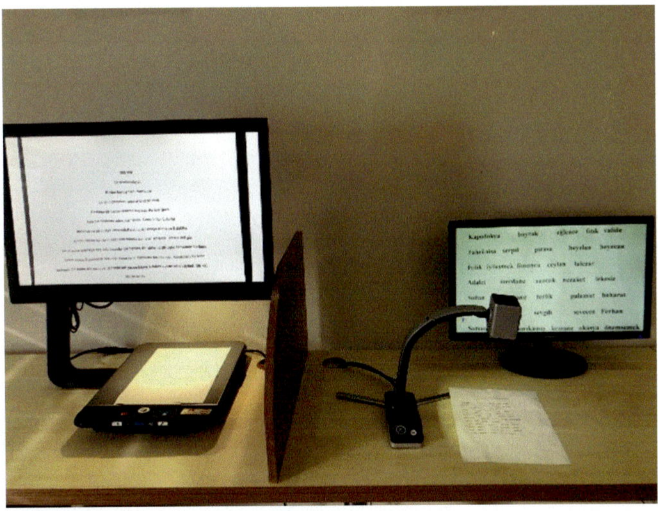

Fig. 71.8 Examples of stand-mounted electro-optic devices

brightness, contrast, and color require cognitive development as well as manual dexterity of the child [6].

The limitations of electro-optic devices such as a lack of portability, poor integration with school information technology networks, and problems with either input or output functions, have been overcome due to the portability of tablet computers and their capability of running a wide range of software and of accessing wireless networks [17]. Because children are quick to follow technology and can learn by trial and error, the accessibility and the acceptability of these devices are high for children. Especially in school-age children, the tablet computer attached to the child's desk with an apparatus can be used as an optical tool to follow the board and read the book. Applications such as Zoom and Magnifier, which can be accessed from the tablet's accessibility settings, are good alternatives to telescopic glasses for suitable children. When this function is used, the child can see the board hands-free through the tablet camera and can scroll the image without the need to move the tablet. For the near tasks, tablet computers make it easier for the child to read by displaying text in enlarged font, better contrast, brightness, and background color. As well as by assistive technologies they can read text out to the user, allow speech to text conversion, and provide access to wide sources of information through the internet (Fig. 71.10).

Electronic reading devices such as the iPad (Apple, Cupertino, CA, USA) and Kindle (Amazon, Seattle, WA, USA) may also be used by children with low vision. These devices include applications that enable the user to increase the size of characters; adjust the contrast, brightness, and color of the display background; magnify; zoom; zoom by taking a photograph of an image; take spoken commands; read text aloud. A prospective study showed that these types of electronic devices increased reading performance in most patients [18]. For those who want to work on a desktop computer, there are also computer speech and text enlargement packages that can be used at home and at school.

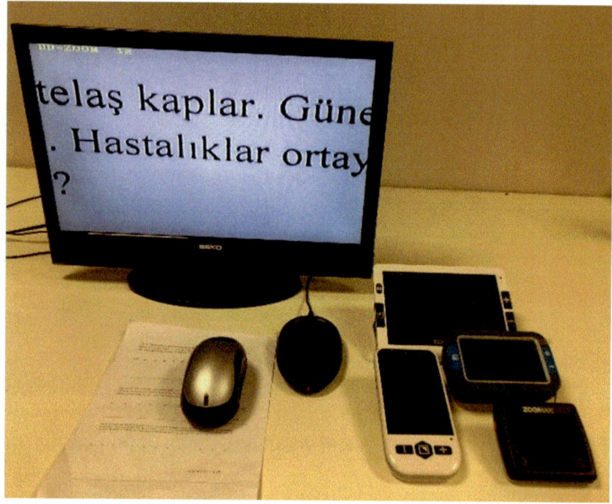

Fig. 71.9 Examples of hand-held electro-optic devices and a mouse-operated electronic magnifier

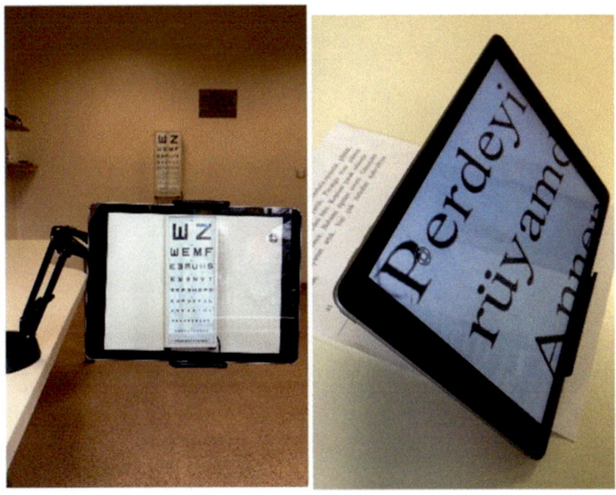

Fig. 71.10 Using an electronic tablet for distant and near view

Smartphone and tablet applications, as well as artificial intelligence technology, have contributed significantly to the available assistive technology for children with severe visual impairment. Applications such as Siri and Alexa, operate using only voice recognition. Audiobooks, computer screen reading software, and audio conversion for text messaging are additional resources that can facilitate the learning process, enhance communication with the world like their peers, and thus improve the quality of life of children with severe vision loss [10, 17, 19].

5. Filtering lenses

Filtering lenses filter certain wavelengths of light while allowing the passage of other wavelengths. This provides a clearer vision by increasing contrast sensitivity and reduces the patient's photophobia. The filtering lenses are in several colors based on the wavelength they filter. According to the patient's needs, different filtering lenses can be prescribed for use indoors and outdoors. Although there are filters recommended for certain diseases, it is more appropriate to try a set of filtering lenses to identify the filter the child is most comfortable with (Fig. 71.11) [10].

Non-optical Aids

Non-optical systems can be used alone or in conjunction with optical systems and increase the patient's residual visual function. Illumination, large-print books, increased contrast, typoscopes, reading stands, and sunglasses or eyeglasses with filtering lenses are some of the non-optical aids for children with low vision. Illumination reduces the need for magnification and increases reading performance, particularly in patients who have reduced contrast sensitivity. The use of a table lamp with a 'goose neck' to control the direction of the light can be helpful for those children who need illumination. The built-in illumination in hand-held and

Fig. 71.11 Filtering glasses

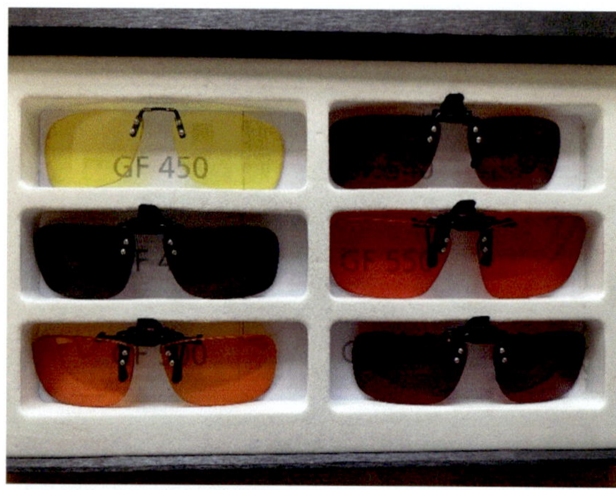

Fig. 71.12 An example of kitchen design for patients with low vision

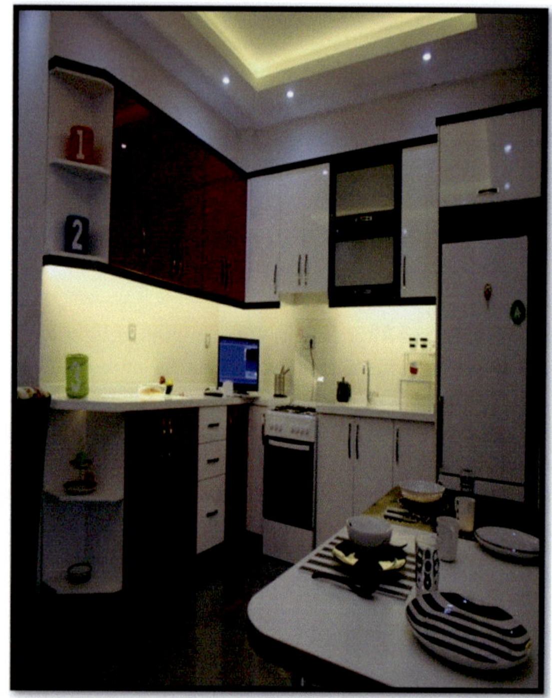

stand magnifiers increases reading performance for most children. On the other hand, patients complaining of excessive glare will benefit from reducing the light level and using hats, sunglasses, and light-blocking glasses. Patients can be advised to use different contrasts such as a light-colored object on dark background in daily life. Organizing the kitchen and other home environments in a contrasting and appropriate way, and accentuating steps and handrails will make daily life easier (Fig. 71.12).

Using typoscope and placing yellow translucent acetate sheet on the page can make print easier to read. Typoscope is a piece of black plastic or cardboard material with a cutout opening that makes patients focus easily on the line they are reading and provides excellent contrast with the reading page. Colored acetate sheets can enhance the contrast between the print and background [10]. As children bring reading materials closer to their eyes, they should be advised to use reading stands that provide better posture and ergonomics. Sloping desks can also be used in the school to help with posture when a child needs to adopt a closer working distance. Another magnification strategy used in education is the enlargement of hardcopy printed material. But, compared with text enlargement, LVAs may have the additional advantage of providing children with more independence of access to printed material [20, 21].

In children with severe vision loss, alternate tools and techniques such as white cane training, use of the Braille alphabet, audiobooks, and voice recording devices, can be offered. It is also very important to modify the children's living conditions. At home, consistent placement of items helps a child develop systems for daily living activities independent of visual cues. At school, large print books, bolded writing, sloped desks for closer working distance, optimal illumination, and even electronic systems can enhance a child's learning experience while at school [12].

Children accept low vision devices more easily than adults and with a higher success rate. Depending on the task, they may often need to use more than one device. It has been shown that the average number of devices prescribed per child with low vision varies from 1.3 to 2.3 [12, 22]. Preschool age 4–6 is the most suitable period for the use of low vision aid devices in rehabilitation. It is important to start low vision aids at the earliest possible age, for the acceptance of the device and its effective use in older ages. In this age group, it is more appropriate to start with telescopic glasses for distance. Generally, low power (such as 2X, 2.2X, 2.5X) Galilean type fixed focus telescopes are preferred. Although Kepler-type focusable telescopes can be used for near activities by focusing, they are not very suitable for this age group as they require dexterity and have a longer anterior–posterior length. Fixed focus telescopes can also be used for near activities by attaching reading caps calculated according to the distance to be studied. However, due to the narrowing effect of the visual field, which is one of the most important disadvantages of telescopic glasses, telescopic glasses are not preferred especially in near activities in children. Another point to be considered in the prescription of fixed focus telescopic glasses is to add the optical value related to the refractive error that children with low vision usually have. In the 4–6 age group, magnifiers and reading glasses are used for near tasks. Stand magnifiers and aspheric bright field and dome magnifiers are ideal for this age group. Studies demonstrated that children older than 3.5 years of age were capable of successfully using a stand magnifier [6]. Depending on the child's choice and eye disease, an illuminated magnifier or focal lighting can be used. Because lighting is a very important factor in children with low vision and can improve the child's functional vision, parents and teachers should be informed and guided in this regard. School-age is the period when LVA is used most effectively. Through these devices, it is possible for the children to participate in educational activities and be independent in their studies. However, due to cosmetic concerns and reactions from the child's peers during this period, children may refuse to use the device. For this reason, appropriate patients can be encouraged to use electro-optic devices after 8 years, when the child's hand–eye coordination also develops. The child and, if the child is young, the parents should be trained for efficient use of the prescribed device, and even home trials of the device should be advised. Good communication with parents and teachers is important to maximize the successful use of low vision devices. Because visual requirements change with age, children should attend follow-up visits at least every six months and the practitioner should change the aids to meet the changing circumstances.

Visual Habilitation

The first years of life are very important as it is the period most visual functions are acquired and improved. Vision loss in this period may cause developmental problems and learning difficulties in perception, cognition, motor function, communication, and visual attention in children [23, 24]. Sonksen first used the phrase 'developmental emergency' to describe the need for immediate care of babies with visual impairment [25]. So, unlike adults, even having light perception only should be considered as a developmental emergency for infants. From the suggestion that everyday visual impressions are not sufficient for optimal visual development, a visual habilitation program should be applied as soon as possible [24–26].

Visual stimulation is mostly applied to children who have difficulty responding to normal visual impressions, while visual training is applied to children who show slightly more visual attention to make them use their visual senses functionally [23, 24, 26]. In the conventional visual stimulation, visual stimuli suitable for the child's visual function such as using lights or objects with bright colors or high-contrast black and white patterns are used systematically and sequentially. (habilitasyon makalesi, 8 Bell) Behaviors aimed in these programs are efficient fixating, following moving objects and improving eye-hand coordination. Ergonomic and adaptive changes to visual stimuli such as adapting the lighting, color, contrast, and movement of visual stimuli are also a kind of visual stimulation [26, 27]. Studies showed that visual functions, electrophysiological response as well as visual acuity can be improved in young children with visual impairment by visual habilitation programs [28–30].

Case

A five-year-old girl with a history of laser treatment for retinopathy of prematurity 3 times before in her right eye. Her left eye was a prosthetic eye. She was born at 26 weeks of gestation and stayed in an incubator for 2 months.

The distant visual acuity was 0.8 log MAR (0.15) with the correction of -1.25 (+4.00 × 90) D and the near vision was 2 M (16 points) in her right eye. Since the child was at the age of starting school, her parents were informed about the choice of school and profession. For distance vision, fixed focus telescopic glasses with 2.5x magnification were tried and her refractive error was added to the glasses. Her distant visual acuity increased to 0.4 log MAR with the telescopic glasses. Her near vision increased to 1 M at 25 cm with the addition of +4.00 D reading cap to her telescopic glasses. Due to the visual field narrowing effect of telescopic glasses, a dome magnifier with 1.8x magnification was prescribed for long-term reading.

The family was informed about the child's legal rights regarding education such as sitting in front desks in the classroom, using low vision aid devices in the lessons, and the right to additional time in the exams. Her visual acuities were similar at her follow-up visits. After primary school, electronic tablet training was given to use at school. Now she continues her high school education with these systems and is an academically successful student.

Conclusion

Low vision in childhood is a significant barrier to the development and learning process. It is important to stimulate the efficient use of vision in early childhood, as this promotes the global development of these children, improves their education and social life. Children with visual impairment face many challenges in school, with orientation and mobility, and with social interactions. The children are not physically active because of a lack of functional independence. Visual impairment can lead to social isolation, which can eventually lead to diminished self-esteem. Children with low vision often fall behind in reading rate [31–33]. Children using devices tend to improve their reading performance while children who use large print tend to have a plateau [34]. They can approach the reading performance of normally sighted children with appropriate devices [33]. LVAs also act as a tool for visual stimulation and are helpful in improving the baseline best-corrected visual acuity after using over a period [35]. Early intervention with low vision rehabilitation will strengthen visual function by reducing visual deprivation at an early age. Low vision devices will provide them with more accurate visual information, which will increase their chances of receiving education in mainstream schools with their sighted peers. Enhanced visual function, improved quality of life and stronger academic performance gains in visually impaired children can be achieved with appropriate and comprehensive low vision management.

Review Questions

1. Which of the following is the most important disadvantage of telescopic glasses in low vision rehabilitation?

a. Reading distance is too short
b. It is not cosmetic
c. Visual field is narrow
d. Not possible to use while walking
e. Binocular use not possible

2. A child who uses 2.2X fixed focus telescopic glasses to see the board wants to read a book from 20 cm with the same glasses. How many diopters (D) should the reading cap be and what would be the total power of the near system?

a. Reading cap + 4 D, magnification power of close system 2.5X
b. Reading cap + 5 D, magnification power of close system 2.75X
c. Reading cap + 5 D, magnification power of close system 2.5X
d. Reading cap + 10 D, magnification power of close system 5X
e. Reading cap + 10 D, magnification power of close system 2.5X

3. A child with low vision who has accommodation lag can read 4 M at 33 cm with +3.00 near glasses. What should be the power (diopter-D) of the system you recommend for 1 M continuous text reading?

a. 12 D
b. 15 D
c. 18 D
d. 20 D
e. 22 D

Answers

1. C
2. B
3. A

References

1. World Health Organization, Blindness and vision impairment. https://www.who.int/news-room/fact-sheets/detail/blindness-and-visual-impairment. Accessed December 2021.
2. Clinical Council for Eye Health Commissioning. Low Vision, Habilitation and Rehabilitation Framework for Adults and Children; July 2017. https://www.rnib.org.uk/sites/default/files/Low%20vision%2C%20habilitation%20and%20rehabilitation%20framework%20for%20adults%20and%20children%20%282%29_0.pdf. Accessed December 2021.

3. Gogate PM, Chottopadhyay T, Kaur H, Narayandas S, Phadke S, Kharat M, et al. Making blind children see: impact of correcting moderate and severe visual impairment in schools for the blind. Middle East Afr J Ophthalmol. 2019;26:216–22.

4. Rahi JS, Gilbert CE, Foster A, Minassian D. Measuring the burden of childhood blindness. Br J Ophthalmol. 1999;83:387–8.

5. Haddad MAO, Sampaio MW, Oltrogge EW, Kara-José N, Betinjane AJ. Visual impairment secondary to congenital glaucoma in children: visual responses, optical correction and use of low vision aids. Clinics. 2009;64(8):725–30.

6. Schurink J, Cox RF, Cillessen AH, van Rens GH, Boonstra FN. Low vision aids for visually impaired children: a perception-action perspective. Res Dev Disabil. 2011;32(3):871–82.

7. Sampaio MW, Haddad MAO, Kara-José N. Auxílios para baixa visão. São Paulo, Laramara;2001

8. Faye EE Padula WV, Gurland JE, Grennberg ML, Hood CM. The low vision child. In: Faye EE. editors. Clinical low vision, 2nd ed. Boston: Little, Brown and Company;1984. p. 437–75.

9. Lindsted E. Accomodation in the visually impaired child. In: Woo G. editor. Low vision. Principles and applications. Waterloo: Springer;1986. p. 425–35.

10. Şahlı E, İdil A. A common approach to low vision: examination and rehabilitation of the patient with low vision. Turk J Ophthalmol. 2019;49:89–98.

11. Wolffsohn JS. Telescopes. In: Jackson AJ, Wolfsohn JS, editors. Low vision manual. 1st ed. Butterworth Heinemann Elsevier, PA: USA;2007. p. 241–56.

12. Lee SM, Cho JC. Low vision devices for children. Community Eye Health. 2007;20(62): 28–9.

13. Rumney NJ. Hand magnifiers. In: Jackson AJ, Wolfsohn JS, editors. Low vision manual. 1st ed. Butterworth Heinemann Elsevier, PA: USA;2007. p. 198–209.

14. Wolffsohn JS. Stand magnifiers. In: Jackson AJ, Wolfsohn JS, editors. Low vision manual. 1st ed. Butterworth Heinemann Elsevier, PA: USA;2007. p. 210–22.

15. Lovie-Kitchin J. Reading with low vision: the impact of research on clinical management. Clin Exp Optom. 2011;94(2):121–32.

16. Rumney NJ. Spectacle magnifiers. In: Jackson AJ, Wolfaohn JS, editors. Low vision manual. 1st ed. Butterworth Heinemann Elsevier, PA: USA;2007. p. 223–40.

17. Crossland MD, Thomas R, Unwin H, et al. Tablet computers versus optical aids to support education and learning in children and young people with low vision: protocol for a pilot randomised controlled trial, CREATE (Children Reading with Electronic Assistance to Educate). BMJ Open. 2017;7:e015939.

18. Morrice E, Johnson AP, Marinier JA, Wittich W. Assessment of the Apple iPad as a low-vision reading aid. Eye. 2017;31:865–71.

19. Alves CC, Monteiro GB, Rabello S, et al. Assistive technology applied to education of students with visual impairment. Rev Panam Salud Publica. 2009;26:148–52.

20. Corn AL, Koenig AJ. Literacy for students with low vision: a framework for delivering instruction. J Vis Impairm Blind. 2002;96(5):305–21.

21. Douglas G, McLinden M, McCall S, Pavey S, Ware J, Farrell AM. Access to print literacy for children and young people with visual impairment: findings from a review of the literature. Eur J Spec Needs Educ. 2011;26(1):25–38.

22. Cho J. The preference of low vision devices of the Hong Kong low vision students. Paper presented in the 12th world conference of the international council for education of people with visual impairment;2006. EA034.

23. Hatton DD. Model registry of early childhood visual impairment: first year results. J Vis Impair Blind. 2001;95:418–33.

24. Dale N, Salt A. Early support developmental journal for children with visual impairment: the case for a new developmental framework for early intervention. Child Care Health Dev. 2007;33(6):684–90.

25. Sonksen PM. Developmental aspects of visual disorders. Curr Paediatr. 1997;7:18–22.

26. Vervloed MPJ, Janssen N, Knoors H. Visual rehabilitation of children with visual impairments. J Dev Behav Pediatr. 2006;27:493–506.
27. Corn AL. Low vision and visual efficiency. In: Scholl GT, editor. Foundations of education for blind and visually handicapped children and youth: theory and practice. New York: American Foundation for the Blind;1986. p. 99Y117.
28. Leguire LE, Fellows RR, Rogers GL, Bremer DL. The CCH vision stimulation program for infants with low vision: preliminary results. J Vis Impair Blind. 1992;86:33–7.
29. Sonksen PM, Petrie A, Drew KJ. Promotion of visual development of severely visually impaired babies: evaluation of a developmentally based programme. Dev Med Child Neurol. 1991;33:320–35.
30. Tsai LT, Hsu JL, Wu CT, Chen CC, Su YC. A new visual stimulation program for improving visual acuity in children with visual impairment: a pilot study. Front Hum Neurosci. 2016;18 (10):157.
31. Lieberman LJ, McHugh E. Health-related fitness of children who are visually impaired. J Vis Impair Blind. 2001;96:272–87.
32. Cochrane G, Lamoureux E, Keeffe J. Defining the content for a new quality of life questionnaire for student with low vision. Ophthal Epidemiol. 2008;15:114–20.
33. Lovie-Kitchin JE, Bevan JD, Hein B. Reading performance in children with low vision. Clin Exp Optom. 2001;84:148–54.
34. Corn AL. Optical devices or large type: Is there a debate. International Conference on Low Vision 1990.
35. Kavitha V, Heralgi MM, Parkar M, Harogoppa S. Quality of life in children with low vision following use of low vision aids. Taiwan J Ophthalmol. 2019;10(3):203–7.

Guidance for Social/School Life and Future Directions

Eric Wei Chen Lai, Janet Alexander, Erin Kenny, and Moran Roni Levin

Abstract

Visual impairment in the children with vitreoretinal disease can greatly impact both academic and social environments. Low vision in children can have ramifications on psychosocial, physical, and mental health that require tailored attention and guidance for each child. Families should be educated and advised on which activities are safest and most beneficial for their child. Affected children require early diagnosis, close monitoring, and prompt referral to visual rehabilitation centers to implement optical aids and low vision devices. These services can increase functional vision and lead to overall improved academic performance and quality of life. It is important for the ophthalmologist to recognize children's individual needs and provide available resources in schools, communities, and local agencies to ensure well-being in both the child and the family.

Keywords

Low vision · Academics · Social development · Visual rehabilitation · Optical aids

E. W. C. Lai · J. Alexander
School of Medicine, University of Maryland, Baltimore, MD, USA
e-mail: WeiChen.Lai@som.umaryland.edu

J. Alexander
e-mail: JAlexander@som.umaryland.edu

E. Kenny
Pennsylvania College of Optometry, Salus University, Philadelphia, PA, USA
e-mail: ekenny@salus.edu

M. R. Levin (✉)
University of Maryland School of Medicine, 419 West Redwood Street, Suite 479, Baltimore, MD 21201, USA
e-mail: rlevin@som.umaryland.edu

© The Author(s), under exclusive license to Springer Nature Switzerland AG 2023
Ş. Özdek et al. (eds.), *Pediatric Vitreoretinal Surgery*,
https://doi.org/10.1007/978-3-031-14506-3_72

1079

Introduction

Background

Infants, children, and teenagers with vitreoretinal disease require continued maintenance of social and academic goals while managing their specific ophthalmic disease. Attention and emphasis must be given to the unique needs of each child. Youth development requires recreation, new experiences and challenges, physical fitness, and academic progress; all of which may be impacted by vitreoretinal disease. It is important for the vitreoretinal specialist to be aware of resources that exist in the community and to work with schools and local agencies to provide social and educational support for pediatric patients and their families.

Low Vision Incidence and Comorbidities

Epidemiology

There are an estimated 1.5 million blind children in the world [1]. The prevalence of childhood blindness ranges from 0.3 in 1000 children aged 0–15 years in highly industrialized regions (i.e. Western Europe, North America, and Japan) to 1.5 in 1000 children in developing countries (i.e., some parts of Asia and Africa) [2].

In a 2012 study evaluating 3070 students across various schools for the blind in the United States, the leading causes of blindness were reported to be cortical visual impairment (CVI) (18%), optic nerve hypoplasia (ONH) (15%), and retinopathy of prematurity (ROP) (14%). Other less common causes include optic atrophy, albinism, coloboma, glaucoma, non-ROP related retinal detachment, Leber congenital amaurosis, retinitis pigmentosa, and congenital cataract [3].

Coexisting disabilities in children with visual impairment are common. Among young children with severe visual impairments such as CVI, ONH, and ROP, approximately 65–75% have disabilities in addition to low vision [4–6]. The most common concurrent disabilities are intellectual deficit and autism spectrum disorder [6]. Careful attention to other disabilities is required to further support developmental needs or visually impaired children.

Psychosocial Impact of Visual Impairment on Quality of Life

Impact on Academics

A cohort study of 8-year-old children with a history of threshold ROP found significant developmental, educational, and social skill differences between those who had favorable versus unfavorable visual status. Children with unfavorable visual status suffered from below-grade-level skills in academic settings, as well as social challenges during independent playtime, peer interaction, and participation in sports settings, requiring additional education resources [7].

Development of fine motor skills is essential for a child's independence of pursuing object manipulation and self-care. A study evaluating children aged 3–7 with altered visual development found that deficits in fine motor skills and slow reading speed were correlated with lower self-perception of academic, athletic, and social competence [8, 9].

Clinical Case

A 12-year-old female presents for ocular evaluation due to difficulty reading in school. Best corrected visual acuity is 20/200 in the right eye and 20/250 in the left eye. There is bilateral pigmentary maculopathy on retinal examination (Figs. 72.1 and 72.2). Fluorescein angiography shows dark choroid with stippled hyperfluorescence (Fig. 72.3). Humphrey visual field shows bilateral central scotomas. Genetic testing indicates a mutation of the ABCA4 gene consistent with a diagnosis of Stargardt disease. You refer the patient to a low vision specialist who recommends the use of a handheld telescope to magnify objects in the distance. The patient returns for follow-up stating that she does not want to use low vision aids in the classroom because she feels embarrassed to stand out among her peers.

Case Discussion

Children with vitreoretinal disease face a unique set of daily challenges that may impact their quality of life. The psychosocial burden of low vision influences many settings including home, school, athletics, and social interaction. It is critical for healthcare providers to recognize the functional abilities and limitations of patients with low vision to better serve their needs. Students may feel stigmatized by the use of visual adaptations such as magnifiers, assistive technology and classroom accommodations. However, given this age of technology, students are becoming

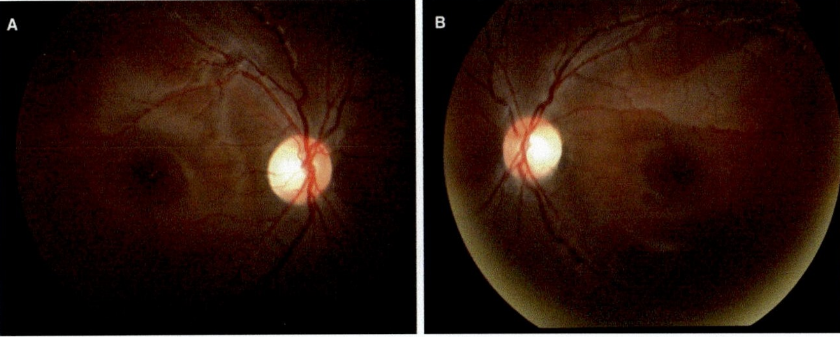

Fig. 72.1 Color fundus photograph of right eye (**A**) and left eye (**B**)

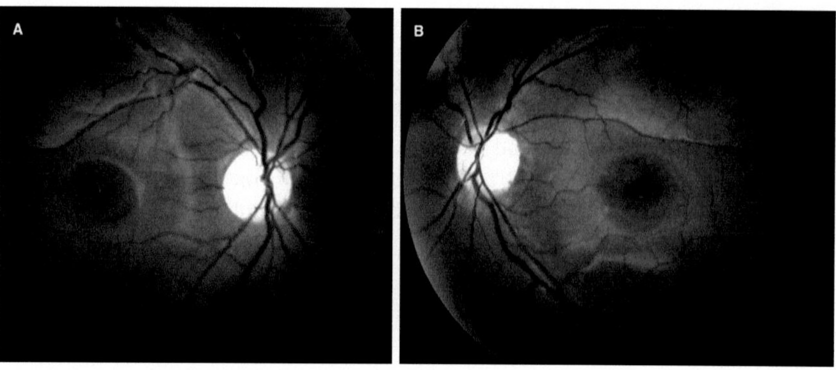

Fig. 72.2 Red free photograph of right eye (**A**) and left eye (**B**)

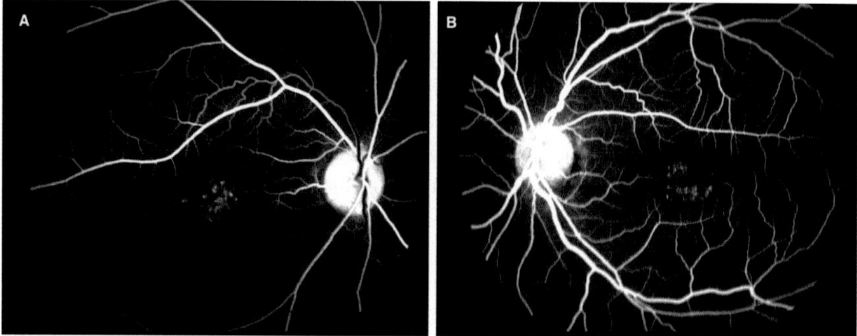

Fig. 72.3 Fluorescein angiogram photograph of right eye in transit (**A**) and left eye (**B**)

more accustomed to using technology and find this socially acceptable. Some students may consider using a laptop or smart phone as an adaptive device, making use of magnification and contrast settings in the classroom. Laptops and smart phones may provide a highly peer-accepted and even desirable low vision aid for young students, in contrast to more bulky or unusual devices.

Impact on Mental Health

Aside from self-perception of physical and emotional competence, studies show that children and young adults with visual impairments also suffer from more mental health issues compared to their peers. Common mood disorders associated among children with vision loss include reduced mobility, loneliness, greater dependency on help, and greater difficulty understanding their peers' facial expressions and associated emotions [10].

Physicians caring for children with low vision should be aware of resources that exist for academic, social, and emotional support. State agencies for the visually impaired can be a great starting point for parents and students to connect them with the resources that a student may need. These include advocacy for the student in the school system, the purchase of low vision devices that benefit the child in and out of the classroom, and referrals to rehabilitation specialists such as orientation and mobility specialist and teachers of the visually impaired. State agencies for the visually impaired may also connect children and parents to support groups and mentorship programs that will aid in social and emotional support.

Additional discussions regarding low vision services in local schools or the potential referral for state schools for the blind should take place with families. Individualized educational plans (IEP) are crucial for the success of a child with visual impairment in the school system. If a public school is not able to provide the accommodations recommended by a low vision specialist, a referral to a state school for the blind should be considered. Common IEP recommendations include increased print size on reading material, the use of low vision devices in the classroom, preferential seating, accessibility features on tablets and laptops, writing in answers instead of filling in bubble sheets, and extended test taking time. In coordination with IEPs, learning media assessments can be performed by teachers of the visually impaired in the school setting to discover the best learning modality for the student—such as visual, auditory or tactile. Teachers of the visually impaired are also trained in teaching Braille if the assessment shows that tactile would be the best reading option. Students will also work with their teachers of the visually impaired throughout their education to make sure they do not fall behind due to visual difficulties. It is also critical to optimize refractive and amblyopia management in children with reduced vision to give them the best possible visual potential. Chapters 1 and 2, Sect. 11 detail the refractive rehabilitation and amblyopia management in children with pediatric retinal disorders.

Key knowledge points

- Safety and wellness are not mutually exclusive. Use advice framed as "I would advise against contact sports such as soccer, but activities like dance and swimming are alternatives that are lower risk"
- Refer children with visual impairment or blindness for low vision evaluation. Remind families that low-vision services will be ongoing as children's needs change rapidly, as do technologic advances
- Co-management between the pediatric retina specialist and the pediatric ophthalmologist is important to optimize refractive and amblyopia management
- Consider referral to state agency for the visually impaired
- Consider referral to sports and arts for the visually impaired child

Table 72.1 Developmental objectives, concerns, and limitations across pediatric age groups in children with reduced vision

Age group	Developmental objectives	Primary concerns	Functional limitations
Ages 0–2 years	Sensory development	Reaching practical milestones, healthy development	Impaired gross motor skills, expressive language, receptive language
Ages 3–6 years	Mobile independence and play	Finding balance between independence and protection	Impaired fine motor skills; slow reading speed
Ages 7–12 years	Communication, social interaction, school life, social-emotional well being	Increasing awareness of visual impairment; worrying about fitting in and asking for help	Reduced mobility; impaired social communication, comprehension, and expression
Ages 13–17 years	Autonomy, acceptance	Keeping up with sighted peers, social isolation; frustration with mobile limitations (i.e., driving), worrying about reaching full independence	Reduced mobility; dependence on caregivers; reliance on visual aids

Physical Activities and Restrictions in Children with Low Vision

Physical activity is important for all children to develop general health, physical fitness, and quality of life. Participation in these activities build confidence and independence in different environments. To guide a child's specific needs, supporting family members and caregivers must recognize the can and can't-do activities in the appropriate age ranges, as different developmental objectives, concerns, and limitations exist within each age group (Table 72.1) [11]. Studies have shown that children and adolescents with low vision tend to adopt a more sedentary lifestyle and have lower physical fitness levels overall compared to their sighted peers [12]. The limitation in physical activity participation in these children is due in part to impaired motor skills and subsequent self-perceptions of physical competence. Furthermore, insufficient instruction and overprotection often prevent children with low vision from engaging in physical activity [13].

Children and young adults with low vision should be encouraged to participate in recreational activities with peers and to pursue independence to reduce the risk of mood disorders and promote physical and psychological wellness (Table 72.2). In a systematic review, higher physical activity and fitness levels were associated with improved retinal microvascular health in children and adults, associating the benefits of exercise with overall eye health [14]. Proper recognition, coordination, and

Table 72.2 Recreational activities for children with low vision

Category	Activities
Nature/outdoors engagement	Walks, hikes, gardening, kite flying, kayaking, camping, mountain biking
Physical activities at school and/or home	Kids fitness videos on YouTube
	Stationary exercise equipment including bicycles, treadmills, and rowing machines
Mental activities at school and/or home	Cards, chess, board games with tactile, large print, or Braille versions
	Journaling, guided imagery meditation
Community recreational activities	Swimming, tennis, cooking classes
Tactile & creative craftwork	Pottery, painting, knitting, basket weaving
Language arts	Books, magazines in large print or Braille formats
	Audio books
Musical arts	Instrument learning and playing using screen-enlarging equipment or Braille system of music notation

teamwork among healthcare providers, parents, and teachers facilitate a safe space for children with low vision to promote wellness through physical activity.

Physical Activity Selection and Safety

Appropriate physical activity restrictions should be considered for children with low vision, as certain sports and activities have higher risks of ocular injury. In a large retrospective cross-sectional study, basketball, baseball, and air guns accounted for approximately half of all primary sports-related eye injuries. Activities that involve projectiles pose the highest risk for accidental visual impairment and should be avoided in children who have low vision [15]. In kids with retinal disease, heavy weightlifting may lead to pressure increases in retinal vasculature, worsening retinopathy and thus should be avoided. Contact sports should also be avoided due to the high risk of retinal tear, hemorrhage, and/or detachment.

Nevertheless, if a child decides to participate in sports, proper eye protection is of the utmost importance. Case reports have described badminton to be the leading cause of racquet sports-related eye injuries in Canada specifically, with traumatic hyphema as a common complication. Ocular injuries from sports can affect all age groups and 90% are preventable with protective eyewear; proper ocular protection is therefore strongly recommended in all children regardless of vision status [16].

Vision Rehabilitation on Pediatric Low Vision: Devices and Specialists

Low vision devices (LVDs) are an important part of low vision rehabilitation in children with reduced visual acuity. Low vision devices (telescopes, magnifiers, etc.) and non-optical devices (lamps, reading stamps, large-printed books, etc.) have been shown to significantly improve functional vision, especially in academic and daily living activities including copying from the blackboard, reading textbook at arm's length, writing along a straight line, and identifying body language from people across a distance [17]. Early intervention with visual rehabilitation strengthens visual abilities and learning abilities and enables children with low vision to function at their best [18].

Assistive technology with smartphones, tablets, and laptops can provide magnification, contrast enhancement, and text to speech options for students. Reverse polarity (black background with white writing) can aid in a student's visual fatigue and glare sensitivity. Applications on these devices may also benefit the student. Apps such as Seeing AI and Visor can turn a smartphone into a video magnifier or reading machine. A student may feel more comfortable with these low vision rehabilitation options in comparison to the use of an optical low vision device such as a handheld magnifier or telescope.

Low vision rehabilitation specialists can be extremely helpful in helping children adapt to their living environment, both at home and in school. These specialists include orientation and mobility specialists, vision rehabilitation therapists, certified low vision therapists, and occupational therapists trained in low vision rehabilitation.

Children with reduced vision may benefit from non-visual cues including tactile and auditory learning. Occupational therapists trained in low vision and vision rehabilitation therapists can assist children in gaining independence and self-care skills such as bathing, dressing, cutting food, pouring liquids, and other activities of daily living. Much of the home environment is low contrast. Caregivers may consider increasing visual contrast in the home environment, and changes such as selecting a plate that will increase contrast with food, enhancing overhead lighting, or adding adjustable LED lamps to desktops can improve visibility for children with low vision at home. These examples enhancing contrast, color, lighting, organization, and other sensory modalities listed below can serve as practical tips to modify the activity or environment for children with low vision and facilitate improved learning and participation (Table 72.3).

Resources for Pediatric Low Vision

Implementation of optical aids has shown to be beneficial in improving reading ability, visual information processing, visual motor skill, and overall visual ability in children with visual impairment [13]. Handheld magnifiers, stand magnifiers,

Table 72.3 Practical tips to enhance the home environment for low children vision

Category goals	Practical examples
Contrast Enhance contrast of objects or important features for the child to understand the action of interest	• Learning to use utensils for food: Use a dark plate to contrast with the lighter colored food to allow the child to use their vision to direct the tines of the fork and learn the concept of pushing the tines into the food • Making a bed: Use a light-colored fitted sheet and a darker-colored top sheet to help align or straighten areas of the sheet when making the bed • Oral hygiene: Choose contrasting colored tooth paste and toothbrush so the student can learn and monitor if they are applying an appropriate amount of toothpaste
Color Enhance important features of objects via color differentiation for easier location in environment	• Locating items: Choose a bright colored container for a personal item so student can efficiently scan the environment to locate items • Tying shoelaces: Use different colored laces so student can better follow the sequence and differentiate orientation and how left and right laces cross and tie
Lighting Enhance adequate lighting and minimize shadows to enhance visibility	• Selecting clothes: Enhance closet or drawer area with lighting to ensure the student has improved color perception of clothing to learn matching skills • Learning to use different sized measuring spoons: Add task lighting for improved visibility when teaching how to level off a spoon for the correct measurement • Moving Goose neck lamps to different locations can be very helpful!
Organization Organize items frequently used to be most accessible. Group items commonly used together and reduce clutter, so less effort is required to visually scan for needed object	• House cleaning: Store glass cleaner with lint-free paper towels, wood cleaner with microfiber towels, and bathroom tile cleaner with a brush. The less visual work to search for materials, the better the cleaning will go • Organizing clothes: Hang nice sweaters on the left side of the closet, then nice pants to the right, then casual shirts to the right, then casual pants on the right side of the closet. A predictable pattern will help with efficiency in locating clothing • Dressing outfits: Remove some clothing from closets and drawers. The less visual clutter to scan to find desired items, the more efficient and success the student will be at the task

(continued)

Table 72.3 (continued)

Category goals	Practical examples
Sensory substitution Encourage participation in tasks by utilizing auditory, tactile, and olfactory senses	• Clothing orientation: Teach the student to find the tag inside the shirt. For tagless shirts, add a line of tactile paint to the inside collar of the shirt • Microwaving food: Add a bump dot or tactile mark for student to locate the "add 30 s" button on the microwave • Boiling water: Teach the child to listen for the rolling boil rather than rely on vision to see the bubbles

Credit Amanda Aaron, OTR/L Occupational Therapist, Maryland School for the Blind

telescopic lenses, Clearview + closed-circuit television (CCTV), etc. are common low vision devices associated with improvement in reading speed. Chapter 11, Sect. 3 outlines pediatric low vision aids in detail. Full time polycarbonate glasses for safety, refractive correction (possibly with tint for improved contrast or comfort) and regular multidisciplinary follow up are the basic needs of most pediatric vitreoretinal patients. Families and specialists should continue to monitor their child's needs and use of vision aids which will change over time with normal developmental progress.

Practical Guidance and Future Directions

In children dealing with ocular conditions requiring vitreoretinal surgery, pediatric-specific information can prove informative in pre-operative and post-operative care for both the patients and their families. Examples include pre-printed child-specific materials that include suggestions for activities including swimming, trampolines, flying on an airplane, or school-related activities during recess or physical education classes. These brief recommendations summarized above are just a couple "tips and tricks" that can provide practical approaches to improve the child's daily life.

Guidance for School

In academic settings, teachers, and staff serve a prominent role in serving the needs of children with low vision. Proper teacher education and training can serve as a tool for teachers to keep track of children with special needs and how they are performing in school (i.e., if they can see the board, participate in peer-to-peer interactions, etc.). Teachers can also remind a child if they are rubbing their eyes excessively, or if a child requires further accommodations in the classroom. For example, during physical education classes, if contact sports are being played, teachers can accommodate students with low vision by replacing these higher risk physical activities with low intensity or safer, kid-friendly fitness videos. School nurses can also provide continued care for children who require eye drops throughout the course of the school day.

Tips and tricks
• Ensure fit and comfort of glasses with accessories
• Provide Peds-specific pre-op and post-op instructions
• Replace contact sports with kids' fitness videos or lower risk activities
• Have eye drops given by school nurses
• Have teachers remind students not to touch eyes and educate on general eye hygiene

The American Association for Pediatric Ophthalmology and Strabismus (AAPOS) has published a wide breadth of resources available for patients, providers, family members, teachers, and anyone involved in the child's care, all with the intention of improving the patient's overall well-being and quality of life (Table 72.4) [19].

Table 72.4 Resources and links for pediatric low vision (adapted from AAPOS)

Resource	Links
Toys, games, and books for pre-literate ages	• LEGO Braille Bricks • Dots for Tots (brailleinstitute.org) • Digital Dots (brailleinstitute.org) • Tactile graphics • Braille "Twister" • Hungry Fingers • Tactile memory game • Braille adapted versions of popular games
Schools	• Hadley School for the Blind Online Courses (www.hadley.edu) • New Mexico School for Blind and Visually Impaired (www.nmsbvi.k12.nm.us) • Perkins School for the Blind (www.perkinselearning.org) • Texas State School for Blind and Visually Impaired (www.tsbvi.edu/about-tsbvi) • Maryland School for the Blind (marylandschoolfortheblind.org)
Low vision aids/resources	• American Printing House for the Blind, Inc. (large-print and Braille books, tapes, low vision aids, tools for teachers and students. www.aph.org) • Learning Ally (audiobooks for blind and dyslexic. www.learningdaily.org) • Learning Sight & Sound (www.learningally.org) • National Library Service for the Blind and Physically Handicapped, Library of Congress (Free library program of Braille and audio materials. www.loc.gov/nls) • Shop Low Vision (supplies a wide range of magnifiers, optical products, professional tools, daily living solutions. www.shoplowvision.com)

(continued)

Table 72.4 (continued)

Resource	Links
Organizations for low vision	• American Council of the Blind (www.acb.org) • American Foundation for the Blind (www.afb.org) • CVI Scotland (www.cviscotland.org) • Pediatric Cortical Visual Impairment Society (www.pcvis.vision) • Family Connect (www.familyconnect.org) • Foundation of Fighting Blindness (www.blindness.org) • National Dissemination Center for Children with Disabilities (NICHCY) (nichcy.org) • Prevent Blindness (www.preventblindness.org)
Where to learn more	• American Association for Pediatric Ophthalmology and Strabismus (https://aapos.org/syndicated/pediatric-low-vision) • Journal articles (https://aapos.org/education/educational-resources/pediatric-low-vision-education/low-vision-references)

Conclusion

Visual impairment in children with vitreoretinal disease can impact children's learning in academic environments. Early referral to visual rehabilitation centers and implementation of optical aids may increase functional vision and comfort in school, leading to improved overall performance and quality of life. Further research on the impact of low vision on psychosocial and cognitive development in children is necessary for pediatric vitreoretinal ophthalmologists to provide optimal guidance and ensure well-being in both the child and the family.

Review Questions

1. A 8-year-old girl with history of Stargardt disease presents for follow up comprehensive eye exam. Visual acuity is stable; however, when asked how school is going, she says she dislikes school because she is having a hard time keeping up in classes and making new friends. Mom is worried about her grades and her not getting enough physical activity. What is the best recommendation you can offer to this family?

a. Refrain from participating in physical activities during school for safety purposes
b. Recommend home schooling for tailored education
c. Refer to vision rehabilitation centers or schools for the blind
d. Reassurance and continue monitoring symptoms

2. A 8-year-old girl with history of Stargardt disease presents for follow up comprehensive eye exam. Visual acuity is stable; however, when asked how school is going, she says she dislikes school because she is having a hard time keeping up in classes and making new friends. Mom is worried about her grades and her not getting enough physical activity. What is the best recommendation you can offer to this family?

a. Autonomy and acceptance
b. Sensory development
c. Mobile independence
d. Social interaction and communication

3. A 12-year-old boy with low vision presents to your office and his father asks what kind of sports he should be allowed to participate in at school. Which of these physical activities would you recommend?

Answers

1. (**C**) Children with low vision may experience psychosocial challenges in academic, home, and social settings that requires further support. Early intervention with visual rehabilitation and optical aids can strengthen visual and learning abilities and enable children with low vision to continue proper education. Discussions regarding low vision services availability or referrals for state schools for the blind should take place with families.

2. (**D**) Children in age group 7–12 years old have the primary objective of developing proper communication, social interaction, and emotional well-being in various settings. A 10-year-old child will start to become more aware of their visual impairment and worry about fitting in at school and asking for help. Children in 0–2 and 3–6 age ranges are focused on sensory development and mobile independence, respectively, while children in 13–17 age range are focused on autonomy and acceptance.

3. (**B**) Contact sports including basketball, baseball, and soccer should be avoided in children with low vision due to high risk of retinal tear, hemorrhage, and/or detachment. Heavy weightlifting may worsen retinopathy due to increased vessel pressure from Valsalva maneuver. Swimming is an example of a non-contact sport that can serve as a healthy aerobic alternative, with obvious exception during the post-operative period.

Acknowledgements We would like to acknowledge Amanda Aaron, OTR/L Occupational Therapist and Sharon Whited, CLVT Low Vision Specialist, from Maryland School for the Blind for their contributions to this chapter.

References

1. Uprety S, Khanal S, Morjaria P, Puri LR. Profile of paediatric low vision population: a retrospective study from Nepal. Clin Exp Optom. 2016;99(1):61–5. https://doi.org/10.1111/cxo.12314.

2. Gilbert CE, Ellwein LB; Refractive Error Study in Children Study Group. Prevalence and causes of functional low vision in school-age children: results from standardized population surveys in Asia, Africa, and Latin America. Invest Ophthalmol Vis Sci. 2008;49(3):877–81. https://doi.org/10.1167/iovs.07-0973.

3. Kong L, Fry M, Al-Samarraie M, Gilbert C, Steinkuller PG. An update on progress and the changing epidemiology of causes of childhood blindness worldwide. J AAPOS. 2012;16(6):501–7. https://doi.org/10.1016/j.jaapos.2012.09.004.

4. Hatton DD, Ivy SE, Boyer C. Severe visual impairments in infants and toddlers in the United States. J Vis Impairm Blind. 2013;107(5):325–36.

5. Hatton DD, Schwietz E, Boyer B, Rychwalski P. Babies count: the national registry for children with visual impairments, birth to 3 years. J Am Assoc Pediatric Ophthalmol Strabismus. 2007;11(4):351–5.

6. de Verdier K, Ulla E, Löfgren S, Fernell E. Children with blindness–major causes, developmental outcomes and implications for habilitation and educational support: a two-decade, Swedish population-based study. Acta Ophthalmologica. 2018;96(3):295–300.

7. Msall ME, Phelps DL, Hardy RJ, Dobson V, Quinn GE, Summers CG, Tremont MR. Educational and social competencies at 8 years in children with threshold retinopathy of prematurity in the CRYO-ROP multicenter study. Pediatrics. 2004;113(4):790–9. https://doi.org/10.1542/peds.113.4.790.

8. Birch EE, Castañeda YS, Cheng-Patel CS, et al. Self-perception in children aged 3 to 7 years with amblyopia and its association with deficits in vision and fine motor skills. JAMA Ophthalmol. 2019;137(5):499–506. https://doi.org/10.1001/jamaophthalmol.2018.7075.

9. Birch EE, Castañeda YS, Cheng-Patel CS, et al. Self-perception of School-aged children with amblyopia and its association with reading speed and motor skills. JAMA Ophthalmol. 2019;137(2):167–74. https://doi.org/10.1001/jamaophthalmol.2018.5527.

10. Augestad LB. Mental health among children and young adults with visual impairments: a systematic review. J Vis Impair Blind. 2017;411–25.

11. Rainey L, Elsman EBM, van Nispen RMA, van Leeuwen LM, van Rens GHMB. Comprehending the impact of low vision on the lives of children and adolescents: a qualitative approach. Qual Life Res. 2016;25(10):2633–43. https://doi.org/10.1007/s11136-016-1292-8.

12. Aslan UB, Calik BB, Kitiş A. The effect of gender and level of vision on the physical activity level of children and adolescents with visual impairment. Res Dev Disabil. 2012;33(6):1799–804. https://doi.org/10.1016/j.ridd.2012.05.005.

13. Qi J, Xu JW, Shao WD. Physical activity of children with visual impairments during different segments of the school day. Int J Environ Res Pub Health. 2020;17(18):6897.

14. Streese L, Guerini C, Bühlmayer L, et al. Physical activity and exercise improve retinal microvascular health as a biomarker of cardiovascular risk: a systematic review. Atherosclerosis. 2020;315:33–42. https://doi.org/10.1016/j.atherosclerosis.2020.09.017.

15. Haring RS, Sheffield ID, Canner JK, Schneider EB. Epidemiology of sports-related eye injuries in the United States. JAMA Ophthalmol. 2016;134(12):1382–90. https://doi.org/10.1001/jamaophthalmol.2016.4253.

16. Wang DN, Luong M, Hanson C. Traumatic hyphema in a 13-year-old girl: eye protection regulation in badminton is needed. CMAJ. 2020;192(27):E778–80. https://doi.org/10.1503/cmaj.191273.

17. Ganesh S, Sethi S, Srivastav S, Chaudhary A, Arora P. Impact of low vision rehabilitation on functional vision performance of children with visual impairment. Oman J Ophthalmol. 2013;6(3):170–4. https://doi.org/10.4103/0974-620X.122271.

18. Lamoureux EL, Pallant JF, Pesudovs K, Rees G, Hassell JB, Keeffe JE. The effectiveness of low-vision rehabilitation on participation in daily living and quality of life. Invest Ophthalmol Vis Sci. 2007;48(4):1476–82. https://doi.org/10.1167/iovs.06-0610.
19. Pediatric Low Vision Rehabilitation Resources. American Association for Pediatric Ophthalmology and Strabismus. https://www.aapos.org/education/educational-resources/pediatric-low-vision-education.